MARKS'
BASIC MEDICAL
BIOCHEMISTRY
A Clinical Approach

5TH EDITION

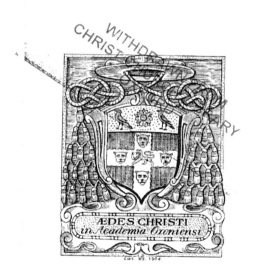

MARKS'
BASIC MEDICAL BIOCHEMISTRY
A Clinical Approach

5TH EDITION

Michael Lieberman, PhD

Distinguished Teaching Professor
Department of Molecular Genetics, Biochemistry and Microbiology
University of Cincinnati College of Medicine
Cincinnati, Ohio

Alisa Peet, MD

Associate Dean Clinical Education
Associate Professor of Clinical Medicine
Lewis Katz School of Medicine at Temple University
Philadelphia, Pennsylvania

Illustrations by Matthew Chansky

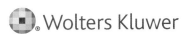 Wolters Kluwer

Philadelphia • Baltimore • New York • London
Buenos Aires • Hong Kong • Sydney • Tokyo

Acquisitions Editor: Shannon Magee
Development Editor: Andrea Vosburgh
Editorial Coordinator: Lauren Pecarich
Marketing Manager: Michael McMahon
Production Project Manager: David Orzechowski
Design Coordinator: Joan Wendt
Prepress Vendor: Absolute Service, Inc.

Fifth Edition

9 8 7 6 5 4 3 2 1

Printed in China

Library of Congress Cataloging-in-Publication Data

Names: Lieberman, Michael, 1950- author. | Peet, Alisa, author.
Title: Marks' basic medical biochemistry : a clinical approach / Michael
   Lieberman, Alisa Peet ; illustrations by Matthew Chansky.
Other titles: Basic medical biochemistry
Description: Fifth edition. | Philadelphia : Wolters Kluwer, [2018] |
   Includes bibliographical references and index.
Identifiers: LCCN 2017016094 | ISBN 9781496324818
Subjects: | MESH: Biochemical Phenomena | Clinical Medicine
Classification: LCC QP514.2 | NLM QU 34 | DDC 612.1/111—dc23 LC record available at
https://lccn.loc.gov/2017016094

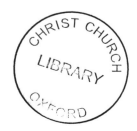

Preface to the 5th Edition

It has been 5 years since the fourth edition was completed. The fifth edition has some significant organizational changes, as suggested by extensive surveys of faculty and students who used the fourth edition in their classes and studies. The major pedagogic features of the text remain. They have been enhanced by the following changes for the fifth edition:

1. Every patient history has been reviewed and revised to reflect current standards of care (as of 2016). The patient names have also been changed to a first name and last initial. A key indicating the "old" names and "new" names is available in the online supplement associated with the text.

2. The Biochemical Comments associated with each chapter have been updated, where appropriate, to allow students to experience where current research efforts are headed.

3. The presentation of metabolism has been altered such that glycolysis is now the first topic discussed, followed by the tricarboxylic acid cycle, and then oxidative phosphorylation. The correlation between fourth edition chapters and fifth edition chapters are as follows:

   a. Chapters 1 through 18, no change

   b. Section IV is now entitled "Carbohydrate Metabolism, Fuel Oxidation, and the Generation of Adenosine Triphosphate" and consists of Chapters 19 through 28.

      i. Chapter 19 of the fifth edition (Basic Concepts in the Regulation of Fuel Metabolism by Insulin, Glucagon, and Other Hormones) is based on Chapter 26 of the fourth edition.

      ii. Chapter 20 of the fifth edition (Cellular Bioenergetics: Adenosine Triphosphate and O_2) is based on Chapter 19 of the fourth edition.

      iii. Chapter 21 of the fifth edition (Digestion, Absorption, and Transport of Carbohydrates) is based on Chapter 27 of the fourth edition.

      iv. Chapter 22 of the fifth edition (Generation of Adenosine Triphosphate from Glucose, Fructose, and Galactose: Glycolysis) is based on Chapter 22 of the fourth edition and also contains parts of Chapter 29 of the fourth edition (Pathways of Sugar Metabolism: Pentose Phosphate Pathway, Fructose, and Galactose Metabolism).

      v. Chapter 23 of the fifth edition (Tricarboxylic Acid Cycle) is based on Chapter 20 of the fourth edition.

      vi. Chapter 24 of the fifth edition (Oxidative Phosphorylation and Mitochondrial Function) is based on Chapter 21 of the fourth edition.

      vii. Chapter 25 of the fifth edition (Oxygen Toxicity and Free-Radical Injury) is based on Chapter 24 of the fourth edition.

      viii. Chapter 26 of the fifth edition (Formation and Degradation of Glycogen) is based on Chapter 28 of the fourth edition.

      ix. Chapter 27 of the fifth edition (Pentose Phosphate Pathway and the Synthesis of Glycosides, Lactose, Glycoproteins, and Glycolipids) is based on Chapter 30 of the fourth edition, along with a section (The Pentose Phosphate Pathway) of Chapter 29 of the fourth edition. This led to the deletion of old Chapter 29 from the Table of Contents of the fifth edition.

         x. Chapter 28 of the fifth edition (Gluconeogenesis and Maintenance of Blood Glucose Levels) is based on Chapter 31 of the fourth edition.

   c. Section V (Lipid Metabolism) now consists of the following chapters:

      i. Chapter 29 of the fifth edition (Digestion and Transport of Dietary Lipids) is based on Chapter 32 of the fourth edition.

     ii. Chapter 30 of the fifth edition (Oxidation of Fatty Acids and Ketone Bodies) is based on Chapter 23 of the fourth edition.

   iii. Chapter 31 of the fifth edition (Synthesis of Fatty Acids, Triacylglycerols, and the Major Membrane Lipids) is based on Chapter 33 of the fourth edition and also contains basic information concerning the eicosanoids from Chapter 35 of the fourth edition. Material from Chapter 35 of the fourth edition that was not incorporated into Chapter 31 of the fifth edition is available as an online supplement. A separate chapter on eicosanoid metabolism is not present in the fifth edition.

    iv. Chapter 32 of the fifth edition (Cholesterol Absorption, Synthesis, Metabolism, and Fate) is based on Chapter 34 of the fourth edition.

     v. Chapter 33 of the fifth edition (Metabolism of Ethanol) is based on Chapter 25 of the fourth edition.

    vi. Chapter 34 of the fifth edition (Integration of Carbohydrate and Lipid Metabolism) is based on Chapter 36 of the fourth edition.

   d. Section VI (Nitrogen Metabolism) has the same chapter order as in the fourth edition, but because two chapters have been deleted previously from the text, the chapter numbers in the fifth edition are two less than in the fourth edition. Section VI in the fifth edition comprises Chapters 35 through 40, whereas in the fourth edition, it is Chapters 37 through 42.

   e. Section VII (Tissue Metabolism) has the same chapter order as in the fourth edition, but the chapter numbers in the fifth edition are two less than in the fourth edition. Section VII in the fifth edition comprises Chapters 41 through 47, whereas in the fourth edition, it is Chapters 43 through 49.

4. The number of printed review questions at the end of each chapter has been increased to 10, up from 5 questions per chapter in the fourth edition (470 total questions). The online question bank associated with the text has also been increased to 560 questions, as compared to 468 questions associated with the fourth edition. Where possible, questions are presented in National Board of Medical Examiners format.

As stated in previous editions, in revising a text geared primarily toward medical students, the authors always struggle with new advances in biochemistry and whether such advances should be included in the text. We have taken the approach of only including advances that will enable the student to better relate biochemistry to medicine and future diagnostic tools. Although providing incomplete, but exciting, advances to graduate students is best for their education, medical students benefit more from a more directed approach—one that emphasizes how biochemistry is useful for the practice of medicine. This is a major goal of this text.

Any errors are the responsibility of the authors, and we would appreciate being notified when such errors are found.

The accompanying website for this edition of *Marks' Basic Medical Biochemistry: A Clinical Approach* contains the aforementioned additional multiple-choice questions for review, a table listing patient names for the fifth edition and how they correspond to those of the fourth edition, summaries of all patients described in the text (patient cases), all chapter references and additional reading (with links to the article in PubMed, where applicable), a listing of diseases discussed in the book (with links to appropriate websites for more information), and a summary of all of the methods described throughout the text.

How to Use This Book

Icons identify the various components of the book: the patients who are presented at the start of each chapter; the clinical notes, methods notes, questions, and answers that appear in the margins; and the Key Concepts, Clinical Comments, and Biochemical Comments that are found at the end of each chapter.

Each chapter starts with an abstract that summarizes the information so that students can recognize the key words and concepts they are expected to learn. The next component of each chapter is The Waiting Room, describing patients with complaints and detailing the events that led them to seek medical help.

 indicates a female patient

 indicates a male patient

 indicates a patient who is an infant or young child

As each chapter unfolds, icons appear in the margin, identifying information related to the material presented in the text:

 indicates a clinical note, usually related to the patients in The Waiting Room for that chapter. These notes explain signs or symptoms of a patient or give some other clinical information relevant to the text.

 indicates a methods note, which elaborates on how biochemistry is required to perform, and interpret, common laboratory tests.

Questions and answers also appear in the margin and should help to keep students thinking as they read the text:

 indicates a question

 indicates the answer to the question. The answer to a question is always located on the next page. If two questions appear on one page, the answers are given in order on the next page.

Each chapter ends with these three sections: Key Concepts, Clinical Comments, and Biochemical Comments:

The Key Concepts summarize the important take-home messages from the chapter.

 The Clinical Comments give additional clinical information, often describing the treatment plan and the outcome.

 The Biochemical Comments add biochemical information that is not covered in the text or explore some facet of biochemistry in more detail or from another angle.

Finally, Review Questions are presented. These questions are written in a United States Medical Licensing Examination–like format, and many of them have a clinical slant. Answers to the review questions, along with detailed explanations, are provided at the end of every chapter.

Acknowledgments

The authors would like to thank Professor Kent Littleton of Bastyr University, for his careful reading of the fourth edition and pointing out mistakes and errors that required correcting for the fifth edition. We greatly appreciate his efforts in improving the text. Dr. Bonnie Brehm was instrumental in helping with the nutrition aspects of the text, and Dr. Rick Ricer was invaluable in writing questions, both for the text and the online supplement. We would also like to acknowledge the initial contributions of Dawn Marks, whose vision of a textbook geared toward medical students led to the first edition of this book. Her vision is still applicable today.

Contents

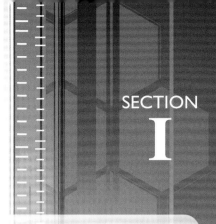

Fuel Metabolism

In order to survive, humans must meet two basic metabolic requirements: We must be able to synthesize everything our cells need that is not supplied by our diet, and we must be able to protect our internal environment from toxins and changing conditions in our external environment. To meet these requirements, we metabolize our dietary components through four basic types of pathways: fuel oxidative pathways, fuel storage and mobilization pathways, biosynthetic pathways, and detoxification or waste disposal pathways. Cooperation between tissues and responses to changes in our external environment are communicated through transport pathways and intercellular signaling pathways (Fig. I.1).

The foods in our diet are the fuels that supply us with energy in the form of calories. This energy is used for carrying out such diverse functions as moving, thinking, and reproducing. Thus, several of our metabolic pathways are *fuel oxidative pathways* that convert fuels into energy that can be used for biosynthetic and mechanical work. But what is the source of energy when we are not eating, such as between meals, and while we sleep? How does a person on a hunger strike that you read about in the morning headlines survive so long? We have other metabolic pathways that are *fuel storage pathways*. The fuels that we store can be mobilized during periods when we are not eating or when we need increased energy for exercise.

Our diet also must contain the compounds we cannot synthesize, as well as all the basic building blocks for compounds we do synthesize in our *biosynthetic pathways*. For example, we have dietary requirements for some amino acids, but we can synthesize other amino acids from our fuels and a dietary nitrogen precursor. The compounds required in our diet for biosynthetic pathways include certain amino acids, vitamins, and essential fatty acids.

Detoxification pathways and *waste disposal pathways* are metabolic pathways devoted to removing toxins that can be present in our diets or in the air we breathe, introduced into our bodies as drugs, or generated internally from the metabolism of dietary components. Dietary components that have no value to the body, and must be disposed of, are called *xenobiotics*.

In general, biosynthetic pathways (including fuel storage) are referred to as *anabolic pathways*; that is, pathways that synthesize larger molecules from smaller components. The synthesis of proteins from amino acids is an example of an anabolic pathway. *Catabolic pathways* are those pathways that break down larger molecules into smaller components. Fuel oxidative pathways are examples of catabolic pathways.

In humans, the need for different cells to carry out different functions has resulted in cell and tissue specialization in metabolism. For example, our adipose tissue is a specialized site for the storage of fat and contains the metabolic pathways that allow it to carry out this function. However, adipose tissue is lacking many of the pathways that synthesize required compounds from dietary precursors. To enable our cells to cooperate in meeting our metabolic needs during changing conditions of diet, sleep, activity, and health, we need *transport pathways* into the blood and between tissues and *intercellular signaling pathways*. One means of communication is for *hormones* to carry signals to tissues about our dietary state. For example, a message that we have just had a meal, carried by the hormone insulin, signals adipose tissue to store fat.

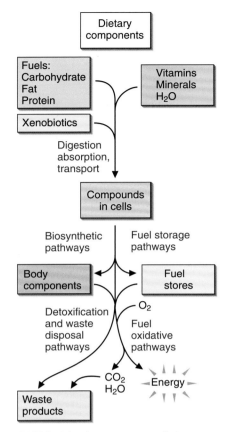

FIGURE I.I An overview of the general metabolic routes for dietary components in the body. The types of pathways are named in *red*.

In the following section, we will provide an overview of various types of dietary components and examples of the pathways involved in using these components. We will describe the fuels in our diet, the compounds produced by their digestion, and the basic patterns of fuel metabolism in the tissues of our bodies. We will describe how these patterns change when we eat, when we fast for a short time, and when we starve for prolonged periods. Patients with medical problems that involve an inability to deal normally with fuels will be introduced. These patients will appear repeatedly throughout the book and will be joined by other patients as we delve deeper into biochemistry.

It is important to note that this section of the book contains an *overview* of basic metabolism, which allows patients to be presented at an elementary level and to whet students' appetites for the biochemistry to come. The goal is to enable the student to taste and preview what biochemistry is all about. It is not designed to be all-inclusive, as all of these topics will be discussed in greater detail in Sections IV through VII of the text. The next section of the text (Section II) begins with the basics of biochemistry and the relationship of basic chemistry to processes that occur in all living cells.

Metabolic Fuels and Dietary Components

Fuel Metabolism. We obtain our fuel primarily from the **macronutrients** (i.e., **carbohydrates**, **fats**, and **proteins**) in our diet. As we eat, our foodstuffs are **digested** and **absorbed**. The products of digestion circulate in the blood, enter various tissues, and are eventually taken up by cells and **oxidized** to produce **energy**. To completely convert our fuels to carbon dioxide (CO_2) and water (H_2O), molecular **oxygen** (O_2) is required. We breathe to obtain this oxygen and to eliminate the CO_2 that is produced by the oxidation of our foodstuffs.

Fuel Stores. Any dietary fuel that exceeds the body's immediate energy needs is stored, mainly as **triacylglycerol** (fat) in adipose tissue, as **glycogen** (a carbohydrate) in muscle, liver, and other cells, and, to some extent, as **protein** in muscle. When we are fasting, between meals and overnight while we sleep, fuel is drawn from these stores and is oxidized to provide energy (Fig. 1.1).

Fuel Requirements. We require enough energy each day to drive the **basic functions** of our bodies and to support our **physical activity**. If we do not consume enough food each day to supply that much energy, the body's fuel stores supply the remainder and we lose weight. Conversely, if we consume more food than required for the energy we expend, our body's fuel stores enlarge and we gain weight.

Other Dietary Requirements. In addition to providing energy, the diet provides **precursors** for the **biosynthesis** of compounds necessary for cellular and tissue structure, function, and survival. Among these precursors are the **essential fatty acids** and essential **amino acids** (those that the body needs but cannot synthesize). The diet must also supply **vitamins**, **minerals**, and **water**.

Waste Disposal. Dietary components that we can use are referred to as nutrients. However, both the diet and the air we breathe contain **xenobiotic compounds**, compounds that have no use or value in the human body and may be toxic. These compounds are excreted in the urine and feces together with metabolic waste products.

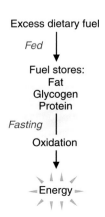

FIGURE 1.1 Fate of excess dietary fuel in fed and fasting states.

Percy V. is a 59-year-old school teacher who was in good health until his wife died suddenly. Since that time, he has experienced an increasing degree of fatigue and has lost interest in many of the activities he previously enjoyed. Shortly after his wife's death, one of his married children moved far from home. Since then, Mr. V. has had little appetite for food. When a neighbor found Mr. V. sleeping in his clothes, unkempt, and somewhat confused, she called an ambulance. Mr. V. was admitted to the hospital psychiatry unit with a diagnosis of mental depression associated with dehydration and malnutrition.

 Otto S. is a 25-year-old medical student who was very athletic during high school and college but is now out of shape. Since he started medical school, he has been gaining weight. He is 5 ft 10 in tall and began medical school weighing 154 lb, within his ideal weight range. By the time he finished his last examination in his first year, he weighed 187 lb. He has decided to consult a physician at the student health service before the problem gets worse, as he would like to reduce his weight (at 187 lb, his body mass index [BMI] is 27) to his previous level of 154 lb (which would reduce his BMI to 23, in the middle of the healthy range of BMI values).

 Ivan A. is a 56-year-old accountant who has been obese for a number of years. He exhibits a pattern of central obesity, called an "apple shape," which is caused by excess adipose tissue being disproportionally deposited in the abdominal area. His major recreational activities are watching TV while drinking scotch and soda and doing occasional gardening. At a company picnic, he became very "winded" while playing softball and decided it was time for a general physical examination. At the examination, he weighed 264 lb at 5 ft 10 in tall. His blood pressure was elevated, 155 mm Hg systolic and 95 mm Hg diastolic (for Ivan's age, hypertension is defined as >140 mm Hg systolic and >90 mm Hg diastolic). For a male of these proportions, a BMI of 18.5 to 24.9 would correspond to a weight between 129 and 173 lb. Mr. A. is almost 100 lb overweight, and his BMI of 37.9 is in the range defined as obesity.

 Ann R. is a 23-year-old buyer for a woman's clothing store. Despite the fact that she is 5 ft 7 in tall and weighs 99 lb, she is convinced she is overweight. Two months ago, she started a daily physical activity program that consists of 1 hour of jogging every morning and 1 hour of walking every evening. She also decided to consult a physician about weight loss. If patients are above (like Ivan A.) or below (like Ann R.) their ideal weight, the physician, often in consultation with a registered dietitian, prescribes a diet designed to bring the weight into the ideal range.

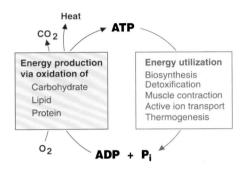

FIGURE 1.2 The ATP–ADP cycle. The energy-generating pathways are shown in *red*; the energy-utilizing pathways in *blue*. *ATP*, adenosine triphosphate; *ADP*, adenosine diphosphate; *P$_i$*, inorganic phosphate.

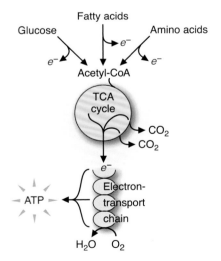

FIGURE 1.3 Generation of ATP from fuel components during respiration. Glucose, fatty acids, and amino acids are oxidized to acetyl coenzyme A (acetyl-CoA), a substrate for the tricarboxylic acid (TCA) cycle. In the TCA cycle, they are completely oxidized to CO_2. As fuels are oxidized, electrons (e^-) are transferred to O_2 by the electron transport chain, and the energy is used to generate ATP.

I. Dietary Fuels

The major fuels we obtain from our diet are the **macronutrients**—namely, **carbohydrates**, **proteins**, and **fats**. When these fuels are oxidized to CO_2 and H_2O in our cells (the process of **catabolism**), energy is released by the transfer of electrons to O_2. The energy from this oxidation process generates heat and **adenosine triphosphate (ATP)** (Fig. 1.2). CO_2 travels in the blood to the lungs where it is expired, and water is excreted in urine, sweat, and other secretions. Although the heat that is generated by fuel oxidation is used to maintain body temperature, the main purpose of fuel oxidation is to generate ATP. ATP provides the energy that drives most of the energy-consuming processes in the cell, including biosynthetic reactions (anabolic pathways), muscle contraction, and active transport across membranes. As these processes use energy, ATP is converted back to adenosine diphosphate (ADP) and inorganic phosphate (P$_i$). The generation and use of ATP is referred to as the *ATP–ADP cycle*.

The oxidation of fuels to generate ATP is called *respiration* (Fig. 1.3). Prior to oxidation, carbohydrates are converted principally to glucose, fat to fatty acids,

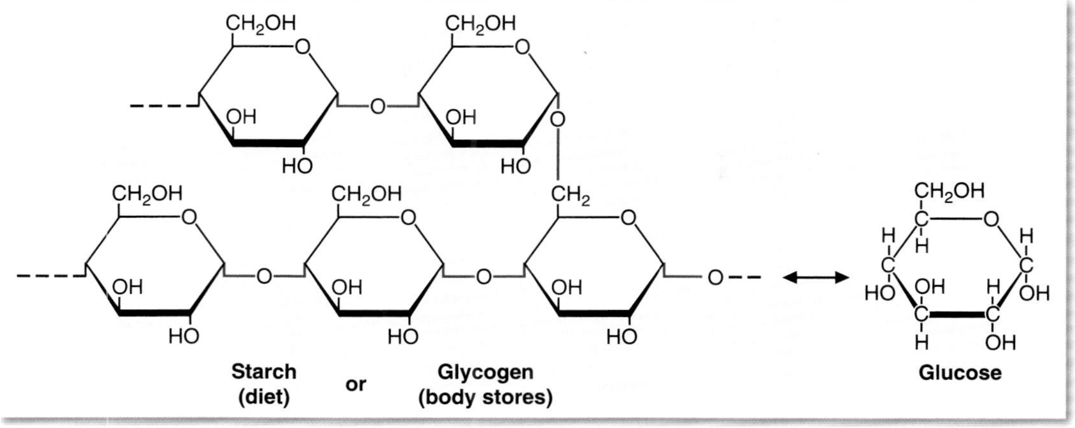

FIGURE 1.4 Structure of starch and glycogen. Starch, our major dietary carbohydrate, and glycogen, the body's storage form of glucose, have similar structures. They are polysaccharides (many sugar units) composed of glucose, which is a monosaccharide (one sugar unit).

and protein to amino acids. The pathways for oxidizing glucose, fatty acids, and amino acids have many features in common. They first oxidize the fuels to **acetyl coenzyme A (acetyl-CoA)**, a precursor of the **tricarboxylic acid (TCA)** cycle. The TCA cycle is a series of reactions that completes the oxidation of fuels to CO_2 (see Chapter 23). Electrons lost from the fuels during oxidative reactions are transferred to O_2 by a series of proteins in the electron transport chain (see Chapter 24). The energy of electron transfer is used to convert ADP and P_i to ATP by a process known as *oxidative phosphorylation*.

In discussions of metabolism and nutrition, energy is often expressed in units of **calories**. A calorie in this context (nutritional calorie) is equivalent to 1 **kilocalorie (kcal)** in energy terms. "Calorie" was originally spelled with a capital C, but the capitalization was dropped as the term became popular. Thus, a 1-cal soft drink actually has 1 kcal of energy. Energy is also expressed in **joules**. One kilocalorie equals 4.18 kilojoules (kJ). Physicians tend to use units of calories, in part because that is what their patients use and understand. One kilocalorie of energy is the amount of energy required to raise the temperature of 1 L of water by 1°C.

A. Carbohydrates

The major carbohydrates in the human diet are starch, sucrose, lactose, fructose, galactose, and glucose. The *polysaccharide starch* is the storage form of carbohydrates in plants. Sucrose (table sugar), maltose, and lactose (milk sugar) are disaccharides, and fructose, galactose, and glucose are monosaccharides. Digestion converts the larger carbohydrates to monosaccharides, which can be absorbed into the bloodstream. Glucose, a monosaccharide, is the predominant sugar in human blood (Fig. 1.4).

Oxidation of carbohydrates to CO_2 and H_2O in the body produces approximately 4 kcal/g (Table 1.1). In other words, every gram of carbohydrate we eat yields approximately 4 kcal of energy. Note that carbohydrate molecules contain a significant amount of oxygen and are already partially oxidized before they enter our bodies (see Fig. 1.4).

TABLE 1.1	**Caloric Content of Fuels**
	kcal/g
Carbohydrate	4
Fat	9
Protein	4
Alcohol	7

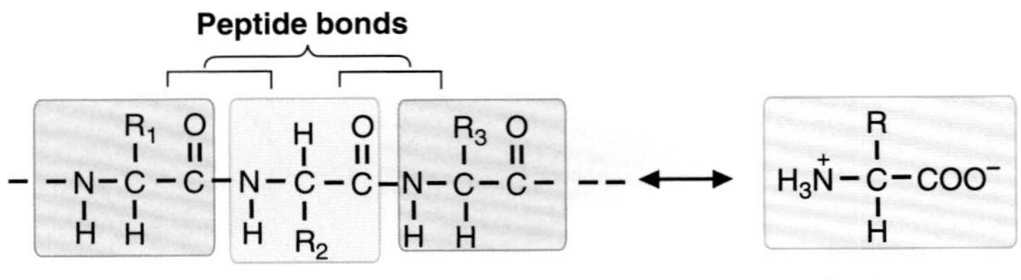

Peptide bonds

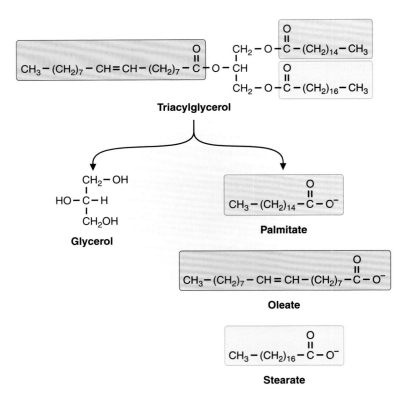

Protein   **Amino acid**

FIGURE 1.5 General structure of proteins and amino acids. Each amino acid in this figure is indicated by a different color. R = side chain. Different amino acids have different side chains. For example, R_1 might be $-CH_3$; R_2, $-CH_2OH$; R_3, $-CH_2-COO^-$. In a protein, the amino acids are linked by peptide bonds.

B. Proteins

Proteins are composed of **amino acids** that are joined to form linear chains (Fig. 1.5). In addition to carbon, hydrogen, and oxygen, proteins contain approximately 16% nitrogen by weight. The digestive process breaks down proteins to their constituent amino acids, which enter the blood. The complete oxidation of proteins to CO_2, H_2O, and NH_4^+ in the body yields approximately 4 kcal/g (see Table 1.1).

C. Fats

Fats are lipids composed of **triacylglycerols** (also called **triglycerides**). A triacylglycerol molecule contains three fatty acids esterified to one glycerol moiety (Fig. 1.6).

   Fats contain much less oxygen than is contained in carbohydrates or proteins. Therefore, fats are more reduced and yield more energy when oxidized. The complete oxidation of triacylglycerols to CO_2 and H_2O in the body releases approximately 9 kcal/g, more than twice the energy yield from an equivalent amount of carbohydrate or protein (see Table 1.1).

An analysis of **Ann R.'s** diet showed that she ate 100 g of carbohydrate, 20 g of protein, and 15 g of fat each day. Approximately how many calories did she consume per day?

Triacylglycerol

Glycerol

Palmitate

Oleate

Stearate

FIGURE 1.6 Structure of a triacylglycerol. Palmitate and stearate are saturated fatty acids (i.e., they have no double bonds in the carbon chain). Oleate is monounsaturated (one double bond). Polyunsaturated fatty acids have more than one double bond.

D. Alcohol

Alcohol (ethanol, in the context of the diet) has considerable caloric content. Ethanol (CH_3–CH_2–OH) is oxidized to CO_2 and H_2O in the body and yields approximately 7 kcal/g; that is, more than carbohydrate or protein but less than fat.

II. Body Fuel Stores

Humans carry supplies of fuel within their bodies (Table 1.2), which are similar to the fuel supplies in the plants and animals we eat. These fuel stores are light in weight, large in quantity, and readily converted into oxidizable substances. Most of us are familiar with fat, our major fuel store, which is located in adipose tissue. Although fat is distributed throughout our bodies, it tends to increase in quantity in our hips, thighs, and abdomens as we advance into middle age. In addition to our fat stores, we also have important, although much smaller, stores of carbohydrate in the form of **glycogen** located primarily in our liver and muscles. Glycogen consists of glucose molecules joined together to form a large, branched polysaccharide (see Fig. 1.4). Body protein, particularly the protein of our large muscle masses, also serves to some extent as a fuel store, and we draw on it for energy when we fast.

A. Fat

Our major fuel store is adipose triacylglycerol (triglyceride), a lipid more commonly known as fat. The average 70-kg man has approximately 15 kg of stored triacylglycerol, which accounts for approximately 85% of his total stored calories (see Table 1.2).

Two characteristics make adipose triacylglycerol a very efficient fuel store: the fact that triacylglycerol contains more calories per gram than carbohydrate or protein (9 kcal/g vs. 4 kcal/g) and the fact that adipose tissue does not contain much water. Adipose tissue contains only about 15% water, compared to tissues such as muscle that contain about 80%. Thus, the 70-kg man with 15 kg of stored triacylglycerol has only about 18 kg of adipose tissue.

B. Glycogen

Our stores of glycogen in liver, muscle, and other cells are relatively small in quantity but are nevertheless important. Liver glycogen is used to maintain blood glucose levels between meals, which is necessary for optimal functioning of the nervous system. Thus, the size of this glycogen store fluctuates during the day; an average 70-kg man might have 200 g or more of liver glycogen after a meal but only 80 g after an overnight fast. Muscle glycogen supplies energy for muscle contraction during exercise. At rest, the 70-kg man has approximately 150 g of muscle glycogen. Almost all cells, including neurons, maintain a small emergency supply of glucose as glycogen.

A **Miss R.** consumed
$100 \times 4 = 400$ calories as carbohydrate
$20 \times 4 = 80$ calories as protein
$15 \times 9 = 135$ calories as fat
for a total of 615 calories/day.

 Ivan A. ate 585 g of carbohydrate, 150 g of protein, and 95 g of fat each day. In addition, he drank 45 g of alcohol daily. How many calories did he consume per day?

TABLE 1.2 Fuel Composition of the Average 70-kg Man[a] after an Overnight Fast		
FUEL	**AMOUNT (kg)**	**PERCENTAGE OF TOTAL STORED CALORIES**
Glycogen		
Muscle	0.15	0.4
Liver	0.08	0.2
Protein	6.0	14.4
Triglyceride	15	85

[a]In biochemistry and nutrition, the standard reference is often the 70-kg (154 lb) man. This standard was probably chosen because in the first half of the 20th century, when many nutritional studies were performed, young healthy medical and graduate students (who were mostly men) volunteered to serve as subjects for these experiments.

It is not practical to store all of the energy in triacylglycerol as glycogen because glycogen is a polar molecule with hydroxyl groups and binds approximately 4 times its weight as water. Storage of energy as triacylglycerol contains much less water weight.

C. Protein

Protein serves many important roles in the body; unlike fat and glycogen, it is not solely a fuel store like fat or glycogen. Muscle protein is essential for body movement. Other proteins serve as **enzymes** (catalysts of biochemical reactions) or as **structural components** of cells and tissues. Only a limited amount of body protein can be degraded, approximately 6 kg in the average 70-kg man, before our body functions are compromised.

III. Daily Energy Expenditure

If we want to stay in energy balance, neither gaining nor losing weight, we must, on average, consume an amount of food equal to our daily energy expenditure. The *daily energy expenditure* (**DEE**) includes the energy to support our basal metabolism (*basal metabolic rate* [BMR] or *resting metabolic rate* [RMR]) and our physical activity, plus the energy required to process the food we eat (*diet-induced thermogenesis* [DIT]). Thus, the DEE, in kilocalories per day, = BMR (or RMR) + the energy needed for physical activity + DIT.

A. Basal Metabolic Rate

Two terms have been used to define the energy required by the body, the BMR and the RMR. The BMR is a measure of the energy required to maintain life: the functioning of the lungs, kidneys, and brain; the pumping of the heart; the maintenance of ionic gradients across membranes; the reactions of biochemical pathways; and so forth. The BMR was originally defined as the energy expenditure of a person mentally and bodily at rest in a thermoneutral environment 12 to 18 hours after a meal. However, when a person is awakened and their heat production or oxygen consumption is measured, they are no longer sleeping or totally at mental rest, and their metabolic rate is called the *resting metabolic rate* (RMR). It is also sometimes called the *resting energy expenditure* (REE). The RMR and BMR differ very little in value, and for the purposes of this text, we will focus on the BMR.

The BMR, which is usually expressed in kilocalories per day, is affected by body size, age, sex, and other factors (Table 1.3). It is proportional to the amount of metabolically active tissue (including the major organs) and to the lean (or fat-free) body mass. Obviously, the amount of energy required for basal functions in a large person is greater than the amount required in a small person. However, the BMR is usually lower for women than for men of the same weight because women usually have more metabolically inactive adipose tissue. Body temperature also affects the BMR, which increases by 12% with each degree centigrade (7% with each degree

TABLE 1.3 Factors Affecting BMR Expressed per Kilogram of Body Weight
Gender (males higher than females)
Body temperature (increased with fever)
Environmental temperature (increased in cold)
Thyroid status (increased in hyperthyroidism)
Pregnancy and lactation (increased)
Age (decreased with age)
Body composition (increased with muscle mass)

TABLE 1.4 The Mifflin-St. Joer Equation for Predicting BMR	
Males	$(10 \times W) + (6.25 \times H) - (5 \times A) + 5$
Females	$(10 \times W) + (6.25 \times H) - (5 \times A) - 161$

Body weight (W) in kilograms, height (H) in centimeters, and age (A) in years; final result is kilocalories per day.
From Mifflin MD, St. Joer ST, Hill LA, Scott BJ, Daugherty SA, Koh XO. A new predictive equation for resting energy expenditure in healthy individuals. *Am J Clin Nutr.* 1990;51:241–247.

Fahrenheit) increase in body temperature (i.e., "feed a fever; starve a cold"). The ambient temperature affects the BMR, which increases slightly in colder climates as thermogenesis is activated. Excessive secretion of thyroid hormone (hyperthyroidism) causes the BMR to increase, whereas diminished secretion (hypothyroidism) causes it to decrease. The BMR increases during pregnancy and lactation. Growing children have a higher BMR per kilogram body weight than adults because a greater proportion of their bodies is composed of brain, muscle, and other more metabolically active tissues. The BMR declines in aging individuals because their metabolically active tissue is shrinking and body fat is increasing. In addition, large variations exist in BMR from one adult to another, determined by genetic factors.

A rough estimate of the BMR may be obtained by assuming it is either 24 or 21.6 kcal/day/kg body weight (for men or for women, respectively) and multiplying by the body weight. An easy way to remember this is 1 kcal/kg/hr for men and 0.9 kcal/kg/hr for women. This estimate works best for young individuals who are near their healthy weight. More accurate methods for calculating the BMR use empirically derived equations for different gender and age groups (Table 1.4). Even these calculations do not take into account variation among individuals.

B. Physical Activity

In addition to the BMR, the energy required for **physical activity** contributes to the DEE. The difference in physical activity between a student and a lumberjack is enormous, and a student who is relatively sedentary during the week may be much more active during the weekend. Table 1.5 gives factors for calculating the approximate energy expenditures associated with typical activities.

TABLE 1.5 Typical Activities with Corresponding Hourly Activity Factors[a]	
ACTIVITY CATEGORY	**HOURLY ACTIVITY FACTOR (FOR TIME IN ACTIVITY)**
Resting: sleeping, reclining	1.0
Very light: seated and standing activities, driving, laboratory work, typing, sewing, ironing, cooking, playing cards, playing a musical instrument	1.5
Light: walking on a level surface at 2.5–3 mph, garage work, electrical trades, carpentry, restaurant trades, house cleaning, golf, sailing, table tennis	2.5
Moderate: walking 3.5–4 mph, weeding and hoeing, carrying loads, cycling, skiing, tennis, dancing	5.0
Heavy: walking uphill with a load, tree felling, heavy manual digging, mountain climbing, basketball, football, soccer	7.0

mph, miles per hour.
[a]The hourly activity factor is multiplied by the BMR per hour times the number of hours engaged in the activity to give the caloric expenditure for that activity. If this is done for all of the hours in a day, the sum over 24 hours will approximately equal the daily energy expenditure.
Reprinted with permission from *Recommended Dietary Allowances.* 10th ed. Washington, DC: The National Academies Press; 1989.

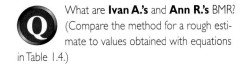

What are **Ivan A.'s** and **Ann R.'s** BMR? (Compare the method for a rough estimate to values obtained with equations in Table 1.4.)

Registered dietitians often use extensive tables for calculating energy requirements, which are based on height, weight, age, gender, and activity level. A more accurate calculation is based on the fat-free mass (FFM), which is equal to the total body mass minus the mass of the person's adipose tissue. With FFM, the BMR is calculated using the equation BMR = 186 + FFM × 23.6 kcal/kg/day. This formula eliminates differences between sexes and between elderly versus young individuals that are attributable to differences in relative adiposity. However, determining FFM is relatively cumbersome—one technique requires weighing the patient underwater and measuring the residual lung volume. More recently, dual-energy X-ray absorptiometry (DXA) is an equally accurate, but simpler, technique that is used to determine the patient's total amount of fat and FFM.

Indirect calorimetry, a technique that measures O_2 consumption and CO_2 production, can be used when more accurate determinations of energy need are required for hospitalized patients. A portable indirect calorimeter is used to measure oxygen consumption and the *respiratory quotient* (RQ), which is the ratio of O_2 consumed to CO_2 produced. The RQ is 1.00 for individuals oxidizing carbohydrates, 0.83 for protein, and 0.71 for fat. From these values, the DEE can be determined.

A simplified method to measure the DEE also uses indirect calorimetry but only measures O_2 production. Because the oxidation of nutrients requires molecular oxygen, through the measurement of the volume of total inspired and expired air, and the amount of O_2 in that air, a very good estimate of the BMR can be determined. The device required for this method is less cumbersome than the device that measures both oxygen and CO_2 consumption and is easier to use, but it is less accurate.

Mr. A. weighs 264 lb or 120 kg (264 lb divided by 2.2 lb/kg). His estimated BMR = 24 calories/kg/day × 120 = 2,880 calories/day. His BMR calculated from Table 1.4 is only 1,992 calories (10 × weight + 6.25 × height − 5 × age + 5, where the weight is in kilograms, the height in centimeters, and the age in years). **Ms. R.** weighs 99 lb or 45 kg (99 divided by 2.2 lb/kg). Her estimated BMR = (21.6 calories/kg/day) × (45 kg) = 972 calories/day. Her BMR from Table 1.4 is above this value (10 × weight + 6.25 × height − 5 × age − 161 = 1,238 calories/day). Thus, for **Ms. R.**, the rough estimate is 78% of the more accurate calculation. For **Mr. A.**, his caloric needs are only 70% that of the rough estimate because a disproportionately larger proportion of his body weight (his adipose tissue) is relatively inactive metabolically.

Based on the activities listed in Table 1.5, the average US citizen is rather sedentary. Sedentary habits correlate strongly with risk for cardiovascular disease, so it is not surprising that cardiovascular disease is the major cause of death in this country.

What are reasonable estimates for **Ivan A.'s** and **Ann R.'s** DEE?

A rough estimate of the energy required per day for physical activity can be made by using a value of 30% of the BMR (per day) for a very sedentary person (such as a medical student who does little but study) and a value of 60% to 70% of the BMR (per day) for a person who engages in about 2 hours of moderate physical activity per day (see Table 1.5). A value of 100% or more of the BMR is used for a person who does several hours of vigorous physical activity per day.

C. Diet-Induced Thermogenesis

Our DEE includes a component related to the intake of food known as *diet-induced thermogenesis* or the *thermic effect of food* (TEF). DIT was formerly called the *specific dynamic action* (SDA). After the ingestion of food, our metabolic rate increases because energy is required to digest, absorb, distribute, and store nutrients.

The energy required to process the types and quantities of food in the typical American diet is probably equal to approximately 10% of the kilocalories ingested. This amount is roughly equivalent to the error involved in rounding off the caloric content of carbohydrate, fat, and protein to 4, 9, and 4, respectively. Therefore, DIT is often ignored and calculations are based simply on the BMR and the energy required for physical activity.

D. Calculations of Daily Energy Expenditure

The total DEE is usually calculated as the sum of the BMR (in kilocalories per day) plus the energy required for the amount of time spent in each of the various types of physical activity (see Table 1.5). An approximate value for the DEE can be determined from the BMR and the appropriate percentage of the BMR required for physical activity (given earlier). For example, a very sedentary medical student would have a DEE equal to the RMR plus 30% of the BMR (or 1.3 × BMR), and an active person's daily expenditure could be two times the BMR.

E. Healthy Body Weight

Ideally, we should strive to maintain a weight consistent with good health. The BMI, calculated as weight divided by height^2 (kg/m^2), is currently the preferred method for determining whether a person's weight is in the healthy range. This formula, in the English system, is (weight [in pounds] × 704)/height^2 (with height in inches).

In general, adults with BMI values <18.5 are considered underweight. Those with BMIs between 18.5 and 24.9 are considered to be in the healthy weight range, between 25 and 29.9 are in the overweight or preobese range, and 30 and above are in the obese range. Class I obesity is defined as a BMI of 30 to 34.9, class II as a BMI of 35 to 39.9, and class III (or extreme obesity) as a BMI of 40 or greater. Degrees of protein-calorie malnutrition (marasmus) are classified according to the BMI. A BMI of 17.0 to 18.4 is degree I; values of 16.0 to 16.9 is degree II; and any value less than 16.0 is degree III, the most severe form of protein-energy malnutrition.

F. Weight Gain and Loss

To maintain our body weight, we must stay in caloric balance. We are in caloric balance if the calories in the food we eat equal our DEE. If we eat less food than we require for our DEE, our body fuel stores supply the additional calories and we lose weight. Conversely, if we eat more food than we require for our energy needs, the excess fuel is stored (mainly in our adipose tissue) and we gain weight.

When we draw on our adipose tissue to meet our energy needs, we lose approximately 1 lb whenever we expend approximately 3,500 calories more than we consume. In other words, if we eat 1,000 calories less than we expend per day, we will lose about 2 lb/week. Because the average individual's food intake is only about

2,000 to 3,000 calories/day, eating one-third to one-half the normal amount will cause a person to lose weight rather slowly. Fad diets that promise a loss of weight much more rapid than this have no scientific merit. In fact, the rapid initial weight loss the fad dieter typically experiences is attributable largely to loss of body water. This loss of water occurs in part because muscle tissue protein and liver glycogen are degraded rapidly to supply energy during the early phase of the diet. When muscle tissue (which is approximately 80% water) and glycogen (approximately 70% water) are broken down, this water is excreted from the body.

IV. Dietary Requirements

In addition to supplying us with fuel and with general purpose building blocks for biosynthesis, our diet also provides us with specific nutrients that we need to remain healthy. We must have a regular supply of vitamins and minerals and of the essential fatty acids and essential amino acids. *Essential* means that they are essential in the diet; the body cannot synthesize these compounds from other molecules and therefore must obtain them from the diet. Nutrients that the body requires in the diet only under certain conditions are called *conditionally essential.*

The **Recommended Dietary Allowance (RDA)** and the **Adequate Intake (AI)** provide quantitative estimates of nutrient requirements. The RDA for a nutrient is the average daily dietary intake level necessary to meet the requirement of nearly all (97% to 98%) healthy individuals in a particular gender and life stage group. *Life stage group* is a certain age range or physiologic status (i.e., pregnancy or lactation). The RDA is intended to serve as a goal for intake by individuals. The AI is a recommended intake value that is used when not enough data are available to establish an RDA.

A. Carbohydrates

The RDA for carbohydrate is 130 g/day for children and adults and is based on the amount of carbohydrate needed to provide the brain with an adequate supply of glucose. Another value, the *acceptable macronutrient distribution range* (AMDR) is the recommended range of intake for a macronutrient that is associated with a reduced risk of disease while providing adequate intake of essential nutrients. The AMDR is expressed as a percentage of caloric intake. For example, according to its AMDR, carbohydrate should provide 45% to 65% of total calories.

Carbohydrates can be synthesized from amino acids, and we can convert one type of carbohydrate to another. However, health problems are associated with the complete elimination of carbohydrate from the diet, partly because a low-carbohydrate diet must contain higher amounts of fat to provide us with the energy we need. High-fat diets are associated with obesity, atherosclerosis, and other health problems.

B. Essential Fatty Acids

The recommended range (AMDR) for dietary fat is 20% to 35% of total calories. Although most lipids required for cell structure, fuel storage, or hormone synthesis can be synthesized from carbohydrates or proteins, we need a minimal level of certain dietary lipids for optimal health. These lipids, known as *essential fatty acids*, are required in our diet because we cannot synthesize fatty acids with these particular arrangements of double bonds. The essential fatty acids α-linoleic and α-linolenic acid are supplied by dietary plant oils, and eicosapentaenoic acid (EPA) and docosahexaenoic acid (DHA) are supplied in fish oils. They are the precursors of the eicosanoids (a set of hormone-like molecules that are secreted by cells in small quantities and have numerous important effects on neighboring cells). The eicosanoids include the prostaglandins, thromboxanes, leukotrienes, and other related compounds.

Mr. A.'s BMR is 1,992 calories/day. He is sedentary, so he only requires approximately 30% more calories for his physical activity. Therefore, his daily expenditure is approximately 1,992 + (0.3 × 1,992) or 1.3 × 1,992 or 2,590 kcal/day. **Ms. R.'s** BMR is 1,238 calories/day. She performs 2 hours of moderate physical activity per day (jogging and walking), so she requires approximately 65% more calories for her physical activity. Therefore, her daily expenditure is approximately 1,238 + (0.65 × 1,238) or 1.65 × 1,238 or 2,043 calories/day.

Ivan A.'s weight is classified as obese. His BMI is (264 lb × 704)/(70 in)^2 = 37.9. **Ann R.** is underweight. Her BMI is (99 lb × 704)/(67 in)^2 = 15.5.

To evaluate a patient's weight, physicians need standards of obesity applicable in a genetically heterogeneous population. Life insurance industry statistics have been used to develop tables, such as the Metropolitan Height and Weight Tables, giving the weight ranges, based on gender, height, and body frame size, that are associated with the greatest longevity. However, these tables are considered inadequate for a number of reasons (e.g., they reflect data from upper-middle-class white groups). The BMI is the classification that is currently used clinically. It is based on two simple measurements, height without shoes and weight with minimal clothing.

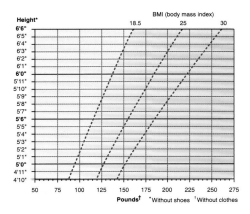

Patients can be shown their BMI in a nomogram and need not use calculations. The healthy weight range coincides with the mortality data derived from life insurance tables. The BMI also shows a good correlation with independent measures of body fat. The major weakness of the use of the BMI is that some very muscular individuals may be classified as obese when they are not. There are also some differences in BMI and risk of certain diseases that vary by race or ethnicity. Other measurements to estimate body fat and other body compartments, such as weighing individuals underwater, are more difficult, expensive, and time-consuming and have generally been confined to research purposes.

If patients are above or below the healthy BMI range (such as **Ivan A.** or **Ann R.**), the physician, often in consultation with a registered dietitian, prescribes a diet designed to bring the weight into the healthy range.

Are **Ivan A.** and **Ann R.** gaining or losing weight?

C. Protein

The RDA for protein is approximately 0.8 g of high-quality protein per kilogram of healthy body weight, or approximately 56 g/day for a 154-lb man and 46 g/day for a 126-lb woman. "High-quality" protein contains all of the essential amino acids in adequate amounts for health. Proteins derived from animal sources (milk, egg, and meat products) and soy are high quality. Most proteins in plant foods are of lower quality, which means they are low in one or more of the essential amino acids. Vegans may obtain adequate amounts of the essential amino acids by eating mixtures of plant-based proteins that complement each other in terms of their amino acid composition. According to its recommended AMDR, protein should contribute 10% to 35% of total caloric intake.

1. Essential Amino Acids

Different amino acids are used in the body as precursors for the synthesis of proteins and other nitrogen-containing compounds. Of the 20 amino acids commonly required in the body for synthesis of protein and other compounds, 9 amino acids are essential in the diet of an adult human because they cannot be synthesized in the body. These are **lysine, isoleucine, leucine, threonine, valine, tryptophan, phenylalanine, methionine,** and **histidine**.

Certain amino acids are conditionally essential—that is, required in the diet only under certain conditions. Children and pregnant women have a high rate of protein synthesis to support growth and require some **arginine** in the diet, although it can be synthesized in the body. Histidine is essential in the adult diet in very small quantities because adults efficiently recycle histidine. The increased requirement of children and pregnant women for histidine is therefore much larger than their increased requirement of other essential amino acids. Tyrosine and cysteine are examples of conditionally essential amino acids. Tyrosine is synthesized from phenylalanine, and it is required in the diet if phenylalanine intake is inadequate or if an individual is congenitally deficient in an enzyme required to convert phenylalanine to tyrosine (the congenital disease phenylketonuria). Cysteine is synthesized by using sulfur from methionine, and it also may be required in the diet under conditions of low methionine intake or malabsorption disorders.

2. Nitrogen Balance

The proteins in the body undergo constant turnover; that is, they are constantly being degraded to amino acids and resynthesized. When a protein is degraded, its amino acids are released into the pool of free amino acids in the body. The amino acids from dietary proteins also enter this pool. Free amino acids can have one of three fates: They are used to make proteins, they serve as precursors for synthesis of essential nitrogen-containing compounds (e.g., heme, DNA, RNA), or they are oxidized as fuel to yield energy. When amino acids are oxidized, their nitrogen atoms are excreted in the urine, principally in the form of urea. The urine also contains smaller amounts of other nitrogenous excretory products (uric acid, creatinine, and NH_4^+) derived from the degradation of amino acids and compounds synthesized from amino acids. Some nitrogen is also lost in sweat, feces, and cells that slough off.

Nitrogen balance is the difference between the amount of nitrogen taken into the body each day (mainly in the form of dietary protein) and the amount of nitrogen in compounds lost (Table 1.6). If more nitrogen is ingested than excreted, a person

TABLE 1.6 Nitrogen Balance		
Positive nitrogen balance	Growth (e.g., childhood, pregnancy)	Dietary N > Excreted N
Nitrogen balance	Normal healthy adult	Dietary N = Excreted N
Negative nitrogen balance	Dietary deficiency of total protein or amino acids: catabolic stress	Dietary N < Excreted N

N refers to nitrogen.

is said to be in positive nitrogen balance. Positive nitrogen balance occurs in growing individuals (e.g., children, adolescents, pregnant women), who are synthesizing more protein than they are breaking down. On the other hand, if less nitrogen is ingested than excreted, a person is said to be in negative nitrogen balance. A negative nitrogen balance develops in a person who is eating either too little protein or protein that is deficient in one or more of the essential amino acids. Amino acids are continuously being mobilized from body proteins. If the diet is lacking an essential amino acid or if the intake of protein is too low, new protein cannot be synthesized and the unused amino acids will be degraded, with the nitrogen appearing in the urine. If a negative nitrogen balance persists for too long, bodily function will be impaired by the net loss of critical proteins. In contrast, healthy adults are in nitrogen balance (neither positive nor negative), and the amount of nitrogen consumed in the diet equals its loss in urine, sweat, feces, and other excretions.

D. Vitamins

Vitamins are a diverse group of organic molecules required in very small quantities in the diet for health, growth, and survival (Latin *vita*, life). The absence of a vitamin from the diet or an inadequate intake results in characteristic deficiency signs and, ultimately, death. Table 1.7 lists the signs or symptoms of deficiency for each vitamin, its RDA or AI for young adults, and common food sources. The amount of each vitamin required in the diet is small (in the microgram or milligram range), compared with essential amino acid requirements (in the gram range). The vitamins often are divided into two classes, **water-soluble vitamins** and **fat-soluble vitamins**. This classification has little relationship to their function but is related to the absorption and transport of fat-soluble vitamins with lipids.

Most vitamins are used for the synthesis of **coenzymes**, complex organic molecules that assist enzymes in catalyzing biochemical reactions, and the deficiency symptoms reflect an inability of cells to carry out certain reactions. However, some vitamins also act as hormones. We will consider the roles played by individual vitamins as we progress through the subsequent chapters of this text.

Although the RDA or AI for each vitamin varies with age and sex, the difference is usually not very large once adolescence is reached. For example, the RDA for riboflavin is 0.9 mg/day for males between 9 and 13 years of age, 1.3 mg/day for males 19 to 30 years of age, still 1.3 mg/day for males older than 70 years, and 1.1 mg/day for females 19 to 30 years. The largest requirements occur during lactation (1.6 mg/day).

Vitamins, by definition, cannot be synthesized in the body or are synthesized from a very specific dietary precursor in insufficient amounts. For example, we can synthesize the vitamin niacin from the essential amino acid tryptophan, but not in sufficient quantities to meet our needs. Niacin is therefore still classified as a vitamin.

Excessive intake of many vitamins, both fat-soluble and water-soluble, may cause deleterious effects. For example, high doses of vitamin A, a fat-soluble vitamin, can cause desquamation of the skin and birth defects. High doses of vitamin C cause diarrhea and gastrointestinal disturbances. One of the sets of values of the Dietary Reference Intakes (DRI) is the **Tolerable Upper Intake Level** (UL), which is the highest level of daily nutrient intake that is likely to pose no risk of adverse effects to almost all individuals in the general population. As intake increases above the UL, the risk of adverse effects increases. Table 1.7 includes the UL for vitamins known to pose a risk at high levels. Intake above the UL occurs most often with dietary or pharmacologic supplements of single vitamins and not from foods.

E. Minerals

Many **minerals** are required in the diet. They are generally divided into macro or major minerals and micro or trace minerals. Electrolytes (inorganic ions that are

Mr. A. expends about 2,590 calories/day and consumes 4,110 calories/day. By this calculation, he consumes 1,520 kcal more than he expends each day and is gaining weight. **Ms. R.** expends 2,043 calories/day while she consumes only 615 calories/day. Therefore, she expends 1,428 calories more than she consumes each day, so she is losing weight.

Malnutrition, which is deficient or excess intake of energy or nutrients, occurs in the United States principally among children of families with incomes below the poverty level, the elderly, individuals whose diet is influenced by alcohol and drug use, and those who make poor food choices. More than 13 million children in the United States live in families with incomes below the poverty level. Of these, approximately 10% have clinical malnutrition, most often anemia resulting from inadequate iron intake. A larger percentage have mild protein and energy malnutrition and exhibit growth retardation, sometimes as a result of parental neglect. Childhood malnutrition also may lead to learning failure and chronic illness later in life. A weight-for-height measurement is one of the best indicators of childhood malnourishment because it is easy to measure, and weight is one of the first parameters to change during malnutrition.

The term *kwashiorkor* refers to a disease originally seen in African children suffering from a protein deficiency (although overall energy intake may be normal). It is characterized by marked hypoalbuminemia (low levels of albumin in the blood), anemia, edema (buildup of fluids in the interstitial spaces), pot belly, loss of hair, and other signs of tissue injury. The term *marasmus* is used for prolonged protein and energy malnutrition, particularly in young children. Marasmus is characterized by loss of weight and body fat, muscle wasting, and poor growth. Children with marasmus usually do not develop edema. The term *protein-energy malnutrition* (PEM) can be used to describe both disorders. The term *severe acute malnutrition* (SAM) includes inadequate intake of vitamins and minerals, as well as energy and protein.

Multiple vitamin deficiencies accompanying malnutrition are far more common in the United States than the characteristic deficiency diseases associated with diets lacking just one vitamin because we generally eat a variety of foods. The characteristic deficiency diseases arising from single vitamin deficiencies often were identified and described in humans through observations of populations consuming a restricted diet because that was all that was available. For example, thiamin deficiency was discovered by a physician in Java who related the symptoms of beriberi to diets composed principally of polished rice. Today, single vitamin deficiencies usually occur as a result of conditions that interfere with the uptake or use of a vitamin or as a result of poor food choices or a lack of variety in the diet. For example, peripheral neuropathy associated with vitamin E deficiency can occur in children with fat malabsorption, and alcohol consumption can result in beriberi. Vegans, individuals who consume diets lacking all animal products, can develop deficiencies in vitamin B_{12}.

In the hospital, it was learned that **Mr. Percy V.** had lost 32 lb in the 8 months since his last visit to his family physician. On admission, his hemoglobin (the iron-containing compound in the blood, which carries O_2 from the lungs to the tissues) was 10.7 g/dL (reference range, males = 12 to 15.5 g/dL), his serum ferritin was 4 ng/mL (reference range, males = 40 to 200 ng/mL), and other hematologic indices that reflect nutritional status were also abnormal. These values are indicative of an iron deficiency anemia. His serum folic acid level was 0.9 ng/mL (reference range = 3 to 20 ng/mL), indicating a low intake of this vitamin. His vitamin B_{12} level was 190 pg/mL (reference range = 180 to 914 pg/mL). A low blood vitamin B_{12} level can be caused by decreased intake, absorption, or transport, but it takes a long time to develop. His serum albumin was 3.2 g/dL (reference range = 3.5 to 5.0 g/dL), which is an indicator of protein malnutrition or liver disease.

TABLE 1.7	Vitamins		
VITAMIN	**DIETARY REFERENCE INTAKES (DRI) FEMALES (F) MALES (M) (18–30 YR OLD)**	**SOME COMMON FOOD SOURCES**	**CONSEQUENCES OF DEFICIENCY (NAMES OF DEFICIENCY DISEASES ARE IN BOLD)**
Water-soluble vitamins			
Vitamin C	**RDA** F: 75 mg M: 90 mg **UL:** 2 g	Citrus fruits; potatoes; peppers, broccoli, spinach; strawberries	**Scurvy:** defective collagen formation leading to subcutaneous hemorrhage, aching bones, joints, and muscle in adults, rigid position and pain in infants
Thiamin	**RDA** F: 1.1 mg M: 1.2 mg	Enriched, fortified, and whole grain cereals and breads; pork; legumes, seeds, nuts	**Beriberi:** (wet) edema; anorexia, weight loss; apathy, decrease in short-term memory, confusion; irritability; muscle weakness; an enlarged heart
Riboflavin	**RDA** F: 1.1 mg M: 1.3 mg	Dairy products; enriched, fortified, and whole grain cereals; meats, poultry, fish; legumes	**Ariboflavinosis:** sore throat, hyperemia, edema of oral mucous membranes; cheilosis, angular stomatitis; glossitis, magenta tongue; seborrheic dermatitis; normochromic normocytic anemia
Niacin[a]	**RDA** F: 14 mg NEQ M: 16 mg NEQ **UL:** 35 mg	Meat, poultry, fish; enriched and whole grain cereals and breads; all protein-containing foods	**Pellagra:** pigmented rash in areas exposed to sunlight; vomiting; constipation or diarrhea; bright red tongue; neurologic symptoms
Vitamin B_6 (pyridoxine)	**RDA** F: 1.3 mg M: 1.3 mg **UL:** 100 mg	Meat, poultry, fish; eggs; fortified cereals, unmilled rice, oats; starchy vegetables; noncitrus fruits; peanuts, walnuts	Seborrheic dermatitis; microcytic anemia; epileptiform convulsions; depression and confusion
Folate	**RDA** F: 400 μg M: 400 μg **UL:** 1,000 μg	Citrus fruits; leafy green vegetables; fortified cereals and breads; legumes	Impaired cell division and growth; **megaloblastic anemia;** neural tube defects
Vitamin B_{12}	**RDA** F: 2.4 μg M: 2.4 μg	Animal products[b]	**Megaloblastic anemia;** neurologic symptoms
Biotin	**AI** F: 30 μg M: 30 μg	Liver Egg yolk	Conjunctivitis; central nervous system abnormalities; glossitis; alopecia; dry, scaly dermatitis
Pantothenic acid	**AI** F: 5 mg M: 5 mg	Wide distribution in foods, especially animal tissues; whole grain cereals; legumes	Irritability and restlessness; fatigue, apathy, malaise; gastrointestinal symptoms; neurologic symptoms
Choline	**AI** F: 425 mg M: 550 mg **UL:** 3.5 g	Milk; liver; eggs; peanuts	Liver damage

(continued)

	DIETARY REFERENCE INTAKES (DRI) FEMALES (F) MALES (M)		CONSEQUENCES OF DEFICIENCY (NAMES OF DEFICIENCY DISEASES ARE IN
VITAMIN	**(18–30 YR OLD)**	**SOME COMMON FOOD SOURCES**	**BOLD)**
Fat-soluble vitamins			
Vitamin A	**RDA** F: 700 μg M: 900 μg **UL**: 3,000 μg	Milk and milk products; dark green and leafy vegetables; broccoli; deep orange fruits and vegetables (carrots, sweet potatoes, squash)	Night blindness; **xerophthalmia**; keratinization of epithelium in gastrointestinal, respiratory, and genitourinary tract; dry and scaly skin
Vitamin K	**RDA** F: 90 μg M: 120 μg	Green leafy vegetables; cabbage family (brassica); vegetable oils; bacterial flora of intestine	Defective blood coagulation; hemorrhagic anemia of the newborn
Vitamin D	**RDA**[c] F: 15 μg M: 15 μg **UL**: 100 μg	Fortified milk; fortified margarine, butter, and cereals; eggs; fatty fish; exposure of skin to sunlight	**Rickets** (in children); inadequate bone mineralization (osteomalacia)
Vitamin E	**RDA** F: 15 mg M: 15 mg **UL**: 1 g	Vegetable oils, margarine; wheat germ; nuts; green leafy vegetables	Muscular dystrophy, neurologic abnormalities

TABLE 1.7 Vitamins *(continued)*

RDA, Recommended Dietary Allowance; AI, Adequate Intake; UL, Tolerable Upper Intake Level.

[a]neq = niacin equivalents. In humans, niacin can be synthesized from tryptophan, and this term takes into account a conversion factor for dietary tryptophan.

[b]Vitamin B$_{12}$ is found only in animal products.

[c]Dietary requirement assumes the absence of sunlight.

Information for this table is adapted from the Dietary Reference Intake series, The National Academies Press, Copyright 1997, 1998, 2000, 2001, 2002, 2004, 2005, 2011 by the National Academies of Sciences. This information can also be obtained via the Web, at http://fnic.nal.usda.gov/; click on Dietary Guidance, then Dietary Reference Intakes, and then DRI Tables.

dissolved in the fluid compartments of the body) are macrominerals. Macrominerals are required in relatively large quantities, whereas microminerals are required in much lower amounts (Table 1.8).

Sodium (Na$^+$), potassium (K$^+$), and chloride (Cl$^-$) are the major electrolytes (ions) in the body. They establish ion gradients across membranes, maintain water balance, and neutralize positive and negative charges on proteins and other molecules.

Calcium and phosphorus serve as structural components of bones and teeth and are thus required in relatively large quantities. Calcium (Ca^{2+}) plays many other roles in the body; for example, it is involved in hormone action and blood clotting. Phosphorus is required for the formation of ATP and of phosphorylated intermediates in metabolism. Magnesium activates many enzymes and also forms a complex with ATP. Iron is a particularly important mineral because it functions as a component of hemoglobin (the oxygen-carrying protein in the blood) and is part of many enzymes. Other minerals, such as zinc or molybdenum, are required in very small quantities (trace or ultratrace amounts).

Sulfur is ingested principally in the amino acids cysteine and methionine. It is found in connective tissue, particularly in cartilage and skin. It has important functions in metabolism, which we will describe when we consider the action of

A dietary deficiency of calcium can lead to *osteoporosis* and *osteomalacia*, a disorder in which bones are insufficiently mineralized and consequently are fragile and easily fractured. Osteoporosis is a particularly common problem among elderly women. Deficiency of phosphorus results in bone loss along with weakness, anorexia, malaise, and pain. Iron deficiencies lead to anemia, a decrease in the concentration of hemoglobin in the blood.

TABLE 1.8 Minerals Required in the Diet	
MAJOR	**TRACE**
Sodium[a]	Iodine
Potassium[a]	Selenium
Chloride[a]	Copper
Calcium	Zinc
Phosphorous	Iron
Magnesium	Manganese[b]
	Fluoride[b]
	Chromium[b]
	Molybdenum[b]

[a]Electrolytes.
[b]Ultratrace minerals.

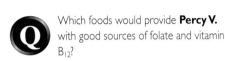

Which foods would provide **Percy V.** with good sources of folate and vitamin B_{12}?

coenzyme A, a compound used to activate carboxylic acids. Sulfur is excreted in the urine as sulfate.

Minerals, like vitamins, have adverse effects if ingested in excessive amounts. Problems associated with dietary excesses or deficiencies of minerals are described in subsequent chapters in conjunction with their normal metabolic functions.

F. Water

Water constitutes one-half to four-fifths of the weight of the human body. The intake of water required per day depends on the balance between the amount produced by body metabolism and the amount lost through the skin, through expired air, and in the urine and feces.

V. Dietary Guidelines

Dietary guidelines or goals are recommendations for food choices that can reduce the risk of developing chronic diseases while maintaining an adequate intake of nutrients. Many studies have shown an association between diet and physical activity and decreased risk of certain diseases, including hypertension, atherosclerosis, stroke, diabetes, certain types of cancer, and osteoarthritis. Thus, the American Heart Institute and the American Cancer Institute, as well as several other groups, have developed diet and physical activity recommendations to decrease the risk of these diseases. The *Dietary Guidelines for Americans (2015–2020)* are prepared by an advisory committee of researchers appointed by the U.S. Department of Agriculture (USDA) and the U.S. Department of Health and Human Services to review the current evidence and revise the guidelines accordingly every 5 years (you can view these at the Web site listed in the references). Recommended servings of different food groups can be customized for individuals accessing the USDA MyPlate Web site (see references). Physicians and dietitians can tailor the dietary guidelines to meet the needs of their patients with specific medical conditions.

A. General Recommendations

- Choose a healthy eating pattern at an appropriate calorie level to help achieve and maintain a healthy body weight. For maintenance of weight, energy intake should balance energy expenditure. Accumulate at least 30 minutes of moderate physical activity (such as walking at a pace of 3 to 4 miles per hour) daily and engage in muscle strengthening exercises at least 2 days per week. A regular physical activity program helps in achieving and maintaining healthy weight, cardiovascular fitness, and strength.

- Choose nutrient-dense foods in the amounts recommended by your personalized plan from MyPlate, including a daily variety of whole grains, fruits, and vegetables; fat-free or low-fat dairy products; and lean protein foods.
- Practice food safety by frequently cleaning hands, cutting boards, and countertops; cooking foods to safe temperatures; and refrigerating leftovers promptly.

B. Carbohydrates

- A diet rich in vegetables, fruits, and grain products should be chosen, providing 45% to 65% of its calories as carbohydrates. A variety of vegetables from all of the subgroups (i.e., dark green, red and orange, legumes, starchy, and other) and whole fruits should be included in a healthy eating pattern. In regard to grains (e.g., starches and other complex carbohydrates in the form of breads, fortified cereals, rice, and pasta), at least half should be whole grains. In addition to energy, vegetables, fruits, and grains supply vitamins, minerals, phytochemicals (protective compounds such as carotenoids, flavonoids, and lycopene), and fiber. Fiber, the indigestible part of plant food, has various beneficial effects, including relief of constipation.
- The consumption of added sugars in foods and beverages should be limited to less than 10% of total calories. Added sugars have no nutritional value other than calories, and they promote tooth decay.

C. Fats

- Dietary fat should account for 20% to 35% of total calories, and saturated fatty acids should account for <10% of total calories. Fats derived from fish, nuts, and vegetables, which are primarily polyunsaturated and monosaturated fatty acids, are preferred. Owing to their saturated fat content, meats such as fatty beef, lamb, pork, and poultry with skin and full-fat dairy products such as cheese, whole milk, butter, and ice cream should be limited. *Trans*-fatty acids, such as the partially hydrogenated vegetable oils found in stick margarines, baked goods, and fried foods, should be avoided.
- Although saturated and trans fats have a greater impact than dietary cholesterol on lowering low-density lipoprotein cholesterol, many organizations recommend that cholesterol intake be <300 mg/day in persons without atherosclerotic disease and <200 mg/day in those with established atherosclerosis. Major sources of dietary cholesterol in the American diet include beef, poultry, processed meats, eggs, cheese, and ice cream.

D. Proteins

- Protein intake for adults should be approximately 0.8 g/kg healthy body weight per day. The protein should be of high quality and should be obtained from sources low in saturated fat (e.g., fish, poultry, beans, lentils, low-fat/fat-free dairy products, soy products). Vegans should eat a mixture of plant proteins that ensures the intake of adequate amounts of the essential amino acids.

E. Alcohol

- Alcohol consumption should not exceed moderate drinking and should only be consumed by adults of legal drinking age. Moderation is defined as no more than one drink per day for women and no more than two drinks per day for men. A drink is defined as 12 oz of beer, 5 oz of wine (a little over 0.5 cup), or 1.5 oz of an 80-proof liquor such as whiskey. Pregnant women should drink no alcohol. The ingestion of alcohol by pregnant women can result in fetal alcohol syndrome (FAS), which is marked by prenatal and postnatal

Folate is found in fruits and vegetables: citrus fruits (e.g., oranges), green leafy vegetables (e.g., spinach and broccoli), fortified cereals, and legumes (e.g., peas) (see Table 1.7). Conversely, vitamin B_{12} is found only in foods of animal origin, including meats, eggs, and milk.

Cholesterol is obtained from the diet and is synthesized in most cells of the body. It is a component of cell membranes and the precursor of steroid hormones and of the bile salts used for fat absorption. High concentrations of cholesterol in the blood, particularly the cholesterol in lipoprotein particles called *low-density lipoproteins* (LDL), contribute to the formation of atherosclerotic plaques inside the lumen of arterial vessels, particularly in the heart and brain. These plaques (fatty deposits on arterial walls) can obstruct blood flow to these vital organs, causing heart attacks and strokes. A high content of saturated fat and trans fat in the diet tends to increase circulatory levels of LDL cholesterol and contributes to the development of atherosclerosis.

growth deficiency; developmental delay; and craniofacial, limb, and cardio-vascular defects.

The high content of sodium (in table salt) in the average American diet appears to be related to the development of hypertension (high blood pressure) in individuals who are genetically predisposed to this disorder.

F. Vitamins and Minerals

- Sodium intake should be decreased in most individuals. Sodium is usually consumed as salt, NaCl. Less than 2.3 g of sodium should be consumed daily, which is equivalent to the sodium in 1 tbsp of salt.
- Many of the required vitamins and minerals can be obtained from eating a variety of fruits, vegetables, and grains (particularly whole grains). Low-fat or fat-free dairy products are an excellent source of calcium; some dark green leafy vegetables provide available calcium. Lean meats, shellfish, poultry, dark meat, cooked dry beans, and some leafy green vegetables provide good sources of iron. Vitamin B_{12} is found only in animal sources.
- Dietary supplementation in excess of the recommended amounts (e.g., mega-vitamin regimens) should be avoided.
- Fluoride should be present in the diet, at least during the years of tooth formation, as a protection against dental caries.

VI. Xenobiotics

In addition to nutrients, our diet also contains a large number of chemicals called *xenobiotics*, which have no nutritional value, are of no use in the body, and can be harmful if consumed in excessive amounts. These compounds occur naturally in foods, can enter the food chain as contaminants, or can be deliberately introduced as food additives.

Dietary guidelines of the American Cancer Society and the American Institute for Cancer Research make recommendations relevant to the ingestion of xenobiotic compounds, particularly carcinogens. The dietary advice that we eat a variety of food helps to protect us against the ingestion of a toxic level of any one xenobiotic compound. It is also suggested that we reduce consumption of salt-cured, smoked, and charred foods, which contain chemicals that can contribute to the development of cancer. Other guidelines encourage the ingestion of fruits and vegetables that contain protective phytochemicals that act as antioxidants.

CLINICAL COMMENTS

Otto S. Otto S. sought help in reducing his weight of 187 lb (BMI of 27) to his previous level of 154 lb (BMI of 22, in the middle of the healthy range).

Otto S. is 5 ft 10 in tall, and he calculated that his maximum healthy weight was 173 lb. He planned on becoming a family physician, and he knew that he would be better able to counsel patients in healthy lifestyle behaviors such as diet and physical activity if he practiced them himself. With this information and assurances from the physician that he was otherwise in good health, Otto embarked on a weight loss program. One of his strategies involved recording all the food he ate and the portions. To analyze his diet for calories, saturated fat, and nutrients, he used the MyPlate personalized Plan (see references), available online from the USDA Center for Nutrition Policy and Promotion (CNPP). As part of his program, Otto met with a registered dietitian who provided the following: tips for buying and cooking nutrient-dense foods at a reasonable cost, tips for modifying eating behavior (e.g., slowing down the pace of eating), the setting of realistic achievable goals (e.g., loss of 10% of initial body weight within 6 months), and tips for dealing with relapse into prior habits.

Ivan A. Ivan A. weighed 264 lb and was 70 in tall with a heavy skeletal frame. For a male of this height, a BMI of 18.5 to 24.9 would correspond to a weight between 129 lb and 173 lb. He is currently almost 100 lb overweight, and his BMI of 37.9 is in the obese range.

Mr. A.'s physician cautioned him that exogenous obesity (caused by overeating) represents a risk factor for atherosclerotic cardiovascular disease, particularly when the distribution of fat is primarily "central" or in the abdominal region (apple shape, in contrast to the pear shape, in which adipose tissue is deposited in the buttocks and hips). In addition, obesity may lead to other cardiovascular risk factors such as hypertension (high blood pressure), hyperlipidemia (high blood lipid levels), and type 2 diabetes mellitus (characterized by hyperglycemia). Mr. A. already has elevated blood pressure. Furthermore, his total serum cholesterol level was 296 mg/dL, well above the desired normal value (200 mg/dL).

Mr. A. was referred to the hospital's weight reduction center, where a team of physicians, dietitians, and psychologists could assist him in reaching a healthy BMI.

 Ann R. Because of her history and physical examination, **Ann R.** was diagnosed as having early *anorexia nervosa*, a psychiatric illness involving a disturbance in body image, which results in low body weight, malnutrition, and other medical complications. Miss R. was referred to a multidisciplinary team that included a psychiatrist with expertise in anorexia nervosa, and a program of psychotherapy and behavior modification was initiated.

 Percy V. Percy V. weighed 125 lb and was 71 in tall (without shoes) with a medium frame. His BMI was 17.5, which is significantly underweight. At the time his wife died, he weighed 147 lb. For his height, a BMI in the healthy weight range corresponds to weights between 132 lb and 178 lb.

Mr. V.'s malnourished state was reflected in his admission laboratory profile. The results of hematologic studies were consistent with an iron deficiency anemia complicated by low levels of folic acid and vitamin B_{12}, two vitamins that can affect the development of normal red blood cells. His low serum albumin level was caused by insufficient protein intake and a shortage of essential amino acids, which result in a reduced ability to synthesize body proteins. The psychiatrist requested a consultation with a hospital dietitian to evaluate the extent of Mr. V.'s severe acute malnutrition caused by inadequate intake of protein, energy, vitamins, and minerals.

BIOCHEMICAL COMMENTS

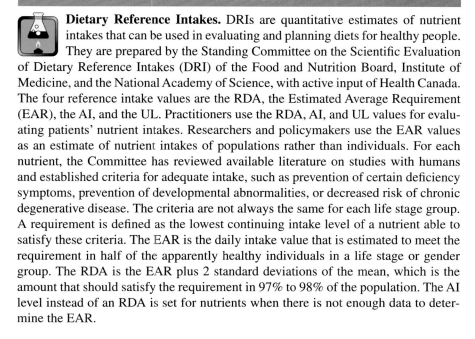 **Dietary Reference Intakes.** DRIs are quantitative estimates of nutrient intakes that can be used in evaluating and planning diets for healthy people. They are prepared by the Standing Committee on the Scientific Evaluation of Dietary Reference Intakes (DRI) of the Food and Nutrition Board, Institute of Medicine, and the National Academy of Science, with active input of Health Canada. The four reference intake values are the RDA, the Estimated Average Requirement (EAR), the AI, and the UL. Practitioners use the RDA, AI, and UL values for evaluating patients' nutrient intakes. Researchers and policymakers use the EAR values as an estimate of nutrient intakes of populations rather than individuals. For each nutrient, the Committee has reviewed available literature on studies with humans and established criteria for adequate intake, such as prevention of certain deficiency symptoms, prevention of developmental abnormalities, or decreased risk of chronic degenerative disease. The criteria are not always the same for each life stage group. A requirement is defined as the lowest continuing intake level of a nutrient able to satisfy these criteria. The EAR is the daily intake value that is estimated to meet the requirement in half of the apparently healthy individuals in a life stage or gender group. The RDA is the EAR plus 2 standard deviations of the mean, which is the amount that should satisfy the requirement in 97% to 98% of the population. The AI level instead of an RDA is set for nutrients when there is not enough data to determine the EAR.

 The prevalence of obesity in the US population is increasing. In 1962, 12.8% of the population had a BMI ≥30 and therefore were clinically obese. That number increased to 14.5% by 1980 and to 22.5% by 1998. An additional 30% were overweight in 1998 (BMI = 25.0 to 29.9). In 2012, based on BMI values, 35.1% of adults were classified as obese, and an additional 33.9% were classified as overweight. It is apparent, therefore, that more than two-thirds of the population is currently overweight or obese.

An elevated BMI increases cardiovascular risk factors, including hypertension, diabetes mellitus, and alterations in blood lipid levels. It also increases the risk for respiratory problems, gallbladder disease, and certain types of cancer.

 When Mr. A. met with the dietitian to discuss his weight loss plans, he received the following advice: tips for devising a meal plan that provides consistent amounts of complex carbohydrates throughout the day for glucose control while limiting calories, saturated and trans fat, and sodium and tips for small, incremental dietary changes to achieve a diet that is lower in trans fat, sodium, and refined carbohydrates while high in essential nutrients via whole grains, fruits, vegetables, lean protein, and nonfat/low-fat dairy products. Mr. A. was also counseled in a manner similar to **Otto S.**, with an emphasis on the importance of losing 10% of initial body weight for improvement in blood pressure, blood lipids, and glucose control.

The UL refers to the highest level of daily nutrient intake consumed over time that is likely to pose no risks of adverse effects for almost all healthy individuals in the general population. Adverse effects are defined as any significant alteration in the structure or function of the human organism. The UL does not mean that most individuals who consume more than the UL will suffer adverse health effects but that the risk of adverse effects increases as intake increases above the UL.

KEY CONCEPTS

- Fuel is provided in the form of carbohydrates, fats, and proteins in our diet.
- Energy is obtained from the fuel by oxidizing it to carbon dioxide and water.
- Unused fuel can be stored as triacylglycerol (fat) or glycogen (carbohydrate) within the body.
- Weight gain or loss is a balance between the energy consumed in our diet and the energy required each day to drive the basic functions of our body and our physical activity. The daily energy expenditure (DEE) is the amount of fuel consumed in a 24-hour period.
- The basal metabolic rate (BMR) is a measure of the energy required to maintain involuntary bodily functions such as respiration, contraction of the heart muscle, biosynthetic processes, and establishment of ion gradients across neuronal membranes.
- The DEE is determined by the BMR and the individual's activity level while awake.
- The body mass index (BMI) is a ratio of weight to height that is used to determine a healthy weight for an individual and to classify a person as underweight, healthy weight, overweight, or obese.
- In addition to macronutrients, the diet provides vitamins, minerals, essential fatty acids, and essential amino acids.
- The Recommended Dietary Allowance (RDA) and the Adequate Intake (AI) provide quantitative estimates of nutrient requirements.
- The Tolerable Upper Intake Level (UL) indicates the highest level of daily nutrient uptake that is likely to pose no risk of adverse effects.
- A summary of the diseases/disorders discussed in this chapter are presented in Table 1.9.

TABLE 1.9	Diseases Discussed in Chapter 1	
DISORDER OR CONDITION	**GENETIC OR ENVIRONMENTAL**	**COMMENTS**
Depression	Both	Diagnosed by behavioral changes, can be treated with a variety of pharmacologic agents and counseling therapy
Obesity	Both	Long-term effects of obesity affect cardiovascular system and may lead to metabolic syndrome.
Anorexia nervosa	Both	Self-induced reduction of food intake, distorted body image, considered at least in part a psychiatric disorder
Kwashiorkor	Environmental	Protein and mineral deficiency yet normal amount of calories in the diet; leads to marked hypoalbuminemia, anemia, edema, pot belly, loss of hair, and other indications of tissue injury
Marasmus	Environmental	Prolonged calorie and protein malnutrition
Osteoporosis/ osteomalacia	Environmental	Calcium-deficient diet leading to insufficient mineralization of the bones, which produces fragile and easily broken bones

Diseases that may have a genetic component are indicated as genetic; disorders caused by environmental factors (with or without genetic influences) are indicated as environmental.

REVIEW QUESTIONS—CHAPTER I

Directions: For each question below, select the single best answer.

1. A dietitian is counseling a patient with celiac sprue (intolerance to gluten, leading to malabsorption issues in the intestine) and describing a diet with appropriate carbohydrate, fat, and protein content. Once properly absorbed, the major fate of these compounds during respiration is which ONE of the following?
   A. They are stored as triacylglycerols.
   B. They are oxidized to generate ATP.
   C. They release energy principally as heat.
   D. They combine with CO_2 and H_2O and are stored.
   E. They combine with other dietary components in anabolic pathways.

2. A dietitian is counseling a patient with celiac sprue (intolerance to gluten, leading to malabsorption issues in the intestine) who has experienced steatorrhea (fatty stools caused by poor absorption of dietary lipids in the intestine) for a number of years. The dietitian, in addition to describing appropriate carbohydrates, lipids, and proteins that will not trigger the malabsorption issue, also encourages the patient to take certain vitamins. Which ONE of the following vitamins is most likely on this list?
   A. Vitamin C
   B. Folic acid
   C. Vitamin B_{12}
   D. Vitamin K
   E. Vitamin B_1

3. Mrs. Jones is a sedentary 83-year-old woman who is 5 ft 4 in tall and weighs 125 lb. She has been at this weight for about a year. She says that a typical diet for her includes a breakfast of toast (white bread, no butter), a boiled egg, and coffee with cream. For lunch she often has a cheese sandwich (white bread) and a glass of whole milk. For supper she prefers cream of chicken soup and a slice of frosted cake. Mrs. Jones's diet is most likely to be inadequate in which one of the following?
   A. Vitamin C
   B. Protein
   C. Calcium
   D. Vitamin B_{12}
   E. Calories

4. A patient is trying to lose weight and wonders what her ideal number of calories per day might be. A dietitian is helping her by estimating the BMR, the DIT, and physical activity. The BMR is best estimated by consideration of which one of the following?
   A. It is equivalent to the caloric requirement of our major organs and resting muscle.
   B. It is generally higher per kilogram of body weight in women than in men.
   C. It is generally lower per kilogram of body weight in children than adults.
   D. It is decreased in a cold environment.
   E. It is approximately equivalent to the DEE.

5. A friend of yours has decided to go on a crash diet, consuming only 700 calories per day. You advise your friend that he is at risk for certain dietary deficiencies and inform him of the RDA, which is best described by which one of the following?
   A. The average amount of a nutrient required each day to maintain normal function in 50% of the US population
   B. The average amount of a nutrient ingested daily by 50% of the US population
   C. The minimum amount of a nutrient ingested daily that prevents deficiency symptoms
   D. A reasonable dietary goal for the intake of a nutrient by a healthy individual
   E. It is based principally on data obtained with laboratory animals.

6. A 35-year-old sedentary male patient weighing 120 kg was experiencing angina (chest pain) and other signs of coronary artery disease. His physician, in consultation with a registered dietitian, conducted a 3-day dietary recall. The patient consumed an average of 585 g of carbohydrate, 150 g of protein, and 95 g of fat each day. In addition, he drank 45 g of alcohol. The patient's diet is best described by which one of the following?
   A. He consumed between 2,500 and 3,000 kcal/day.
   B. He had a fat intake within the range recommended in current dietary guidelines (i.e., year 2010).
   C. He consumed 50% of his calories as alcohol.
   D. He was deficient in protein intake.
   E. He was in negative caloric balance.

7. A sedentary 75-kg male is trying to lose weight and has begun a calorie-restricted diet. He has reduced his daily intake by 10 g of carbohydrates, 10 g of fat, 10 g of protein, and 10 g of ethanol. By what percentage has this man reduced his daily intake as compared to what he would require to maintain his current weight?
   A. 5%
   B. 10%
   C. 15%
   D. 20%
   E. 25%

8. A 45-year old man developed deep vein thrombosis and subsequently a pulmonary embolism. After recovery, the patient was placed on warfarin to prevent future blood clots. The patient was counseled by a dietitian to limit his consumption of which one of the following foods because of the finding that eating the food could interfere with the action of warfarin?
   A. Egg yolks
   B. Yellow vegetables
   C. Citrus fruits
   D. Green leafy vegetables
   E. Skinless chicken

9. A 25-year-old female with Hashimoto's thyroiditis is being treated with thyroid hormone replacement and is now euthyroid. She wishes to lose some of the weight she gained while she was in a hypothyroid state. In order to help her lose weight, her dietitian must determine her daily energy expenditure in order to determine a diet with fewer calories than her DEE. The patient weighs 70 kg, is moderately active (1 to 2 hours of exercise 5 days per week), and is currently consuming 2,700 calories per day. If the patient is to lose 1 lb per week, she would need to reduce her daily consumption by how many calories per day?
   A. 200
   B. 400

C. 600
D. 800
E. 1,000

10. A patient with cirrhosis is having mental status changes owing to elevated ammonia levels in his blood. In prescribing a diet to reduce ammonia production in this patient, which class of nutrients should be most restricted?
   A. Ethanol
   B. Lipids
   C. Proteins
   D. Carbohydrates
   E. Water-soluble vitamins

ANSWERS TO REVIEW QUESTIONS

1. **The answer is B.** In the process of respiration, O_2 is consumed and fuels are oxidized to CO_2 and H_2O. The energy from the oxidation reactions is used to generate ATP from ADP and P_i. However, a small amount of energy is also released as heat (thus, C is incorrect). Although fuels can be stored as triacylglycerols, this is not part of respiration (thus, A is incorrect). Respiration is a catabolic pathway (fuels are degraded), as opposed to an anabolic pathway (compounds combine to make larger molecules) (thus, E is incorrect).

2. **The answer is D.** Vitamin K is a fat-soluble vitamin, and it is absorbed from the small intestine in the presence of lipids. If lipids cannot be absorbed, the fat-soluble vitamins (vitamins A, D, E, and K) also will not be absorbed. The other vitamins listed (vitamins B_1, C, folic acid, B_{12}) are all water-soluble vitamins that do not require the presence of lipid for absorption from the intestinal lumen.

3. **The answer is A.** Mrs. Jones's diet lacks fruits and vegetables, both of which are good sources of vitamin C. Her diet is adequate in protein, as eggs, milk, cheese and cream contain significant levels of protein. Her calcium levels should be fine owing to the milk, cream, and cheese in her diet. Vitamin B_{12} is derived from foods of animal origin, such as eggs, milk, and cheese. As the patient's weight has been stable for a year, her diet contains sufficient calories to allow her to maintain this weight, which is in the normal range for a patient who is 5 ft 4 in tall, as her BMI is 21.5.

4. **The answer is A.** The BMR is the calories being expended by a recently awakened resting person who has fasted 12 to 18 hours and is at 20°C. It is equivalent to the energy expenditure of our major organs and resting skeletal muscle. Women generally have a lower BMR per kilogram of body weight because more of their body weight is usually metabolically less-active adipose tissue. Children have a higher BMR per kilogram of body weight because more of their body weight is metabolically active organs like the brain. The BMR increases in a cold environment because more energy is being

expended to generate heat. The BMR is not equivalent to our DEE, which includes BMR, physical activity, and DIT.

5. **The answer is D.** The RDA of a nutrient is determined from the EAR plus 2 standard deviations of the mean (SD) and should meet the needs for 97% to 98% of the healthy population. It is therefore a reasonable goal for the intake of a healthy individual. The EAR is the amount that prevents development of established signs of deficiency in 50% of the healthy population. Although data with laboratory animals have been used to establish deficiency symptoms, RDAs are based on data collected on nutrient ingestion by humans.

6. **The answer is B.** The recommended total fat intake is <30% of total calories. His total caloric consumption was 4,110 calories/day (carbohydrate, $4 \times 585 = 2,340$ calories; protein $150 \times 4 = 600$ calories; fat, $95 \times 9 = 855$ calories; alcohol, $45 \times 7 = 315$ calories) (thus, A is incorrect). His fat intake was 21% ($855 \div 4,110$) of his total caloric intake. His alcohol intake was 7.7% ($315 \div 4,110$) (thus, C is incorrect). His protein intake was well above the RDA of 0.8 g/kg body weight (thus, D is incorrect). His BMR is roughly 24 calories/day/kg body weight, or 2,880 calories/day (it will actually be less because he is obese and has a greater proportion of metabolically less-active tissue than the average 70-kg man). His DEE is about 3,744 calories/day ($1.3 \times 2,880$) or less. Thus, his intake is greater than his expenditure, and he is in positive caloric balance and is gaining weight (thus, E is incorrect).

7. **The answer is B.** The man weighs 75 kg, so a rough estimate of his daily caloric need (to maintain his weight) is $75 \times 24 \times 1.3 = 2,340$ calories/day (1.3 is the sedentary activity factor). The man has reduced his daily intake by 240 calories (10 g of carbohydrates is 40 calories; 10 g of protein is 40 calories; 10 g of lipid is 90 calories; 10 g of ethanol is 70 calories; $40 + 40 + 90 + 70 = 240$). Thus, the man has reduced his daily intake by approximately 10% of that needed to maintain his weight (240/2,340).

8. **The answer is D.** Warfarin acts by inhibiting the ability of vitamin K to participate in reactions required by clotting factors. If one's diet contains additional vitamin K, the efficacy of the warfarin could be reduced. Green leafy vegetables are an excellent source of vitamin K, and their consumption should be limited while on warfarin therapy.

9. **The answer is D.** The patient's DEE is calculated as $70 \times 21.6 \times 1.6 = 2,420$ (70 kg weight, times 21.6 kcal/kg/day, times 1.6 activity factor for being moderately active). Because the patient is currently consuming 2,700 calories/day, she is gaining weight despite her activity. To lose 1 lb of weight, a loss of 3,500 calories must occur. Over a 1-week period, that is 500 calories/day. Thus, the patient should be consuming 1,920 calories/day to lose 1 lb per week, which is approximately 800 fewer calories/day based on her current consumption.

10. **The answer is C.** Ethanol, lipids (triglycerides), and carbohydrates do not contain a nitrogen group that is converted to ammonia during its catabolism—only proteins do. Water-soluble vitamins are present at low levels and are not appreciably catabolized, so their contribution to ammonia production is low as compared to protein catabolism.

2

The Fed or Absorptive State

The Fed State. During a **meal**, we ingest carbohydrates, lipids, and proteins, which are subsequently **digested** and **absorbed**. Some of this food is **oxidized** to meet the immediate **energy** needs of the body. The amount consumed in **excess** of the body's energy needs is transported to the **fuel depots**, where it is stored. During the period from the start of absorption until absorption is completed, we are in the **fed**, or absorptive, state. Whether a fuel is oxidized or stored in the fed state is determined principally by the concentration of two **endocrine hormones** in the blood, **insulin** and **glucagon**.

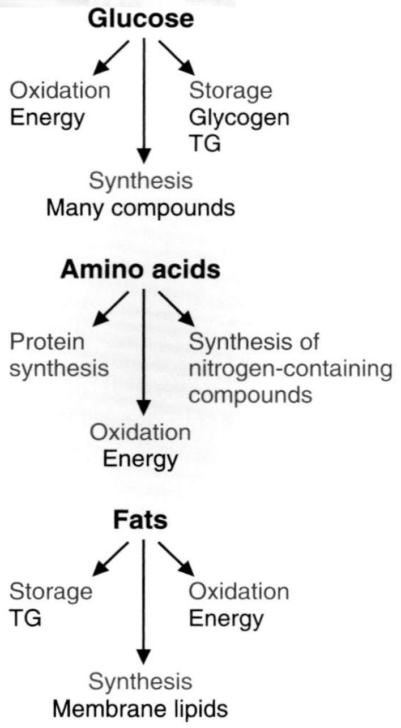

Fate of Carbohydrates. Dietary carbohydrates are digested to monosaccharides, which are absorbed into the blood. The major monosaccharide in the blood is **glucose** (Fig. 2.1). After a meal, glucose is **oxidized** by various tissues for energy, enters biosynthetic pathways, and is **stored** as **glycogen**, mainly in liver and muscle. Glucose is the major biosynthetic precursor in the body, and the carbon skeletons of most of the compounds we synthesize can be synthesized from glucose. Glucose is also converted to **triacylglycerols**. The liver packages triacylglycerols, made from glucose or from fatty acids obtained from the blood, into **very low-density lipoproteins (VLDL)** and releases them into the blood. The fatty acids of the VLDL are stored mainly as triacylglycerols in adipose tissue, but some may be used to meet the energy needs of cells.

Fate of Proteins. Dietary proteins are digested to **amino acids**, which are absorbed into the blood. In cells, the amino acids are converted to **proteins** or used to make various **nitrogen-containing compounds** such as neurotransmitters and heme. The carbon skeleton may also be **oxidized** for energy directly or converted to glucose.

Fate of Fats. Triacylglycerols are the major lipids in the diet. They are digested to fatty acids and 2-monoacylglycerols, which are resynthesized into **triacylglycerols** in intestinal epithelial cells, packaged in **chylomicrons**, and secreted by way of the lymph into the blood. The **fatty acids** of the chylomicron triacylglycerols are stored mainly as triacylglycerols in **adipose** cells. They are subsequently oxidized for energy or used in biosynthetic pathways, such as synthesis of membrane lipids.

Glucose

Oxidation
Energy

Storage
Glycogen
TG

Synthesis
Many compounds

Amino acids

Protein
synthesis

Synthesis of
nitrogen-containing
compounds

Oxidation
Energy

Fats

Storage
TG

Oxidation
Energy

Synthesis
Membrane lipids

FIGURE 2.1 Major fates of fuels in the fed state. *TG*, triacylglycerol.

THE WAITING ROOM -------------------------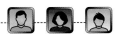

 Ivan A. returned to his doctor for a second visit. His initial efforts to lose weight and follow the dietitian's recommendations had failed dismally. In fact, he now weighed 270 lb, an increase of 6 lb since his first visit 2 months ago (see Chapter 1). He reported that the recent death of his 45-year-old brother of a heart attack had made him realize that he must pay more attention to his health. Because Mr. A.'s brother had a history of hypercholesterolemia and because Mr. A.'s serum total cholesterol had been significantly elevated (296 mg/dL) at his first visit, his blood lipid profile was determined, he was screened for type 2 diabetes, and a few other blood tests were ordered. (The *blood lipid profile* is a test that measures the content of the various triacylglycerol- and cholesterol-containing particles in the blood.) His blood pressure was 162 mm Hg systolic and 98 mm Hg diastolic, or 162/98 mm Hg (normal is ≤120/80 mm Hg, with prehypertension 120 to 139/80 to 89 mm Hg and hypertension is defined as >140/90 mm Hg). His waist circumference was 48 in (healthy values for men, <40 in; for women, <35 in).

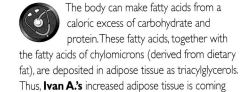

The body can make fatty acids from a caloric excess of carbohydrate and protein. These fatty acids, together with the fatty acids of chylomicrons (derived from dietary fat), are deposited in adipose tissue as triacylglycerols. Thus, **Ivan A.'s** increased adipose tissue is coming from his intake of all fuels in excess of his caloric need.

I. Digestion and Absorption

A. Carbohydrates

Dietary carbohydrates are converted to monosaccharides. *Starch*, a polymer of glucose, is the major carbohydrate of the diet. It is digested by the enzyme salivary α-amylase and then by pancreatic α-amylase, which acts in the small intestine. *Enzymes* are proteins that catalyze biochemical reactions (usually they increase the speed at which the reactions occur). Di-, tri-, and oligosaccharides (*disaccharide* refers to two linked sugars; a *trisaccharide* to three linked sugars, and an *oligosaccharide* to *n* linked sugars) produced by these α-amylases are cleaved to glucose by digestive enzymes located on the surface of the brush border of the intestinal epithelial cells. Dietary disaccharides also are cleaved by enzymes in this brush border. Sucrase converts the disaccharide sucrose (table sugar) to glucose and fructose, and lactase converts the disaccharide lactose (milk sugar) to glucose and galactose. Monosaccharides produced by digestion and dietary monosaccharides are absorbed by the intestinal epithelial cells and released into the hepatic portal vein, which carries them to the liver.

B. Proteins

Proteins contain amino acids that are linked through peptide bonds (see Chapter 1). Dipeptides contain two amino acids, tripeptides contain three amino acids, and so on. Dietary proteins are cleaved to amino acids by enzymes known as *proteases* (Fig. 2.2, circle 3), which cleave the peptide bond between amino acids (see Fig. 1.5). Pepsin acts in the stomach, and the proteolytic enzymes produced by the pancreas (trypsin, chymotrypsin, elastase, and the carboxypeptidases) act in the lumen of the small intestine. Aminopeptidases and di- and tripeptidases associated with the intestinal epithelial cells complete the conversion of dietary proteins to amino acids, which are absorbed into the intestinal epithelial cells and released into the hepatic portal vein.

C. Fats

The digestion of fats is more complex than that of carbohydrates or proteins because fats are not very soluble in water. The triacylglycerols of the diet are emulsified in the intestine by bile salts, which are synthesized in the liver and stored in the gallbladder. The enzyme pancreatic lipase converts the triacylglycerols in the lumen of the intestine to fatty acids and 2-monoacylglycerols (glycerol with a fatty acid esterified at carbon 2), which interact with bile salts to form tiny microdroplets called *micelles*. The fatty acids and 2-monoacylglycerols are absorbed from these micelles into the intestinal epithelial cells, where they are resynthesized

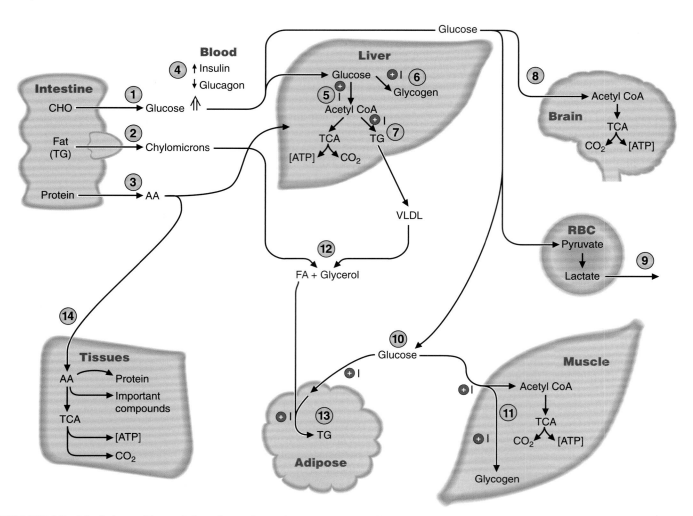

FIGURE 2.2 The fed state. The *circled numbers* indicate the approximate order in which the processes occur. *TG*, triacylglycerols; *FA*, fatty acid; *AA*, amino acid; *RBC*, red blood cell; *VLDL*, very low-density lipoprotein; *I*, insulin; *CHO*, carbohydrate; *acetyl CoA*, acetyl coenzyme A; *ATP*, adenosine triphosphate; *TCA*, tricarboxylic acid; ⊕, stimulated by.

into triacylglycerols. The triacylglycerols are packaged with proteins, phospholipids, cholesterol, and other compounds into the lipoprotein complexes known as *chylomicrons*, which are secreted into the lymph and ultimately enter the bloodstream (see Fig. 2.2, circle 2). Fats must be transported in the blood bound to protein or in lipoprotein complexes because they are insoluble in water. Thus, both triacylglycerols and cholesterol are found in lipoprotein complexes.

II. Changes in Hormone Levels after a Meal

After a typical high-carbohydrate meal, the **pancreas** is stimulated to release the hormone **insulin**, and release of the hormone **glucagon** is inhibited (see Fig. 2.2, circle 4). **Endocrine hormones** are released from endocrine glands, such as the pancreas, in response to a specific stimulus. They travel in the blood, carrying messages between tissues concerning the overall physiologic state of the body. At their target tissues, they adjust the rate of various metabolic pathways to meet the changing conditions. The endocrine hormone insulin, which is secreted from the β-cells of the pancreas in response to a high-carbohydrate meal, carries the message that dietary glucose is available and can be transported into the cell, used, and stored. The release of another hormone, glucagon, from the α-cells of the pancreas, is suppressed by glucose and insulin. Glucagon carries the message that glucose must be generated from endogenous fuel stores. The subsequent changes in circulating hormone levels cause changes in the body's metabolic patterns, involving several different tissues and metabolic pathways.

III. Fate of Glucose

A. Conversion to Glycogen, Triacylglycerols, and Carbon Dioxide in the Liver

Because glucose leaves the intestine via the hepatic portal vein (a blood vessel that carries blood from the intestine to the liver), the liver is the first tissue it passes through. The liver extracts a portion of this glucose from the blood. Some of the glucose that enters **hepatocytes** (liver cells) is oxidized in adenosine triphosphate (ATP)-generating pathways to meet the immediate energy needs of these cells, and the remainder is converted to glycogen and triacylglycerols or used for biosynthetic reactions. In the liver, insulin promotes the uptake of glucose by increasing its use as a fuel and its storage as glycogen and triacylglycerols (see Fig. 2.2, circles 5 to 7).

As glucose is being oxidized to CO_2, it is first oxidized to pyruvate in the pathway of glycolysis (discussed in more detail in Chapter 22) and consists of a series of reactions common to the metabolism of many carbohydrates. Pyruvate is then oxidized to acetyl coenzyme A (acetyl-CoA). The acetyl group enters the tricarboxylic acid (TCA) cycle, where it is completely oxidized to CO_2. Energy from the oxidative reactions is used to generate ATP. The ATP that is generated is used for anabolic and other energy-requiring processes in the cell. Coenzyme A (CoA), which makes the acetyl group more reactive, is a cofactor derived from the vitamin pantothenic acid.

Liver glycogen stores reach a maximum of approximately 200 to 300 g after a high-carbohydrate meal, whereas the body's fat stores are relatively limitless. As the glycogen stores begin to fill, the liver also begins converting some of the excess glucose it receives to triacylglycerols. Both the glycerol and the fatty acid moieties of the triacylglycerols can be synthesized from glucose. The fatty acids are also obtained preformed from the blood (these are the dietary fatty acids). The liver does not store triacylglycerols, however, but packages them along with proteins, *phospholipids*, and *cholesterol* into the lipoprotein complexes known as *VLDL*, which are secreted into the bloodstream. Some of the fatty acids from the VLDL are taken up by tissues for their immediate energy needs, but most are stored in adipose tissue as triacylglycerols.

B. Glucose Metabolism in Other Tissues

The glucose from the intestine that is not metabolized by the liver travels in the blood to peripheral tissues (most other tissues), where it can be oxidized for energy. Glucose is the one fuel that can be used by all tissues. Many tissues store small amounts of glucose as glycogen. Muscle has relatively large glycogen stores.

Insulin greatly stimulates the transport of glucose into the two tissues that have the largest mass in the body, muscle and adipose tissue. It has much smaller effects on the transport of glucose into other tissues.

Fuel metabolism often is discussed as though the body consisted only of brain, skeletal and cardiac muscle, liver, adipose tissue, red blood cells, kidney, and intestinal epithelial cells ("the gut"). These are the dominant tissues in terms of overall fuel economy, and they are the tissues we describe most often. Of course, all tissues require fuels for energy, and many have very specific fuel requirements.

1. Brain and Other Neural Tissues

The brain and other neural tissues are very dependent on glucose for their energy needs. They generally oxidize glucose, via glycolysis and the TCA cycle, completely to CO_2 and H_2O, generating ATP (see Fig. 2.2, circle 8). Except under conditions of starvation, glucose is their only major fuel. Glucose is also a major precursor of

 The laboratory studies ordered at the time of his second office visit show that **Ivan A.** has hyperglycemia, an elevation of blood glucose above normal values. At the time of this visit, his blood glucose determined after an overnight fast was 162 mg/dL (normal, 80 to 100 mg/dL). Because this blood glucose measurement was significantly above normal, a hemoglobin A1c (glycosylated hemoglobin) level was ordered, which was also elevated. This led to a diagnosis of type 2 diabetes mellitus. In this disease, liver, muscle, and adipose tissue are relatively resistant to the action of insulin in promoting glucose uptake into cells and storage as glycogen and triacylglycerols. Therefore, more glucose remains in his blood. The registered dietitian met with Ivan to assess his current nutrient intake and to counsel him about a heart-healthy diet with a moderate amount of carbohydrate and an emphasis on high-fiber, minimally processed foods. Based on Ivan's metabolic needs, the dietitian then developed a meal plan that allowed for four to five carbohydrate portions at each meal, and two carbohydrate portions each for an afternoon and evening snack. Note that a carbohydrate portion equals 15 g of carbohydrate (60 kcal).

neurotransmitters, the chemicals that convey electrical impulses (as ion gradients) between neurons. If our blood glucose drops much below normal levels, we become dizzy and light-headed. If blood glucose continues to drop, we become comatose and ultimately die. Under normal, nonstarving conditions, the brain and the rest of the nervous system require roughly 150 g of glucose each day.

2. Red Blood Cells

Glucose is the only fuel used by red blood cells because they lack *mitochondria*. Fatty acid oxidation, amino acid oxidation, the TCA cycle, the electron-transport chain, and oxidative phosphorylation (ATP generation that is dependent on oxygen and the electron-transport chain) occur principally in mitochondria. Glucose, in contrast, generates ATP from anaerobic glycolysis in the cytosol, and thus, red blood cells obtain all their energy by this process. In anaerobic glycolysis, the pyruvate formed from glucose is converted to *lactate* and then released into the blood (see Fig. 2.2, circle 9).

Without glucose, red blood cells could not survive. Red blood cells carry O_2 from the lungs to the tissues. Without red blood cells, most of the tissues of the body would suffer from a lack of energy because they require O_2 to completely convert their fuels to CO_2 and H_2O.

3. Muscle

Exercising skeletal muscles can use glucose from the blood or from their own glycogen stores, converting glucose to lactate through glycolysis or oxidizing it completely to CO_2 and H_2O. Muscle also uses other fuels from the blood, such as fatty acids (Fig. 2.3). After a meal, glucose is used by muscle to replenish the glycogen stores that were depleted during exercise. Glucose is transported into muscle cells and converted to glycogen by processes that are stimulated by insulin.

4. Adipose Tissue

Insulin stimulates the transport of glucose into adipose cells as well as into muscle cells. Adipocytes oxidize glucose for energy, and they also use glucose as the source of the glycerol moiety of the triacylglycerols they store (see Fig. 2.2, circle 10).

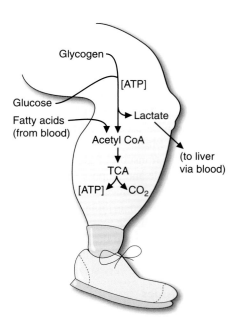

FIGURE 2.3 Oxidation of fuels in exercising skeletal muscle. Exercising muscle uses more energy than resting muscle, and therefore fuel use is increased to supply more adenosine triphosphate (ATP). *Acetyl CoA*, acetyl coenzyme A; *TCA*, tricarboxylic acid.

IV. Lipoproteins

Two types of *lipoproteins*, *chylomicrons* and *VLDL*, are produced in the fed state. The major function of these lipoproteins is to provide a blood transport system for triacylglycerols, which are very insoluble in water. However, these lipoproteins also contain the lipid cholesterol, which is also somewhat insoluble in water. The triacylglycerols of chylomicrons are formed in intestinal epithelial cells from the products of digestion of dietary triacylglycerols. The triacylglycerols of VLDL are synthesized in the liver.

When these lipoproteins pass through blood vessels in adipose tissue, their triacylglycerols are degraded to fatty acids and glycerol (see Fig. 2.2, circle 12). The fatty acids enter the adipose cells and combine with a glycerol moiety that is produced from blood glucose. The resulting triacylglycerols are stored as large fat droplets in the adipose cells. The remnants of the chylomicrons are cleared from the blood by the liver. The remnants of the VLDL can be cleared by the liver, or they can form **low-density lipoprotein (LDL)**, which is cleared by the liver or by peripheral cells.

Most of us have not even begun to reach the limits of our capacity to store triacylglycerols in adipose tissue. The ability of humans to store fat appears to be limited only by the amount of tissue we can carry without overloading the heart.

 Ivan A.'s total cholesterol level is now 315 mg/dL, slightly higher than his previous level of 296 mg/dL. His triacylglycerol level is 250 mg/dL (normal, between 60 and 150 mg/dL), LDL is 210 mg/dL, and HDL is 27 mg/dL (normal for a male, >40 mg/dL). These lipid levels clearly indicate that Mr. A. has a hyperlipidemia (high level of lipoproteins in the blood) and therefore is at risk for the future development of atherosclerosis and its consequences such as heart attacks and strokes.

V. Amino Acids

The amino acids derived from dietary proteins travel from the intestine to the liver in the hepatic portal vein (see Fig. 2.2, circle 3). The liver uses amino acids for the synthesis of serum proteins as well as its own proteins, and for the biosynthesis of nitrogen-containing compounds that need amino acid precursors, such as the nonessential amino acids, *heme*, hormones, neurotransmitters, and *purine* and *pyrimidine* bases (which are required for the synthesis of the nucleic acids RNA and DNA). The liver also may oxidize the amino acids or convert them to glucose or ketone bodies and dispose of the nitrogen as the nontoxic compound urea.

Many of the amino acids will go into the peripheral circulation, where they can be used by other tissues for protein synthesis and various biosynthetic pathways, or they can be oxidized for energy (see Fig. 2.2, circle 14). Proteins undergo *turnover*; they are constantly being synthesized and degraded. The amino acids released by protein breakdown enter the same pool of free amino acids in the blood as the amino acids from the diet. This free amino acid pool in the blood can be used by all cells to provide the right ratio of amino acids for protein synthesis or for biosynthesis of other compounds. In general, each individual biosynthetic pathway using an amino acid precursor is found in only a few tissues in the body.

VI. Summary of the Fed (Absorptive) State

After a meal, the macronutrients that we eat are oxidized to meet our immediate energy needs. Glucose is the major fuel for most tissues. Excess glucose and fatty acids are stored as glycogen mainly in muscle and liver and as triacylglycerols in adipose tissue. Amino acids from dietary proteins are converted to body proteins or oxidized as fuels.

CLINICAL COMMENTS

 Ivan A. Mr. A. was advised that his obesity represents a risk factor for future heart attacks and strokes. He was told that his body has to maintain a larger volume of circulating blood to service his extra fat tissue. This expanded blood volume not only contributes to his elevated blood pressure

Ivan A.'s waist circumference indicates that he has the android pattern of obesity (apple shape). Fat stores are distributed in the body in two different patterns—android and gynecoid. After puberty, men tend to store fat within their abdominal cavity (an android pattern), whereas women tend to store fat subcutaneously in their hips and thighs (a gynecoid pattern). Thus, the typical overweight male tends to have more of an apple shape than the typical overweight female, who is more pear-shaped. Abdominal fat carries a greater risk for hypertension, cardiovascular disease, hyperinsulinemia, diabetes mellitus, gallbladder disease, stroke, and cancer of the breast and endometrium. It also carries a greater risk of overall mortality. Because more men than women have the android distribution, they are more at risk for most of these conditions. Likewise, women who deposit their excess fat in a more android manner have a greater risk than women whose fat distribution is more gynecoid.

Upper-body fat deposition tends to occur more by hypertrophy of the existing cells, whereas lower-body fat deposition is by differentiation of new fat cells (hyperplasia). This may partly explain why many women with lower-body obesity have difficulty losing weight.

The constellation of symptoms exhibited by Mr. A.—abdominal obesity, hyperglycemia, hypertriglyceridemia, and high blood pressure—can all be related to the disorder known as metabolic syndrome or "syndrome X." We will discuss more aspects of metabolic syndrome as Mr. A.'s case progresses.

To obtain reliable measures of SFT, procedures are carefully defined. For example, in the triceps measurement, a fold of skin in the posterior aspect of the nondominant arm midway between shoulder and elbow is grasped gently and pulled away from the underlying muscle. The SFT reading is taken at a precise time, 4 seconds after applying the caliper, because the caliper compresses the skin. Even when these procedures are performed by trained dietitians, reliable measurements are difficult to obtain.

(itself a risk factor for vascular disease) but also puts an increased workload on his heart. This increased load will cause his heart muscle to thicken and eventually to fail.

Mr. A.'s increasing adipose mass has also contributed to his development of type 2 diabetes mellitus, characterized by hyperglycemia (high blood glucose levels). The mechanism behind this breakdown in his ability to maintain normal levels of blood glucose is, at least in part, a resistance by his triacylglycerol-rich adipose cells to the action of insulin.

In addition to type 2 diabetes mellitus, Mr. A. has a hyperlipidemia (high blood lipid level—elevated cholesterol and triacylglycerols), another risk factor for cardiovascular disease. A genetic basis for Mr. A.'s disorder is inferred from a positive family history of hypercholesterolemia and premature coronary artery disease in a brother.

At this point, the first therapeutic steps should be nonpharmacologic. Mr. A.'s obesity should be treated with caloric restriction and a carefully monitored program of exercise. A reduction of dietary fat (particularly saturated fat and trans fat) and sodium would be advised in an effort to correct his hyperlipidemia and his hypertension, respectively. He should also control his carbohydrate intake because of his type 2 diabetes.

BIOCHEMICAL COMMENTS

Anthropometric Measurements. Anthropometry uses body measurements to monitor growth and nutritional health in individuals and to detect nutritional inadequacies or excesses. In adults, the measurements most commonly used are height, weight, triceps skinfold thickness (SFT), arm muscle circumference (AMC), and waist circumference. In infants and young children, length and head circumference are also measured.

Weight and Height. Weight should be measured by using a calibrated beam, lever-balance-type scale, or electronic scale, and the patient should be in minimal clothing (i.e., gown or underwear). Height for adults should be measured while the patient stands against a straight surface, without shoes, with the heels together, and with the head erect and level. The weight and height are used in calculation of the body mass index (BMI).

Skinfold Thickness. Over half of the fat in the body is deposited in subcutaneous tissue under the skin, and the percentage increases with increasing weight. To provide an estimate of the amount of total body fat, a standardized caliper is used to pinch a fold of the skin, usually at more than one site (e.g., the thigh, triceps, subscapular, and suprailiac areas). Obesity by this physical anthropometric technique is defined as a fatfold thickness greater than the 85th percentile for young adults; that is, 18.6 mm for males and 25.1 mm for females.

Midarm Anthropometry. The AMC, also called the mid-upper arm muscle circumference (MUAMC), reflects both caloric adequacy and muscle mass and can serve as a general index of marasmic-type malnutrition. The AMC is measured at the midpoint of the left upper arm by a flexible fiberglass-type tape. The AMC can be calculated from a formula that subtracts a factor related to the SFT from the AMC:

$$\text{MUAMC (cm)} = \text{AMC (cm)} - (3.14 \times \text{SFT [mm]})/10$$

where MUAMC is the mid-upper arm muscle circumference in centimeters and SFT is the skinfold thickness expressed in millimeters.

MUAMC values can be compared with reference graphs available for both sexes and all ages. Protein-calorie malnutrition and negative nitrogen balance induce muscle wasting and decrease muscle circumference.

Waist Circumference. The waist circumference is another anthropometric measurement that serves as an indicator of body composition but is used as a measure of obesity and body fat distribution (the "apple shape"), not malnutrition. The measurement is made by placing a measuring tape around the abdomen at the level of the iliac crest of a standing individual. A high-risk waistline is larger than 35 in (88 cm) for women and larger than 40 in (102 cm) for men.

 The waist-to-hip ratio has been used instead of the waist circumference as a measure of abdominal obesity in an attempt to correct for differences between individuals with respect to body type or bone structure. In this measurement, the waist circumference is divided by the hip circumference (measured at the iliac crest). The average waist-to-hip ratio for men is 0.93 (range = 0.75 to 1.10), and the average for women is 0.83 (range = 0.70 to 1.00). However, the waist circumference may actually correlate better with intra-abdominal fat and the associated risk factors than the waist-to-hip ratio.

KEY CONCEPTS

- During a meal, we ingest carbohydrate, lipids, and proteins.
- Two endocrine hormones—insulin and glucagon—primarily regulate fuel storage and retrieval.
- The predominant carbohydrate in the blood is glucose. Blood glucose levels regulate the release of insulin and glucagon from the pancreas.
- Under the influence of insulin (fed state), glucose can be used as a fuel and also as a precursor for storage via conversion to glycogen or triacylglycerol.
- Insulin stimulates the uptake of glucose into adipose and muscle cells.
- Triacylglycerol obtained from the diet is released into circulation in the form of chylomicrons. Triacylglycerol synthesized from glucose in the liver is released as VLDL. Adipose tissue is the storage site for triacylglycerol.
- The brain and red blood cells use glucose as their primary energy source under normal conditions.
- Amino acids obtained from the diet are used for the biosynthesis of proteins and nitrogen-containing molecules and as an energy source.
- Diseases discussed in this chapter are summarized in Table 2.1.

TABLE 2.1 Diseases Discussed in Chapter 2

DISORDER OR CONDITION	GENETIC OR ENVIRONMENTAL	COMMENTS
Hypercholesterolemia	Both	Elevated cholesterol caused by mutation within a specific protein or excessive cholesterol intake
Hyperglycemia	Both	High blood glucose levels caused by either mutations in specific proteins or tissue resistance to insulin
Hyperlipidemia	Both	High levels of blood lipids may be caused by mutations in specific proteins or ingestion of high-fat diets.

REVIEW QUESTIONS—CHAPTER 2

1. A patient with celiac sprue needs advice on which foods and in what proportions he should ingest them because he still requires a diet containing all essential components. When he eats and digests a mixed meal (containing carbohydrates, lipids, and proteins), which one of the following is most likely to occur?
   A. Starch and other polysaccharides are transported to the liver.
   B. Proteins are converted to dipeptides, which enter the blood.
   C. Dietary triacylglycerols are transported in the portal vein to the liver.
   D. Monosaccharides are transported to adipose tissue via the lymphatic system.
   E. Glucose levels increase in the blood.

2. A marathon runner is training for a race. Two days before the race, the runner exhausts her glycogen stores through an extensive training session and then goes out and eats a large helping of pasta, a process known as "carb loading," which is designed to do which ONE of the following?
   A. To induce the release of glucagon from the pancreas
   B. To release insulin to stimulate glucose entry into the nervous system
   C. To stimulate glycogen synthesis in liver and muscles
   D. To stimulate the oxidation of glucose to carbon dioxide in the muscle
   E. To stimulate red blood cell production of carbon dioxide from glucose

3. A type 2 diabetic, whose diabetes is well controlled (as determined by his hemoglobin A1c levels), has taken his insulin and 15 minutes later eats his evening meal. Which of the following changes will occur as he digests his meal? Choose the ONE best answer.

	Increased Glucose Transport by Muscle	VLDL Synthesis by the Liver	Fatty Acid Synthesis in Fat Cells	Glycogen Synthesis in the Liver	Triacylglycerol Storage in Adipose Tissue
A	Yes	Yes	Yes	No	Yes
B	Yes	No	Yes	No	No
C	Yes	Yes	No	Yes	Yes
D	No	No	Yes	Yes	No
E	No	Yes	Yes	Yes	Yes
F	No	Yes	No	Yes	No

4. Elevated levels of chylomicrons were measured in the blood of a patient. To lower chylomicron levels most effectively, you would prescribe a diet that is restricted in which one of the following?
   A. Overall calories
   B. Fat
   C. Cholesterol
   D. Starch
   E. Sugar

5. A male patient exhibited a BMI of 33 kg/m^2 and a waist circumference of 47 in. What nutrition therapy would be most helpful?
   A. Decreased intake of total calories because all fuels can be converted to adipose tissue triacylglycerols
   B. The same amount of total calories but substitution of carbohydrate calories for fat calories
   C. The same amount of total calories but substitution of protein calories for fat calories
   D. A pure-fat diet because only fatty acids synthesized by the liver can be deposited as adipose triacylglycerols
   E. A limited food diet such as the ice cream and sherry diet

6. A 2-month-old baby is exclusively breastfed. Which ONE of the following anatomic locations contains the most important enzyme needed by this baby for absorption of carbohydrate from this diet?
   A. Salivary gland
   B. Pancreas
   C. Stomach
   D. Small intestine
   E. Liver

7. A "lipid panel" is ordered for a patient as a screening tool to help determine cardiovascular disease risk. The patient is told to fast for 12 hours before the blood draw so that which ONE of the following would be in significantly reduced amounts in the blood?
   A. Cholesterol
   B. Triglycerides
   C. Serum albumin
   D. Chylomicrons
   E. Fatty acids

8. A patient with type 2 diabetes mellitus takes his insulin shot and then 15 minutes later ingests a meal of bread, potatoes, and milk. Which ONE of the following proteins is suppressed during the absorption of this meal?
   A. Glucagon
   B. Insulin
   C. Salivary amylase
   D. Pancreatic amylase
   E. Lactase

9. An athlete is competing in a 400-meter dash. Which ONE of the following is the major source of energy for the muscles used in this competition?
   A. Muscle glycogen stores
   B. Muscle triacylglycerol stores
   C. Muscle amino acid oxidation
   D. Lactic acid from the red blood cells
   E. Liver triacylglycerol stores

10. A patient with type 1 diabetes has neglected to take his insulin before eating a carbohydrate-rich meal. Which of the following tissues will metabolize glucose under these conditions? Choose the ONE best answer.

	Red Blood Cells	Brain	Skeletal Muscle	Adipose Tissue
A	Yes	Yes	No	Yes
B	No	Yes	No	No
C	Yes	Yes	No	No
D	No	No	Yes	No
E	Yes	No	Yes	Yes
F	No	No	Yes	Yes

ANSWERS

1. **The answer is E.** During digestion of a mixed meal, starch and other carbohydrates, proteins, and dietary triacylglycerols are broken into their monomeric units (carbohydrates into simple monosaccharides, protein into amino acids, and triacylglycerols into fatty acids and 2-monacylglycerol) in the small intestine. Glucose is the principal sugar in dietary carbohydrates, and thus, it increases in the blood. Amino acids and monosaccharides enter the portal vein and go to the liver first. After digestion of fats and absorption of the fatty acids by the intestinal epithelial cells, most of the fatty acids are converted back into triacylglycerols and subsequently into chylomicrons by the intestinal cells. Chylomicrons go through lymphatic vessels to

reach the blood, where the triacylglycerol content is principally stored in adipose tissue.

2. **The answer is C.** After a high-carbohydrate meal, glucose is the major fuel for most tissues, including skeletal muscle, adipose tissue, and liver. The increase in blood glucose levels stimulates the release of insulin, not glucagon. Insulin stimulates the transport of glucose in skeletal muscle and adipose tissue, not brain. Liver, not skeletal muscle, converts glucose to fatty acids. Although the red blood cell uses glucose as its only fuel at all times, it generates ATP from conversion of glucose to lactate, not CO_2. When the muscle totally depletes its glycogen stores through exercise and then a meal containing carbohydrate is ingested, the muscle and liver will synthesize glycogen to replete those stores; in the case of muscle, the amount of glycogen synthesized is greater than normal, leading to higher-than-normal glycogen stores in the muscle and an advantage for the muscle during exercise.

3. **The answer is C.** In the fed state, and in the presence of insulin, glucose transport into both the adipocyte and muscle cell will be increased. Insulin will also stimulate the liver to synthesize both glycogen and fatty acids, which leads to enhanced triglyceride synthesis and VLDL production to deliver the fatty acids to other tissues of the body. Insulin will stimulate glucose uptake in fat cells but does not stimulate fatty acid synthesis in the fat cells (that is unique to the liver) but will lead to enhanced triglyceride synthesis in the fat cells.

4. **The answer is B.** Chylomicrons are the lipoprotein particles formed in intestinal epithelial cells from dietary fats and contain principally triacylglycerols formed from components of dietary triacylglycerols. A decreased intake of calories in general would include a decreased consumption of fat, carbohydrate, and protein, which might not lower chylomicron levels. Dietary cholesterol, although found in chylomicrons, is not their principal component.

5. **The answer is A.** The patient's BMI is in the obese range, with large abdominal fat deposits. He needs to decrease his intake of total calories because an excess of calories ingested as carbohydrate, fat, or protein results in deposition of triacylglycerols in adipose tissue. If he keeps his total caloric intake the same, substitution of one type of food for another will help very little with weight loss. (However, a decreased intake of fat may be advisable for other reasons.) Limited food diets, such as the ice cream and sherry diet or a high-protein diet of shrimp, work if they decrease appetite and therefore ingestion of total calories.

6. **The answer is D.** Milk contains lactose (milk sugar) that is converted by the enzyme lactase (located on the brush border of intestinal epithelial cells) to glucose and galactose. The salivary glands produce amylase, which digests starch but not lactose. The pancreas also produces amylase but not an enzyme that can digest lactose. The pancreas does produce insulin, which is not needed for the absorption of lactose but is needed for the absorption of glucose into muscle and fat cells. The stomach produces hydrochloric acid and pepsin for protein digestion but does not digest disaccharides. The liver does not synthesize any enzymes that digest dietary carbohydrates.

7. **The answer is D.** The purpose of fasting is to measure circulating triglycerides and cholesterol without complication from recently ingested food. Upon eating a mixed meal (protein, lipid, and carbohydrate), the intestine synthesizes chylomicrons to distribute the recently ingested lipid throughout the body. Upon fasting, chylomicrons are not present, and what the lipid panel is measuring is the cholesterol content of the blood, the subset of particles carrying the cholesterol (high-density lipoprotein [HDL] and LDL), and the triglyceride content (primarily from VLDL). Serum albumin is the major serum protein and will bind to free fatty acids, but its levels are not measured in a lipid panel (measurement of albumin is done to check liver function). The fatty acids are a part of the triacylglycerol in the circulating lipoprotein particles in the blood and would not be reduced under fasting conditions.

8. **The answer is A.** Bread and potatoes are high in starch/carbohydrates. A high-carbohydrate meal stimulates the release of insulin from the β-cells of the pancreas to help use and store this available glucose. Glucose and insulin suppress the release of glucagon from the α-cells of the pancreas. Glucagon helps to generate glucose from endogenous stores, which is unnecessary with such high levels of glucose from dietary sources. Salivary and pancreatic amylase are both required in the breakdown of dietary starches to glucose. Lactase is required to convert lactose to glucose and galactose (from the milk sugar in the meal).

9. **The answer is A.** The 400-meter dash is primarily an anaerobic activity, and the major source of energy for the muscle is glucose from its own glycogen stores (this pathway is also the one that produces energy at the fastest rate). The muscle does not store triacylglycerol (adipose tissue does). During the exercise, the muscle will generate lactic acid, which will be secreted in the blood. The muscle will not use lactate as an energy source. The muscle will not degrade its own proteins to generate amino acids to use as an energy source.

10. **The answer is C.** Insulin is required for glucose transport into both skeletal muscle and adipose tissue but is not required for glucose uptake into the red blood cells or brain (nervous tissue). The tissues that cannot transport glucose will be unable to metabolize it under these conditions. The inability of skeletal muscle and adipose tissue to take up glucose in the absence of insulin contributes to the high blood glucose levels seen in people with type 1 diabetes who have neglected to take their insulin.

Fasting

The Fasting State. Fasting begins approximately 2 to 4 hours after a meal, when blood glucose levels return to basal levels, and continues until blood glucose levels begin to rise after the start of the next meal. Within about 1 hour after a meal, blood glucose levels begin to fall. Consequently, **insulin** levels decline and **glucagon** levels rise. These changes in hormone levels trigger the **release of fuels** from the body stores. **Liver glycogen** is **degraded** by the process of **glycogenolysis,** which supplies glucose to the blood. **Adipose triacylglycerols** are **mobilized** by the process of **lipolysis,** which releases fatty acids and glycerol into the blood. Use of **fatty acids** as a fuel increases with the length of the fast; they are the **major fuel** oxidized during overnight fasting.

Fuel Oxidation. During fasting, glucose continues to be **oxidized** by **glucose-dependent tissues** such as the brain and red blood cells, and **fatty acids** are oxidized by tissues such as muscle and liver. Muscle and most other tissues oxidize fatty acids completely to CO_2 and H_2O. However, the **liver** partially oxidizes fatty acids to smaller molecules called **ketone bodies**, which are released into the blood. Muscle, kidney, and certain other tissues derive energy from completely oxidizing ketone bodies in the tricarboxylic acid (TCA) cycle.

Maintenance of Blood Glucose. As fasting progresses, the **liver produces glucose** not only by **glycogenolysis** (the release of glucose from glycogen) but also by a second process called **gluconeogenesis** (the synthesis of glucose from noncarbohydrate compounds). The major **sources of carbon** for gluconeogenesis are **lactate**, **glycerol**, and **amino acids.** When the carbons of the amino acids are converted to glucose by the liver, their **nitrogen** is converted to **urea**.

Starvation. When we fast for 3 or more days, we are in the starved state. **Muscle** continues to burn fatty acids but **decreases** its use of **ketone bodies.** As a result, the concentration of ketone bodies rises in the blood to a level at which the **brain** begins to **oxidize** them for energy. The brain then needs less glucose, so the liver decreases its rate of gluconeogenesis. Consequently, less **protein** in muscle and other tissues is degraded to supply amino acids for gluconeogenesis. Protein sparing preserves vital functions for as long as possible. Because of these changes in the fuel use patterns of various tissues, humans can survive for extended periods without ingesting food.

THE WAITING ROOM

Percy V. had been admitted to the hospital with a diagnosis of mental depression associated with malnutrition (see Chapter 1). At the time of admission, his body weight of 125 lb gave him a body mass index (BMI) of 17.5 (healthy range = 18.5 to 24.9). His serum albumin was 10% below the low end of the normal range, and he exhibited signs of iron and vitamin deficiencies.

Additional tests were made to help evaluate Mr. V.'s degree of malnutrition and his progress toward recovery. His arm circumference and triceps skinfold were measured, and his mid-upper arm muscle circumference (MUAMC) was calculated (see Chapter 2, Anthropometric Measurements). His serum prealbumin and serum albumin levels were measured. Fasting blood glucose and serum ketone body concentration were determined on blood samples drawn the next day before breakfast. A 24-hour urine specimen was collected to determine ketone body excretion and creatinine excretion for calculation of the creatinine–height index (CHI), a measure of protein depletion from skeletal muscle.

Ann R. was receiving psychological counseling for anorexia nervosa but with little success (see Chapter 1). She continues to want to lose weight despite being underweight. She saw her gynecologist because she had not had a menstrual period for 5 months. She also complained of becoming easily fatigued. The physician recognized that Ann's body weight of 85 lb was now <65% of her ideal weight, and he calculated that her BMI was now 13.7. The physician recommended immediate hospitalization. The admission diagnosis was severe malnutrition (grade III protein-energy malnutrition [PEM]) secondary to anorexia nervosa. Clinical findings included decreased body core temperature, blood pressure, and pulse (adaptive responses to malnutrition). Her physician ordered measurements of blood glucose as well as other blood tests to check electrolytes and her kidney function and an electrocardiogram to see any effects on the electrical activity of the heart.

Percy V. has grade I PEM. At his height of 71 inches, his body weight would have to be >132 lb to achieve a BMI >18.5. **Ann R.** has grade III malnutrition. At 67 inches, she needs a body weight >118 lb to achieve a BMI of 18.5. Degrees of PEM are classified as grades I, II, and III, according to BMI. Grade I refers to a BMI in the range of 17.0 to 18.4, grade II to a BMI in the range of 16.0 to 16.9, and grade III is designated for a BMI <16.0.

Creatinine is usually released from the muscles at a constant rate, and it is proportional to muscle mass. The creatinine is removed from the circulation by the kidneys and appears in the urine. Thus, elevated creatinine in the blood relates to impaired renal function. To measure creatinine in biologic specimens, the Jaffe reaction is used. Creatinine is reacted with picric acid in an alkaline solution to form a red-orange product, which can be quantitated via spectrophotometry. To increase specificity, a kinetic Jaffe reaction is run and the rate of formation of the product is determined. Creatinine can be measured in plasma, serum, and urine.

I. The Fasting State

Blood glucose levels peak at about 1 hour after eating (the postprandial state) and then decrease as tissues oxidize glucose or convert it to storage forms of fuel. By 2 hours after a meal, the level returns to the fasting range (between 80 and 100 mg/dL). This decrease in blood glucose causes the pancreas to decrease its secretion of insulin and the serum insulin level decreases. The liver responds to this hormonal signal by starting to degrade its glycogen stores (glycogenolysis) and release glucose into the blood.

If we eat another meal within a few hours, we return to the fed state. However, if we continue to fast for a 12-hour period, we enter the basal state (also known as the postabsorptive state). A person is generally considered to be in the basal state after an overnight fast, when no food has been eaten since dinner the previous evening. By this time, the serum insulin level is low and glucagon is rising. Figure 3.1 illustrates the main features of the basal state.

A. Blood Glucose and the Role of the Liver during Fasting

The liver maintains blood glucose levels during fasting, and its role is thus critical. Glucose is the major fuel for tissues such as the brain and neural tissue and is the sole fuel for red blood cells. Most neurons lack enzymes required for oxidation of fatty acids, but they can use ketone bodies to a limited extent. Red blood cells lack mitochondria, which contain the enzymes of fatty acid and ketone body oxidation, and can use only glucose as a fuel. Therefore, it is imperative that blood glucose not decrease too rapidly nor fall too low.

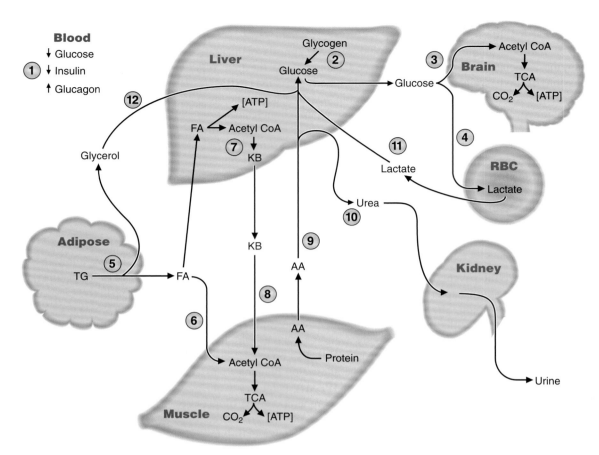

FIGURE 3.1 Basal state. This state occurs after an overnight (12 hours) fast. The *circled numbers* serve as a guide indicating the approximate order in which the processes begin to occur. *KB*, ketone bodies; *TG*, triacylglycerols; *FA*, fatty acids; *AA*, amino acid; *RBC*, red blood cells; *ATP*, adenosine triphosphate; *acetyl CoA*, acetyl coenzyme A; *TCA*, tricarboxylic acid.

$$O$$
$$\|$$
$$NH_2 - C - NH_2$$

Urea

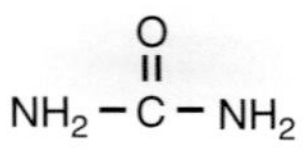

FIGURE 3.2 The structure of urea, the highly soluble nitrogen disposal molecule.

Initially, liver glycogen stores are degraded to supply glucose to the blood, but these stores are limited. This pathway is known as *glycogenolysis* (the lysis, or splitting, of glycogen, to form glucose subunits). Although liver glycogen levels may increase to 200 to 300 g after a meal, only approximately 80 g remain after an overnight fast. Fortunately, the liver has another mechanism for producing blood glucose, known as *gluconeogenesis*. Gluconeogenesis means formation (genesis) of new (neo) glucose and, by definition, converts new (noncarbohydrate) precursors to glucose. In gluconeogenesis, lactate, glycerol, and amino acids are used as carbon sources to synthesize glucose. As fasting continues, gluconeogenesis progressively adds to the glucose produced by glycogenolysis in the liver.

Lactate is a product of glycolysis in red blood cells and exercising muscle, *glycerol* is obtained from lipolysis of adipose triacylglycerols, and *amino acids* are generated by the breakdown of protein. Because our muscle mass is so large, most of the amino acid is supplied from degradation of muscle protein. These compounds travel in the blood to the liver, where they are converted to glucose by gluconeogenesis. Because the nitrogen of the amino acids can form ammonia, which is toxic to the body, the liver converts this nitrogen to urea. Urea has two amino groups for just one carbon (Fig. 3.2). It is a very soluble, nontoxic compound that can be readily excreted by the kidneys and thus is an efficient means for disposing of excess ammonia.

As fasting progresses, gluconeogenesis becomes increasingly more important as a source of blood glucose. After a day or so of fasting, liver glycogen stores are depleted and gluconeogenesis is the only source of blood glucose.

B. Role of Adipose Tissue during Fasting

Adipose triacylglycerols are the major source of energy during fasting. They supply fatty acids, which are quantitatively the major fuel for the human body. Fatty acids are oxidized not only directly by various tissues of the body, but they are also partially oxidized in the liver to four-carbon products called *ketone bodies*. Ketone bodies are subsequently oxidized as a fuel by other tissues.

As blood insulin levels decrease and blood glucagon levels rise, adipose triacylglycerols are mobilized by a process known as *lipolysis* (lysis of triacylglycerol). They are converted to fatty acids and glycerol, which enter the blood.

It is important to recognize that most fatty acids cannot provide carbon for gluconeogenesis. Thus, of the vast store of food energy in adipose tissue triacylglycerols, only the small glycerol portion travels to the liver to enter the gluconeogenic pathway.

Fatty acids serve as a fuel for muscle, kidney, and most other tissues. They are oxidized to acetyl coenzyme A (acetyl-CoA) and subsequently to CO_2 and H_2O in the TCA cycle, producing energy in the form of adenosine triphosphate (ATP). In addition to the ATP required to maintain cellular integrity, muscle uses ATP for contraction and the kidney uses it for urinary transport processes.

Most of the fatty acids that enter the liver are converted to ketone bodies rather than being completely oxidized to CO_2. The process of conversion of fatty acids to acetyl-CoA produces a considerable amount of energy (ATP), which drives the reactions of the liver under these conditions. The acetyl-CoA is converted to the ketone bodies *acetoacetate* and *β-hydroxybutyrate*, which are released into the blood (Fig. 3.3).

The liver lacks an enzyme required for ketone body oxidation. However, ketone bodies can be further oxidized by most other cells with mitochondria, such as muscle and kidney. In these tissues, acetoacetate and β-hydroxybutyrate are converted to acetyl-CoA and then oxidized in the TCA cycle, with subsequent generation of ATP.

C. Summary of the Metabolic Changes during a Brief Fast

In the initial stages of fasting, stored fuels are used for energy (see Fig. 3.1). The liver plays a key role by maintaining blood glucose levels in the range of 80 to 100 mg/dL, first by glycogenolysis (Fig. 3.1, circle 2) and subsequently by gluconeogenesis (Fig. 3.1, circles 9, 11, and 12). Lactate, glycerol, and amino acids serve as carbon sources for gluconeogenesis. Amino acids are supplied by muscle (via *proteolysis*, lysis of proteins to individual amino acids). Their nitrogen is converted in the liver to urea (Fig. 3.1, circle 10), which is excreted by the kidneys.

Fatty acids, which are released from adipose tissue by the process of lipolysis (Fig. 3.1, circle 5), serve as the body's major fuel during fasting. The liver oxidizes most of its fatty acids only partially, converting them to ketone bodies (Fig. 3.1, circle 7), which are released into the blood. Thus, during the initial stages of fasting, blood levels of fatty acids and ketone bodies begin to increase. Muscle uses fatty acids, ketone bodies (Fig. 3.1, circles 6 and 8), and (when exercising and while supplies last) glucose from muscle glycogen. Many other tissues use either fatty acids or ketone bodies. However, red blood cells, the brain, and other neural tissues use mainly glucose (Fig. 3.1, circles 3 and 4). The metabolic capacities of different tissues with respect to pathways of fuel metabolism are summarized in Table 3.1.

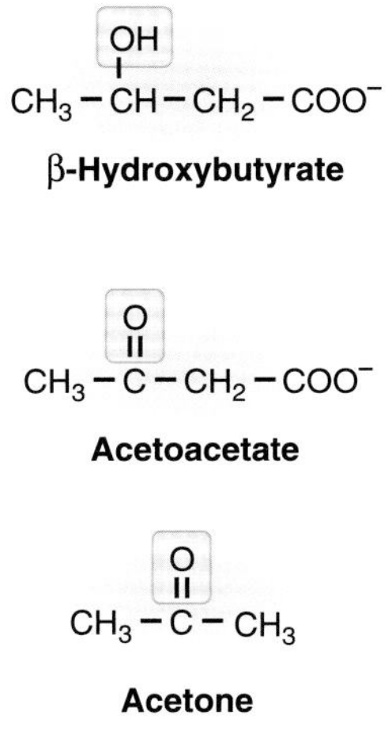

II. Metabolic Changes during Prolonged Fasting

If the pattern of fuel use that occurs during a brief fast were to persist for an extended period, the body's protein would be quite rapidly consumed to the point at which critical functions would be compromised. Fortunately, metabolic changes occur during prolonged fasting that conserve (spare) muscle protein by causing muscle protein turnover to decrease. Figure 3.4 shows the main features of metabolism during prolonged fasting (starvation).

 Percy V. had not eaten much on his first day of hospitalization. His fasting blood glucose determined on the morning of his second day of hospitalization was 72 mg/dL (normal, overnight fasting = 80 to 100 mg/dL). Thus, in spite of his malnutrition and his overnight fast, his blood glucose was being maintained at nearly normal levels through gluconeogenesis using amino acid precursors. If his blood glucose had decreased to <50 to 60 mg/dL during fasting, his brain would have been unable to absorb glucose fast enough to obtain the glucose needed for energy and neurotransmitter synthesis, resulting in coma and eventual death. Although many other tissues, such as red blood cells, are also totally or partially dependent on glucose for energy, they are able to function at lower concentrations of blood glucose than is the brain.

On his second day of hospitalization, **Percy V.'s** serum ketone body level was 110 μM (normal value after a 12-hour fast is ~70 μM). No ketone bodies were detectable in his urine. At this early stage of PEM, Mr. V. still has remaining fat stores. After 12 hours of fasting, most of his tissues are using fatty acids as a major fuel and the liver is beginning to produce ketone bodies from fatty acids. As these ketone bodies increase in the blood, their use as a fuel will increase.

FIGURE 3.3 The ketone bodies β-hydroxybutyrate, acetoacetate, and acetone. β-Hydroxybutyrate and acetoacetate are formed in the liver. Acetone is produced by nonenzymatic decarboxylation of acetoacetate. However, acetone is expired in the breath and is not metabolized to a significant extent in the body, whereas β-hydroxybutyrate and acetoacetate are used by muscle and the nervous system as an energy source.

TABLE 3.1 Metabolic Capacities of Various Tissues

PROCESS	LIVER	ADIPOSE TISSUE	KIDNEY CORTEX	MUSCLE	BRAIN	RED BLOOD CELLS
TCA cycle (acetyl-CoA → CO_2 + H_2O)	+++	++	+++	+++	+++	− −
β-Oxidation of fatty acids	+++	− −	++	+++	− −	− −
Ketone body formation	+++	− −	+	− −	− −	− −
Ketone body use	− −	+	+	+++	+++ (Prolonged starvation)	− −
Glycolysis (glucose → CO_2 + H_2O)	+++	++	++	+++	+++	− −
Lactate production (glucose → lactate)	+	+	− − −	+++ (Exercise)	+	+++
Glycogen metabolism (synthesis and degradation)	+++	+	+	+++	+	− −
Gluconeogenesis (lactate, amino acids, glycerol → glucose)	+++	− −	+	− −	− −	− −
Urea cycle (ammonia → urea)	+++	− −	− −	− −	− −	− −
Lipogenesis (glucose → fatty acids)	+++	+	− −	− −	− −	− −

Acetyl-CoA, acetyl coenzyme A; TCA, tricarboxylic acid.
++ indicates use of the fuel; +++ is maximal use, whereas + is minimal use. − − indicates no use of the fuel.

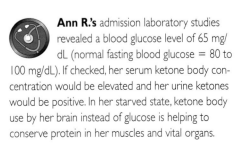

The liver synthesizes several serum proteins and releases them into the blood. The synthesis of these proteins decreases during protein malnutrition, leading to a decrease in their concentration in the blood. Two of these serum proteins, albumin and prealbumin (a liver-derived protein that transports thyroid hormone), are often measured to assess the state of protein malnutrition. A measurement of serum albumin levels is the traditional standard used to assess protein malnutrition, but serum albumin levels respond slowly to changes in protein status because of its relatively long half-life of 14 to 20 days. Prealbumin, however, has a half-life of 2 to 3 days and its levels are a more sensitive indicator of changes in protein status. Neither measurement is specific for protein malnutrition. Serum albumin and prealbumin levels decrease with hepatic disease (although prealbumin levels are less affected by liver disease than are albumin levels), certain renal diseases, surgery, and several other conditions, in addition to protein malnutrition. **Percy V.'s** values were below the normal range for both of these proteins, indicating that his muscle mass was unable to supply sufficient amino acids to sustain both gluconeogenesis and the synthesis of serum proteins by the liver.

Ann R.'s admission laboratory studies revealed a blood glucose level of 65 mg/dL (normal fasting blood glucose = 80 to 100 mg/dL). If checked, her serum ketone body concentration would be elevated and her urine ketones would be positive. In her starved state, ketone body use by her brain instead of glucose is helping to conserve protein in her muscles and vital organs.

A. Role of Liver during Prolonged Fasting

After 3 to 5 days of fasting, when the body enters the starved state, muscle decreases its use of ketone bodies and depends mainly on fatty acids for its fuel. The liver, however, continues to convert fatty acids to ketone bodies. The result is that the concentration of ketone bodies rises in the blood (Fig. 3.5). The brain begins to take up these ketone bodies from the blood and to oxidize them for energy. Therefore, the brain needs less glucose than it did after an overnight fast (Table 3.2).

Glucose is still required, however, as an energy source for red blood cells, and the brain continues to use a limited amount of glucose, which it oxidizes for energy and uses as a source of carbon for the synthesis of neurotransmitters. Overall, however, glucose is "spared" (conserved). Less glucose is used by the body, and therefore, the liver needs to produce less glucose per hour during prolonged fasting than during shorter periods of fasting.

Because the stores of glycogen in the liver are depleted by approximately 30 hours of fasting, gluconeogenesis is the only process by which the liver can supply glucose to the blood if fasting continues. The amino acid pool, produced by the breakdown of protein, continues to serve as a major source of carbon for gluconeogenesis. A fraction of this amino acid pool is also used for biosynthetic functions (e.g., synthesis of heme and neurotransmitters) and new protein synthesis, processes that must continue during fasting. However, as a result of the decreased rate of gluconeogenesis during prolonged fasting, protein is "spared"; less protein is degraded to supply amino acids for gluconeogenesis.

While converting amino acid carbon to glucose in gluconeogenesis, the liver also converts the nitrogen of these amino acids to urea. Consequently, because glucose production decreases during prolonged fasting compared with early fasting, urea production also decreases.

B. Role of Adipose Tissue during Prolonged Fasting

During prolonged fasting, adipose tissue continues to break down its triacylglycerol stores, providing fatty acids and glycerol to the blood. These fatty acids serve as the major source of fuel for the body. The glycerol is converted to glucose, whereas the fatty acids are oxidized to CO_2 and H_2O by tissues such as muscle. In the liver, fatty

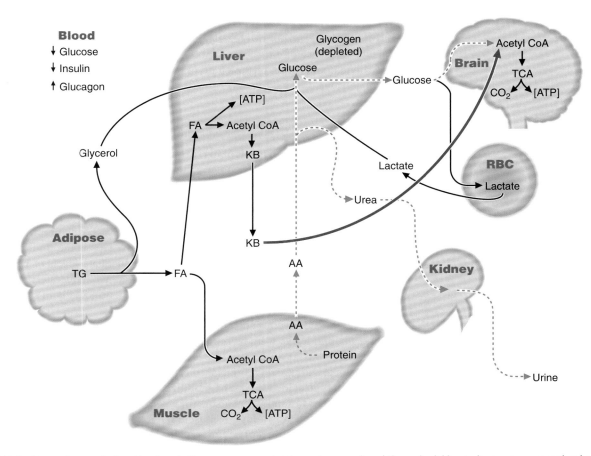

FIGURE 3.4 Starved state. *Broken blue lines* indicate processes that have decreased, and the *red solid line* indicates a process that has increased relative to the fasting state. *KB*, ketone bodies; *TG*, triacylglycerols; *FA*, fatty acids; *AA*, amino acid; *RBC*, red blood cells. *KB*, ketone bodies; *TG*, triacylglycerols; *FA*, fatty acids; *AA*, amino acid; *RBC*, red blood cells; *ATP*, adenosine triphosphate; *acetyl CoA*, acetyl coenzyme A; *TCA*, tricarboxylic acid.

acids are converted to ketone bodies that are oxidized by many tissues, including the brain.

Several factors determine how long we can fast and still survive. The amount of adipose tissue is one factor because adipose tissue supplies the body with its major source of fuel. However, body protein levels can also determine the length of time we can fast. Glucose is still used during prolonged fasting (starvation) but in significantly reduced amounts. Although we degrade protein to supply amino acids for gluconeogenesis at a slower rate during starvation than during the first days of a fast, we are still losing protein that serves vital functions for our tissues. Protein can become so depleted that the heart, kidney, and other vital tissues stop functioning, or we can develop an infection and not have adequate reserves to mount an

 Death by starvation occurs with loss of roughly 40% of body weight, when approximately 30% to 50% of body protein, or 70% to 95% of body fat stores, has been lost. Generally, this occurs at BMI of approximately 13 for men and 11 for women.

TABLE 3.2 **Metabolic Changes during Prolonged Fasting Compared with Fasting for 24 Hours**	
Muscle use of ketone bodies	Decreases
Brain use of ketone bodies	Increases
Brain use of glucose	Decreases
Liver gluconeogenesis	Decreases
Muscle protein degradation	Decreases
Liver production of urea	Decreases

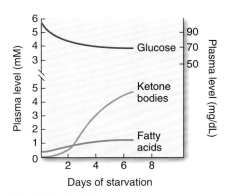

FIGURE 3.5 Changes in the concentration of fuels in the blood during prolonged fasting.

immune response. In addition to fuel problems, we are also deprived of the vitamin and mineral precursors of coenzymes and other compounds necessary for tissue function. Because of either a lack of ATP or a decreased intake of electrolytes, the electrolyte composition of the blood or cells could become incompatible with life. Ultimately, we die of starvation.

CLINICAL COMMENTS

Percy V. As a result of his severely suppressed appetite for food, **Percy V.** developed a mild degree (grade I) of PEM. When prolonged, this type of protein malnutrition can cause changes in the villi of the small intestine that reduce its absorptive capacity for what little food is ingested.

Despite his insufficient intake of dietary carbohydrates, Mr. V.'s blood glucose level was 72 mg/dL, close to the lower limit (80 mg/dL) of the normal range for a well-nourished, healthy person after a 12-hour fast. This is the finding you would expect; it reflects the liver's capacity to maintain adequate levels of blood glucose by means of gluconeogenesis, even during prolonged and moderately severe caloric restriction. Amino acids from degradation of protein, principally in skeletal muscle, supply most of the precursors for gluconeogenesis.

Percy V. had several indicators of his protein malnutrition: His serum albumin and prealbumin levels were below normal, his MUAMC was at the 12th percentile, and his CHI was at 85%. The low levels of serum proteins reflect a low dietary protein intake and possibly diminished capacity to absorb dietary amino acids. Consequently, amino acids were being mobilized from degradation of protein in muscle and other tissues to supply precursors for new protein synthesis as well as gluconeogenesis. The result was a loss of muscle mass, indicated by the MUAMC and the CHI, and decreased levels of serum proteins.

Fatty acids mobilized from adipose tissue are the major source of energy for most tissues. Because Percy was eating, and not in total starvation, his ketone bodies were only moderately elevated in the blood (110 μM vs. normal of 70 μM) and did not appear in the urine.

Percy had several psychological counseling sessions as well as several discussions with a registered dietitian to help him improve and maintain his nutrient uptake. The dietitian suggested that Percy add nutritional drinks (such as Boost [Nestlé S.A., Vevey, Switzerland], Ensure [Abbott Laboratories, Chicago, Illinois], or an instant breakfast drink) to provide essential nutrients. Percy was advised that small frequent feedings (three meals and two snacks) can provide adequate calories, proteins, and other nutrients throughout the day. The dietitian also suggested that Percy (1) use frozen dinners in combination with a fresh salad and a glass of milk and (2) engage in physical activity to enhance mood and increase appetite.

After several psychological counseling sessions, and the promise of an extended visit from his grandchild, Mr. V. resumed his normal eating pattern.

Ann R. Ann R. meets the diagnostic criteria for *anorexia nervosa*. She has low body weight with continual fear of gaining weight. Patients with anorexia nervosa also have body image disturbance or a lack of recognition of the seriousness of their illness.

Amenorrhea (lack of menses) usually develops during anorexia nervosa and other conditions when a woman's body fat content falls to approximately 22% of her total body weight. The immediate cause of amenorrhea is a reduced production of the gonadotropic protein hormones (luteinizing hormone and follicle-stimulating hormone) by the anterior pituitary; the connection between this hormonal change and body fat content is not yet understood.

Ms. R. is suffering from the consequences of prolonged and severe protein and caloric restriction. Fatty acids, released from adipose tissue by lipolysis, are being converted to ketone bodies in the liver, and the level of ketone bodies in the blood

Ⓜ Creatinine–height index. The most widely used biochemical marker for estimating body muscle mass is the 24-hour urinary creatinine excretion. Creatinine is a degradation product formed in active muscle at a constant rate, in proportion to the amount of muscle tissue present in a patient. In a protein-malnourished individual, urinary creatinine will decrease in proportion to the decrease in muscle mass. To assess depletion of muscle mass, the amount of creatinine excreted is expressed relative to the height of the patient, yielding a CHI. The amount of creatinine (in milligrams) excreted by the subject in 24 hours is divided by the amount of creatinine excreted by a normal, healthy subject of the same height and sex. The resulting ratio is multiplied by 100 to express it as a percentage. **Percy V.'s** CHI was 85% (80% to 90% of normal indicates a mild deficit, 60% to 80% of normal indicates a moderate deficit, and <60% of normal indicates a severe deficit of muscle mass).

can be extremely elevated. The fact that her kidneys are excreting ketone bodies can be reflected in a positive urine test for ketone bodies.

Although Ms. R.'s blood glucose is below the normal fasting range (65 mg/dL vs. normal of 80 mg/dL), she is experiencing only a moderate degree of hypoglycemia (low blood glucose) despite her severe, near-starvation diet. Her blood glucose level reflects the ability of the brain to use ketone bodies as a fuel when they are elevated in the blood, thereby decreasing the amount of glucose that must be synthesized from amino acids provided by protein degradation.

Ms. R.'s BMI showed that she is close to death through starvation (grade III PEM). She was therefore hospitalized and placed on enteral nutrition (nutrients provided through tube feeding). The general therapeutic plan, outlined in Chapter 1, of nutritional restitution and identification and treatment of those emotional factors leading to the patient's anorectic behavior was continued. She slowly started to eat small amounts of food while hospitalized. As part of Ann's eating disorder team, the dietitian's role included helping the patient to recognize and address disordered eating patterns and guiding Ann to focus on health rather than weight gain. The dietitian also determined the proper amount of calories needed for a slow, gradual weight gain to prevent the complications of refeeding syndrome and devised an individualized eating plan for Ann to reach her target goals.

BIOCHEMICAL COMMENTS

 Clinical Use of Metabolite Measurements in Blood and Urine. When a patient develops a metabolic problem, it is difficult to examine cells to determine the cause. To obtain tissue for metabolic studies, biopsies must be performed. These procedures can be difficult, dangerous, or even impossible, depending on the tissue. Cost is an additional concern. However, both blood and urine can be obtained readily from patients, and measurements of substances in the blood and urine can help in diagnosing a patient's problem. Concentrations of substances that are higher or lower than normal indicate which tissues are malfunctioning. For example, if blood urea nitrogen (BUN) levels are low, a problem centered in the liver might be suspected because urea is produced in the liver. Conversely, high blood levels of urea suggest that the kidney is not excreting this compound normally. Decreased urinary and blood levels of creatinine indicate diminished production of creatinine by skeletal muscle. However, high blood creatinine levels could indicate an inability of the kidney to excrete creatinine, resulting from renal disease. If high levels of ketone bodies are found in the blood or urine, the patient's metabolic pattern is that of the starved state. If the high levels of ketone bodies are coupled with elevated levels of blood glucose, the problem is most likely a deficiency of insulin; that is, the patient probably has type 1 diabetes (these patients are usually young). Without insulin, fuels are mobilized from tissues rather than being stored.

These relatively easy and inexpensive tests on blood and urine can be used to determine which tissues need to be studied more extensively to diagnose and treat the patient's problem. A solid understanding of fuel metabolism helps in the interpretation of these simple tests.

KEY CONCEPTS

- During fasting, when blood glucose levels drop, glucagon is released from the α-cells of the pancreas. Glucagon signals the liver to use its stored carbohydrate to release glucose into the circulation, primarily for use by the brain and red blood cells.
- After fasting for about 3 days, the liver releases ketone bodies (derived from fat oxidation) as an alternative fuel supply for the brain. Liver glycogen stores are depleted and gluconeogenesis provides glucose to the body.

- Glucagon also signals the fat cells to degrade triacylglycerol, supplying the body with fatty acids for energy and glycerol for gluconeogenesis.
- The substrates for liver gluconeogenesis are lactate (from the red blood cells), amino acids (from muscle protein degradation), and glycerol.
- In prolonged starvation, the brain can adapt to using ketone bodies for energy, which reduces the body's demand for glucose. This reduces the rate of muscle protein degradation to provide precursors for gluconeogenesis and allows extended survival times under starvation conditions.
- The major disease discussed in this chapter is summarized in Table 3.3.

TABLE 3.3 Disease Discussed in Chapter 3		
DISORDER OR CONDITION	**GENETIC OR ENVIRONMENTAL**	**COMMENTS**
Malnutrition	Both	Reduced nutrient uptake may be caused by genetic mutation in specific proteins or to dietary habits leading to reduced nutrient intake. May lead to increased ketone body production and reduced liver protein synthesis.

REVIEW QUESTIONS—CHAPTER 3

You will need some information from Chapters 1 and 2, as well as Chapter 3, to answer these questions.

1. A hiker has become lost on the Appalachian Trail and has consumed the last of his rations and has only water to drink. By 24 hours after his last meal, which one of the following is most likely to occur?
   A. Gluconeogenesis in the liver will be the major source of blood glucose.
   B. Muscle glycogenolysis provides glucose to the blood.
   C. Muscles convert amino acids to blood glucose.
   D. Fatty acids released from adipose tissue provide carbon for synthesis of glucose.
   E. Ketone bodies provide carbon for gluconeogenesis.
2. A physician is treating a type 1 diabetic who has neglected to take her insulin for 5 days. The patient demonstrates elevated blood glucose and ketone body levels. Ketone bodies are elevated because of which one of the following?
   A. Elevated glucose levels
   B. Reduced BUN
   C. Decreased fatty acid release from the adipocyte
   D. Inhibition of liver oxidation of ketone bodies
   E. Reduced muscle use of fatty acids
3. In a well-nourished individual, as the length of fasting increases from overnight to 1 week, which one of the following is most likely to occur?
   A. Blood glucose levels decrease by approximately 50%.
   B. Red blood cells switch to using ketone bodies.
   C. Muscles decrease their use of ketone bodies, which increase in the blood.
   D. The brain begins to use fatty acids as a major fuel.
   E. Adipose tissue triacylglycerols are nearly depleted.

4. A hospitalized patient had low levels of serum albumin and high levels of blood ammonia. His CHI was 98%. His BMI was 20.5. BUN was in the normal range, consistent with normal kidney function. The diagnosis most consistent with these findings is which one of the following?
   A. A loss of hepatic function (e.g., alcohol-induced cirrhosis)
   B. Anorexia nervosa
   C. Kwashiorkor (protein malnutrition)
   D. Marasmus (PEM)
   E. Decreased absorption of amino acids by intestinal epithelial cells (e.g., celiac disease)
5. **Otto S.**, an overweight medical student (see Chapter 1), discovered that he could not exercise enough during his summer clerkship rotations to lose 2 to 3 lb/wk. He decided to lose weight by eating only 300 calories/day of a dietary supplement that provided half the calories as carbohydrate and half as protein. In addition, he consumed a multivitamin supplement. During the first 3 days on this diet, which statement best represents the state of Otto's metabolism?
   A. His protein intake met the Recommended Dietary Allowance (RDA) for protein.
   B. His carbohydrate intake met the fuel needs of his brain.
   C. Both his adipose mass and his muscle mass decreased.
   D. He remained in nitrogen balance.
   E. He developed severe hypoglycemia.

6. A pregnant woman is having an oral glucose tolerance test done to diagnose gestational diabetes. The test consists of ingesting a concentrated solution of glucose (75 g of glucose) and then having her blood glucose levels measured at various times after ingesting the sugar. Her test results come back normal. At what time after her oral sugar solution in consumed will she have the highest blood glucose level?
   A. Immediately
   B. 1 hour
   C. 2 hours
   D. 3 hours
   E. 4 hours

7. A patient with frequent sweating and tremors is diagnosed with "reactive hypoglycemia" and has been prescribed a small meal every 4 hours throughout the day. The patient most likely is impaired in carrying out which one of the following?
   A. Glycogenesis of liver glycogen stores
   B. Glycogenolysis of muscle glycogen stores
   C. Glycogenolysis of liver glycogen stores
   D. Glycogenesis of muscle glycogen stores
   E. Glycogenesis of adipose tissue glycogen stores

8. An activist is on a hunger strike to bring attention to her latest cause, and she has only consumed H$_2$O and vitamins for the past 5 days. Which ONE of the following organs/structures has begun to use ketone bodies as a major secondary fuel source?
   A. Red blood cells
   B. Brain
   C. Liver
   D. Heart
   E. All of the above

9. You are evaluating a patient who has a mutation that hinders his ability to carry out liver glycogenolysis. One initial finding shortly after entering the fasting state in this patient would be which ONE of the following?
   A. Hyperglycemia
   B. Ketosis (elevated levels of ketone bodies)
   C. Significantly increased urea synthesis
   D. Reduced blood lactate levels
   E. Hypoglycemia

10. A prisoner has gone on a hunger strike, drinking only water. Careful monitoring of the prisoner demonstrated a drop in BUN during the second week of the fast. This occurred because of which one of the following?
    A. Enhanced glycogenolysis
    B. Reduced ketone body formation
    C. A decrease in the rate of gluconeogenesis
    D. An increase in the rate of gluconeogenesis
    E. Enhanced glucose metabolism in the brain

ANSWERS

1. **The answer is A.** By 24 hours after a meal, hepatic (liver) gluconeogenesis is the major source of blood glucose because hepatic glycogen stores have been nearly depleted. Muscle and other tissues lack an enzyme necessary to convert glycogen or amino acids to glucose for export (thus, B is incorrect). The liver is the only significant source of blood glucose. Glucose is synthesized in the liver from amino acids (provided by protein degradation), from glycerol (provided by hydrolysis of triacylglycerols in adipose tissue), and from lactate (provided by anaerobic glycolysis in red blood cells and other tissues). Glucose cannot be synthesized from fatty acids or ketone bodies (thus, D and E are incorrect).

2. **The answer is A.** The liver will produce ketone bodies when fatty acid oxidation is increased, which occurs when glucagon is the predominant hormone (glucagon leads to fatty acid release from the fat cells for oxidation in the liver and muscle). This would be the case in an individual who cannot produce insulin and is not taking insulin injections. However, in this situation, the ketone bodies are not being used by the nervous system (brain) because of the high levels of glucose in the circulation. This leads to severely elevated ketone levels because of non-use. The glucose is high because, in the absence of insulin, muscle and fat cells are not using the glucose in circulation as an energy source. Recall that although the liver produces ketone bodies, it lacks a necessary enzyme to use ketone bodies as an energy source. There is no relation between BUN levels and the rate of ketone body production. The muscle reduces its use of ketone bodies under these conditions but not its use of fatty acids.

3. **The answer is C.** The major change during prolonged fasting is that as muscles decrease their use of ketone bodies, ketone bodies increase enormously in the blood and are used by the brain as a fuel. However, even during starvation, glucose is still required by the brain, which cannot oxidize fatty acids to an appreciable extent (thus, D is incorrect). Red blood cells can use only glucose as a fuel (thus, B is incorrect). Because the brain, red blood cells, and certain other tissues are glucose-dependent, the liver continues to synthesize glucose, and blood glucose levels are maintained at only slightly less than fasting levels (thus, A is incorrect). Adipose tissue stores ($\sim$135,000 kcal) are not depleted in a well-nourished individual after 1 week of fasting (thus, E is incorrect).

4. **The answer is A.** Decreased serum albumin could have several causes, including hepatic disease, which decreases the ability of the liver to synthesize serum proteins; protein malnutrition; marasmus; or diseases that affect the ability of the intestine to digest protein and absorb amino acids. However, his BMI is in the healthy weight range (thus, B and D are incorrect). His normal

CHI indicates that he has not lost muscle mass and is therefore not suffering from protein malnutrition (thus, B, C, D, and E are incorrect).

5. **The answer is C.** His protein intake of 150 calories is about 37 g of protein (150 calories ÷ 4 calories/g = 37 g), below the RDA of 0.8 g of protein/kg of body weight (thus, A is incorrect because Otto weighs ~88 kg). His carbohydrate intake of 150 calories is below the glucose requirements of his brain and red blood cells (~150 g/day; see Chapter 2) (thus, B is incorrect). Therefore, he will be breaking down muscle protein to synthesize glucose for the brain and other glucose-dependent tissues and adipose tissue mass to supply fatty acids for muscle and tissues able to oxidize fatty acids. Because he will be breaking down muscle protein to amino acids and converting the nitrogen from both these amino acids and his dietary amino acids to urea, his nitrogen excretion will be greater than his intake and he will be in negative nitrogen balance (thus, D is incorrect). It is unlikely that he will develop hypoglycemia while he is able to supply gluconeogenic precursors.

6. **The answer is B.** Blood glucose levels peak approximately 1 hour after eating and return to the fasting range by about 2 hours. If the blood glucose levels remain elevated for an extended period of time, it is an indication of impaired glucose transport (insulin stimulates glucose transport into muscle and adipose tissue). If the blood glucose levels are <140 mg/dL at 2 hours after the test, the result is considered normal. If the levels are between 140 and 200 mg/dL, the patient is considered to have "impaired glucose tolerance." If the levels are >200 mg/dL after 2 hours, a diagnosis of diabetes is confirmed.

7. **The answer is C.** Blood glucose levels return to the fasting range about 2 hours after a meal. The decrease in blood glucose causes a decrease in insulin and an increase in glucagon production. Glucagon stimulates the liver to degrade its glycogen stores (glycogenolysis) and release glucose into the bloodstream. If the patient eats another meal within a few hours, the patient returns to the fed state. Glycogenesis is the synthesis of glycogen. While the muscle contains glycogen stores, degradation of muscle glycogen only benefits the muscle; the muscle cannot export glucose to maintain blood glucose levels. Adipose tissue does not contain significant levels of glycogen.

8. **The answer is B.** After 24 to 48 hours of the fast, the activist's liver has run out of glycogen and all glucose is being produced from gluconeogenesis. The liver is oxidizing fatty acids as an energy source and producing ketone bodies as an alternative fuel source for the nervous system (brain). Muscle continues to use fatty acids as a fuel source but decreases its use of ketone bodies, thereby raising the blood concentration of ketone bodies. At the higher concentration of ketone bodies in the blood, the brain can use the ketone bodies and does not need as much glucose. Up to 40% of the brain's energy needs can be met by ketone bodies, but the other 60% still needs to be met by glucose as an energy source. As the brain uses ketone bodies, the liver can reduce gluconeogenesis, thereby reducing the need for amino acids as precursors and preserving muscle protein. Red blood cells have no mitochondria so they must use glucose only as an energy source (ketone bodies are oxidized in mitochondria). The liver cannot use ketone bodies because it lacks a key enzyme for their degradation, and the heart uses lactate as an energy source along with fatty acids.

9. **The answer is E.** As blood glucose levels begin to drop, glucagon is released from the pancreas, which stimulates glycogenolysis in the liver. The glucose produced from liver glycogen is used initially to maintain blood glucose levels during the early stages of a fast. Gluconeogenesis will kick in later because this process requires more energy than glycogenolysis, and fatty acid oxidation must be under way before glucose can be produced from lactate, glycerol, and amino acids. Ketone bodies will not be evident after initiating a fast (the levels of ketones will not be significant until 24 to 48 hours after a fast is initiated). Significant protein degradation will not occur until the liver runs out of glycogen, about 24 to 36 hours after the start of the fast (and without protein degradation, urea synthesis will remain normal). The red blood cells will still be metabolizing glucose, so blood lactate levels (the end product of red cell glucose metabolism) will remain relatively constant.

10. **The answer is C.** As a fast increases in length, the liver will begin to produce ketone bodies from the oxidation of fatty acids obtained from the adipocyte. As the ketone bodies are released from the liver, the brain will begin to use them, reducing its need for glucose by approximately 40%. This, in turn, reduces the need of the liver to produce glucose by gluconeogenesis (recall that glycogen stores are depleted by 36 hours of the fast), which, in turn, reduces the rate of protein degradation in the muscle. The overall effect is to spare muscle protein for as long as possible.

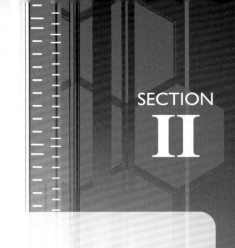

Chemical and Biologic Foundations of Biochemistry

The discipline of biochemistry developed as chemists began to study the molecules of cells, tissues, and body fluids and physicians began to look for the molecular basis of various diseases. Today, the practice of medicine depends on understanding the roles and interactions of the enormous number of different chemicals that enable our bodies to function. The task is less overwhelming if one knows the properties, nomenclature, and functions of classes of compounds, such as carbohydrates and enzymes. The intent of this section is to review some of this information in a context relevant to medicine. Students enter medical school with different scientific backgrounds, and some of the information in this section will therefore be familiar to many students.

We begin by discussing the relationship of metabolic acids and buffers to blood pH in Chapter 4. Chapter 5 focuses on the nomenclature, structure, and some of the properties of the major classes of compounds found in the human body. The structure of a molecule determines its function and its fate, and the common name of a compound can often tell you something about its structure.

Proteins are linear chains of amino acids that fold into complex three-dimensional structures. They function in the maintenance of cellular and tissue structure and the transport and movement of molecules. Some proteins are enzymes, which are catalysts that enormously increase the rate of chemical reactions in the body. Chapters 6 and 7 describe the amino acids and their interactions within proteins that provide proteins with a flexible and functional three-dimensional structure. Chapters 8 and 9 describe the properties, functions, and regulation of enzymes.

Our proteins and other compounds function within a specialized environment defined by their location in cells or body fluids. Their ability to function is partially dependent on membranes that restrict the free movement of molecules. Chapter 10 includes a brief review of the components of cells, their organization into subcellular organelles, and the manner in which various types of molecules move into cells and between compartments within a cell.

In a complex organism such as a human, different cell types carry out different functions. This specialization of function requires cells to communicate with each other. One of the ways they communicate is through secretion of chemical messengers that carry a signal to another cell. In Chapter 11, we consider some of the principles of cell signaling and describe some of the chemical messenger systems.

Both in this book and in medical practice, you will need to interconvert different units used for the weight and size of compounds and for their concentration in blood and other fluids. Table II.1 provides definitions of some of the units used for these interconversions.

The nomenclature used to describe patients may include the name of a class of compounds. For example, a patient with diabetes mellitus who has hyperglycemia has hyper (high) concentrations of carbohydrates (glyc) in her blood (emia).

From a biochemist's point of view, most metabolic diseases are caused by enzymes and other proteins that malfunction, and the pharmacologic drugs used to treat these diseases correct that malfunction. For example, individuals with atherosclerosis, who have elevated blood cholesterol levels, are treated with a drug that inhibits an enzyme in the pathway for cholesterol synthesis. Even a bacterial infection can be considered a disease of protein function, if one considers the bacterial toxins that are proteins, the enzymes in our cells affected by these toxins, and the proteins involved in the immune response when we try to destroy these bacteria.

Dianne A. had an elevated blood glucose level of 684 mg/dL. What is the molar concentration of glucose in Dianne's blood? (Hint: The molecular weight of glucose [$C_6H_{12}O_6$] is 180 g/mol.)

SECTION II

Milligrams per deciliter (mg/dL) is the common way clinicians in the United States express blood glucose concentration. A concentration of 684 mg/dL is 684 mg per 100 mL of blood, or 6,480 mg/L, or 6.48 g/L. If 6.84 g/L is divided by 180 g/mol, one obtains a value of 0.038 mol/L, which is 0.038 M, or 38 mM.

TABLE II.1	Common Units Expressed in Equivalent Ways	
1 M	1 mol/L	MOLECULAR WEIGHT IN g/L
1 mM	1 millimol/L	10^{-3} mol/L
1 μM	1 micromol/L	10^{-6} mol/L
1 nM	1 nanomol/L	10^{-9} mol/L
1 mL	1 milliliter	10^{-3} L
1 mg%	1 mg/100 mL	10^{-3} g/100 mL
1 mg/dL	1 mg/100 mL	10^{-3} g/100 mL
1 mEq/L	1 milliequivalent/L	mM $\times$ valence of ion
1 kg	1,000 g	2.2 lb
1 cm	10^{-2} m	0.394 in

Water, Acids, Bases, and Buffers

Approximately 60% of our body is water. It acts as a solvent for the substances we need, such as K$^+$, glucose, adenosine triphosphate (ATP), and proteins. It is important for the transport of molecules and heat. Many of the compounds produced in the body and dissolved in water contain chemical groups that act as acids or bases, releasing or accepting hydrogen ions. The hydrogen ion content and the amount of body water are controlled to maintain a constant environment for the cells called homeostasis (same state) (Fig. 4.1). Significant deviations from a constant environment, such as acidosis or dehydration, may be life threatening. This chapter describes the role of water in the body and the buffer systems used by the body to protect itself from acids and bases produced from metabolism.

Water. Water is distributed between intracellular and extracellular compartments, the latter comprising interstitial fluids, blood, and lymph. Because water is a **dipolar molecule** with an uneven distribution of electrons between the hydrogen and oxygen atoms, it forms hydrogen bonds with other polar molecules and acts as a **solvent**.

The pH of Water. Water **dissociates** to a slight extent to form **hydrogen (H$^+$)** and hydroxyl (OH$^-$) ions. The concentration of hydrogen ions determines the acidity of the solution, which is expressed in terms of **pH**. The pH of a solution is the negative log of its hydrogen ion concentration.

Acids and Bases. An **acid** is a substance that can **release hydrogen ions** (protons), and a **base** is a substance that can **accept hydrogen ions**. When dissolved in water, almost all the molecules of a **strong acid** dissociate and release their hydrogen ions, but only a small percentage of the total molecules of a weak acid dissociate. A **weak acid** has a characteristic **dissociation constant**, K_a. The relationship between the pH of a solution, the K_a of an acid, and the extent of its dissociation are given by the **Henderson-Hasselbalch equation**.

Buffers. A buffer is a mixture of an **undissociated acid** and its **conjugate base** (the form of the acid that has lost its proton). It causes a solution to resist changes in pH when either H$^+$ or OH$^-$ is added. A buffer has its greatest buffering capacity in the pH range near its **pK_a** (the negative log of its K_a). Two factors determine the effectiveness of a buffer: its pK_a relative to the pH of the solution and its concentration.

Metabolic Acids and Bases. Normal metabolism generates **CO$_2$**, **metabolic acids** (e.g., **lactic acid** and **ketone bodies**), and **inorganic acids** (e.g., **sulfuric acid**). The major source of acid is **CO$_2$**, which reacts with water to produce **carbonic acid**. To maintain the pH of body fluids in a range compatible with life, the body has **buffers** such as **bicarbonate, phosphate**, and **hemoglobin** (see Fig. 4.1). Ultimately, **respiratory mechanisms** remove carbonic acid through the **expiration of CO$_2$**, and the **kidneys excrete acid** as **ammonium ion** (NH$_4^+$) and other ions.

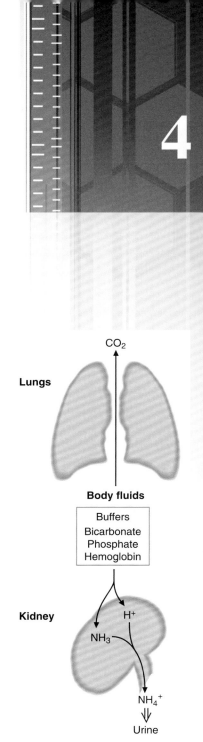

FIGURE 4.1 Maintenance of body pH. The body produces approximately 13 to 22 mol/day of acid from normal metabolism. The body protects itself against this acidity by buffers that maintain a neutral pH and by the expiration of CO$_2$ through the lungs and the excretion of NH$_4^+$ and other ions through the kidneys.

Dianne A. has a ketoacidosis. When the amount of insulin she injects is inadequate, she remains in a condition similar to a fasting state even though she ingests food (see Chapters 2 and 3). Her liver continues to metabolize fatty acids to the ketone bodies acetoacetic acid and β-hydroxybutyric acid. These compounds are weak acids that dissociate to produce anions (acetoacetate and β-hydroxybutyrate, respectively) and hydrogen ions, thereby lowering her blood and cellular pH below the normal range. Because the dissociation of the ketone bodies is causing the acidosis, it is classified as a ketoacidosis.

 Dianne (Di) A. is a 26-year-old woman who was diagnosed with type 1 diabetes mellitus at the age of 12 years. She has an absolute insulin deficiency resulting from autoimmune destruction of the β-cells of her pancreas. As a result, she depends on daily injections of insulin to prevent severe elevations of glucose and ketone bodies in her blood. When Dianne A. could not be aroused from an afternoon nap, her roommate called an ambulance and Di was brought to the emergency department of the hospital in a coma. Her roommate reported that Di had been feeling nauseated and drowsy and had been vomiting for 24 hours. Di is clinically dehydrated, and her blood pressure is low. Her respirations are deep and rapid and her pulse rate is rapid. Her breath has the "fruity" odor of acetone.

Blood samples are drawn for measurement of her arterial blood pH, arterial partial pressure of carbon dioxide ($Paco_2$), serum glucose, and serum bicarbonate (HCO_3^-). In addition, serum and urine are tested for the presence of ketone bodies, and Di is treated with intravenous normal saline and insulin. The laboratory reports that her blood pH is 7.08 (reference range = 7.36 to 7.44) and that ketone bodies are present in both blood and urine. Her blood glucose level is 648 mg/dL (reference range = 80 to 110 mg/dL after an overnight fast, and no higher than 200 mg/dL in a casual glucose sample taken without regard to the time of a last meal).

 Dennis V., age 3 years, was brought to the emergency department by his grandfather, **Percy V.** While Dennis was visiting his grandfather, he climbed up on a chair and took a half-full 500-tablet bottle of 325-mg aspirin (acetylsalicylic acid) tablets from the kitchen counter. Mr. V. discovered Dennis with a mouthful of aspirin, which he removed, but he could not tell how many tablets Dennis had already swallowed. When they arrived at the emergency department, the child appeared bright and alert, but Mr. V. was hyperventilating.

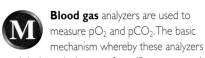 **Blood gas** analyzers are used to measure pO_2 and pCO_2. The basic mechanism whereby these analyzers work is through the use of specific gas-permeable membranes. For oxygen, a Clark electrode is used; oxygen diffuses through a membrane specific for oxygen permeability, and once oxygen passes through the membrane, it diffuses to the cathode. When oxygen reaches the cathode, electrons are attracted from the anode, thereby reducing the oxygen to water. Because it requires four electrons to reduce molecular oxygen (forming two molecules of water), measurement of the current flow can quantitate the amount of oxygen that has reached the cathode. pCO_2 is determined using a Severinghaus electrode, which consists of an outer gas-permeable membrane, specific for CO_2, and a bicarbonate buffer within the electrode. Once the CO_2 crosses the membrane, the gas interacts with bicarbonate, altering the equilibrium among CO_2, carbonic acid, and bicarbonate. This alters the pH in direct proportion to the amount of CO_2 gas that has entered the electrode, and the change in pH can be used to calculate the pCO_2. Improved manufacturing techniques have allowed microelectrodes and tiny circuit boards to be used in these machines, thereby greatly increasing their portability.

I. Water

Water is the solvent of life. It bathes our cells, dissolves and transports compounds in the blood, provides a medium for movement of molecules into and throughout cellular compartments, separates charged molecules, dissipates heat, and participates in chemical reactions. Most compounds in the body, including proteins, must interact with an aqueous medium in order to function. In spite of the variation in the amount of water we ingest each day and produce from metabolism, our body maintains a nearly constant amount of water that is approximately 60% of our body weight (Fig. 4.2).

A. Fluid Compartments in the Body

Total body water is roughly 50% to 60% of body weight in adults and 75% of body weight in children. Because fat has relatively little water associated with it, obese people tend to have a lower percentage of body water than thin people, women tend to have a lower percentage than men, and older people have a lower percentage than younger people.

Approximately 60% of the total body water is intracellular and 40% extracellular (see Fig. 4.2). The extracellular water includes the fluid in plasma (blood after the cells have been removed) and interstitial water (the fluid in the tissue spaces, lying between cells). Transcellular water is a small, specialized portion of extracellular water that includes gastrointestinal secretions, urine, sweat, and fluid that has leaked through capillary walls because of such processes as increased hydrostatic pressure or inflammation.

B. Hydrogen Bonds in Water

The dipolar nature of the water (H_2O) molecule allows it to form hydrogen bonds, a property that is responsible for the role of water as a solvent. In H_2O, the oxygen atom has two unshared electrons that form an electron-dense cloud around it. This cloud lies above and below the plane formed by the water molecule (Fig. 4.3). In the covalent bond formed between the hydrogen and oxygen atoms, the shared electrons are attracted toward the oxygen atom, thus giving the oxygen atom a partial negative charge and the hydrogen atom a partial positive charge. As a result, the oxygen side of the molecule is much more electronegative than the hydrogen side, and the molecule is dipolar.

Both the hydrogen and oxygen atoms of the water molecule form hydrogen bonds and participate in hydration shells. A hydrogen bond is a weak noncovalent interaction between the hydrogen of one molecule and the more electronegative atom of an acceptor molecule. The oxygen of water can form hydrogen bonds with two other water molecules, so that each water molecule is hydrogen-bonded to approximately four close neighboring water molecules in a fluid three-dimensional lattice (see Fig. 4.3).

1. Water as a Solvent

Polar organic molecules and inorganic salts can readily dissolve in water because water also forms hydrogen bonds and electrostatic interactions with these molecules. Organic molecules containing a high proportion of electronegative atoms (generally oxygen or nitrogen) are soluble in water because these atoms participate in hydrogen bonding with water molecules (Fig. 4.4A). Chloride (Cl^-), bicarbonate (HCO_3^-), and other anions are surrounded by a hydration shell of water molecules arranged with their hydrogen atoms closest to the anion. In a similar fashion, the oxygen atom of water molecules interacts with inorganic cations such as Na^+ and K^+ to surround them with a hydration shell (see Fig. 4.4B).

Although hydrogen bonds are strong enough to dissolve polar molecules in water and to separate charges, they are weak enough to allow movement of water and solutes. The strength of the hydrogen bond between two water molecules is only approximately 4 kcal, roughly 1/20th of the strength of the covalent O–H bond in the water molecule. Thus, the extensive water lattice is dynamic and has many strained bonds that are continuously breaking and re-forming. The average hydrogen bond between water molecules lasts only about 10 picoseconds (1 picosecond is 10^{-12} second), and each water molecule in the hydration shell of an ion stays only 2.4 nanoseconds (1 nanosecond = 10^{-9} second). As a result, hydrogen bonds between water molecules and polar solutes continuously dissociate and re-form, thereby permitting solutes to move through water and water to pass through channels in cellular membranes.

2. Water and Thermal Regulation

The structure of water also allows it to resist temperature change. Its heat of fusion is high, so a large drop in temperature is needed to convert liquid water to the solid state of ice. The thermal conductivity of water is also high, thereby facilitating heat dissipation from high energy-using areas such as the brain into the blood and the total body water pool. Its heat capacity and heat of vaporization are remarkably high; as liquid water is converted to a gas and evaporates from the skin, we feel a cooling effect. Water responds to the input of heat by decreasing the extent of hydrogen bonding and to cooling by increasing the bonding between water molecules.

C. Electrolytes

Both extracellular fluid (ECF) and intracellular fluid (ICF) contain *electrolytes*, a general term applied to bicarbonate and inorganic anions and cations. The electrolytes are unevenly distributed between compartments; Na^+ and Cl^- are the major electrolytes in the ECF (plasma and interstitial fluid), and K^+ and phosphates such as HPO_4^{2-} are the major electrolytes in cells (Table 4.1). This distribution is maintained principally by energy-requiring transporters that pump Na^+ out of cells in exchange for K^+ (see Chapter 10).

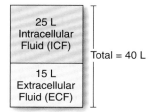

A. Total body water

25 L Intracellular Fluid (ICF)

15 L Extracellular Fluid (ECF)

Total = 40 L

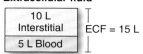

B. Extracellular fluid

10 L Interstitial

5 L Blood

ECF = 15 L

FIGURE 4.2 Fluid compartments in the body based on an average 70-kg man.

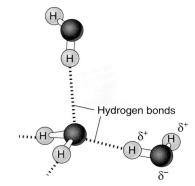

Hydrogen bonds

FIGURE 4.3 Hydrogen bonds between water molecules. The oxygen atoms are shown in *black*.

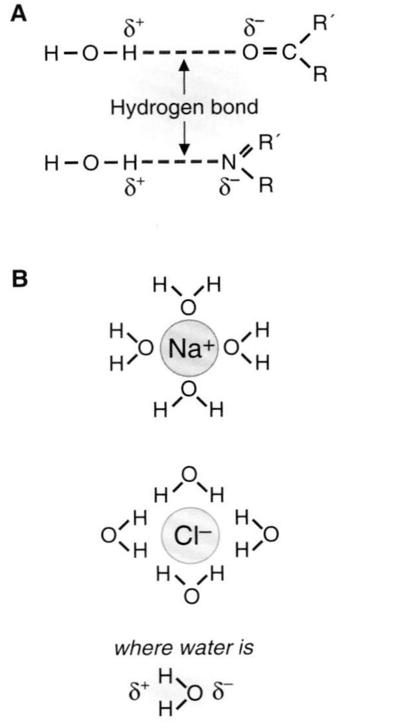

A

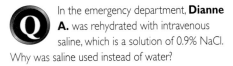

Hydrogen bond

B

where water is

$$\delta^+ \; H{>}O \; \delta^-$$

FIGURE 4.4 A. Hydrogen bonds between water and polar molecules. *R* denotes additional atoms. **B.** Hydration shells surrounding anions and cations.

Q In the emergency department, **Dianne A.** was rehydrated with intravenous saline, which is a solution of 0.9% NaCl. Why was saline used instead of water?

Dianne A. has an osmotic diuresis. Because her blood levels of glucose and ketone bodies are so high, these compounds are passing from the blood into the glomerular filtrate in the kidneys and then into the urine. As a consequence of the high osmolality of the glomerular filtrate, much more water than usual is being excreted in the urine. Thus, Di has polyuria (increased urine volume). As a result of water lost from the blood into the urine, water passes from inside cells into the interstitial space and into the blood, resulting in intracellular dehydration. The dehydrated cells in the brain are unable to carry out their normal functions. As a result, Di is in a coma.

$$H_2O \; \rightleftharpoons \; H^+ + OH^-$$

FIGURE 4.5 Dissociation of water.

TABLE 4.1	**Distribution of Ions in Body Fluids**	
	ECF^a (mmol/L)	**ICF (mmol/L)**
Cations		
Na$^+$	145	12
K$^+$	4	150
Anions		
Cl$^-$	105	5
HCO$_3^-$	25	12
Inorganic phosphate	2	100

ECF, extracellular fluid; ICF, intracellular fluid.
^{a}The content of inorganic ions is very similar in plasma and interstitial fluid, the two components of the extracellular fluid.

D. Osmolality and Water Movement

Water distributes between the different fluid compartments according to the concentration of solutes, or osmolality, of each compartment. The osmolality of a fluid is proportional to the total concentration of all dissolved molecules, including ions, organic metabolites, and proteins, and is usually expressed as milliosmoles (mOsm)/kg water. The semipermeable cellular membrane that separates the extracellular and intracellular compartments contains a number of ion channels through which water can move freely, but other molecules cannot. Likewise, water can move freely through the capillaries separating the interstitial fluid and the plasma. As a result, water will move from a compartment with a low concentration of solutes (lower osmolality) to one with a higher concentration to achieve an equal osmolality on both sides of the membrane. The force it would take to keep the same amount of water on both sides of the membrane is called the *osmotic pressure.*

As water is lost from one fluid compartment, it is replaced with water from another compartment to maintain a nearly constant osmolality. The blood contains a high content of dissolved negatively charged proteins and the electrolytes needed to balance these charges. As water is passed from the blood into the urine to balance the excretion of ions, the blood volume is repleted with water from interstitial fluid. When the osmolality of the blood and interstitial fluid is too high, water moves out of the cells. The loss of cellular water also can occur in hyperglycemia because the high concentration of glucose increases the osmolality of the blood.

II. Acids and Bases

Acids are compounds that donate a hydrogen ion (H$^+$) to a solution, and bases are compounds (such as the OH$^-$ ion) that accept hydrogen ions. Water itself dissociates to a slight extent, generating H$^+$, which are also called *protons*, and hydroxide ions (OH$^-$) (Fig. 4.5). The hydrogen ions are extensively hydrated in water to form species such as H$_3$O$^+$ but nevertheless are usually represented as simply H$^+$. Water itself is neutral, neither acidic nor basic.

A. The pH of Water

The extent of dissociation by water molecules into H$^+$ and OH$^-$ is very slight, and the hydrogen ion concentration of pure water is only 0.0000001 M, or 10^{-7} mol/L. The concentration of hydrogen ions in a solution is usually denoted by the term *pH*, which is the negative log$_{10}$ of the hydrogen ion concentration expressed in moles per liter (mol/L) (Equation 4.1). Therefore, the pH of pure water is 7.

$$pH = -\log[H^+] \qquad \textbf{Equation 4.1. Definition of pH.}$$

The dissociation constant for water, K_d, expresses the relationship between the hydrogen ion concentration [H$^+$], the hydroxide ion concentration [OH$^-$], and the concentration of water [H_2O] at equilibrium (Equation 4.2). Because water dissociates to such a small extent, [H_2O] is essentially constant at 55.5 M. Multiplication of the K_d for water ($\sim1.8 \times 10^{-16}$ M) by 55.5 M gives a value of approximately 10^{-14} (mol/L)^2, which is called the *ion product of water* (K_w) (Equation 4.3). Because K_w, the product of [H^+] and [OH^-], is always constant, a decrease of [H^+] must be accompanied by a proportionate increase of [OH^-].

$$K_d = \frac{[H^+][OH^-]}{[H_2O]}$$ **Equation 4.2. Dissociation of water.**

$$K_w = [H^+][OH^-] = 1 \times 10^{-14}$$ **Equation 4.3. Ion product of water.**

A pH of 7 is termed *neutral* because [H^+] and [OH^-] are equal. Acidic solutions have a greater hydrogen ion concentration and a lower hydroxide ion concentration than pure water (pH <7.0), and basic solutions have a lower hydrogen ion concentration and a greater hydroxide ion concentration (pH >7.0).

B. Strong and Weak Acids

During metabolism, the body produces a number of acids that increase the hydrogen ion concentration of the blood or other body fluids and tend to lower the pH (Table 4.2). These metabolically important acids can be classified as weak acids or strong acids by their degree of dissociation into a hydrogen ion and a base (the anion component). Inorganic acids such as sulfuric acid (H_2SO_4) and hydrochloric acid (HCl) are strong acids that dissociate completely in solution (Fig. 4.6). Organic acids containing carboxylic acid groups (e.g., the ketone bodies acetoacetic acid and β-hydroxybutyric acid) are weak acids that dissociate to only a limited extent in water. In general, a weak acid (HA), called the *conjugate acid*, dissociates into a hydrogen ion and an anionic component (A^-), called the *conjugate base*. The name of an undissociated acid usually ends in "ic acid" (e.g., acetoacetic acid), and the name of the dissociated anionic component ends in "ate" (e.g., acetoacetate).

The tendency of the acid (HA) to dissociate and donate a hydrogen ion to solution is denoted by its K_a, the equilibrium constant for dissociation of a weak acid (Equation 4.4). The higher the K_a, the greater is the tendency to dissociate a proton.

For the reaction   **Equation 4.4. The K_a of an acid.**

$$HA \leftrightarrow A^- + H^+$$

$$K_a = \frac{[H^+][A^-]}{[HA]}$$

A solution of 0.9% NaCl is 0.9 g NaCl/100 mL, equivalent to 9 g/L. NaCl has a molecular weight of 58 g/mol, so the concentration of NaCl in isotonic saline is 0.155 M, or 155 mM. If all of the NaCl were dissociated into Na^+ and Cl^- ions, the osmolality would be 310 mOsm/kg water. Because NaCl is not completely dissociated and some of the hydration shells surround undissociated NaCl molecules, the osmolality of isotonic saline is approximately 290 mOsm/kg H_2O. The osmolality of plasma, interstitial fluids, and ICF is also approximately 290 mOsm/kg water, so no large shifts of water or swelling occurs when isotonic saline is given intravenously. In some cases, glucose is added to this at a 5% concentration (5 g/100 mL). The glucose provides fuel for the individual. If this is done, the saline solution has the designation of *D5*, for 5% dextrose.

TABLE 4.2	Acids in the Blood of a Healthy Individual		
ACID	**ANION**	**pK_a**	**MAJOR SOURCES**
Strong acid			
Sulfuric acid (H_2SO_4)	Sulfate (SO_4^{2-})	Completely dissociated	Dietary sulfate and S-containing amino acids
Weak acid			
Carbonic acid (R–COOH)	Bicarbonate (R–COO$^-$)	3.80	CO_2 from TCA cycle
Lactic acid (R–COOH)	Lactate (R–COO$^-$)	3.73	Anaerobic glycolysis
Pyruvic acid (R–COOH)	Pyruvate (R–COO$^-$)	2.39	Glycolysis
Citric acid (R–3COOH)	Citrate (R–3COO$^-$)	3.13; 4.76; 6.40	TCA cycle and diet (e.g., citrus fruits)
Acetoacetic acid (R–COOH)	Acetoacetate (R–COO$^-$)	3.62	Fatty acid oxidation to ketone bodies
β-Hydroxybutyric acid (R–COOH)	β-Hydroxybutyrate (R–COO$^-$)	4.41	Fatty acid oxidation to ketone bodies
Acetic acid (R–COOH)	Acetate (R–COO$^-$)	4.76	Ethanol metabolism
Dihydrogen phosphate ($H_2PO_4^-$)	Monohydrogen phosphate (HPO_4^{2-})	6.8	Dietary organic phosphates
Ammonium ion (NH_4^+)	Ammonia (NH_3)	9.25	Dietary nitrogen-containing compounds

pK_a, the pH at which 50% dissociation occurs; TCA, tricarboxylic acid.

Dennis V. has ingested an unknown number of acetylsalicylic acid (aspirin) tablets. Acetylsalicylic acid is rapidly converted to salicylic acid in the body. The initial effect of aspirin is to produce a respiratory alkalosis caused by a stimulation of the "metabolic" central respiratory control center in the medulla. This increases the rate of breathing and the expiration of CO_2. This is followed by a complex metabolic acidosis caused partly by the dissociation of salicylic acid (salicylic acid $\leftrightarrow$ salicylate$^-$ + H$^+$, pK_a = ~3.5).

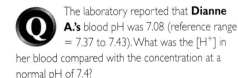

Acetylsalicylate

Salicylate also interferes with mitochondrial ATP production (acting as an uncoupler; see Chapter 24), resulting in increased generation of CO_2 and accumulation of lactate (caused by stimulation of glycolysis; see Chapter 22) and other organic acids in the blood. Subsequently, salicylate may impair renal function, resulting in the accumulation of strong acids of metabolic origin, such as sulfuric acid and phosphoric acid. Usually, children who ingest toxic amounts of aspirin are acidotic by the time they arrive in the emergency department.

Q The laboratory reported that **Dianne A.'s** blood pH was 7.08 (reference range = 7.37 to 7.43). What was the [H$^+$] in her blood compared with the concentration at a normal pH of 7.4?

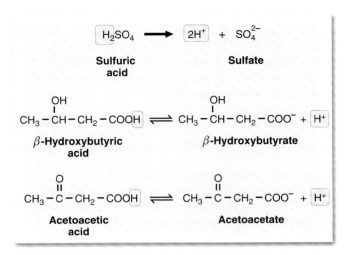

FIGURE 4.6 Dissociation of acids. Sulfuric acid is a strong acid that dissociates into H$^+$ ions and sulfate. The ketone bodies acetoacetic acid and β-hydroxybutyric acid are weak acids that partially dissociate into H$^+$ and their conjugate bases.

In the Henderson-Hasselbalch equation, the formula for the dissociation constant of a weak acid is converted to a convenient logarithmic equation (Equation 4.5). The term pK_a represents the negative log of K_a. If the pK_a for a weak acid is known, this equation can be used to calculate the ratio of the unprotonated to the protonated form at any pH. From this equation, you can see that a weak acid is 50% dissociated at a pH equal to its pK_a.

For the weak acid HA,

$$pH = pK_a + \log\frac{[A^-]}{[HA]}$$

Equation 4.5. The Henderson-Hasselbalch equation.

Most of the metabolic carboxylic acids have a pK_a between 2 and 5, depending on the other groups on the molecule (see Table 4.2). The pK_a reflects the strength of an acid. Acids with a pK_a of 2 are stronger acids than those with a pK_a of 5 because, at any pH, a greater proportion is dissociated.

III. Buffers

Buffers consist of a weak acid and its conjugate base. Buffers allow a solution to resist changes in pH when hydrogen ions or hydroxide ions are added. In Figure 4.7, the pH of a solution of the weak acid acetic acid is graphed as a function of the amount of OH$^-$ that has been added. The OH$^-$ is expressed as equivalents of total acetic acid present in the dissociated and undissociated forms. At the midpoint of this curve, 0.5 equivalents of OH$^-$ have been added and half of the conjugate acid has dissociated, so [A$^-$] equals [HA]. This midpoint is expressed in the Henderson-Hasselbalch equation as the pK_a, defined as the pH at which 50% dissociation occurs. As you add more OH$^-$ ions and move to the right on the curve, more of the conjugate acid molecules (HA) dissociate to generate H$^+$ ions, which combine with the added OH$^-$ ions to form water. Consequently, only a small increase in pH results. If you add hydrogen ions to the buffer at its pK_a (moving to the left of the midpoint in Fig. 4.7), conjugate base molecules (A$^-$) combine with the added hydrogen ions to form HA, and there is almost no fall in pH.

As can be seen from Figure 4.7, a buffer can only compensate for an influx or removal of hydrogen ions within approximately 1 pH unit of its pK_a. As the pH of a buffered solution changes from the pK_a to 1 pH unit below the pK_a, the ratio of [A$^-$] to HA changes from 1:1 to 1:10. If more hydrogen ions were added, the

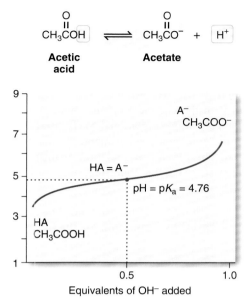

FIGURE 4.7 Titration curve for acetic acid. *HA*, weak acid; pK_a, the pH at which 50% dissociation occurs.

From inspection, you can tell that her [H$^+$] is greater than normal, but it is <10 times higher. A 10-fold change in [H$^+$] changes the pH by 1 unit. For Di, the pH of 7.08 = $-$log[H$^+$], and therefore her [H$^+$] is 1 × 10$^{-7.08}$. To calculate her [H$^+$], express $-$7.08 as $-8 + 0.92$. The antilog to the base 10 of 0.92 is 8.3. Thus, her [H$^+$] is 8.3 × 10^{-8} compared to 4.0 × 10^{-8} at pH 7.4, or slightly more than double the normal value.

pH would fall rapidly because relatively little conjugate base remains. Likewise, at 1 pH unit above the pK_a of a buffer, relatively little undissociated acid remains. More concentrated buffers are more effective simply because they contain a greater total number of buffer molecules per unit volume that can dissociate or recombine with hydrogen ions.

IV. Metabolic Acids and Buffers

An average rate of metabolic activity produces roughly 22,000 mEq of acid per day. If all of this acid were dissolved at one time in unbuffered body fluids, their pH would be <1. However, the pH of the blood is normally maintained between 7.36 and 7.44 and intracellular pH at approximately 7.1 (between 6.9 and 7.4). The widest range of extracellular pH over which the metabolic functions of the liver, the beating of the heart, and conduction of neural impulses can be maintained is 6.8 to 7.8. Thus, until the acid produced from metabolism can be excreted as CO_2 in expired air and as ions in the urine, it needs to be buffered in the body fluids. The major buffer systems in the body are the bicarbonate–carbonic acid buffer system, which operates principally in ECF; the hemoglobin buffer system in red blood cells; the phosphate buffer system in all types of cells; and the protein buffer system of cells and plasma.

A. The Bicarbonate Buffer System

The major source of metabolic acid in the body is the gas CO_2, produced principally from fuel oxidation in the tricarboxylic acid (TCA) cycle. Under normal metabolic conditions, the body generates >13 mol of CO_2 per day (~0.5 to 1 kg). CO_2 dissolves in water and reacts with water to produce carbonic acid, H_2CO_3, a reaction that is accelerated by the enzyme carbonic anhydrase (Fig. 4.8). Carbonic acid is a weak acid that partially dissociates into H$^+$ and bicarbonate anion, HCO_3^-.

Carbonic acid is both the major acid produced by the body and its own buffer. The pK_a of carbonic acid itself is only 3.8, so at the blood pH of 7.4, it is almost completely dissociated and theoretically unable to buffer and generate bicarbonate. However, carbonic acid can be replenished from CO_2 in body fluids and air because the concentration of dissolved CO_2 in body fluids is approximately 400 times greater than that of carbonic acid. As base is added and H$^+$ is

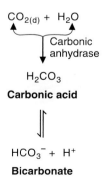

FIGURE 4.8 The bicarbonate buffer system. $CO_{2(d)}$ refers to carbon dioxide dissolved in water and not in the gaseous state.

$PaCO_2$ in **Dianne A.'s** arterial blood was 28 mm Hg (reference range = 37 to 43 mm Hg) and her serum bicarbonate level was 8 mEq/L (reference range = 24 to 28 mEq/L). Elevated levels of ketone bodies had produced a ketoacidosis, and Di was exhaling increased amounts of CO_2 by breathing deeply and frequently (Kussmaul breathing) to compensate. Why does this occur? Ketone bodies are weak acids that partially dissociate, increasing H^+ levels in the blood and the interstitial fluid surrounding the "metabolic" respiratory center in the hypothalamus that controls the rate of breathing. A drop in pH elicits an increase in the rate of breathing. Bicarbonate combines with protons, forming H_2CO_3, thereby lowering bicarbonate levels. The H_2CO_3 is converted to CO_2 and H_2O, which increase the CO_2 concentration, which is exhaled. The increase in CO_2 concentration leads to an increase in the respiratory rate, causing a fall in the $PaCO_2$. As shown by Di's low arterial blood pH of 7.08, the Kussmaul breathing was unable to fully compensate for the high rate of acidic ketone body production.

removed, H_2CO_3 dissociates into hydrogen and bicarbonate ions, and dissolved CO_2 reacts with H_2O to replenish the H_2CO_3 (see Fig. 4.8). Dissolved CO_2 is in equilibrium with the CO_2 in air in the alveoli of the lungs, and thus, the availability of CO_2 can be increased or decreased by an adjustment in the rate of breathing and the amount of CO_2 expired. The pK_a for the bicarbonate buffer system in the body thus combines K_h (the hydration constant for the reaction of water and CO_2 to form H_2CO_3) with the chemical pK_a to obtain a modified version of the Henderson-Hasselbalch equation (Equation 4.6). To use the terms for blood components measured in the emergency department, the dissolved CO_2 is expressed as a fraction of $PaCO_2$. The pK_a for dissociation of bicarbonate anion (HCO_3^-) into H^+ and carbonate (CO_3^{2+}) is 9.8; therefore, only trace amounts of carbonate exist in body fluids.

$$pH = pK_a + \log \frac{[HCO_3^-]}{[H_2CO_3]}$$

Equation 4.6. The Henderson-Hasselbalch equation for the bicarbonate buffer system.

The $pK_a = 3.5$, so

$$pH = 3.5 + \log \frac{[HCO_3^-]}{[H_2CO_3]}$$

$[H_2CO_3]$ is best estimated as $[CO_2]_d/400$, where $[CO_2]_d$ is the concentration of dissolved CO_2, so substituting this value for $[H_2CO_3]$ we get

$$pH = 3.5 + \log 400 + \log \frac{[HCO_3^-]}{[CO_2]_d}$$

or

$$pH = 6.1 + \log \frac{[HCO_3^-]}{[CO_2]_d}$$

Because only 3% of the gaseous CO_2 is dissolved, $[CO_2]_d = 0.03 \ PaCO_2$, so

$$pH = 6.1 + \log \frac{[HCO_3^-]}{0.03 \ PaCO_2}$$

The concentration of HCO_3^- is expressed as milliequivalents per milliliter (mEq/mL) and $PaCO_2$ as millimeters of mercury (mm Hg).

B. Bicarbonate and Hemoglobin in Red Blood Cells

The bicarbonate buffer system and hemoglobin in red blood cells cooperate in buffering the blood and transporting CO_2 to the lungs. Most of the CO_2 produced from tissue metabolism in the TCA cycle diffuses into the interstitial fluid and the blood plasma and then into red blood cells (Fig. 4.9, circle 1). Although no carbonic anhydrase can be found in blood plasma or interstitial fluid, the red blood cells contain high amounts of this enzyme, and CO_2 is rapidly converted to carbonic acid (H_2CO_3) within these cells (Fig. 4.9, circle 2). As the carbonic acid dissociates (Fig. 4.9, circle 3), the H^+ released is also buffered by combination with hemoglobin (Hb; Fig. 4.9, circle 4). The side chain of the amino acid histidine in hemoglobin has a pK_a of 6.7 and is thus able to accept a proton. The bicarbonate anion is transported out of the red blood cells into the blood in exchange for chloride anions, and thus, bicarbonate is relatively high in the plasma (Fig. 4.9, circle 5) (see Table 4.1).

As the red blood cells approach the lungs, the direction of the equilibrium reverses. CO_2 is released from the red blood cells, causing more carbonic acid to dissociate into CO_2 and water and more hydrogen ions to combine with bicarbonate. Hemoglobin loses some it of its hydrogen ions, a feature that allows it to bind oxygen more readily (see Chapter 7). Thus, the bicarbonate buffer system is intimately linked to the delivery of oxygen to tissues.

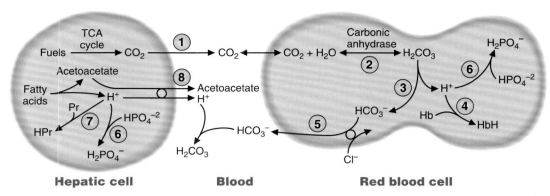

FIGURE 4.9   Buffering systems of the body. CO_2 produced from cellular metabolism is converted to bicarbonate and H^+ in the red blood cells. Within the red blood cells, the H^+ is buffered by hemoglobin (Hb) and phosphate (HPO_4^{2-}) (*circles 4 and 6*). The bicarbonate is transported into the blood to buffer H^+ generated by the production of other metabolic acids such as the ketone body acetoacetic acid (*circle 5*). Other proteins (*Pr*) also serve as intracellular buffers. *Numbers* refer to the text discussion. *TCA*, tricarboxylic acid.

Bicarbonate and carbonic acid, which diffuse through the capillary wall from the blood into interstitial fluid, provide a major buffer for both plasma and interstitial fluid. However, blood differs from interstitial fluid in that the blood contains a high content of extracellular proteins, such as albumin, which contribute to its buffering capacity through amino acid side chains that are able to accept and release protons. The protein content of interstitial fluid is too low to serve as an effective buffer.

C. Intracellular pH

Phosphate anions and proteins are the major buffers involved in maintaining a constant pH of ICF. The inorganic phosphate anion $H_2PO_4^-$ dissociates to generate H^+ and the conjugate base HPO_4^{2-} with a pK_a of 7.2 (see Fig. 4.9, circle 6). Thus, phosphate anions play a major role as an intracellular buffer in the red blood cell and in other types of cells, where their concentration is much higher than in blood and interstitial fluid (see Table 4.1, extracellular fluid). Organic phosphate anions, such as glucose-6-phosphate and ATP, also act as buffers. ICF contains a high content of proteins that contain histidine and other amino acids that can accept protons in a fashion similar to hemoglobin (see Fig. 4.9, circle 7).

The transport of hydrogen ions out of the cell is also important for maintenance of a constant intracellular pH. Metabolism produces a number of other acids in addition to CO_2. For example, the metabolic acids acetoacetic acid and β-hydroxybutyric acid are produced from fatty acid oxidation to ketone bodies in the liver, and lactic acid is produced by glycolysis in muscle and other tissues. The pK_a for most metabolic carboxylic acids is <5, so these acids are completely dissociated at the pH of blood and cellular fluid. Metabolic anions are transported out of the cell together with H^+ (see Fig. 4.9, circle 8). If the cell becomes too acidic, more H^+ is transported out in exchange for Na^+ ions by a different transporter. If the cell becomes too alkaline, more bicarbonate is transported out in exchange for Cl^- ions.

D. Urinary Hydrogen, Ammonium, and Phosphate Ions

The nonvolatile acid that is produced from body metabolism cannot be excreted as expired CO_2 and is excreted in the urine. Most nonvolatile acid hydrogen ion is excreted as undissociated acid that generally buffers the urinary pH between 5.5 and 7.0. A pH of 5.0 is the minimum urinary pH. The acid secretion includes inorganic acids such as phosphate and ammonium ions, as well as uric acid, dicarboxylic acids, and TCAs such as citric acid (see Table 4.2). One of the major sources of nonvolatile acid in the body is sulfuric acid (H_2SO_4). Sulfuric acid is generated from the sulfate-containing compounds ingested in foods and from metabolism of

 Both **Dianne A.** and **Percy V.** were hyperventilating when they arrived at the emergency department: Ms. A. in response to her primary metabolic acidosis and Mr. V. in response to anxiety. Hyperventilation raised blood pH in both cases: In Ms. A.'s case, it partially countered the acidosis, and in Mr. V.'s case, it produced a respiratory alkalosis (abnormally high arterial blood pH).

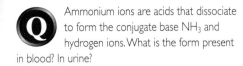

Ammonium ions are acids that dissociate to form the conjugate base NH_3 and hydrogen ions. What is the form present in blood? In urine?

the sulfur-containing amino acids cysteine and methionine. It is a strong acid that is dissociated into H^+ and sulfate anion (SO_4^-) in the blood and urine (see Fig. 4.6). Urinary excretion of $H_2PO_4^-$ helps to remove acid. To maintain metabolic homeostasis, we must excrete the same amount of phosphate in the urine that we ingest with food as phosphate anions or organic phosphates such as phospholipids. Whether the phosphate is present in the urine as $H_2PO_4^-$ or $HPO4^-$ depends on the urinary pH and the pH of the blood.

Ammonium ions are major contributors to buffering urinary pH but not blood pH. Ammonia (NH_3) is a base that combines with protons to produce ammonium (NH_4^+) ions ($NH_3 + H^+ \leftrightarrow NH_4^+$), a reaction that occurs with a pK_a of 9.25. NH_3 is produced from amino acid catabolism or absorbed through the intestine and is kept at very low concentrations in the blood because it is toxic to neural tissues. Cells in the kidney generate NH_4^+ and excrete it into the urine in proportion to the acidity (proton concentration) of the blood. As the renal tubular cells transport H^+ into the urine, they return bicarbonate anions to the blood.

E. Hydrochloric Acid

HCl, also called *gastric acid*, is secreted by parietal cells of the stomach into the stomach lumen, where the strong acidity denatures ingested proteins so they can be degraded by digestive enzymes. When the stomach contents are released into the lumen of the small intestine, gastric acid is neutralized by bicarbonate secreted from pancreatic cells and by cells in the intestinal lining.

CLINICAL COMMENTS

Dianne A. Dianne A. has type 1 diabetes mellitus. Because the β-cells of her pancreas have a very limited ability to synthesize and secrete insulin, she maintains her insulin level by giving herself several subcutaneous (under the skin) injections of insulin every day. If her blood insulin levels fall too low, she remains in a condition similar to a fasting state even though she ingests food (see Chapters 2 and 3). Free fatty acids leave her adipocytes (fat cells) and are converted by the liver to the ketone bodies acetoacetic acid and β-hydroxybutyric acid. These compounds are weak acids that dissociate to produce anions (acetoacetate and β-hydroxybutyrate, respectively) and hydrogen ions, thereby lowering her blood and cellular pH below the normal range. As these acids accumulate in the blood, a metabolic acidosis known as *diabetic ketoacidosis* (DKA) develops.

Once DKA develops, until insulin is administered to reverse this trend, several compensatory mechanisms operate to minimize the extent of the acidosis. One of these mechanisms is a stimulation of the respiratory center in the hypothalamus induced by the acidosis, which leads to deeper and more frequent respiration (Kussmaul breathing). CO_2 is expired more rapidly than normal, and the blood pH rises toward normal. The results of the laboratory studies performed on **Dianne A.** in the emergency department were consistent with a moderately severe DKA. Her arterial blood pH and serum bicarbonate were low, and ketone bodies were present in her blood and urine (normally, ketone bodies are not present in the urine). In addition, her serum glucose level was 648 mg/dL (reference range = 80 to 110 mg/dL fasting and no higher than 200 mg/dL in a random glucose sample). Her hyperglycemia, which induces an osmotic diuresis, contributed to her dehydration and the hyperosmolality of her body fluids.

Treatment was initiated with intravenous saline solutions to replace fluids lost with the osmotic diuresis and hyperventilation. The osmotic diuresis resulted from increased urinary water volume required to dilute the large amounts of glucose and ketone bodies excreted in the urine. Hyperventilation increased the water of respiration lost with expired air. A loading dose of regular insulin was given as an intravenous bolus followed by an insulin drip, giving her continuous insulin. The patient's metabolic response to the treatment was monitored closely.

Diabetes mellitus is diagnosed by the concentration of plasma glucose (plasma is blood from which the red blood cells have been removed by centrifugation). Because plasma glucose normally increases after a meal, the normal reference ranges and the diagnostic level are defined relative to the time of consumption of food or to consumption of a specified amount of glucose during an oral glucose tolerance test. After an overnight fast, values for the fasting plasma glucose <100 mg/dL are considered normal; a level >126 mg/dL defines diabetes mellitus. Fasting plasma glucose values ≥100 and <126 mg/dL define an intermediate condition termed *impaired fasting glucose* or *prediabetes*. Normal random plasma glucose levels (random is defined as any time of day without regard to the time since a last meal) should not be >200 mg/dL. Normal subjects generally do not increase their blood sugar >140 mg/dL, even after a meal. Thus, a 2-hour postprandial (after a meal or after an oral glucose load) plasma glucose level between 140 and 199 mg/dL defines a condition known as *impaired glucose tolerance*, or *prediabetes*, where a level >200 mg/dL defines overt diabetes mellitus. Diabetes mellitus is also diagnosed by measuring the hemoglobin A_{IC} (HbA_{IC}) value, which is a measure of glycosylated hemoglobin in the red blood cells. This is a nonenzymatic reaction that is dependent upon glucose concentration; thus, as the glucose concentration increases, the levels of HbA_{IC} increase. Normal levels of HbA_{IC} are 4% to 6% of total hemoglobin, and a value of >6.5% HbA_{IC} defines diabetes mellitus.

Dennis V. Dennis remained alert in the emergency department. While awaiting the report of his initial serum salicylate level, his stomach was lavaged, and several white tablets were found in the stomach aspirate. He was examined repeatedly and showed none of the early symptoms of salicylate toxicity, such as respiratory stimulation, upper abdominal distress, nausea, or headache.

His serum salicylate level was reported as 92 μg/mL (usual level in an adult on a therapeutic dosage of 4 to 5 g/day is 120 to 350 μg/mL, and a level of 800 μg/mL is considered potentially lethal). He was admitted for overnight observation and continued to do well. A serum salicylate level the following morning was 24 μg/mL. He was discharged later that day.

Percy V. At the emergency department, Mr. V. complained of light-headedness and "pins and needles" (paresthesias) in his hands and around his lips. These symptoms resulted from an increase in respiratory drive mediated in this case through the "behavioral" rather than the "metabolic" central respiratory control system (as seen in **Dianne A.** when she was in DKA). The behavioral system was activated in Mr. V.'s case by his anxiety over his grandson's potential poisoning. His alveolar hyperventilation caused Mr. V.'s $PaCO_2$ to decrease below the normal range of 37 to 43 mm Hg. The alkalemia caused his neurologic symptoms. After being reassured that his grandson would be fine, Mr. V. was asked to breathe slowly into a small paper bag placed around his nose and mouth, allowing him to reinhale the CO_2 being exhaled through hyperventilation. Within 20 minutes, his symptoms disappeared.

BIOCHEMICAL COMMENTS

Body Water and Dehydration. Dehydration, or loss of water, occurs when salt and water intake is less than the combined rates of renal plus extrarenal volume loss (Fig. 4.10). In a true hypovolemic state, total body water, functional ECF volume, and ICF volume are decreased. One of the causes of hypovolemia is an intake of water that is inadequate to resupply the daily excretion volume (maintenance of fluid homeostasis). The amount of water lost by the kidneys is determined by the amount of water necessary to dilute the ions, acids, and other solutes excreted. Both urinary solute excretion and water loss in expired air, which amount to almost 400 mL/day, occur during fasting as well as during periods of normal food intake. Thus, people who are lost in the desert or shipwrecked continue to lose water in air and urine, in addition to their water loss through the skin and sweat glands. Comatose patients and patients who are debilitated and unable to swallow also continue to lose water and become dehydrated. Anorexia (loss of appetite), such as **Percy V.** experienced during his depression (see Chapters 1 and 3), can result in dehydration because food intake is normally a source of fluid. Cerebral injuries that cause a loss of thirst response also can lead to dehydration.

Dehydration also can occur secondary to excessive water loss through the kidneys, lungs, and skin. Excessive renal loss could be the result of impaired kidney function or impaired response to the hormones that regulate water balance (e.g., antidiuretic hormone [ADH] and aldosterone). However, in individuals who have normal kidney function, such as **Dianne A.**, dehydration can occur as a response to water dilution of the high concentrations of ketone bodies, glucose, and other solutes excreted in the urine (osmotic diuresis). If the urinary water loss is associated with an acidosis, hyperventilation occurs, increasing the amount of water lost in expired air. Water loss in expired air (pulmonary water loss) could occur also as a result of a tracheotomy or cerebral injury. An excessive loss of water and electrolytes through the skin can result from extensive burns.

Gastrointestinal water losses also can result in dehydration. We secrete approximately 8 to 10 L of fluid per day into our intestinal lumen. Normally, >90% of this fluid is reabsorbed in the intestines. The percentage reabsorbed can be decreased by vomiting, diarrhea, tube drainage of gastric contents, or loss of water into tissues around the gut via bowel fistulas.

A The pK_a for dissociation of ammonium ions is 9.25. Thus, the undissociated conjugate acid form NH_4^+ predominates at the physiologic pH of 7.4 and urinary pH of 5.5 to 7.0. NH_3 is an unusual conjugate base because it is not an anion.

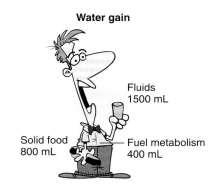

Water gain

Fluids
1500 mL

Solid food
800 mL

Fuel metabolism
400 mL

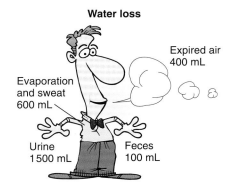

Water loss

Expired air
400 mL

Evaporation
and sweat
600 mL

Urine
1500 mL

Feces
100 mL

FIGURE 4.10 Body fluid homeostasis (constant body water balance). Intake is influenced by availability of fluids and food, thirst, hunger, and the ability to swallow. The rates of breathing and evaporation and urinary volume influence water loss. The body adjusts the volume of urinary excretion to compensate for variations in other types of water loss and for variations in intake. The hormones aldosterone and antidiuretic hormone (ADH) help to monitor blood volume and osmolality through mechanisms that regulate thirst as well as sodium and water balance.

KEY CONCEPTS

- Approximately 60% of our body weight is water.
- Water is distributed between intracellular and extracellular (interstitial fluids, blood, lymph) compartments.
- Because water is a dipolar molecule with an uneven distribution of electrons between the hydrogen and oxygen atoms, it forms hydrogen bonds with other polar molecules and acts as a solvent.
- Many of the compounds produced in the body and dissolved in water contain chemical groups that act as acids or bases, releasing or accepting hydrogen ions.
- The hydrogen ion content and the amount of body water are controlled to maintain homeostasis, a constant environment for our cells.
- The pH of a solution is the negative log of its hydrogen ion concentration.
- Acids release hydrogen ions; bases accept hydrogen ions.
- Strong acids dissociate completely in water, whereas only a small percentage of the total molecules of a weak acid dissociate.
- The dissociation constant of a weak acid is designated as K_a.
- The Henderson-Hasselbalch equation defines the relationship between the pH of a solution, the K_a of the acid, and the extent of acid dissociation.
- A buffer, a mixture of an undissociated acid and its conjugate base, resists changes in pH when either H^+ or OH^- is added.
- Buffers work best within a range of 1 pH unit either above or below the pK_a of the buffer, where the pK_a is the negative log of the K_a.
- Normal metabolism generates metabolic acids (lactate, ketone bodies), inorganic acids (sulfuric acid, hydrochloric acid), and carbon dioxide.
- Carbon dioxide reacts with water to form carbonic acid, which will dissociate to form bicarbonate and a proton.
- Physiologic buffers include bicarbonate, phosphate, and the protein hemoglobin.
- Diseases discussed in this chapter are described in Table 4.3.

TABLE 4.3 Diseases Discussed in Chapter 4		
DISORDER OR CONDITION	**GENETIC OR ENVIRONMENTAL**	**COMMENTS**
Type I diabetes	Genetic and environmental	Lack of insulin production leads to type I diabetes. Consequences of untreated type I diabetes include polydipsia (increased thirst), polyuria (increased urination) and ketoacidosis (elevated levels of ketone bodies in the blood).
Salicylate overdose	Environmental	Complex effects on respiratory center and basic metabolism, causing alterations in acid/base management, among other effects. Leads to impaired renal function.
Hyperventilation	Environmental	Complex effects on respiratory center and acid/base management. Leads to a respiratory alkalosis.

REVIEW QUESTIONS—CHAPTER 4

1. A patient attempted suicide by ingesting 50 aspirin tablets. This led to a fairly severe metabolic acidosis. A decrease of blood pH from 7.5 to 6.5 would be accompanied by which one of the following changes in ion concentration?
   A. A 10-fold increase in hydrogen ion concentration
   B. A 10-fold increase in hydroxyl ion concentration
   C. An increase in hydrogen ion concentration by a factor of 7.5/6.5
   D. A decrease in hydrogen ion concentration by a factor of 6.5/7.5
   E. A shift in concentration of buffer anions, with no change in hydrogen ion concentration

2. A medical student is attempting to understand the buffering system of the human body and has set up the following experiment in the lab to help with his understanding. Consider a biochemical reaction that is taking place in a 0.1 M buffer. The initial pH is 7.4, and the pK_a of the buffer is 7.2. If, in a final reaction volume of 1.0 mL, 10 μmol of protons are generated, what would be the final pH of the solution?
   A. 7.59
   B. 7.25
   C. 7.22
   D. 7.20
   E. 7.15

3. A patient with an enteropathy (intestinal disease) produced large amounts of ammonia (NH_3) from bacterial overgrowth in the intestine. The NH_3 was absorbed through the intestine into the portal vein and entered the circulation. Which of the following is a likely consequence of his NH_3 absorption?
   A. A decrease of blood pH
   B. Conversion of NH_3 to ammonium ion in the blood
   C. A decreased concentration of bicarbonate in the blood
   D. Kussmaul respiration
   E. Increased expiration of CO_2

4. Which of the following physiologic/pathologic conditions is most likely to result in an alkalosis, provided the body could not fully compensate?
   A. Production of lactic acid by muscles during exercise
   B. Production of ketone bodies by a patient with diabetes mellitus
   C. Repeated vomiting of stomach contents, including HCl
   D. Diarrhea with loss of the bicarbonate anions secreted into the intestine
   E. An infection resulting in a fever and hypercatabolism

5. Laboratory tests on the urine of a patient identified the presence of methylmalonate ($^-OOC–CH(CH_3)–COO^-$). Methylmalonate is best described as which one of the following?
   A. A strong acid
   B. The conjugate base of a weak acid
   C. It is 100% dissociated at its pK_a.
   D. It is 50% dissociated at the pH of the blood.
   E. It is a major intracellular buffer.

6. A patient with influenza has a fever of 101.8°F orally. The excess heat is dissipated throughout the body via a substance that can be best described by which one of the following?
   A. It is a dipolar molecule.
   B. It is composed mostly of amino acids.
   C. It is a weak acid.
   D. It is a weak base.
   E. It is composed mostly of carbohydrates.

7. A patient with hypertension is being treated with hydrochlorothiazide, a diuretic medication that can cause some dehydration and major intracellular electrolyte imbalances. Which one of the following electrolytes might be in imbalance under these conditions?
   A. Na^+
   B. K^+
   C. Cl^-
   D. HCO_3^-
   E. H_2O

8. A patient with panic attacks and hyperventilation is in a respiratory alkalosis. The excess hydroxide ions were able to overcome which one of the following buffers, which has the greatest buffering capacity in and near to normal blood pH?
   A. Carbonic acid
   B. Dihydrogen phosphate
   C. Ammonium ion
   D. Acetoacetic acid
   E. Ascetic acid

9. A patient is in early DKA. Which one of the following would this patient be expected to exhibit upon examination?
   A. Excess fluid in the tissues of the lower extremity
   B. Increased respiratory rate
   C. Low blood glucose
   D. Decreased respiratory rate
   E. Decreased urine output as an attempt to preserve water

10. A patient with severe anemia (reduced number of red blood cells in circulation) has a decreased capacity to use the bicarbonate buffer system to help maintain blood pH in the normal range. Which one of the following statements best describes the reason for this decreased capacity?
    A. The total amount of carbonic anhydrase in blood plasma is decreased in anemia.
    B. The total amount of carbonic anhydrase in blood plasma is increased in anemia.
    C. The total amount of carbonic anhydrase in red blood cells is decreased in anemia.
    D. The total amount of carbonic anhydrase in red blood cells is increased in anemia.
    E. The total amount of carbonic anhydrase in interstitial fluid is decreased.
    F. The total amount of carbonic anhydrase in interstitial fluid is increased.

ANSWERS

1. **The answer is A.** The pH is the negative log of the hydrogen ion concentration, $[H^+]$. Thus, at a pH of 7.5, $[H^+]$ is $10^{-7.5}$, and at pH 6.5, it is $10^{-6.5}$. The $[H^+]$ has changed by a factor of $10^{-6.5}/10^{-7.5}$, which is 10^1, or 10. Any decrease of 1 pH unit is a 10-fold increase of $[H^+]$, or a 10-fold decrease of $[OH^-]$. A shift in the concentration of buffer anions has definitely occurred, but the change in pH reflects the increase in hydrogen ion concentration in excess of that absorbed by buffers. A drop of 1 pH unit in a metabolic acidosis is a very severe condition.

2. **The answer is C.** In order to solve this problem, one first needs to calculate the concentration of the conjugate base and acid of the buffer at pH 7.4. Using the Henderson-Hasselbalch equation, one can calculate that the concentration of the conjugate base is 0.061 M and that of the acid is 0.039 M. At this point, the reaction occurs, generating 0.01 M protons (10 μmol/mL is a concentration of 10 mM, or 0.01 M). As the protons are generated, they will combine with the conjugate base, producing the acid. This will change the concentration of conjugate base to 0.051 M and the concentration of the acid to 0.049 M. Plugging those values into the Henderson-Hasselbalch equation leads to a pH value of 7.22. Recall that if the concentration of the conjugate base equaled the concentration of the acid, the pH would be the pK value (in this case, 7.2). Because protons are being generated, the pH will drop, not rise, so answer A cannot be correct.

3. **The answer is B.** NH_3 is a weak base that associates with a proton to produce the ammonium ion ($NH_3 + H^+ \rightarrow NH_4^+$), which has a p$K_a$ of 9.5. Thus, at pH 7.4, most of the NH_3 will be present as ammonium ion. The absorption of hydrogen ions will tend to increase, not decrease, the pH of the blood (thus, A is incorrect). With the decrease of hydrogen ions, carbonic acid will dissociate to produce more bicarbonate ($H_2CO_3 \rightarrow HCO_3^- + H^+$), and more CO_2 will go toward carbonic acid (thus, C is incorrect). Kussmaul respiration, an increased expiration of CO_2, occurs under an acidosis, the opposite condition.

4. **The answer is C.** Vomiting expels the strong acid gastric acid (HCl). As cells in the stomach secrete more HCl, they draw on H^+ ions in interstitial fluid and blood, thereby tending to increase blood pH and cause an alkalosis. The other conditions tend to produce an acidosis (thus, A, B, D, and E are incorrect). Lactic acid is a weak acid secreted into the blood by muscles during exercise. A patient with increased ketone body production can exhibit a fall of pH because the ketone bodies acetoacetate and β-hydroxybutyrate are dissociated acids. As bicarbonate in the intestinal lumen is lost in the watery diarrhea, more bicarbonate is secreted by intestinal cells. As intestinal cells produce bicarbonate, more

H^+ is also generated ($H_2CO_3 \rightarrow HCO_3^- + H^+$). While the bicarbonate produced by these cells is released into the intestinal lumen, the protons accumulate in blood, resulting in an acidosis. Hypercatabolism (see E), an increased rate of catabolism, generates additional CO_2, which produces more acid ($CO_2 + H_2O \rightarrow H_2CO_3 \rightarrow HCO_3^- + H^+$).

5. **The answer is B.** Methylmalonic acid contains two carboxylic acid groups and is, therefore, a weak acid. According to the Henderson-Hasselbalch equation, the carboxylic acid groups are 50% dissociated at their pK_a (thus, C is incorrect). Carboxylic acid groups usually have a pK_a between 2 and 5, so this acid would be nearly fully dissociated at a blood pH of 7.4 and cannot buffer intracellularly at neutral pH (thus, D and E are incorrect). (Although you do not need to know anything about methylmalonate to answer this question, methylmalonate is an organic acid generated in patients with a problem in metabolism of methylmalonyl coenzyme A, such as a deficiency in vitamin B_{12}. Its acidity may contribute to the development of symptoms involving the nervous system. Its appearance in the urine can be classified as an organic aciduria.)

6. **The answer is A.** Water has high thermal conductivity and is the main transporter of molecules and heat in the body. It is a dipolar molecule (H_2O). It has a neutral pH with the same amount of H^+ and OH^- ions so it is neither a weak acid nor a weak base. Water is neither a protein nor a carbohydrate, although water can transport both proteins and carbohydrates.

7. **The answer is B.** Electrolyte is a general term applied to bicarbonate and inorganic anions and cations. Water is not an electrolyte. The major extracellular electrolytes are Na^+, Cl^-, and HCO_3^-. The major intracellular electrolytes are K^+ and inorganic phosphate.

8. **The answer is B.** A buffer has its greatest buffering capacity in the pH ranges near its pK_a. Normal blood pH is 7.4. The pK_a of dihydrogen phosphate ($H_2PO_4^-$) is 6.80. The pK_a of carbonic acid is 3.80. The pK_a of ammonium ion (NH_4^+) is 9.25, whereas that of acetoacetic acid (a ketone body) is 3.62. Acetic acid has a pK_a of 4.76. The pK_a of dihydrogen phosphate is thus the closest to normal blood pH (7.4) and of the buffers listed would exhibit the greatest buffering ability at that pH. This is because of the other acids and ammonium ion exhibiting a pK_a >1 pH unit from normal blood and thereby containing relatively little undissociated acid or conjugate base, at that pH, to be an effective buffer.

9. **The answer is B.** Because of the high concentration of ketone bodies (acid) in the blood, the patient would have a lower blood pH and a metabolic acidosis. To help compensate for this acidosis, the respiratory rate would increase to "blow off CO_2." The decrease of blood CO_2 would increase the formation of carbonic

acid from bicarbonate and a proton, thereby reducing the proton concentration and raising the blood pH. Decreasing respiration would do the opposite and actually increase the proton concentration to further decrease pH and worsen the acidosis. A patient with DKA has abnormally high blood glucose and ketone body levels, which greatly increase blood osmolality; this leads to water leaving the tissues and entering the blood to help balance the increased osmolality, which results in intracellular dehydration. The kidney normally would decrease urine output in dehydration, but the high osmolality of the glomerular filtrate increases the water content of the filtrate in order to dilute these ions. This movement of water increases urine output, leading to the patient becoming even more dehydrated.

10. **The answer is C.** Carbonic anhydrase is not normally found in blood plasma or interstitial fluid, but the red blood cells contain high amounts of this enzyme, which helps to rapidly convert CO_2 to carbonic acid within the red blood cells. In a person with severe anemia, the number of red blood cells is greatly decreased so that the total amount of carbonic anhydrase available would be decreased and the bicarbonate buffer system, as well as the hemoglobin buffer system, would be less effective than in someone who was not anemic.

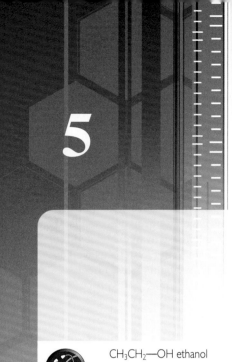

5

Structures of the Major Compounds of the Body

CH₃CH₂—OH ethanol
CH₃—OH methanol
The names of chemical groups are often incorporated into the common name of a compound and denote important differences in chemical structure. For example, in the name "ethanol," the "eth" denotes the ethyl group (CH₃CH₂—), the "ol" denotes the alcohol group (OH), and the "an" denotes the single bonds between the carbon atoms. Methanol contains a methyl group (CH₃) instead of the ethyl group. Methanol (also called *wood alcohol*) is much more toxic to humans than ethanol, the alcohol in alcoholic beverages. Ingestion of methanol results in visual disturbances, bradycardia (slow heart beat), coma, and seizures.

The body contains compounds of great structural diversity, ranging from relatively simple sugars and amino acids to enormously complex polymers such as proteins and nucleic acids. Many of these compounds have common structural features related to their names, their solubility in water, the pathways in which they participate, or their physiologic function. Thus, learning the terminology used to describe individual compounds and classes of compounds can greatly facilitate learning biochemistry.

In this chapter, we describe the major classes of carbohydrates and lipids and some of the classes of nitrogen-containing compounds. The structures of amino acids, proteins, the nucleic acids, and vitamins are covered in more detail in subsequent chapters.

Functional Groups on Molecules. Organic molecules are composed principally of carbon and hydrogen. However, their unique characteristics are related to structures termed **functional groups**, which involve **oxygen, nitrogen, phosphorus,** or **sulfur**.

Carbohydrates. Carbohydrates, commonly known as sugars, can be classified by their carbonyl group (**aldo-** or **ketosugars**), the number of carbons they contain (e.g., pentoses, hexoses), or the positions of the hydroxyl groups on their asymmetric carbon atoms (**D-** *or* **L-sugars, stereoisomers,** or **epimers**). They also can be categorized according to their substituents (e.g., **amino sugars**) or the number of monosaccharides (such as glucose) joined through **glycosidic bonds** (**disaccharides, oligosaccharides,** and **polysaccharides**). **Glycoproteins** and **proteoglycans** have sugars attached to their protein components.

Lipids. Lipids are a group of structurally diverse compounds defined by their **hydrophobicity**; they are not very soluble in water. The major lipids of the human body are the **fatty acids**, which are esterified to **glycerol** to form **triacylglycerols** (triglycerides) or **phosphoacylglycerols** (phosphoglycerides). In the **sphingolipids**, a fatty acid is attached to sphingosine, which is derived from the amino acid serine and another fatty acid. **Glycolipids** contain lipids attached to a sugar hydroxyl group. Specific **polyunsaturated fatty acids** are precursors of **eicosanoids**. The lipid **cholesterol** is a component of membranes and the precursor of other compounds that contain the steroid nucleus, such as the **bile salts** and **steroid hormones**. Cholesterol is one of the compounds synthesized from a five-carbon precursor called the **isoprene** unit.

Nitrogen-Containing Compounds. Nitrogen in **amino groups** or **heterocyclic ring** structures often carries a positive charge at neutral pH. **Amino acids** contain a carboxyl group, an amino group, and one or more additional carbons. **Purines, pyrimidines,** and **pyridines** have heterocyclic nitrogen-containing ring structures. **Nucleosides** comprise one of these ring structures attached to a sugar. The addition of a phosphate to a nucleoside produces a **nucleotide**.

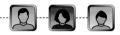

THE WAITING ROOM

 Dianne A. recovered from her bout of diabetic ketoacidosis (DKA) and was discharged from the hospital (see Chapter 4). She has returned for a follow-up visit as an outpatient. She reports that she has been compliant with her recommended diet and that she faithfully gives herself insulin by subcutaneous injection several times daily. She self-monitors her blood glucose levels at least four times a day and reports the results to her physician.

Lotta T. is a 54-year-old woman who came to her physician's office complaining of a severe throbbing pain in the right great toe that began 8 hours earlier. The toe has suffered no trauma but appears red and swollen. It is warmer than the surrounding tissue and is exquisitely tender to even light pressure. Ms. T. is unable to voluntarily flex or extend the joints of the digit, and passive motion of the joints causes great pain.

I. Functional Groups on Biologic Compounds

A. Biologic Compounds

The organic molecules of the body consist principally of carbon, hydrogen, oxygen, nitrogen, sulfur, and phosphorus joined by covalent bonds. The key element is carbon, which forms four covalent bonds with other atoms. Carbon atoms are joined through double or single bonds to form the carbon backbone for structures of varying size and complexity (Fig. 5.1). Groups containing one, two, three, four, and five carbons plus hydrogen are referred to as *methyl*, *ethyl*, *propionyl*, *butyl*, and *pentanyl* groups, respectively. If the carbon chain is branched, the prefix "iso-" is used. If the compound contains a double bond, "ene" is sometimes incorporated into the name. Carbon structures that are straight or branched with single or double bonds, but do not contain a ring, are called *aliphatic*.

Carbon-containing rings are found in several biologic compounds. One of the most common is the six-membered carbon-containing benzene ring, sometimes called a *phenyl group* (see Fig. 5.1B). This ring has three double bonds, but the electrons are shared equally by all six carbons and delocalized in planes above and below the ring. Compounds containing the benzene ring, or a similar ring structure with benzene-like properties, are called *aromatic*.

B. Functional Groups

Biochemical molecules are defined both by their carbon skeleton and by structures called *functional groups* that usually involve bonds between carbon and oxygen, carbon and nitrogen, carbon and sulfur, or carbon and phosphate groups (Fig. 5.2). In carbon–carbon and carbon–hydrogen bonds, the electrons are shared equally between atoms, and the bonds are nonpolar and relatively unreactive. In carbon–oxygen and carbon–nitrogen bonds, the electrons are shared unequally, and the bonds are polar and more reactive. Thus, the properties of the functional groups usually determine the types of reactions that occur and the physiologic role of the molecule.

Functional group names are often incorporated into the common name of a compound. For example, a ke**tone** might have a name that ends in "-one," such as ace**tone**, and the name of a compound that contains a hydroxyl (alcoh**ol** or OH group) might end in "-ol" (e.g., ethan**ol**). The acyl group is the portion of the molecule that provides the carbonyl (—C═O) group in an ester or amide linkage. It is denoted in a name by an "-yl" ending. For example, the fat stores of the body are tri**acyl**glycerols. Three acyl (fatty acid) groups are esterified to glyc**erol**, a compound that contains three alcohol groups. In the remainder of this chapter, the portions of names of compounds that refer to a class of compounds or a structural feature are shown in **bold** type.

Dianne A. had a metabolic acidosis resulting from increased hepatic production of ketone bodies. Her initial workup included screening tests for ketone bodies in her urine that employed a paper strip containing nitroprusside, a compound that reacts with keto groups. Her blood glucose was measured with an enzymatic assay that is specific for the sugar D-glucose and will not react with other sugars.

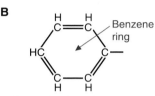

FIGURE 5.1 Examples of aliphatic and aromatic compounds. **A.** An **isoprene** group, which is an aliphatic group. The "iso-" prefix denotes branching, and the "-ene" denotes a double bond. **B.** A benzene ring (or phenyl group), which is an aromatic group.

The ketone bodies synthesized in the liver are β-hydroxybutyrate and acetoacetate. A third ketone body, acetone, is formed by the nonenzymatic decarboxylation of acetoacetate (see Figure 3.3). Acetone is volatile and accounts for the sweet mousy odor in the breath of patients such as **Dianne A.** when they have a ketoacidosis. What functional groups are present in each of these ketone bodies?

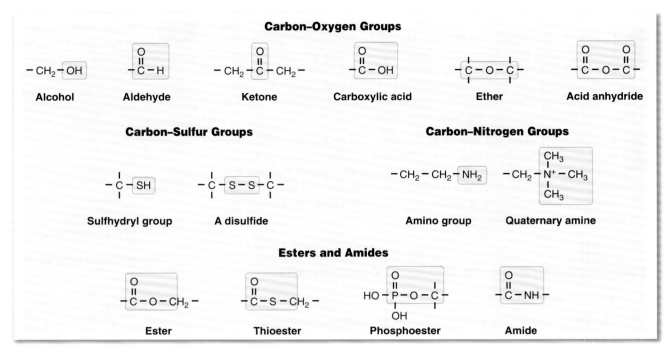

FIGURE 5.2 Major types of functional groups found in biochemical compounds of the human body.

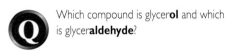

β-Hydroxybutyr**ate** and acetoacet**ate** are carboxyl**ates** (dissociated carboxylic acids). Acet**o**acetate and acet**one** contain ket**o**/ket**one** groups. Because β-**hydroxy**butyrate contains an alcohol (**hydroxyl**) group and not a keto group, the general name of ketone bodies for these compounds is really a misnomer.

Which compound is glycer**ol** and which is glycer**aldehyde**?

$$
\begin{array}{cc}
\text{CH}_2\text{OH} & \overset{\text{O}}{\underset{\displaystyle}{\text{H}-\text{C}}} \\
\text{H}-\text{C}-\text{OH} & \text{H}-\text{C}-\text{OH} \\
\text{CH}_2\text{OH} & \text{CH}_2\text{OH} \\
\textbf{A} & \textbf{B}
\end{array}
$$

Judging from the structures of the ketone bodies shown in Figure 3.3, which compound is more oxidized, β-hydroxybutyrate or acetoacetate? Which is more reduced?

I. Oxidized and Reduced Groups

The carbon–carbon and carbon–oxygen groups are described as "oxidized" or "reduced" according to the number of electrons around the carbon atom. *Oxidation* is the loss of electrons and results in the loss of hydrogen atoms together with one or two electrons, or the gain of an oxygen atom or hydroxyl group. *Reduction* is the gain of electrons and results in the gain of hydrogen atoms or loss of an oxygen atom. Thus, the carbon becomes progressively more oxidized (and less reduced) as we go from an alcohol to an aldehyde or a ketone to a carboxyl group (see Fig. 5.2). Carbon–carbon double bonds are more oxidized (and less reduced) than carbon–carbon single bonds.

2. Groups that Carry a Charge

Acidic groups contain a proton that can dissociate, usually leaving the remainder of the molecule as an anion with a negative charge (see Chapter 4). In biomolecules, the major anionic substituents are carboxyl**ate** groups, phosph**ate** groups, or sulf**ate** groups (the "-ate" suffix denotes a negative charge) (Fig. 5.3). Phosphate groups attached to metabolites are often abbreviated as P with a circle around it, or just as "P," as in glucose 6-**P**.

Compounds that contain nitrogen are usually basic and can acquire a positive charge (Fig. 5.4). Nitrogen has five electrons in its valence shell. If only three of these electrons form covalent bonds with other atoms, the nitrogen has no charge. If the remaining two electrons form a bond with a hydrogen ion or a carbon atom, the nitrogen carries a positive charge. Amines consist of nitrogen attached through single bonds to hydrogen atoms and to one or more carbon atoms. Primary amines, such as dop**amine**, have one carbon–nitrogen bond. These amines are weak acids with a pK_a value of approximately 9, so that at pH 7.4 they carry a positive charge. Secondary, tertiary, and quaternary amines have two, three, and four nitrogen–carbon bonds, respectively (see Fig. 5.4).

C. Polarity of Bonds and Partial Charges

Polar bonds are covalent bonds in which the electron cloud is more dense around one atom (the atom with the greater electronegativity) than the other. Oxygen is more electronegative than carbon, and a carbon–oxygen bond is therefore polar, with the oxygen atom carrying a partial negative charge and the carbon atom carrying a partial positive charge (Fig. 5.5). In nonpolar carbon–carbon bonds and carbon–hydrogen bonds, the two electrons in the covalent bond are shared almost equally. Nitrogen, when it has only three covalent bonds, also carries a partial negative charge relative to carbon, and the carbon–nitrogen bond is polarized. Sulfur can carry a slight partial negative charge.

1. Solubility

Water is a dipolar molecule in which the oxygen atom carries a partial negative charge and the hydrogen atoms carry partial positive charges (see Chapter 4). For molecules to be soluble in water, they must contain charged or polar groups that can associate with the partial positive and negative charges of water. Thus, the solubility of organic molecules in water is determined by both the proportion of polar to nonpolar groups attached to the carbon–hydrogen skeleton and to their relative positions in the molecule. Polar groups or molecules are called *hydrophilic* (water-loving), and nonpolar groups or molecules are *hydrophobic* (water-fearing). Sugars such as glucose 6-phosphate, for example, contain so many polar groups (many hydroxyl and one phosphate) that they are very hydrophilic and almost infinitely water-soluble (Fig. 5.6). The water molecules interacting with a polar or ionic compound form a hydration shell around the compound, which includes hydrogen bonds and/or ionic interactions between water and the compound.

Compounds that have large nonpolar regions are relatively water-insoluble. They tend to cluster together in an aqueous environment and form weak associations through van der Waals interactions and hydrophobic interactions. Hydrophobic compounds are essentially pushed together (the hydrophobic effect) as the water molecules maximize the number of energetically favorable hydrogen bonds they can form with each other in the water lattice. Thus, lipids form droplets or separate layers in an aqueous environment (e.g., vegetable oils in a salad dressing).

2. Reactivity

Another consequence of bond polarity is that atoms that carry a partial (or full) negative charge are attracted to atoms that carry a partial (or full) positive charge and vice versa. These partial or full charges dictate the course of biochemical reactions, which follow the same principles of electrophilic and nucleophilic attack that are characteristic of organic reactions in general. The partial positive charge on the carboxyl carbon attracts more negatively charged groups and accounts for many of the reactions of carboxylic acids. An ester is formed when a carboxylic acid and an alcohol combine, releasing water (Fig. 5.7). Similarly, a thioester is formed when an acid combines with a sulfhydryl group, and an amide is formed when an acid combines with an amine. Similar reactions result in the formation of a phosphoester from phosphoric acid and an alcohol and in the formation of an anhydride from two acids.

D. Nomenclature

Biochemists use two systems for the identification of the carbons in a chain. In the first system, the carbons in a compound are numbered, starting with the carbon in the most oxidized group (e.g., the carboxyl group). In the second system, the carbons are given Greek letters, starting with the carbon next to the most oxidized group. Hence, the compound shown in Figure 5.8 is known as *3-hydroxybutyrate* or β-*hydroxybutyrate*.

Compound A contains three **alcohol** groups and is called *glycerol*. Compound B contains an **aldehyde group** and is called *glyceraldehyde*.

Acetoacetate is more oxidized than β-hydroxybutyrate. The carbon in the keto group contains one less hydrogen than the carbon to which the –OH group is attached. It has lost an electron.

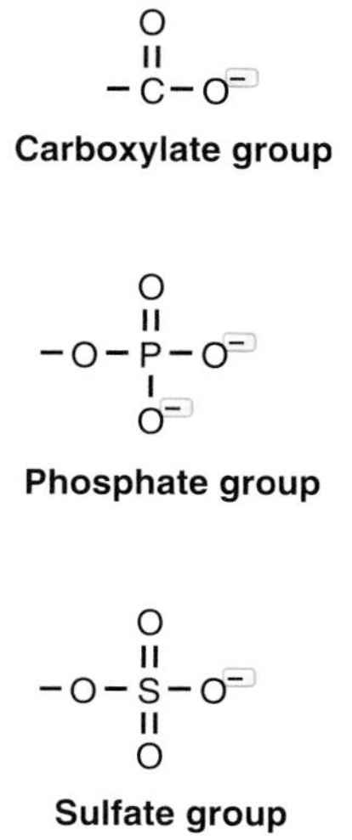

Carboxylate group

Phosphate group

Sulfate group

FIGURE 5.3 Examples of anions formed by dissociation of acidic groups. At physiologic pH, carboxylic acids, phosphoric acid, and sulfuric acid are dissociated into hydrogen ions and negatively charged anions.

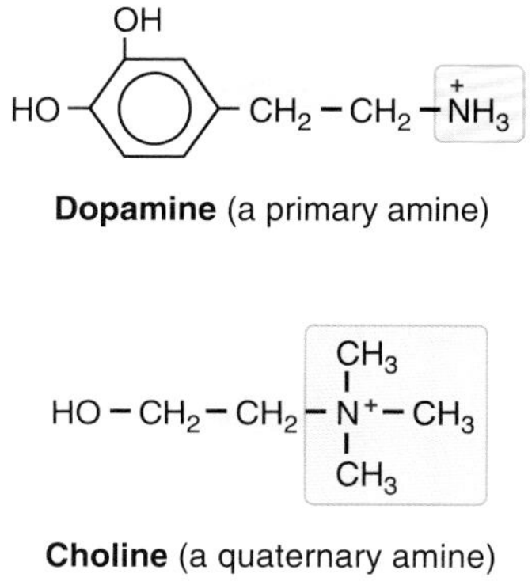

Dopamine (a primary amine)

Choline (a quaternary amine)

FIGURE 5.4 Examples of amines. At physiologic pH, many amines carry positive charges.

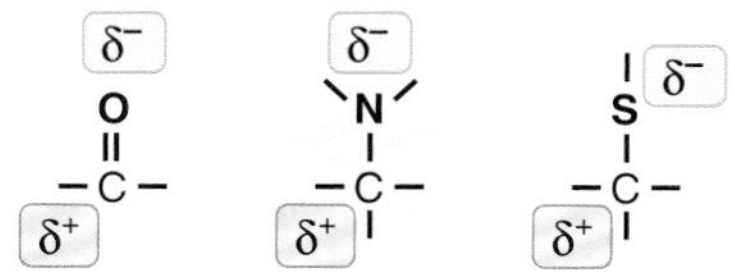

FIGURE 5.5 Partial charges on carbon–oxygen, carbon–nitrogen, and carbon–sulfur bonds.

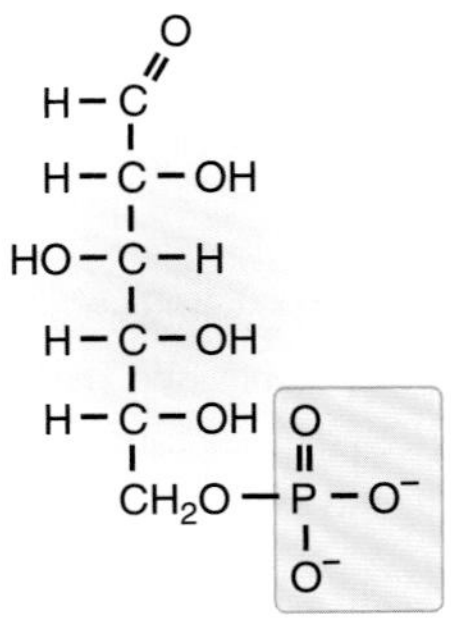

FIGURE 5.6   Glucose 6-phosphate, a very polar and water-soluble molecule.

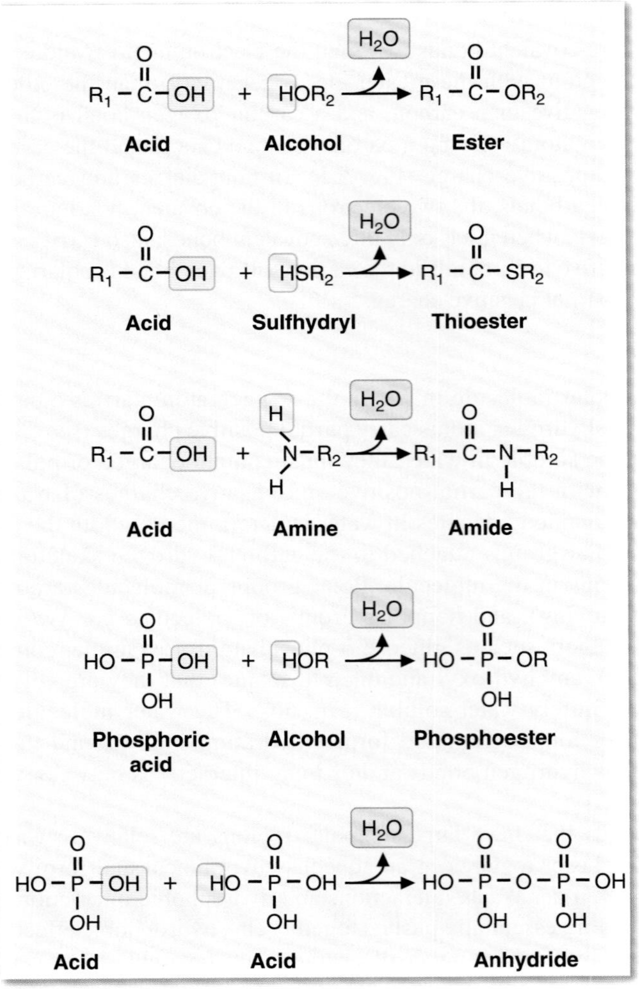

FIGURE 5.7   Formation of esters, thioesters, amides, phosphoesters, and anhydrides.

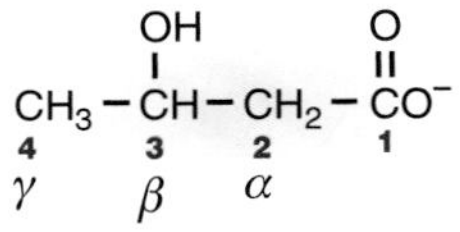

FIGURE 5.8   Two systems for identifying the carbon atoms in a compound. This compound is called 3-hydroxybutyrate or β-hydroxybutyrate.

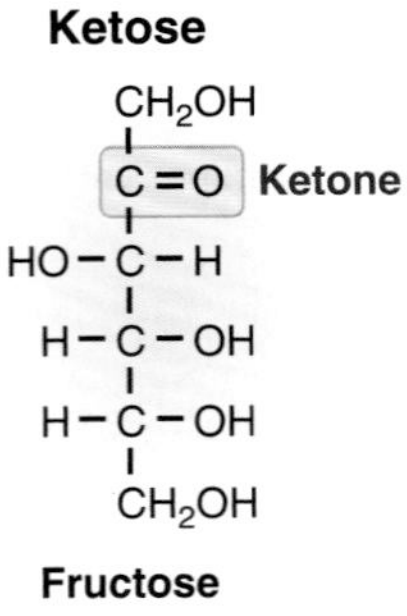

FIGURE 5.9   Fructose is a ketohexose.

II. Carbohydrates

A. Monosaccharides

Simple monosaccharides consist of a linear chain of three or more carbon atoms, one of which forms a carbonyl group through a double bond with oxygen (Fig. 5.9). The other carbons of an unmodified monosaccharide contain hydroxyl groups, resulting in the general formula for an unmodified sugar of $C_nH_{2n}O_n$. The suffix "-ose" is used in the names of sugars. If the carbonyl group is an aldehyde, the sugar is an aldose; if the carbonyl group is a ketone, the sugar is a ketose. Monosaccharides are also classified according to their number of carbons: Sugars containing three, four, five, six, and seven carbons are called *trioses*, *tetroses*, *pentoses*, *hexoses*, and *heptoses*, respectively. Fructose is therefore a ketohexose (see Fig. 5.9), and glucose is an aldohexose (see Fig. 5.6).

1. D- and L-Sugars

A carbon atom that contains four different chemical groups forms an asymmetric (or chiral) center (Fig. 5.10A). The groups attached to the asymmetric carbon atom can be arranged to form two different isomers that are mirror images of each other and not superimposable. Monosaccharide stereoisomers are designated D or L based on whether the position of the hydroxyl group farthest from the carbonyl carbon matches D- or L-glyceraldehyde (see Fig. 5.10B). Such mirror image compounds are known as *enantiomers*. Although a more sophisticated system of nomenclature using the designations (R) and (S) is generally used to describe the positions of groups on complex molecules such as drugs, the D and L designations are still used in medicine for describing sugars and amino acids. Because glucose (the major sugar in human blood) and most other sugars in human tissues belong to the D series, sugars are assumed to be D unless L is specifically added to the name.

2. Stereoisomers and Epimers

Stereoisomers have the same chemical formula but differ in the position of the hydroxyl group on one or more of their asymmetric carbons (Fig. 5.11). A sugar with n asymmetric centers has 2^n stereoisomers unless it has a plane of symmetry. Epimers are stereoisomers that differ in the position of the hydroxyl group at only one of their asymmetric carbons. D-Glucose and D-galactose are epimers of each other, differing only at position 4, and can be interconverted in human cells by enzymes called *epimerases*. D-Mannose and D-glucose are also epimers of each other, differing only at position 2.

3. Ring Structures

Monosaccharides exist in solution mainly as ring structures in which the carbonyl (aldehyde or ketone) group has reacted with a hydroxyl group in the same molecule to form a five- or six-membered ring (Fig. 5.12). The oxygen that was on the hydroxyl group is now part of the ring, and the original carbonyl carbon, which now contains an —OH group, has become the anomeric carbon atom. A hydroxyl group on the anomeric carbon drawn down below the ring is in the α-position; drawn up above the ring, it is in the β position. In the actual three-dimensional structure, the ring is not planar but usually takes a "chair" conformation in which the hydroxyl groups are located at a maximal distance from each other.

In solution, the hydroxyl group on the anomeric carbon spontaneously (nonenzymatically) changes from the α to the β position through a process called *mutarotation*. When the ring opens, the straight-chain aldehyde or ketone is formed. When the ring closes, the hydroxyl group may be in either the α or the β position (Fig. 5.13). This process occurs more rapidly in the presence of cellular enzymes called *mutarotases*. However, if the anomeric carbon forms a bond with another molecule, that bond is fixed in the α or β position and the sugar cannot mutarotate. Enzymes are specific for α or β-bonds between sugars and other molecules and react with only one type.

4. Substituted Sugars

Sugars frequently contain phosphate groups, amino groups, sulfate groups, or *N*-acetyl groups. Most of the free monosaccharides within cells are phosphorylated

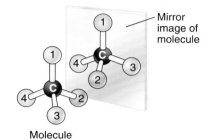

FIGURE 5.10 A. D- and L-Glyceraldehyde. The carbon in the center contains four different substituent groups arranged around it in a tetrahedron. A different arrangement creates an isomer that is a nonsuperimposable mirror image. If you rotate the mirror image structure so that groups 1 and 2 align, group 3 will be in the position of group 4, and group 4 will be in position 3. **B.** D-Glyceraldehyde and D-glucose. These sugars have the same configuration at the asymmetric carbon atom farthest from the carbonyl group. Both belong to the D series. Asymmetric carbons are shown in *red*.

FIGURE 5.11   Examples of stereoisomers. These compounds have the same chemical formula ($C_6H_{12}O_6$) but differ in the positions of the hydroxyl groups on their asymmetric carbons (in *red*).

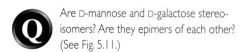

Are D-mannose and D-galactose stereoisomers? Are they epimers of each other? (See Fig. 5.11.)

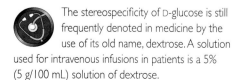

The stereospecificity of D-glucose is still frequently denoted in medicine by the use of its old name, dextrose. A solution used for intravenous infusions in patients is a 5% (5 g/100 mL) solution of dextrose.

A They are stereoisomers but not epimers of each other. They have the same chemical formula but differ in the position of two hydroxyl groups.

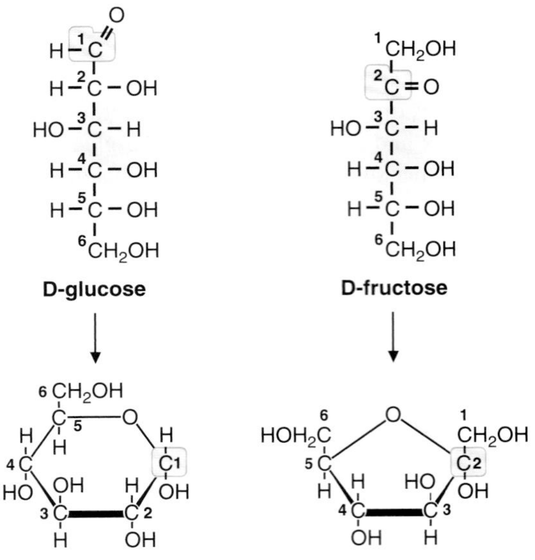

D-glucose

D-fructose

α-D-glucopyranose

α-D-fructofuranose

FIGURE 5.12 Pyranose and furanose rings formed from glucose and fructose. The anomeric carbons are *highlighted* (carbon 1 of glucose and carbon 2 of fructose).

at their terminal carbons, which prevents their transport out of the cell (see glucose 6-phosphate in Fig. 5.6). Amino sugars such as galactos**amine** and glucos**amine** contain an amino group instead of a hydroxyl group on one of the carbon atoms, usually carbon 2 (Fig. 5.14). Frequently, this amino group has been acetylated to form an *N*-acetylated sugar. In complex molecules termed *proteoglycans*, many of the *N*-acetylated sugars also contain negatively charged sulfate groups attached to a hydroxyl group on the sugar.

5. Oxidized and Reduced Sugars

Sugars can be oxidized at the aldehyde carbon to form an acid. Technically, the compound is no longer a sugar, and the ending on its name is changed from "-ose" to "-onic acid" or "-onate" (e.g., gluc**onic** acid, Fig. 5.15). If the carbon containing the terminal hydroxyl group is oxidized, the sugar is called a *uronic acid* (e.g., gluc**uronic** acid).

If the aldehyde of a sugar is reduced, all of the carbon atoms contain alcohol (hydroxyl) groups, and the sugar is a poly**ol** (e.g., sorbit**ol**) (see Fig. 5.15). If one of the hydroxyl groups of a sugar is reduced so that the carbon contains only hydrogen, the sugar is a deoxysugar, such as the **deoxy**ribose in DNA.

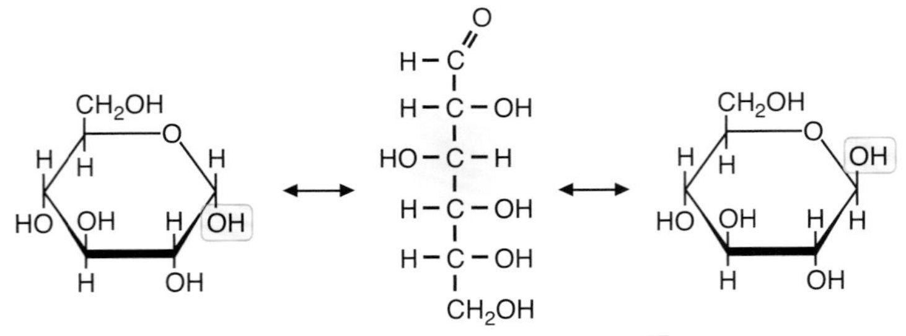

α-D-glucopyranose
(36%)

D-glucose
(<0.1%)

β-D-glucopyranose
(63%)

FIGURE 5.13 Mutarotation of glucose in solution, with percentages of each form at equilibrium.

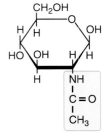

N-acetyl-β-D-glucosamine

FIGURE 5.14 An *N*-acetylated amino sugar. The "*N-*" denotes the amino group to which the acetyl group is attached, shown in the *shaded box*.

Proteoglycans contain many long unbranched polysaccharide chains attached to a core protein. The polysaccharide chains, called *glycosaminoglycans*, are composed of repeating disaccharide units containing oxidized acid sugars (such as glucuronic acid), sulfated sugars, and *N*-acetylated amino sugars. The large number of negative charges causes the glycosaminoglycan chains to radiate out from the protein so that the overall structure resembles a bottle brush. The proteoglycans are essential parts of the extracellular matrix, the aqueous humor of the eye, secretions of mucus-producing cells, and cartilage and are described in further detail in Chapter 47.

B. Glycosides

1. N- and O-Glycosidic Bonds

The hydroxyl group on the anomeric carbon of a monosaccharide can react with an —OH or an —NH group of another compound to form a glyc**osidic** bond. The linkage may be either α or β, depending on the position of the atom attached to the anomeric carbon of the sugar. *N*-Glycosidic bonds are found in nucle**osides** and nucle**otides**. For example, in the adenosine moiety of adenosine triphosphate (ATP), the nitrogenous base adenine is linked to the sugar ribose through a β-*N*-glycosidic bond (Fig. 5.16). In contrast, *O*-glycosidic bonds, such as those found in lactose, join sugars to each other or attach sugars to the hydroxyl group of an amino acid on a protein.

2. Disaccharides, Oligosaccharides, and Polysaccharides

A disaccharide contains two monosaccharides joined by an *O*-glycosidic bond. Lactose, which is the sugar in milk, consists of galactose and glucose linked through a β(1→4) bond formed between the β–OH group of the anomeric carbon of galactose and the hydroxyl group on carbon 4 of glucose (see Fig. 5.16). Oligosaccharides contain from 3 to roughly 12 monosaccharides linked together. They are often found attached through *N*- or *O*-glycosidic bonds to proteins to form **glyco**proteins (see Chapter 6). Polysaccharides contain tens to thousands of monosaccharides joined by glycosidic bonds to form linear chains or branched structures. Amylopectin (a form of starch) and glycogen (the storage form of glucose in human cells) are branched polymers of glucosyl residues linked through α(1→4) and α(1→6) bonds.

III. Lipids

A. Fatty Acids

Fatty acids are usually straight aliphatic chains with a methyl group at one end (called the ω-*carbon*) and a carboxyl group at the other end (Fig. 5.17A). Most fatty acids in the human have an even number of carbon atoms, usually between 16 and 20. Saturated fatty acids have single bonds between the carbons in the chain, and unsaturated fatty acids contain one or more double bonds. The most common saturated fatty acids present in the cell are palmitic acid (C16) and stearic acid (C18). Although these two fatty acids are generally called by their common names, shorter fatty acids are often called by the Latin word for the number of carbons, such as octanoic acid (8 carbons) and decanoic acid (10 carbons).

The melting point of a fatty acid increases with chain length and decreases with the degree of unsaturation. Thus, fatty acids with many double bonds, such as those in vegetable oils, are liquid at room temperature; and saturated fatty acids, such as those in butterfat, are solids. Lipids with lower melting points are more fluid at body temperature and contribute to the fluidity of our cellular membranes.

Monounsaturated fatty acids contain one double bond, and polyunsaturated fatty acids contain two or more double bonds (see Fig. 5.17). The position of a double bond is designated by the number of the carbon in the double bond that is closest to the carboxyl group. For example, oleic acid, which contains 18 carbons and a double bond between positions 9 and 10, is designated 18:1, Δ^9. The number 18 denotes the number of carbon atoms, 1 (one) denotes the number of

Oxidized Sugars

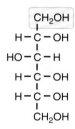

β-D-glucuronate

D-gluconate

Reduced Sugars

CH$_2$OH
|
H − C − OH
|
HO − C − H
|
H − C − OH
|
H − C − OH
|
CH$_2$OH

D-sorbitol

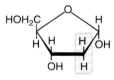

Deoxyribose

FIGURE 5.15 Oxidized and reduced sugars. The affected group is shown in the *shaded box*. Glucuronic acid is formed by oxidation of the glucose terminal —OH group. Gluconic acid (D-gluconate) is formed by oxidation of the glucose aldehyde carbon. Sorbitol, a sugar alcohol, is formed by reduction of the glucose aldehyde group. Deoxyribose is formed by reduction of ribose.

 Palmitoleic acid, oleic acid, and arachidonic acid are the most common unsaturated fatty acids in the cell. Palmitoleic acid is a 16:1, Δ^9 fatty acid. How would you name it as an ω fatty acid?

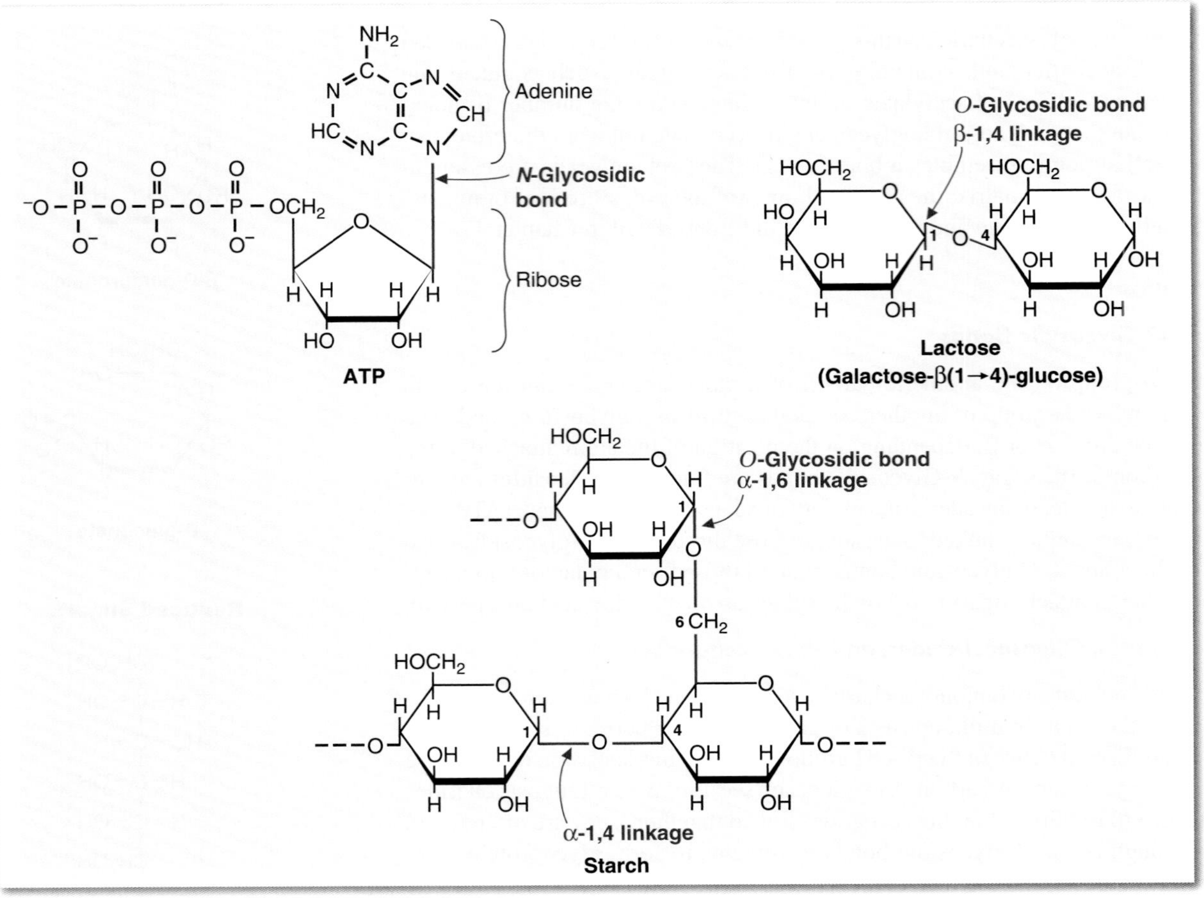

FIGURE 5.16 *N*- and *O*-Glycosidic bonds. Adenosine triphosphate (ATP) contains a β-*N*-glycosidic bond. Lactose contains an *O*-glycosidic β(1→4) bond. Starch contains α-1,4 and α-1,6 *O*-glycosidic bonds. The glycosidic bonds are shown in *red*.

Palmitoleic acid is an ω7 fatty acid. It has one double bond between the 9th and 10th carbons. It has 16 carbons, like palmitic acid, so the double bond is at the 7th carbon from the ω end.

Trans-fatty acids (partially hydrogenated fat) were used by restaurants as an oil that had a longer shelf life than polyunsaturated fatty acids. However, the presence of *trans* fats in food has been linked in some studies to an increased risk of heart disease. These findings, however, have been challenged by the food industry. The U.S. Food and Drug Administration now mandates the labeling of foods with *trans*-fatty acid content, and the use of *trans*-fatty acids in commercial food preparations has been banned in certain localities in the United States.

double bonds, and Δ^9 denotes the position of the double bond between the 9th and 10th carbon atoms. Oleic acid can also be designated 18:1(9), without the Δ. Fatty acids are also classified by the distance of the double bond closest to the ω end (the methyl group at the end farthest from the carboxyl group). Thus, oleic acid is an ω9 fatty acid, and linolenic acid is an ω3 fatty acid. Arachidonic acid, a polyunsaturated fatty acid with 20 carbons and 4 double bonds, is an ω6 fatty acid that is completely described as 20:4, $\Delta^{5,8,11,14}$. The eicosanoids are a group of hormone-like compounds produced by many cells in the body. They are derived from polyunsaturated fatty acids such as arachidonic acid that contain 20 carbons (eicosa) and have 3, 4, or 5 double bonds. The prostaglandins, thromboxanes, and leukotrienes belong to this group of compounds.

The double bonds in most naturally occurring fatty acids are in the *cis* configuration (Fig. 5.17B). The designation *cis* means that the hydrogens are on the same side of the double bond and the acyl chains are on the other side. In *trans*-fatty acids, the acyl chains are on opposite sides of the double bond. *Trans*-fatty acids are produced by the chemical hydrogenation of polyunsaturated fatty acids in vegetable oils and are not a natural food product.

B. Acylglycerols

An **acyl**glycerol comprises glycerol with one or more fatty acids (the **acyl** group) attached through ester linkages (Fig. 5.18). Monoacylglycerols, diacylglycerols, and triacylglycerols contain one, two, or three fatty acids esterified to glycerol,

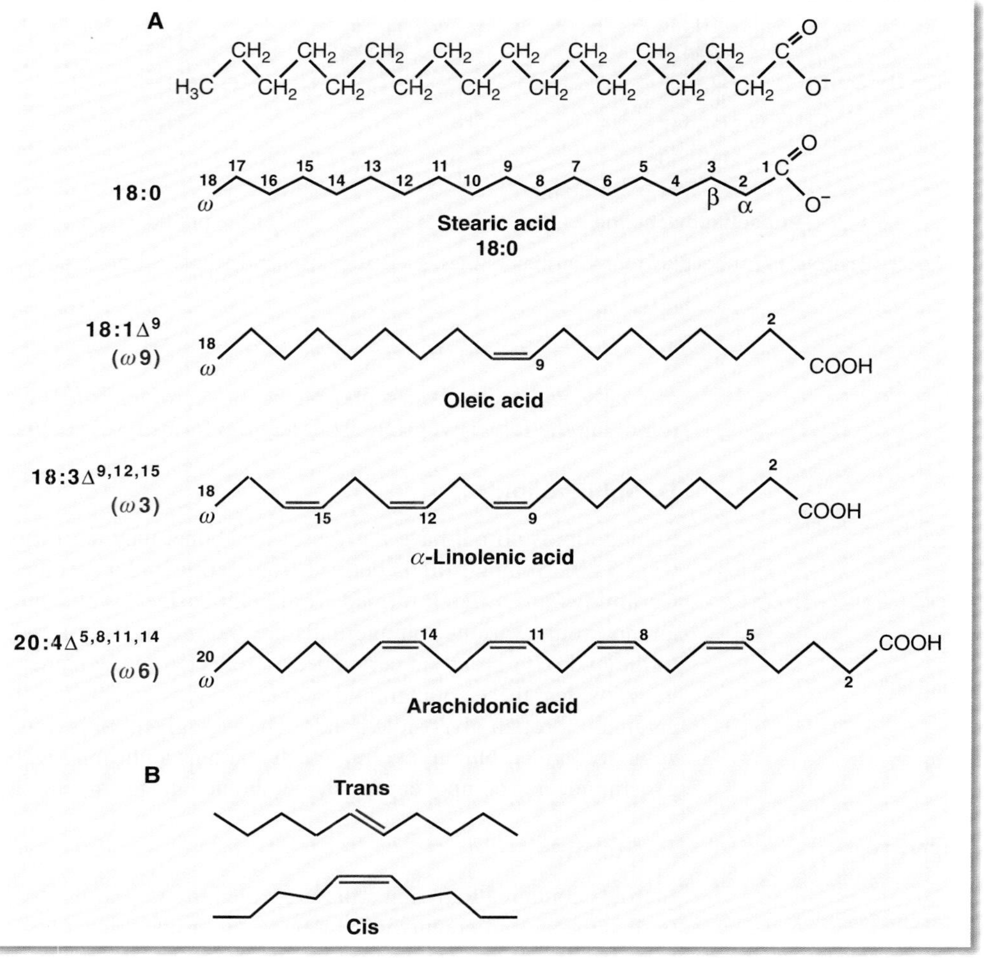

A

18:0

Stearic acid
18:0

18:1Δ^9
(ω9)

Oleic acid

18:3Δ^{9,12,15}
(ω3)

α-Linolenic acid

20:4Δ^{5,8,11,14}
(ω6)

Arachidonic acid

B

Trans

Cis

FIGURE 5.17 A. Saturated fatty acids and unsaturated fatty acids. In stearic acid (*top*), a saturated fatty acid, all the atoms are shown. A more common way of depicting the same structure is shown below the numbered structure. The carbons are either numbered starting with the carboxyl group or given Greek letters starting with the carbon next to the carboxyl group. The methyl (or ω) carbon at the end of the chain is always called the ω-carbon, regardless of the chain length. The symbol 18:0 refers to the number of carbon atoms (18) and the number of double bonds (0). In the unsaturated fatty acids shown, not all of the carbons are numbered, but note that the double bonds are *cis* and spaced at three-carbon intervals. Both ω3 and ω6 fatty acids are required in the diet. **B.** *Cis* and *trans* double bonds in fatty-acid side chains. Note that the *cis* double bond causes the chain to bend.

respectively. Tri**acyl**glycerols rarely contain the same fatty acid at all three positions and are therefore called *mixed triacylglycerols*. Unsaturated fatty acids, when present, are most often esterified to carbon 2. In the three-dimensional configuration of glycerol, carbons 1 and 3 are not identical, and enzymes are specific for one or the other carbon.

C. Phosphoacylglycerols

Phosphoacylglycerols contain fatty acids esterified to positions 1 and 2 of glycerol and a phosphate (alone or with a substituent) attached to carbon 3. If only a phosphate group is attached to carbon 3, the compound is **phospha**tidic acid (Fig. 5.19). Phosphatidic acid is a precursor for the synthesis of the other phosphoacylglycerols.

Phosphatidylchol**ine** is one of the major phosphoacylglycerols found in membranes (see Fig. 5.19). The am**ine** is positively charged at neutral pH, and the phosphate is negatively charged. Thus, the molecule is amphipathic: It contains large polar and nonpolar regions. Phosphatidylcholine is also called *lecithin*. Removal

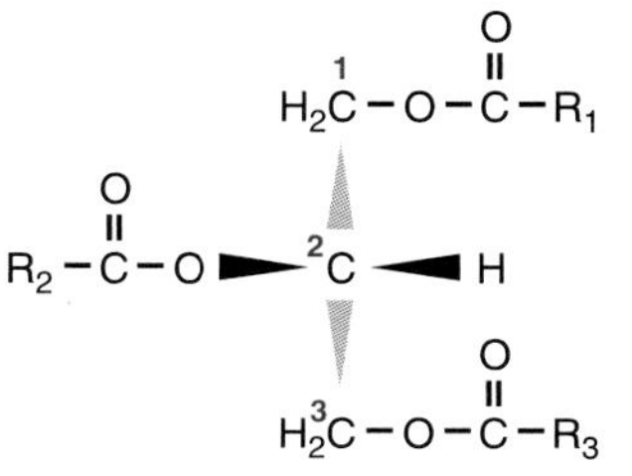

Triacyl-*sn*-glycerol

FIGURE 5.18 A triacylglycerol. Note that carbons 1 and 3 of the glycerol moiety are not identical. The broad end of each *arrowhead* is closer to the reader than the narrow, pointed end.

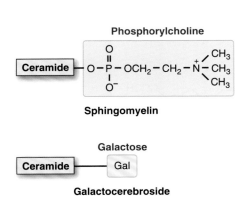

FIGURE 5.19   Phosphoacylglycerols. Phospholipids found in membranes, such as phosphatidylcholine, have a polar group attached to the phosphate.

of a fatty acyl group from a phosphoacylglycerol leads to a lysolipid; for example, removing the fatty acyl group from lecithin forms lysolecithin.

D. Sphingolipids

Sphingolipids do not have a glycerol backbone; they are formed from sphingosine (Fig. 5.20). Sphingos**ine** is derived from ser**ine** and a specific fatty acid, palmitate. Cer**amides** are **amides** formed from sphingosine by attaching a fatty acid to the amino group. Various sphingolipids are then formed by attaching different groups to the hydroxyl group on ceramide. As reflected in the names for cerebr**osides** and gangli**osides**, these sphingolipids contain sugars attached to the hydroxyl group of ceramide through glycosidic bonds. They are glycolipids (more specifically, glycosphingolipids). Sphingomyelin, which contains a phosphorylcholine group attached to ceramide, is a component of cell membranes and the myelin sheath around neurons.

E. Steroids

Steroids contain a four-ring structure called the *steroid nucleus* (Fig. 5.21). Cholesterol is the steroid precursor in human cells from which all of the steroid hormones are synthesized by modifications to the ring or C-20 side chain. Although cholesterol is not very water-soluble, it is converted to amphipathic water-soluble bile salts such as cholic acid. Bile salts line the surfaces of lipid droplets called *micelles* in the lumen of the intestine, where they keep the droplets emulsified in the aqueous environment.

Cholesterol is one of the compounds synthesized in the human from branched five-carbon units with one double bond called an *isoprenyl unit* (see Fig. 5.1A). Isoprenyl units are combined in long chains to form other structures such as the side chains of coenzyme Q in humans and vitamin A in plants. Isoprene units form polymers to generate geranyl groups (10 carbons) and farnesyl groups (15 carbons) (see Chapter 32). The geranyl and farnesyl groups, because of their highly hydrophobic nature, are often covalently attached to proteins to allow the proteins to associate with cellular membranes.

IV. Nitrogen-Containing Compounds

Nitrogen, as described in Section I.B.2, is an electronegative atom with two unshared electrons in its outer valence shell. At neutral pH, the nitrogen in amino groups is usually bonded to four other atoms and carries a positive charge. However, the presence of a nitrogen atom in an organic compound will increase its solubility in water, whether the nitrogen is charged or uncharged.

A. Amino Acids

Amino acids are compounds that contain an amino group and a carboxylic acid group. In proteins, the amino acids are always L-α-amino acids (the amino group

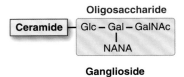

FIGURE 5.20   Sphingolipids, derivatives of ceramide. The structure of ceramide is shown at the bottom of the figure. The portion of ceramide shown in *red* is sphingosine. The — NH and —OH were contributed by serine. Different groups are added to the hydroxyl group of ceramide to form sphingomyelin, galactocerebrosides, and gangliosides. *NANA*, N-acetylneuraminic acid, also called *sialic acid*; *Glc*, glucose; *Gal*, galactose; *GalNAc*, N-acetylgalactosamine.

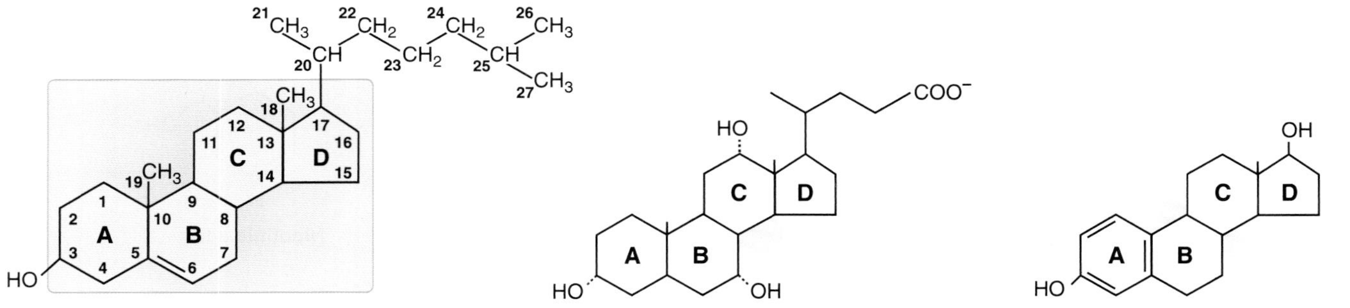

FIGURE 5.21 Cholesterol and its derivatives. The steroid nucleus is shown in the *green box*. The bile salt cholic acid and the steroid hormone 17β-estradiol are derived from cholesterol and contain the steroid ring structure.

is attached to the α-carbon in the L-configuration) (Fig. 5.22). These same amino acids also serve as precursors of nitrogen-containing compounds in the body, such as phosphatidylcholine (see Fig. 5.19) and are the basis of most human amino acid metabolism. However, our metabolic reactions occasionally produce an amino acid that has a β- or γ-amino group, such as the neurotransmitter γ-aminobutyric acid (see Fig. 5.22). However, only L-α-amino acids are incorporated into proteins. Although D-amino acids are not usually incorporated into proteins in living organisms, they serve many other functions in bacteria, such as synthesis of cross-links in cell walls.

Q What structural features account for the differences in the solubility of choles-**terol**, estra**diol**, and chol**ic acid** in the body? (See Fig. 5.21.)

B. Nitrogen-Containing Ring Structures

I. Purines, Pyrimidines, and Pyridines

Nitrogen is also a component of ring structures referred to as *heterocyclic rings* or *nitrogenous bases*. The three most common types of nitrogen-containing rings in the body are pur**ines** (e.g., aden**ine**), pyrimid**ines** (e.g., thym**ine**), and pyrid**ines** (e.g., the vitamins nicot**ine** acid, also called *niacin*, and pyridox**ine**, also called *vitamin B6*) (Fig. 5.23). The suffix "-ine" denotes the presence of nitrogen (am**ine**) in the ring. The pyrimidine uracil is an exception to this general type of nomenclature. The utility of these nitrogen-containing ring structures lies in the ability of the nitrogen to form hydrogen bonds and to accept and donate electrons while still part of the ring. In contrast, the unsubstituted aromatic benzene ring, in which electrons are distributed equally among all six carbons (see Fig. 5.1), is nonpolar, hydrophobic, and relatively unreactive.

2. Nucleosides and Nucleotides

Nitrogenous bases form nucleosides and nucleotides. A nucleoside consists of a nitrogenous base joined to a sugar, usually ribose or deoxyribose, through an

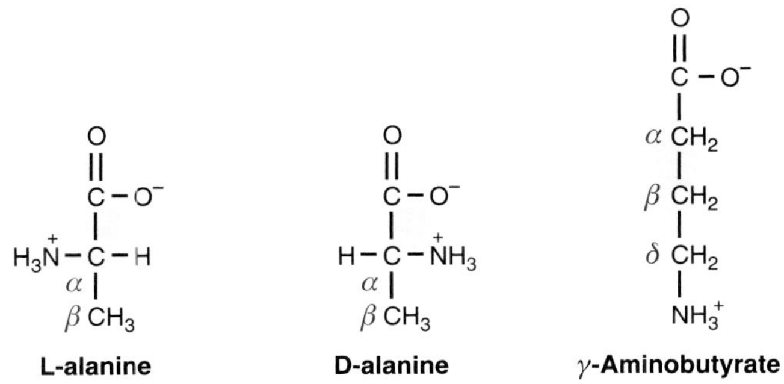

FIGURE 5.22 The structure of the α-amino acid alanine (both the D- and L-configuration) and the γ-amino acid γ-aminobutyrate.

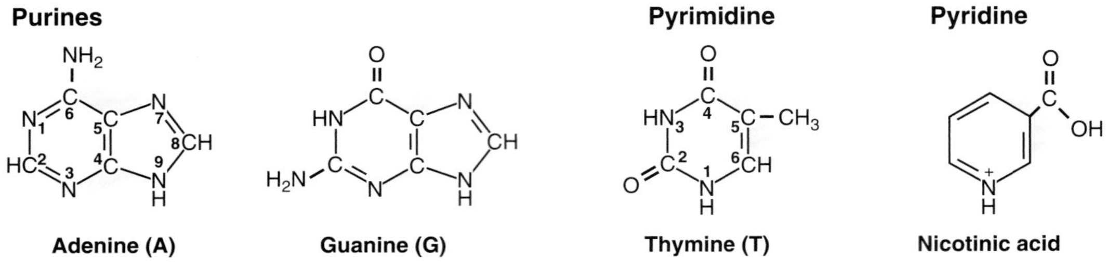

FIGURE 5.23 The nitrogenous bases.

Cholesterol is composed almost entirely of –CH_2 groups and is therefore water-insoluble. Estradiol is likewise relatively water-insoluble. However, cholic acid contains a hydrophilic carboxyl group and three hydroxyl groups. As shown by the *dashed lines*, the three hydroxyl groups all lie on one side of the molecule, thus creating a hydrophilic surface.

N-glycosidic bond (see Fig. 5.16). If phosphate groups are attached to the sugar, the compound becomes a nucleotide. In the name of the nucleotide ATP, the addition of the ribose is indicated by the name change from adenine to aden**osine** (for the gly**cosidic** bond). Monophosphate, diphosphate, or triphosphate is added to the name to indicate the presence of one, two, or three phosphate groups in the nucleotide. The structures of the nucleotides that serve as precursors of DNA and RNA are discussed in more detail in Section III, Chapter 12.

3. Tautomers

In many of the nitrogen-containing rings, the hydrogen can shift to produce a tautomer, a compound in which the hydrogen and double bonds have changed position (i.e., —N=C—OH → —NH—C=O) (Fig. 5.24). Tautomers are considered the same compound, and the structure may be represented either way. Generally, one tautomeric form is more reactive than the other. For example, in the two tautomeric forms of uric acid, a proton can dissociate from the enol form to produce urate.

Lotta T. has gouty arthritis (podagra) involving her great right toe. Polarized light microscopy of the fluid aspirated from the joint space showed crystals of monosodium urate phagocytosed by white blood cells. The presence of the relatively insoluble urate crystals within the joint space activates an inflammatory cascade leading to the classic components of joint inflammation (pain, redness, warmth, swelling, and limitation of joint motion). Uric acid is produced from the degradation of purines (adenine and guanine). At a blood pH of 7.4, all of the uric acid has dissociated a proton to form urate, which is not very water-soluble and forms crystals of the Na^+ salt. In the more acidic urine generated by the kidney, the acidic form, uric acid, may precipitate to form kidney stones.

V. Free Radicals

Radicals are compounds that have a single electron, usually in an outer orbital. Free radicals are radicals that exist independently in solution or in a lipid environment. Although many enzymes generate radicals as intermediates in reactions, these are not usually released into the cell to become free radicals.

Many of the compounds in the body are capable of being converted to free radicals by natural events that remove one of their electrons or by radiation. Radiation, for example, dissociates water into the hydrogen atom and the hydroxyl radical:

$$H_2O \leftrightarrow H\bullet + OH\bullet$$

In contrast, water normally dissociates into a proton and the negatively charged hydroxyl ion. The hydroxyl radical forms organic radicals by taking one electron (as H•) from a compound such as an unsaturated membrane lipid, which then has a single unpaired electron and is a new radical.

Compounds that are radicals may be written with, or without, the radical showing. For example, nitrogen dioxide, a potent, reactive, toxic radical present in smog and cigarette smoke, may be designated in medical and lay literature as NO_2

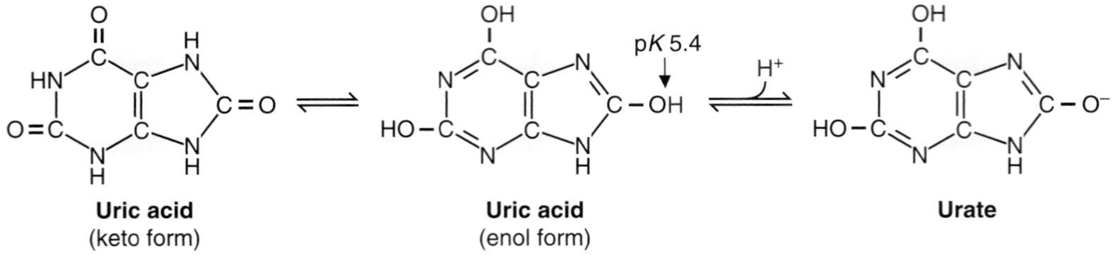

FIGURE 5.24 Tautomers of uric acid. The tautomeric form affects the reactivity. The enol form dissociates a proton to form urate.

rather than $NO_2\bullet$. Superoxide, a radical produced in the cell and that is the source of much destruction, is correctly written as the superoxide anion, O_2^-. However, to emphasize its free radical nature, the same compound is sometimes written as $O_2^-\bullet$. If a compound is designated as a radical in the medical literature, you can be certain that it is a reactive radical and that its radical nature is important for the pathophysiology under discussion. Reactive oxygen- and nitrogen-containing free radicals are discussed in more detail in Chapter 25.

 Free radicals are not just esoteric reactants; they are the agents of cell death and destruction. They are involved in many chronic disease states (e.g., coronary artery disease, diabetes mellitus, arthritis, emphysema) as well as acute injury (e.g., radiation, strokes, myocardial infarction, spinal cord injury). Through free radical defense mechanisms in our cells, we can often restrict the damage attributed to the "normal" aging process.

CLINICAL COMMENTS

 Dianne A. The severity of clinical signs and symptoms in patients with DKA, such as **Dianne A.**, is correlated directly with the concentration of ketone bodies in the blood. Direct quantitative methods for measuring acetoacetate and β-hydroxybutyrate are not routinely available. As a result, clinicians usually rely on semiquantitative reagent strips (Ketostix, Bayer Corporation, Pittsburgh, PA) or tablets (Acetest, Bayer Corporation) to estimate the level of acetoacetate in the blood and the urine. The nitroprusside on the strips and in the tablets reacts with acetoacetate and to a lesser degree with acetone (both of which have ketone groups) but does not react with β-hydroxybutyrate (which does not have a ketone group). β-Hydroxybutyrate is the predominant ketone body present in the blood of a patient in DKA, and its concentration could decline at a disproportionately rapid rate compared with that of acetoacetate and acetone. Therefore, tests employing the nitroprusside reaction to monitor the success of therapy in such a patient may be misleading. As a result, clinicians will follow the "anion gap" in the blood, which in DKA represents the increase in ketone bodies.

In contrast to the difficulty of ketone body measurements, patients with diabetes can self-monitor blood glucose levels at home, thereby markedly decreasing the time and expense of the many blood glucose determinations they need. Capillary blood obtained from a finger prick is placed on the pad of a plastic strip. The strip has been impregnated with an enzyme (usually the bacterial enzyme glucose oxidase) that specifically converts the glucose in the blood to an oxidized sugar (gluconate) and a reduced compound (hydrogen peroxide, H_2O_2). The H_2O_2 reacts with a dye to produce a color. The intensity of the color, which is directly proportionate to the concentration of glucose in the patient's blood, is read on an instrument called a *blood glucose monitor*.

 The anion gap refers to the difference in concentration between routinely measured anions (chloride and bicarbonate) and cations (sodium and potassium) in the blood. Because these cations are in most cases in greater concentration than the measured anions, the difference in value is known as the *anion gap*. The normal value for the anion gap is 12 (range = 8–16). If the anion gap is greater than normal, it is indicative of unknown anions being present in excess and, in the case of type 1 diabetes, most often reflects the production of ketone bodies.

 Lotta T. Ms. T. has acute gouty arthritis (podagra) involving her right great toe. Lotta was treated with colchicine (acetyltrimethyl colchinic acid methyl ether) for the acute attack of gout affecting her great right toe. After having two doses of colchicine, the throbbing pain in her toe had abated significantly. The redness and swelling also seemed to have lessened slightly. Colchicine will reduce the effects of the inflammatory response to the urate crystals. Several weeks later, Lotta was started on allopurinol (150 mg twice daily), which inhibits the enzyme that produces uric acid. Within several days of starting allopurinol therapy, Lotta's uric acid levels began to decrease.

BIOCHEMICAL COMMENTS

Chlorinated Aromatic Hydrocarbon Environmental Toxins. As a result of human endeavor, toxic compounds containing chlorinated benzene rings have been widely distributed in the environment. The pesticide dichlorodiphenyltrichloroethane (DDT), the class of chemicals called *dioxins*, and polychlorinated biphenyls (PCBs) provide examples of chlorinated aromatic hydrocarbons and structurally related compounds that are very hydrophobic and poorly biodegraded (Fig. 5.25). As a consequence of their persistence and lipophilicity, these chemicals are concentrated in the adipose tissue of fish, fish-eating birds, and carnivorous mammals, including humans.

 The reducing sugar test. The reducing sugar test was used for detection of sugar in the urine long before specific enzymatic assays for glucose and galactose became available. In this test, the aldehyde group of a sugar is oxidized as it donates electrons to copper; the copper becomes reduced and produces a blue color. In alkaline solution, keto sugars (e.g., fructose) also react in this test because they form tautomers that are aldehydes. Ring structures of sugars also react but only if the ring can open (i.e., it is not attached to another compound through a glycosidic bond). Until a specific test for fructose becomes available, a congenital disease resulting in the presence of fructose in the urine is indicated by a positive reducing sugar test and negative results in the specific enzymatic assays for glucose or galactose.

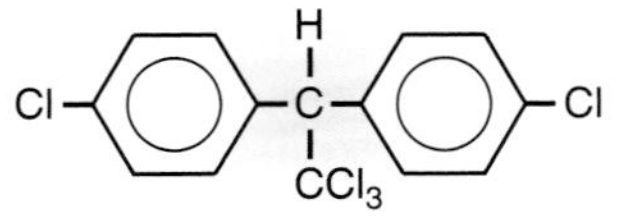

DDT

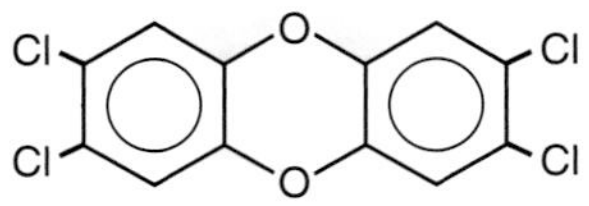

Chlorodibenzo-p-dioxin

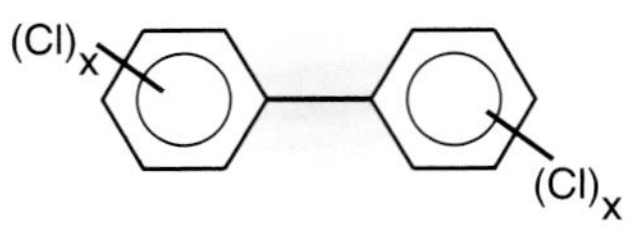

PCB

FIGURE 5.25 Environmental toxins. Dichlorodiphenyltrichloroethane (DDT) is a member of a class of aromatic hydrocarbons that contains two chlorinated benzene (phenyl) rings joined by a chlorinated ethane molecule. Chlorodibenzo-p-dioxins (CDDs) are a related class of more than 75 chlorinated hydrocarbons that all contain a dibenzo-p-dioxin (DD) molecule comprising two benzene rings joined via two oxygen bridges at adjacent carbons on each of the benzene rings. The compound 2,3,7,8-tetrachlorodibenzo-p-dioxin is one of the most toxic and the most extensively studied. Chlorinated dibenzofurans (CDFs) are structurally and toxicologically related. Polychlorinated biphenyls (PCBs) consist of two benzene rings linked by a bond with 2 to 10 of the remaining carbons containing a chlorine atom. There are >200 different varieties of PCBs.

 The accumulation of DDT in adipose tissue may be protective in humans because it decreases the amount of DDT available to pass through nonpolar lipid membranes to reach neurons in the brain or to pass through placental membranes to reach the fetus. Eventually, we convert DDT to more polar metabolites that are excreted in the urine. However, some may pass with lipid into the breast milk of nursing mothers.

Most of what is known about the toxicity of dioxins in humans comes from individuals exposed incidentally or chronically to higher levels (e.g., industrial accidents or presence in areas sprayed with Agent Orange or other herbicides contaminated with dioxins). The lowest dose effects are probably associated with thymic atrophy and decreased immune response, chloracne and related skin lesions, and neoplasia (cancer). Dioxins can cross into the placenta to cause developmental and reproductive effects, decreased prenatal growth, and prenatal mortality.

DDT, a chlorinated biphenyl, was widely used in the United States as a herbicide from the 1940s through the 1960s (see Fig. 5.25). Although it has not been used in this country since 1972, the chlorinated benzene rings are resistant to biodegradation, and US soil and water are still contaminated with small amounts. DDT continues to be used in other parts of the world. Because this highly lipophilic molecule is stored in the fat of animals, organisms accumulate progressively greater amounts of DDT at each successive stage of the food chain. Fish-eating birds, one of the organisms at the top of the food chain, have declined in population because of the effect of DDT on the thickness of their eggshells. DDT is not nearly as toxic in the human, although long-term exposure or exposure to high doses may cause reversible neurologic symptoms, hepatotoxic effects, or cancer.

Dioxins, specifically polychlorinated dibenzo-p-dioxins (PCDDs), constitute another class of environmental toxins that are currently of great concern (see Fig. 5.25). They have been measured at what is termed background levels in the blood, adipose tissue, and breast milk of all humans tested. PCDDs are formed as a by-product during the production of other chlorinated compounds and herbicides and from the chlorine bleaching process used by pulp and paper mills. They are released during the incineration of industrial, municipal, and domestic waste and during the combustion of fossil fuels, and they are found in cigarette smoke and the exhaust from engines that burn gasoline and diesel fuels. PCDDs can also be formed from the combustion of organic matter during forest fires. They enter the atmosphere as particulate matter, are vaporized, and can spread large distances to enter soil and water.

PCBs were originally synthesized for use as nonflammable material for cooling and insulating industrial transformers and capacitors. As a result of accidents in the chemical plants producing the PCBs, it became evident that these chemicals can cause adverse health effects in humans. Production of PCBs stopped in the United States in 1979, although they may still be found in enclosed containers for electrical transformers. All of the chlorinated compounds thus far discussed may have as their mechanism of action an alteration of gene expression via binding to the cytoplasmic arylhydrocarbon receptor (see Section III of this text). PCB exposure has been linked to cancer and to disorders of the immune, reproductive, nervous, and endocrine systems.

All of the polychlorinated derivatives are difficult to remove from the environment. One promising approach is to use genetically engineered bacteria that can use these compounds as a food source and safely metabolize the toxins. This approach, however, has the drawback of introducing genetically engineered organisms into the environment, which has its own potential problems (see Chapter 17).

As humans at the top of the food chain, we have acquired our background levels of dioxins principally through the consumption of food—primarily meat, dairy products, and fish. Once in the human body, dioxins are stored in human fat and adipose tissue and have an average half-life of approximately 5 to 15 years. They are unreactive, poorly degraded, and not readily converted to more water-soluble compounds that can be excreted in the urine. They are slowly excreted in the bile and feces and together with lipids enter the breast milk of nursing mothers.

KEY CONCEPTS

- Carbohydrates, commonly known as *sugars*, can be classified by several criteria:
  - Type of carbonyl group (aldo- or ketosugars)
  - Number of carbons (pentoses [five carbons], hexoses [six carbons])
  - Positions of hydroxyl groups on asymmetric carbon atoms (D- or L-configuration, stereoisomers, epimers)
  - Substituents (amino sugars)
  - Number of monosaccharides joined through glycosidic bonds (disaccharides, oligosaccharides, polysaccharides)

- Lipids are structurally diverse compounds that are not very soluble in water (i.e., they are hydrophobic).
  - The major lipids are fatty acids.
  - Triacylglycerols (triglycerides) consist of three fatty acids esterified to the carbohydrate glycerol.
  - Phosphoacylglycerols (phosphoglycerides or phospholipids) are similar to triacylglycerol but contain a phosphate in place of a fatty acid.
  - Sphingolipids are built on sphingosine.
  - Cholesterol is a component of membranes and a precursor for molecules that contain the steroid nucleus, such as bile salts and steroid hormones.
- Nitrogen is found in a variety of compounds, in addition to amino sugars.
  - Amino acids and heterocyclic rings contain nitrogens, which carry a positive charge at neutral pH.
  - Amino acids contain a carboxyl group, an amino group, and a side chain attached to a central carbon.
  - Proteins consist of a linear chain of amino acids.
  - Purines, pyrimidines, and pyridines have heterocyclic nitrogen-containing ring structures.
  - Nucleosides consist of a heterocyclic ring attached to a sugar.
  - A nucleoside plus phosphate is a nucleotide.
- Glycoproteins and proteoglycans have sugars attached to protein components.
- Diseases discussed in this chapter are summarized in Table 5.1.

TABLE 5.1 Diseases Discussed in Chapter 5		
DISORDER OR CONDITION	**GENETIC OR ENVIRONMENTAL**	**COMMENTS**
Gout	Both	May be the result of mutations in specific proteins or dietary habits; leads to a buildup of uric acid in the blood and precipitates of urate crystals in the joints
Type I diabetes	Both	Appropriate management of type I diabetes requires insulin injections and frequent monitoring of blood glucose levels throughout the day. Without such careful monitoring, ketone bodies may be produced inappropriately.

REVIEW QUESTIONS—CHAPTER 5

Select the single best answer for each of the following questions. Base your answers on your knowledge of nomenclature. You need not recognize any of the structures shown to answer the questions.

1. A component of a "lipid panel" for a patient is triglyceride, which is best described by which one of the following?
   A. Contains a steroid nucleus
   B. Three fatty acids esterified to sphingosine
   C. Three fatty acids esterified to a carbohydrate
   D. Two fatty acids and a phosphate esterified to a sphingosine
   E. Two fatty acids and a phosphate esterified to a carbohydrate

2. A patient was admitted to the hospital emergency department in a coma. Laboratory tests found high levels of the compound shown below in her blood:

$$CH_2OH—CH_2—CH_2—COO^-$$

   On the basis of its structure (and your knowledge of the nomenclature of functional groups), you identify the compound as which one of the following?
   A. Methanol (wood alcohol)
   B. Ethanol (alcohol)
   C. Ethylene glycol (antifreeze)
   D. β-Hydroxybutyrate (a ketone body)
   E. γ-Hydroxybutyrate (the "date rape" drug)

3. A patient was diagnosed with a deficiency of the lyso-somal enzyme α-glycosidase. The name of the deficient enzyme suggests that it hydrolyzes a glycosidic bond, which is best described as a bond formed via which one of the following?
    A. Through multiple hydrogen bonds between two sugar molecules
    B. Between the anomeric carbon of a sugar and an O—H (or N) of another molecule
    C. Between two anomeric carbons in polysaccharides
    D. Internal bond formation between the anomeric carbon of a monosaccharide and its own fifth carbon hydroxyl group
    E. Between the carbon containing the aldol or keto group and the α-carbon of the sugar
4. In the congenital disease galactosemia, high concentrations of galactose and galactitol accumulate in the blood. On the basis of their names, you would expect which one of the following statements to be correct?
    A. Galactitol is an aldehyde formed from the keto sugar galactose.
    B. Galactitol is the oxidized form of galactose.
    C. Galactitol is the sugar alcohol of galactose.
    D. Both galactose and galactitol are sugars.
    E. Both galactose and galactitol would give a positive reducing sugar test.
5. A patient was diagnosed with one of the types of sphingolipidoses, which are congenital diseases involving the inability to degrade sphingolipids. All sphingolipids have in common which one of the following?
    A. A glycerol backbone
    B. Ceramide
    C. Phosphorylcholine
    D. N-Acetylneuraminic acid (NANA)
    E. A steroid ring structure to which sphingosine is attached
6. In DKA, a metabolic acidosis results from increased hepatic production of ketone bodies (β-hydroxybutyrate, acetoacetate, and acetone). Which one of the following terms best describes all three of these ketone bodies?
    A. Butyl structure
    B. Aromatic structure
    C. Aliphatic structure
    D. Hydroxyl-containing structure
    E. Amine-containing structure

7. Omega-3 fatty acids are found in "oily" fish and are considered beneficial for heart health. A food containing which one of the following would fall into this category?
    A. Cis, $\Delta^{9,12,15}$, C18:3
    B. Cis, $\Delta^{9,12}$, C18:2
    C. Cis, $\Delta^{6,9,12}$, C18:3
    D. Cis, $\Delta^{9,12,15}$, C20:3
    E. Cis, $\Delta^{6,9}$, C16:2
8. A patient has had viral gastroenteritis for 3 days and has been unable to keep any oral intake down, such that the patient is now dehydrated. In the emergency department, he is given 2 L of intravenous (IV) D5 0.9% NaCl solution. Which of the following best describes this IV solution?
    A. It is hypotonic.
    B. It is hypertonic.
    C. It contains D-glucose.
    D. It contains L-glucose.
    E. It contains D-galactose.
9. A patient with hyperlipidemia has been counseled to reduce the saturated fats in his diet, so he has replaced butter with a butter substitute that he knows is made from a polyunsaturated oil. The manufacturer of this butter substitute has partially hydrogenated this product. Which one of the following is the best description of why this product was partially hydrogenated?
    A. The trans-fatty acids produced by commercial hydrogenation are very healthy in humans.
    B. Hydrogenation reduces the double bonds, creating a more saturated product, which is more marketable.
    C. Hydrogenation makes the product less expensive to produce.
    D. Hydrogenation reduces the cholesterol content of the oil.
    E. Hydrogenation increases the cholesterol content of the oil.
10. A researcher is trying to design an antibiotic to kill bacteria but not harm any human cells. Which one of the following theoretically could be used for this purpose?
    A. A medication that inhibits reactions using only D-amino acids
    B. A medication that inhibits reactions using only L-amino acids
    C. A medication that inhibits reactions using only amino acids containing a β-amino group
    D. A medication that inhibits reactions using only amino acids containing a γ-amino group
    E. A medication that only inhibits reactions using only aromatic amino acids

ANSWERS

1. **The answer is C.** Triglyceride (triacylglycerol) consists of three fatty acids esterified to the carbohydrate glycerol. Phosphoacylglycerols are similar to triacylglycerol but contain a phosphate in place of a fatty acid. Cholesterol contains a steroid nucleus. Sphingolipids are built on sphingosine, but triglycerides are not.

2. **The answer is E.** The compound contains an —OH group, which should appear in the name as an "-ol" or a "hydroxyl-" group. All answers fit this criterion. The structure also contains a carboxylate group (—COO⁻), which should appear in the name as an "-ate" or "acid." Only D and E fit this criterion. Counting backward from

the carboxylate group (carbon 1), the second carbon is α, the third carbon is β, and the fourth carbon, containing the hydroxyl group, is γ. Thus, the compound is γ-hydroxybutyrate. A, B, and C can also be eliminated because "meth-" denotes a single carbon, "eth-" denotes two carbons, and the "-ene" in ethylene denotes a double bond.

3. **The answer is B.** The term "glycosidic bond" refers to a *covalent* bond formed between the anomeric carbon of one sugar, when it is in a ring form, and a hydroxyl group or nitrogen of another compound (see Fig. 5.16) (thus, A, D, and E are incorrect). Disaccharides can be linked through their anomeric carbons, but polysaccharides cannot because there would be no anomeric carbon left to form a link with the next sugar in the chain (thus, C is incorrect).

4. **The answer is C.** The keto or aldehyde group is necessary for a positive reducing sugar test (a nonspecific test used to identify the presence of sugar in the urine). Because galactitol has had its aldehyde group already reduced to form the alcohol group, it would no longer give a positive result in a reducing sugar test. An "**ol**" in the name denotes that the compound is an alcoh**ol** (has an —OH group) and an "**ose**" denotes a sugar. Thus, the alcohol that is derived from galact**ose** is galactit**ol**. All sugars have a keto or aldehyde group, which is reduced when the compound becomes an alcohol (a gain of electrons, as indicated by an increase of hydrogen relative to oxygen). Oxidation of the keto or aldehyde group would lead to an acid group being generated, not an alcohol group. Galactose is an aldose sugar, not a keto sugar.

5. **The answer is B.** Sphingolipids contain a ceramide group, which is sphingosine with an attached fatty acid. They do not contain a glycerol moiety (thus, A is incorrect). However, different sphingolipids have different substituents on the —CH₂OH group of ceramide. For example, sphingomyelin contains phosphorylcholine, and gangliosides contain NANA (thus, C and D are incorrect). No known sphingolipids contain a steroid (thus, E is incorrect).

6. **The answer is C.** None of these ketone bodies contains a benzene or similar ring (aromatic), so they are all defined as aliphatic. Two of these have four carbons (butyl), but acetone has only three carbons (propyl structure). Only β-hydroxybutyrate contains a hydroxyl group (—OH), and none contains a nitrogen atom or group (amine).

7. **The answer is A.** The ω-series of fatty acids refers to counting carbons from the ω-end of the fatty acid (usually the methyl carbon end) until a double bond is reached. For the *cis* $\Delta^{9,12,15}$ C18:3 fatty acid, the double bonds are between carbons 9 and 10, 12 and 13, and 15 and 16. If one counts backward from carbon 18, one counts three carbons (18, 17, and 16) before the double bond is reached, indicating that this fatty acid belongs to the ω-3 family. The *cis* $\Delta^{,12}$ C18:2 fatty acid belongs to the ω-6 group, as does the *cis* $\Delta^{6,9,12}$ C18:3 fatty acid. The *cis* $\Delta^{9,12,15}$ C20:3 fatty acid belongs to the ω-5 group, whereas the *cis* $\Delta^{6,9}$ C16:2 fatty acid belongs to the ω-7 group.

8. **The answer is C.** Saline 0.9% is considered "normal" saline (NS) and is isotonic. This is a very common solution in IV fluids used to treat dehydration. *D5* refers to 5% dextrose solution or 50 g/L dextrose given as a means of parenteral nutrition because the patient cannot take oral nutrition. Dextrose is another name for D-glucose. L-Glucose is not commonly found in the human body. The glucose is completely metabolized and does not contribute to tonicity. Galactose is not present in this type of solution.

9. **The answer is B.** Polyunsaturated fatty acids have a lower melting point than more saturated fats. Butter is a highly saturated fat and is a solid around room temperature. Polyunsaturated fats melt at room temperature. Most consumers do not want a butter substitute that melts at room temperature, so such a product would not sell as well as natural butter. Hydrogenation reduces the double bonds in the polyunsaturated fats and makes the product more saturated, which raises the melting point of the oil as well as increasing the shelf life of the product. Hydrogenated oils are less expensive to produce than animal fats, but hydrogenation introduces an extra step in manufacturing and increases costs as compared to not changing the product at all. Unfortunately, commercial hydrogenation creates *trans* double bonds in the fats, whereas all naturally occurring unsaturated fatty acids contain double bonds in the *cis*-configuration. The presence of *trans* fats in American diets has been linked to the development of cardiovascular disease. Hydrogenation of fatty acids has nothing to do with cholesterol.

10. **The answer is A.** In human proteins, the amino acids are always L-α-amino acids (in the L-configuration). D-Amino acids are not used for synthesizing proteins in humans but are used to generate products in bacteria. Inhibiting the use of D-amino acids would inhibit bacterial growth but does not affect human cell growth. Some human products contain β- and γ-amino groups, so drugs inhibiting their production would not be beneficial for human use.

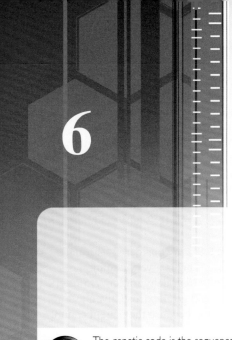

6 Amino Acids in Proteins

 The genetic code is the sequence of three bases (nucleotides) in DNA that contains the information for the linear sequence of amino acids in a polypeptide chain (its primary structure). A gene is the portion of DNA that encodes a functional product, such as a polypeptide chain. Mutations, which are changes in the nucleotides in a gene, result in a change in the products of that gene that may be inherited. The inherited disease sickle cell anemia, for example, is caused by a mutation in the gene that encodes one of the subunits of hemoglobin. Hemoglobin is the protein present in red blood cells that reversibly binds O_2 and transports it to tissues. The adult hemoglobin protein comprises four polypeptide chains, 2α and 2β. The α and β subunits differ in primary structure (i.e., they have different sequences of amino acids and are encoded by different genes). Sickle cell anemia is caused by a single nucleotide mutation in DNA that changes just one amino acid in the hemoglobin β-chains from a glutamic acid to a valine.

Proteins have many functions in the body. They serve as transporters of hydrophobic compounds in the blood, as cell adhesion molecules that attach cells to each other and to the extracellular matrix, as hormones that carry signals from one group of cells to another, as ion channels through lipid membranes, and as enzymes that increase the rate of biochemical reactions. The unique characteristics of a protein are dictated by its linear sequence of amino acids, termed its **primary structure**. The primary structure of a protein determines how it can fold and how it interacts with other molecules in the cell to perform its function. The primary structures of all of the diverse human proteins are synthesized from 20 amino acids arranged in a linear sequence determined by the genetic code.

General Properties of Amino Acids. Each of the amino acids used for protein synthesis has the same general structure (Fig. 6.1A). It contains a **carboxylic acid** group, an **amino group** attached to the **α-carbon** in an **L-configuration**, a **hydrogen atom**, and a chemical group called a **side chain** that is different for each amino acid. In solution, at physiologic pH, the free amino acids exist as **zwitterions**: ions in which the amino group is positively charged and the carboxylate group is negatively charged (see Fig. 6.1B). In proteins, these amino acids are joined into linear polymers called **polypeptide chains** through **peptide bonds** between the carboxylic acid group of one amino acid and the amino group of the next amino acid.

Classification of Amino Acids according to Chemical Properties of the Side Chains. The chemical properties of the side chain determine the types of bonds and interactions each amino acid in a polypeptide chain can make with other molecules. Thus, amino acids are often grouped by polarity of the side chain (**charged**, **nonpolar hydrophobic**, or **uncharged polar**) or by structural features (**aliphatic**, **cyclic**, or **aromatic**). The side chains of the **nonpolar hydrophobic** amino acids (alanine, valine, leucine, isoleucine, phenylalanine, and methionine) cluster together to exclude water in the **hydrophobic effect**. The **uncharged polar** amino acids (serine, threonine, tyrosine, asparagine, and glutamine) participate in **hydrogen bonding**.

Cysteine, which contains a sulfhydryl group, forms **disulfide bonds**. The negatively charged **acidic** amino acids (aspartate and glutamate) form **ionic (electrostatic) bonds** with positively charged molecules such as the **basic** amino acids (lysine, arginine, and histidine). The charge on the amino acid at a particular pH is determined by the pK_a ($-$log of the acid **dissociation constant**) of each group that has a dissociable proton.

Amino Acid Substitutions in the Primary Structure. Mutations in the genetic code result in proteins with an altered **primary structure**. Mutations resulting in single amino acid substitutions can affect the functioning of a protein or can confer an advantage specific to a tissue or a set of circumstances. Many proteins, such as **hemoglobin**, exist in the human population as **polymorphisms** (genetically determined variations in primary structure).

Within the same individual, the primary structure of many proteins varies with the stage of development and is present in **fetal** and **adult isoforms** such as fetal and adult hemoglobin. The primary structure of some proteins, such as

creatine kinase, can also vary between tissues (**tissue-specific isozymes**) or between intracellular locations in the same tissue. **Electrophoretic separation** of tissue-specific isozymes has been useful in medicine as a means of identifying the tissue site of injury.

Modified Amino Acids. In addition to the amino acids encoded by DNA that form the primary structure of proteins, many proteins contain specific amino acids that have been modified by **phosphorylation, oxidation, carboxylation**, or other reactions. When these reactions are catalyzed by enzymes, they are referred to as **posttranslational modifications**.

THE WAITING ROOM

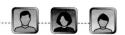

 Will S. is a 17-year-old boy who presented to the hospital emergency department with severe pain in his lower back, abdomen, and legs, which began after a 2-day history of nausea and vomiting caused by gastroenteritis. He was diagnosed as having sickle cell disease at age 3 years and has been admitted to the hospital on numerous occasions for similar vaso-occlusive sickle cell crises.

On admission, the patient's hemoglobin level in peripheral venous blood was 7.8 g/dL (reference range = 12 to 16 g/dL). The hematocrit or packed cell volume (the percentage of the total volume of blood made up of red blood cells) was 23.4% (reference range = 41% to 53%). His serum total bilirubin level (a pigment derived from hemoglobin degradation) was 2.3 mg/dL (reference range = 0.2 to 1.0 mg/dL). A radiograph of his abdomen showed radiopaque stones in his gallbladder. With chronic hemolysis (red blood cell destruction), the amount of heme degraded to bilirubin is increased. These stones are the result of the chronic excretion of excessive amounts of bilirubin from the liver into the bile, leading to bilirubinate crystal deposition in the gallbladder lumen.

 David K. is an 18-year-old boy who was brought to the hospital by his mother because of the sudden onset of severe pain in his left flank, radiating around his left side toward his pubic area. His urine was reddish-brown in color, and a urinalysis showed the presence of many red blood cells. When his urine was acidified with acetic acid, clusters of flat hexagonal transparent crystals of cystine were noted. There was no family history of kidney stone disease.

 Dianne A., who has type 1 diabetes mellitus, has to give herself subcutaneous injections of insulin several times a day to try to mimic what her pancreas would do if she could produce insulin. Insulin was initially purified from animals, and then synthetic human insulin was developed. There is now modified synthetic insulin, which allows the onset of action to be adjusted. Dianne A. takes long-acting insulin (glargine) once a day and rapid-acting insulin (lispro) with meals. Her physician will adjust the doses to keep her blood glucose levels controlled.

 Anne J. is a 54-year-old woman who is 68 in tall and weighs 198 lb. She has a history of high blood pressure and elevated serum cholesterol levels. Following a heated argument with a neighbor, Mrs. J. experienced a "tight pressure-like band of pain" across her chest, associated with shortness of breath, sweating, and a sense of light-headedness.

After 5 hours of intermittent chest pain, she went to the hospital emergency department, where her electrocardiogram showed changes consistent with an acute infarction of the anterior wall of her heart. She was admitted to the cardiac care unit. Blood was sent to the laboratory for various tests, including a determination of cardiac troponin T (cTnT) levels.

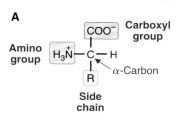

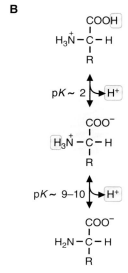

FIGURE 6.1 A. General structure of the amino acids found in proteins. **B.** Dissociation of the α-carboxyl and α-amino groups of amino acids. At physiologic pH (~7), a form in which both the α-carboxyl and α-amino groups are charged predominates. Some amino acids also have ionizable groups on their side chains. pK, −log acid dissociation constant; R, side chain.

 The term *calculus* is used to describe any abnormal concretion (concretelike precipitate) of mineral salts. These almost always form within the cavity of a hollow organ, such as the kidney (kidney or renal stones) or the lumen of a duct (e.g., common bile duct stones).

 The term *angina* describes a crushing or compressive pain. The term *angina pectoris* is used when this pain is located in the center of the chest or pectoral region, often radiating to the neck or arms. The most common mechanism for the latter symptom is a decreased supply of oxygen to the heart muscle caused by atherosclerotic coronary artery disease, which results in obstruction of the vessels that supply arterial blood to cardiac muscle.

I. General Structure of the Amino Acids

Twenty different amino acids are commonly found in proteins. They are all α-amino acids—amino acids in which the amino group is attached to the α-carbon (the carbon atom next to the carboxylate group) (see Fig 6.1A). The α-carbon has two additional substituents, a hydrogen atom and an additional chemical group called a *side chain* (–R). The side chain is different for each amino acid.

At a physiologic pH of 7.4, the amino group on these amino acids carries a positive charge and the carboxylic acid group is negatively charged (see Fig. 6.1B). The pK_a of the primary carboxylic acid groups for all of the amino acids is approximately 2 (1.8 to 2.4). At pH values much lower than the pK_a (higher hydrogen ion concentrations), all of the carboxylic acid groups are protonated. At the pK_a, 50% of the molecules are dissociated into carboxylate anions and protons, and at a pH of 7.4, >99% of the molecules are dissociated (see Chapter 4). The pK_a for all of the α-amino groups is approximately 9.5 (8.8 to 11.0), so that at the lower pH of 7.4, most of the amino groups are fully protonated and carry a positive charge. The form of an amino acid that has both a positive and a negative charge is called a *zwitterion*. Because these charged chemical groups can form hydrogen bonds with water molecules, all of these amino acids are water-soluble at physiologic pH.

In all of the amino acids but glycine (where the side chain is a hydrogen), the α-carbon is an asymmetric carbon atom that has four different substituents and can exist in either the D- or L-configuration (Fig. 6.2). The amino acids in mammalian proteins are all L-amino acids represented with the amino group to the left if the carboxyl group is at the top of the structure. These same amino acids serve as precursors of nitrogen-containing compounds that are synthesized in the body, and thus, human amino acid metabolism is also centered on L-amino acids. The amino acid glycine is neither D nor L because the α-carbon atom contains two hydrogen atoms and is not an asymmetric carbon.

The chemical properties of the amino acids give each protein its unique characteristics. Proteins are composed of one or more linear *polypeptide chains* and may contain hundreds of amino acids. The sequence of amino acids, termed the *primary structure*, is determined by the genetic code for the protein. In the polypeptide chains, amino acids are joined through *peptide bonds* between the carboxylic acid of one amino acid and

Bilirubin is a degradation product of hemoglobin, and its levels are elevated in **Will S**. Bilirubin can be present in serum either conjugated to glucuronic acid (which is determined by the direct measurement) or free (which is very hydrophobic and is determined by indirect measurement). Measurement of bilirubin in serum is dependent on the reaction of bilirubin with a diazotized sulfonic acid, which generates, after appropriate treatments, a blue azobilirubin. The intensity of the blue color can be determined spectrophotometrically at 600 nm. Total bilirubin is measured in the presence of caffeine-benzoate, which separates the hydrophobic nonconjugated bilirubin from its binding partners. A second measurement is done in the absence of caffeine-benzoate, which will only determine the conjugated, soluble forms of bilirubin (the direct measurement). Unconjugated bilirubin is then calculated by determining the difference in values obtained in the presence and absence of caffeine-benzoate (the indirect measurement). Recently, a transcutaneous device has been developed to determine bilirubin levels in newborns. The instrument is pressed against the infant's forehead, and light at various wavelengths is transmitted through the forehead, generating a reflective multiwavelength spectrum. Analysis of the spectrum allows the instrument to determine the levels of bilirubin, hemoglobin, and melanin in the infant's skin.

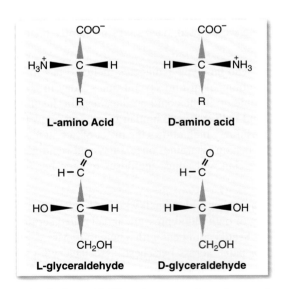

FIGURE 6.2 L- and D-Amino acids. The L-forms are the only ones found in human proteins. Bonds coming out of the paper are shown by *black arrows*; those going in, by *shaded arrows*. The α-amino groups and H atoms come toward the reader, and the α-carboxyl and side chains go away from the reader. The L- and D-forms are mirror images that cannot be superimposed by rotating the molecule. The reference for the L- and D-forms is the stereoisomers of glyceraldehyde (see Fig. 5.10A). R, side chain.

the amino group of the adjacent amino acid (Fig. 6.3, see also Fig. 1.5). Thus, the amino group, the α-carbon, and the carboxyl groups form the peptide backbone, and the side chains of the amino acids extend outward from this backbone. The side chains interact with the peptide backbone of other regions of the chain or with the side chains of other amino acids in the protein to form hydrophobic regions, electrostatic bonds, hydrogen bonds, or disulfide bonds. These interactions dictate the folding pattern of the molecule. The three-dimensional folding of the protein forms distinct regions called *binding sites* that are lined with amino acid side chains that interact specifically with another molecule termed a *ligand* (e.g., the heme in hemoglobin). Thus, the chemical properties of the side chains determine how the protein folds, how it binds specific ligands, and how it interacts with its environment (e.g., the aqueous medium of the cytoplasm). Each chain will have a *carboxyl terminal* and an *amino terminal*. The amino terminal is the first amino acid in the chain, which contains a free amino group. The carboxyl terminal is the last amino acid in the chain, which contains a free carboxylate group.

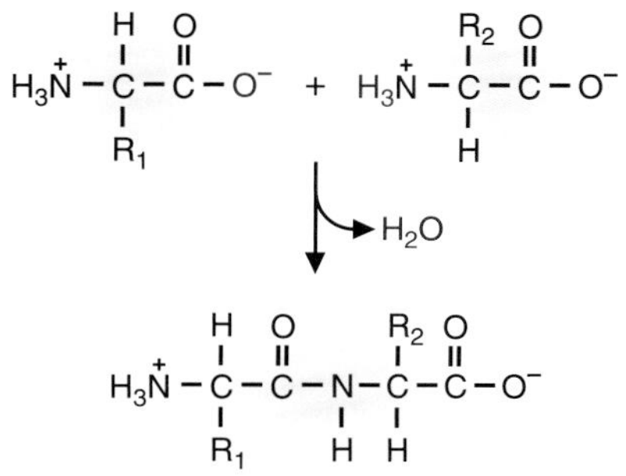

FIGURE 6.3 Peptide bonds. Amino acids in a polypeptide chain are joined through peptide bonds between the carboxyl group of one amino acid and the amino group of the next amino acid in the sequence. *R*, side chain.

II. Classification of Amino Acid Side Chains

As seen in Figure 6.4, the 20 amino acids used for protein synthesis are grouped into different classifications according to the polarity and structural features of the side chains. These groupings can be helpful in describing common functional roles or metabolic pathways of the amino acids. However, some amino acid side chains fit into several different classifications and are therefore grouped differently in different textbooks. Two of the characteristics of the side chain that are useful for classification are its pK_a and its hydropathic index, listed in Table 6.1. The *hydropathic index* is a scale used to denote the hydrophobicity of the side chain; the more positive the hydropathic index, the greater is the tendency to cluster with other nonpolar molecules and exclude water in the hydrophobic effect. These hydrophobic side chains tend to occur in membranes or in the center of a folded protein, where water is excluded. The more negative the hydropathic index of an amino acid, the more hydrophilic is its side chain.

The names of the different amino acids have been given three-letter and one-letter abbreviations (see Fig. 6.4). The three-letter abbreviations use the first two letters in the name plus the third letter of the name or the letter of a characteristic sound, such as "trp" for tryptophan. The one-letter abbreviations use the first letter of the name of the most frequent amino acid in proteins (e.g., "A" for alanine). If the first letter has already been assigned, the letter of a characteristic sound is used (e.g., "R" for arginine). Single-letter abbreviations are commonly used to denote the amino acids in a polypeptide sequence.

A. Nonpolar, Aliphatic Amino Acids

Glycine is the simplest amino acid, and it does not fit well into any classification because its side chain is just a hydrogen atom. Because the side chain of glycine is so small compared with that of other amino acids, it causes the least amount of steric hindrance in a protein (i.e., it does not significantly impinge on the space occupied by other atoms or chemical groups). Therefore, glycine often is found in bends or in the tightly packed chains of fibrous proteins.

Alanine and the branched-chain amino acids (valine, leucine, and isoleucine) have bulky, nonpolar, *aliphatic* (open-chain hydrocarbons) side chains and exhibit a high degree of hydrophobicity (see Table 6.1). Electrons are shared equally between the carbon and hydrogen atoms in these side chains, so that they cannot hydrogen bond with water. Within proteins, these amino acid side chains will cluster together to form hydrophobic cores. Their association is also promoted by van der Waals forces between the positively charged nucleus of one atom and the electron cloud of another. This force is effective over short distances when many atoms pack closely together.

The role of proline in amino acid structure differs from those of the nonpolar amino acids. The amino acid proline contains a ring involving its α-carbon and its α-amino group, which are part of the peptide backbone. It is an *imino acid*. This

Q The proteolytic digestive enzyme chymotrypsin cleaves the peptide bonds formed by the carboxyl groups of large, bulky uncharged amino acids. Which amino acids fall into this category?

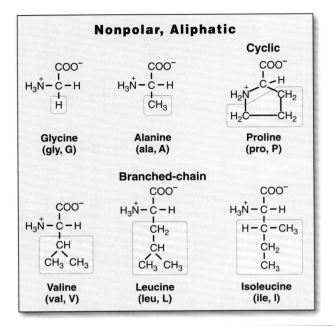

Nonpolar, Aliphatic

Glycine (gly, G)

Alanine (ala, A)

Cyclic

Proline (pro, P)

Branched-chain

Valine (val, V)

Leucine (leu, L)

Isoleucine (ile, I)

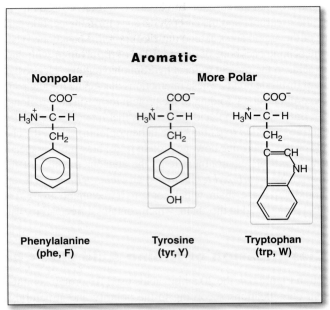

Aromatic

Nonpolar

Phenylalanine (phe, F)

More Polar

Tyrosine (tyr, Y)

Tryptophan (trp, W)

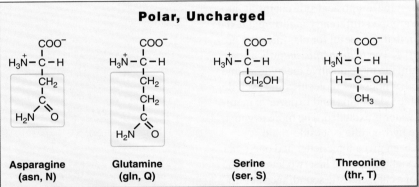

Polar, Uncharged

Asparagine (asn, N)

Glutamine (gln, Q)

Serine (ser, S)

Threonine (thr, T)

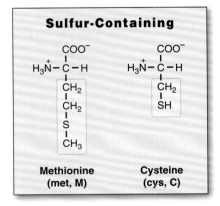

Sulfur-Containing

Methionine (met, M)

Cysteine (cys, C)

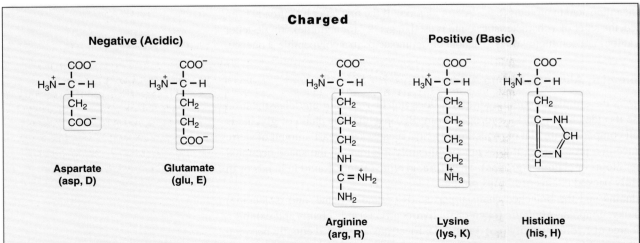

Charged

Negative (Acidic)

Aspartate (asp, D)

Glutamate (glu, E)

Positive (Basic)

Arginine (arg, R)

Lysine (lys, K)

Histidine (his, H)

FIGURE 6.4   The side chains of the amino acids. The side chains are *highlighted*. The amino acids are grouped by the polarity and structural features of their side chains. These groupings are not absolute, however. Tyrosine and tryptophan, often listed with the nonpolar amino acids, are more polar than other aromatic amino acids because of their phenolic and indole rings, respectively. The single-letter and three-letter codes are also indicated for each amino acid.

TABLE 6.1 Properties of the Common Amino Acids

AMINO ACID	PK$_{a1}$^{a} (CARBOXYL)	PK$_{a2}$ (AMINO)	PK$_{aR}$ (R GROUP)	HYDROPATHY INDEX^b
Nonpolar aliphatic				
Glycine	2.4	9.8		−0.4
Proline	2.0	11.0		−1.6
Alanine	2.3	9.7		1.8
Leucine	2.4	9.6		3.8
Valine	2.3	9.6		4.2
Isoleucine	2.4	9.7		4.5
Aromatic				
Phenylalanine	1.8	9.1		2.8
Tyrosine	2.2	9.1	10.5	−1.3
Tryptophan	2.4	9.4		−0.9
Polar uncharged				
Threonine	2.1	9.6	13.6	−0.7
Serine	2.2	9.2	13.6	−0.8
Asparagine	2.0	8.8		−3.5
Glutamine	2.2	9.1		−3.5
Sulfur-containing				
Cysteine	2.0	10.3	8.4	2.5
Methionine	2.3	9.2		1.9
Charged negative				
Aspartate	1.9	9.6	3.9	−3.5
Glutamate	2.2	9.7	4.1	−3.5
Charged positive				
Histidine	1.8	9.3	6.0	−3.2
Lysine	2.2	9.0	10.5	−3.9
Arginine	2.2	9.0	12.5	−4.5
Average	2.2	9.5		

^{a}When these amino acids reside in proteins, the pK$_a$ values for the side chains may vary to some extent from the value for the free amino acid, depending on the local environment of the amino acid in the three-dimensional structure of the protein.

^{b}The hydropathy index is a measure of the hydrophobicity of the amino acid (the higher the number, the more hydrophobic). Values based on Kyte J, Doolittle RF. A simple method for displaying the hydropathic character of a protein. J Mol Biol. 1982;157:105–132.

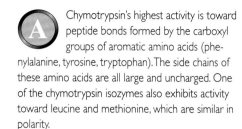

Chymotrypsin's highest activity is toward peptide bonds formed by the carboxyl groups of aromatic amino acids (phenylalanine, tyrosine, tryptophan). The side chains of these amino acids are all large and uncharged. One of the chymotrypsin isozymes also exhibits activity toward leucine and methionine, which are similar in polarity.

rigid ring causes a kink in the peptide backbone that prevents it from forming its usual configuration, and it will restrict the conformation of the protein at that point.

B. Aromatic Amino Acids

The *aromatic* amino acids have been grouped together because they all contain ring structures with similar properties, but their polarities differ a great deal. The aromatic ring is a six-membered carbon–hydrogen ring with three conjugated double bonds (the benzene ring or phenyl group). These hydrogen atoms do not participate in hydrogen bonding. The substituents on this ring determine whether the amino acid side chain engages in polar or hydrophobic interactions. In the amino acid phenylalanine, the ring contains no substituents and the electrons are shared equally between the carbons in the ring, resulting in a very nonpolar hydrophobic structure in which the rings can stack on each other (Fig. 6.5). In tyrosine, a hydroxyl group on the phenyl

A. Hydrophobic interaction

FIGURE 6.5 Hydrophobic and hydrogen bonds. **A.** Strong hydrophobic interactions occur with the stacking of aromatic groups in phenylalanine side chains. **B.** Examples of hydrogen bonds in which a hydrogen atom is shared by a nitrogen in the peptide backbone and an oxygen atom in an amino acid side chain or between an oxygen in the peptide backbone and an oxygen in an amino acid side chain. R, side chain.

Will S. has sickle cell anemia caused by a point mutation in his DNA that changes the sixth amino acid in the β-globin chain of hemoglobin from glutamate to valine. What difference would you expect to find in the chemical bonds formed by these two amino acids?

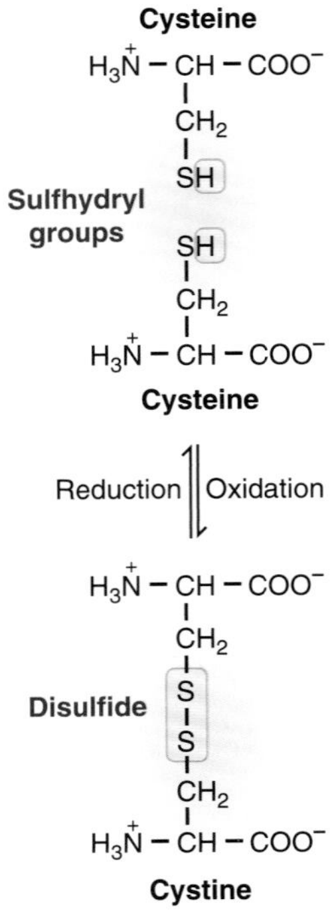

Cysteine

$$H_3\overset{+}{N} - CH - COO^-$$
$$|$$
$$CH_2$$
$$|$$
$$SH$$

Sulfhydryl groups

$$SH$$
$$|$$
$$CH_2$$
$$|$$
$$H_3\overset{+}{N} - CH - COO^-$$

Cysteine

Reduction ‖ Oxidation

$$H_3\overset{+}{N} - CH - COO^-$$
$$|$$
$$CH_2$$
$$|$$
Disulfide $$S$$
$$|$$
$$S$$
$$|$$
$$CH_2$$
$$|$$
$$H_3\overset{+}{N} - CH - COO^-$$

Cystine

FIGURE 6.6 A disulfide bond. Covalent disulfide bonds may be formed between two molecules of cysteine or between two cysteine residues in a protein. The disulfide compound is called cystine. The hydrogens of the cysteine sulfhydryl groups are removed during oxidation.

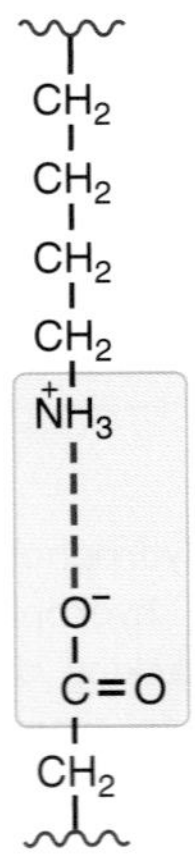

$$CH_2$$
$$|$$
$$CH_2$$
$$|$$
$$CH_2$$
$$|$$
$$CH_2$$
$$|$$
$$\overset{+}{N}H_3$$
$$\vdots$$
$$O^-$$
$$|$$
$$C = O$$
$$|$$
$$CH_2$$

FIGURE 6.7 Electrostatic interaction between the positively charged side chain of lysine and the negatively charged side chain of aspartate.

ring engages in hydrogen bonds, and the side chain is therefore more polar and more hydrophilic. The more complex ring structure in tryptophan is an indole ring with a nitrogen that can engage in hydrogen bonds. Tryptophan is therefore also more polar than phenylalanine.

C. Aliphatic, Polar, Uncharged Amino Acids

Amino acids with side chains that contain an amide group (asparagine and glutamine) or a hydroxyl group (serine and threonine) can be classified as aliphatic, polar, uncharged amino acids. Asparagine and glutamine are amides of the amino acids aspartate and glutamate. The hydroxyl groups and the amide groups in the side chains allow these amino acids to form hydrogen bonds with water, with each other and the peptide backbone, or with other polar compounds in the binding sites of the proteins (see Fig. 6.5). As a consequence of their hydrophilicity, these amino acids are frequently found on the surface of water-soluble globular proteins. Cysteine, which is sometimes included in this class of amino acids, has been separated into the class of sulfur-containing amino acids.

D. Sulfur-Containing Amino Acids

Both cysteine and methionine contain sulfur. The side chain of cysteine contains a sulfhydryl group that has a pK_a of approximately 8.4 for dissociation of its hydrogen, so cysteine is predominantly undissociated and uncharged at the physiologic pH of 7.4. The free cysteine molecule in solution can form a covalent disulfide bond with another cysteine molecule through spontaneous (nonenzymatic) oxidation of their sulfhydryl groups. The resultant amino acid, cystine, is present in blood and tissues and is not very water-soluble. In proteins, the formation of a cystine disulfide bond between two appropriately positioned cysteine sulfhydryl groups often plays an important role in holding two polypeptide chains or two different regions of a chain together (Fig. 6.6). *Methionine*, although it contains a sulfur group, is a nonpolar amino acid with a large, bulky side chain that is hydrophobic. It does not contain a sulfhydryl group and cannot form disulfide bonds. Its important and central role in metabolism is related to its ability, when appropriately activated, to transfer the methyl group attached to the sulfur atom to other compounds.

E. The Acidic and Basic Amino Acids

The amino acids aspartate and glutamate have carboxylic acid groups that carry a negative charge at physiologic pH (see Fig. 6.4). The basic amino acids histidine, lysine, and arginine have side chains containing nitrogen that can be protonated and positively charged at physiologic and lower pH values. Histidine has a nitrogen-containing imidazole ring for a side chain, lysine has a primary amino group on the ε-carbon (from the sequence α, β, γ, δ, ε), and arginine has a guanidinium group.

The positive charges on the basic amino acids enable them to form ionic bonds (electrostatic bonds) with negatively charged groups, such as the side chains of acidic amino acids or the phosphate groups of coenzymes (Fig. 6.7). In addition, lysine and arginine side chains often form ionic bonds with negatively charged compounds bound to the protein binding sites, such as the phosphate groups in adenosine triphosphate (ATP). The acidic and basic amino acid side chains also participate in hydrogen bonding and the formation of salt bridges (e.g., the binding of an inorganic ion such as Na$^+$ between two partially or fully negatively charged groups).

The charge on these amino acids at physiologic pH is a function of their pK_a for dissociation of protons from the α-carboxylic acid groups, the α-amino groups, and the side chains. The titration curve of histidine illustrates the changes in amino acid structure that occurs as the pH of the solution is changed from <1 to 14 by the addition of hydroxide ions (Fig. 6.8). At low pH, all groups carry protons, amino groups have a positive charge, and carboxylic acid groups have zero charge. As the pH is increased by the addition of alkali (OH$^-$), the proton dissociates from the carboxylic

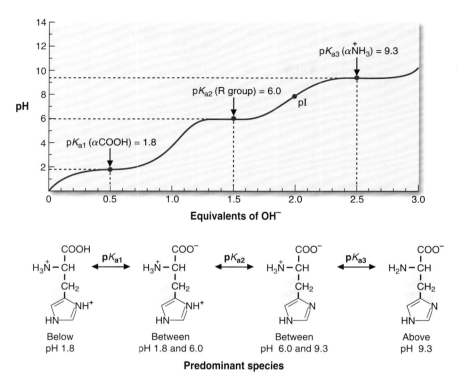

Predominant species

FIGURE 6.8 Titration curve of histidine. The ionic species that predominates in each region is shown below the graph. *pI* is the isoelectric point (the pH at which there is no net charge on the molecule). pK, −log acid dissociation constant; R, side chain.

acid group and its charge changes from 0 to −1 with a pK_a of approximately 2, the pH at which 50% of the protons have dissociated.

The histidine side chain is an imidazole ring with a pK_a of approximately 6 that changes from a predominantly protonated positively charged ring to an uncharged ring at this pH. The amino group on the α-carbon titrates at a much higher pH (between 9 and 10), and the charge changes from +1 to 0 as the pH rises. The pH at which the net charge on the molecules in solution is 0 is called the *isoelectric point* (pI). At this pH, the molecules will not migrate in an electric field toward either a positive pole (cathode) or a negative pole (anode) because the number of negative charges on each molecule is equal to the number of positive charges.

Amino acid side chains change from uncharged to negatively charged, or positively charged to uncharged as they release protons (Fig. 6.9). The acidic amino acids lose a proton from their carboxylic acid side chains at a pH of approximately 4 and are thus negatively charged at pH 7.4. Cysteine and tyrosine lose protons at their pK_a (~8.4 and 10.5, respectively), so their side chains are uncharged at physiologic pH. Histidine, lysine, and arginine side chains change from positively charged to neutral at their pK_a. The side chains of the two basic amino acids arginine and lysine have pK_a values >10, so that the positively charged form always predominates at physiologic pH. The side chain of histidine (pK_a ~6.0) dissociates near physiologic pH, so only a portion of the histidine side chains carries a positive charge (see Fig. 6.8).

In proteins, only the amino acid side chains, the amino group at the amino terminal, and the carboxyl group at the carboxyl terminal have dissociable protons. All of the other carboxylic acid and amino groups on the α-carbons are joined in peptide bonds that have no dissociable protons. The amino acid side chains might have very different pK_a values than those of the free amino acids if they are involved in hydrogen or ionic bonds with other amino acid side chains. The pK_a of the imidazole group of histidine, for example, is often shifted to a higher value between 6 and 7 so that it adds and releases a proton in the physiologic pH range.

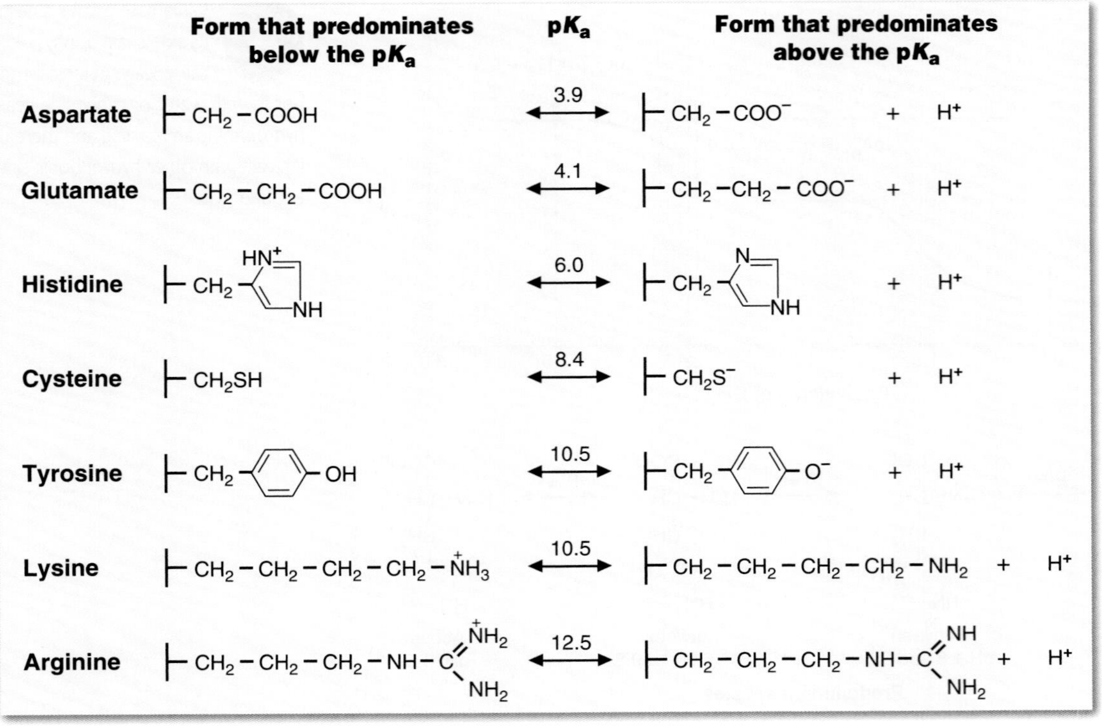

	Form that predominates below the pK_a	pK_a	Form that predominates above the pK_a
Aspartate	—CH$_2$—COOH	3.9	—CH$_2$—COO$^-$ + H$^+$
Glutamate	—CH$_2$—CH$_2$—COOH	4.1	—CH$_2$—CH$_2$—COO$^-$ + H$^+$
Histidine	—CH$_2$—(HN$^+$ ring, NH)	6.0	—CH$_2$—(N ring, NH) + H$^+$
Cysteine	—CH$_2$SH	8.4	—CH$_2$S$^-$ + H$^+$
Tyrosine	—CH$_2$—(ring)—OH	10.5	—CH$_2$—(ring)—O$^-$ + H$^+$
Lysine	—CH$_2$—CH$_2$—CH$_2$—CH$_2$—$\overset{+}{N}$H$_3$	10.5	—CH$_2$—CH$_2$—CH$_2$—CH$_2$—NH$_2$ + H$^+$
Arginine	—CH$_2$—CH$_2$—CH$_2$—NH—C$\overset{\overset{+}{N}H_2}{\diagdown NH_2}$	12.5	—CH$_2$—CH$_2$—CH$_2$—NH—C$\overset{NH}{\diagdown NH_2}$ + H$^+$

FIGURE 6.9   Dissociation of the side chains of the amino acids. As the pH increases, the charge on the side chain goes from 0 to negative (−) or from positive (+) to 0. The pK_a is the pH at which half the molecules of an amino acid in solution have side chains that are charged. Half are uncharged. pK_a, −log acid dissociation constant.

Is the substitution of a glutamate for a valine in sickle cell hemoglobin a conservative replacement? What about the substitution of an aspartate for a glutamate?

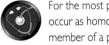

For the most part, human chromosomes occur as homologous pairs, with each member of a pair containing the same genetic information. One member of the pair is inherited from the mother and one from the father. Genes are arranged linearly along each chromosome. A genetic locus is a specific position or location on a chromosome. Alleles are alternative versions of a gene at a given locus. For each locus (site), we have two alleles of each gene, one from our mother and one from our father. If both alleles of a gene are identical, the individual is homozygous for this gene; if the alleles are different, the individual is heterozygous for this gene. **Will S.** has two identical alleles for the sickle variant of the β-globin gene that results in substitution of a valine for a glutamate residue at the sixth position of the β-globin chain. He is therefore homozygous for the sickle cell allele and has sickle cell anemia. Individuals with one normal gene and one sickle cell allele are heterozygous. They are carriers of the disease and have sickle cell trait.

Electrophoresis, a technique used to separate proteins on the basis of charge, has been extremely useful in medicine to identify proteins with different amino acid compositions. The net charge on a protein at a certain pH is a summation of all of the positive and negative charges on all of the ionizable amino acid side chains plus the *N*-terminal amino and *C*-terminal carboxyl groups. Theoretically, the net charge of a protein at any pH could be determined from its amino acid composition by calculating the concentration of positively and negatively charged groups from the Henderson-Hasselbalch equation (see Chapter 4). However, hydrogen bonds and ionic bonds between amino acid side chains in the protein, which can alter pK_a values, make this calculation unrealistic.

III. Variations in Primary Structure

The primary structure of a protein is its linear sequence of amino acids. Although almost every amino acid in the primary structure of a protein contributes to its conformation (three-dimensional structure), the primary structure of a protein can vary to some degree between species. Even within the human species, the amino acid sequence of a normal functional protein can vary somewhat among individuals, tissues of the same individual, and the stage of development. These variations in the primary structure of a functional protein are tolerated if they are confined to noncritical regions (called *variant regions*), if they are conservative substitutions (replace one amino acid with one of similar structure), or if they confer an advantage. If many different amino acid residues are tolerated at a position, the region is called *hypervariable*. In contrast, the regions that form binding sites or are critical for forming a functional three-dimensional structure are usually *invariant* regions that have exactly the same amino acid sequence from individual to individual, tissue to tissue, or species to species.

A. Polymorphism in Protein Structure

Within the human population, the primary structure of a protein may vary slightly among individuals. The variations generally arise from mutations in DNA that are passed to the next generation. The mutations can result from the substitution of one base for another in the DNA sequence of nucleotides (a point mutation), from deletion or insertions of bases into DNA, or from larger changes (see Chapter 14). For many alleles, the variation has a distinct phenotypic consequence that contributes to our individual characteristics, produces an obvious dysfunction (a congenital or inherited disease), or increases susceptibility to certain diseases. A defective protein may differ from the most common allele by as little as a single amino acid that is a nonconservative substitution (replacement of one amino acid with another of a different polarity or very different size) in an invariant region. Such mutations might affect the ability of the protein to carry out its function, catalyze a particular reaction, reach the appropriate site in a cell, or be degraded. For other proteins, the variations appear to have no significance.

Variants of an allele that occur with a significant frequency in the population are referred to as *polymorphisms*. Thus far in studies of the human genome, almost one-third of the genetic loci appear to be polymorphic. When a particular variation of an allele, or polymorphism, increases in the general population to a frequency of $>1\%$, it is considered stable. The sickle cell allele is an example of a point mutation that is stable in the human population. Its persistence is probably the result of selective pressure for the heterozygous mutant phenotype, which confers some protection against malaria.

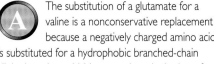 The substitution of a glutamate for a valine is a nonconservative replacement because a negatively charged amino acid is substituted for a hydrophobic branched-chain aliphatic amino acid. However, the substitution of an aspartate for a glutamate is a conservative replacement because the two amino acids have the same polarity and are nearly the same size.

B. Protein Families and Superfamilies

A homologous family of proteins is composed of proteins related to the same ancestral protein. Groups of proteins with similar, but not identical, structure and function that have evolved from the same gene after the gene was duplicated are called *paralogs* and are considered members of the same protein family. Once a gene has duplicated, one gene can continue to perform the original function, and the second copy can mutate into a protein with another function or another type of regulation. This process is called *divergent evolution*. Very large families of homologous proteins are called a *superfamily*, which is subdivided by name into families of proteins with the most similarity in structure.

The paralogs of a protein family are considered to be different proteins and have different names because they have different functions. They are all present in the same individual. Myoglobin and the different chains of hemoglobin, for example, are paralogs and members of the same globin family that have similar, but not identical, structures and functions. Myoglobin, an intracellular heme protein present in most cells that stores and transports O_2 to mitochondria, is a single polypeptide chain containing one heme oxygen-binding site. In contrast, hemoglobin is composed of four globin chains, each with a heme oxygen-binding site that is present in red blood cells; hemoglobin transports O_2 from the lungs to tissues. The gene for myoglobin is assumed to have evolved from gene duplication of the α-chain for hemoglobin, which evolved from duplication of the β-chain. Figure 6.10 compares a region of the structure of myoglobin and the α- and β-chains of hemoglobin. Among these three proteins, only 15 invariant (identical) residues are present, but many of the other amino acid residues are conservative substitutions.

C. Tissue and Developmental Variations in Protein Structure

Within the same individual, different *isoforms* or *isozymes* of a protein may be synthesized during different stages of fetal and embryonic development, may be present in different tissues, or may reside in different intracellular locations. Isoforms of a protein all have the same function. If they are isozymes (isoforms of enzymes), they catalyze the same reactions. However, isoforms have somewhat different properties and amino acid structure.

Will S.'s hemoglobin, HbS, is composed of two normal α-chains and two β-globin chains with the sickle cell variant ($\alpha_2\beta_2^S$). The change in amino acid composition from a glutamate to a valine in the β-chain allows sickle hemoglobin to be separated from normal adult hemoglobin (HbA, or $\alpha_2\beta_2^A$) by electrophoresis. In electrophoresis, an aliquot of blood or other solution containing proteins is applied to a support, such as paper or a gel. An electrical field is applied and the proteins migrate a distance toward the anode (negative pole) or cathode (positive pole) depending on their net charge. Because β^S contains one less negative charge than β^A, it will migrate differently in an electric field. Individuals with sickle cell trait are heterozygous and express both HbA and HbS, plus small amounts of HbF (fetal hemoglobin, $\alpha_2\gamma_2$).

In heterozygous individuals with sickle cell trait, the sickle cell allele provides some protection against malaria. Malaria is caused by the parasite *Plasmodium falciparum*, which spends part of its life cycle in red blood cells. The infected red blood cells of individuals with normal hemoglobin (HbA) develop protrusions that attach to the lining of capillaries. This attachment occludes the vessels and prevents oxygen from reaching cells in the affected region, resulting in cell death. In heterozygous individuals, HbS in infected cells aggregates into long fibers that cause the cell to become distorted. These distorted cells containing the malarial parasite are preferentially recognized by the spleen and are rapidly destroyed, thus ending the life of the parasite.

In **Will S.** and other homozygous individuals with sickle cell anemia, the red blood cells sickle more frequently than in heterozygotes, especially under conditions of low oxygen tension (see Chapter 7). The result is a vaso-occlusive crisis in which the sickled cells clog capillaries and prevent oxygen from reaching cells (ischemia), thereby causing pain. The enhanced destruction of the sickled cells by the spleen results in anemia. Consequently, the sickle cell allele is of little advantage to homozygous individuals.

Because heterozygous individuals occur more frequently in a population than homozygous individuals, a selective advantage in a heterozygous state can outweigh a disadvantage in a homozygous state, causing the mutation to become a stable polymorphism in a population. As a consequence, the frequency of sickle cell anemia in parts of equatorial Africa in which malaria was endemic in the past is 1 in 25 births. Migration from Africa accounts for the high frequency of sickle cell anemia among African Americans in the United States, which is approximately 1/400 at birth.

	1		5			10			15	
Myoglobin	gly-----leu-ser-asp-gly-glu-trp-gln-leu-val-leu-asn-val-trp-gly-lys-val-
β-chain hemoglobin	val-his-leu-thr-pro-glu-glu-lys-ser-ala-val-thr-ala-leu-trp-gly-lys-val-
α-chain hemoglobin	val-----leu-ser-pro-ala-asp-lys-thr-asn-val-lys-ala-ala-trp-gly-lys-val-
ζ-chain hemoglobin	met-ser-leu-thr-lys-thr-glu-arg-thr-ile-ile-val-ser-met-trp-ala-lys-ile-
γ-chain hemoglobin	met-gly-his-phe-thr-glu-glu-asp-lys-ala-thr-ile-thr-ser-leu-trp-gly-lys-val-

FIGURE 6.10 The primary structures of a region in human globin proteins. To compare the primary structure of two homologous polypeptide chains, the sequences are written left to right from the amino terminal to the carboxyl terminal. The sequences are aligned with computer programs that maximize the identity of amino acids and minimize the differences caused by segments that are present in one protein and not in the other. Gaps in the structure, indicated with *dashes*, are introduced to maximize the alignment between proteins in structure comparisons. They are assumed to coincide with mutations that caused a deletion. Regions of sequence similarity (identity and conservative substitution) are indicated by *colored bars*. Within these regions are smaller regions of invariant residues that are exactly the same from protein to protein. Myoglobin is a single polypeptide chain. The α- and β-chains are part of hemoglobin A ($\alpha_2\beta_2$). The ζ-chain is part of embryonic hemoglobin ($\zeta_2\varepsilon_2$). The γ-chain is part of fetal hemoglobin (HbF), $\alpha_2\gamma_2$.

1. Developmental Variation

Hemoglobin isoforms provide an example of variation during development. Hemoglobin (Hb) is expressed as the fetal isozyme HbF during the last trimester of pregnancy until after birth, when it is replaced with HbA. HbF is composed of two hemoglobin α and two hemoglobin γ polypeptide chains, in contrast to the adult hemoglobin, HbA, which has two α- and two β-chains. During the embryonic stages of development, chains with a different amino acid composition, the embryonic ε- and ζ-chains, are produced (see Fig. 6.10). These differences are believed to arise evolutionarily from mutation of a duplicated α gene to produce ζ, and mutation of a duplicate α gene to produce ε. The fetal and embryonic forms of hemoglobin have a much higher affinity for O_2 than the adult forms and thus confer an advantage at the low O_2 tensions to which the fetus is exposed. At different stages of development, the globin genes specific for that stage are expressed and translated. (This is discussed in more detail in Chapter 42, Section V.)

2. Tissue-Specific Isoforms

Proteins that differ somewhat in primary structure and properties from tissue to tissue, but that retain essentially the same function, are called *tissue-specific isoforms* or *isozymes*. The enzyme creatine kinase (CK) is an example of a protein that exists as tissue-specific isozymes, each composed of two subunits with 60% to 72% sequence homology (similarity between sequences). Of the two CKs that bind to the muscle sarcomere, the M form is produced in skeletal muscle and the B polypeptide chains are produced in the brain. The protein is composed of two subunits; therefore, skeletal muscle produces an MM creatine kinase and the brain produces a BB form. The heart produces both types of chains and thus forms a heterodimer, MB, as well as the homodimers. Two more CK isozymes are found in mitochondria—a heart mitochondrial CK and the "universal" isoform found in other tissues. In general, most proteins that are present in both the mitochondria and cytosol will be present as different isoforms. The advantage conferred on different tissues by having their own isoform of CK is unknown. However, tissue-specific isozymes such as MB creatine kinase are useful in diagnosing sites of tissue injury and cell death.

The structure of proteins involved in the response to hormones has been studied in greater depth than many other types of proteins, and most of these proteins are present as several tissue-specific isoforms that help different tissues respond

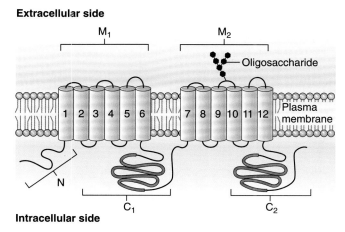

Extracellular side

FIGURE 6.11 Invariant regions in the isoforms of adenylyl cyclase. The invariant regions are on the cytosolic side of the membrane in the C_1 and C_2 loops shown in *red*. These amino acid residues participate in the catalytic function of the enzyme, synthesis of 3′,5′-cyclic adenosine monophosphate. The protein also has several helical regions that span the membrane (M_1 and M_2 helices), represented as *tubes*. An oligosaccharide chain is attached to an extracellular domain. *N* is the amino terminus. (From Taussig R, Gilman AG. Mammalian membrane-bound adenylyl cyclases. *J Biol Chem.* 1995;270:1–4.)

differently to the same hormone. One of these proteins present in cell membranes is *adenylyl cyclase*, an enzyme that catalyzes the synthesis of intracellular 3′,5′-cyclic adenosine monophosphate (cAMP) (Fig. 6.11). In human tissues, at least nine different isoforms of adenylyl cyclase are coded by different genes in different tissues. Although they have an overall sequence homology of 50%, the two intracellular regions involved in the synthesis of cAMP are an invariant consensus sequence with a 93% identity. The different isoforms help cells respond differently to the same hormone.

D. Species Variations in the Primary Structure of Insulin

Species variations in primary structure are also important in medicine, as illustrated by the comparison of human, beef, and pork insulins. *Insulin* is one of the hormones that are highly conserved between species, with very few amino acid substitutions and none in the regions that affect activity. Insulin is a polypeptide hormone of 51 amino acids that is composed of two polypeptide chains (Fig. 6.12). It is synthesized as a single polypeptide chain but is cleaved in three places before secretion to form the C peptide and the active insulin molecule containing the A and B chains. The folding of the A and B chains into the correct three-dimensional structure is promoted by the presence of one intrachain and two interchain disulfide bonds formed by cysteine residues. The invariant residues consist of the cysteine residues engaged in disulfide bonds and the residues that form the surface of the insulin molecule that binds to the insulin receptor. The amino acid substitutions in bovine and porcine insulins (shown in *red* in Fig. 6.12) are not in amino acids that affect its activity. Consequently, insulins from beef and pork were used for many years for the treatment of diabetes mellitus. However, even with only a few different amino acids, some patients developed an immune response to these forms of insulin.

IV. Modified Amino Acids

After synthesis of a protein has been completed, a few amino acid residues in the primary sequence may be further modified in enzyme-catalyzed reactions that add a chemical group, oxidize, or otherwise modify specific amino acids in the protein. Because protein synthesis occurs by a process known as *translation*, these changes

 A myocardial infarction (heart attack) is caused by an atheromatous obstruction and/or a severe spasm in a coronary artery that prevents the flow of blood to an area of heart muscle distal to the obstruction. Thus, heart cells in this region suffer from a lack of oxygen and blood-borne fuel. Because the cells cannot generate ATP, the membranes become damaged, and enzymes leak from the cells into the blood.

The blood test of choice to determine whether cell damage has occurred is the cTnT level. Creatine kinase (see next paragraph) was originally used for this determination, but the introduction of very sensitive assays for troponin led to the recommendation of using cTnT measurements to follow the course of heart damage.

Creatine kinase (CK or CPK) assays are still performed at some hospitals. The protein is composed of two subunits, which may be either of the muscle (M) or the brain (B) type. The MB form, containing one M and one B subunit, is found primarily in cardiac muscle. It can be separated electrophoretically from other CK isozymes and the amount in the blood used to determine whether a myocardial infarction has occurred. On admission to the hospital, **Anne J.'s** total CK was 182 U/L (reference range = 38 to 174 U/L).

 Although bovine (beef) insulin is identical to human insulin in those amino acid residues essential for activity, the amino acid residues that are in the variable regions can act as antigens and stimulate the formation of antibodies against bovine insulin. Consequently, recombinant DNA techniques have been used for the synthesis of human insulins, such as Humulin (intermediate acting) or Humalog (rapid acting, also known as *lispro*) (see Chapter 17 for information on recombinant DNA technology.) There are no longer animal-sourced insulins manufactured in the United States.

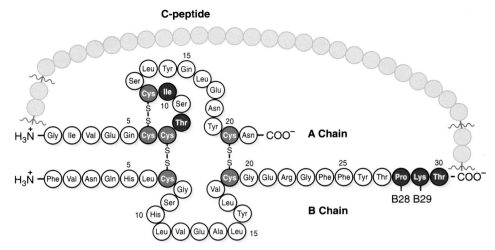

FIGURE 6.12 The primary structure of human insulin. The substituted amino acids in bovine (beef) and porcine (pork) insulin are shown in *red*. Threonine 30 at the carboxyl terminal of the B chain is replaced by alanine in both beef and pork insulin. In beef insulin, threonine 8 on the A chain is also replaced with alanine, and isoleucine 10 with valine. The cysteine residues, which form the disulfide bonds (shown in *blue*) holding the chains together, are invariant. In the bioengineered insulin Humalog (lispro insulin), the positions of proline at B28 and lysine at B29 are switched. Insulin is synthesized as a longer precursor molecule, proinsulin, which is one polypeptide chain. Proinsulin is converted to insulin by proteolytic cleavage of certain peptide bonds (*wavy lines* in the figure). The cleavage removes a few amino acids and the 31-amino acid C-peptide that connects the A and B chains. The active insulin molecule thus has two nonidentical chains.

are called *posttranslational modification*. More than 100 different posttranslationally modified amino acid residues have been found in human proteins. These modifications change the structure of one or more specific amino acids on a protein in a way that may serve a regulatory function, target or anchor the protein in membranes, enhance a protein's association with other proteins, or target it for degradation (Fig. 6.13). Posttranslational modifications usually occur once the protein has already folded into its three-dimensional conformation.

A. Glycosylation

Glycosylation refers to the addition of carbohydrates to a molecule. In *O*-glycosylation, oligosaccharides (small carbohydrate chains) are bound to serine or threonine residues in proteins by *O*-linkages. In *N*-glycosylation, the carbohydrates are bound by *N*-linkage to the amide nitrogen of asparagine (see Fig. 6.13). *N*-Linked oligosaccharides are found attached to cell surface proteins, where they protect the cell from proteolysis or an immune attack. In contrast, an *O*-glycosidic link is a common way of attaching oligosaccharides to the serine or threonine hydroxyl groups in secreted proteins. The intracellular polysaccharide glycogen is attached to a protein through an *O*-glycosidic linkage to a tyrosine. Adenylyl cyclase is an example of an enzyme that is posttranslationally modified (see Fig. 6.11). It has an oligosaccharide chain attached to the external portion of the protein.

B. Fatty Acylation or Prenylation

The addition of lipids to a molecule is called *fatty acylation*. Many membrane proteins contain a covalently attached lipid group that interacts hydrophobically with lipids in the membrane. Palmitoyl groups (C16) often are attached to plasma membrane proteins, and the myristoyl group (C14) often is attached to proteins in the lipid membranes of intracellular vesicles (myristoylation; see Fig. 6.13). Prenylation involves the addition of the farnesyl group (C15) or geranylgeranyl groups (C20), which are synthesized from the five-carbon isoprene unit (isopentenyl pyrophosphate; see Fig. 5.1A). These are attached in thioether linkage to a specific cysteine residue of certain membrane proteins, particularly proteins involved in regulation.

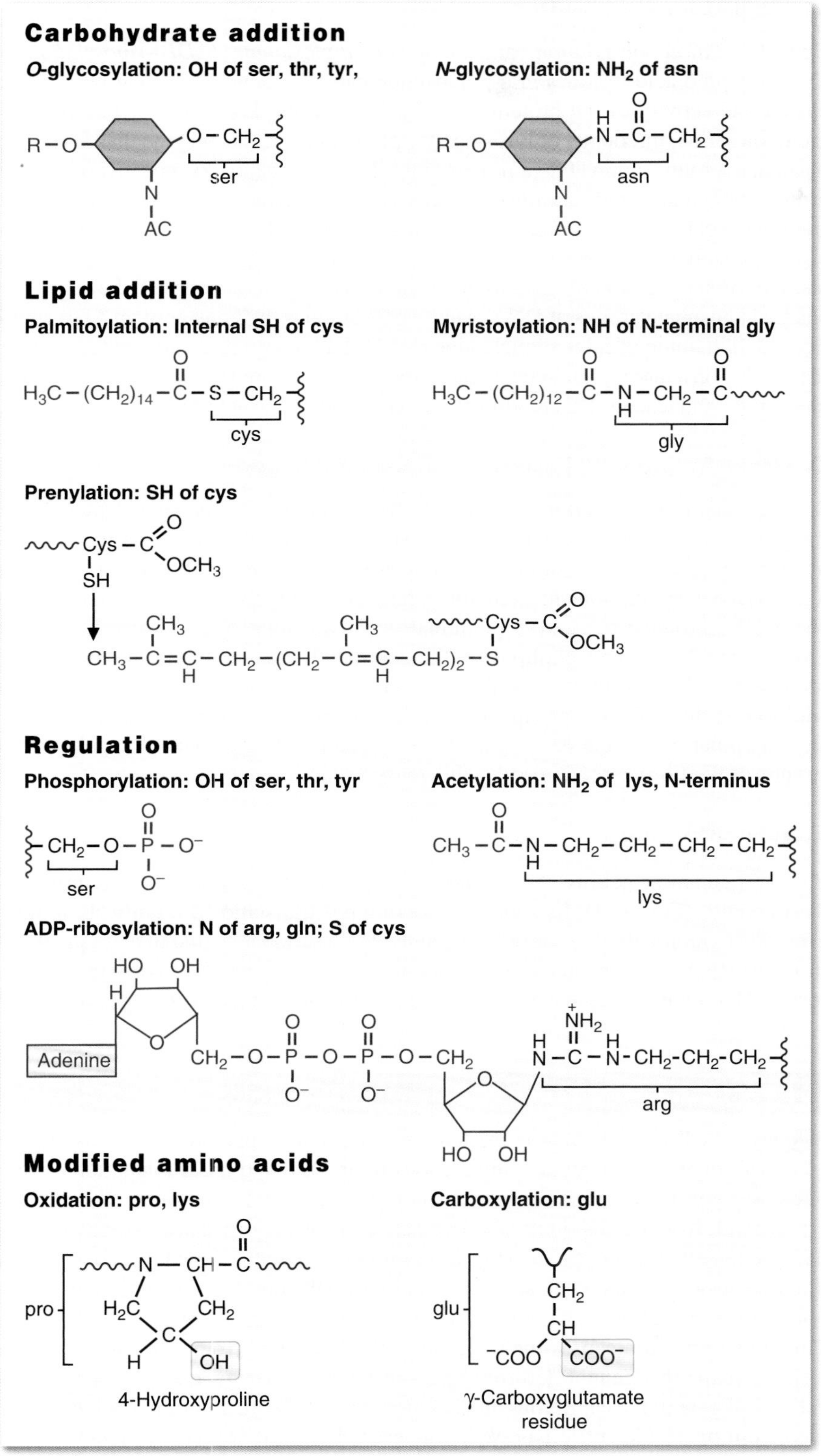

Carbohydrate addition

O-glycosylation: OH of ser, thr, tyr,

N-glycosylation: NH₂ of asn

Lipid addition

Palmitoylation: Internal SH of cys

Myristoylation: NH of N-terminal gly

Prenylation: SH of cys

Regulation

Phosphorylation: OH of ser, thr, tyr

Acetylation: NH₂ of lys, N-terminus

ADP-ribosylation: N of arg, gln; S of cys

Modified amino acids

Oxidation: pro, lys

4-Hydroxyproline

Carboxylation: glu

γ-Carboxyglutamate
residue

FIGURE 6.13 Posttranslational modifications of amino acids in proteins. Some of the common amino acid modifications and the sites of attachment are illustrated. The added group is shown in *red*. Because these modifications are catalyzed by enzymes, only a specific amino acid in the primary sequence is altered. *R–O–* represents additional carbohydrates attached to the first carbohydrate. In *N*-glycosylation, the attached sugar is usually *N*-acetylglucosamine (*N*-Ac).

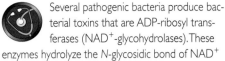

Several pathogenic bacteria produce bacterial toxins that are ADP-ribosyl transferases (NAD⁺-glycohydrolases). These enzymes hydrolyze the N-glycosidic bond of NAD⁺ and transfer the ADP-ribose portion to a specific amino acid residue on a protein in the affected human cell. Cholera AB toxin, a pertussis toxin, and a diphtheria toxin are all ADP-ribosyl transferases.

C. Regulatory Modifications

Phosphorylation, acetylation, and *adenosine diphosphate (ADP)-ribosylation* of specific amino acid residues in a polypeptide can alter bonding by that residue and change the activity of the protein (see Fig. 6.13). Phosphorylation of the hydroxyl group on serine, threonine, or tyrosine by a protein kinase (an enzyme that transfers a phosphate group from ATP to a protein) introduces a large, bulky, negatively charged group that can alter the structure and activity of a protein. Some of the isozymes of adenylyl cyclase contain serine residues on the intracellular portion of the protein that can be phosphorylated by a protein kinase. Reversible acetylation occurring on lysine residues of histone proteins in chromatin changes their interaction with the negatively charged phosphate groups of DNA. ADP-ribosylation is the transfer of an ADP-ribose from nicotinamide adenine dinucleotide (NAD⁺) to an arginine, glutamine, or cysteine residue on a target protein in the membrane (primarily in leukocytes, skeletal muscles, brain, and testes). This modification may regulate the activity of these proteins.

D. Other Amino Acid Posttranslational Modifications

Several other posttranslational modifications of amino acid side chains alter the activity of the protein in the cell (see Fig 6.13). Carboxylation of the γ-carbon of glutamate (carbon 4) in certain blood-clotting proteins is important for attaching the clot to a surface. Calcium ions mediate this attachment by binding to the two negatively charged carboxyl groups of γ-glutamate and two additional negatively charged groups provided by phospholipids in the cell membrane. Collagen, an abundant fibrous extracellular protein, contains the oxidized amino acid hydroxyproline. The addition of the hydroxyl group (hydroxylation) to the proline side chain provides an extra polar group that can engage in hydrogen bonding between the polypeptide strands of the fibrous protein and stabilize its structure.

E. Selenocysteine

The unusual amino acid *selenocysteine* is found in a few enzymes and is required for their activity (Fig. 6.14). Its synthesis is not a posttranslational modification, however, but a modification to serine that occurs while serine is bound to a unique tRNA (transfer RNA; see Chapter 15). A selenium atom replaces the hydroxyl group of serine. The selenocysteine is then inserted into the protein as it is being synthesized.

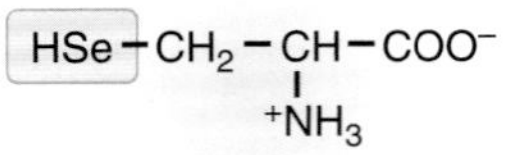

$$HSe-CH_2-\underset{\underset{^+NH_3}{|}}{CH}-COO^-$$

Selenocysteine

FIGURE 6.14 Selenocysteine.

CLINICAL COMMENTS

Will S. Will S. was treated for 3 days with parenteral (not by mouth/digestion) narcotics, intravenous hydration, and nasal inhalation of oxygen for his vaso-occlusive crisis. The diffuse severe pains of sickle cell crises result from occlusion of small vessels in a variety of tissues, thereby causing damage to cells from ischemia (low blood flow) or hypoxia (low levels of oxygen). Vaso-occlusion occurs when sickle hemoglobin (HbS) molecules in red blood cells polymerize in the lumen of capillaries, where the partial pressure of O_2 (pO_2) is low. This polymerization causes the red blood cells to change from a biconcave disc to a sickle shape that cannot deform to pass through the narrow capillary lumen. The cells aggregate in the capillaries and occlude blood flow. In addition, once he recovered from his sickle cell crisis, Will was treated with hydroxyurea therapy, which increases the production of red blood cells containing HbF. HbF molecules cannot participate in sickling and can decrease the frequency at which sickle crises occur.

Will's acute symptoms gradually subsided. Patients with sickle cell anemia periodically experience sickle cell crises, and Will's physician urged him to seek medical help whenever symptoms reappeared. He also counseled him to try to avoid triggers of sickle cell crisis: overexertion, dehydration, extremely cold weather, and exposure to tobacco.

David K. David has cystinuria, a relatively rare disorder, with a prevalence that ranges between 1 in 2,500 and 1 in 15,000 births, depending on the population studied. It is a genetically determined disease with a complex recessive mode of inheritance resulting from allelic mutations. These mutations lead to a reduction in the activity of renal tubular cell transport proteins that normally carry cystine from the tubular lumen into the renal tubular cells. The transport of the basic amino acids (lysine, arginine, and ornithine, an amino acid found in the urea cycle but not in proteins) also is often compromised, and they appear in the urine.

Because cystine is produced by oxidation of cysteine, conservative treatment of cystinuria includes decreasing the amount of cysteine within the body and, therefore, the amount of cystine eventually filtered by the kidneys. Reduction of cysteine levels is accomplished by restricting dietary methionine, which contributes its sulfur to the pathway for cysteine formation. To increase the amount of cystine that remains in solution, the volume of fluid ingested daily is increased. Crystallization of cystine is further prevented by chronically alkalinizing the urine. Finally, drugs may be administered to enhance the conversion of urinary cystine to more soluble compounds. If these conservative measures fail to prevent continued cystine stone formation, existing stones may be removed by a surgical technique that involves sonic fracture of the stones. The fragmented stones may then pass spontaneously or may be more easily extracted surgically because of their smaller size.

Dianne A. Dianne A.'s treatment was initially changed from beef insulin to Humulin (synthetic human insulin; Lilly USA, LLC, Indianapolis, IN). Humulin is mass-produced by recombinant DNA techniques that insert the human DNA sequences for the insulin A and B chains into the *Escherichia coli* or yeast genome (see Chapter 17). The insulin chains that are produced are then extracted from the media and treated to form the appropriate disulfide bonds between the chains. As costs have fallen for production of the synthetic human insulins, they have replaced pork insulin and the highly antigenic beef insulin.

Dianne's physician then recommended that she take Humalog (Lilly USA, LLC), an insulin preparation containing lispro, an ultrafast-acting bioengineered insulin analog in which lysine at position B29 has been moved to B28 and proline at B28 has been moved to B29 (hence, lispro) (see Fig. 6.12). With lispro, Dianne will be able to time her injections of this rapidly acting insulin minutes before her consumption of carbohydrate-containing meals rather than having to remember to give herself an insulin injection 1 hour before a meal. Dianne will also take a long-acting insulin shot once a day (Lantus; Sanofi US, Bridgewater, NJ), along with her Humalog shots prior to meals each day.

Anne J. Mrs. J. continued to be monitored in the cardiac care unit. The physicians followed the trends of TnT in her blood. Historically, physicians would also follow the total CK and CK-MB levels. Within 2 hours of the onset of an acute myocardial infarction, the MB form of CK begins leaking from heart cells that were injured by the ischemic process. These rising serum levels of the MB fraction (and, therefore, of the total CK) reach their peak 12 to 36 hours later and usually return to normal within 3 to 5 days from the onset of the infarction (Fig. 6.15).

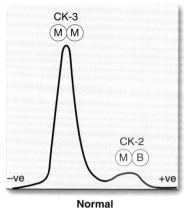

Creatine kinase isozymes in blood

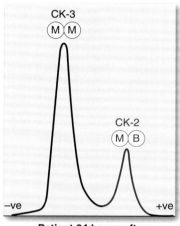

FIGURE 6.15 Electrophoretic separation of serum creatine kinase (CK) enzymes from a normal healthy adult and from a patient who had a myocardial infarction 24 hours previously. CK catalyzes the reversible transfer of a phosphate from ATP to creatine to form phosphocreatine and adenosine diphosphate. The reaction is an important part of energy metabolism in heart muscle, skeletal muscle, and brain. Three different forms of the dimer exist: BB (or CK-1) found in brain, MB (or CK-2) found only in heart (indicated in *red*), and MM (or CK-3), found only in skeletal and heart muscle. −ve, cathode; +ve, anode.

BIOCHEMICAL COMMENTS

Nucleic Acid, Enzyme, and Protein Databases. Large databases of nucleic acid sequences and protein structure have been assembled to collate data from various laboratories around the world. The National Library of Medicine maintains a Web site, PubMed, which catalogs the medical literature, and a search engine allows you to search for reference articles by topic or author (www.ncbi.nlm .nih.gov/pubmed). From the menu, you can enter a nucleic acid, protein, or a structure

The switch in position of amino acids in lispro does not affect the action of this synthetic insulin on cells because it is not in a critical invariant region, but it does affect the ability of insulin to bind zinc. Normally, human insulin is secreted from the pancreas as a zinc hexamer in which six insulin molecules are bound to the zinc atom. When zinc insulin is injected, the binding to zinc slows the absorption from the subcutaneous (under the skin) injection site. Lispro cannot bind zinc to form a hexamer, and thus, it is absorbed much more quickly than other forms of insulin.

database directly. These databases are linked, so you can type in the name of a protein, such as *human hemoglobin chain A*, obtain a list of contributors to sequence data, and retrieve a complete amino acid sequence for many proteins. You can link to PubMed to find recent articles about the protein, or you can link to the structure database. A program called *Cn3D* can be downloaded from this site that allows you to view three-dimensional versions of the protein structures.

These databases are only a few of more than 500 biologic databases that have been assembled to collate and exchange biologic information in the areas of DNA, RNA, genomics, gene mapping, and protein structure. The first issue of the *Journal of Nucleic Acid Research* each year provides a description of currently available biologic databases. Their goal is to provide information that can relate a particular DNA sequence or mutation to the protein involved, to its function, and to the pathologic consequences of a particular amino acid substitution by comparing proteins that have similar functional elements.

Two of the very useful databases accessible to scientists are GenBank (https://www.ncbi.nlm.nih.gov/genbank/) and the RCSB (Research Collaboratory for Structural Bioinformatics) protein data bank (www.rcsb.org/pdb/home/home.do). GenBank is a nucleic acid sequence database, which is linked to the DNA Data Bank of Japan (DDBJ) and the European Molecular Biology Laboratory (EMBL) database. The three databases exchange information every day, so all are current. GenBank allows for submission of new sequences as well as searches for existing sequences. One can also perform a BLAST search (Basic Logical Alignment Search Tool) to compare a nucleic acid sequence of unknown origin with those in the database to detect comparable sequences in existing genes and to garner an understanding of what the gene from which the unknown sequence was obtained may do.

The RCSB protein data bank allows one to search for proteins, to examine the amino acid sequence of the protein (and the nucleic acid sequence which led to the protein sequence; see Section III of this text), and to visualize the protein's structure in a three-dimensional format. One can also search the database with an amino acid sequence from a protein with no known function to determine if other proteins contain similar sequences, which will give clues as to the function of the unknown protein.

The field of bioinformatics is developing new tools for scientists to appropriately mine the large amount of data becoming available through nucleic acid and protein structure databases. Will these databases be of any use to the practicing physician or to the practice-oriented medical student? Very few students will ever want to do protein modeling. However, students and physicians may wish to use the literature search in PubMed as part of their approach to evidence-based medicine. They also may wish to use it to track definitions or fundamental knowledge about particular topics. Thus, biomedical and basic science textbooks are also being linked to PubMed.

KEY CONCEPTS

- A protein's unique characteristics, including its three-dimensional folded structure, are dictated by its linear sequence of amino acids, termed its primary structure.
- The primary structures of all of the diverse human proteins are synthesized from 20 amino acids arranged in a linear sequence determined by the genetic code.
- Each three-base (nucleotide) sequence within the coding region of a gene (the genetic code) specifies which amino acid should be present in a protein. The genetic code is discussed further in Chapter 12.
- All amino acids contain a central α-carbon joined to a carboxylic acid group, an amino group, a hydrogen, and a side chain, which varies among the 20 different amino acids.
- At physiologic pH, the amino acids are zwitterions; the amino group is positively charged, and the carboxylate is negatively charged.

- In proteins, amino acids are joined into linear polymers called *polypeptide chains* via peptide bonds, which are formed between the carboxylic acid of one amino acid and the amino group of the next amino acid.
- Amino acid side chains can be classified either by polarity (charged, nonpolar hydrophobic, or uncharged polar) or structural features (aliphatic, cyclic, or aromatic).
- Depending on their side-chain characteristics, certain amino acids cluster together to exclude water (hydrophobic effect), whereas others participate in hydrogen bonding. Cysteine can form disulfide bonds, whereas charged amino acids can form ionic bonds.
- Amino acids in proteins can be modified by phosphorylation, carboxylation, or other reactions after the protein is synthesized (posttranslational modifications).
- Alterations in the genetic code may lead to mutations in the protein's primary structure, which can affect the protein's function.
- Proteins with the same function but different primary structures (isoforms and isozymes) can exist in different tissues or during different phases of development.
- Diseases discussed in this chapter are summarized in Table 6.2.

TABLE 6.2   Diseases Discussed in Chapter 6

DISORDER OR CONDITION	GENETIC OR ENVIRONMENTAL	COMMENTS
Sickle cell anemia	Genetic	Single amino acid replacement at the sixth position of the β-chain of hemoglobin, leading to an E6V alteration (instead of glutamic acid at position 6, a valine is in its place)
Cystinuria	Genetic	Inability to appropriately transport cystine, leading to its accumulation in the kidney and the formation of kidney stones
Type I diabetes	Both	Understanding the structure of insulin, and how it is absorbed at injection sites, allows various forms of insulin to be synthesized that are either rapidly or slowly absorbed. This provides patients who have type I diabetes with a variety of treatment options.
Myocardial infarction	Both	Primarily environmental factors, which can be exacerbated by genetic conditions. The release of heart-specific isozymes into the circulation is diagnostic for a heart attack.

REVIEW QUESTIONS—CHAPTER 6

1. Sickle cell anemia is caused by a single nucleotide change in DNA that leads to the substitution of one amino acid (E6V) in the β-chain. This one change in the primary sequence leads to the ability of the deoxygenated form of HbS to form polymers. As the polymers grow in size, the shape of the red blood cell is altered to accommodate the chains of hemoglobin. Which one of the following primarily dictates the polymerization of deoxygenated HbS?
   A. The peptide backbone
   B. Ionic interactions
   C. Hydrophobic interactions
   D. Hydrogen bonds
   E. Peptide bonds

2. One of the main sources of nonvolatile acid in the body is sulfuric acid generated from the sulfur-containing compounds in ingested food or from the metabolism of the sulfur-containing amino acids. Which of the following amino acids would lead to sulfuric acid formation?
   A. Cysteine and isoleucine
   B. Cysteine and alanine
   C. Cysteine and methionine
   D. Methionine and isoleucine
   E. Isoleucine and alanine

3. Dianne A.'s different preparations of insulin contain some insulin complexed with protamine that is absorbed slowly after injection. Protamine is a protein preparation from rainbow trout sperm containing arginine-rich peptides that bind insulin. Which one of the following provides the best explanation for complex formation between protamine and insulin?
   A. Arginine is a basic amino acid that binds to negatively charged amino acid side chains in insulin.
   B. Arginine is a basic amino acid that binds to the α-carboxylic acid groups at the N-terminals of insulin chains.
   C. Arginine is a large, bulky hydrophobic amino acid that complexes with leucine and phenylalanine in insulin.
   D. Arginine forms disulfide bonds with the cysteine residues that hold the A and B chains together.
   E. Arginine has a side chain that forms peptide bonds with the carboxyl terminals of the insulin chains.

4. Phosphorylation of proteins is an important component of signal transduction. Protein kinases phosphorylate proteins only at certain hydroxyl groups on amino acid side chains. Which of the following groups of amino acids contain side-chain hydroxyl groups and could be a potential substrate for a protein kinase?
   A. Aspartate, glutamate, and serine
   B. Serine, threonine, and tyrosine
   C. Threonine, phenylalanine, and arginine
   D. Lysine, arginine, and proline
   E. Alanine, asparagine, and serine

5. A protein's activity is altered when a particular serine side chain is phosphorylated. Which of the following amino acid substitutions at this position could lead to a permanent alteration in normal enzyme activity?
   A. S→E
   B. S→T
   C. S→Y
   D. S→K
   E. S→L

6. Proteins, which are composed of amino acids, help transport lipids in the bloodstream. These proteins need to be able to cluster with other nonpolar molecules and exclude water. Which of the following would best describe the side chains of these amino acids in the lipid transport proteins?
   A. A more positive hydropathic index
   B. A more negative hydropathic index
   C. A neutral hydropathic index
   D. A pK_a of the primary carboxylic acid group of approximately 2
   E. A pK_a of the α-amino group of approximately 9.5

7. A patient with high cholesterol begins taking a statin medication and develops myalgias (muscle soreness and aches). The physician orders CK (creatine kinase) levels to check for muscle damage, a known side effect of statins. Lab results show a higher than normal level of CK-MM. Which one of the following best describes CK-MM?
   A. Heterodimer
   B. Isozyme
   C. Produced by the brain
   D. Produced by the heart
   E. Produced by the liver

8. All of the amino acids that are used to synthesize human proteins (with the exception of glycine) have which one of the following in common?
   A. An aromatic group
   B. A hydroxyl group
   C. An asymmetric carbon in the D-configuration
   D. An asymmetric carbon in the L-configuration
   E. An asymmetric β-carbon

9. Questions 9 and 10 refer to the following patient:
   A patient with recurrent kidney stones is found to have an inherited amino acid substitution in a transport protein that reabsorbs certain amino acids from the glomerular filtrate so they are not lost in the urine.
   Which of the following amino acid groups are not reabsorbed from the glomerular filtrate in this disease process?
   A. Cysteine, methionine, and arginine
   B. Cysteine, methionine, and lysine
   C. Cysteine, arginine, and lysine
   D. Methionine, arginine, and lysine
   E. Methionine, arginine, and histidine

10. Which one of the following amino acids is most responsible for this patient's recurrent kidney stones?
    A. Cysteine
    B. Methionine
    C. Arginine
    D. Lysine
    E. Histidine

ANSWERS

1. **The answer is C.** In the sickle version of hemoglobin, a valine has replaced a glutamate in the sixth position of the β-chain. In the deoxygenated state, the valine forms hydrophobic interactions with a hydrophobic patch on another sickle hemoglobin molecule, leading to polymerization of the hemoglobin molecules. The primary interaction is not the result of ionic interactions or hydrogen bonding; it is the hydrophobic interactions between molecules that initiate the polymerization. The peptide backbone, along with peptide bonds, can participate in hydrogen bonding but does not play a role in polymerization.

2. **The answer is C.** Cysteine and methionine are the sulfur-containing amino acids. Isoleucine and alanine are both nonpolar hydrophobic amino acids, and neither contains sulfur.

3. **The answer is A.** Arginine is a basic amino acid that has a positively charged side chain at neutral pH. It can, therefore, form tight electrostatic bonds with negatively charged asp and glu side chains in insulin. The α-carboxylic acid groups at the *N*-terminals of proteins are bound through peptide bonds (thus, B is incorrect). The arginine side chain is not hydrophobic, and it cannot form disulfide bonds because it has no sulfhydryl group (thus, C and D are incorrect). Its basic group is a ureido group that cannot form peptide bonds (see E).

4. **The answer is B.** Only these amino acids—serine, threonine, and tyrosine—have side-chain hydroxyl groups. As a general rule, serine–threonine protein kinases form one group of protein kinases, and tyrosine protein kinases form another.

5. **The answer is A.** Adding a phosphate group to the serine side chain adds negative charges to the side chain, allowing ionic interactions to develop. These new ionic interactions allow the protein to change shape and to alter its activity. Substituting a glutamate for the serine adds a negative charge to this location within the protein, which may participate in ionic interactions and lead to a shape change in the protein. None of the other suggested mutations (serine to either threonine [which adds a hydroxyl group, just as serine has], to tyrosine [again, another hydroxyl containing amino acid side-chain], to lysine [adding a positive charge rather than a negative charge], or to leucine [a totally hydrophobic side chain]) will lead to the insertion of negative charges at this location in the protein.

6. **The answer is A.** The hydropathic index is a scale that denotes the hydrophobicity of the side chains. The more positive the hydropathic index, the greater the hydrophobicity of the side chain. The pK_a of the primary carboxylic acid group for all the amino acids is around 2 and the pK_a of the α-amino groups of all the amino acids is approximately 9.5, but these elements of the protein do not contribute to the protein's hydrophobic nature.

7. **The answer is B.** Proteins that differ somewhat in primary structure from tissue to tissue but retain essentially the same function are called *tissue-specific isoforms* or *isozymes*. CK is a classic example of this. Muscle produces the M form, brain the B form, and heart both, leading to an MB form (a heterodimer). Because the protein consists of two subunits, muscle produces CK-MM, a homodimer. By measuring specific isozymes of CK one can determine if there is skeletal muscle damage (CK-MM) or heart-specific damage (elevated levels of CK-MB).

8. **The answer is D.** Each of the amino acids used for protein synthesis has the same general structure. Each contains a carboxylic acid group, an amino group attached to the α-carbon, a hydrogen atom, and a side chain. When the α-carbon is asymmetric, the configuration about that carbon is in the L-configuration. Glycine is excluded because its side chain is a hydrogen atom, and there is no asymmetric carbon atom in glycine.

9. **The answer is C.** The patient described has cystinuria, an inherited amino acid substitution in the transport protein that reabsorbs cysteine, arginine, and lysine from the glomerular filtrate. Therefore, these amino acids cannot be returned to the blood and the urine contains large amounts of these amino acids.

10. **The answer is A.** Cysteine will be oxidized to form cystine (a dimer of cysteine linked by a disulfide bond). Cystine is less soluble than the other amino acids indicated as answers and precipitates in the kidney, forming renal stones (kidney stones or calculi). Cystine also is found in the urine in elevated amounts, leading to cystinuria.

7 Structure–Function Relationships in Proteins

Diseases can be caused by changes in protein structure that affect the protein's ability to bind other molecules and carry out its function. They also can be caused by conformational changes in proteins that affect their solubility and degradability. In amyloidosis/AL, immunoglobulin chains form an insoluble protein aggregate called *amyloid* in organs and tissues. Alzheimer disease and familial amyloid polyneuropathy are neurodegenerative diseases characterized by the deposition of amyloid. Prion diseases result from misfolding and aggregation of a normal cellular protein. Even in sickle cell anemia, the mutation in hemoglobin principally affects the quaternary structure of hemoglobin and its solubility and not its ability to bind oxygen.

A multitude of different proteins can be formed from only 20 common amino acids because these amino acids can be linked together in an enormous variety of sequences determined by the genetic code. The sequence of amino acids, its primary structure, determines the way a protein folds into a unique three-dimensional structure, which is its native conformation. Once it is folded, the three-dimensional structure of a protein forms binding sites for other molecules, thereby dictating the function of the protein in the body. In addition to creating binding sites, a protein must fold in such a way that it is flexible, stable, able to function in the correct site in the cell, and capable of being degraded by cellular enzymes.

Levels of Protein Structure. Protein structure is described in terms of four different levels: primary, secondary, tertiary, and quaternary (Fig. 7.1). The **primary structure** of a protein is the linear sequence of amino acids in the polypeptide chain. **Secondary structure** consists of local regions of polypeptide chains formed into structures that are stabilized by a repeating pattern of hydrogen bonds, such as the regular structures called α-helices and β-sheets. The **rigidity of the peptide backbone** determines the types of secondary structure that can occur. The **tertiary structure** involves folding of the secondary structural elements into an overall three-dimensional conformation. In **globular proteins** such as **myoglobin**, the tertiary structure generally forms a densely packed **hydrophobic core** with polar amino acid side chains on the outside. Some proteins exhibit **quaternary structure**, the combination of two or more **subunits**, each composed of a polypeptide chain.

Domains and Folds. The tertiary structure of a globular protein can be made up of structural **domains**, regions of structure that fold independently. Multiple domains can be linked together to form a functional protein. Within a domain, a combination of secondary structural elements forms a fold, such as the **nucleotide binding fold** or an **actin fold**. Folds are defined by their similarity in several different proteins.

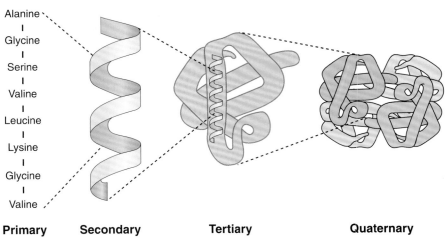

Alanine
|
Glycine
|
Serine
|
Valine
|
Leucine
|
Lysine
|
Glycine
|
Valine

Primary   **Secondary**   **Tertiary**   **Quaternary**

FIGURE 7.1   Levels of structure in a protein.

Quaternary Structure. Assembly of globular polypeptide subunits into a multisubunit complex can provide the opportunity for **cooperative binding** of ligands (e.g., O_2 binding to hemoglobin), form **binding sites** for complex molecules (e.g., antigen binding to immunoglobulin), and increase **stability** of the protein. The polypeptide chains of **fibrous proteins** such as **collagen** are aligned along an axis, have repeating elements, and are extensively linked to each other through hydrogen and covalent bonds.

Ligand Binding. Proteins form binding sites for specific molecules, called **ligands** (e.g., adenosine triphosphate [ATP] or O_2), or for another protein. The affinity of a binding site for its ligand is characterized quantitatively by an **association** or **affinity constant, K_a (or its dissociation constant [K_d], in which $K_d = 1/K_a$).**

Folding of Proteins. The primary structure of a protein dictates the way that it folds into its tertiary structure, which is a **stable conformation** that is identical to the shape of other molecules of the same protein (i.e., its **native conformation**). **Chaperonins** act as templates to overcome the kinetic and thermodynamic barrier to reaching a stable conformation. **Prion proteins** cause neurodegenerative diseases by acting as a template for misfolding. Heat, acid, and other agents cause proteins to **denature**; that is, to unfold or refold and lose their native three-dimensional conformation.

THE WAITING ROOM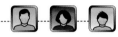

 Will S., who has sickle cell anemia, was readmitted to the hospital with symptoms indicating that he was experiencing another sickle cell crisis (see Chapter 6). Sickle cell disease is a result of improper aggregation of hemoglobin within red blood cells.

 Anne J. is a 54-year-old woman who arrived in the hospital 4 days ago, about 5 hours after she began to feel chest pain (see Chapter 6). In the emergency department, the physician drew blood for the measurement of cardiac troponin T subunit (cTnT), and the muscle–brain fraction (CK-MB) of creatine kinase. The results from these tests had supported the diagnosis of an acute myocardial infarction (MI), and Mrs. J. was hospitalized. Subtle differences in the structure of similar proteins in different tissues were used diagnostically to come to this conclusion.

 Amy L. is a 62-year-old woman who presented with weakness, fatigue, an enlarged tongue (macroglossia), and edema. She had signs and symptoms of cardiac failure, including electrocardiographic abnormalities. Initial laboratory studies showed a serum creatinine of 1.9 mg/dL (reference range [females] = 0.5 to 1.1 mg/dL), indicating mild renal failure. A urinalysis indicated the presence of a moderate proteinuria. She was subsequently diagnosed with amyloidosis/AL secondary to a plasma cell dyscrasia. *Amyloidosis* is a term that encompasses many diseases that share as a common feature the extracellular deposition of pathologic insoluble fibrillar proteins called *amyloid* in organs and tissues. In **Amy L.'s** disease, amyloidosis/AL, the amyloid is derived from immunoglobulin light chains (AL-5 amyloidosis, light-chain–related) and is the most common form of amyloidosis.

 Dianne A. returned to her physician's office for a routine visit to monitor her treatment (see Chapters 4, 5, and 6). Her physician drew blood for an HbA1c (pronounced "hemoglobin A-1-c") determination. Her HbA1c was 8.5%, which was above the normal level of <6.0% for a person without diabetes, and <7.0% for a person with controlled diabetes.

The simplest test to detect protein in the urine is the use of specific reagent test strips. The strips are coated with tetrabromophenol blue, buffered at pH 3.0. In the presence of protein, the indicator dye is no longer as responsive to changes in pH as in the absence of protein. A yellow color indicates that protein is not detectable; as protein levels increase, the yellow color changes, going to green and then bluish-green. This is a useful qualitative test (which detects primarily serum albumin), but to be more quantitative, different dyes, which react specifically with particular amino acid side chains, are used. Different tests are required to detect the presence of a specific protein in the urine or sera, and these will be discussed in subsequent chapters.

I. General Characteristics of Three-Dimensional Structure

The overall conformation of a protein, the particular position of the amino acid side chains in three-dimensional space, determines the function of the protein.

A. Descriptions of Protein Structure

Proteins are generally grouped into major structural classifications: globular proteins, fibrous proteins, and transmembrane proteins. *Globular proteins* are usually soluble in aqueous medium and resemble irregular balls. The *fibrous proteins* are geometrically linear, arranged around a single axis, and have a repeating unit structure. Another general classification, *transmembrane proteins*, consists of proteins that have one or more regions aligned to cross the lipid membrane (see Fig. 6.11). *DNA-binding proteins*, although a member of the globular protein family, are sometimes classified separately and are considered in Chapter 16.

The structure of proteins is often described according to levels called *primary*, *secondary*, *tertiary*, and *quaternary structure* (see Fig. 7.1). The *primary structure* is the linear sequence of amino acid residues joined through peptide bonds to form a polypeptide chain. The *secondary structure* refers to recurring structures (e.g., the regular structure of the α-helix) that form in short localized regions of the polypeptide chain. The overall three-dimensional conformation of a protein is its *tertiary structure*, the summation of its secondary structural elements. The *quaternary structure* is the association of polypeptide subunits in a geometrically specific manner. The forces involved in a protein folding into its final conformation are primarily noncovalent interactions. These interactions include the attraction between positively and negatively charged molecules (ionic interactions), the hydrophobic effect, hydrogen bonding, and van der Waals interactions (the nonspecific attraction between closely packed atoms).

B. Requirements of the Three-Dimensional Structure

The overall three-dimensional structure of a protein must meet certain requirements to enable the protein to function in the cell or extracellular medium of the body. The first requirement is the creation of a binding site that is specific for just one molecule or a group of molecules with similar structural properties. The specific binding sites of a protein usually define its role. The three-dimensional structure must also exhibit the degrees of flexibility and rigidity appropriate to its specific function. Some rigidity is essential for the creation of binding sites and for a stable structure (i.e., a protein that is excessively flexible would have the potential to be dysfunctional). However, flexibility and mobility in structure enables the protein to fold as it is synthesized and to adapt as it binds other proteins and small molecules. The three-dimensional structure must have an external surface that is appropriate for its environment (e.g., cytoplasmic proteins need to keep polar amino acids on the surface to remain soluble in an aqueous environment). In addition, the conformation must also be stable, with little tendency to undergo refolding into a form that cannot fulfill its function or that precipitates in the cell. Finally, the protein must have a structure that can de degraded when it is damaged or no longer needed in the cell.

II. The Three-Dimensional Structure of the Peptide Backbone

The amino acids in a polypeptide chain are joined sequentially by peptide bonds between the carboxyl group of one amino acid and the amide group of the next amino acid in the sequence (Fig. 7.2). Usually, the peptide bond assumes a *trans* configuration in which successive α-carbons and their R groups are located on opposite sides of the peptide bond.

The polypeptide backbone can bend in a very restricted way. The peptide bond itself is a hybrid of two *resonance structures*, one of which has double-bond character, so that the carboxyl and amide groups that form the bond must remain planar (see Fig. 7.2). However, rotation within certain allowed angles (torsion angles) can occur around the bond between the α-carbon and the α-amino group and around the bond between the α-carbon and the carbonyl group. This rotation is subject to steric

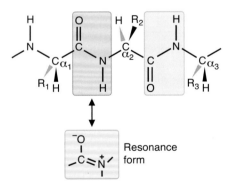

FIGURE 7.2 The peptide backbone. Because of the resonant nature of the peptide bond, the C and N of the peptide bonds form a series of rigid planes. Rotation within allowed torsion angles can occur around the bonds attached to the α-carbon. The side chains are *trans* to each other and alternate above and below the peptide chain. The actual peptide bond is a hybrid between the resonance forms shown, resulting in a partial negative charge on the carbonyl oxygen, a partial positive charge on the nitrogen, and partial double-bond character for the peptide bond itself.

constraints that maximize the distance between atoms in the different amino acid side chains and prohibit torsion (rotation) angles that place the side-chain atoms too close to each other. These folding constraints, which depend on the specific amino acids present, limit the secondary and tertiary structures that can be formed from the polypeptide chain.

III. Secondary Structure

Regions within polypeptide chains form recurring, localized structures known as *secondary structures*. The two regular secondary structures called the *α-helix* and the *β-sheet* contain repeating elements formed by hydrogen bonding between atoms of the peptide bonds. Other regions of the polypeptide chain form nonregular, nonrepetitive secondary structures such as loops and coils.

A. The α-Helix

The α-helix is a common secondary structural element of globular proteins, membrane-spanning domains, and DNA-binding proteins. It has a rigid, stable conformation that maximizes hydrogen bonding while staying within the allowed rotation angles of the polypeptide backbone. The peptide backbone of the α-helix is formed by hydrogen bonds between each carbonyl oxygen atom and the amide hydrogen (N–H) of an amino acid residue located four residues farther down the chain (Fig. 7.3). Thus, each peptide bond is connected by hydrogen bonds to the peptide bond four amino acid residues ahead of it and four amino acid residues behind it in the amino acid sequence. The core of the helix is tightly packed, thereby maximizing association energies between atoms. The *trans* side chains of the amino acids project backward and outward from the helix, thereby avoiding steric hindrance with the polypeptide backbone and with each other (Fig. 7.4). The amino acid proline, because of its ring structure, cannot form the necessary bond angles to fit within an α-helix. Thus, proline is known as a "helix breaker" and is not found in α-helical regions of proteins.

B. β-Sheets

β-Sheets are a second type of regular secondary structure that maximizes hydrogen bonding between the peptide backbones while maintaining the allowed torsion angles. In β-sheets, the hydrogen bonding usually occurs between regions of separate neighboring polypeptide strands aligned parallel to each other (Fig. 7.5A). Thus, the carbonyl oxygen of one peptide bond is hydrogen-bonded to the amide hydrogen of a peptide bond on an adjacent strand. This pattern contrasts with the α-helix, in which the peptide backbone hydrogen bonds are located within the same strand. Optimal hydrogen bonding occurs when the sheet is bent (pleated) to form β-pleated sheets.

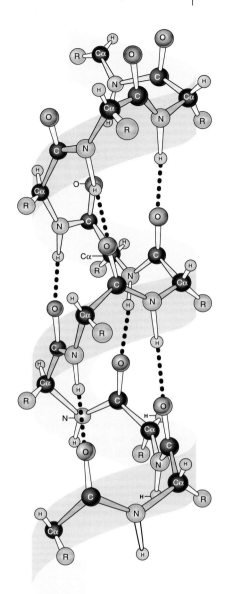

FIGURE 7.3 The α-helix. Each oxygen atom of a carbonyl group of a peptide bond forms a hydrogen bond (indicated by the *black dots*) with the hydrogen atom attached to a nitrogen atom in a peptide bond four amino acids further along the chain. The result is a highly compact and rigid structure.

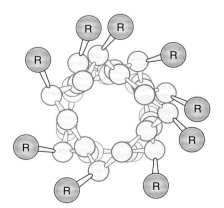

FIGURE 7.4 A view down the axis of an α-helix. The side chains (*R*) jut out from the helix. Steric hindrance occurs if they come within their van der Waals radii of each other, and a stable helix cannot form.

A

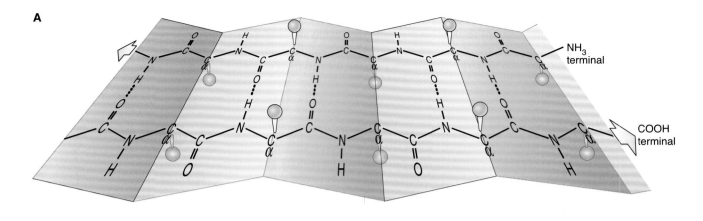

B

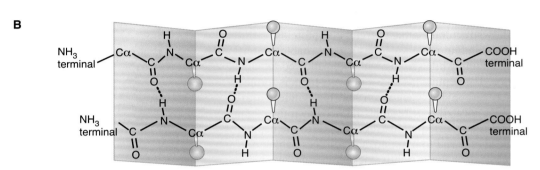

FIGURE 7.5 **A.** A β-pleated sheet. In this case, the chains are oriented in opposite directions (antiparallel). The *large arrows* show the direction of the carboxyl terminus. The amino acid side chains (R) in one strand are *trans* to each other and alternate above and below the plane of the sheet, which can have a hydrophobic face and a polar face that engages in hydrogen bonding. **B.** Hydrogen bonding pattern with parallel β-strands.

The β-pleated sheet is described as parallel if the polypeptide strands run in the same direction (as defined by their amino and carboxyl terminals) and antiparallel if they run in opposite directions. Antiparallel strands are often the same polypeptide chain folded back on itself, with simple hairpin turns or long runs of polypeptide chain connecting the strands. The amino acid side chains of each polypeptide strand alternate between extending above and below the plane of the β-sheet (see Fig. 7.5). Parallel sheets tend to have hydrophobic residues on both sides of the sheets; antiparallel sheets usually have a hydrophobic side and a hydrophilic side. Frequently, sheets twist in one direction.

The hydrogen-bonding pattern is slightly different depending on whether one examines a parallel or antiparallel β-sheet (see Fig. 7.5B). In an antiparallel sheet, the atoms involved in hydrogen bonding are directly opposite each other; in a parallel β-sheet, the atoms involved in the hydrogen bonding are slightly skewed from one another, such that one amino acid is hydrogen-bonded to two others in the opposite strand.

C. Nonrepetitive Secondary Structures

α-Helices and β-pleated sheets are patterns of regular structure with a repeating element—the ordered formation of hydrogen bonds. In contrast, bends, loops, and turns are nonregular secondary structures that do not have a repeating element of hydrogen bond formation. They are characterized by an abrupt change of direction and are often found on the protein surface. For example, β-turns are short regions that usually involve four successive amino acid residues. They often connect strands of antiparallel β-sheets (Fig. 7.6). The surface of large globular proteins usually has at least one omega loop: a structure with a neck like the capital Greek letter omega (Ω).

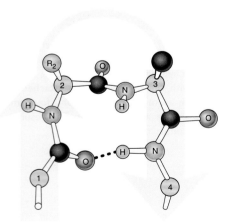

FIGURE 7.6 β-Turn. The four amino acid residues that form the β-turn (also called a *hairpin loop*) are held together by hydrogen bonds, which make this an extremely stable structure. The Cα carbons of the amino acids are *numbered* in the figure.

D. Patterns of Secondary Structure

Figure 7.7 is a three-dimensional drawing of a globular domain in the soluble enzyme lactate dehydrogenase (LDH). It illustrates the combination of secondary structural elements to form patterns. This LDH domain is typical of globular proteins, which average approximately 31% α-helical structure and approximately 28% β-pleated sheets (with a wide range of variation). The helices of globular domains have an average span of approximately 12 residues, corresponding to approximately three to four helical turns, although many are much longer. The β-sheets, represented in diagrams by an *arrow* for each strand, are an average of six residues long and six strands wide (2 to 15 strands). Like the β-sheet in the LDH domain, they generally twist to the right rather than lie flat (see Fig. 7.7). Most globular domains, such as this LDH domain, also contain motifs. *Motifs* are relatively small arrangements of secondary structure that are recognized in many different proteins. For example, certain of the β-strands are connected with α-helices to form the βα βα β structural motif.

The remaining polypeptide segments connecting the helices and β-sheets are said to have a coil or loop conformation (see Fig. 7.7). Although some of the connecting segments recognized in many proteins have been given names (like the Ω-loops), other segments such as those in this LDH domain appear disordered or irregular. These nonregular regions, generally called *coils*, should never be referred to as "random coils." They are neither truly disordered nor random; they are stabilized through specific hydrogen bonds dictated by the primary sequence of the protein and do not vary from one molecule of the protein to another of the same protein.

The nonregular coils, loops, and other segments are usually more flexible than the relatively rigid helices and β-pleated sheets. They often form hinge regions that allow segments of the polypeptide chain to move as a compound binds or to move as the protein folds around another molecule.

IV. Tertiary Structure

The tertiary structure of a protein is the pattern of the secondary structural elements folding into a three-dimensional conformation, as shown for the LDH domain in Figure 7.7. The three-dimensional structure is flexible and dynamic, with rapidly fluctuating movement in the exact positions of amino acid side chains and domains. These fluctuating movements take place without unfolding of the protein. They allow ions and water to diffuse through the structure and provide alternative conformations for ligand binding. As illustrated with examples later in this chapter, this three-dimensional structure is designed to serve all aspects of the protein's function. It creates specific and flexible binding sites for *ligands* (the compounds that bind), illustrated with actin and myoglobin. The tertiary structure also maintains residues on the surface appropriate for the protein's cellular location, polar residues for cytosolic proteins, and hydrophobic residues for transmembrane proteins (illustrated with the β₂-adrenergic receptor). Flexibility is one of the most important features of protein structure. The forces that maintain tertiary structure are hydrogen bonds, ionic bonds, van der Waals interactions, the hydrophobic effect, and disulfide bond formation.

A. Domains in the Tertiary Structure

The tertiary structure of large complex proteins is often described in terms of physically independent regions called *structural domains*. You can usually identify domains from visual examination of a three-dimensional figure of a protein, such as the three-dimensional figure of G-actin shown in Figure 7.8. Each domain is formed from a continuous sequence of amino acids in the polypeptide chain that are folded into a three-dimensional structure independently of the rest of the protein, and two

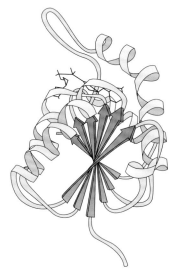

Lactate dehydrogenase domain 1

FIGURE 7.7 Ribbon drawing showing the arrangement of secondary structures into a three-dimensional pattern in domain 1 of lactate dehydrogenase. The individual polypeptide strands in the six-stranded β-sheet are shown with *arrows*. Different strands are connected by helices and by nonrepetitive structures (turns, coils, and loops). This domain is the nucleotide binding fold. Nicotinamide adenine dinucleotide (NAD⁺) is bound to a site created by the helices (*upper left* of figure). (Modified from Richardson JS. The anatomy and taxonomy of protein structure. *Adv Protein Chem*. 1981;34:167.)

A renal biopsy used in the diagnosis of **Amy L.'s** disease showed amorphous deposits in the glomeruli. When stained with Congo red dye, these deposits appeared red with ordinary light microscopy and exhibited apple-green fluorescence when viewed in polarized light. This staining is characteristic of the amyloid fibril structure, which is composed of repeated β-sheets aligned orthogonally (perpendicular) to the axis of the fiber.

Several diseases involve deposition of a characteristic amyloid fiber. However, in each of these diseases, the amyloid is derived from a different protein that has changed its conformation (three-dimensional structure) to that of the amyloid repeated β-sheet structure. Once amyloid deposition begins, it seems to proceed rapidly, as if the fibril itself were promoting formation and deposition of more fibrils (a phenomenon called "seeding"). The different clinical presentations in each of these diseases result from differences in the function of the native protein and the site of amyloid deposition.

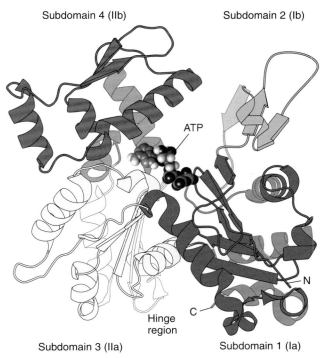

Subdomain 4 (IIb) Subdomain 2 (Ib)

ATP

N

C

Hinge region

Subdomain 3 (IIa) Subdomain 1 (Ia)

FIGURE 7.8 G-actin. ATP binds in the center of the cleft. The two domains that form the cleft are further subdivided into subdomains 1 through 4. The overall structure is found in many ATP-binding proteins and is called the *actin fold*. The *arrows* represent regions of β-sheet, whereas the *coils* represent α-helical regions of the protein.

domains are connected through a simpler structure such as a loop (e.g., the hinge region of Fig. 7.8). The structural features of each domain can be discussed independently of another domain in the same protein, and the structural features of one domain may not match that of other domains in the same protein.

B. Folds in Globular Proteins

Folds are relatively large patterns of three-dimensional structure that have been recognized in many proteins, including proteins from different branches of the phylogenetic tree. A characteristic activity is associated with each fold, such as ATP binding and hydrolysis (the actin fold) or nicotinamide adenine dinucleotide (NAD^+) binding (the nucleotide binding fold). Examples of these folding patterns are discussed in the following sections.

I. The Actin Fold

In the three-dimensional drawing of G-actin shown in Figure 7.8, all four subdomains contribute to a folding pattern called the *actin fold*, named for the first protein in which it was described. ATP is bound into the middle of the cleft of the actin fold by amino acid residues contributed by domains on both sides; thus, ATP binding promotes a conformational change that closes the cleft. Once it is bound, ATP is cleaved to adenosine diphosphate (ADP) and phosphate.

The actin fold is found in proteins as diverse as actin, which polymerizes to form the cytoskeleton, heat-shock protein 70 (hsp70), which uses ATP energy in changing the conformation of other proteins, and hexokinase, which catalyzes phosphorylation of glucose (see Chapter 8 for further discussion of hexokinase). Although these proteins have very little sequence identity, three-dimensional drawings of their actin folds are almost superimposable. The amount of sequence identity they do have is consistent with their membership in the same fold family and establishes that they are all homologs of the same ancestral protein. In all of these proteins, ATP binding results in large conformational changes that contribute to the function of the protein.

2. The Nucleotide Binding Fold

A fold also can be formed by one domain. In the example of secondary structures provided by LDH (see Fig. 7.7), domain 1 alone forms the nucleotide binding fold. This fold is a binding site for NAD^+ or, in other proteins, molecules with a generally similar structure (e.g., riboflavin). However, many proteins that bind NAD^+ or NAD^+ phosphate ($NADP^+$) contain a very different fold from a separate fold family. These two different NAD^+ binding folds arise from different ancestral lines and have different structures, but they have similar properties and function. They are believed to be the product of convergent evolution.

C. The Solubility of Globular Proteins in an Aqueous Environment

Most globular proteins are soluble in the cell. In general, the core of a globular domain has a high content of amino acids with nonpolar side chains (valine, leucine, isoleucine, methionine, and phenylalanine), out of contact with the aqueous medium (the hydrophobic effect). This hydrophobic core is densely packed to maximize attractive van der Waals forces, which exert themselves over short distances. The charged polar amino acid side chains (arginine, histidine, lysine, aspartate, and glutamic acid) are generally located on the surface of the protein, where they form ion pairs (salt bridges, ionic interactions) or are in contact with aqueous solvent. Charged side chains often bind inorganic ions (e.g., K^+, PO_4^{3-}, or Cl^-) to decrease repulsion between like charges. When charged amino acids are located on the interior, they are generally involved in forming specific binding sites. The polar uncharged amino acid side chains of serine, threonine, asparagine, glutamine, tyrosine, and tryptophan are also usually found on the surface of the protein, but they may occur in the interior, hydrogen-bonded to other side chains. Cystine disulfide bonds (the bond formed by two cysteine sulfhydryl groups) are sometimes involved in the formation of tertiary structure, where they add stability to the protein. However, their formation in soluble globular proteins is infrequent.

D. Tertiary Structure of Transmembrane Proteins

Transmembrane proteins, such as the β_2-adrenergic receptor, contain membrane-spanning domains and intra- and extracellular domains on either side of the membrane (Fig. 7.9). Many ion channel proteins, transport proteins, neurotransmitter receptors, and hormone receptors contain similar membrane-spanning segments that are α-helices with hydrophobic residues exposed to the lipid bilayer. These rigid helices are connected by loops containing hydrophilic amino acid side chains that extend into the aqueous medium on both sides of the membrane. In the β_2-adrenergic receptor, the helices clump together so that the extracellular loops form a surface that acts as a binding site for the hormone adrenaline (epinephrine)—our fight-or-flight hormone. The binding site is sometimes referred to as a *binding domain* (a functional domain), even though it is not formed from a continuous segment of the polypeptide chain. Once adrenaline binds to the receptor, a conformational change in the arrangement of rigid helical structures is transmitted to the intracellular domains that form a binding site for another signaling protein, a heterotrimeric G-protein (a guanosine triphosphate [GTP]-binding protein composed of three different subunits, which is described further in Chapter 11). Thus, receptors require both rigidity and flexibility to transmit signals across the cell membrane.

As discussed in Chapter 6, transmembrane proteins usually have several posttranslational modifications that provide additional chemical groups to fulfill requirements of the three-dimensional structure. As shown in Figure 7.9 (and see Fig. 6.13), the amino terminus of the β_2-adrenergic receptor (residues 1 to 34) extends out

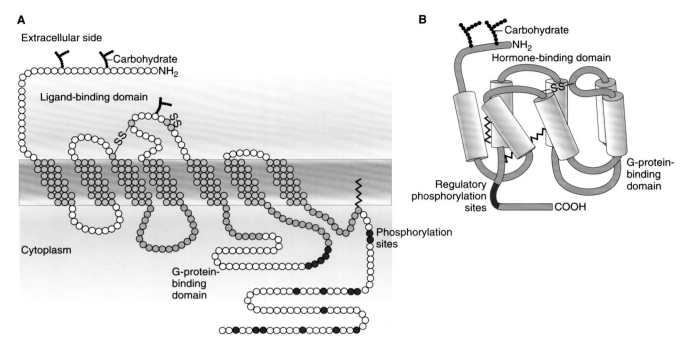

FIGURE 7.9 β₂-Adrenergic receptor. The receptor has seven α-helical domains that span the membrane and is therefore a member of the heptahelical class of receptors. **A.** The transmembrane domains are drawn in an extended form. The amino terminus (residues 1 through 34) extends out of the membrane and has branched high-mannose oligosaccharides linked through N-glycosidic bonds to the amide of asparagine. Part of the receptor is anchored in the lipid plasma membrane by a palmitoyl group (shown as *squiggle*) that forms a thioester with the –SH residue of a cysteine. The –COOH terminus, which extends into the cytoplasm, has several serine and threonine phosphorylation sites (shown as *red circles*). **B.** The seven transmembrane helices (shown as *tubes*) form a cylindrical structure. Loops connecting helices form the hormone-binding site on the external side of the plasma membrane, and a binding site for a G-protein is on the intracellular side.

of the membrane and has branched high-mannose oligosaccharides linked through N-glycosidic bonds to the amide of asparagine. Part of the receptor is anchored in the lipid plasma membrane by a palmitoyl group that forms a thioester with the –SH residue of a cysteine. The carboxyl terminus, which extends into the cytoplasm, has several serine and threonine phosphorylation sites (shown as *red circles* in Fig. 7.9) that regulate receptor activity.

V. Quaternary Structure

The quaternary structure of a protein refers to the association of individual polypeptide chain subunits in a geometrically and stoichiometrically specific manner. Many proteins function in the cell as dimers, tetramers, or oligomers, proteins in which two, four, or more subunits, respectively, have combined to make one functional protein. The subunits of a particular protein always combine in the same number and in the same way because the binding between the subunits is dictated by the tertiary structure, which is dictated by the primary structure, which in turn is determined by the genetic code.

Several different terms are used to describe subunit structure. The prefixes *homo-* and *hetero-* are used to describe identical or different subunits, respectively, of two-, three-, or four-subunit proteins (e.g., heterotrimeric G-proteins have three different subunits). A *protomer* is the unit structure composed of nonidentical subunits. For example, adult hemoglobin consists of two a- and two b-chains and is a tetramer (a₂b₂). One a-b pair can be considered a protomer. In contrast, F-actin is an *oligomer*, a multisubunit protein composed of identical G-actin subunits. *Multimer* is sometimes used as a more generic term to designate a complex with many subunits of more than one type.

The contact regions between the subunits of globular proteins resemble the interior of a single subunit protein; they contain closely packed nonpolar side chains, hydrogen bonds involving the polypeptide backbones and their side chains, and occasional ionic bonds or salt bridges. The subunits of globular proteins are very rarely held together by interchain disulfide bonds and never by other covalent bonds. In contrast, fibrous and other structural proteins may be extensively linked to other proteins through covalent bonds.

Assembly into a multisubunit structure increases the stability of a protein. The increase in size increases the number of possible interactions between amino acid residues and therefore makes it more difficult for a protein to unfold and refold. As a result, many soluble proteins are composed of two or four identical or nearly identical subunits with an average size of approximately 200 amino acids. The forming of multisubunit proteins also aids in the function of the protein.

A multisubunit structure has many advantages besides increased stability. It may enable the protein to exhibit cooperativity between subunits in binding ligands (illustrated later with hemoglobin) or to form binding sites with a high affinity for large molecules (illustrated with antigen binding to the immunoglobulin molecule immunoglobulin G [IgG]). An additional advantage of a multisubunit structure is that the different subunits can have different activities and cooperate in a common function. Examples of enzymes that have regulatory subunits or exist as multiprotein complexes are provided in Chapter 9.

 Insulin is composed of two nonidentical polypeptide chains attached to each other through disulfide bonds between the chains (see Chapter 6, Fig. 6.12). The subunits of globular proteins are generally not held together by disulfide bonds, but regions of the same chain may be connected by disulfide bonds that form as the chain folds. Insulin actually fits this generalization because it is synthesized as a single polypeptide chain, which forms the disulfide bonds. Subsequently, a proteolytic enzyme in secretory vesicles clips the polypeptide chain into two nonidentical subunits. Generally, each subunit of most protomers and oligomers is synthesized as a separate polypeptide chain. In fibrous proteins, which have a regular, sometimes repeating sequence of amino acids, inter- and intrachain covalent binding serves different functions. In collagen, for example, extensive interchain binding provides great tensile strength. Collagen is discussed in more detail in Chapter 47.

VI. Quantitation of Ligand Binding

In the examples of tertiary structure we have discussed, the folding of a protein created a three-dimensional binding site for a ligand (NAD^+ for the LDH domain 1, ATP for G-actin, or adrenaline for the β_2-adrenergic receptor). The binding affinity of a protein for a ligand is described quantitatively by its *association constant*, K_a, which is the equilibrium constant for the binding reaction of a ligand (L) with a protein (P) (Equation 7.1).

Equation 7.1. The association constant (K_a) for a binding site on a protein. Consider a reaction in which a ligand (L) binds to a protein (P) to form a ligand–protein complex (LP) with a rate constant of k_1. LP dissociates with a rate constant of k_2:

$$L + P \underset{k_2}{\overset{k_1}{\rightleftharpoons}} LP$$

then,

$$K_{eq} = \frac{k_1}{k_2} = \frac{[LP]}{[L][P]} = K_a = \frac{1}{K_d}$$

The equilibrium constant, K_{eq}, is equal to the association constant (K_a) or $1/K_d$, the dissociation constant. Unless otherwise given, the concentrations of L, P, and LP are expressed as moles per liter (mol/L), and K_a has the units of $(mol/L)^{-1}$.

K_a is equal to the rate constant (k_1) for association of the ligand with its binding site divided by the rate constant (k_2) for dissociation of the ligand–protein complex (LP). K_d, the *dissociation constant* for ligand–protein binding, is the reciprocal of K_a. The tighter the binding of the ligand to the protein, the higher the K_a and the lower the K_d. The K_a is useful for comparing proteins produced by different alleles or for describing the affinity of a receptor for different drugs.

Q Two different ligands (A and B) bind to the same receptor on the cell surface. The K_d for ligand A is 10^{-7} M; for ligand B, it is 10^{-9} M. Which ligand has the higher affinity for the receptor?

VII. Structure–Function Relationships in Myoglobin and Hemoglobin

Myoglobin and hemoglobin are two oxygen-binding proteins with a very similar primary structure (Fig. 7.10). However, myoglobin is a globular protein composed of a single polypeptide chain that has one oxygen-binding site. Hemoglobin is a tetramer composed of two different types of subunits (2α- and 2β-polypeptide chains, referred

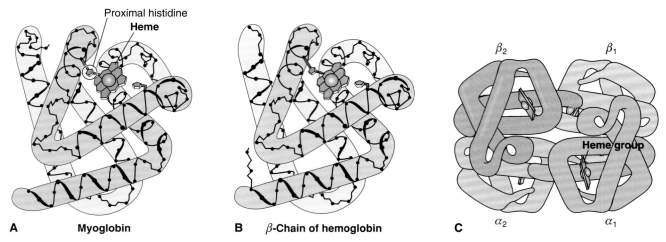

FIGURE 7.10 Myoglobin and hemoglobin. Myoglobin **(A)** consists of a single polypeptide chain, which is similar in structure to the α- and β-subunits of hemoglobin **(B)**. In all of the subunits, heme is tightly bound in a hydrophobic binding pocket. The proximal histidine extends down from a helix to bind to the Fe^{2+} atom. The oxygen binds between the distal histidine and the heme. **(C)** displays the quaternary structure of hemoglobin (which consists of two α- and two β-chains). (From Frescht A. *Structure and Mechanism in Protein Science*. New York, NY: WH Freeman; 1999. Used with permission.)

A The K_a (association constant) is equal to the reciprocal of the dissociation constant (K_d). The K_a for ligand A is 10^7 M^{-1}, whereas for ligand B, it is 10^9 M^{-1}. Ligand B has the higher affinity for the receptor by 100-fold as compared to ligand A.

to as *two αβ-protomers*). Each subunit has a strong sequence homology to myoglobin and contains an oxygen-binding site. A comparison between myoglobin and hemoglobin illustrates some of the advantages of a multisubunit quaternary structure.

The tetrameric structure of hemoglobin facilitates saturation with O_2 in the lungs and release of O_2 as it travels through the capillary beds (Fig. 7.11). When the amount of oxygen bound to myoglobin or hemoglobin is plotted against the partial pressure of oxygen (Po_2), a hyperbolic curve is obtained for myoglobin, whereas that for hemoglobin is sigmoidal. These curves show that when the Po_2 is high, as in the lungs, both myoglobin and hemoglobin are saturated with oxygen. However, at the lower levels of Po_2 in oxygen-using tissues, hemoglobin cannot bind oxygen as well as myoglobin (i.e., its percentage saturation is much lower). Myoglobin, which is present in heart and skeletal muscle, can bind the O_2 released by hemoglobin, which it stores to meet the demands of contraction. As O_2 is used in the muscle cell for generation of ATP during contraction, it is released from myoglobin and picked up by cytochrome oxidase, a heme-containing enzyme in the electron transport chain that has an even higher affinity for oxygen than myoglobin.

A. Oxygen Binding and Heme

The tertiary structure of myoglobin consists of eight α-helices connected by short coils, a structure that is known as the *globin fold* (see Fig. 7.10). This structure is unusual for a globular protein in that it has no β-sheets. The helices create a hydrophobic O_2 binding pocket containing tightly bound heme with an iron atom (ferrous [Fe^{2+}]) in its center.

Heme consists of a planar porphyrin ring composed of four pyrrole rings linked by methenyl bridges that lie with their nitrogen atoms in the center, binding a Fe^{2+} atom (Fig. 7.12). Negatively charged propionate groups on the porphyrin ring interact with arginine and histidine side chains from the hemoglobin, and the hydrophobic methyl and vinyl groups that extend out from the porphyrin ring interact with hydrophobic amino acid side chains from hemoglobin, positioning the heme group within the protein. All together, there are about 16 different interactions between myoglobin amino acids and different groups in the porphyrin ring.

Organic ligands that are tightly bound to proteins, such as the heme of myoglobin, are called *prosthetic groups*. A protein with its attached prosthetic group is called a *holoprotein*; without the prosthetic group, it is called an *apoprotein*. The tightly bound prosthetic group is an intrinsic part of the protein and does not dissociate until the protein is degraded.

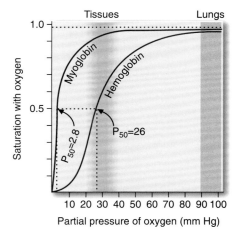

FIGURE 7.11 Oxygen saturation curves for myoglobin and hemoglobin. Note that the curve for myoglobin is hyperbolic, whereas that for hemoglobin is sigmoidal. The effect of the tetrameric structure is to inhibit O_2 binding at low O_2 concentrations. P_{50} is the partial pressure of O_2 (Po_2) at which the protein is half-saturated with O_2. P_{50} for myoglobin is 2.8 torr and that for hemoglobin is 26 torr, where 1 torr is equal to 1 mm Hg.

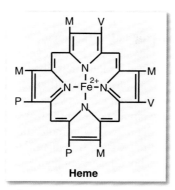

FIGURE 7.12 Heme. The Fe^{2+} is bound to four nitrogen atoms in the center of the heme porphyrin ring. Methyl (M, $-CH_3$), vinyl (V, $-CH = CH_2$), and propionate (P, $-CH_2CH_3COO-$) side chains extend out from the four pyrrole rings that comprise the porphyrin ring.

Within the binding pocket of myoglobin and hemoglobin, O_2 binds directly to the Fe^{2+} atom on one side of the planar porphyrin ring (Fig. 7.13A). The Fe^{2+} atom is able to chelate (binds to) six different ligands; four of the ligand positions are in a plane and taken by the central nitrogens in the planar porphyrin ring. There are two ligand positions perpendicular to this plane. One of these positions is taken by the nitrogen atom on a histidine, called the *proximal histidine*, which extends down from a myoglobin or hemoglobin α-helix. The other position is taken by O_2, by CO (carbon monoxide), or remains empty.

The proximal histidine of myoglobin and hemoglobin is sterically repelled by the heme porphyrin ring. Thus, when the histidine binds to the Fe^{2+} in the middle of the ring, it pulls the Fe^{2+} above the plane of the ring (see Fig. 7.13A). When oxygen binds on the other side of the ring, it pulls the Fe^{2+} back into the plane of the ring (see Fig. 7.13B). The pull of O_2 binding moves the proximal histidine toward the porphyrin ring, which moves the helix containing the proximal histidine. This conformational change has no effect on the function of myoglobin. However, in hemoglobin, the movement of one helix leads to the movement of other helices in that subunit, including one in a corner of the subunit that is in contact with a different subunit through ionic interactions (salt bridges). The loss of these salt bridges then induces conformational changes in all other subunits, and all four subunits may change in a concerted manner from their original conformation to a new conformation (see "Biochemical Comments").

 Myoglobin is readily released from skeletal muscle or cardiac tissue when the cell is damaged. It has a low molecular weight, 17,000 Da and is not complexed to other proteins in the cell. (*Da* is the abbreviation for the dalton, which is a unit of mass approximately equal to one H atom. Thus, a molecular weight of 17,000 Da is equal to approximately 17,000 g/mol.) Large injuries to skeletal muscle that result from physical crushing or lack of ATP production result in cellular swelling and the release of myoglobin and other proteins into the blood. Myoglobin passes into the urine (myoglobinuria) and turns the urine red because the heme (which is red) remains covalently attached to the protein. During an acute MI, myoglobin is one of the first proteins released into the blood from damaged cardiac tissue; however, the amount released is not high enough to cause myoglobinuria. Laboratory measurements of serum myoglobin were used in the past for early diagnosis in patients such as **Anne J.** Because myoglobin is not present in skeletal muscle and the heart as tissue-specific isozymes, and the amount released from the heart is much smaller than the amount that can be released from a large skeletal muscle injury, myoglobin measurements are not specific for an MI. Owing to the lack of specificity in myoglobin measurements, the cardiac marker of choice for detection of an MI is the heart isozyme of the troponins (I and/or T).

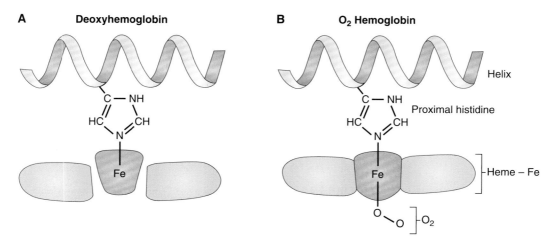

FIGURE 7.13 **A.** Oxygen binding to the Fe^{2+} of heme in hemoglobin. A histidine residue called the proximal histidine binds to the Fe^{2+} on one side of the porphyrin ring and slightly pulls the Fe^{2+} out of the plane of the ring; O_2 binds to Fe^{2+} on the other side. **B.** O_2 binding causes a conformational change that pulls the Fe^{2+} back into the plane of the ring. As the proximal histidine moves, it moves the helix (the F-helix) that contains it.

Sickle cell anemia is really a disease caused by an abnormal quaternary structure. The painful vaso-occlusive crises experienced by **Will S.** are caused by the polymerization of sickle cell hemoglobin (HbS) molecules into long fibers that distort the shape of the red blood cells into sickle cells. The substitution of a hydrophobic valine for a glutamate in the β_2-chain of hemoglobin creates a knob on the surface of deoxygenated hemoglobin that fits into a hydrophobic binding pocket on the β_1-subunit of a different hemoglobin molecule. A third hemoglobin molecule, which binds to the first and second hemoglobin molecules through aligned polar interactions, binds a fourth hemoglobin molecule through its valine knob. Thus, the polymerization continues until long fibers are formed.

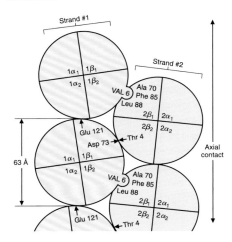

Polymerization of the hemoglobin molecules is highly dependent on the concentration of HbS and is promoted by the conformation of the deoxygenated molecules. At 100% oxygen saturation, even high concentrations of HbS will not polymerize. A red blood cell spends the longest amount of time at the lower oxygen concentrations of the venous capillary bed, where polymerization is most likely initiated.

B. Cooperativity of O_2 Binding in Hemoglobin

The cooperativity in oxygen binding in hemoglobin comes from conformational changes in tertiary structure that takes place when O_2 binds (Fig. 7.14). The conformational change of hemoglobin is usually described as changing from a T (tense) state with low affinity for O_2 to an R (relaxed) state with a high affinity for O_2. Breaking the salt bridges in the contacts between subunits is an energy-requiring process, and consequently, the binding rate for the first oxygen is very low. When the next oxygen binds, many of the hemoglobin molecules containing one O_2 will already have all four subunits in the R state, and therefore, the rate of binding is much higher. With two O_2 molecules bound, an even higher percentage of the hemoglobin molecules will have all four subunits in the R state. This phenomenon, known as *positive cooperativity*, is responsible for the sigmoidal oxygen saturation curve of hemoglobin (see Fig. 7.11).

C. Agents that Affect O_2 Binding

The major agents that affect O_2 binding to hemoglobin are shown in Figure 7.15.

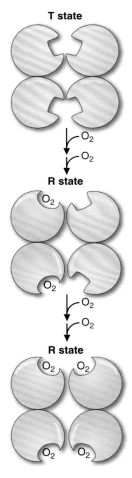

FIGURE 7.14   Equilibria for binding of O_2 molecules to hemoglobin according to the concerted model of Monod, Wyman, and Changeux. Hemoglobin exists in two alternate conformations, the T (tense) state with a low affinity for O_2 and the R (relaxed) state with a higher affinity. In the T subunits, the binding sites are hindered, and in the R state, the binding sites are open. Each successive addition of O_2 shifts the equilibrium further toward the R state. Because the conformation of all the subunits can change when O_2 binds to one subunit, oxygen binding is said to follow the concerted model. Most of the molecules change to the R state when two O_2 molecules have bound.

I. 2,3-Bisphosphoglycerate

2,3-Bisphosphoglycerate (2,3-BPG) is formed in red blood cells from the glycolytic intermediate 1,3-bisphosphoglycerate (see Chapters 22 and 42). 2,3-BPG binds to hemoglobin in the central cavity formed by the four subunits, increasing the energy required for the conformational changes that facilitate the binding of O_2. Thus, 2,3-BPG lowers the affinity of hemoglobin for oxygen. Therefore, O_2 is less readily bound (i.e., is more readily released in tissues) when hemoglobin has bound 2,3-BPG. Red blood cells can modulate O_2 affinity for hemoglobin by altering the rate of synthesis or degradation of 2,3-bisphosphoglycerate.

2. Proton Binding (Bohr Effect)

The binding of protons by hemoglobin lowers its affinity for oxygen (Fig. 7.16), contributing to a phenomenon known as the *Bohr effect* (Fig. 7.17). The pH of the

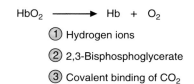

$$HbO_2 \longrightarrow Hb + O_2$$

① Hydrogen ions

② 2,3-Bisphosphoglycerate

③ Covalent binding of CO_2

FIGURE 7.15 Agents that affect oxygen binding by hemoglobin (*Hb*). Binding of hydrogen ions, 2,3-bisphosphoglycerate, and carbon dioxide to Hb decreases its affinity for oxygen.

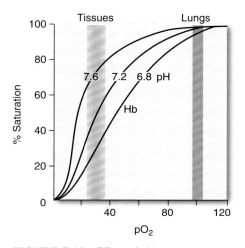

FIGURE 7.16 Effect of pH on oxygen saturation curves. As the pH decreases, the affinity of hemoglobin (*Hb*) for oxygen decreases, producing the Bohr effect.

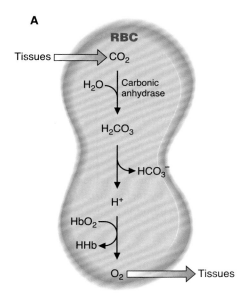

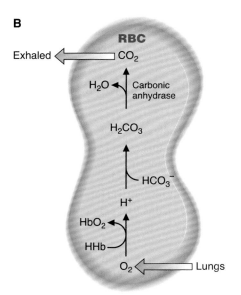

FIGURE 7.17 Effect of H^+ on oxygen binding by hemoglobin (Hb). **A.** In the tissues, CO_2 is released. In the red blood cell, this CO_2 forms carbonic acid, which releases protons. The protons bind to Hb, causing it to release oxygen to the tissues. **B.** In the lungs, the reactions are reversed. O_2 binds to protonated Hb, causing the release of protons. They bind to bicarbonate (HCO_3^-), forming carbonic acid, which is cleaved to water and CO_2, which is exhaled. *RBC*, red blood cells; *HHb*, protonated hemoglobin.

Amy L.'s serum protein electrophoresis indicated the presence of a sharp narrow peak or homogeneous "spike" in the characteristic γ-globulin zone known as an *M protein* (monoclonal protein) component. A narrow peak or spike in electrophoresis, which separates proteins according to charge distribution of the side chains, suggests an elevation of proteins with a similar or identical structure. Subsequently, it was shown that Amy L.'s immunoglobulin M component was composed of a single homogeneous type of immunoglobulin (just one amino acid sequence in the *N*-terminal variable region). Thus, the M protein was produced by a single clone of antibody-secreting cells (cells that all arose from proliferation of one cell) in the bone marrow (called *plasma cell dyscrasia*).

In amyloidosis/AL, amyloid is formed from degradation products of the λ- or κ-light chains that deposit most frequently in the extracellular matrix (ECM) of the kidney and the heart but also may deposit in the tongue. In other types of amyloidosis, the amyloid arises from other proteins and deposits in a characteristic organ. For example, the amyloid associated with chronic inflammatory conditions, such as rheumatoid arthritis, is derived from the serum protein called *serum amyloid A* that is produced by the liver in response to inflammation. It deposits most frequently in the kidney.

The treatment of AL is multifactorial and only partially successful. Initially, alkylating agents were used to reduce the synthesis of immunoglobulin light chains by plasma cells but were found to be too toxic for routine use. The most efficacious approach involves the use of stem cell transplantation in concert with melphalan (an antineoplastic agent). If the patient is not a candidate for transplantation, then melphalan (an antineoplastic agent) and dexamethasone (a steroid) can be used.

Renal transplantation and cardiac transplantation have been performed in patients with renal and cardiac amyloidosis, respectively, with some success.

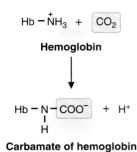

Hemoglobin

Carbamate of hemoglobin

FIGURE 7.18 Binding of CO_2 to hemoglobin. CO_2 forms carbamates with the *N*-terminal amino groups of hemoglobin (*Hb*) chains. Approximately 15% of the CO_2 in blood is carried to the lungs bound to Hb. The reaction releases protons, which contribute to the Bohr effect. The overall effect is the stabilization of the deoxy form of hemoglobin.

blood decreases as it enters the tissues (and the proton concentration rises) because the CO_2 produced by metabolism is converted to carbonic acid by the reaction catalyzed by carbonic anhydrase in red blood cells. Dissociation of carbonic acid produces protons that react with several amino acid residues in hemoglobin, causing conformational changes that promote the release of oxygen.

In the lungs, this process is reversed. Oxygen binds to hemoglobin (because of the high oxygen concentration in the lung), causing a release of protons, which combine with bicarbonate to form carbonic acid. This decrease of protons causes the pH of the blood to rise. Carbonic anhydrase cleaves the carbonic acid to H_2O and CO_2, and the CO_2 is exhaled. Thus, in tissues in which the pH of the blood is low because of the CO_2 produced by metabolism, O_2 is released from hemoglobin. In the lungs, where the pH of the blood is higher because CO_2 is being exhaled, O_2 binds to hemoglobin.

C. Carbon Dioxide

Although most of the CO_2 produced by metabolism in the tissues is carried to the lungs as bicarbonate, some of the CO_2 is covalently bound to hemoglobin (Fig. 7.18). In the tissues, CO_2 forms carbamate adducts with the *N*-terminal amino groups of deoxyhemoglobin and stabilizes the deoxy conformation. In the lungs, where the P_{O_2} is high, O_2 binds to hemoglobin and this bound CO_2 is released.

VIII. Structure–Function Relationships in Immunoglobulins

The *immunoglobulins* (or antibodies) are one line of defense against invasion of the body by foreign organisms. In this capacity, they function by binding to ligands called *antigens* on the invading organisms, thereby initiating the process by which these organisms are inactivated or destroyed.

Immunoglobulins all have a similar structure; each antibody molecule contains two identical small polypeptide chains (the light or L chains) and two identical large polypeptide chains (the heavy or H chains) (Fig. 7.19). The chains are joined to each other by disulfide bonds.

The body has five major classes of immunoglobulins. The most abundant immunoglobulins in human blood are the γ-globulins, which belong to the IgG class. The γ-globulins have approximately 220 amino acids in their light chains and 440 in their heavy chains. Like most serum proteins, they have attached oligosaccharides that participate in targeting the protein for clearance from the blood. Both the light and heavy chains consist of domains known as the *immunoglobulin fold*, which is a collapsed number of β-sheets, known as a β-*barrel* (Fig. 7.20).

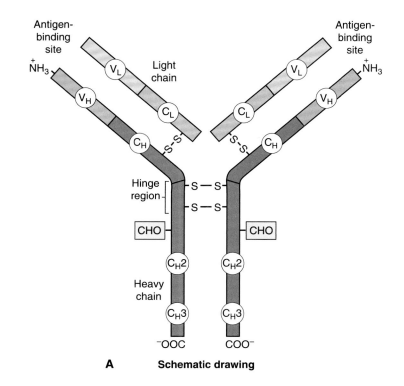

A   **Schematic drawing**

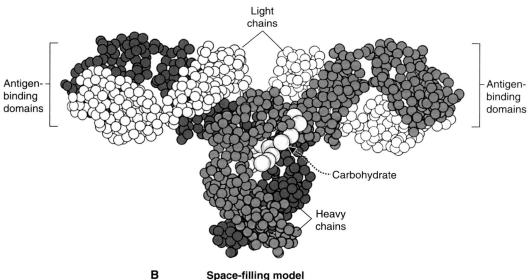

B   **Space-filling model**

FIGURE 7.19   Structure of immunoglobulins. **A.** Each IgG molecule contains two light (L) and two heavy (H) chains joined by disulfide bonds. Each light chain contains two domains, a variable domain (V_L) and a region of constant amino acid sequence (C_L). Each heavy chain has four domains: one variable domain (V_H) and three constant domains (C_H). The conformation of the constant domain contains the β-sheets that are called the *immunoglobulin fold.* The variable domains are specific for the antigen that is bound, whereas the constant regions are the same for all antibody molecules of a given class. Carbohydrate ($-CHO$) is bound as indicated within the constant region of the heavy chains. The hinge region allows flexibility when the molecule binds antigen. **B.** In the space-filling model, the light chains are *light in color* and the heavy chains are *two different shades of orange.* (Modified from Silverton EW, Navia MA, Davies DR, et al. Three-dimensional structure of an intact human immunoglobulin. *Proc Natl Acad Sci U S A.* 1977;11:5142.)

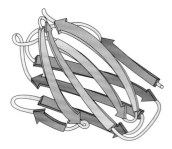

V$_L$ domain

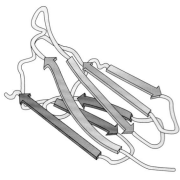

C$_L$ domain

FIGURE 7.20 Structure of the light chain variable domain (V_L) and constant domain (C_L) of IgG. Layers of antiparallel β-sheets are stacked in these domains, which have been referred to as *collapsed β-barrels* (one can envision a hollow space between the β-sheets, which define the barrel). The antigen binds between the heavy chain V$_H$ and V$_L$ immunoglobulin folds and *not* in the barrel. The C$_L$ domain is also called the *immunoglobulin fold*. (Top modified from Richardson JS. The anatomy and taxonomy of protein structure. *Adv Protein Chem.* 1981;34:167; bottom reprinted in part with permission from Edmundson AB, Ely KR, Abola EE, et al. Rational allomerism and divergent evolution of domains in immunoglobulin light chains. *Biochemistry.* 1975;14:3954. Copyright © 1975 American Chemical Society.)

The tight binding affinity of immunoglobulins for their specific antigen makes them useful for the measurement of small amounts of other compounds in various radioimmunoassays. The principle of the radioimmunoassay is that the immunoglobulin will specifically bind the compound being measured, and an additional component of the system that is labeled with a radioactive or fluorescent chemical will bind the immunoglobulin. The complex is then separated from the solution and the bound radioactivity or fluorescence measured. The different isozymes of CK and TnT used to track **Anne J.'s** MI are measured with a type of radioimmunoassay by using antibodies specific for each isozyme. This method is much faster than the laborious separation of isozymes by electrophoresis. Radioimmunoassays are also useful for measuring the small amounts of hormones present in the blood for diagnosis of endocrine diseases.

Both the light and heavy chains contain regions termed *variable* (V) and *constant* (C) regions. The variable regions of the L and H chains (V$_L$ and V$_H$, respectively) interact to produce a single antigen-binding site at each branch of the Y-shaped molecule. Each population (clone) of B cells produces an antibody with a different amino acid composition in the variable region that is complementary to the structure of the antigen that elicits the response. The K_d of antibodies for their specific antigens is extremely small and varies from approximately 10^{-7} to 10^{-11} M. The antigen thus binds very tightly with almost no tendency to dissociate and can be removed from circulation as the antigen–antibody complex is ingested by macrophages. The constant domains that form the Fc (fragment, crystallizable) part of the antibody are important for binding of the antigen–antibody complex to phagocytic cells for clearance and for other aspects of the immune response.

IX. Protein Folding

Although the peptide bonds in a protein are rigid, flexibility around the other bonds in the peptide backbone allows an enormous variety of possible conformations for each protein. However, every molecule of the same protein folds into the same stable three-dimensional structure. This shape is known as the *native conformation*.

A. Primary Structure Determines Folding

The primary structure of a protein determines its three-dimensional conformation. More specifically, the sequence of amino acid side chains dictates the fold pattern of the three-dimensional structure and the assembly of subunits into quaternary structure. Proteins become denatured when they lose their overall structure. However, under certain conditions, denatured proteins can refold into their native conformation, regaining their original function. Proteins can be denatured with organic molecules such as urea that disrupt hydrogen bonding patterns (both of the protein and of water) and convert the protein to a soluble random coil. Many simple single-subunit proteins such as ribonuclease that are denatured in this way refold spontaneously into their native conformation if they are carefully brought back to physiologic conditions. Even complex multisubunit proteins containing bound cofactors can sometimes renature spontaneously under the right conditions. Thus, the primary structure essentially specifies the folding pattern. If misfolded proteins do not precipitate into aggregates, they can be degraded in the cell by proteolytic reactions, or even refolded.

In the cell, not all proteins fold into their native conformation on their own. As the protein folds and refolds while it is searching for its native low-energy state, it passes through many high-energy conformations that slow the process (called *kinetic barriers*). These kinetic barriers can be overcome by heat-shock proteins (some of which are also called *chaperonins*), which use energy provided by ATP hydrolysis to assist in the folding process (Fig. 7.21). Heat-shock proteins were named for the fact that their synthesis in bacteria increased when the temperature was raised suddenly. They are present in human cells as different families of proteins with different activities. For example, the hsp70 proteins bind to nascent polypeptide chains as their synthesis is being completed to keep the uncompleted chains from folding prematurely. They also unfold proteins before their insertion through the membrane of mitochondria and other organelles. The multisubunit barrel-shaped hsp60 family of proteins are called *chaperonins*. The unfolded protein fits into the barrel cavity that excludes water and serves as a template for the folding process. The hydrolysis of several ATP molecules is used to overcome the energy barriers to reaching the native conformation.

A *cis–trans isomerase* and a *protein disulfide isomerase* also participate in folding. The *cis–trans* isomerase converts a *trans* peptide bond preceding a proline into the *cis* conformation, which is well suited for making hairpin turns. The protein disulfide isomerase breaks and reforms disulfide bonds between the –SH groups of two cysteine residues in transient structures formed during the folding process. After the protein has folded, cysteine–SH groups in close contact in the tertiary structure can react to form the final disulfide bonds.

It is important to note that there is very little difference in the energy state of the native conformation and several other stable conformations that a protein might assume. This enables the protein to have the flexibility to change conformation when modifiers are bound to the protein, which enables a protein's activity to be regulated (similar to 2,3-bisphosphoglycerate binding to hemoglobin and stabilizing the deoxy form of hemoglobin).

B. Fibrous Proteins—Collagen

Collagen, a family of fibrous proteins, is produced by a variety of cell types but principally by fibroblasts (cells found in interstitial connective tissue), muscle cells, and epithelial cells. Type I collagen, or *collagen(I)*, the most abundant protein in mammals, is a fibrous protein that is the major component of connective tissue. It is found in the ECM (see Chapter 47) of loose connective tissue, bone, tendons, skin, blood vessels, and the cornea of the eye. Collagen(I) contains about 33% glycine and 21% proline and hydroxyproline. Hydroxyproline is an amino acid produced by posttranslational modification of peptidyl proline residues.

 Treatment of mature insulin (see Fig. 6.12) with denaturing agents, followed by renaturation, does not restore mature insulin activity (a result distinct from that which occurred when the experiment was done with ribonuclease). Why does renaturation of denatured mature insulin not result in restoration of biologic activity?

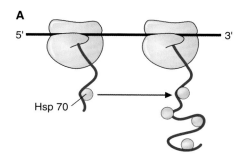

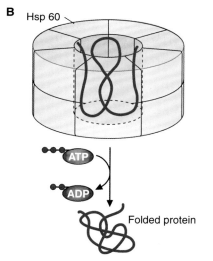

FIGURE 7.21 Role of heat-shock proteins in folding. **A.** The hsp70 family of proteins prevent folding of the nascent chain and promote unfolding. The adenosine triphosphatase (ATPase) domain of the protein has the actin fold. This figure depicts the synthesis of protein from ribosomes bound to messenger RNA in the cytoplasm (see Chapter 15). **B.** The hsp60 class of protein has a barrel shape into which the protein fits. It acts as a template, binding and rebinding portions of the unfolded protein until folding is completed. It hydrolyzes many adenosine triphosphate (ATP) bonds (generating adenosine diphosphate [ADP]) to provide energy for the process. *Hsp*, heat-shock proteins.

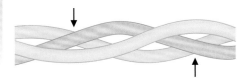

FIGURE 7.22 The triple helix of collagen. Glycines are present in the three chains where they come into close contact with each other (*arrows*).

A Recall that the primary structure of a protein dictates the folding pattern of the protein. The primary structure of mature insulin is different than that of its precursor, preproinsulin. Proinsulin forms the three-dimensional structure, and then the C-peptide is removed from the protein by proteolytic cleavage, thereby altering the primary structure of the protein. This change in primary structure (the loss of the C-peptide) does not allow the denatured mature insulin to refold into an active conformation.

Procollagen(I), the precursor of collagen(I), is a triple helix composed of three polypeptide (pro-α) chains that are twisted around each other, forming a ropelike structure (Fig. 7.22). Polymerization of collagen(I) molecules forms collagen fibrils, which provide great tensile strength to connective tissues. The individual polypeptide chains each contain approximately 1,000 amino acid residues. The three polypeptide chains of the triple helix are linked by interchain hydrogen bonds. Each turn of the triple helix contains three amino acid residues, such that every third amino acid is in close contact with the other two strands in the center of the structure. Only glycine, which lacks a side chain, can fit in this position, and indeed, every third amino acid residue of collagen is glycine. Thus, collagen is a polymer of (Gly-X-Y) repeats, where Y is frequently proline or hydroxyproline and X is any other amino acid found in collagen.

Procollagen(I) is an example of a protein that undergoes extensive posttranslational modifications. Hydroxylation reactions produce hydroxyproline residues from proline residues and hydroxylysine from lysine residues. These reactions occur after the protein has been synthesized (Fig. 7.23) and require vitamin C (ascorbic acid) as a cofactor of the enzymes prolyl hydroxylase and lysyl hydroxylase. Hydroxyproline residues are involved in hydrogen bond formation that helps to stabilize the triple helix, whereas hydroxylysine residues are the sites of attachment of disaccharide moieties (galactose–glucose). The role of carbohydrates in collagen structure is still controversial. In the absence of vitamin C (*scurvy*), the melting temperature of collagen drops from 42°C to 24°C because of the loss of interstrand hydrogen bond formation, which is in turn caused by the lack of hydroxyproline residues.

The side chains of lysine residues also may be oxidized to form the aldehyde *allysine*. These aldehyde residues produce covalent cross-links between collagen molecules to further stabilize the collagen fibril (Fig. 7.24). An allysine residue on one collagen molecule reacts with the amino group of a lysine residue on another molecule, forming a covalent Schiff base (a nitrogen–carbon double bond) that is converted to more stable covalent cross-links. Aldol condensation also may occur between two allysine residues, which form the structure lysinonorleucine.

The synthesis and secretion of collagen, as well as its multiple types, is discussed further in Chapter 47.

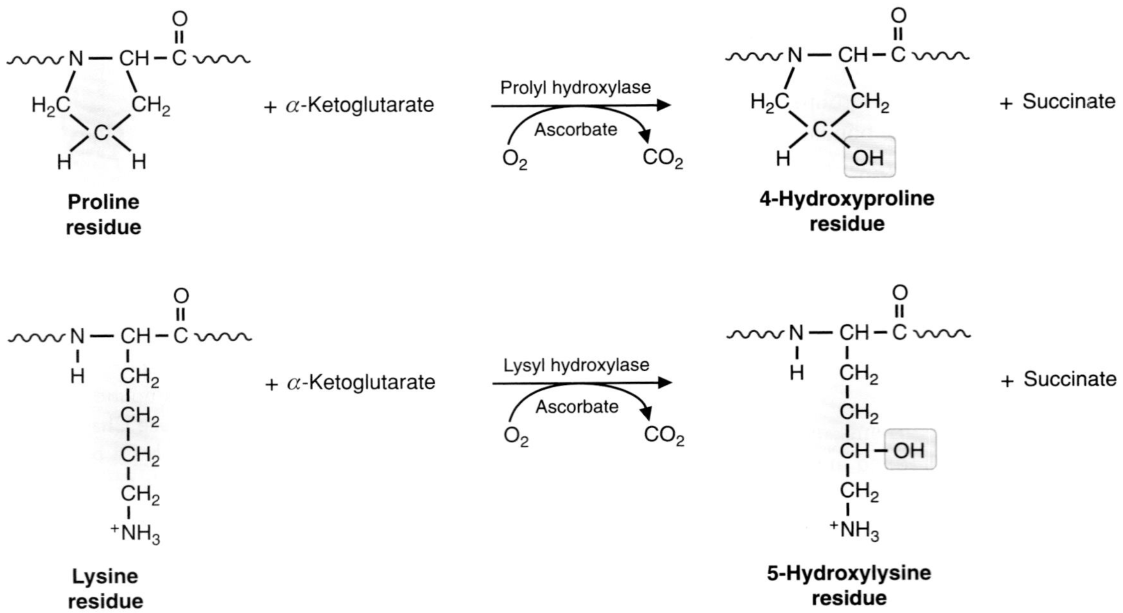

FIGURE 7.23 Hydroxylation of proline and lysine residues in collagen. Proline and lysine residues within the collagen chains are hydroxylated by reactions that require vitamin C.

C. Protein Denaturation

A protein's quaternary, tertiary, and secondary structures can be destroyed by several processes, and when this occurs, the protein is considered to be *denatured*. Denaturation can occur by a variety of means.

1. Denaturation through Nonenzymatic Modification of Proteins

Amino acids on proteins can undergo a wide range of chemical modifications that are not catalyzed by enzymes, such as nonenzymatic glycosylation or oxidation. Such modifications may lead to a loss of function and denaturation of the protein, sometimes to a form that cannot be degraded in the cell. In nonenzymatic glycosylation, glucose that is present in blood, or in interstitial or intracellular fluid, binds to an exposed amino group on a protein (Fig. 7.25). The two-step process forms an irreversibly glycosylated protein. Proteins that turn over very slowly in the body, such as collagen or hemoglobin, exist with a significant fraction present in the glycosylated form. Because the reaction is nonenzymatic, the rate of glycosylation is proportionate to the concentration of glucose present, and individuals with hyperglycemia have much higher levels of glycosylated proteins than individuals with normal blood glucose levels. Collagen and other glycosylated proteins in tissues are further modified by nonenzymatic oxidation and form additional cross-links. The net result is the formation of large protein aggregates referred to as *advanced glycosylation end products* (AGEs). AGE is a particularly meaningful acronym because AGEs accumulate with age, even in individuals with normal blood glucose levels.

2. Protein Denaturation by Temperature, pH, and Solvent

Proteins can be denatured by changes of pH, temperature, or solvent that disrupt ionic, hydrogen, and hydrophobic bonds. At a low pH, ionic bonds and hydrogen bonds formed by carboxylate groups would be disrupted; at a very alkaline pH, hydrogen and ionic bonds formed by the basic amino acids would be disrupted. Thus, the pH of the body must be maintained within a range compatible with three-dimensional structure.

Physiologically, proteins are denatured by the gastric juice of the stomach, which has a pH of 1 to 2. Although this pH cannot break peptide bonds, disruption of the native conformation makes the protein a better substrate for digestive enzymes. Temperature increases vibrational and rotational energies in the bonds, thereby affecting the energy balance that goes into making a stable three-dimensional conformation. Thermal denaturation is often illustrated by the process of cooking an egg. With heat, the protein albumin converts from its native translucent state to a denatured white precipitate. Protein precipitates can sometimes be dissolved by amphipathic agents such as urea, guanidine hydrochloride (HCl), or sodium dodecylsulfate (SDS) that form extensive hydrogen bonds and hydrophobic interactions with the protein.

Hydrophobic molecules can also denature proteins by disturbing hydrophobic interactions in the protein. For example, long-chain fatty acids can inhibit many enzyme-catalyzed reactions by binding nonspecifically to hydrophobic pockets in proteins and disrupting hydrophobic interactions. Thus, long-chain fatty acids and other highly hydrophobic molecules have their own binding proteins in the cell.

3. Protein Misfolding and Prions

Prion proteins are believed to cause a neurodegenerative disease by acting as a template to misfold other cellular prion proteins into a form that cannot be degraded. The word *prion* stands for "proteinaceous infectious agent." The prion diseases may be acquired either through infection (e.g., Creutzfeldt-Jakob disease [CJD], also called "mad cow disease") or from sporadic (majority of cases) or inherited mutations (e.g., familial CJD [fCJD]). Although the infectious prion diseases represent <1% of human cases, their link to mad cow disease in the United Kingdom (new variant CJD), to cadaveric human growth hormone use in the United States and

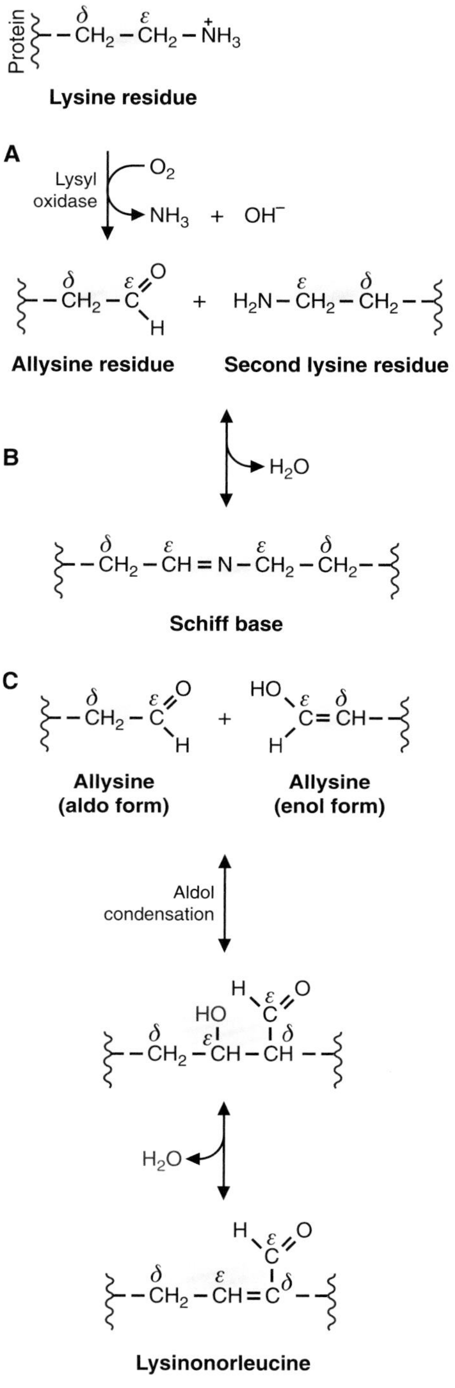

FIGURE 7.24 Formation of cross-links in collagen. **A.** Lysine residues are oxidized to allysine (an aldehyde). Allysine may react with an unmodified lysine residue to form a Schiff base **(B)**, or two allysine residues may undergo an aldol condensation **(C)** to form lysinonorleucine.

Dianne A.'s physician used her glycosylated hemoglobin levels, specifically the HbA1c fraction, to determine the control of her blood glucose and whether she had sustained hyperglycemia over a long period of time. The rate of irreversible nonenzymatic glycosylation of hemoglobin and other proteins is directly proportional to the glucose concentration to which they are exposed over the last 4 months (the life span of the red blood cell). The danger of sustained hyperglycemia is that, over time, many proteins become glycosylated and subsequently oxidized, affecting their solubility and ability to function. The glycosylation of collagen in the heart, for example, is believed to result in a cardiomyopathy in patients with chronic uncontrolled diabetes mellitus. In contrast, glycosylation of hemoglobin has little effect on its function.

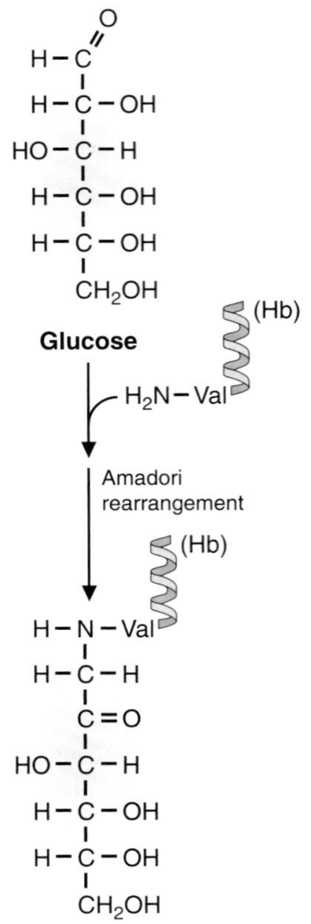

FIGURE 7.25   Nonenzymatic glycosylation of hemoglobin (*Hb*). Glucose forms a Schiff base with the *N*-terminal amino group of the protein, which rearranges to form a stable glycosylated product. Similar nonenzymatic glycosylation reactions occur on other proteins. Four minor components of adult hemoglobin (HbA) result from posttranslational, nonenzymatic glycosylation of different amino acid residues (HbA1a1, HbA1a2, HbA1b1, and HbA1c). In HbA1c, the fraction that is usually measured, the glycosylation occurs on an *N*-terminal valine.

Prion diseases are categorized as transmissible spongiform encephalopathies, which are neurodegenerative diseases characterized by spongiform degeneration and astrocytic gliosis in the central nervous system. Frequently, protein aggregates and amyloid plaques are seen. These aggregates are resistant to proteolytic degradation.

France (iatrogenic or "doctor-induced" CJD), and to ritualistic cannibalism in the Fore tribespeople of Papua New Guinea (Kuru) have received the most publicity.

The prion protein is normally found in the brain and is encoded by a gene that is a normal component of the human genome. The disease-causing form of the prion protein has the same amino acid composition but is folded into a different conformation that aggregates into multimeric protein complexes resistant to proteolytic degradation (Fig. 7.26). The normal conformation of the prion protein has been designated PrP^c and the disease-causing form as PrP^{Sc} (*Sc* for the prion disease known as scrapie in sheep). Although PrP^{Sc} and PrP^c have the same amino acid composition, the PrP^{Sc} conformer is substantially enriched in β-sheet structure compared with the normal PrP^c conformer, which has little or no β-sheet structure and is approximately 40% α-helix. This difference favors the aggregation of PrP^{Sc} into multimeric complexes. These two conformations presumably have similar energy levels. Fortunately, spontaneous refolding of PrP proteins into the PrP^{Sc} conformation is prevented by a large activation energy barrier that makes this conversion extremely slow. Thus, very few molecules of PrP^{Sc} are normally formed during a lifetime.

The infectious disease occurs with the ingestion of PrP^{Sc} dimers in which the prion protein is already folded into the high β-structure. These PrP^{Sc} proteins are thought to act as a template to lower the activation energy barrier for the conformational change, causing native proteins to refold into the PrP^{Sc} conformation much more rapidly (much like the role of chaperonins). The refolding initiates a cascade as each new PrP^{Sc} formed acts as a template for the refolding of other molecules. As the

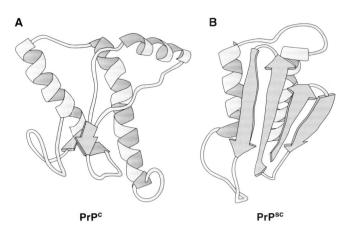

A   **B**

PrP^c   **PrP^sc**

FIGURE 7.26 The conformation of PrP^c (normal) and PrP^Sc (disease form). **A.** The prion proteins have two domains, an *N*-terminal region that binds four Cu^{2+} per chain, and a *C*-terminal region. **B.** In PrP^c, the *C*-terminal regions contain three substantial helices and two three-residue β-strands joined by two to three hydrogen bonds (~40% α-helix and almost no β-sheet structure). It exists as a monomer. In PrP^Sc, the *C*-terminal region is folded into an extensive β-sheet. The overall structure is approximately 40% to 50% β-sheet and 20% to 30% α-helices. This conformation promotes aggregation.

 Familial prion diseases are caused by point mutations in the gene encoding the Pr protein (point mutations are changes in one base in the DNA nucleotide sequence). The diseases have a various names related to the different mutations and the clinical syndrome (e.g., Gerstmann-Straüssler-Scheinker disease and fCJD). fCJD arises from an inherited mutation and has an autosomal dominant pedigree. It typically presents in the fourth decade of life. The mutation lowers the energy required for the protein to fold into the PrP^Sc conformation; thus, the conversion occurs more readily. It is estimated that the rate of generating prion disease by refolding of PrP^c in the normal cell is about 3,000 to 4,000 years. Lowering of the activation energy for refolding by mutation presumably decreases this time to the observed 30- to 40-year prodromal period. Sporadic CJD may arise from somatic cell mutation or rare spontaneous refoldings that initiate a cascade of refolding into the PrP^Sc conformation. The sporadic form of the disease accounts for 85% of all cases of CJD.

number of PrP^Sc molecules increases in the cell, they aggregate into a multimeric assembly that is resistant to proteolytic digestion. Once an aggregate begins to form, the concentration of free PrP^Sc decreases, thereby shifting the equilibrium between PrP and PrP^Sc to produce more PrP^Sc. This leads to further aggregate formation through the shift in equilibrium.

CLINICAL COMMENTS

 Will S. Will S. continues to experience severe low back and lower extremity pain for many hours after admission. The diffuse pains of sickle cell crises are believed to result from occlusion of small vessels in a variety of tissues, thereby depriving cells of oxygen and cause ischemic or anoxic damage to the tissues. In a *sickle cell crisis*, long hemoglobin polymers form, causing the red blood cells to become distorted and change from a biconcave disc to an irregular shape, such as a sickle (for which the disease was named) or a stellate structure (Fig. 7.27). The aggregating Hb polymers damage the red blood cell membrane and promote aggregation of membrane proteins, leading to increased permeability of the red blood cell and dehydration. Surface charge and antigens of red blood cells are carried on the transmembrane proteins glycophorin and band 3 (the erythrocyte anion exchange channel, see Chapter 10). Hemoglobin S binds tightly to the cytoplasmic portion of band 3, contributing to further polymer aggregation and uneven distribution of negative charge on the sickle cell surface. As a result, the affected cells adhere to endothelial cells in capillaries, occluding the vessel and decreasing blood flow to the distal tissues. The subsequent hypoxia in these tissues causes cellular damage, severe ischemic pain, and even death.

The sickled cells are sequestered and destroyed mainly by phagocytic cells, particularly those in the spleen. An anemia results as the number of circulating red blood cells decreases and bilirubin levels rise in the blood as hemoglobin is degraded.

After a few days of treatment, Will's crisis was resolved. In the future, should Will S. suffer a cerebrovascular accident (stroke) as a consequence of sickle cell disease causing damage to one of the large cerebral arteries, or have recurrent life-threatening episodes of generalized vaso-occlusion in microvessels, a course of long-term maintenance blood transfusions to prevent cerebrovascular accidents may

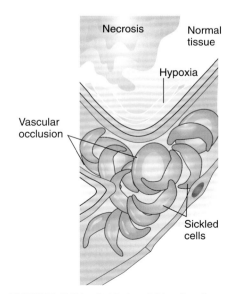

FIGURE 7.27 Sickled red blood cells occlude a blood vessel, causing hypoxia (low O$_2$ in cells) and necrosis (cell death).

Troponin is a heterotrimeric protein involved in the regulation of striated and cardiac muscle contraction. Most troponin in the cell is bound to the actin–tropomyosin complex in the muscle fibril. The three subunits of troponin consist of TnC, TnT, and TnI, each with a specific function in the regulatory process. TnT and TnI exist as different isoforms in cardiac and skeletal muscle (sequences with a different amino acid composition), thus allowing the development of specific antibodies against each form. As a consequence, either cTnT or cTnI may be rapidly measured in blood samples by immunoassay with a high degree of specificity.

be indicated. Iron chelation would likely have to accompany such a program to prevent or delay the development of iron overload. Although a few individuals with this disease have survived into the sixth decade, mean survival is probably into the fourth decade. Death usually results from infection, renal failure, and/or cardiopulmonary disease.

 Anne J. Mrs. J.'s diagnosis of an acute MI was partly based on measurements of cTnT (the cardiac isozyme of TnT, a subunit of the regulatory protein troponin). Early diagnosis is critical for a decision on the type of therapeutic intervention to be used. Serum cTnT is a highly specific marker of myocardial injury. It is typically detected in an acute MI within 3 to 5 hours after onset of symptoms, is positive in most cases within 8 hours, and approaches 100% sensitivity at 10 to 12 hours. It remains elevated for 5 to 10 days.

Mrs. J. stayed in the hospital until she had recovered from her catheterization and was stable on her medication. She was discharged on a low-fat diet and medications for her heart disease and was asked to participate in the hospital's cardiac rehabilitation program for patients recovering from a recent heart attack. Her physician scheduled regular examinations for her.

 Amy L. Amy L. has amyloidosis/AL, which is characterized by deposition of amyloid fibers derived principally from the variable region of λ- or κ-immunoglobulin light chains. Increased amounts of the fragments of the light chains called *Bence-Jones proteins* appeared in her urine. Fibril deposition in the ECM of her kidney glomeruli has resulted in mild renal failure. Deposition of amyloid in the ECM of her heart muscle resulted in thickened heart muscle seen on an echocardiogram. In addition to other signs of right-sided heart failure, she had peripheral edema. The loss of weight may have been caused by infiltrations of amyloid in the gastrointestinal tract or by constipation and diarrhea resulting from involvement of the autonomic nervous system. Treatment may be directed against the plasma cell proliferation and against the symptomatic results of organ dysfunction and is only partially successful. The most effective approach involves the use of stem cell transplantation in concert with melphalan (an antineoplastic agent). If the patient is not a candidate for transplantation, then melphalan with dexamethasone (a steroid) can be used. Renal transplantation and cardiac transplantation have been performed in patients with renal and cardiac amyloidosis, respectively, with some success.

During Amy's evaluation, she developed a cardiac arrhythmia that was refractory to treatment. The extensive amyloid deposits in her heart had disrupted the flow of electrical impulses in the conduction system of the heart, ultimately resulting in cardiac arrest. On autopsy, amyloid deposits were found within the heart, tongue, liver, adipose tissue, and every organ examined except the central nervous system, which had been protected by the blood–brain barrier.

 Dianne A. Dianne A.'s HbA1c of 8.5% was above the normal level of <6.0% of total hemoglobin. Glycosylation is a nonenzymatic reaction that occurs with a rate directly proportionate to the concentration of glucose in the blood. In the normal range of blood glucose concentrations (~80 to 140 mg/dL, depending on time after a meal), up to 6% of the hemoglobin is glycosylated to form HbA1c. Hemoglobin turns over in the blood as red blood cells are phagocytosed and their hemoglobin degraded and new red blood cells enter the blood from the bone marrow. The average lifespan of a red blood cell is 120 days. Thus, the extent of hemoglobin glycosylation is a direct reflection of the average serum glucose concentration to which the cell has been exposed over its 120-day lifespan. Dianne A.'s elevated HbA1c indicates that her average blood glucose level has been elevated over the preceding 3 to 4 months. An increase of Dianne A.'s insulin dosage would decrease her hyperglycemia and, over time, decrease her HbA1c level.

BIOCHEMICAL COMMENTS

The Basics of Hemoglobin Cooperativity. Using X-ray diffraction to study both the oxygenated and deoxygenated forms of hemoglobin, it is now possible to describe the change in conformation at the molecular level when oxygen binds to hemoglobin. We will present a simplistic approach here, looking at interactions that the β-subunit experiences and having oxygen bind initially to one of the two β-subunits in the hemoglobin tetramer. All of the subunits of hemoglobin contain eight helices, labeled A through H, with A representing the helix at the amino-terminal end. The deoxygenated form of hemoglobin is stabilized by the following interactions, which are also depicted in Figure 7.28:

1. Asp94 (of the F helix of the β-chain), through its carboxylate side chain, forms a salt bridge (ionic interaction) with the charged imidazole group of His146, which is the carboxy-terminal amino acid in the β-chain. Part of the Bohr effect is realized through this interaction because as the pH is reduced, the possibility that His146 is protonated is increased.
2. The carbonyl carbon of Val98 forms a hydrogen bond with the tyrosine hydroxyl group at position 145 (the next-to-last amino acid in the β-chain). The effect of these first two interactions is to position helices F and H in close proximity to each other.
3. The free carboxylate group of His146 (of the β-chain) forms a salt bridge with the ε-amino group of the side chain of Lys40 of the corresponding α-chain. This salt bridge allows communication between these two subunits and places the β-chain H helix close to the α-subunit.

A. No oxygen

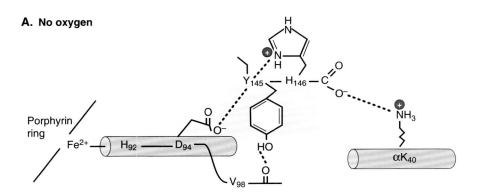

B. Plus oxygen

FIGURE 7.28 Molecular changes that occur when oxygen binds to hemoglobin. See the text for details. **A.** Interactions in the absence of oxygen. **B.** The loss of stabilizing interactions when oxygen binds.

In the β-chain, the proximal His92 (the eighth amino acid of the F helix [F8]) forms a coordinate covalent bond with the iron in heme and, in so doing, pulls the iron slightly out of the plane of the heme ring. These interactions are all occurring in the deoxygenated state.

So what happens when oxygen binds to a β-subunit? Oxygen binds to the iron in a bent conformation. The binding event triggers the movement of the iron into the plane of the heme ring. Because the iron is also covalently linked to histidine F8, the entire F helix, and the FG corner (where the F and G helices meet), also move.

1. Asp94 is in the F helix. As it is moved (because of the movement of the F helix), it can no longer form a salt bridge with the imidazole of His146, which weakens the interactions between the F and H helices.
2. Valine 98 is in the FG corner of the β-subunit, so as that moves, the hydrogen bond formed between Val98 and Tyr145 (at the end of the H helix) is also broken.
3. Due in part to the loss of interactions between the F and H helices, the H helix moves and, in so doing, breaks the ionic interaction between His146 and Lys40 of the α-subunit. This, along with the steric hindrance of the heme ring and His92, leads to a rotation of one αβ-dimer relative to the other αβ-dimer and will allow oxygen to bind more readily to the other subunits. The rotation of dimers also forces 2,3-BPG to leave its binding site on hemoglobin, which will favor oxygen binding.

The disruption of the bonds listed previously has to occur for oxygen to bind. This is why it takes a high concentration of oxygen to get the first oxygen bound to hemoglobin. At low oxygen levels, the oxygen can dissociate from the iron, which allows the T form to re-form and allow the salt bridges and hydrogen bonds, which stabilize the deoxygenated form, to re-form. If the oxygen concentration is high, such that the iron is continuously occupied with oxygen, the events described earlier are more likely to occur, and the oxygenation of hemoglobin will occur.

KEY CONCEPTS

- There are four levels of protein structure:
  - The primary structure (linear sequence of amino acids within the protein)
  - The secondary structure (a regular, repeating pattern of hydrogen bonds that stabilize a particular structure)
  - The tertiary structure (the folding of the secondary structure elements into a three-dimensional conformation)
  - The quaternary structure (the association of subunits within a protein)
- The primary structure of a protein determines the way a protein folds into a unique three-dimensional structure, called its *native conformation*.
- When globular proteins fold, the tertiary structure generally forms a densely packed hydrophobic core with polar amino acid side chains on the outside, facing the aqueous environment.
- The tertiary structure of a protein consists of structural domains, which may be similar between different proteins, and performs similar functions for the different proteins.
- Certain structural domains are binding sites for specific molecules, called a *ligand*, or for other proteins.
- The affinity of a binding site for its ligand is quantitatively characterized by an association or affinity constant, K_a (or dissociation constant, K_d).
- Protein denaturation is the loss of tertiary (and/or secondary) structure within a protein, which can be caused by heat, acid, or other agents that interfere with hydrogen bonding and usually causes a decrease in solubility (precipitation).
- Diseases discussed in this chapter are summarized in Table 7.1.

TABLE 7.1 Diseases Discussed in Chapter 7		
DISORDER OR CONDITION	**GENETIC OR ENVIRONMENTAL**	**COMMENTS**
Myocardial infarction	Both	Specific heart proteins analyzed include creatine kinase MB (heart-specific isozyme) and cardiac troponin T (cTnT, cardiac-specific isozyme). Myoglobin release is also elevated after a heart attack, but it is the least specific marker, whereas cTnT is the most specific marker for evidence of heart muscle damage.
Amyloidosis	Both	A generic name for the extracellular deposition of pathologic insoluble proteins, called amyloid, which are located in organs and tissues. In this chapter, the amyloid is derived from the immunoglobulin light chain. In this disorder, the amyloid will accumulate in the kidney and heart, leading to renal and cardiac related symptoms.
Sickle cell disease	Genetic	Hemoglobin S polymerization under deoxygenated conditions, owing to hydrophobic interactions caused by the valine in position 6 of the β-chain, instead of glutamic acid. This leads to alterations in red blood cell shape, which causes occluded capillaries. The lack of blood flow through the capillaries will lead to hypoxia and tissue damage, which generates some of the pain endured during a sickle-cell crisis.
Diabetes, types 1 and 2	Both	The use of glycosylated hemoglobin (HbA1c) to determine glycemic control in the diabetic patient. HbA1c is generated by the non-enzymatic glycosylation of hemoglobin. The extent of this reaction is dependent on the glucose levels in the circulation. The higher the blood glucose levels, the greater the extent of glycosylation.
Prion diseases	Both	Protein aggregation diseases due to altered tertiary structure for proteins with the same, or slightly altered, primary structure; the aggregates which form precipitate in the brain, leading to eventual neural degeneration and loss of function

REVIEW QUESTIONS—CHAPTER 7

1. One theory of amyloid fibril formation is that sections of α-helical structure are converted to β-sheets. Such regions of the amyloid proteins would most likely lack which one of the following amino acids?
   A. Cysteine
   B. Methionine
   C. Proline
   D. Leucine
   E. Isoleucine

2. In order for lipid-based hormones such as testosterone or estrogen to be transported in the bloodstream, they are bound to and transported by water-soluble proteins. In order to be water-soluble, the transporting protein contains which one of the following amino acids on its surface in contact with aqueous blood?
   A. Valine
   B. Arginine
   C. Leucine
   D. Isoleucine
   E. Phenylalanine

3. A patient has wheezing and shortness of breath, which are his typical asthma symptoms, so he takes a "rescue inhalant" which is a β_2-adrenergic receptor agonist. The active ingredient of the inhalant relaxes the smooth muscle of the bronchi and allows him to breathe more normally. The receptor to which the agonist binds can be best described by which one of the following?
   A. A globular protein
   B. A transmembrane protein
   C. A protein containing a nucleotide binding fold
   D. An exclusively β-pleated sheet protein
   E. A protein containing an actin fold

4. Autopsies of patients with Alzheimer disease show protein aggregates called *neurofibrillary tangles* and *neuritic plaques* in various regions of the brain. These plaques exhibit the characteristic staining of amyloid. Which of the following structural features is the most likely characteristic of at least one protein in these plaques?
   A. A high content of β-pleated sheet structure
   B. A high content of α-helical structure
   C. A high content of random coils
   D. Disulfide bond cross-links between polypeptide chains
   E. A low-energy native conformation

5. While studying a novel pathway in a remote species of bacteria, you discover a new globular protein that phosphorylates a substrate, using ATP as the phosphate donor. This protein most likely contains which one of the following structures?
   A. An actin fold
   B. An immunoglobulin fold
   C. A nucleotide binding fold
   D. A globin fold
   E. A β-barrel

6. β_2-Adrenergic agonists used as treatments for acute asthma attacks were formulated to have a higher affinity for the β_2-adrenergic receptor than epinephrine. Which one of the following would be true of the β_2-agonist as compared to epinephrine?
   A. The K_a of the agonist is higher than that of adrenaline.
   B. The K_a of the agonist is lower than that of adrenaline.
   C. The K_a of the agonist is the same as adrenaline.
   D. The K_d of the agonist is higher than that of adrenaline.
   E. The K_d of the agonist is equal to adrenaline.

7. A patient is exposed to hepatitis A and as a preventative measure is given hepatitis A immune globulin to prevent the patient from contracting the disease. The vaccine is an IgG immunoglobulin specific for coat proteins of the hepatitis A virus. The target of the immunoglobulin binds to which of the following locations in the immunoglobulin? Choose the one best answer.
   A. A site consisting of the constant regions of the heavy chains
   B. A site consisting of the constant regions of the light chains
   C. A site consisting of the variable regions of the light chains
   D. A site consisting of the variable regions of the heavy chains
   E. A site consisting of variable regions of both the light and heavy chains

8. Each IgG molecule (like hepatitis A immunoglobulin) contains two light and two heavy chains, which can be separated by the loss of which one of the following types of interactions?
   A. Hydrogen bonds
   B. Disulfide bonds
   C. Ionic bonds
   D. Van der Waals interactions
   E. The hydrophobic effect

9. A patient with type 1 diabetes was able to lower her HbA1c value from 8.2% to 5.9%. This occurred because of a reduction of which one of the following processes?
   A. Enzymatic oxidation
   B. Nonenzymatic oxidation
   C. Enzymatic glycosylation
   D. Nonenzymatic glycosylation
   E. Enzymatic reduction
   F. Nonenzymatic reduction

10. In amyloidosis, α-helices may form alternative β-sheets of amyloid fibrils. The α-helices in these proteins can be characterized by which one of the following?
   A. They all have the same primary structure.
   B. They are formed principally by hydrogen bonds between a carbonyl oxygen atom in one peptide bond and the amide hydrogen from a different peptide bond.
   C. They are formed principally by hydrogen bonds between a carbonyl atom in one peptide bond and the hydrogen atoms on the side chain of another amino acid.
   D. They are formed by hydrogen bonding between two adjacent amino acids in the primary sequence.
   E. They require a high content of proline and glycine.

ANSWERS

1. **The answer is C.** In the α-helix, the oxygen atom of a carbonyl group forms a hydrogen bond with the nitrogen atom four amino acids farther along the chain. Because proline's nitrogen is part of its cyclic structure, when proline is in a peptide bond, its nitrogen group lacks a proton and cannot form a hydrogen bond with the appropriate carbonyl oxygen atom. The bond angles within the proline ring are also incompatible with α-helix formation, such that proline is known as a "helix breaker." None of the other amino acids listed has its nitrogen in a cyclic structure, so all can form the bond angles and hydrogen bonds necessary for an α-helix.

2. **The answer is B.** Arginine is a charged polar amino acid and is water-soluble, whereas the others listed are non-polar and hydrophobic and are not expected to be on the surface of a protein exposed to an aqueous environment.

3. **The answer is B.** The β_2-adrenergic receptor is a transmembrane protein that contains seven membrane-spanning domains and has intracellular and extracellular domains on either side of the membrane. It is composed primarily of α-helices but not β-sheets. It does not contain an actin fold and is neither a globular protein nor a protein containing a nucleotide binding fold. The receptor is coupled to a GTP-binding protein (a G-protein), which does bind GTP or guanosine diphosphate (GDP). The receptor itself, however, does not bind nucleotides.

4. **The answer is A.** The characteristic staining of amyloid arises from fibrils of β-pleated sheet structure perpendicular to the axis of the fiber (thus, B, C, and D are incorrect). The native conformation of a protein is generally the most stable and lowest energy conformation, and the lower its energy state, the more readily a protein folds into its native conformation and the less likely it will assume the insoluble β-pleated sheet structure of amyloid (thus, E is incorrect).

5. **The answer is A.** The protein hydrolyzes ATP, which is a characteristic of the actin fold. None of the other folds described will hydrolyze ATP.

6. **The answer is A.** The binding affinity is described quantitatively by its association constant, K_a. The higher the K_a, the higher the affinity. Because K_d is the reciprocal of K_a ($1/K_a$), the higher the affinity, the lower the K_d. Because the β-agonist has a higher affinity than adrenaline, its K_a would be higher and its K_d would be lower than that of adrenaline.

7. **The answer is E.** The variable regions of the light and heavy chains interact to produce a single antigen-specific binding site (in this case, for the hepatitis A virus) at each branch of the Y-shaped immunoglobulin. The constant regions are not involved with specific immunity. The variable regions are physically separated such that they are not able to interact with each other (variable L with variable L or variable H with variable H). The variable region of a light chain is immediately adjacent to the variable region of a heavy chain, and they interact to form a single binding site.

8. **The answer is B.** Each IgG molecule contains two light and two heavy chains joined by disulfide bonds. Reduction of the disulfide bonds will lead to the separation of the light and heavy chains.

9. **The answer is D.** In nonenzymatic glycosylation, glucose present in blood binds to amino acids on hemoglobin forming an irreversible glycosylated protein through the lifetime of that red blood cell. Because the reaction is nonenzymatic, the rate of glycosylation is proportional to the concentration of the glucose present. Patients with consistently high blood glucose will have a high HbA1c, a marker of poor diabetic control. Oxidation and/or reduction is not involved with the formation of HbA1c.

10. **The answer is B.** The regular repeating structure of an α-helix is possible because it is formed by hydrogen bonds within the peptide backbone of a single strand. Thus, α-helices can be formed from a variety of primary structures. However, proline cannot accommodate the bends for an α-helix because the atoms involved in the peptide backbone are part of a ring structure and glycine cannot provide the space-filling required for a stable structure.

8 Enzymes as Catalysts

Enzymes are proteins that act as **catalysts**, which are compounds that increase the rate of chemical reactions (Fig. 8.1). Enzyme catalysts bind reactants (substrates), convert them to products, and release the products. Although enzymes may be modified during their participation in this reaction sequence, they return to their original form at the end. In addition to increasing the speed of reactions, enzymes provide a means for regulating the rate of metabolic pathways in the body. This chapter describes the properties of enzymes that allow them to function as catalysts. The next chapter explains the mechanisms of enzyme regulation.

Enzyme-Binding Sites. An enzyme binds the **substrates** of the reaction and converts them to **products**. The substrates are bound to specific **substrate-binding sites** on the enzyme through interactions with the amino acid residues of the enzyme. The spatial geometry required for all the interactions between the substrate and the enzyme makes each enzyme **selective for** its **substrates** and ensures that only **specific products** are formed.

Active Catalytic Sites. The substrate-binding sites overlap in the **active catalytic site** of the enzyme, the region of the enzyme where the reaction occurs. Within the catalytic site, **functional groups** provided by **coenzymes**, **tightly bound metals**, and, of course, **amino acid residues** of the enzyme, participate in catalysis.

Activation Energy and the Transition State. The functional groups in the catalytic site of the enzyme activate the substrate and decrease the energy needed to form the high-energy intermediate stage of the reaction known as the **transition-state complex**. Some of the catalytic strategies employed by enzymes, such as **general acid–base catalysis**, formation of **covalent intermediates**, and **stabilization of the transition state**, are illustrated by **chymotrypsin**.

pH and Temperature Profiles. Enzymes have a functional pH range determined by the **pK_a** of the functional groups in the active site and the interactions required for three-dimensional structure. Increases of temperature, which do not lead to protein denaturation, increase the reaction rate.

Mechanism-Based Inhibitors. The effectiveness of many **drugs** and **toxins** depends on their ability to inhibit an enzyme. The strongest inhibitors are **covalent inhibitors**, compounds that form covalent bonds with a reactive group in the enzyme active site, or **transition-state analogs** that mimic the transition-state complex.

Enzyme Names. Most enzyme names end in "-ase." Enzymes usually have both a common name and a systematic classification that includes a name and an Enzyme Commission (EC) number.

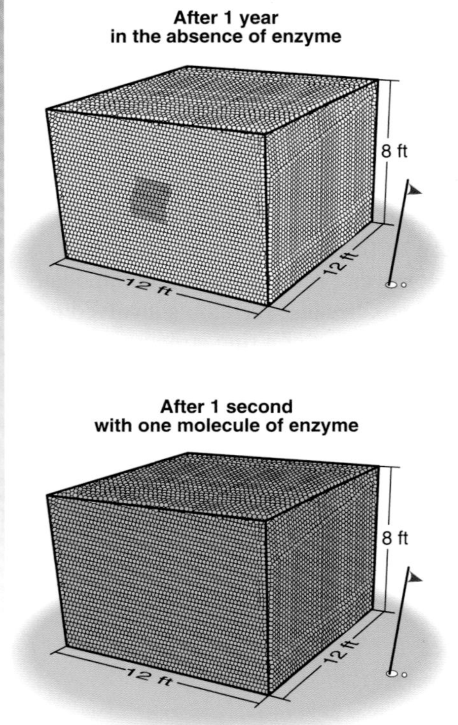

After 1 year in the absence of enzyme

After 1 second with one molecule of enzyme

FIGURE 8.1 Catalytic power of enzymes. Many enzymes increase the rate of a chemical reaction by a factor of 10^{11} or higher. To appreciate an increase in reaction rate by this order of magnitude, consider a room-sized box of golf balls that "react" by releasing energy and turning brown. The 12 ft × 12 ft × 8 ft box contains 380,000 golf balls. If the rate of the reaction in the absence of enzyme were 100 golf balls per year, the presence of 1 molecule of enzyme would turn the entire box of golf balls brown in 1 second (assuming a 10^{11} increase in reaction rate).

THE WAITING ROOM

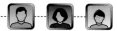

A year after recovering from salicylate poisoning (see Chapter 4), **Dennis V.** was playing in his grandfather's basement. Dennis drank an unknown amount of the insecticide malathion, which is sometimes used for killing fruit flies and other insects (Fig. 8.2). Sometime later, when he was not feeling well, Dennis told his grandfather what he had done. Mr. V. retrieved the bottle and rushed Dennis to the emergency department of the local hospital. On the way, Dennis vomited repeatedly and complained of abdominal cramps. At the hospital, he began salivating and had an uncontrollable defecation.

In the emergency department, physicians passed a nasogastric tube for stomach lavage, started intravenous fluids, and recorded vital signs. Dennis's pulse rate was 48 beats/minute (slow), and his blood pressure was 78/48 mm Hg (low). The physicians noted involuntary twitching of the muscles in his extremities.

Lotta T. was diagnosed with acute gouty arthritis involving her right great toe (see Chapter 5). The presence of insoluble urate crystals within the joint space confirmed the diagnosis. Several weeks after her acute gout attack subsided, Ms. T. was started on allopurinol therapy in an oral dose of 150 mg twice per day. Allopurinol therapy is effective because the drug inhibits the activity of a specific enzyme.

Al M., a 44-year-old man who has been an alcoholic for the past 5 years, has a markedly diminished appetite for food. One weekend, he became unusually irritable and confused after drinking two 750-mL bottles of scotch and eating very little. His landlady convinced him to visit his doctor. Physical examination indicated a heart rate of 104 beats/minute. His blood pressure was slightly low, and he was in early congestive heart failure. He was poorly oriented to time, place, and person.

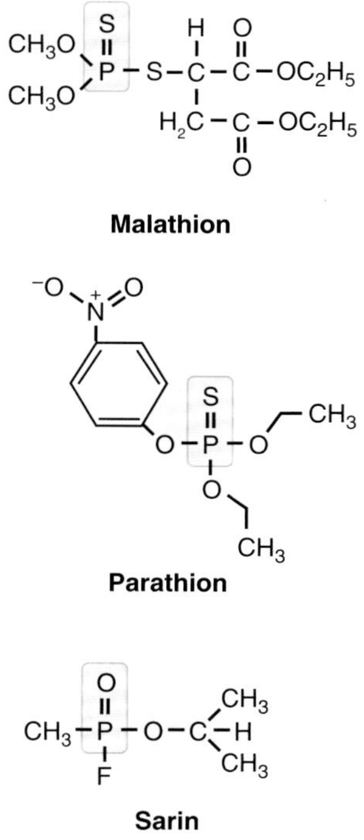

I. The Enzyme-Catalyzed Reaction

Enzymes, in general, provide speed, specificity, and regulatory control to reactions in the body. Enzymes are usually proteins that act as catalysts, compounds that increase the rate of chemical reactions. Enzyme-catalyzed reactions have three basic steps:

1. Binding of substrate (a reactant): $\mathbf{E + S \leftrightarrow ES}$
2. Conversion of bound substrate to bound product: $\mathbf{ES \leftrightarrow EP}$
3. Release of product: $\mathbf{EP \leftrightarrow E + P}$

An enzyme binds the substrates of the reaction it catalyzes and brings them together at the right orientation to react. The enzyme then participates in the making and breaking of bonds required for product formation, releases the products, and returns to its original state once the reaction is completed.

Enzymes do not invent new reactions; they simply make reactions occur faster. The catalytic power of an enzyme (the rate of the catalyzed reaction divided by the rate of the uncatalyzed reaction) is usually in the range of 10^6 to 10^{14}. Without the catalytic power of enzymes, reactions such as those involved in nerve conduction, heart contraction, and digestion of food would occur too slowly for life to exist.

Each enzyme usually catalyzes a specific biochemical reaction. The ability of an enzyme to select just one substrate and distinguish this substrate from a group of very similar compounds is referred to as *specificity* (Fig. 8.3). The enzyme converts this substrate to just one product. The specificity as well as the speed of enzyme-catalyzed reactions result from the unique sequence of specific amino acids that form the three-dimensional structure of the enzyme.

A. The Active Site

To catalyze a chemical reaction, the enzyme forms an enzyme–substrate complex in its active catalytic site (Fig. 8.4). The *active site* is usually a cleft or crevice in the

Malathion

Parathion

Sarin

FIGURE 8.2 Organophosphorus compounds. Malathion and parathion are organophosphorus insecticides. Nausea, coma, convulsions, respiratory failure, and death have resulted from the use of parathion by farmers who have gotten it on their skin. Malathion is similar in structure to parathion but is not nearly as toxic. The nerve gas sarin, another organophosphorus compound, was used in a terrorist attack in a subway in Japan.

Most, if not all, of the tissues and organs in the body are adversely affected by chronic ingestion of excessive amounts of alcohol, including the liver, pancreas, heart, reproductive organs, central nervous system, and the fetus. Some of the effects of alcohol ingestion, such as the psychotropic effects on the brain or inhibition of vitamin transport, are direct effects caused by ethanol itself. However, many of the acute and chronic pathophysiologic effects of alcohol relate to the pathways of ethanol metabolism (see Chapter 33).

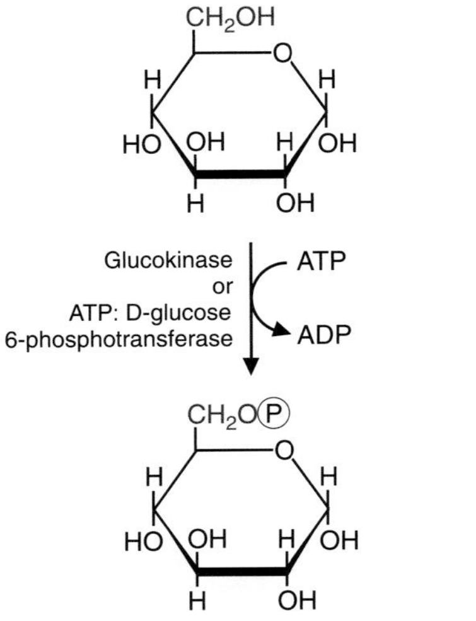

FIGURE 8.3 Reaction catalyzed by glucokinase, an example of enzyme reaction specificity. Glucokinase catalyzes the transfer of a phosphate (*P*) from adenosine triphosphate (ATP) to carbon 6 of glucose. It cannot rapidly transfer a phosphate from other nucleotides to glucose, or from ATP to closely related sugars such as galactose, or from ATP to any other carbon on glucose. The only products formed are glucose 6-phosphate and adenosine diphosphate (ADP).

enzyme formed by one or more regions of the polypeptide chain. Within the active site, cofactors and functional groups from the polypeptide chain participate in transforming the bound substrate molecules into products.

Initially, the substrate molecules bind to their substrate-binding sites, also called the *substrate-recognition sites* (see Fig. 8.4B). The three-dimensional arrangement of binding sites in a crevice of the enzyme allows the reacting portions of the substrates to approach each other from the appropriate angles. The proximity of the bound substrate molecules and their precise orientation toward each other contribute to the catalytic power of the enzyme.

The active site also contains functional groups that participate directly in the reaction (see Fig. 8.4C). The functional groups are donated by the polypeptide chain, or by bound cofactors (metals or complex organic molecules called *coenzymes*). As the substrate binds, it induces conformational changes in the enzyme that promote further interactions between the substrate molecules and the enzyme functional groups. (For example, a coenzyme might form a covalent intermediate with the substrate, or an amino acid side chain might abstract a proton from the reacting substrate.) The activated substrates and the enzyme form a *transition-state complex*, an unstable high-energy complex with a strained electronic configuration that is intermediate between substrate and product. Additional bonds with the enzyme stabilize the transition-state complex and decrease the energy required for its formation.

The transition-state complex decomposes to products, which dissociate from the enzyme (see Fig. 8.4D). The enzyme generally returns to its original form. The free enzyme then binds another set of substrates and repeats the process.

B. Substrate-Binding Sites

Enzyme specificity (the enzyme's ability to react with just one substrate) results from the three-dimensional arrangement of specific amino acid residues in the enzyme that form binding sites for the substrates and activate the substrates during the course of the reaction. The "lock-and-key" and the "induced-fit" models for substrate binding describe two aspects of the binding interaction between the enzyme and substrate.

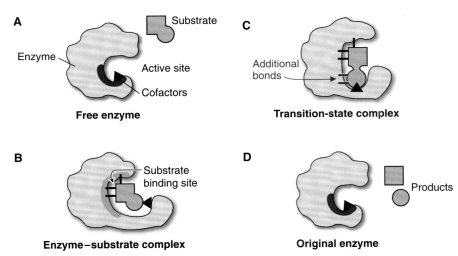

FIGURE 8.4 Reaction in the enzyme active catalytic site. **A.** The enzyme contains an active catalytic site, shown in *dark red*, with a region or domain where the substrate binds. The active site also may contain cofactors—nonprotein components that assist in catalysis. **B.** The substrate forms bonds with amino acid residues in the substrate-binding site. Substrate binding induces a conformational change in the active site. **C.** Functional groups of amino acid residues and cofactors in the active site participate in forming the transition-state complex, which is stabilized by additional noncovalent bonds with the enzyme, shown in *red*. **D.** Because the products of the reaction dissociate, the enzyme returns to its original conformation.

I. Lock-and-Key Model for Substrate Binding

The substrate-binding site contains amino acid residues arranged in a complementary three-dimensional surface that "recognizes" the substrate and binds it through multiple hydrophobic interactions, electrostatic interactions, or hydrogen bonds. The amino acid residues that bind the substrate can come from very different parts of the linear amino acid sequence of the enzyme, as seen in glucokinase. The binding of compounds with a structure that differs from the substrate even to a small degree may be prevented by steric hindrance and charge repulsion. In the lock-and-key model, the complementarity between the substrate and its binding site is compared to that of a key fitting into a rigid lock.

2. Induced-Fit Model for Substrate Binding

Complementarity between the substrate and the binding site is only part of the picture. As the substrate binds, enzymes undergo a conformational change ("induced fit") that repositions the side chains of the amino acids in the active site and increases the number of binding interactions (see Fig. 8.4). The induced-fit model for substrate binding recognizes that the substrate-binding site is not a rigid "lock" but rather a dynamic surface created by the flexible overall three-dimensional structure of the enzyme.

The function of the conformational change induced by substrate binding, the induced fit, is usually to reposition functional groups in the active site in a way that promotes the reaction, improves the binding site of a cosubstrate, or activates an adjacent subunit through cooperativity. For example, consider the large conformational changes that occur in the actin fold of glucokinase when glucose binds. First, the substrate glucose binds in a manner resembling a lock and key (Fig. 8.5). As glucose binds, the induced fit results. The induced fit involves changes in the conformation of the whole enzyme that close the cleft of the fold, thereby improving the binding site for adenosine triphosphate (ATP) and excluding water (which

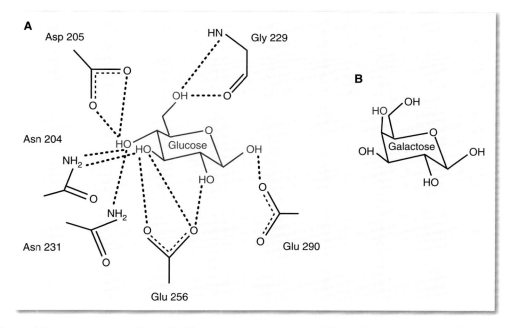

FIGURE 8.5 Glucose-binding site in glucokinase. **A.** Glucose, shown in *red*, is held in its binding site by multiple hydrogen bonds between each hydroxyl group and polar amino acids from different regions of the enzyme amino acid sequence in the actin fold (see Chapter 7). The position of the amino acid residue in the linear sequence is given by its number. The multiple interactions enable glucose to induce large conformational changes in the enzyme (induced fit). (Modified from Pilkis SJ, Weber IT, Harrison RW, Bell GI. Glucokinase: structural analysis of a protein involved in susceptibility to diabetes. *J Biol Chem.* 1994;269:21925–21928.) **B.** Enzyme specificity is illustrated by the comparison of galactose and glucose. Galactose differs from glucose only in the position of the –OH group shown in *red*. However, it is not phosphorylated at a significant rate by the enzyme. Cells therefore require a separate galactokinase for the metabolism of galactose.

A

D-glucose

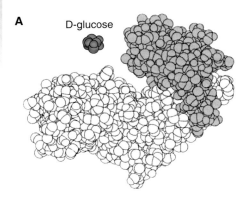

B

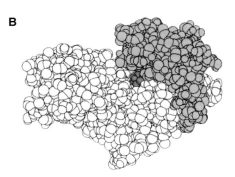

FIGURE 8.6 Conformational change resulting from the binding of glucose to hexokinase. (The figure is actually yeast hexokinase, which is more similar to human glucokinase than it is to the other human hexokinase isozymes.) The *shaded* and *unshaded areas* show the two domains (four subdomains) that form the actin fold with its adenosine triphosphate (ATP)-binding cleft. **A.** Free enzyme. **B.** With glucose bound, the cleft closes, forming the ATP-binding site. The closure of the cleft when glucose binds to hexokinase (or human glucokinase) is one of the largest "induced fits" known. The combination of secondary structures in the actin fold that give hexokinase the flexibility required for this shift are discussed in Chapter 7, Section IV.B.I, "The Actin Fold." (From Bennett WS, Steitz TA. Structure of a complex between yeast hexokinase A and glucose II. Detailed comparisons of conformation and active site configuration with the native hexokinase B monomer and dimer. *J Mol Biol.* 1980;140:211–230.)

might interfere with the reaction) from the active site (Fig. 8.6). Thus, the multiple interactions between the substrate and the enzyme in the catalytic site serve both for substrate recognition and for initiating the next stage of the reaction, formation of the transition-state complex.

C. The Transition-State Complex

In order for a reaction to occur, the substrates undergoing the reaction need to be activated. If the energy levels of a substrate are plotted as the substrate is progressively converted to product, the curve will show a maximum energy level that is higher than that of either the substrate or the product (Fig. 8.7). This high energy level occurs at the transition state. For some enzyme-catalyzed reactions, the transition state is a condition in which bonds in the substrate are maximally strained. For other enzyme-catalyzed reactions, the electronic configuration of the substrate becomes very strained and unstable as it enters the transition state. The highest energy level corresponds to the most unstable substrate configuration and the condition in which the changing substrate molecule is most tightly bound to participating functional groups in the enzyme. The difference in energy between the substrate and the transition-state complex is called the *activation energy*.

According to transition-state theory, the overall rate of the reaction is determined by the number of molecules acquiring the activation energy necessary to form the transition-state complex. Enzymes increase the rate of the reaction by decreasing this activation energy. They use various catalytic strategies, such as electronic stabilization of the transition-state complex or *acid–base catalysis*, to obtain this decrease.

Once the transition-state complex is formed, it can collapse back to substrates or decompose to form products. The enzyme does not change the initial energy level of the substrates or the final energy level of the products.

Because the transition-state complex binds more tightly to the enzyme than does the substrate, compounds that resemble its electronic and three-dimensional surface (*transition-state analogs*) are more potent inhibitors of an enzyme than are substrate analogs. Consequently, a drug developed as a transition-state analog would be highly specific for the enzyme it is designed to inhibit. However, transition-state analogs are highly unstable when they are not bound to the enzyme and would have great difficulty making it from the digestive tract or injection site to the site of action. Some of the approaches in drug design that are being used to deal with the

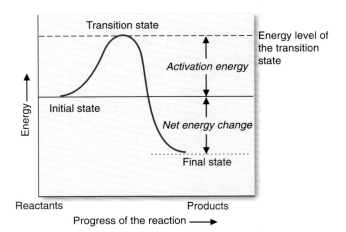

FIGURE 8.7 Energy diagram showing the energy levels of the substrates as they progress toward products in the absence of enzyme. The substrates must pass through the high-energy transition state during the reaction. Although a favorable loss of energy occurs during the reaction, the rate of the reaction is slowed by the energy barrier to forming the transition state. The energy barrier is referred to as the *activation energy*.

instability problem include designing drugs that are almost transition-state analogs but have a stable modification, designing a prodrug that is converted to a transition-state analog at the site of action, and using the transition-state analog to design a complementary antibody.

If the structure of a transition state can be modeled, it can be used as an antigen for the production of *abzymes* (catalytic antibodies). These antibodies have an arrangement of amino acid side chains in their variable regions that is similar to the active site of the enzyme in the transition state. Consequently, they can act as artificial enzymes. For example, abzymes have been developed against analogs of the transition-state complex of cocaine esterase, the enzyme that degrades cocaine in the body. These abzymes have esterase activity, and monthly injections of the abzyme drug can be used to rapidly destroy cocaine in the blood, thereby decreasing the dependence of addicted individuals. (See Chapter 7 for antibody structure.)

II. Strategies for Catalysis

There are five major strategies used by enzymes to enable catalysis: general acid–base catalysis, covalent catalysis, metal-ion catalysis, catalysis by approximation, and cofactor catalysis. Some enzymes will use a combination of these strategies.

A. General Acid–Base Catalysis

In *general acid–base catalysis*, a functional group on the protein either donates a proton (acid catalysis) or accepts a proton (general base catalysis) during the course of the reaction. An example of general acid–base catalysis is seen in the mechanism of chymotrypsin (see the chymotrypsin online module). During the course of this reaction, histidine 57 acts as a general base catalyst and accepts a proton from serine 195, activating the serine to act as a nucleophile. Later on in the reaction sequence, the protonated histidine 57 acts as a general acid catalyst and donates a proton to a product leaving the reaction.

B. Covalent Catalysis

In *covalent catalysis*, the substrate is covalently linked during the course of the reaction to an amino acid side chain at the active site of the enzyme. *Chymotrypsin* (a protease, an enzyme that breaks peptide bonds) also exhibits covalent catalysis. Once histidine 57 activates serine 195 by removing its proton from the hydroxyl group on the side chain, the negatively charged oxyanion attacks the carbonyl group of the peptide bond to be cleaved by the enzyme, forming a covalent bond and tetrahedral intermediate. The substrate stays covalently linked to the enzyme through the course of the reaction.

C. Metal-Ion Catalysis

Many enzymes contain required metal ions to allow catalysis to occur. In the case of carbonic anhydrase, an enzyme-bound zinc at the active site binds and orients water appropriately so it can participate in the reaction. In the absence of the active site zinc, the reaction occurs very slowly, if at all.

D. Catalysis by Approximation

Catalysis by approximation refers to the enzyme forcing (through the formation of hydrogen bonds and ionic interactions between the enzyme and substrate) substrates to bind in a manner that places reactive groups in the appropriate orientation so a reaction can take place. Nucleoside monophosphate kinases use this type of mechanism to transfer a phosphate from a nucleoside triphosphate to a nucleoside monophosphate, producing two nucleoside diphosphates.

E. Cofactor Catalysis

In *cofactor catalysis*, a required cofactor for an enzyme usually forms a covalent bond with the substrate during the course of the reaction. Enzymes involved in amino acid metabolism use pyridoxal phosphate (derived from vitamin B_6) to form a covalent bond during the course of the reaction.

III. Functional Groups in Catalysis

The catalytic strategies as described in the previous section to increase the reaction rate are common to many enzymes. A variety of functional groups are used by different enzymes to carry out these catalytic strategies. Some enzymes, such as chymotrypsin, rely on amino acid residues within the active site. Other enzymes increase their repertoire by employing cofactors (nonprotein compounds that participate in the catalytic process) to provide a functional group with the right size, shape, and properties. They are generally divided into three categories: coenzymes (e.g., pyridoxal phosphate), metal ions (e.g., Fe^{2+}, Mg^{2+}, or Zn^{2+}), and metallocoenzymes (similar to the Fe^{2+}-heme in hemoglobin; see Chapter 7).

A. Functional Groups on Amino Acid Side Chains

Almost all of the polar amino acids participate directly in catalysis in one or more enzymes (Table 8.1). Serine, cysteine, lysine, and histidine can participate in covalent catalysis. Histidine, because it has a pK_a that can donate and accept a proton at neutral pH, often participates in acid–base catalysis. Most of the polar amino acid side chains are nucleophilic and participate in nucleophilic catalysis by stabilizing more positively charged groups that develop during the reaction.

B. Coenzymes in Catalysis

Coenzymes (cofactors) are complex nonprotein organic molecules that participate in catalysis by providing functional groups, much like the amino acid side chains. In humans, they are usually (but not always) synthesized from vitamins. Each coenzyme is involved in catalyzing a specific type of reaction for a class of substrates with certain structural features. Coenzymes can be divided into two general classes: activation-transfer coenzymes and oxidation–reduction coenzymes.

Q In the stomach, gastric acid decreases the pH to 1 to 2 to denature proteins through disruption of hydrogen bonding. The protease in the stomach, pepsin, is a member of the aspartate protease superfamily, enzymes that use two aspartate residues in the active site for acid–base catalysis of the peptide bond. Why can they not use histidine like chymotrypsin?

Because most vitamins function as coenzymes, the symptoms of vitamin deficiencies reflect the loss of specific enzyme activities that depend on the coenzyme form of the vitamin. Thus, drugs and toxins that inhibit proteins required for coenzyme synthesis (e.g., vitamin transport proteins or biosynthetic enzymes) can cause the symptoms of a vitamin deficiency. This type of deficiency is called a *functional deficiency*, whereas an inadequate intake is called a *dietary deficiency*.

Most coenzymes are tightly bound to their enzymes and do not dissociate during the course of the reaction. However, a functional or dietary vitamin deficiency that decreases the level of a coenzyme will result in the presence of the apoenzyme in cells (an enzyme devoid of cofactor).

Ethanol is an "antivitamin" that decreases the cellular content of almost every coenzyme. For example, ethanol inhibits the absorption of thiamine, and acetaldehyde produced from ethanol oxidation displaces pyridoxal phosphate from its protein-binding sites, thereby accelerating its degradation.

Q Although coenzymes look as though they should be able to catalyze reactions autonomously (on their own), they have almost no catalytic power when not bound to the enzyme. Why?

TABLE 8.1 Some Functional Groups in the Active Site	
FUNCTION OF AMINO ACID	**ENZYME EXAMPLE**
Covalent intermediates	
Cysteine–SH	Glyceraldehyde 3-phosphate dehydrogenase
Serine–OH	Acetylcholinesterase, chymotrypsin
Lysine–NH$_2$	Aldolase
Histidine–NH	Phosphoglucomutase
Acid–base catalysis	
Histidine–NH	Chymotrypsin
Aspartate–COOH	Pepsin
Stabilization of anion formed during the reaction	
Peptide backbone–NH	Chymotrypsin
Arginine–NH	Carboxypeptidase A
Serine–OH	Alcohol dehydrogenase

I. Activation-Transfer Coenzymes

Activation-transfer coenzymes usually participate directly in catalysis by forming a covalent bond with a portion of the substrate; the tightly held substrate moiety is then activated for transfer, addition of water, or some other reaction. The portion of the coenzyme that forms a covalent bond with the substrate is its functional group. A separate portion of the coenzyme binds tightly to the enzyme. In general, coenzymes are nonprotein organic cofactors that participate in reactions. They may be covalently bound to enzymes (e.g., biotin), noncovalently bound such that they dissociate from the enzyme under cofactor deficiency conditions (e.g., thiamin), or become incorporated into a product of the reaction (e.g., coenzyme A [CoA], which is derived from pantothenic acid). Cofactors that are covalently or very tightly bound to nonenzyme proteins are usually called *prosthetic groups*. A prosthetic group, such as the heme in hemoglobin, usually does not dissociate from a protein until the protein is degraded.

Thiamine pyrophosphate (TPP) provides a good illustration of the manner in which coenzymes participate in catalysis (Fig. 8.8). It is synthesized in human cells from the vitamin thiamine by the addition of a pyrophosphate. This pyrophosphate provides negatively charged oxygen atoms that chelate Mg^{2+}, which then binds

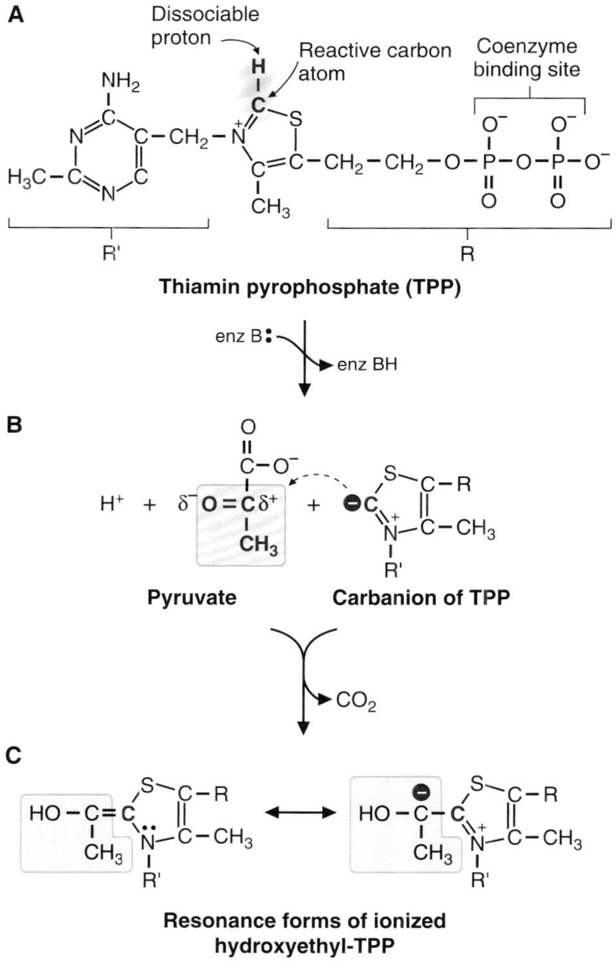

A To participate in general acid–base catalysis, the amino acid side chain must be able to extract a proton at one stage of the reaction and donate it back at another. Histidine (pK_a = 6.0) would be protonated at this low pH and could not extract a proton from a potential nucleophile. However, aspartic acid, with a pK_a of ~2 can release protons at a pH = 2. The two aspartates work together to activate water through the removal of a proton to form the hydroxyl nucleophile.

A In order for a substrate to react with a coenzyme, it must collide with a coenzyme at exactly the right angle. The probability of the substrate and coenzyme in free solution colliding in exactly the right place at the exactly right angle is very small. In addition to providing this proximity and orientation, enzymes contribute in other ways, such as activating the coenzyme by extracting a proton (e.g., TPP and CoA) or polarizing the substrate to make it more susceptible to nucleophilic attack.

FIGURE 8.8 The role of the functional group of thiamin pyrophosphate (*TPP*; the reactive carbon shown in *red*) in formation of a covalent intermediate. **A.** A base on the enzyme (*enzB*) abstracts a proton from thiamine, creating a carbanion (general acid–base catalysis). **B.** The carbanion is a strong nucleophile and attacks the partially positively charged keto group on the substrate. **C.** A covalent intermediate is formed, which, after decarboxylation, is stabilized by resonance forms. The uncharged intermediate is the stabilized transition-state complex.

tightly to the enzyme. The functional group that extends into the active site is the reactive carbon atom with a dissociable proton (see Fig. 8.8). In all of the enzymes that use thiamin pyrophosphate, this reactive thiamin carbon forms a covalent bond with a substrate keto group while cleaving the adjacent carbon–carbon bond. However, each thiamin-containing enzyme catalyzes the cleavage of a different substrate (or group of substrates with very closely related structures).

Coenzymes have very little activity in the absence of the enzyme and very little specificity. The enzyme provides *specificity*, *proximity*, and *orientation* in the substrate-recognition site, as well as other functional groups for stabilization of the transition state, acid–base catalysis, and so forth. For example, thiamin is made into a better nucleophilic attacking group by a basic amino acid residue in the enzyme that removes the dissociable proton (*EnzB* in Fig. 8.8), thereby generating a negatively charged thiamin carbon anion. Later in the reaction, the enzyme returns the proton.

CoA, biotin, and pyridoxal phosphate are also activation-transfer coenzymes synthesized from vitamins. CoA (CoASH), which is synthesized from the vitamin pantothenate, contains an adenosine $3',5'$-bisphosphate that binds reversibly, but tightly, to a site on an enzyme (Fig. 8.9A). Its functional group, a sulfhydryl group at the other end of the molecule, is a nucleophile that always attacks carbonyl groups and forms acyl thioesters (in fact, the "A" in Co*A* stands for the *a*cyl group that becomes attached). Most coenzymes, such as functional groups on the enzyme amino acids, are regenerated during the course of the reaction. However, CoASH and a few of the oxidation–reduction coenzymes are transformed during the reaction into products that dissociate from the enzyme at the end of the reaction (e.g., CoASH is converted to an acyl-CoA derivative, and nicotinamide adenine dinucleotide [NAD^+] is reduced to NADH). These dissociating coenzymes are nonetheless classified as coenzymes rather than substrates because they are common to so many reactions, the original form is regenerated by subsequent reactions in a metabolic pathway, they are synthesized from vitamins, and the amount of coenzyme in the cell is nearly constant.

Biotin, which does not contain a phosphate group, is covalently bonded to a lysine in enzymes called *carboxylases* (see Fig. 8.9B). Its functional group is a nitrogen atom that covalently binds a CO_2 group in an energy-requiring reaction. This bound CO_2 group is activated for addition to another molecule. In humans, biotin functions only in carboxylation reactions.

Pyridoxal phosphate is synthesized from the vitamin pyridoxine, which is also called *vitamin B_6* (see Fig. 8.9C). The reactive aldehyde group usually functions in enzyme-catalyzed reactions by forming a covalent bond with the amino groups on amino acids. The positively charged ring nitrogen withdraws electrons from a bond in the bound amino acid, resulting in cleavage of that bond. The enzyme participates by removing protons from the substrate and by keeping the amino acid and the pyridoxal group in a single plane to facilitate shuttling of electrons.

These coenzymes illustrate three features all activation-transfer coenzymes have in common: (1) a specific chemical group involved in binding to the enzyme, (2) a separate and different functional or reactive group that participates directly in the catalysis of one type of reaction by forming a covalent bond with the substrate, and (3) dependence on the enzyme for additional specificity of substrate and additional catalytic power.

2. Oxidation–Reduction Coenzymes

Oxidation–reduction coenzymes are involved in oxidation–reduction reactions catalyzed by enzymes categorized as *oxidoreductases*. When a compound is oxidized, it loses electrons. As a result, the oxidized carbon has fewer H atoms or gains an O atom. The reduction of a compound is the gain of electrons, which shows in its structure as the gain of H, or loss of O. Some coenzymes, such as NAD^+ and flavin adenine dinucleotide (FAD), can transfer electrons together with hydrogen and have unique roles in the generation of ATP from the oxidation of fuels.

Many people with alcoholism, like **Al M.**, develop thiamin deficiency because alcohol inhibits the transport of thiamine through the intestinal mucosal cells. In the body, thiamine is converted to TPP. TPP acts as a coenzyme in the decarboxylation of α-keto acids such as pyruvate and α-ketoglutarate (see Fig. 8.9) and in the use of pentose phosphates in the pentose phosphate pathway. As a result of thiamin deficiency, the oxidation of α-keto acids is impaired. Dysfunction occurs in the central and peripheral nervous system, the cardiovascular system, and other organs, which require a large amount of energy.

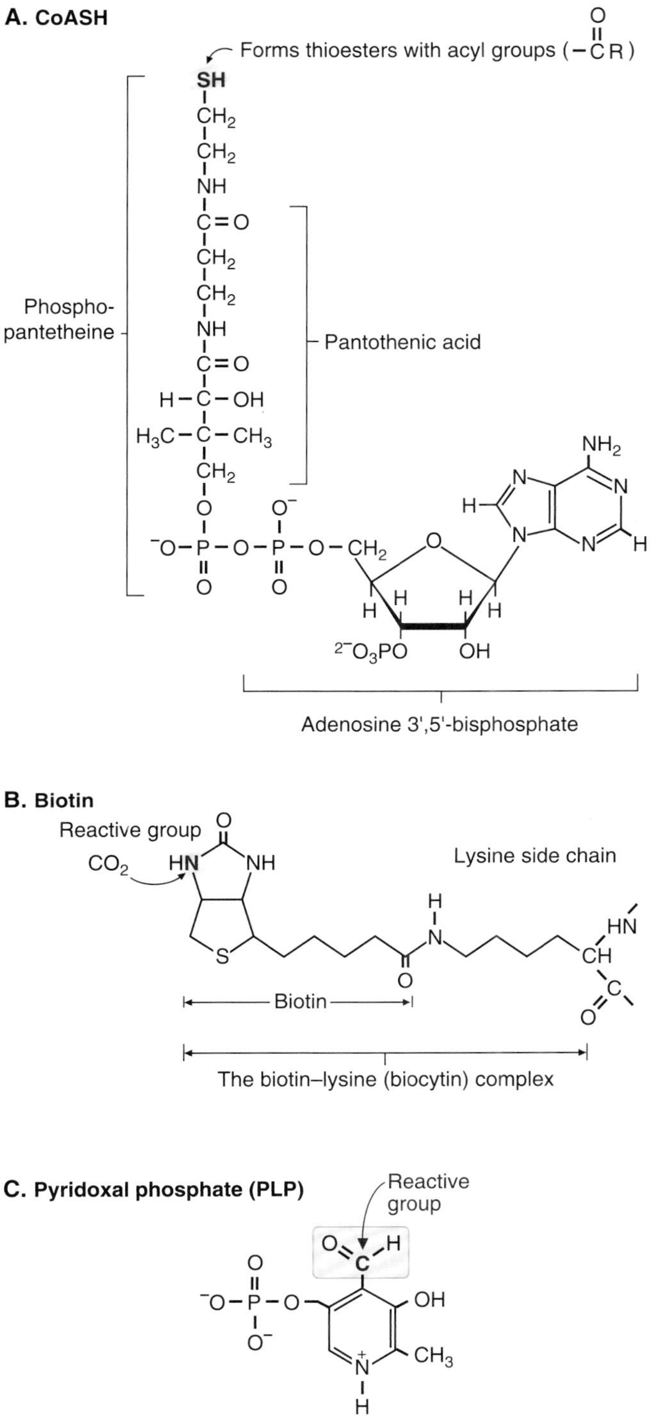

A. CoASH

B. Biotin

C. Pyridoxal phosphate (PLP)

FIGURE 8.9 Activation-transfer coenzymes. **A.** Coenzyme A (CoA or CoASH) and phosphopantetheine are synthesized from the vitamin pantothenate (pantothenic acid). The active sulfhydryl group, shown in *red*, binds to acyl groups (e.g., acetyl, succinyl, or fatty acyl) to form thioesters. **B.** Biotin activates and transfers CO_2 to compounds in carboxylation reactions. The reactive N is shown in *red*. Biotin is covalently attached to a lysine residue in the carboxylase enzyme. **C.** Reactive sites of pyridoxal phosphate. The functional group of pyridoxal phosphate (PLP) is a reactive aldehyde (shown in the *yellow box*) that forms a covalent intermediate with amino groups of amino acids (a Schiff base). The positively charged pyridine ring is a strong electron-withdrawing group that can pull electrons into it (electrophilic catalysis).

Other oxidation–reduction coenzymes work with metals to transfer single electrons to oxygen. Vitamin E and vitamin C (ascorbic acid) are oxidation–reduction coenzymes that can act as antioxidants and protect against oxygen free radical injury. The different functions of oxidation–reduction coenzymes in metabolic pathways are explained in Chapters 20 through 24. A subclass of oxidoreductases is given the name *dehydrogenases* because they transfer hydrogen (hydrogen atoms or hydride ions) from the substrate to an electron-accepting coenzyme such as NAD$^+$.

Oxidation–reduction coenzymes follow the same principles as activation-transfer coenzymes, except that they do not form covalent bonds with the substrate. Each coenzyme has a unique functional group that accepts and donates electrons and is specific for the form of electrons it transfers (e.g., hydride ions, hydrogen atoms, oxygen). A different portion of the coenzyme binds the enzyme. Like activation-transfer coenzymes, oxidation–reduction coenzymes are not good catalysts without participation from amino acid side chains on the enzyme.

The enzyme lactate dehydrogenase, which catalyzes the transfer of electrons from lactate to NAD$^+$, illustrates these principles (Fig. 8.10). In the oxidation of lactate to pyruvate, lactate loses two electrons as a hydride ion, and a proton (H$^+$) is released. NAD$^+$, which accepts the hydride ion, is reduced to NADH. The carbon atom with the keto group in pyruvate is not at a higher oxidation state than in lactate because both of the electrons in bonds between carbon and oxygen are counted as

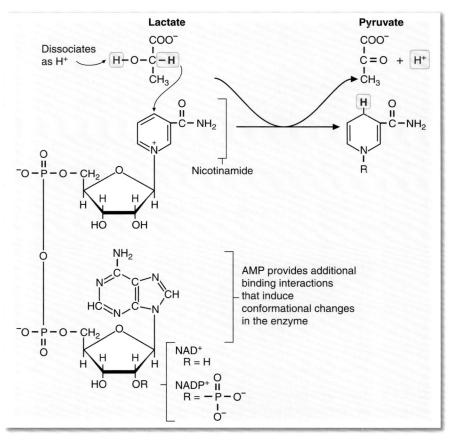

FIGURE 8.10 The coenzyme nicotinamide adenine dinucleotide (NAD$^+$) accepting a hydride ion, shown in *red*, from lactate. NAD$^+$-dependent dehydrogenases catalyze the transfer of a hydride ion (H$^-$) from a carbon to NAD$^+$ in oxidation reactions such as the oxidation of alcohols to ketones or aldehydes to acids. The positively charged pyridine ring nitrogen of NAD$^+$ increases the electrophilicity of the carbon opposite it in the ring. This carbon then accepts the negatively charged hydride ion. The proton from the alcohol group is released into water. NADP$^+$ functions by the same mechanism, but it is usually involved in pathways of reductive synthesis.

belonging to oxygen, whereas the two electrons in the carbon–hydrogen bond are shared equally between carbon and hydrogen.

The coenzyme NAD^+ is synthesized from the vitamin niacin (which forms the nicotinamide ring), and from ATP (which contributes an adenosine monophosphate [AMP]). The adenosine diphosphate (ADP) portion of the molecule binds tightly to the enzyme and causes conformational changes in the enzyme. The functional group of NAD^+ is the carbon on the nicotinamide ring opposite the positively charged nitrogen. This carbon atom accepts the hydride ion (a hydrogen atom that has two electrons) transferred from a specific carbon atom on the substrate. The H^+ from the substrate alcohol (–OH) group then dissociates, and a keto group (C=O) is formed. One of the roles of the enzyme is to contribute a histidine nitrogen that can bind the dissociable proton on lactate, thereby making it easier for NAD^+ to pull off the other hydrogen with both electrons. Finally, NADH dissociates.

C. Metal Ions in Catalysis (see also Section II.C)

Metal ions, which have a positive charge, contribute to the catalytic process by acting as *electrophiles* (electron-attracting groups). They assist in binding of the substrate, or they stabilize developing anions in the reaction. They can also accept and donate electrons in oxidation–reduction reactions.

The ability of certain metals to bind multiple ligands in their coordination sphere enables them to participate in binding substrates or coenzymes to enzymes. For example, Mg^{2+} plays a role in the binding of the negatively charged phosphate groups of TPP to anionic or basic amino acids in the enzyme (see Fig. 8.8). The phosphate groups of ATP are usually bound to enzymes through Mg^{2+} chelation.

The metals of some enzymes bind anionic substrates or intermediates of the reaction to alter their charge distribution, thereby contributing to catalytic power. The enzyme alcohol dehydrogenase (ADH), which transfers electrons from ethanol to NAD^+ to generate acetaldehyde and NADH, illustrates this role (Fig. 8.11). In the active site of ADH, an activated serine pulls a proton off the ethanol –OH group, leaving a negative charge on the oxygen that is stabilized by zinc. This electronic configuration allows the transfer of a hydride ion to NAD^+. Zinc is essentially fulfilling the same function in ADH that histidine fulfills in lactate dehydrogenase.

D. Noncatalytic Roles of Cofactors

Cofactors sometimes play a noncatalytic structural role in certain enzymes, binding different regions of the enzyme together to form the tertiary structure. They also can serve as substrates that are cleaved during the reaction.

IV. Optimal pH and Temperature

If the activity of most enzymes is plotted as a function of the pH of the reaction, an increase of reaction rate is usually observed as the pH goes from a very acidic level to the physiologic range; a decrease of reaction rate occurs as the pH goes from the physiologic range to a very basic range (Fig. 8.12). The reason for the increased activity as the pH is raised to physiologic levels usually reflects the ionization of specific functional groups in the active site (or in the substrate) by the increase of pH, and the more general formation of hydrogen bonds important for the overall conformation of the enzyme. The loss of activity on the basic side usually reflects the inappropriate ionization of amino acid residues in the enzyme.

Most human enzymes function optimally at a temperature of around 37°C. An increase of temperature from 0°C to 37°C increases the rate of the reaction by increasing the vibrational energy of the substrates. The maximum activity for most human enzymes occurs near 37°C because denaturation (loss of secondary and tertiary structure) occurs at higher temperatures.

 In humans, most of ingested ethanol is oxidized to acetaldehyde in the liver by ADH:

Ethanol + NAD^+ ↔ acetaldehyde + NADH + H^+

ADH is active as a dimer, with an active site containing zinc present in each subunit. The human has at least seven genes that encode isozymes of ADH, each with a slightly different range of specificities for the alcohols it oxidizes.

The acetaldehyde produced from ethanol is highly reactive, toxic, and immunogenic. In **Al M.** and other patients with chronic alcoholism, acetaldehyde is responsible for much of the liver injury associated with this addiction.

 In the clinical laboratory, ethanol (in serum) is usually analyzed by coupling its oxidation to the formation of NADH using the enzyme ADH. NAD^+ has a low extinction coefficient at 340 nm; NADH has a much higher one. Thus, the increase in absorbance at 340 nm that occurs during the reaction indicates how much NADH was produced, which is directly proportional to the ethanol concentration in the serum. These reactions have been fully automated for the clinical lab.

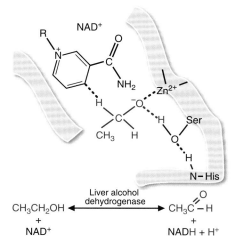

FIGURE 8.11 Liver alcohol dehydrogenase (ADH) catalyzes the oxidation of ethanol (shown in *red*) to acetaldehyde. The active site of liver ADH contains a bound zinc atom, and a serine side chain –OH, and a histidine nitrogen that participate in the reaction. The histidine pulls an H^+ off the active site serine, which pulls the H^+ off of the substrate –OH group, leaving the oxygen with a negative charge that is stabilized by zinc.

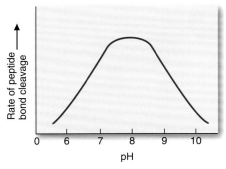

FIGURE 8.12 pH profile of an enzyme. The rate of the reaction increases as the pH increases from 6 to 7.4. The exact shape of the curve depends on the protonation state of active-site amino acid residues or on the hydrogen bonding required for maintenance of three-dimensional structure in the enzyme. For the enzyme shown in the figure, the increase of reaction rate corresponds to deprotonation of the active-site histidine. At pH >8.5, deprotonation of an amino-terminal $-NH_3^+$ alters the conformation at the active site and the activity decreases. Other enzymes might have a lower pH maximum, a broader peak, or retain their activity in the basic side of the curve.

The symptoms experienced by **Dennis V.** resulted from inhibition of acetylcholinesterase. Acetylcholinesterase cleaves the neurotransmitter acetylcholine to acetate and choline in the postsynaptic terminal, thereby terminating the transmission of the neural signal (see Fig. 8.13). Malathion is metabolized in the liver to a toxic derivative (malaoxon) that binds to the active-site serine in acetylcholinesterase and other enzymes, an action similar to that of DFP. As a result, acetylcholine accumulates and overstimulates the autonomic nervous system (the involuntary nervous system, including the heart, blood vessels, and glands), thereby accounting for Dennis's vomiting, abdominal cramps, salivation, and sweating. Acetylcholine is also a neurotransmitter for the somatic motor nervous system, where its accumulation resulted in Dennis's involuntary muscle twitching (muscle fasciculations).

V. Mechanism-Based Inhibitors

Inhibitors are compounds that decrease the rate of an enzymatic reaction. Mechanism-based inhibitors mimic or participate in an intermediate step of the catalytic reaction. The term includes transition-state analogs (see Section I.C) and compounds that can react irreversibly with functional groups in the active site.

A. Covalent Inhibitors

Covalent inhibitors form covalent or extremely tight bonds with functional groups in the active catalytic site. These functional groups are activated by their interactions with other amino acid residues and are therefore far more likely to be targeted by drugs and toxins than amino acid residues outside the active site.

The lethal compound *diisopropylphosphofluoridate* (diisopropylfluorophosphate [DFP]) is an organophosphorus compound that served as a prototype for the development of the nerve gas Sarin and other organophosphorus toxins, such as the insecticides malathion and parathion (Fig. 8.13). DFP exerts its toxic effect by forming a covalent intermediate in the active site of acetylcholinesterase, thereby preventing the enzyme from degrading the neurotransmitter acetylcholine. Once the covalent bond is formed, the inhibition by DFP is essentially irreversible and activity can only be recovered as new enzyme is synthesized. DFP also inhibits many other enzymes that use serine for hydrolytic cleavage, but the inhibition is not as lethal.

Aspirin (acetylsalicylic acid) provides an example of a pharmacologic drug that exerts its effect through the covalent acetylation of an active site serine in the enzyme prostaglandin endoperoxide synthase (cyclooxygenase). Aspirin resembles a portion of the prostaglandin precursor that is a physiologic substrate for the enzyme.

B. Transition-State Analogs and Compounds that Resemble Intermediate Stages of the Reaction

Transition-state analogs are extremely potent and specific inhibitors of enzymes because they bind so much more tightly to the enzyme than do substrates or products. Drugs cannot be designed that precisely mimic the transition state because of its highly unstable structure. However, substrates undergo progressive changes in their overall electrostatic structure during the formation of a transition-state complex, and effective drugs often resemble an intermediate stage of the reaction more closely than they resemble the substrate. Medical literature often refers to such compounds as *substrate analogs*, even though they bind more tightly than substrates.

1. Penicillin

The antibiotic *penicillin* is a transition-state analog that binds very tightly to glycopeptidyl transferase, an enzyme required by bacteria for synthesis of the cell wall (Fig. 8.14). Glycopeptidyl transferase catalyzes a partial reaction with penicillin that covalently attaches penicillin to its own active-site serine. The reaction is favored by the strong resemblance between the peptide bond in the β-lactam ring of penicillin and the transition-state complex of the natural transpeptidation reaction. Active-site inhibitors like penicillin that undergo partial reaction to form irreversible inhibitors in the active site are sometimes termed *suicide inhibitors*.

2. Allopurinol

Allopurinol, a drug used to treat gout, decreases urate production by inhibiting xanthine oxidase. This inhibition provides an example of an enzyme that commits suicide by converting a drug to a transition-state analog. The normal physiologic

A. Normal reaction of acetylcholinesterase

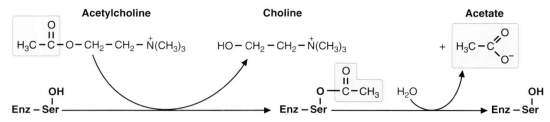

B. Reaction with organophosphorus inhibitors

FIGURE 8.13 **A.** Acetylcholinesterase normally catalyzes inactivation of the neurotransmitter acetylcholine in a hydrolysis reaction. The active-site serine forms a covalent intermediate with a portion of the substrate during the course of the reaction. **B.** Diisopropyl phosphofluoridate (DFP), the ancestor of current organophosphorus nerve gases and pesticides, inactivates acetylcholinesterase by forming a covalent complex with the active-site serine that cannot be hydrolyzed by water. The result is that the enzyme (*Enz*) cannot carry out its normal reaction, and acetylcholine accumulates.

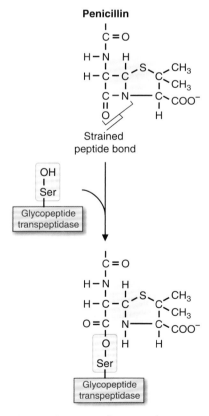

FIGURE 8.14 The antibiotic penicillin inhibits the bacterial enzyme glycopeptide transpeptidase. The transpeptidase is a serine protease involved in cross-linking components of bacterial cell walls and is essential for bacterial growth and survival. It normally cleaves the peptide bond between two D-alanine residues in a polypeptide. Penicillin contains a strained peptide bond within the β-lactam ring that resembles the transition state of the normal cleavage reaction, and thus, penicillin binds very readily in the enzyme active site. As the bacterial enzyme attempts to cleave this penicillin peptide bond, penicillin becomes irreversibly covalently attached to the enzyme's active-site serine, thereby inactivating the enzyme.

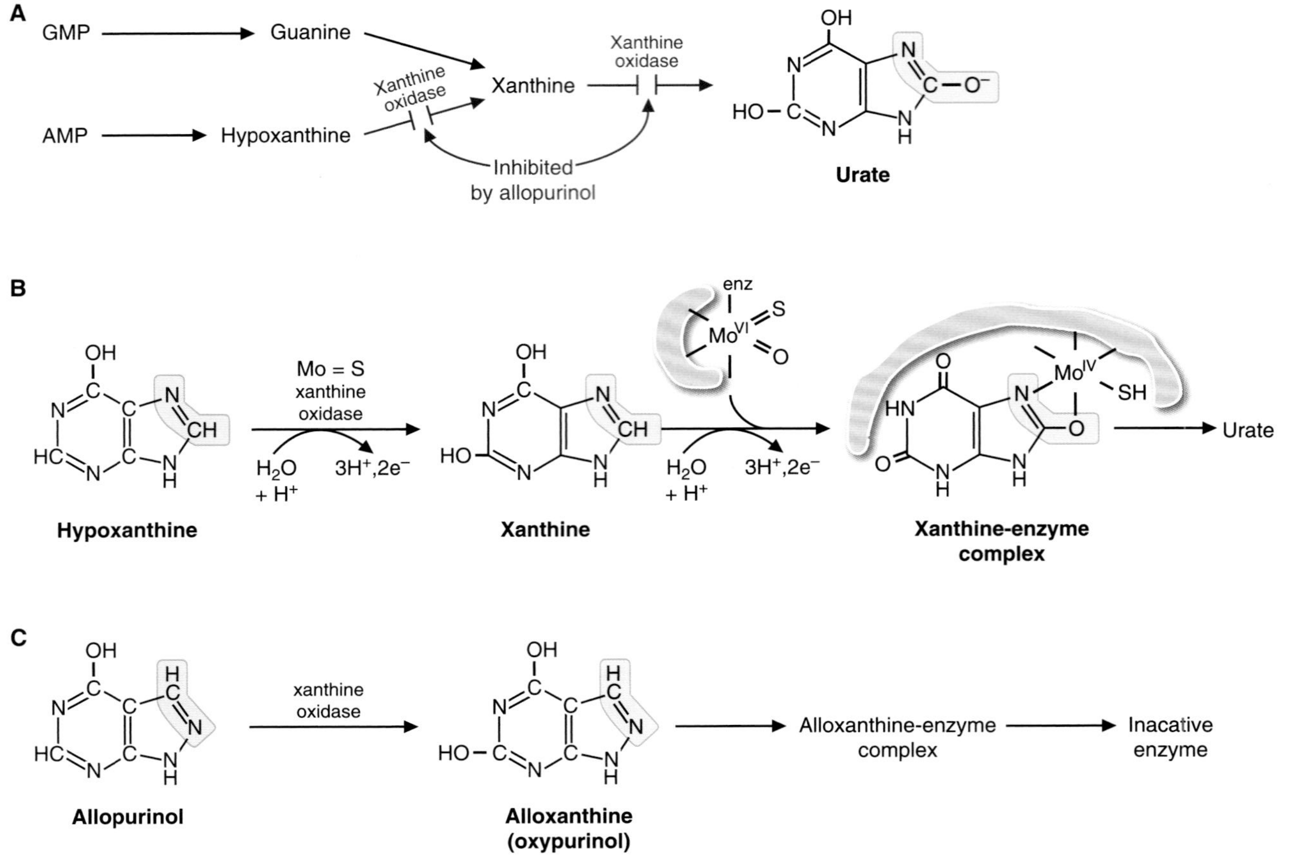

A

GMP ⟶ Guanine
AMP ⟶ Hypoxanthine

Xanthine oxidase

Xanthine ⟶ Xanthine oxidase ⟶ Urate

Inhibited by allopurinol

Urate

B

Hypoxanthine — Mo = S xanthine oxidase — $H_2O + H^+$ — $3H^+, 2e^-$ — **Xanthine** — $H_2O + H^+$ — $3H^+, 2e^-$ — enz Mo^{VI} = S, = O — **Xanthine-enzyme complex** — Mo^{IV} — SH — ⟶ Urate

C

Allopurinol — xanthine oxidase ⟶ **Alloxanthine (oxypurinol)** ⟶ Alloxanthine-enzyme complex ⟶ Inacative enzyme

FIGURE 8.15 Allopurinol is a suicide inhibitor of xanthine oxidase. **A.** Xanthine oxidase catalyzes the oxidation of hypoxanthine to xanthine, and xanthine to uric acid (urate) in the pathway for degradation of purine nucleotides. **B.** The oxidations are performed by a molybdenum–oxo–sulfide coordination complex in the active site that complexes with the group being oxidized. Oxygen is donated from water. The enzyme (*enz*) can work either as an oxidase (O_2 accepts the $2e^-$ and is reduced to H_2O_2) or as a dehydrogenase (NAD^+ accepts the $2e^-$ and is reduced to NADH). The figure only indicates that $2e^-$ are generated during the course of the reaction. **C.** Xanthine oxidase is able to perform the first oxidation step and convert allopurinol to alloxanthine (oxypurinol). As a result, the enzyme has committed suicide; the oxypurinol remains bound in the molybdenum coordination sphere, where it prevents the next step of the reaction. The portion of the purine ring in *green* indicates the major structural difference between hypoxanthine, xanthine, and allopurinol.

Lotta T. is being treated with allopurinol for gout, which is caused by an accumulation of sodium urate crystals in joints and joint fluid, particularly in the ankle and great toe. Allopurinol is a suicide inhibitor of the enzyme xanthine oxidase, which is involved in the degradation of purine nucleotides AMP and GMP to uric acid (urate). Although both hypoxanthine and xanthine levels increase in the presence of allopurinol, neither compound forms crystals nor precipitates at this concentration. They are excreted in the urine.

function of xanthine oxidase is the oxidation of hypoxanthine to xanthine and xanthine to uric acid (urate) in the pathway for degradation of purines (Fig. 8.15). The enzyme contains a molybdenum–sulfide (Mo-S) complex that binds the substrates and transfers the electrons required for the oxidation reactions. Xanthine oxidase oxidizes the drug allopurinol to oxypurinol, a compound that binds very tightly to a Mo-S complex in the active site. As a result, the enzyme has committed suicide and is unable to carry out its normal function, the generation of uric acid (urate).

C. Heavy Metals

Heavy-metal toxicity is caused by tight binding of a metal such as mercury (Hg), lead (Pb), aluminum (Al), or iron (Fe) to a functional group in an enzyme. Heavy metals are relatively nonspecific for the enzymes they inhibit, particularly if the metal is associated with high dose toxicity. Mercury, for example, binds to so many enzymes, often at reactive sulfhydryl groups in the active site, that it has been difficult to determine which of the inhibited enzymes is responsible for mercury toxicity. Lead provides an example of a metal that inhibits through replacing the normal functional metal in an enzyme, such as calcium, iron, or zinc. Its developmental and neurologic toxicity may be caused by its ability to replace Ca^{2+} in two regulatory proteins important in the central nervous system and other tissues—Ca^{2+}–calmodulin and protein kinase C.

CLINICAL COMMENTS

Dennis V. Dennis V. survived his malathion intoxication because he had ingested only a small amount of the chemical, vomited shortly after the agent was ingested, and was treated rapidly in the emergency department. Lethal doses of oral malathion are estimated at 1 g/kg of body weight for humans, although the correlation between dose and severity of toxicity is poor. Once it has been ingested, the liver converts malathion to the toxic reactive compound malaoxon by replacing the sulfur with an oxygen (Fig. 8.16). Malaoxon then binds to the active site of acetylcholinesterase and reacts to form the covalent intermediate. Unlike the complex formed between DFP and acetylcholinesterase, this initial acyl enzyme intermediate is reversible. However, with time, the enzyme–inhibitor complex "ages" (dealkylation of the inhibitor and enzyme modification) to form an irreversible complex.

Emergency department physicians used intravenous atropine, an anticholinergic (antimuscarinic) agent, to antagonize the action of the excessive amounts of acetylcholine accumulating in cholinergic receptors throughout Dennis's body. They also used the drug pralidoxime (an oxime) to reactivate the acetylcholinesterase before aged complexes formed. Although this therapy has not been shown to be consistently effective in clinical trials, it is still used.

After several days of intravenous therapy, the signs and symptoms of acetylcholine excess abated, and therapy was slowly withdrawn. Dennis made an uneventful recovery.

Lotta T. Within several days of starting allopurinol therapy, Ms. T.'s serum uric acid level began to fall. Several weeks later, the level in her blood was normal. In order to prevent an acute attack of gouty arthritis, Ms. T. was given a daily dose of colchicine when she was started on the allopurinol (see Chapter 10).

Al M. Al M. was admitted to the hospital and intravenous thiamin was initiated at a dose of 100 mg/day (compared with the Recommended Dietary Allowance of 1.4 mg/day). His congestive heart failure was believed to be the result, in part, of the cardiomyopathy (heart-muscle dysfunction) of acute thiamin deficiency known as *beriberi heart disease*. The cardiac and peripheral nerve dysfunction that result from this nutritional deficiency usually responds to thiamin replacement. However, an alcoholic cardiomyopathy can also occur in well-nourished patients with adequate thiamin levels. Exactly how ethanol, or its toxic metabolite acetaldehyde, causes alcoholic cardiomyopathy in the absence of thiamin deficiency is not completely understood.

 At low concentrations of ethanol, liver ADH is the major route of ethanol oxidation to form acetaldehyde, a highly toxic chemical. Acetaldehyde not only damages the liver but it can also enter the blood and potentially damage the heart and other tissues. At low ethanol intakes, much of the acetaldehyde produced is safely oxidized to acetate in the liver by aldehyde dehydrogenases.

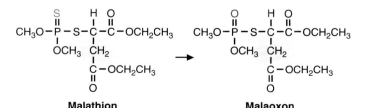

FIGURE 8.16 The liver converts malathion to malaoxon by replacing a sulfur with an oxygen. Malaoxon will interact with acetylcholinesterase, inhibiting the enzyme. The initial inhibition is reversible with pralidoxime, but if not treated in time, the enzyme–inhibitor complex becomes resistant to oxime treatment.

BIOCHEMICAL COMMENTS

 Basic Reactions and Classes of Enzymes. In the following chapters, students will be introduced to a wide variety of reaction pathways and enzyme names. Although it may seem that the number of reactions is infinite, many of these reactions are similar and occur frequently in different pathways. Recognition of the type of reaction can aid in remembering the pathways and enzyme names, thereby reducing the amount of memorization required. You may wish to use this section for reference as you go through your first biochemical pathways.

The Enzyme Commission (EC) has divided the basic reaction types and the enzymes catalyzing them into six broad numbered classes: (1) oxidoreductases, (2) transferases, (3) hydrolases, (4) lyases, (5) isomerases, and (6) ligases. Each broad class of enzymes includes subsets of enzymes with a systematic name and a common name (e.g., dehydrogenases and kinases). For example, glucokinase (common name) has the systematic name ATP:D-hexose 6-phosphotransferase, and its EC number is EC 2.7.1.2. The first "2" refers to the general class (transferase) of enzyme, followed by a period. The "7" refers to the specific number of subclasses within the transferase family of enzymes (in this case, the class that transfers a phosphate). The "1" denotes transfer to an alcohol receptor; and the final "2" yields a specific enzyme number for glucokinase.

 Oxidoreductases. Oxidation–reduction reactions are very common in biochemical pathways and are catalyzed by a broad class of enzymes called *oxidoreductases*. Whenever an oxidation–reduction reaction occurs, at least one substrate gains electrons and becomes reduced, and another substrate loses electrons and becomes oxidized. One subset of reactions is catalyzed by dehydrogenases, which accept and donate electrons in the form of hydride ions (H^-) or hydrogen atoms. Usually an electron-transferring coenzyme, such as NAD^+/NADH, acts as an electron donor or acceptor (e.g., see Figs. 8.10 and 8.11).

In another subset of reactions, O_2 donates either one or both of its oxygen atoms to an acceptor (e.g., see xanthine oxidase, Fig. 8.15). When this occurs, O_2 becomes reduced and an electron donor is oxidized. Enzymes participating in reactions with O_2 are called *hydroxylases* and *oxidases* when one oxygen atom is incorporated into a substrate and the other oxygen atom into water, or both atoms are incorporated into water. They are called *oxygenases* when both atoms of oxygen are incorporated into the acceptor. Most hydroxylases and oxidases require metal ions, such as Fe^{2+}, for electron transfer.

 Transferases. Transferases catalyze group transfer reactions—the transfer of a functional group from one molecule to another. If the transferred group is a high-energy phosphate (as shown in Fig. 8.3), the enzyme is a kinase; if the transferred group is a carbohydrate residue, the enzyme is a glycosyltransferase; if it is a fatty acyl group, the enzyme is an acyltransferase. A common feature of these reactions is that the group being transferred exists as a good leaving group on the donor molecule.

Another subset of group transfer reactions consists of transaminations (Fig. 8.17A). In this type of reaction, the nitrogen group from an amino acid is donated to an α-keto acid, forming a new amino acid and the α-keto acid corresponding to the donor amino acid. Enzymes that catalyze this last type of reaction are called *transaminases* or *aminotransferases*. The coenzyme pyridoxal phosphate is required for all transaminases (see Fig. 8.9C).

When the physiologically important aspect of the reaction is the compound synthesized, the transferase may be called a *synthase*. For example, the enzyme commonly called *glycogen synthase* transfers a glucosyl residue from uridine diphosphate (UDP) glucose to the end of a glycogen molecule. Its systematic name is UDP-glucose-glycogen glycosyltransferase.

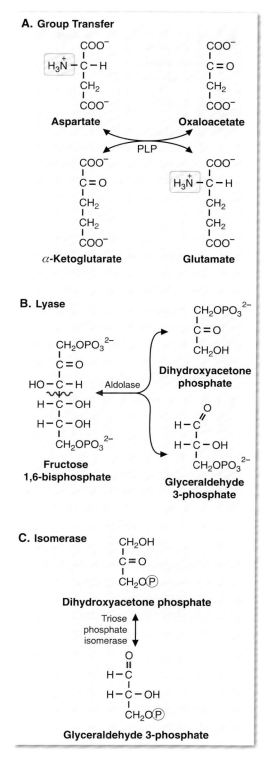

FIGURE 8.17 **A.** An example of a group transfer reaction—a transamination. Pyridoxal phosphate (PLP) on aspartate aminotransferase transfers an amino group from aspartate to the α-keto acid (α-ketoglutarate) to form a new amino acid (glutamate). The enzyme was formerly called *glutamate-oxaloacetate transaminase*. **B.** An example of a lyase. Aldolases catalyze carbon–carbon bond cleavage in reactions that are usually reversible. In glycolysis, the enzyme fructose 1,6-bisphosphate aldolase cleaves a carbon–carbon bond in fructose 1,6-bisphosphate. Aldolases have a lysine ε-amino group in the active site that participates in the reaction. **C.** An example of an isomerase. Isomerases rearrange atoms within a molecule. In the pathway of glycolysis, triose phosphate isomerase converts dihydroxyacetone phosphate to glyceraldehyde 3-phosphate by rearranging hydrogen atoms. No other substrates or products of the reaction exist.

Hydrolases. In hydrolysis reactions, C–O, C–N, or C–S bonds are cleaved by the addition of H_2O in the form of OH^- and H^+ to the atoms forming the bond. The enzyme class names specify the group being cleaved (e.g., the enzyme commonly named chymotrypsin is a protease, a hydrolase that cleaves peptide bonds in proteins).

 Lyases. The lyase class of enzymes consists of a diverse group of enzymes that cleave C–C, C–O, and C–N bonds by means other than hydrolysis or oxidation. Some of the enzymes that catalyze C–C bond cleavage are called *aldolases*, decarboxylases (when carbon dioxide is released from a substrate), and thiolases (when the sulfur-containing nucleophile of cysteine or CoASH is used to break a carbon–carbon bond) (see Fig. 8.17B). The structures amenable to carbon–carbon bond cleavage usually require a carbonyl carbon that can act as an electron sink to stabilize the carbanion formed transiently when the carbon–carbon bond breaks.

This broad class of enzymes also includes dehydratases and many synthases. Dehydratases remove the elements of water from two adjacent carbon–carbon bonds to form a double bond. Certain enzymes in this group, such as certain group transferases, are commonly called *synthases* when the physiologically important direction of the reaction favors the formation of a carbon–carbon bond (e.g., citrate synthase).

 Isomerases. Many biochemical reactions simply rearrange the existing atoms of a molecule; that is, create isomers of the starting material (see Fig. 8.17C). Enzymes that rearrange the bond structure of a compound are called *isomerases*, whereas enzymes that catalyze movement of a phosphate from one atom to another are called *mutases*.

 Ligases. Ligases synthesize C–C, C–S, C–O, and C–N bonds in reactions coupled to the cleavage of a high-energy phosphate bond in ATP or another nucleotide. Carboxylases, for example, add CO_2 to another compound in a reaction that requires ATP cleavage to provide energy (see Fig. 8.9B). Most carboxylases require the coenzyme biotin. Other ligases are named synthetases (e.g., fatty acyl-CoA synthetase). Synthetases differ from the synthases mentioned under "Lyases" and "Group Transferases" in that synthetases derive the energy for new bond formation from cleavage of high-energy phosphate bonds, and synthases use a different source of energy.

KEY CONCEPTS

- Enzymes are proteins that act as catalysts—molecules that can accelerate the rate of a reaction.
- Enzymes are specific for various substrates because of the selective nature of the binding sites on the enzyme.
- The catalytic (active) site is the portion of the enzyme molecule at which the reaction occurs.
- Enzymes accelerate reaction rates by decreasing the amount of energy required to reach a high-energy intermediate stage of the reaction known as the *transition-state complex*. This is referred to as *lowering the energy of activation*.
- Enzymes use functional groups at the active site, provided by coenzymes, metals, or amino acid residues, to perform catalysis.
- Enzymes use general acid–base catalysis, formation of covalent intermediates, metal ions, cofactor catalysis, and transition-state stabilization as various mechanisms to accelerate reaction rates.
- Many drugs and toxins act by inhibiting enzymes.
- Enzymes can be regulated to control reaction rates through a variety of mechanisms.
- Diseases discussed in this chapter are summarized in Table 8.2.

TABLE 8.2 Diseases Discussed in Chapter 8

DISORDER OR CONDITION	GENETIC OR ENVIRONMENTAL	COMMENTS
Malathion poisoning	Environmental	Inhibition of acetylcholinesterase at neuromuscular junctions. This leads to acetylcholine accumulation at the junction and overstimulation of the autonomic nervous system.
Gout	Both	Accumulation of uric acid in blood, leading to precipitation in joints, accompanied by severe pain and discomfort
Thiamin deficiency (beriberi heart disease)	Environmental	Leads to lack of energy production because of reduced activity of key enzymes and can lead to disease in the nervous system (Wernicke's encephalopathy/Wernicke-Korsakoff syndrome) and cardiovascular system (beriberi heart disease). It is most often brought about by alcoholism, as manifest by a poor diet, and by ethanol inhibition of thiamin transport through the intestinal mucosa.

REVIEW QUESTIONS—CHAPTER 8

The following questions below cover material from Chapters 6 and 7 as well as Chapter 8 (including Biochemical Comments).

1. A patient was born with a congenital mutation in an enzyme that severely affected its ability to bind an activation-transfer coenzyme. As a consequence, which one of the following is most likely to occur?
   A. The enzyme will be unable to bind the substrate of the reaction.
   B. The enzyme will be unable to form the transition-state complex.
   C. The enzyme will normally use a different activation-transfer coenzyme.
   D. The enzyme will normally substitute the functional group of an active-site amino acid residue for the coenzyme.
   E. The reaction may be carried out by the free coenzyme, provided the diet carries an adequate amount of its vitamin precursor.

2. An individual had a congenital mutation in glucokinase in which a proline was substituted for a leucine on a surface helix far from the active site but within the hinge region of the actin fold. This mutation would be expected to have which one of the following effects?
   A. It would have no effect on the rate of the reaction because it is not in the active site.
   B. It would have no effect on the rate of the reaction because proline and leucine are both nonpolar amino acids.

   C. It would have no effect on the number of substrate molecules reaching the transition state.
   D. It would probably affect the binding of ATP or a subsequent step in the reaction sequence.
   E. It would probably cause the reaction to proceed through an alternate mechanism.

3. Lysozyme is an important component of the human innate immune system. Lysozyme is an enzyme that cleaves glycosidic linkages in bacterial cell walls. The pH optimum of the purified enzyme is 5.2. There are two acidic residues at the active site of lysozyme (E35 and D52) that are required for enzyme activity. The pK_a of E35 is 5.9, whereas the pK_a of D52 is 4.5. What are the primary ionization states of these two residues at the pH optimum of the enzyme?
   A. E35 is protonated; D52 is ionized.
   B. E35 is protonated; D52 is protonated.
   C. E35 is ionized; D52 is protonated.
   D. E25 is ionized; D52 is ionized.
   E. This cannot be determined from the information provided.

Questions 4 and 5 refer to the following reaction:

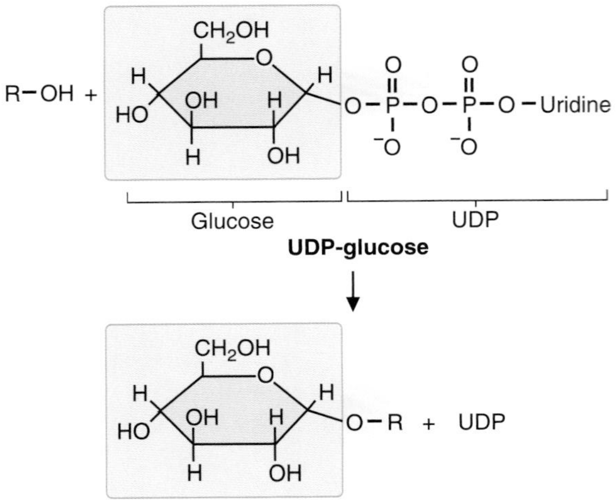

UDP-glucose

UDP-glucose is a key intermediate in carbohydrate metabolism and serves as a precursor for glycogen synthesis and glycosylation of lipids and protein.

4. The type of reaction shown fits into which one of the following classifications?
    A. Group transfer
    B. Isomerization
    C. Carbon–carbon bond breaking
    D. Carbon–carbon bond formation
    E. Oxidation–reduction

5. The type of enzyme that catalyzes this reaction is which one of the following?
    A. Kinase
    B. Dehydrogenase
    C. Glycosyltransferase
    D. Transaminase
    E. Isomerase

6. A patient has accidentally ingested the insecticide malathion, leading to symptoms of an overstimulated autonomic nervous system. Which one of the following best describes malathion in this context?
    A. Enzyme
    B. Coenzyme
    C. Inhibitor
    D. Cofactor
    E. Coactivator

7. Penicillin is an antibiotic used to treat certain infections. It is a transition-state analog and suicide inhibitor. The use of penicillin affects which one of the following in susceptible targets?
    A. Viral cell wall
    B. Bacterial cell wall
    C. Viral nucleus
    D. Bacterial nucleus
    E. Protozoan nucleus

8. Vitamins can act as coenzymes that participate in catalysis by providing functional groups. Therefore, vitamin deficiencies reflect the loss of specific enzyme activities that depend on those coenzymes. Coenzymes are best described by which one of the following?
    A. In humans, they are always synthesized from vitamins.
    B. They are proteins.
    C. They participate in only one reaction, like enzymes.
    D. They are complex, nonprotein organic molecules.
    E. They are all carbohydrates.

Questions 9 and 10 are linked.

9. Many chronic alcoholics develop thiamin deficiency because of a poor diet and an inability to absorb thiamin from the intestine in the presence of ethanol. Which one of the following cofactors, synthesized from a vitamin, or a vitamin itself, exhibits a mechanism of action similar to thiamin?
    A. NAD^+
    B. FAD
    C. Ascorbic acid
    D. γ-Tocopherol
    E. CoA

10. Which one of the following vitamins is the precursor for the correct answer to the previous question?
    A. Pantothenate
    B. Niacin
    C. Pyridoxine (vitamin B_6)
    D. Folate
    E. Biotin

ANSWERS

1. **The answer is B.** In most reactions, the substrate binds to the enzyme before its reaction with the coenzyme occurs. Thus, the substrate may bind, but it cannot react with the coenzyme to form the transition-state complex. Each coenzyme carries out a single type of reaction, so no other coenzyme can substitute (thus, C is incorrect). The three-dimensional geometry of the reaction is so specific that functional groups on amino acid side chains cannot substitute (thus, D is incorrect). Free coenzymes are not very reactive because amino acid side chains in the active site are required to activate the coenzyme or the reactants (thus, E is incorrect). However, increasing the supply of vitamins to increase the amount of coenzyme bound to the enzyme can sometimes help.

2. **The answer is D.** The patient was diagnosed with maturity-onset diabetes of the young (MODY) caused by this mutation. In glucokinase, binding of glucose normally causes a huge conformational change in the actin fold that creates the binding site for ATP. Although proline and leucine are both nonpolar amino acids, B is incorrect—proline creates kinks in helices and thus would be expected to disturb the large conformational change required (see Chapter 7). In general, binding of the first substrate to an enzyme creates conformational changes that increases the binding of the second substrate or brings functional groups into position for further steps in the reaction. Thus, a mutation need not be in the active site to impair the reaction, and A is incorrect. It would probably take more energy to fold the enzyme into the form required for the transition-state complex, and fewer molecules would acquire the energy necessary (thus, C is incorrect). The active site lacks the functional groups required for an alternate mechanism (thus, E is incorrect).

3. **The answer is A.** When the pK_a of an ionizable group is below the pH value, the group will be deprotonated. When the pK_a of an ionizable group is above the pH value, the group will be protonated. Thus, at pH 5.2, glutamate 35 (with a $pK_a = 5.9$, which is >5.2) will remain protonated, and aspartate 52 (with a $pK_a = 4.5$, which is <5.2) will be ionized (because the side chain carries a negative charge when deprotonated). Therefore, E35 is protonated and D52 is ionized. There is sufficient information presented to answer this question.

4. **The answer is A.** The glucose residue from UDP-glucose is being transferred to the alcohol group of another compound. In isomerization reactions, groups are transferred within the same molecule (thus, B is incorrect). There is no cleavage or synthesis of carbon–carbon bonds (thus, C and D are incorrect). Oxidation-reduction has not occurred because no hydrogens or oxygen atoms have been removed or added in the conversion of substrate to product.

5. **The answer is C.** Transfer of a carbohydrate residue from one molecule to another is a glycosyltransferase reaction. Kinases transfer phosphate groups, dehydrogenases transfer electrons as hydrogen atoms or hydride ions, transaminases transfer amino groups, and isomerases transfer atoms within the same molecule.

6. **The answer is C.** Malathion is a covalent inhibitor and forms an extremely tight bond with the active site of acetylcholinesterase (the enzyme) preventing its function. It does not help the enzyme as a coenzyme would and does not assist catalysis as a cofactor would.

7. **The answer is B.** Penicillin irreversibly binds to glycopeptidyl transferase, an enzyme required by bacteria for synthesis of the cell wall. Neither bacteria nor viruses have nuclei. Viruses have no cell wall. Protozoans have a nucleus but no cell wall. The enzyme inhibited is for cell wall synthesis and is only in bacteria. This is why penicillin is not useful in treating a viral or protozoan infection.

8. **The answer is D.** Most, but not all, coenzymes in humans are synthesized from vitamins. They are neither proteins nor carbohydrates but are complex organic molecules. They assist in the catalysis of a type of reaction, not just one reaction (coenzymes can associate with several different enzymes).

9. **The answer is E.** Thiamin acts via an activation-transfer mechanism, as does CoA. All the other listed coenzymes are of the oxidation–reduction group (tocopherol is vitamin E, niacin is part of NAD^+, riboflavin part of FAD, and ascorbic acid is vitamin C).

10. **The answer is A.** CoA, an activation-transfer coenzyme, is synthesized from the vitamin pantothenate. NAD^+ is synthesized from niacin and pyridoxal phosphate from vitamin B_6. Folate and biotin are themselves vitamins.

Regulation of Enzymes

In the human body, thousands of diverse enzymes are regulated to fulfill their individual functions without waste of dietary components. Thus, with changes in our physiologic state, time of eating, environment, diet, or age, the rates of some enzymes must increase and those of others decrease. In this chapter, we describe the mechanisms for regulating enzyme activity and the strategies used to regulate the metabolic pathways in which they reside.

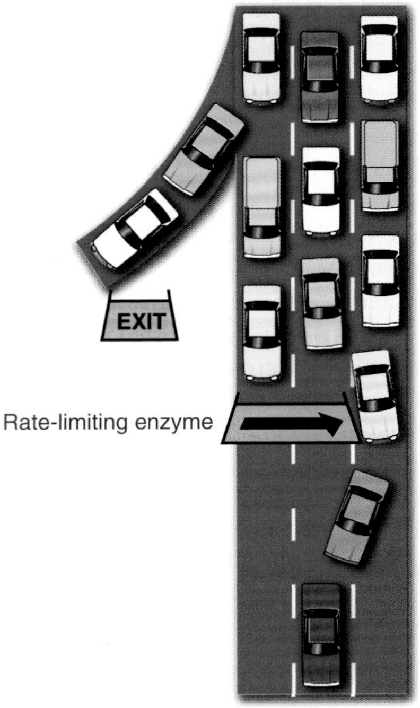

Regulation Matches Function. Changes in the rate of a metabolic pathway occur because at least one enzyme in that pathway, the regulatory enzyme, has been activated or inhibited, or the amount of enzyme has increased or decreased. Regulatory enzymes usually catalyze the rate-limiting, or slowest, step in the pathway, so that increasing or decreasing their rate changes the rate of the entire pathway (Fig. 9.1). The mechanisms used to regulate the rate-limiting enzyme in a pathway reflect the function of the pathway.

Substrate Concentration. The rate of all enzymes depends on substrate concentration. Enzymes exhibit **saturation kinetics**; their rate increases with increasing substrate concentration [S], but it reaches a maximum velocity (V_{max}) when the enzyme is saturated with substrate. For many enzymes, the **Michaelis-Menten equation** describes the relationship between v_i (the initial velocity of a reaction), [S], V_{max}, and the K_m (the substrate concentration at which $v_i = \frac{1}{2}V_{max}$).

Reversible Inhibition. Enzymes are reversibly inhibited by **structural analogs** and **products**. These inhibitors are classified as **competitive, noncompetitive,** or **uncompetitive**, depending on their effect on formation of the **enzyme–substrate complex**.

Allosteric Enzymes. Allosteric activators or **inhibitors** are compounds that bind at sites other than the active catalytic site and regulate the enzyme through **conformational changes** that affect the catalytic site.

Covalent Modification. Enzyme activity may also be regulated by a covalent modification such as **phosphorylation** of a serine, threonine, or tyrosine residue by a **protein kinase**.

Protein–Protein Interactions. Enzyme activity can be modulated through the reversible binding of a **modulator protein** such as Ca^{2+}**-calmodulin. Monomeric G-proteins** (guanosine triphosphate [GTP]-binding proteins) activate target proteins through reversible binding.

Zymogen Cleavage. Some enzymes are synthesized as inactive precursors, called zymogens, that are activated by **proteolysis** (e.g., the digestive enzyme chymotrypsin).

Changes in Enzyme Concentration. The concentration of an enzyme can be regulated by changes in the rate of enzyme synthesis (e.g., induction of gene transcription) or the rate of degradation.

Regulation of Metabolic Pathways. The regulatory mechanisms for the rate-limiting enzyme of a pathway always reflects the **function of the pathway in a particular tissue**. In **feedback regulation**, the end product of a pathway directly or indirectly controls its own rate of synthesis; in **feed-forward regulation**, the substrate controls the rate of the pathway. **Biosynthetic** and **degradative** pathways are controlled through different but **complementary regulation**. Pathways are also regulated through **compartmentation** of enzymes unique to specific pathways.

FIGURE 9.1 The flux of substrates down a metabolic pathway is analogous to cars traveling down a highway. The rate-limiting enzyme is the portion of the highway that is narrowed to one lane by a highway barrier. This single portion of the highway limits the rate at which cars can arrive at their final destination miles later. Cars will back up before the barrier (similar to the increase in concentration of a precursor when a rate-limiting enzyme is inhibited). Some cars may exit and take an alternate route (similar to precursors entering another metabolic pathway). Moving the barrier just a little to open an additional lane is like activating a rate-limiting enzyme: It increases flow through the entire length of the pathway.

Rate-limiting enzyme

EXIT

THE WAITING ROOM

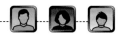

Al M. is a 44-year-old man who has had a severe alcohol use disorder for the past 5 years. He was recently admitted to the hospital for congestive heart failure (see Chapter 8). After being released from the hospital, he continued to drink. One night he arrived at a friend's house at 7:00 P.M. Between his arrival and 11:00 P.M., he drank four beers and five martinis (for a total ethanol consumption of 9.5 oz). His friends encouraged him to stay an additional hour to try and sober up. Nevertheless, he ran his car off the road on his way home. He was taken to the emergency department of the local hospital and arrested for driving under the influence of alcohol. His blood alcohol concentration at the time of his arrest was 240 mg/dL, compared with the legal limit of ethanol for driving of 80 mg/dL (0.08% blood alcohol).

Ann R., a 23-year-old woman, 5 ft 7 in tall, is being treated for anorexia nervosa (see Chapters 1 through 3). She has been gaining weight and is now back to 99 lb from a low of 85 lb. Her blood glucose is still below normal (fasting blood glucose = 72 mg/dL, compared with a normal range = 80 to 100 mg/dL). She complains to her physician that she feels tired when she jogs, and she is concerned that the "extra weight" she has gained is slowing her down. Regulation of various metabolic pathways is critical as Ann gains weight and strives to restore normal activity levels.

I. General Overview

Although the regulation of metabolic pathways is an exceedingly complex subject, dealt with in most of the subsequent chapters of this text, several common themes are involved. Physiologic regulation of a metabolic pathway depends on the ability to alter flux through the pathway by activating the enzyme catalyzing the rate-limiting step in the pathway (see Fig. 9.1). The type of regulation employed always reflects the function of the pathway and the need for that pathway in a particular tissue or cell type. Pathways that produce a necessary product are usually feedback-regulated through a mechanism that involves concentration of product (e.g., allosteric inhibition or induction/repression of enzyme synthesis), either directly or indirectly. The concentration of the product signals when enough of the product has been synthesized. Storage and toxic disposal pathways are usually regulated directly or indirectly through a feed-forward mechanism that reflects the availability of precursor. Regulatory enzymes are often tissue-specific isozymes whose properties reflect the different functions of a pathway in particular tissues. Pathways are also regulated through compartmentation, collection of enzymes with a common function within a particular organelle or at a specific site in the cell.

The mechanisms employed to regulate enzymes have been organized into three general categories: regulation by compounds that bind reversibly in the active site (including the dependence of velocity on substrate concentration and product levels), regulation by changing the conformation of the active site (including allosteric regulators, covalent modification, protein–protein interactions, and zymogen cleavage), and regulation by changing the concentration of enzyme (enzyme synthesis and degradation). We will generally be using the pathways of fuel oxidation to illustrate the role of various mechanisms of enzyme regulation in metabolic pathways (see Chapters 1 through 3 for a general overview of these pathways).

II. Regulation by Substrate and Product Concentration

A. Velocity and Substrate Concentration

The velocity (rate of formation of product per unit of time) of all enzymes is dependent on the concentration of substrate. This dependence is reflected in conditions

When **Al M.** was stopped by police, he was required to take a Breathalyzer test. The Breathalyzer analyzes ethanol levels in expired air (assuming a ratio of 1 part ethanol in expired air to 2,100 parts ethanol in the blood). Once the sample enters the Breathalyzer, it is mixed with sulfuric acid, silver nitrate, and potassium dichromate. If ethanol is present, it will react with the potassium dichromate to form potassium sulfate, chromium sulfate, acetic acid, and water. Potassium dichromate generates a reddish-brown color, whereas chromium sulfate is light green. In the Breathalyzer device, the reacted sample is compared to a nonreacted sample, and the difference in light absorption (because of the different colors) is converted to an electrical current. The extent of current generated will lead to a determination of blood alcohol level (i.e., if there is no ethanol in the sample, no current will be generated). Other forms of gaseous ethanol determination use infrared spectroscopy or a fuel cell.

Al M. was not able to clear his blood ethanol rapidly enough to stay within the legal limit for driving. Ethanol is cleared from the blood at about 0.5 oz/hr (15 mg/dL/hr). Liver metabolism accounts for more than 90% of ethanol clearance from the blood. The major route of ethanol metabolism in the liver is the enzyme liver alcohol dehydrogenase (ADH), which oxidizes ethanol to acetaldehyde with generation of NADH.

$$\text{Ethanol} + NAD^+ \rightarrow \text{acetaldehyde} + NADH + H^+$$

The multienzyme complex MEOS (microsomal ethanol oxidizing system), which is also called *cytochrome P450-2E1*, provides an additional route for ethanol oxidation to acetaldehyde in the liver and is used when ethanol levels are elevated.

One of the fuels used for jogging by **Ann R.'s** skeletal muscles is glucose, which is converted to glucose 6-phosphate by the enzymes hexokinase and glucokinase. Glucose 6-phosphate is metabolized in the pathway of glycolysis to generate adenosine triphosphate (ATP). This pathway is feedback-regulated, so that as her muscles use ATP, the rate of glycolysis will increase to generate more ATP.

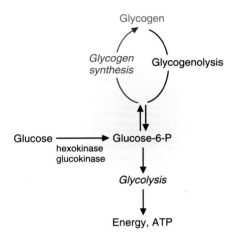

When she is resting, her muscles and liver will convert glucose 6-phosphate to glycogen (a fuel storage pathway, shown in red). Glycogen synthesis is feed-forward–regulated by the supply of glucose and by insulin and other hormones that signal glucose availability. Glycogenolysis (glycogen degradation) is activated during exercise to supply additional glucose 6-phosphate for glycolysis. Unless Ann consumes sufficient calories, her glycogen stores will not be replenished after exercise and she will tire easily.

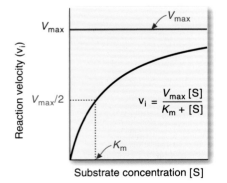

FIGURE 9.2 A graph of the Michaelis-Menten equation. V_{max} (*solid red line*) is the initial velocity extrapolated to infinite substrate concentration ([S]). K_m (*dotted red line*) is the concentration of S at which $v_i = V_{max}/2$.

such as starvation, in which several pathways are deprived of substrate. In contrast, storage pathways (e.g., glucose conversion to glycogen in the liver) and toxic-waste disposal pathways (e.g., the urea cycle, which prevents NH_3 toxicity by converting NH_3 to urea) are normally regulated to speed up when more substrate is available. In the following sections, we use the *Michaelis-Menten equation* to describe the response of an enzyme to changes in substrate concentration, and we use glucokinase to illustrate the role of substrate supply in regulation of enzyme activity.

I. The Michaelis-Menten Equation

The equations of enzyme kinetics provide a quantitative way of describing the dependence of enzyme rate on substrate concentration. The simplest of these equations, the Michaelis-Menten equation, relates the initial velocity (v_i) to the concentration of substrate [S] (the *brackets* denote concentration) and the two parameters K_m and V_{max} (Equation. 9.1). The V_{max} of the enzyme is the maximal velocity that can be achieved at an infinite concentration of substrate, and the K_m of the enzyme for a substrate is the concentration of substrate required to reach ½V_{max}. The Michaelis-Menten model of enzyme kinetics applies to a simple reaction in which the enzyme and substrate form an enzyme–substrate complex (ES) that can dissociate back to the free enzyme and substrate. The initial velocity of product formation, v_i, is proportional to the concentration of ES complexes, [ES]. As substrate concentration is increased, the concentration of ES complexes increases, and the reaction rate increases proportionately. The total amount of enzyme present is represented by E_t.

For the reaction   **Equation 9.1. The Michaelis-Menten equation.**

$$E + S \underset{k_2}{\overset{k_1}{\rightleftharpoons}} ES \overset{k_3}{\longrightarrow} E + P$$

the Michaelis-Menten equation is given by

$$v_i = \frac{V_{max}[S]}{K_m + [S]}$$

where $K_m = (k_2 + k_3)/k_1$

and $V_{max} = k_3 [E_t]$

The graph of the Michaelis-Menten equation (v_i as a function of substrate concentration) is a rectangular hyperbola that approaches a finite limit, V_{max}, as the fraction of total enzyme present as ES complex increases (Fig. 9.2). At a hypothetical infinitely high substrate concentration, all of the enzyme molecules contain bound substrate, and the reaction rate is at V_{max}. The approach to the finite limit of V_{max} is called *saturation kinetics* because velocity cannot increase any further once the enzyme is saturated with substrate. Saturation kinetics is a characteristic property of all rate processes that depend on the binding of a compound to a protein.

The K_m of the enzyme for a substrate is defined as the concentration of substrate at which v_i equals ½V_{max}. The velocity of an enzyme is most sensitive to changes in substrate concentration over a concentration range below its K_m (see Fig. 9.2). As an example, at substrate concentrations less than one-tenth of the K_m, a doubling of substrate concentration nearly doubles the velocity of the reaction; at substrate concentrations 10 times the K_m, doubling the substrate concentration has little effect on the velocity.

The K_m of an enzyme for a substrate is related to the dissociation constant, K_d, which is the rate of substrate release divided by the rate of substrate binding (k_2/k_1). For example, a genetic mutation that decreases the rate of substrate binding to the enzyme decreases the affinity of the enzyme for the substrate and increases the K_d

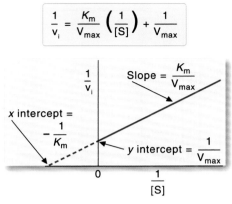

$$\frac{1}{v_i} = \frac{K_m}{V_{max}}\left(\frac{1}{[S]}\right) + \frac{1}{V_{max}}$$

FIGURE 9.3 The Lineweaver-Burk transformation (shown in the *green box*) for the Michaelis-Menten equation converts it to a straight line of the form $y = mx + b$. When the concentration of substrate ([S]) is infinite, $1/[S] = 0$, and the line crosses the ordinate (y-axis) at $1/v = 1/V_{max}$. The slope of the line is K_m/V_{max}. Where the line intersects the abscissa (x-axis), $1/[S] = -1/K_m$.

and K_m of the enzyme for that substrate. The higher the K_m, the higher is the substrate concentration required to reach $\frac{1}{2}V_{max}$.

2. The Lineweaver-Burk Transformation

The K_m and V_{max} for an enzyme can be visually determined from a plot of $1/v_i$ versus $1/S$ called a *Lineweaver-Burk* plot or a *double-reciprocal* plot. The reciprocal of both sides of the Michaelis-Menten equation generates an equation that has the form of a straight line, $y = mx + b$ (Fig. 9.3). K_m and V_{max} are equal to the reciprocals of the intercepts on the abscissa and ordinate, respectively. Although double-reciprocal plots are often used to illustrate certain features of enzyme reactions, they are not used directly for the determination of K_m and V_{max} values by researchers.

3. Hexokinase Isozymes Have Different K_m Values for Glucose

A comparison between the isozymes of hexokinase found in red blood cells and in the liver illustrates the significance of the K_m of an enzyme for its substrate. Hexokinase catalyzes the first step in glucose metabolism in most cells—the transfer of a phosphate from ATP to glucose to form glucose 6-phosphate. Glucose 6-phosphate may then be metabolized in glycolysis, which generates energy in the form of ATP, or it can be converted to glycogen, a storage polymer of glucose. Hexokinase I, the isozyme in red blood cells (erythrocytes), has a K_m for glucose of approximately 0.05 mM (Fig. 9.4). The isozyme of hexokinase called *glucokinase*, which is found in the liver and pancreas, has a much higher K_m of approximately 5 to 6 mM. The red blood cell is totally dependent on glucose metabolism to meet its needs for ATP. At the low K_m of the erythrocyte hexokinase, blood glucose could fall drastically below its normal fasting level of approximately 5 mM, and the red blood cell could still phosphorylate glucose at rates near V_{max}. The liver, however, stores large amounts of "excess" glucose as glycogen or converts it to fat. Because glucokinase has a K_m of approximately 5 mM, the rate of glucose phosphorylation in the liver will tend to increase as blood glucose increases after a high-carbohydrate meal and decrease as blood glucose levels fall. The high K_m of hepatic glucokinase thus promotes the storage of glucose as liver glycogen or as fat but only when glucose is in excess supply.

4. Velocity and Enzyme Concentration

The rate of a reaction is directly proportional to the concentration of enzyme; if you double the amount of enzyme, you will double the amount of product

Patients with maturity-onset diabetes of the young (MODY) have a rare genetic form of diabetes mellitus in which the amount of insulin being secreted from the pancreas is too low, resulting in hyperglycemia. There are several forms of the disease, all caused by a mutation in a single gene. One of the mutations in the gene for pancreatic glucokinase (a closely related isozyme of liver glucokinase) affects its kinetic properties (K_m or V_{max}). Glucokinase is part of the mechanism that controls release of insulin from the pancreas. Decreased glucokinase activity results in lower insulin secretion for a given blood glucose level.

 As **Ann R.** eats a high-carbohydrate meal, her blood glucose will rise to approximately 20 mM in the portal vein, and much of the glucose from her high-carbohydrate meal will enter the liver. How will the activity of glucokinase in the liver change as glucose is increased from 4 to 20 mM? (Hint: Calculate v_i as a fraction of V_{max} for both conditions, using a K_m for glucose of 5 mM and the Michaelis-Menten equation.)

Glucokinase, which has a high K_m for glucose, phosphorylates glucose to glucose 6-phosphate about twice as fast after a carbohydrate meal as during fasting. Substitute the values for S and K_m into the Michaelis-Menten equation. The initial velocity will be $0.44 \times V_{max}$ when blood glucose is at 4 mM and about $0.80 \times V_{max}$ when blood glucose is at 20 mM. In the liver, glucose 6-phosphate is a precursor for both glycogen and fat synthesis. Thus, these storage pathways are partially regulated through a direct effect of substrate supply. They are also partially regulated through an increase of insulin and a decrease of glucagon, two hormones that signal the supply of dietary fuel.

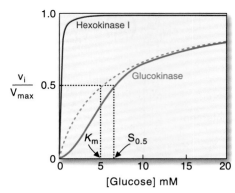

FIGURE 9.4 A comparison between hexokinase I and glucokinase. The initial velocity (v_i) as a fraction of maximum velocity (V_{max}) is graphed as a function of glucose concentration. The plot for glucokinase (*heavy blue line*) is slightly sigmoidal (S-shaped), possibly because the rate of an intermediate step in the reaction is so slow that the enzyme does not follow Michaelis-Menten kinetics. The *dashed blue line* has been derived from the Michaelis-Menten equation fitted to the data for concentrations of glucose >5 mM. For S-shaped curves, the concentration of substrate (S) required to reach $\frac{1}{2}V_{max}$, or half-saturation, is sometimes called the $S_{0.5}$ or $K_{0.5}$ rather than K_m. At $v_i/V_{max} = 0.5$, for glucokinase, the K_m is 5 mM and the $S_{0.5}$ is 6.7 mM.

produced per minute, whether you are at low or at saturating concentrations of substrate. This important relationship between velocity and enzyme concentration is not immediately apparent in the Michaelis-Menten equation because the concentration of total enzyme present (E_t) has been incorporated into the term V_{max} (i.e., V_{max} is equal to the rate constant $k_3 \times E_t$). However, V_{max} is most often expressed as product produced per minute per milligram of enzyme and is meant to reflect a property of the enzyme that is not dependent on its concentration.

5. Multisubstrate Reactions

Most enzymes have more than one substrate, and the substrate-binding sites overlap in the catalytic (active) site. When an enzyme has more than one substrate, the sequence of substrate binding and product release affect the rate equation. As a consequence, an apparent value of K_m ($K_{m,app}$) depends on the concentration of cosubstrate or product present.

6. Rates of Enzyme-Catalyzed Reactions in the Cell

Equations for the initial velocity of an enzyme-catalyzed reaction, such as the Michaelis-Menten equation, can provide useful parameters for describing or comparing enzymes. However, many multisubstrate enzymes such as glucokinase have kinetic patterns that do not fit the Michaelis-Menten model (or do so under nonphysiologic conditions). The Michaelis-Menten model is also inapplicable to enzymes present in a higher concentration than their substrates. Nonetheless, the term K_m is still used for these enzymes to describe the approximate concentration of substrate at which velocity equals $\frac{1}{2}V_{max}$.

B. Reversible Inhibition within the Active Site

One of the ways of altering enzyme activity is through compounds binding in the active site. If these compounds are not part of the normal reaction, they inhibit the enzyme. An *inhibitor* of an enzyme is defined as a compound that decreases the velocity of the reaction by binding to the enzyme. It is a *reversible inhibitor* if it is not covalently bound to the enzyme and can dissociate at a significant rate. Reversible inhibitors are generally classified as competitive, noncompetitive,

The liver ADH that is most active in oxidizing ethanol has a very low K_m for ethanol, approximately 0.04 mM, and is at >99% of its V_{max} at the legal limit of blood alcohol concentration for driving (80 mg/dL or ~17 mM). In contrast, the MEOS isozyme that is most active toward ethanol has a K_m of approximately 11 mM. Thus, MEOS makes a greater contribution to ethanol oxidation and clearance from the blood at higher ethanol levels than at lower ones. Liver damage, such as cirrhosis, results partly from toxic by-products of ethanol oxidation generated by MEOS. **AI M.**, who has a blood alcohol level of 240 mg/dL (~52 mM), is drinking enough to potentially cause liver damage, as well as his car accident and arrest for driving under the influence of alcohol. The various isozymes and polymorphisms of ADH and MEOS are discussed in more detail in Chapter 33.

or uncompetitive with respect to their relationship to a substrate of the enzyme. In most reactions, the products of the reaction are reversible inhibitors of the enzyme producing them.

1. Competitive Inhibition

A *competitive inhibitor* "competes" with a substrate for binding at the enzyme's substrate-recognition site and therefore is usually a close structural analog of the substrate (Fig. 9.5A). An increase of substrate concentration can overcome competitive inhibition; when the substrate concentration is increased to a sufficiently high level, the substrate-binding sites are occupied by substrate, and inhibitor molecules cannot bind. Competitive inhibitors, therefore, increase the apparent K_m of the enzyme ($K_{m,app}$) because they raise the concentration of substrate necessary to saturate the enzyme. They have no effect on V_{max}.

2. Noncompetitive and Uncompetitive Inhibition

If an inhibitor does not compete with a substrate for its binding site, the inhibitor is either a *noncompetitive* or an *uncompetitive inhibitor* with respect to that particular substrate (see Fig. 9.5B). Uncompetitive inhibition is almost never encountered in medicine and will not be discussed further. To illustrate noncompetitive inhibition, consider a multisubstrate reaction in which substrates A and B react in the presence of an enzyme to form a product. An inhibitor (*NI* in Fig. 9.5B) that is a structural analog of substrate B would fit into substrate B's binding site, but the inhibitor would be a noncompetitive inhibitor with regard to the other substrate, substrate A. An increase of A will not prevent the inhibitor from binding to substrate B's binding site. The inhibitor, in effect, lowers the concentration of the active enzyme and therefore changes the V_{max} of the enzyme. If the inhibitor has absolutely no effect on the binding of substrate A, it will not change the K_m for substrate A (a pure noncompetitive inhibitor).

Lineweaver-Burk plots provide a good illustration of competitive inhibition and pure noncompetitive inhibition (Fig. 9.6). In competitive inhibition, plots of $1/v_i$ versus $1/[S]$ at a series of inhibitor concentrations intersect on the y-axis. Thus, at infinite substrate concentration, or $1/[S] = 0$, there is no effect of the inhibitor. In pure noncompetitive inhibition, the inhibitor decreases the velocity even when [S] has been extrapolated to an infinite concentration. However, if the inhibitor has no effect on the binding of the substrate, the K_m is the same for every concentration of inhibitor, and the lines intersect on the x-axis.

Some inhibitors, such as metals, might not bind at either substrate-recognition site. In this case, the inhibitor would be noncompetitive with respect to both substrates.

3. Simple Product Inhibition in Metabolic Pathways

All products are reversible inhibitors of the enzymes that produce them and may be competitive or noncompetitive relative to a particular substrate. *Simple product inhibition*, a decrease in the rate of an enzyme caused by the accumulation of its own product, plays an important role in metabolic pathways: It prevents one enzyme in a sequence of reactions from generating a product faster than it can be used by the next enzyme in that sequence. As an example, product inhibition of hexokinase by glucose 6-phosphate conserves blood glucose for tissues that need it. Tissues take up glucose from the blood and phosphorylate it to glucose 6-phosphate, which can then enter several different pathways (including glycolysis and glycogen synthesis). As these pathways become more active, glucose 6-phosphate concentration decreases, and the rate of hexokinase increases. When these pathways are less active, glucose 6-phosphate concentration increases, hexokinase is inhibited, and glucose remains in the blood for other tissues to use.

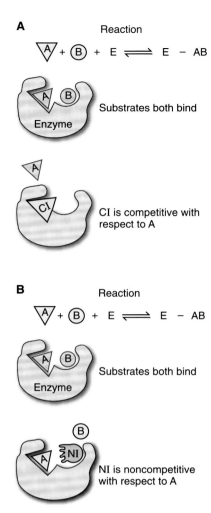

FIGURE 9.5 A. Competitive inhibition with respect to substrate A. A and B are substrates for the reaction that forms the enzyme–substrate complex (*E–AB*). The enzyme has separate binding sites for each substrate, which overlap in the active site. The competitive inhibitor (*CI*) competes for the binding site of A, the substrate it most closely resembles. **B.** *NI* is a noncompetitive inhibitor with respect to substrate A. A can still bind to its binding site in the presence of NI. However, NI is competitive with respect to B because it binds to the B-binding site. In contrast, an inhibitor that is uncompetitive with respect to A might also resemble B, but it could only bind to the B site after A is bound.

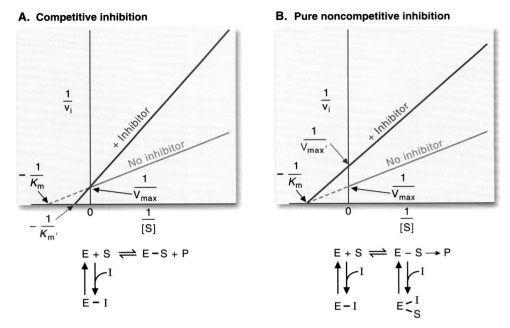

FIGURE 9.6 Lineweaver-Burk plots of competitive and pure noncompetitive inhibition. **A.** $1/v_i$ versus $1/[S]$ in the presence of a competitive inhibitor. The competitive inhibitor alters the intersection on the x-axis. The new intersection is $1/K_{m,app}$ (also called $1/K_m'$). A competitive inhibitor does not affect V_{max}. **B.** $1/v_i$ versus $1/[S]$ in the presence of a pure noncompetitive inhibitor. The noncompetitive inhibitor alters the intersection on the y-axis, $1/V_{max,app}$ or $1/V_{max}'$, but does not affect $1/K_m'$. A pure noncompetitive inhibitor binds to E and ES with the same affinity. If the inhibitor has different affinities for E and ES, the lines will intersect to either side of the y-axis, and the noncompetitive inhibitor will change both the K_m' and the V_{max}'. *I*, inhibitor; *P*, product; *E*, enzyme; *S*, substrate; v_i, initial velocity; V_{max}, maximum velocity.

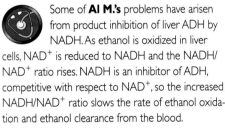

Some of **Al M.'s** problems have arisen from product inhibition of liver ADH by NADH. As ethanol is oxidized in liver cells, NAD^+ is reduced to NADH and the NADH/NAD^+ ratio rises. NADH is an inhibitor of ADH, competitive with respect to NAD^+, so the increased NADH/NAD^+ ratio slows the rate of ethanol oxidation and ethanol clearance from the blood.

NADH is also a product inhibitor of enzymes in the pathway that oxidizes fatty acids. Consequently, these fatty acids accumulate in the liver, eventually contributing to the alcoholic fatty liver.

III. Regulation through Conformational Changes

In substrate response and product inhibition, the rate of the enzyme is affected principally by the binding of a substrate or a product within the catalytic site. Most rate-limiting enzymes are also controlled through regulatory mechanisms that change the conformation of the enzyme in a way that affects the catalytic site. These regulatory mechanisms include (1) allosteric activation and inhibition, (2) phosphorylation or other covalent modification, (3) protein–protein interactions between regulatory and catalytic subunits or between two proteins, and (4) proteolytic cleavage. These types of regulation can rapidly change an enzyme from an inactive form to a fully active conformation.

In the following sections, we describe the general characteristics of these regulatory mechanisms and illustrate the first three with glycogen phosphorylase, glycogen phosphorylase kinase, and protein kinase A.

A. Conformational Changes in Allosteric Enzymes

Allosteric activators and **inhibitors** (**allosteric effectors**) are compounds that bind to the *allosteric site* (a site separate from the catalytic site) and cause a conformational change that affects the affinity of the enzyme for the substrate. Usually, an allosteric enzyme has multiple interacting subunits that can exist in active and inactive conformations, and the allosteric effector promotes or hinders conversion from one conformation to another.

I. Cooperativity in Substrate Binding to Allosteric Enzymes

Allosteric enzymes usually contain two or more subunits and exhibit positive cooperativity; the binding of substrate to one subunit facilitates the binding of substrate to another subunit (Fig. 9.7). The first substrate molecule has difficulty in binding to the enzyme because all of the subunits are in the conformation with a low affinity for substrate (the taut "T" conformation) (see "Cooperativity of O_2 Binding in Hemoglobin" in Chapter 7, Section VII.B). The first substrate molecule to bind changes its own subunit and at least one adjacent subunit to the high-affinity conformation (the relaxed "R" state). In the example of the tetramer hemoglobin, discussed in Chapter 7, the change in one subunit facilitated changes in all four subunits, and the molecule generally changed to the new conformation in a concerted fashion. However, most allosteric enzymes follow a more stepwise (sequential) progression through intermediate stages (see Fig. 9.7).

2. Allosteric Activators and Inhibitors

Allosteric enzymes bind activators at the allosteric site, a site physically separate from the catalytic site. The binding of an allosteric activator changes the conformation of the catalytic site in a way that increases the affinity of the enzyme for the substrate.

In general, activators of allosteric enzymes bind more tightly to the high-affinity R state of the enzyme than the T state (i.e., the allosteric site is open only in the R enzyme) (Fig. 9.8). Thus, the activators increase the amount of enzyme in the active state, thereby facilitating substrate binding in their own and other subunits. In contrast, allosteric inhibitors bind more tightly to the T state, so either substrate concentration or activator concentration must be increased to overcome the effects of the allosteric inhibitor.

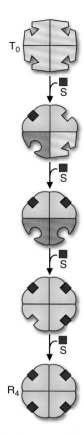

FIGURE 9.7 A sequential model for an allosteric enzyme. The sequential model is actually the preferred path from the T_0 (taut, with 0 substrate, S, bound) low-affinity conformation to the R_4 (relaxed, with four substrate molecules bound) conformation, taken from an array of all possible equilibrium conformations that differ by the conformation of only one subunit. The final result is a stepwise path in which intermediate conformations exist, and subunits may change conformations independently, depending on their geometric relationship to the subunits already containing bound substrate.

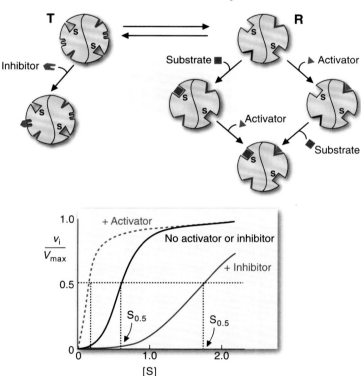

FIGURE 9.8 Activators and inhibitors of an allosteric enzyme (simplified model). This enzyme has two identical subunits, each containing three binding sites: one for the substrate (S), one for the allosteric activator (*green triangle*), and one for the allosteric inhibitor (*two-pronged red shape*). The enzyme has two conformations, a relaxed active conformation (R) and an inactive conformation (T). The activator binds only to its activator site when the enzyme is in the R configuration. The inhibitor-binding site is open only when the enzyme is in the T state.

A plot of velocity (v_i/V_{max}) versus substrate concentration reveals that binding of the substrate at its binding site stabilizes the active conformation so that the second substrate binds more readily, resulting in an S (sigmoidal)-shaped curve. The graph of v_i/V_{max} becomes hyperbolic in the presence of activator (which stabilizes the high-affinity R form) and more sigmoidal with a higher $S_{0.5}$ in the presence of inhibitor (which stabilizes the low-affinity form).

In the absence of activator, a plot of velocity versus substrate concentration for an allosteric enzyme usually results in a sigmoid or S-shaped curve (rather than the rectangular hyperbola of Michaelis-Menten enzymes) as the successive binding of substrate molecules activates additional subunits (see Fig. 9.8). In plots of velocity versus substrate concentration, the effect of an allosteric activator generally makes the sigmoidal S-shaped curve more like the rectangular hyperbola, with a substantial decrease in the $S_{0.5}$ (K_m) of the enzyme, because the activator changes all of the subunits to the high-affinity state. These allosteric effectors alter the K_m but not the V_{max} of the enzyme. An allosteric inhibitor makes it more difficult for substrate or activators to convert the subunits to the most active conformation, and, therefore, inhibitors generally shift the curve to the right, either increasing the $S_{0.5}$ alone or increasing it together with a decrease in the V_{max}.

Some of the rate-limiting enzymes in the pathways of fuel oxidation (e.g., muscle glycogen phosphorylase in glycogenolysis, phosphofructokinase-1 in glycolysis, and isocitrate dehydrogenase in the tricarboxylic acid [TCA] cycle) are allosteric enzymes regulated by changes in the concentration of adenosine diphosphate (ADP) or adenosine monophosphate (AMP) which are allosteric activators. The function of fuel oxidation pathways is the generation of ATP. When the concentration of ATP in a muscle cell begins to decrease, ADP and AMP increase; ADP activates isocitrate dehydrogenase, and AMP activates glycogen phosphorylase and phosphofructokinase-1. The response is very fast, and small changes in the concentration of activator can cause large changes in the rate of the reaction.

3. Allosteric Enzymes in Metabolic Pathways

Regulation of enzymes by allosteric effectors provides several advantages over other methods of regulation. Allosteric inhibitors usually have a much stronger effect on enzyme velocity than competitive and noncompetitive inhibitors in the active catalytic site. Because allosteric effectors do not occupy the catalytic site, they may function as activators. Thus, allosteric enzymes are not limited to regulation through inhibition. Furthermore, the allosteric effector need not bear any resemblance to substrate or product of the enzyme. Finally, the effect of an allosteric effector is rapid, occurring as soon as its concentration changes in the cell. These features of allosteric enzymes are often essential for feedback regulation of metabolic pathways by end products of the pathway or by signal molecules that coordinate multiple pathways.

B. Conformational Changes from Covalent Modification

1. Phosphorylation

The activity of many enzymes is regulated through *phosphorylation* by a *protein kinase* or *dephosphorylation* by a *protein phosphatase* (Fig. 9.9). Serine/threonine protein kinases transfer a phosphate from ATP to the hydroxyl group of a specific serine (and sometimes threonine) on the target enzyme; tyrosine kinases transfer a phosphate to the hydroxyl group of a specific tyrosine residue. Phosphate is a bulky, negatively charged residue that interacts with other nearby amino acid residues of the protein to create a conformational change at the catalytic site. The conformational change is caused by alterations in ionic interactions and/or hydrogen bond patterns resulting from the presence of the phosphate group. The conformational change makes certain enzymes more active and other enzymes less active. The effect is reversed by a specific protein phosphatase that removes the phosphate by hydrolysis.

2. Muscle Glycogen Phosphorylase

Muscle glycogen phosphorylase, the rate-limiting enzyme in the pathway of glycogen degradation, degrades glycogen to glucose 1-phosphate. It is regulated by the allosteric activator AMP, which increases in the cell as ATP is used for muscular contraction (Fig. 9.10) Thus, a rapid increase in the rate of glycogen degradation to glucose 1-phosphate is achieved when an increase of AMP signals that more fuel is needed for ATP generation in the glycolytic pathway.

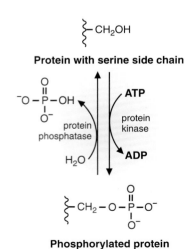

FIGURE 9.9 Protein kinases and protein phosphatases. *ATP*, adenosine triphosphate; *ADP*, adenosine diphosphate.

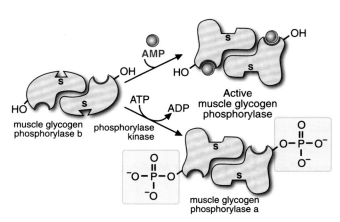

When **Ann R.** begins to jog, AMP activates her muscle glycogen phosphorylase, which degrades glycogen to glucose 1-phosphate. This compound is converted to glucose 6-phosphate, which feeds into the glycolytic pathway to generate ATP for muscle contraction. As she continues to jog, her adrenaline (epinephrine) levels rise, producing the signal that activates glycogen phosphorylase kinase. This enzyme phosphorylates glycogen phosphorylase, causing it to remain active even as AMP levels may drop (see Fig. 9.10).

FIGURE 9.10 Activation of muscle glycogen phosphorylase by adenosine monophosphate (AMP) and by phosphorylation. Muscle glycogen phosphorylase is composed of two identical subunits. The substrate-binding sites in the active catalytic site are denoted by S. AMP binds to the allosteric site, a site separate from the active catalytic site. Glycogen phosphorylase kinase can transfer a phosphate from adenosine triphosphate (ATP) to one serine residue in each subunit. Either phosphorylation or binding of AMP causes a change in the active site that increases the activity of the enzyme. The first event at one subunit facilitates the subsequent events that convert the enzyme to the fully active form. *ADP*, adenosine diphosphate.

Glycogen phosphorylase also can be activated through phosphorylation by glycogen phosphorylase kinase. Either phosphorylation or AMP binding can change the enzyme to a fully active conformation. The phosphate is removed by protein phosphatase-1. Glycogen phosphorylase kinase links the activation of muscle glycogen phosphorylase to changes in the level of the hormone adrenaline (epinephrine) in the blood. It is regulated through phosphorylation by protein kinase A and by activation of Ca^{2+}–calmodulin (a modulator protein) during contraction.

3. Protein Kinase A

Some protein kinases, called *dedicated protein kinases*, are tightly bound to a single protein and regulate only the protein to which they are tightly bound. However, other protein kinases and protein phosphatases simultaneously regulate several rate-limiting enzymes in a cell to achieve a coordinated response. For example, *protein kinase A*, a serine/threonine protein kinase, phosphorylates several enzymes that regulate different metabolic pathways. One of these enzymes is glycogen phosphorylase kinase (see Fig. 9.10).

Protein kinase A provides a means for hormones to control metabolic pathways. Epinephrine and many other hormones increase the intracellular concentration of the allosteric regulator 3′,5′-cyclic AMP (cAMP), which is referred to as a *hormonal second messenger* (Fig. 9.11A). cAMP binds to regulatory subunits of protein kinase A, which dissociate and release the activated catalytic subunits (see Fig. 9.11B). Dissociation of inhibitory regulatory subunits is a common theme in enzyme regulation. The active catalytic subunits phosphorylate glycogen phosphorylase kinase and other enzymes at serine and threonine residues.

In the example shown in Figure 9.10, epinephrine indirectly increases cAMP, which activates protein kinase A, which phosphorylates and activates glycogen phosphorylase kinase, which phosphorylates and activates glycogen phosphorylase. The sequence of events in which one kinase phosphorylates another kinase is called a *phosphorylation cascade*. Because each stage of the phosphorylation cascade is associated with one enzyme molecule activating many enzyme molecules, the initial activating event is greatly amplified.

4. Other Covalent Modifications

Many proteins are modified covalently by the addition of groups such as acetyl, ADP-ribose, or lipid moieties (see Chapter 6). These modifications may activate

A

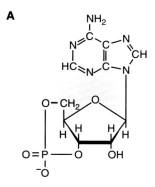

B Inactive protein kinase A

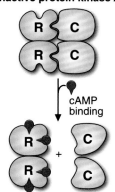

Active protein kinase A

FIGURE 9.11 **A.** Structure of 3′,5′-cyclic adenosine monophosphate (cAMP). The phosphate group is attached to hydroxyl groups on both the third (3′) and fifth (5′) carbons of ribose, forming a cyclic molecule. **B.** Protein kinase A. When the regulatory subunits (R) of protein kinase A bind the allosteric activator cAMP, they dissociate from the enzyme, thereby releasing active catalytic subunits (C).

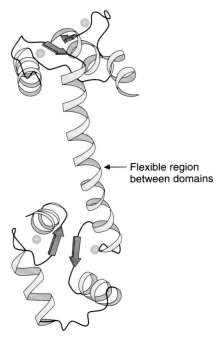

← Flexible region between domains

FIGURE 9.12 Calcium–calmodulin has four binding sites for calcium (shown in *green*). Each calcium forms a multiligand coordination sphere by simultaneously binding several amino acid residues on calmodulin. Thus, calmodulin can create large conformational changes in proteins to which it is bound when calcium binds. Calmodulin has a flexible region in the middle connecting the two domains.

or inhibit the enzyme directly. However, they also may modify the ability of the enzyme to interact with other proteins or to reach its correct location in the cell.

C. Conformational Changes Regulated by Protein–Protein Interactions

Changes in the conformation of the active site can also be regulated by direct protein–protein interaction. This type of regulation is illustrated by Ca^{2+}–calmodulin and small (monomeric) GTP-binding proteins (G-proteins).

1. The Calcium–Calmodulin Family of Modulator Proteins

Modulator proteins bind to other proteins and regulate their activity by causing a conformational change at the catalytic site or by blocking the catalytic site (steric hindrance). They are protein allosteric effectors that can either activate or inhibit the enzyme or protein to which they bind.

Ca^{2+}–calmodulin is an example of a dissociable modulator protein that binds to several different proteins and regulates their function in either a positive or negative manner. It also exists in the cytosol and functions as a Ca^{2+}–binding protein (Fig. 9.12). The center of the symmetric molecule is a hinge region that bends as Ca^{2+}–calmodulin folds over the protein it is regulating.

One of the enzymes activated by Ca^{2+}–calmodulin is muscle glycogen phosphorylase kinase (see Fig. 9.10), which is also activated by protein kinase A. When a neural impulse triggers Ca^{2+} release from the sarcoplasmic reticulum, Ca^{2+} binds to the calmodulin subunit of muscle glycogen phosphorylase kinase, which undergoes a conformational change. This conformational change leads to the activation of glycogen phosphorylase kinase, which then phosphorylates glycogen phosphorylase, ultimately increasing the synthesis of ATP to supply energy for muscle contraction. Simultaneously, Ca^{2+} binds to troponin C, a member of the Ca^{2+}–calmodulin superfamily that serves as a nondissociable regulatory subunit of troponin, a regulator of muscle contraction. Calcium binding to troponin prepares the muscle for contraction. Thus, the supply of energy for contraction is activated simultaneously with the contraction machinery.

2. G-Proteins

The masters of regulation through reversible protein association in the cell are the *monomeric G-proteins*, small single-subunit proteins that bind and hydrolyze GTP. GTP is a purine nucleotide that, like ATP, contains high-energy phosphoanhydride bonds that release energy when hydrolyzed. When G-proteins bind GTP, their conformation changes so that they can bind to a target protein, which is then either activated or inhibited in carrying out its function (Fig. 9.13, Step 1).

G-proteins are said to possess an internal clock because they are GTPases that slowly hydrolyze their own bound GTP to guanosine diphosphate (GDP) and phosphate. As they hydrolyze GTP, their conformation changes and the complex they have formed with the target protein disassembles (see Fig. 9.13, Step 2). The bound GDP on the inactive G-protein is eventually replaced by GTP, and the process can begin again (see Fig. 9.13, Step 3).

The activity of many G-proteins is regulated by accessory proteins (GAPs [*GT*Pase-*a*ctivating *p*roteins], GEFs [*g*uanine nucleotide *e*xchange *f*actors], and GDIs [*G*DP *d*issociation *i*nhibitors]), which may, in turn, be regulated by allosteric effectors. GAPs increase the rate of GTP hydrolysis by the G-protein and therefore the rate of dissociation of the G-protein–target protein complex (see Fig. 9.13, Step 2). When a GEF protein binds to a G-protein, it increases the rate of GTP exchange for a bound GDP and therefore activates the G-protein (see Fig. 9.13, Step 3). GDI proteins bind to the GDP–G-protein complex and inhibit dissociation of GDP, thereby keeping the G-protein inactive.

The Ras superfamily of small G-proteins is divided into five families: Ras, Rho, Arf, Rab, and Ran. These monomeric G-proteins play major roles in the regulation of cell growth, morphogenesis, cell motility, axonal guidance, cytokinesis, and trafficking through the Golgi, nucleus, and endosomes. They are generally bound to a lipid membrane through a lipid anchor, such as a myristoyl group or farnesyl group, and regulate the assembly and activity of protein complexes at these sites. The functions of some of these G-proteins will be discussed further in Chapters 10 and 11.

D. Proteolytic Cleavage

Although many enzymes undergo some cleavage during synthesis, others enter lysosomes, secretory vesicles, or are synthesized as proenzymes, which are precursor proteins that must undergo proteolytic cleavage to become fully functional. Unlike most other forms of regulation, proteolytic cleavage is irreversible.

The precursor proteins of proteases (enzymes that cleave specific peptide bonds) are called *zymogens*. To denote the inactive zymogen form of an enzyme, the name is modified by addition of the suffix "-ogen" or the prefix "pro-." The synthesis of zymogens as inactive precursors prevents them from cleaving proteins prematurely at their sites of synthesis or secretion. Chymotrypsinogen, for example, is stored in vesicles within pancreatic cells until secreted into ducts leading to the intestinal lumen. In the digestive tract, chymotrypsinogen is converted to chymotrypsin by the proteolytic enzyme trypsin, which cleaves off a small peptide from the *N*-terminal region (and two internal peptides). This cleavage activates chymotrypsin by causing a conformational change in the spacing of amino acid residues around the binding site for the denatured protein substrate and around the catalytic site.

Most of the proteases involved in blood clotting are zymogens, such as fibrinogen and prothrombin, which circulate in blood in the inactive form. They are cleaved to the active form (fibrin and thrombin, respectively) by other proteases, which have been activated by their attachment to the site of injury in a blood vessel wall. Thus, clots form at the site of injury and not randomly in the circulation (see Chapter 43).

IV. Regulation through Changes in Amount of Enzyme

Tissues continuously adjust the rate at which proteins are synthesized to vary the amount of different enzymes present. The expression for V_{max} in the Michaelis-Menten equation incorporates the concept that the rate of a reaction is proportional to the amount of enzyme present. Thus, the maximal capacity of a tissue can change with increased protein synthesis or with increased protein degradation.

A. Regulated Enzyme Synthesis

Protein synthesis begins with the process of gene transcription, transcribing the genetic code for that protein from DNA into messenger RNA. The code in messenger RNA is then translated into the primary amino acid sequence of the protein. Generally, the rate of enzyme synthesis is regulated by increasing or decreasing the rate of gene transcription, processes that are generally referred to as *induction* (increase) and *repression* (decrease). However, the rate of enzyme synthesis is sometimes regulated through stabilization of the messenger RNA. (These processes are covered in Section III of this text.) Compared with the more immediate types of regulation discussed previously, regulation by means of induction/repression of enzyme synthesis is usually slow in humans, occurring over hours to days.

B. Regulated Protein Degradation

The content of an enzyme in the cell can be altered through selective regulated degradation as well as through regulated synthesis. For example, during fasting

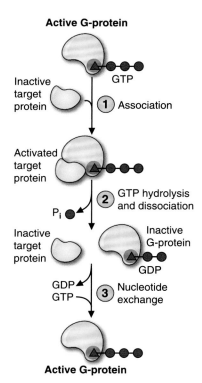

Active G-protein

FIGURE 9.13 Monomeric guanosine triphosphate (GTP)-binding proteins (G-proteins). Step 1: When GTP is bound, the conformation of the G-protein allows it to bind target proteins, which are then activated (as shown), or inhibited. Step 2: The G-protein hydrolyzes a phosphate from GTP to form guanosine diphosphate (GDP), which changes the G-protein conformation and causes it to dissociate from the target protein. Step 3: GDP is exchanged for GTP, which reactivates the G-protein.

 The maximum capacity of MEOS (cytochrome P450-2E1) is increased in the liver with continued ingestion of ethanol through a mechanism involving induction of gene transcription. Thus, **AI M.** has a higher capacity to oxidize ethanol to acetaldehyde than a naive drinker (a person not previously subjected to alcohol). Nevertheless, the persistence of his elevated blood alcohol level shows that he has saturated his capacity for ethanol oxidation (i.e., the enzyme is always running at V_{max}). Once his enzymes are operating near V_{max}, any additional ethanol he drinks will not appreciably increase the rate of ethanol clearance from his blood.

or infective stress, protein degradation in skeletal muscle is activated to increase the supply of amino acids in the blood for gluconeogenesis or for the synthesis of antibodies and other components of the immune response. Under these conditions, synthesis of ubiquitin, a protein that targets proteins for degradation in proteosomes, is increased by the steroid hormone cortisol. Although all proteins in the cell can be degraded with a characteristic half-life within lysosomes, protein degradation via two specialized systems, proteosomes and caspases, is highly selective and regulated. Protein degradation is discussed in more detail in Chapter 35.

V. Regulation of Metabolic Pathways

The different means of regulating enzyme activity described earlier are used to control metabolic pathways, cellular events, and physiologic processes to match the body's requirements. Although there are hundreds of metabolic pathways in the body, there are a few common themes or principles are involved in their regulation. The overriding principle is that regulation of a pathway matches its *function*.

A. Principles of Pathway Regulation

Metabolic pathways are a series of sequential reactions in which the product of one reaction is the substrate of the next reaction (Fig. 9.14). Each step or reaction is usually catalyzed by a separate enzyme. The enzymes of a pathway have a common function—conversion of substrate to the final end products of the pathway. A pathway also may have a branch point at which an intermediate becomes the precursor for another pathway.

1. Role of the Rate-Limiting Step in Regulation

Pathways are principally regulated at one key enzyme, the regulatory enzyme, which catalyzes the rate-limiting step in the pathway. This is the slowest step and usually is not readily reversible. Thus, changes in the rate-limiting step can influence flux through the rest of the pathway (see Fig. 9.1). The rate-limiting step is usually the first committed step in a pathway or a reaction that is related to or influenced by the first committed step. Additional regulated enzymes occur after each metabolic branchpoint to direct flow into the branch (e.g., in Fig. 9.14, feedback inhibition of

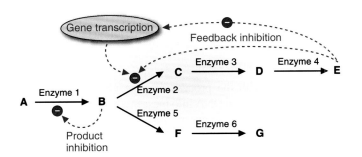

FIGURE 9.14 A common pattern for feedback inhibition of metabolic pathways. The *letters* represent compounds formed from different enzymes in the reaction pathway. Compound B is at a metabolic branch point: It can go down one pathway to E or down an alternate pathway to G. The end product of the pathway, E, might control its own synthesis by allosterically inhibiting enzyme 2, the first committed step of the pathway, or by inhibiting transcription of the gene for enzyme 2. As a result of the feedback inhibition, B accumulates and more B enters the pathway for conversion to G, which could be a storage pathway or a disposal pathway. In this hypothetical pathway, B is a product inhibitor of enzyme 1, competitive with respect to A. Precursor A might induce the synthesis of enzyme 1, which would allow more A to go to G.

enzyme 2 results in accumulation of B, which enzyme 5 then uses for synthesis of compound G). Inhibition of the rate-limiting enzyme in a pathway usually leads to accumulation of the pathway precursor.

2. Feedback Regulation

Feedback regulation refers to a situation in which the end product of a pathway controls its own rate of synthesis (see Fig. 9.14). Feedback regulation usually involves allosteric regulation of the rate-limiting enzyme by the end product of a pathway (or a compound that reflects changes in the concentration of the end product). The end product of a pathway may also control its own synthesis by inducing or repressing the gene for transcription of the rate-limiting enzyme in the pathway. This type of regulation is much slower to respond to changing conditions than allosteric regulation.

3. Feed-Forward Regulation

Certain pathways, such as those involved in the disposal of toxic compounds, are feed-forward–regulated. *Feed-forward regulation* may occur through an increased supply of substrate to an enzyme with a high K_m, allosteric activation of a rate-limiting enzyme through a compound related to substrate supply, substrate-related induction of gene transcription (e.g., induction of cytochrome P450-2E1 by ethanol), or increased concentration of a hormone that stimulates a storage pathway by controlling the enzyme phosphorylation state.

4. Tissue Isozymes of Regulatory Proteins

The human body is composed of several different cell types that perform specific functions unique to that cell type and synthesize only the proteins consistent with their functions. Because regulation matches function, regulatory enzymes of pathways usually exist as tissue-specific isozymes with somewhat different regulatory properties unique to their function in different cell types. For example, hexokinase and glucokinase are tissue-specific isozymes with different kinetic properties. These different isozymes arose through gene duplication. Glucokinase, the low-affinity enzyme found in liver, is a single polypeptide chain with a molecular weight of 55 kDa that contains one active catalytic site. The hexokinases found in erythrocytes, skeletal muscles, and most other tissues are 110 kDa and are essentially two mutated glucokinase molecules synthesized as one polypeptide chain. However, only one catalytic site is functional. All of the tissue-specific hexokinases except glucokinase have a K_m for glucose that is <0.2 mM.

5. Counterregulation of Opposing Pathways

A pathway for the synthesis of a compound usually has one or more enzymatic steps that differ from the pathway for degradation of that compound. A biosynthetic pathway can therefore have a different regulatory enzyme than the opposing degradative pathway, and one pathway can be activated, whereas the other is inhibited (e.g., glycogen synthesis is activated while glycogen degradation is inhibited).

6. Substrate Channeling through Compartmentation

In the cell, compartmentation of enzymes into multienzyme complexes or organelles provides a means of regulation either because the compartment provides unique conditions or because it limits or channels access of the enzymes to substrates. Enzymes or pathways with a common function are often assembled into organelles. For example, enzymes of the TCA cycle are all located within the mitochondrion. The enzymes catalyze sequential reactions, and the product of one reaction is the substrate for the next reaction. The concentration of the pathway intermediates remains much higher within the mitochondrion than in the surrounding cellular cytoplasm.

 When **Ann R.** jogs, the increased use of ATP for muscle contraction results in an increase of AMP, which allosterically activates both the key enzyme phosphofructokinase-1, the rate-limiting enzyme of glycolysis, and muscle glycogen phosphorylase, the rate-limiting enzyme of glycogenolysis. These pathways both provide for a means to increase ATP production. This is an example of feedback regulation by the ATP/AMP ratio. Unfortunately, Ann's low caloric consumption has not allowed feed-forward activation of the rate-limiting enzymes in her fuel storage pathways, and she has very low glycogen stores. Consequently, she has inadequate fuel stores to support the increased energy demands of exercise.

Another type of compartmentation involves the assembly of enzymes that catalyze sequential reactions into multienzyme complexes so that intermediates of the pathway can be transferred directly from the active site on one enzyme to the active site on another enzyme, thereby preventing loss of energy and information. One example of this is the MEOS, which is composed of two different subunits with different enzyme activities. One subunit transfers electrons from reduced nicotinamide dinucleotide phosphate (NADPH) to a cytochrome Fe-heme group on the second subunit, which then transfers the electrons to O_2.

7. Levels of Complexity

You may have noticed by now that regulation of metabolic pathways in humans is exceedingly complex; this might be called the *second principle of metabolic regulation*. As you study different pathways in subsequent chapters, it may help to develop diagrams such as Fig. 9.14 to keep track of the function and rationale behind different regulatory interactions.

CLINICAL COMMENTS

Al M. In the emergency department, **Al M.** was evaluated for head injuries. From the physical examination and blood alcohol levels, it was determined that his mental state resulted from his alcohol consumption. Although his chronic ethanol consumption had increased his level of MEOS (and, therefore, the rate of ethanol oxidation in his liver), his excessive drinking resulted in a blood alcohol level higher than the legal limit of 80 mg/dL. He suffered bruises and contusions but was otherwise uninjured. He left in the custody of the police officer and his driving license was suspended.

Ann R. Ann R.'s physician explains that she had inadequate fuel stores for her exercise program. To jog, her muscles require an increased rate of fuel oxidation to generate the ATP for muscle contraction. The fuels used by muscles for exercise include glucose from muscle glycogen, fatty acids from adipose-tissue triacylglycerols, and blood glucose supplied by liver glycogen. These fuel stores were depleted during her prolonged bout of starvation. In addition, starvation resulted in the loss of muscle mass as muscle protein was degraded to supply amino acids for other processes, including gluconeogenesis (the synthesis of glucose from amino acids and other noncarbohydrate precursors). Therefore, Ann will need to increase her caloric consumption to rebuild her fuel stores. Her physician helps her calculate the additional amount of calories her jogging program will need, and they discussed which foods she will eat to meet these increased caloric requirements. He also helps her visualize the increase of weight as an increase in strength.

The hormones epinephrine (released during stress and exercise) and glucagon (released during fasting) activate the synthesis of cAMP in several tissues. cAMP activates protein kinase A. Because protein kinase A is able to phosphorylate key regulatory enzymes in many pathways, these pathways can be regulated coordinately. In muscle, for example, glycogen degradation is activated, whereas glycogen synthesis is inhibited. At the same time, fatty-acid release from adipose tissue is activated to provide more fuel for muscle. The regulation of glycolysis, glycogen metabolism, and other pathways of metabolism is much more complex than we have illustrated here and is discussed in many subsequent chapters of this text.

BIOCHEMICAL COMMENTS

The catalytic rate constant, k_{cat} and fractional occupancy of an enzyme can also be determined by enzyme kinetics. Enzymes will typically, at maximal velocity, convert substrate to product as fast as the reaction can proceed. But how fast is that? Every enzyme has its own unique turnover number—that is, the number of reactions the enzyme can catalyze per unit of time (i.e., reactions per second). For example, the turnover number of carbonic anhydrase is about 4×10^5 reactions per second, whereas for the enzyme lysozyme the turnover number is 0.5 reaction per second (it takes 2 seconds to complete one reaction).

One can estimate the turnover number, or catalytic constant, from the rate constant k_3 in equation 1 (see the next paragraph). Recall that $v = k_3[ES]$; at maximal velocity, all of the enzyme is in the ES form, so $ES = E_t$, where E_t is the total enzyme concentration. Thus, $V_{max} = k_3E_t$. If the concentration of enzyme is known, and the maximal velocity at that concentration of enzyme, then k_3 (the catalytic constant) can be calculated. The turnover number of an enzyme is dependent on the enzyme's structure and the rate at which it can bind substrate and approach and allow the transition state of the reaction to form.

Michael-Menten kinetics can also allow one to determine the fractional occupancy of an enzyme at any given reaction velocity. The fraction of an enzyme, E, with bound substrate, S, can be represented as f_{ES}. f_{ES} is equal to the velocity in the presence of S divided by the maximal velocity of the reaction:

$$f_{ES} = (v)/(V_{max}) \qquad \text{(equation 1)}$$

Recall that the velocity of a reaction is equal to the following:

$$v = (V_{max})([S])/([S] + K_m) \qquad \text{(equation 2)}$$

If one substitutes the value of v in equation 2 for v in equation 1, one obtains:

$$f_{ES} = (V_{max})([S])/(V_{max})([S] + K_m) \qquad \text{(equation 3)}$$

If one cancels out the V_{max} in the numerator and denominator of equation 3, one obtains:

$$f_{ES} = [S]/([S] + K_m)$$

Thus, when $[S] = K_m$, $f_{ES} = \frac{1}{2}$. Knowing the concentration of substrate, and the K_m value, one can determine what percentage of enzyme has bound substrate at that time.

KEY CONCEPTS

- Enzyme activity is regulated to reflect the physiologic state of the organism.
- The rate of an enzyme-catalyzed reaction is dependent on substrate concentration and can be represented mathematically by the Michaelis-Menten equation.
- The Lineweaver-Burk transformation of the Michaelis-Menten equation allows a rapid differentiation between competitive and noncompetitive inhibitors of enzyme activity.
- Allosteric activators or inhibitors are compounds that bind at sites other than the active catalytic site and regulate the enzyme through conformational changes that affect the catalytic site.
- Several different mechanisms are available to regulate enzyme activity. These include the following:
  - Feedback inhibition, which often occurs at the first committed step of a metabolic pathway
  - Covalent modification of an amino acid residue (or residues) within the protein
  - Interactions with modulator proteins which, when bound to the enzyme, alter the conformation of the enzyme and hence activity
  - Altering the primary structure of the protein via proteolysis
  - Increasing or decreasing the amount of enzyme available in the cell via alterations in the rate of synthesis or degradation of the enzyme
- Metabolic pathways are frequently regulated at the slowest, or rate-limiting, step of the pathway.
- Diseases discussed in this chapter are summarized in Table 9.1.

TABLE 9.1	Diseases Discussed in Chapter 9	
DISORDER OR CONDITION	**GENETIC OR ENVIRONMENTAL**	**COMMENTS**
Alcohol use disorder (alcoholism)	Both	Both alcohol dehydrogenase (ADH) and the microsomal ethanol oxidizing system (MEOS) are active in detoxifying ethanol. High nicotinamide adenine dinucleotide (NADH) can inhibit ADH, allowing toxic metabolites to accumulate.
Anorexia nervosa	Both	Effects of malnutrition on energy production were discussed.
Maturity-onset diabetes of the young (MODY)	Genetic	Mutations in various proteins can lead to this form of diabetes, which is manifest by hyperglycemia but without other complications associated with either type 1 or 2 diabetes. Specifically, mutations in pancreatic glucokinase were discussed.

REVIEW QUESTIONS—CHAPTER 9

1. Salivary amylase is an enzyme that digests dietary starch. Assume that salivary amylase follows Michaelis-Menten kinetics. Which one of the following best describes a characteristic feature of salivary amylase?
   A. The enzyme velocity is at one-half the maximal rate when 100% of the enzyme molecules contain bound substrate.
   B. The enzyme velocity is at one-half the maximal rate when 50% of the enzyme molecules contain bound substrate.
   C. The enzyme velocity is at its maximal rate when 50% of the enzyme molecules contain bound substrate.
   D. The enzyme velocity is at its maximal rate when all of the substrate molecules in solution are bound by the enzyme.
   E. The velocity of the reaction is independent of the concentration of enzyme.

2. The pancreatic glucokinase of a patient with MODY had a mutation replacing a leucine with a proline. The result was that the K_m for glucose was decreased from a normal value of 6 mM to a value of 2.2 mM, and the V_{max} was changed from 93 U/mg protein to 0.2 U/mg protein. Which one of the following best describes the patient's glucokinase compared with the normal enzyme?
   A. The patient's enzyme requires a lower concentration of glucose to reach $\frac{1}{2}V_{max}$.
   B. The patient's enzyme is faster than the normal enzyme at concentrations of glucose <2.2 mM.
   C. The patient's enzyme is faster than the normal enzyme at concentrations of glucose >2.2 mM.
   D. At near-saturating glucose concentration, the patient would need 90 to 100 times more enzyme than normal to achieve normal rates of glucose phosphorylation.
   E. As blood glucose levels increase after a meal from a fasting value of 5 to 10 mM, the rate of the patient's enzyme will increase more than the rate of the normal enzyme.

3. Methanol (CH_3OH) is converted by ADHs to formaldehyde (CH_2O), a compound that is highly toxic to humans. Patients who have ingested toxic levels of methanol are sometimes treated with ethanol (CH_3CH_2OH) to inhibit methanol oxidation by ADH. Which one of the following statements provides the best rationale for this treatment?
   A. Ethanol is a structural analog of methanol and might therefore be an effective noncompetitive inhibitor.
   B. Ethanol is a structural analog of methanol that can be expected to compete with methanol for its binding site on the enzyme.
   C. Ethanol can be expected to alter the V_{max} of ADH for the oxidation of methanol to formaldehyde.
   D. Ethanol is an effective inhibitor of methanol oxidation regardless of the concentration of methanol.
   E. Ethanol can be expected to inhibit the enzyme by binding to the formaldehyde-binding site on the enzyme, even though it cannot bind at the substrate-binding site for methanol.

4. A runner's muscles use glucose as a source of energy. Muscle contains glycogen stores that are degraded into glucose 1-phosphate via glycogen phosphorylase, which is an allosteric enzyme. Assume that an allosteric enzyme has the follow-

ing kinetic properties: a V_{max} of 25 U/mg enzyme and a $K_{m,app}$ of 1.0 mM. These kinetic parameters were then measured in the presence of an allosteric activator. Which one of the following would best describe the findings of that experiment?

A. A V_{max} of 25 U/mg enzyme and a $K_{m,app}$ of 0.2 mM
B. A V_{max} of 15 U/mg enzyme with a $K_{m,app}$ of 2.0 mM
C. A V_{max} of 25 U/mg enzyme with a $K_{m,app}$ of 2.0 mM
D. A V_{max} of 50 U/mg enzyme with a $K_{m,app}$ of 5.0 mM
E. A V_{max} of 50 U/mg enzyme with a $K_{m,app}$ of 10.0 mM

5. A rate-limiting enzyme catalyzes the first step in the conversion of a toxic metabolite to a urinary excretion product. Which of the following mechanisms for regulating this enzyme would provide the most protection to the body?

A. The product of the pathway should be an allosteric inhibitor of the rate-limiting enzyme.
B. The product of the pathway should act through gene transcription to decrease synthesis of the enzyme.
C. The toxin should act through gene transcription to increase synthesis of the enzyme.
D. The enzyme should have a high K_m value for the toxin.
E. The toxin allosterically activates the last enzyme in the pathway.

6. In thyroid hormone production, thyrotropin-releasing hormone (TRH) from the hypothalamus stimulates thyroid-stimulating hormone (TSH) release from the anterior pituitary, which stimulates the thyroid to produce thyroid hormones (triiodothyronine [T_3] and thyroxine [T_4]). Normal or high levels of thyroid hormone then suppress release of TRH. The regulation of this pathway is best described by which one of the following?

A. Complementary regulation
B. Feedback regulation
C. Compartmentation
D. Feed-forward regulation
E. Negative regulation

7. A patient with alcoholic liver disease has profound mental status changes caused by a buildup of ammonia (NH_4^+) and is suffering from hepatic encephalopathy. The conversion of NH_4^+ to urea is an example of which one of the following types of pathway regulation?

A. Complementary
B. Feedback

C. Compartmentation
D. Feed-forward
E. Negative

8. Pathway regulation can occur via the expression of tissue-specific isozymes. Glucose metabolism differs in red blood cells and liver in that red blood cells need to metabolize glucose, whereas the liver prefers to store glucose. The first step of glucose metabolism requires either glucokinase (liver) or hexokinase I (red blood cells), which are isozymes. Which one of the following best describes these different isozymes and their K_m for glucose?

A. The K_m of hexokinase I is higher than the K_m of glucokinase.
B. The K_m of hexokinase I is lower than the K_m of glucokinase.
C. The K_m of hexokinase I is the same as the K_m of glucokinase.
D. Hexokinase I is found in liver.
E. Glucokinase is found in red blood cells.

Questions 9 and 10 are linked.

9. An antibiotic is developed that is a close structural analog of a substrate of an enzyme that participates in cell wall synthesis in bacteria. This binding of the antibiotic reduces overall enzyme activity, but such activity can be restored if more substrate is added. The binding of the antibiotic to the enzyme is not via a covalent bond, nor does the enzyme alter the structure of the antibiotic. Which one of the following would best describe this antibiotic?

A. It is a suicide inhibitor.
B. It is an irreversible inhibitor.
C. It is a competitive inhibitor.
D. It is a noncompetitive inhibitor.
E. It is an uncompetitive inhibitor.

10. Which one of the following is true for the inhibitor described in the previous question?

A. It increases the apparent K_m of the enzyme.
B. It decreases the apparent K_m of the enzyme.
C. It has no effect on the apparent K_m of the enzyme.
D. It increases the V_{max} of the enzyme.
E. It decreases the V_{max} of the enzyme.

ANSWERS

1. **The answer is B.** The rate of an enzyme-catalyzed reaction is directly proportional to the proportion of enzyme molecules that contain bound substrate. Thus, it is at 50% of its maximal rate when 50% of the molecules contain bound substrate (thus, A, C, and D are incorrect). The rate of the reaction is directly proportional to the amount of enzyme present, which is incorporated into the term V_{max} (where $V_{max} = k$[total enzyme]) (thus, E is incorrect).

2. **The answer is A.** The patient's enzyme has a lower K_m than the normal enzyme and therefore requires a lower glucose concentration to reach $\frac{1}{2}V_{max}$. Thus, the mutation may have increased the affinity of the enzyme for glucose, but it has greatly decreased the subsequent steps of the reaction leading to formation of the transition-state complex, and thus, V_{max} is much slower. The difference in V_{max} is so great that the patient's enzyme

is much slower whether you are above or below its K_m for glucose. You can test this by substituting 2 mM glucose and 4 mM glucose into the Michaelis-Menten equation, $v = V_{max} S/(K_m + S)$ for the patient's enzyme and for the normal enzyme. The values are 0.0095 and 0.0129 for the patient's enzyme versus 23.2 and 37.2 for the normal enzyme, respectively (thus, B and C are incorrect). At near-saturating glucose concentrations, both enzymes will be near V_{max}, which is equal to k_{cat} times the enzyme concentration. Thus, it will take nearly 500 times as much of the patient's enzyme to achieve the normal rate (93 ÷ 0.2), and so C is incorrect. E is incorrect because rates change most as you decrease substrate concentration below the K_m. Thus, the enzyme with the highest K_m will show the largest changes in rate.

3. **The answer is B.** Ethanol has a structure very similar to methanol (a structural analog) and thus can be expected to compete with methanol at its substrate-binding site. This inhibition is competitive with respect to methanol, and, therefore, V_{max} for methanol will not be altered and ethanol inhibition can be overcome by high concentrations of methanol (thus, A, C, and D are incorrect). E is illogical because the substrate methanol stays in the same binding site as it is converted to its product, formaldehyde.

4. **The answer is A.** Allosteric activators will shift the sigmoidal kinetic curve for the enzyme to the left, thereby reducing the $K_{m,app}$ (so ½V_{max} will be reached at a lower substrate concentration) without affecting the maximum velocity (although in some cases, V_{max} can also be increased). Allosteric inhibitors will shift the curve to the right, increasing the $K_{m,app}$ and sometimes also decreasing the V_{max}.

5. **The answer is C.** The most effective regulation should be a feed-forward type of regulation in which the toxin activates the pathway. One of the most common ways this occurs is through the toxin acting to increase the amount of enzyme by increasing transcription of its gene. A and B describe mechanisms of feedback regulation, in which the end product of the pathway decreases its own rate of synthesis and are, therefore, incorrect. D is incorrect because a high K_m for the toxin might prevent the enzyme from working effectively at low toxin concentrations, although it would allow the enzyme to respond to increases of toxin concentration. It would do little good for the toxin to allosterically activate any enzyme but the rate-limiting enzyme (thus, E is incorrect).

6. **The answer is B.** In feedback regulation, the end product (thyroid hormone) directly controls its own rate of synthesis by suppressing earlier stimulating hormones. This is called a *feedback loop*. Feed-forward mechanisms reflect the availability of a precursor to

activate a downstream step of a pathway, such as with toxin disposal pathways (only activated when toxin is present, and the rate of toxin removal increases as the level of toxin increases). Compartmentation is a collection of enzymes within a specific compartment of the cell (e.g., cytoplasm, peroxisome, lysosome, mitochondria). Although negative regulation refers to an inhibitor of an enzyme, the best answer to this question is feedback regulation, as the end product of the pathway is the effector that is regulating the pathway. Complementary regulation refers to several factors acting similarly (complementing each other) in regulating a pathway, which is not the case in this example.

7. **The answer is D.** Ammonia is a toxin and needs to be removed from the body by converting it to urea. If no ammonia is present, the pathway does not function. When arginine is present (a component of the cycle that generates urea), the disposal pathway becomes functional, and the higher the concentration of arginine, the faster the pathway—a great example of feed-forward regulation. Urea does not feedback to slow production of more urea. The enzymes of the urea cycle are not compartmentalized (they exist both in the mitochondria and in cytoplasm).

8. **The answer is B.** Red blood cells rely solely on glucose for energy needs and must have an isoenzyme with a much lower K_m (hexokinase I), so that at even low levels of substrate (glucose), glucose can still be phosphorylated at rates near the V_{max} to allow the red blood cells to survive. With a K_m near the normal fasting level of blood glucose, liver glucokinase can convert elevated levels of glucose (after a meal) into glycogen, a glucose storage molecule.

9. **The answer is C.** Because the antibiotic is not covalently bound to the enzyme, it is a reversible inhibitor. The antibiotic is not a suicide inhibitor because the enzyme does not alter the structure of the antibiotic. Because adding excess substrate can overcome the effects of the inhibitor, the inhibitor is acting in a competitive manner, competing with substrate for binding to the active site of the enzyme. Excess substrate cannot overcome the effects of a noncompetitive inhibitor. Uncompetitive or anticompetitive inhibitors bind to the complex formed between the enzymes and substrate and are not overcome by adding excess substrate.

10. **The answer is A.** A competitive inhibitor increases the apparent K_m of the enzyme because it raises the concentration of substrate necessary to saturate the enzyme. They have no effect on V_{max}. In the example of the antibiotic, a higher dose of the antibiotic would be expected to be more effective (up to maximal saturation of the enzyme). Noncompetitive inhibitors change V_{max} with no effect on the K_m of the substrate.

Relationship between Cell Biology and Biochemistry

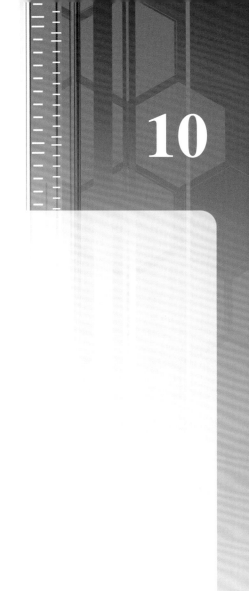

The basic unit of a living organism is the cell. In humans, each tissue is composed of a variety of cell types, which differ from those cell types in other tissues. The diversity of cell types serves the function of the tissue and organs in which they reside, and each cell type has unique structural features that reflect its role. In spite of their diversity in structure, human cell types have certain architectural features in common, such as the plasma membrane, membranes around the nucleus and organelles, and a cytoskeleton (Fig. 10.1). In this chapter, we review some of the chemical characteristics of these common features, the functions of organelles, and the transport systems for compounds into cells and between organelles.

Plasma Membrane. The cell membrane consists of a **lipid bilayer** that serves as a selective barrier; it restricts the entry and exit of compounds. Within the plasma membrane, different **integral membrane proteins** facilitate the **transport** of compounds by **energy-requiring active transport, facilitated diffusion,** or by forming **pores** or **gated channels**. The plasma membrane is supported by a **membrane skeleton** composed of proteins.

Organelles and Cytoplasmic Membrane Systems. Most organelles within the cell are compartments surrounded by a membrane system that restricts exchange of compounds and information with other compartments (see Fig. 10.1). In general, each organelle has unique functions that are served by the enzymes and other compounds it contains, or the environment it maintains. **Lysosomes** contain **hydrolytic enzymes** that degrade proteins and other large molecules. The **nucleus** contains the genetic material and carries out **gene replication** and **transcription** of **DNA**, the first step of protein synthesis. The last phase of protein synthesis occurs on **ribosomes**. For certain proteins, the ribosomes become attached to the complex membrane system called the **endoplasmic reticulum**; for other proteins, synthesis is completed on ribosomes that remain in the cytoplasm. The **endoplasmic reticulum** is also involved in lipid synthesis and transport of molecules to the Golgi. The **Golgi** forms vesicles for transport of molecules to the plasma membrane and other membrane systems, and for secretion. **Mitochondria** are organelles committed to **fuel oxidation** and **adenosine triphosphate (ATP) generation. Peroxisomes** contain many enzymes that use or produce **hydrogen peroxide**. The **cytosol** is the intracellular compartment free of organelles and membrane systems.

Cytoskeleton. The **cytoskeleton** is a flexible fibrous protein support system that maintains the geometry of the cell, fixes the position of organelles, and moves compounds within the cell. The cytoskeleton also facilitates movement of the cell itself. It is composed primarily of **actin microfilaments, intermediate filaments, tubulin microtubules,** and their attached proteins.

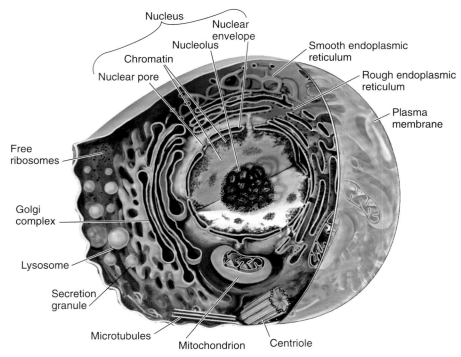

FIGURE 10.1 Common components of human cells.

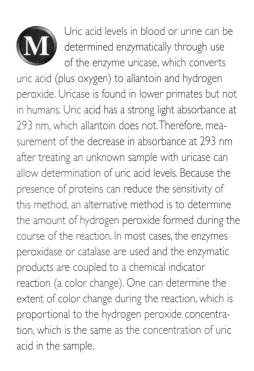

V. cholerae epidemics are rare in the United States. However, these bacteria grow well under the alkaline conditions found in seawater and attach to chitin in shellfish. Thus, sporadic cases occur in the southeast United States associated with the ingestion of contaminated shellfish.

Uric acid levels in blood or urine can be determined enzymatically through use of the enzyme uricase, which converts uric acid (plus oxygen) to allantoin and hydrogen peroxide. Uricase is found in lower primates but not in humans. Uric acid has a strong light absorbance at 293 nm, which allantoin does not. Therefore, measurement of the decrease in absorbance at 293 nm after treating an unknown sample with uricase can allow determination of uric acid levels. Because the presence of proteins can reduce the sensitivity of this method, an alternative method is to determine the amount of hydrogen peroxide formed during the course of the reaction. In most cases, the enzymes peroxidase or catalase are used and the enzymatic products are coupled to a chemical indicator reaction (a color change). One can determine the extent of color change during the reaction, which is proportional to the hydrogen peroxide concentration, which is the same as the concentration of uric acid in the sample.

THE WAITING ROOM

 Al M. had been drinking heavily when he drove his car off the road and was taken to the hospital emergency department (see Chapters 8 and 9). Although he suffered only minor injuries, his driving license was suspended.

 Two years after **Dennis V.** recovered from his malathion poisoning, he visited his grandfather, **Percy V.** Mr. V. took Dennis with him to a picnic at the shore, where they ate steamed crabs. Early the next morning, Dennis experienced episodes of profuse watery diarrhea and vomiting. Mr. V. rushed him to the hospital emergency department. Dennis's hands and feet were cold, he appeared severely dehydrated, and he was approaching hypovolemic shock (a severe drop in blood pressure). He was diagnosed with cholera, caused by the bacteria *Vibrio cholerae*. Dennis was placed on intravenous rehydration therapy, followed by oral rehydration therapy with high glucose and sodium (Na^+)-containing fluids and given antibiotics.

 Before **Lotta T.** was treated with allopurinol for prevention of an attack of gout (see Chapter 8), her physician administered colchicine (acetyltrimethylcolchicinic acid) for the acute attack of gout affecting her great toe. After taking two doses of colchicine divided over 1 hour (1.2 mg for the first dose, followed 1 hour later by 0.6 mg), the throbbing pain in her toe had abated significantly. The redness and swelling also seemed to have lessened slightly.

I. Compartmentation in Cells

Membranes are lipid structures that separate the contents of the compartment they surround from its environment. An outer plasma membrane separates the cell from the external environment. Organelles (such as the nucleus, mitochondria, lysosomes, and peroxisomes) are also surrounded by membrane systems that separate the internal compartment of the organelle from the cytosol. The function of these membranes is to allow the organelle to collect or concentrate enzymes and other molecules serving a common function into a compartment within a localized environment. The transporters and receptors in each membrane system control this localized environment and facilitate communication of the cell or organelle with the surrounding milieu.

The following sections describe the various organelles and membrane systems found in most human cells and outline the relationship between their properties and function. Each organelle contains different enzymes and carries out different general functions. For example, the nucleus contains the enzymes for DNA and RNA synthesis. The cells of humans and other animals are eukaryotes (*eu*, good; *karyon*, nucleus) because the genetic material is organized into a membrane-enclosed nucleus. In contrast, bacteria are prokaryotes (*pro*, before; *karyon*, nucleus); they do not contain nuclei or other organelles found in eukaryotic cells.

Not all cells in humans are alike. Different cell types differ quantitatively in their organelle content, and their organelles may contain vastly different amounts of a particular enzyme, *consistent with the function of the cell*. For example, liver mitochondria contain a key enzyme for synthesizing ketone bodies, but they lack a key enzyme required for their use. The reverse is true in muscle mitochondria. Thus, the enzyme content of the organelles varies somewhat from cell type to cell type.

II. Plasma Membrane

A. Structure of the Plasma Membrane

All mammalian cells are enclosed by a plasma membrane composed of a *lipid bilayer* (two layers) containing embedded proteins (Fig. 10.2). The membrane layer facing the "inside" of the organelle or cell is termed the *inner leaflet*; the other layer is the *outer*, or *external leaflet*. The membranes are continuous and sealed so that the hydrophobic lipid bilayer selectively restricts the exchange of polar compounds between the external fluid and the intracellular compartment. The membrane is referred to as a *fluid mosaic* because it consists of a mosaic of proteins and lipid molecules that can for the most part move laterally in the plane of the membrane. The proteins are classified as *integral proteins*, which span the cell membrane, or *peripheral proteins*, which are attached to the membrane surface through electrostatic bonds to

 Bacteria are single cells surrounded by a cell membrane and a cell wall exterior to the membrane. They are prokaryotes, which do not contain nuclei or other organelles (i.e., membrane-surrounded subcellular structures) found in eukaryotic cells. Nonetheless, bacteria carry out many similar metabolic pathways, with the enzymes located in either the intracellular compartment or the cell membrane.

The *V. cholerae* responsible for **Dennis V.'s** cholera are gram-negative bacteria. Their plasma membrane is surrounded by a thin cell wall composed of a protein–polysaccharide structure called *peptidoglycan* and an outer membrane. In contrast, gram-positive bacteria have a plasma membrane and a thick peptidoglycan cell wall that retains the Gram stain. *Vibrio* grow best under aerobic conditions but also can grow under low-oxygen conditions. They possess enzymes similar to those in human cells for glycolysis, the tricarboxylic acid (TCA) cycle, and oxidative phosphorylation. They have a low tolerance for acid, which partially accounts for their presence in slightly basic seawater and shellfish.

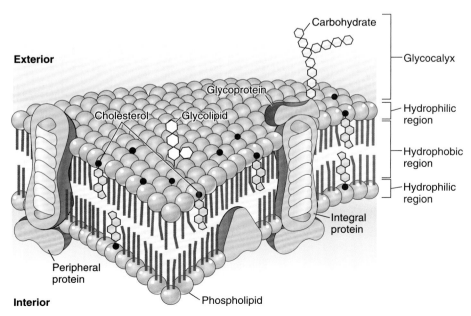

FIGURE 10.2   Basic structure of a mammalian cell membrane.

lipids or integral proteins. Many of the proteins and lipids on the external leaflet of the plasma membrane contain covalently bound carbohydrate chains and therefore are *glycoproteins* and *glycolipids*. This layer of carbohydrate on the outer surface of the cell is called the *glycocalyx*. The variable carbohydrate components of the glycolipids on the cell surface function, in part, as cell recognition markers for small molecules or other cells.

I. Lipids in the Plasma Membrane

One of the bacterial toxins secreted by *Clostridium perfringens*, the bacteria that cause gas gangrene, is a lipase that hydrolyzes phosphocholine from phosphatidylcholine and from sphingomyelin. The resulting lysis (breakage) of the cell membrane releases intracellular contents that provide the bacteria with nutrients for rapid growth. These bacteria are strict anaerobes and grow only in the absence of oxygen. As their toxins lyse membranes in the endothelial cells of blood vessels, the capillaries are destroyed, and the bacteria are protected from oxygen transported by the red blood cells. They are also protected from antibiotics and components of the immune system carried in the blood.

Each layer of the plasma membrane lipid bilayer is formed primarily by *phospholipids*, which are arranged with their hydrophilic head groups facing the aqueous medium and their fatty acyl tails forming a hydrophobic membrane core (see Fig. 10.2). The principal phospholipids in the membrane are the glycerol lipids *phosphatidylcholine* (also named lecithin), *phosphatidylethanolamine*, and *phosphatidylserine*, and the sphingolipid *sphingomyelin* (Fig. 10.3). Sphingosine also forms the base for the glycosphingolipids, which are membrane-anchored lipids with carbohydrates attached. The lipid composition varies among different cell types, with phosphatidylcholine being the major plasma membrane phospholipid in most cell types and glycosphingolipids the most variable.

The lipid composition of the bilayer is asymmetric, with a higher content of phosphatidylcholine and sphingomyelin in the outer leaflet and a higher content of phosphatidylserine and phosphatidylethanolamine in the inner leaflet. Phosphatidylinositol, which can function in the transfer of information from hormones and neurotransmitters across the cell membrane (see Chapter 11), is also primarily found

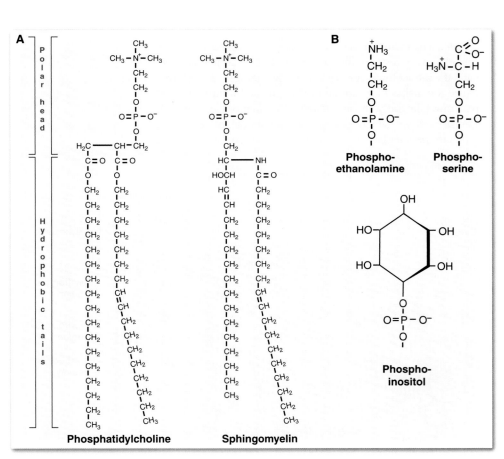

FIGURE 10.3 Common phospholipids in the mammalian cell membrane. **A.** Phosphatidylcholine (a glycerol-based lipid) and sphingomyelin (a sphingosine-based lipid). Note the similarity in structures. **B.** Different head groups for the phospholipids. These head groups replace the choline in phosphatidylcholine and form, respectively, phosphatidylethanolamine, phosphatidylserine, and phosphatidylinositol.

in the inner leaflet. Phosphatidylserine contains a net negative charge that contributes to the membrane potential and may be important for binding positively charged molecules within the cell.

Cholesterol, which is interspersed between the phospholipids, maintains membrane fluidity. In the glycerol-based phospholipids, unsaturated fatty-acid chains bent into the *cis* conformation form a pocket for cholesterol, which binds with its hydroxyl group in the external hydrophilic region of the membrane and its hydrophobic steroid nucleus in the hydrophobic membrane core (Fig. 10.4). The presence of cholesterol and the *cis* unsaturated fatty acids in the membrane prevent the hydrophobic chains from packing too closely together. As a consequence, lipid and protein molecules that are not bound to external or internal structural proteins can rotate and move laterally in the plane of the leaflet. This movement enables the plasma membrane to partition between daughter cells during cell division, to deform as cells pass through capillaries, and to form and fuse with vesicle membranes. Cholesterol can also stabilize very fluid membranes by increasing interactions between the fatty acids of phospholipids. The fluidity of the membrane is also partially determined by the unsaturated fatty acid content of the diet.

The composition of the membrane is dynamic. Sections of membrane form buds that pinch off into vesicles, and membrane vesicles formed in the Golgi and elsewhere bring new and recycled components back to the membrane. Individual fatty acyl chains turn over as they are hydrolyzed from the lipids and replaced, and enzymes called *flippases* transfer lipids between leaflets.

2. Proteins in the Plasma Membrane

Integral proteins contain transmembrane domains with hydrophobic amino acid side chains that interact with the hydrophobic portions of the lipids to seal the membrane (see Fig. 10.2). Hydrophilic regions of the proteins protrude into the aqueous medium on both sides of the membrane. Many of these proteins function as either channels or transporters for the movement of compounds across the membrane, as receptors for the binding of hormones and neurotransmitters, or as structural proteins (Fig. 10.5).

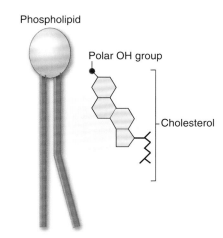

FIGURE 10.4 Cholesterol in the plasma membrane. The polar hydroxyl group of cholesterol is oriented toward the surface. The hydrocarbon tail and the steroid nucleus (*orange*) lie in the hydrophobic core. A *cis* double bond in the fatty acyl chain of a phospholipid bends the chain to create a hydrophobic binding site for cholesterol.

 Al M. is suffering from both short-term and long-term effects of ethanol on his central nervous system. Data support the theory that the short-term effects of ethanol on the brain arise partly from an increase in membrane fluidity caused when ethanol intercalates between the membrane lipids. The changes in membrane fluidity may affect proteins that span the membrane (integral proteins), such as ion channels and receptors for neurotransmitters involved in conducting the nerve impulse.

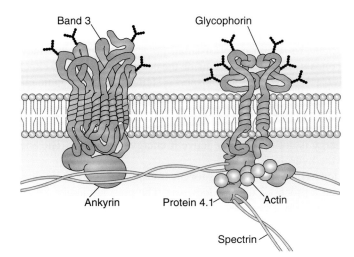

FIGURE 10.5 Proteins in the red blood cell membrane. The proteins named *Band 3* (the bicarbonate–chloride exchange transporter) and *glycophorin* (provides an external negative charge that repels other cells) both contain nonpolar α-helical segments spanning the lipid bilayer. These proteins contain a large number of polar and charged hydrophilic amino acids in the intracellular and extracellular domains. On the inside of the cell, they are attached to peripheral proteins comprising the inner membrane skeleton. Band 3 is connected to spectrin filaments via the protein ankyrin. Glycophorin is connected to short actin filaments and spectrin via protein 4.1. Band 3 allows the transport of bicarbonate into the red blood cell in exchange for chloride. This allows bicarbonate transport to the lung, where it is expired as carbon dioxide.

All cells contain an inner membrane skeleton of spectrin-like proteins. Red blood cell spectrin was the first member of the spectrin family to be described. The protein dystrophin, present in skeletal muscle cells, is a member of the spectrin family. Genetic defects in the dystrophin gene are responsible for Duchenne and Becker muscular dystrophies.

 The prion protein, present in neuronal membranes, provides an example of a protein attached to the membrane through a GPI anchor. This is the protein that develops an altered pathogenic conformation in both mad cow disease and Creutzfeldt-Jakob disease (see Chapter 7, Section IX.C.3).

Peripheral membrane proteins, which were originally defined as those proteins that can be released from the membrane by ionic solvents, are bound through weak electrostatic interactions with the polar head groups of lipids or with integral proteins. One of the best characterized classes of peripheral proteins is the *spectrin* family of proteins, which are bound to the intracellular membrane surface and provide mechanical support for the membrane. Spectrin is bound to actin, which together form a structure that is called the *inner membrane skeleton* or the *cortical skeleton* (see Fig. 10.5).

A third classification of membrane proteins consists of *lipid-anchored proteins* bound to the inner or outer surface of the membrane. The *glycophosphatidylinositol (GPI) glycan anchor* is a covalently attached lipid that anchors proteins to the external surface of the membrane (Fig. 10.6). Several proteins involved in hormonal regulation are anchored to the internal surface of the membrane through palmityl (C16) or myristyl (C14) fatty acyl groups or through geranylgeranyl (C20) or farnesyl (C15) isoprenyl groups (see Fig. 6.13). However, many integral proteins also contain attached lipid groups to increase their stability in the membrane.

3. The Glycocalyx of the Plasma Membrane

Some of the proteins and lipids on the external surface of the membrane contain short chains of carbohydrates (oligosaccharides) that extend into the aqueous medium. Carbohydrates constitute 2% to 10% of the weight of plasma membranes. This hydrophilic carbohydrate layer, called the *glycocalyx*, protects the cell from digestion and restricts the uptake of hydrophobic compounds.

The glycoproteins generally contain branched oligosaccharide chains of approximately 15 sugar residues that are attached through *N*-glycosidic bonds to the amide nitrogen of an asparagine side chain (*N*-glycosidic linkage), or through a glycosidic bond to the oxygen of serine (*O*-glycoproteins). The membrane glycolipids are usually gangliosides or cerebrosides. Specific carbohydrate chains on the glycolipids serve as cell-recognition molecules (see Chapter 5 for structures of these compounds).

B. Transport of Molecules across the Plasma Membrane

Membranes form hydrophobic barriers around cells to control the internal environment by restricting the entry and exit of molecules. As a consequence, cells require *transport systems* to permit entry of small polar compounds that they need (e.g., glucose) to concentrate compounds inside the cell (e.g., K^+) and to expel other compounds (e.g., Ca^{2+} and Na^+). The transport systems for small organic molecules and inorganic ions generally fall into four categories: First is *simple diffusion* through the lipid bilayer, second is *facilitative diffusion*, third is *gated channels*, and fourth is *active transport pumps* (Fig. 10.7). These transport mechanisms are classified as passive if energy is not required or active if energy is required. The energy is often provided by the hydrolysis of ATP.

In addition to these mechanisms for the transport of small individual molecules, cells engage in a process called *endocytosis*. The plasma membrane extends or invaginates to surround a particle, a foreign cell, or extracellular fluid, which then closes into a vesicle that is released into the cytoplasm (see Fig. 10.7).

I. Simple Diffusion

Gases such as O_2 and CO_2 and lipid-soluble substances (such as steroid hormones) can cross membranes by simple diffusion (see Fig. 10.7). In simple diffusion (free diffusion), molecules move by engaging in random collisions with other like molecules. There is a net movement from a region of high concentration to a region of low concentration because molecules keep bumping into each other where their concentration is highest. Energy is not required for diffusion, and compounds that are uncharged eventually reach the same concentrations on both sides of the membrane.

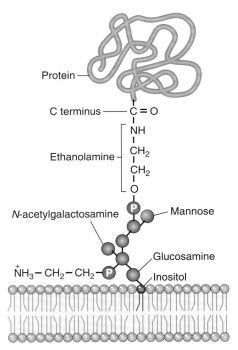

FIGURE 10.6 An example of a glycosylphosphatidylinositol (GPI) glycan anchor. The carboxyl terminus of the protein is attached to phosphoethanolamine, which is bound to a branched oligosaccharide that is attached to the inositol portion of phosphatidylinositol. The hydrophobic fatty acyl chains of the phosphatidylinositol portion are bound in the hydrophobic core of the membrane.

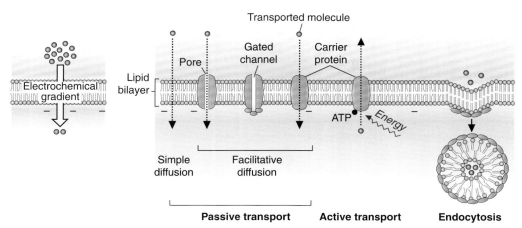

FIGURE 10.7 Common types of transport mechanisms for human cells. The electrochemical gradient consists of the concentration gradient of the compound and the distribution of charge on the membrane, which affects the transport of charged ions such as Cl^-. Both protein amino acid residues and lipid polar head groups contribute to the net negative charge on the inside of the membrane. Generally, the diffusion of uncharged molecules (passive transport) is net movement from a region of high concentration to a region of low concentration, and active transport (energy-requiring) is net movement from a region of low concentration to one of high concentration. *ATP*, adenosine triphosphate.

Water is considered to diffuse through membranes by nonspecific movement through ion channels, pores, or around proteins embedded in the lipids. Certain cells (e.g., renal tubule cells) also contain large protein pores, called *aquaporins*, which permit a high rate of water flow from a region of a high water concentration (low solute concentration) to one of low water concentration (high solute concentration).

2. Facilitative Diffusion through Binding to Transporter Proteins

Facilitative diffusion requires that the transported molecule bind to a specific carrier or transport protein in the membrane (Fig. 10.8A). The transporter protein then undergoes a conformational change that allows the transported molecule to be released on the other side of the membrane. Although the transported molecules are bound to proteins, the transport process is still classified as diffusion because energy is not required, and the compound equilibrates (achieves a balance of concentration and charge) on both sides of the membrane.

Transporter proteins, like enzymes, exhibit saturation kinetics; when all the binding sites on the transporter proteins in the membrane are occupied, the system is saturated and the rate of transport reaches a plateau (the maximum velocity). By analogy to enzymes, the concentration of a transported compound required to reach one-half of the maximum velocity is often called the K_m (see Fig. 10.8B). Facilitative transporters are similar to enzymes with respect to two additional features: They are relatively specific for the compounds they bind, and they can be inhibited by compounds that block their binding sites or change their conformation.

3. Gated Channels in Plasma Membranes

In the case of gated channels, transmembrane proteins form a pore for ions that is either opened or closed in response to a stimulus. These stimuli can be voltage changes across the membrane (voltage-gated channels), the binding of a compound (ligand-gated channels), or a regulatory change in the intracellular domain (phosphorylation-gated and pressure-gated channels). For example, the conduction of a nerve impulse along an axon depends on the passive flux of Na^+ ions through a voltage-gated channel that is opened by depolarization of the membrane. Cystic *f*ibrosis *t*ransmembrane conductance *r*egulator (CFTR) is a Cl^- channel that provides an example of a ligand-gated channel regulated through

The A, B, and O blood groups are determined by the carbohydrate composition of the glycolipids on the surface of red blood cells. Glycolipids on other cell surfaces may also serve as binding sites for viruses and bacterial toxins before penetrating the cell. For example, the cholera AB toxin (which is affecting **Dennis V.**) binds to GM_1-gangliosides on the surface of the intestinal epithelial cells. The toxin is then endocytosed in caveolae (invaginations or "caves" that can form in specific regions of the membrane). Once inside the cell, the toxin will alter normal cellular metabolism.

Dennis V. has become dehydrated because he has lost so much water through vomiting and diarrhea (see Chapter 4). Cholera toxin increases the efflux of sodium and chloride ions from his intestinal mucosal cells into the intestinal lumen. The increase of water in his stools results from the passive transfer of water from inside the cell and body fluids, where it is in high concentration (i.e., intracellular Na^+ and Cl^- concentrations are low), to the intestinal lumen and bowel, where water is in lower concentration (relative to high Na^+ and Cl^-). The watery diarrhea is also high in K^+ ions and bicarbonate. All of the signs and symptoms of cholera generally derive from this fluid loss.

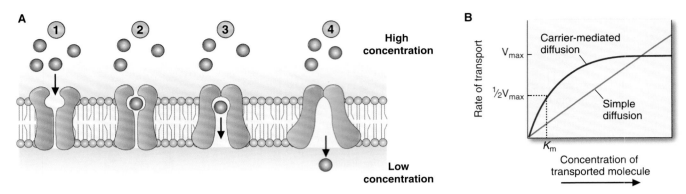

FIGURE 10.8 A. Facilitative transport. Although the molecule being transported must bind to the protein transporter, the mechanism is passive diffusion and the molecule moves from a region of high concentration to one of low concentration. "Passive" refers to the lack of an energy requirement for the transport. **B.** Saturation kinetics of transporter proteins. When a compound must bind to a protein to be transported across a membrane, the velocity of transport depends on the amount of compound bound. It reaches a maximum rate when the compound's concentration is raised so high that all of the transporter-binding sites are occupied. The curve is a rectangular hyperbola that approaches maximum velocity (V_{max}) at infinite substrate concentration, identical to that of Michaelis-Menten enzymes. The K_m of transport is the concentration of compound required for $\frac{1}{2}V_{max}$. In contrast, simple diffusion of a compound does not require its binding to a protein, and the rate of transport increases linearly with increasing concentration of the compound.

All of the cells in the body have facilitative glucose transporters that transport glucose across the plasma membrane down an electrochemical (concentration) gradient as it is rapidly metabolized in the cell. In muscle and adipose tissue, insulin increases the content of facilitative glucose transporters in the cell membrane, thus increasing the ability of these tissues to take up glucose. Patients with type 1 diabetes mellitus, who do not produce insulin (e.g., **Dianne A.**; see Chapter 7), have a decreased ability to transport glucose into these tissues, thereby contributing to hyperglycemia (high blood glucose).

phosphorylation (phosphorylation-gated) (Fig. 10.9). CFTR is a member of the *a*denine nucleotide–*b*inding *c*assette, or ATP-binding cassette (ABC) superfamily of transport proteins and is the protein mutated in cystic fibrosis. CFTR consists of two transmembrane domains that form a closed channel, each connected to an ATP-binding site, and a regulatory domain that sits in front of the channel. When the regulatory domain is phosphorylated by a kinase, its conformation changes and it moves away from the ATP-binding domains. As ATP binds and is hydrolyzed, the transmembrane domains change conformation and open the channel, and chloride ions diffuse through. As the conformation reverts back to its original form, the channel closes.

Transport through a ligand-gated channel can be considered simple diffusion, although ATP is involved, because only a few ATP molecules are being used to open and close the channel through which many, many chloride ions diffuse. However, the distinction between ligand-gated channels and facilitative transporters is not always as clear. Many gated channels show saturation kinetics at very high concentrations of the compounds being transported, which is why Figure 10.7 characterizes ligand-gated channels as facilitative transport.

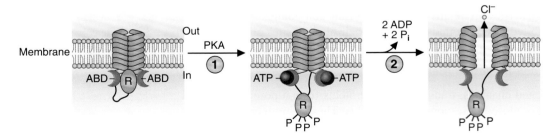

FIGURE 10.9 The cystic fibrosis transmembrane conductance regulator (CFTR), a ligand-gated channel controlled by phosphorylation. Two intracellular binding domains control opening of the channel, an adenine nucleotide–binding domain (ABD) and a regulatory domain (R). (*1*) Phosphorylation of the regulatory subunit by protein kinase A (PKA) causes a conformational change that allows adenosine triphosphate (ATP) to bind to the adenine nucleotide–binding domain (ABD). (2) Hydrolysis of bound ATP opens the channel so that chloride ions can diffuse through. *ADP*, adenosine diphosphate; *P$_i$*, inorganic phosphate.

4. Active Transport Requires Energy and Transporter Proteins

Both active transport and facilitative transport are mediated by protein transporters (carriers) in the membrane. However, in facilitative transport, the compound is transported down an electrochemical gradient (the balance of concentration and charge across a membrane), usually from a high concentration to a low concentration, to equilibrate between the two sides of the membrane. In active transport, energy is used to concentrate the compound on one side of the membrane. If energy is applied directly to the transporter (e.g., ATP hydrolysis by Na^+, K^+-ATPase), the transport is called *primary active transport*; if energy is used to establish an ion gradient (e.g., the Na^+ gradient), and the gradient is used to concentrate another compound, the transport is called *secondary active transport*. Protein-mediated transport systems, whether facilitative or active, are classified as *antiports* if they specifically exchange compounds of similar charge across a membrane; they are called *symports* or *cotransporters* if they simultaneously transport two molecules across the membrane in the same direction. Band 3 in the red blood cell membrane, which exchanges chloride ion for bicarbonate, provides an example of an antiport.

The Na^+,K^+-ATPase spans the plasma membrane, much like a gated pore, with a binding site for three Na^+ ions open to the intracellular side (Fig. 10.10). Energy from ATP hydrolysis is used to phosphorylate an internal domain and change the transporters' conformation so that bound Na^+ ions are released to the outside and two external K^+ ions bind. K^+ binding triggers hydrolysis of the bound phosphate group and a return to the original conformation, accompanied by release of K^+ ions inside the cell. As a consequence, cells are able to maintain a much lower intracellular Na^+ concentration and a much higher intracellular K^+ ion concentration than are present in the external fluid.

The Na^+ gradient, which is maintained by primary active transport, is used to power the transport of glucose, amino acids, and many other compounds into the cell through secondary active transport. An example is provided by the transport of glucose into cells of the intestinal epithelium in conjunction with Na^+ ions (Fig. 10.11). These cells create a gradient in Na^+ and then use this gradient to drive the transport of glucose from the intestinal lumen into the cell against its concentration gradient.

The Ca^{2+}-ATPase, a calcium pump, uses a mechanism similar to that of Na^+,K^+-ATPase to maintain intracellular Ca^{2+} concentration below 10^{-7} M in spite of the high extracellular concentration of 10^{-3} M. This transporter is inhibited by binding

 The CFTR was named for its role in cystic fibrosis. Individuals homozygous for mutations in CFTR display cystic fibrosis; heterozygotes for the mutated gene are thought to have protection against cholera. An inactive CFTR leads to an inability to release chloride ions from cells into the extracellular space, with a concomitant reduced diffusion of water into the same space. Thus, a consequence of the CFTR mutation is the dehydration of respiratory and interstitial mucosal linings, leading to a plugging of airways and ducts with a thick mucus. The CFTR is also involved in the dehydration experienced by cholera patients such as **Dennis V.** In intestinal mucosal cells, the cholera A-subunit indirectly promotes phosphorylation of the regulatory domain of CFTR by protein kinase A. Thus, the channel stays open and Cl^- and H_2O flow from the cell into the intestinal lumen, resulting in dehydration.

 The dehydration of cholera is often treated first with an intravenous rehydration solution followed by an oral rehydration solution containing Na^+,K^+, and glucose. or a diet of rice (which contains glucose and amino acids). Glucose is absorbed from the intestinal lumen via the Na^+-dependent glucose cotransporters, which cotransport Na^+ into the cells together with glucose. Many amino acids are also absorbed by Na^+-dependent cotransport. With the return of Na^+ to the cytoplasm, the release of water from the cell into the intestinal lumen decreases.

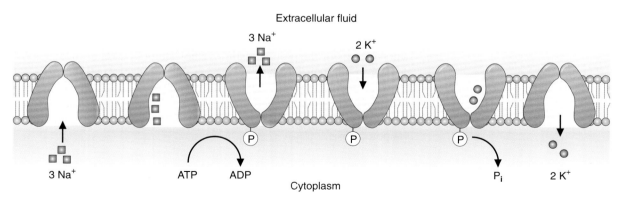

FIGURE 10.10   Active transport by Na^+,K^+-ATPase. Three sodium ions bind to the transporter protein on the cytoplasmic side of the membrane. When adenosine triphosphate (ATP) is hydrolyzed to adenosine diphosphate (ADP), the carrier protein is phosphorylated and undergoes a change in conformation that causes the sodium ions to be released into the extracellular fluid. Two potassium ions then bind on the extracellular side. Dephosphorylation of the carrier protein produces another conformational change, and the potassium ions are released on the inside of the cell membrane. The transporter protein then resumes its original conformation, ready to bind more sodium ions.

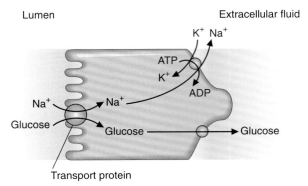

FIGURE 10.11 Secondary active transport of glucose by the Na⁺-glucose cotransporter. One sodium ion binds to the carrier protein in the luminal membrane, stimulating the binding of glucose. After a conformational change, the protein releases Na⁺ and glucose into the cell and returns to its original conformation. Na⁺,K⁺-ATPase in the basolateral membrane pumps Na⁺ against its concentration gradient into the extracellular fluid. Thus, the Na⁺ concentration in the cell is low, and Na⁺ moves from the lumen down its concentration gradient into the cell and is pumped against its gradient into the extracellular fluid. Glucose, consequently, moves against its concentration gradient from the lumen into the cell by traveling on the same carrier as Na⁺. Glucose then passes down its concentration gradient into the extracellular fluid on a passive transporter protein.

of the regulatory protein calmodulin. When the intracellular Ca^{2+} concentration increases, Ca^{2+} binds to calmodulin, which dissociates from the transporter, thereby activating it to pump Ca^{2+} out of the cell (see Fig. 9.12 for the structure of calmodulin). High levels of intracellular Ca^{2+} are associated with irreversible progression from cell injury to cell death.

C. Vesicular Transport across the Plasma Membrane

Vesicular transport occurs when a membrane completely surrounds a compound, particle, or cell and encloses it into a vesicle, which buds from the membrane. When the released vesicle fuses with another membrane system, the entrapped compounds are released. *Endocytosis* refers to vesicular transport into the cell, and *exocytosis* refers to transport out of the cell. Endocytosis is further classified as phagocytosis if the vesicle forms around particulate matter (such as whole bacterial cells or metals and dyes from a tattoo), and pinocytosis if the vesicle forms around fluid containing dispersed molecules. *Receptor-mediated endocytosis* is the name given to the formation of *clathrin-coated vesicles* that mediate the internalization of membrane-bound receptors in vesicles coated on the intracellular side with subunits of the protein clathrin. Cholesterol uptake, as mediated by the low-density lipoprotein receptor, occurs via this mechanism. *Potocytosis* is the name given to endocytosis that occurs via caveolae (small invaginations or "caves"), which are regions of the cell membrane with a unique lipid and protein composition (including the protein caveolin-1). The transport of the vitamin folate occurs via potocytosis.

III. Lysosomes

Lysosomes are the intracellular organelles of digestion and are enclosed by a single membrane that prevents the release of its digestive enzymes into the cytosol. They are central to a wide variety of body functions that involve elimination of unwanted material and recycling their components, including destruction of infectious bacteria and yeast, recovery from injury, tissue remodeling, involution of tissues during development, and normal turnover of cells and organelles.

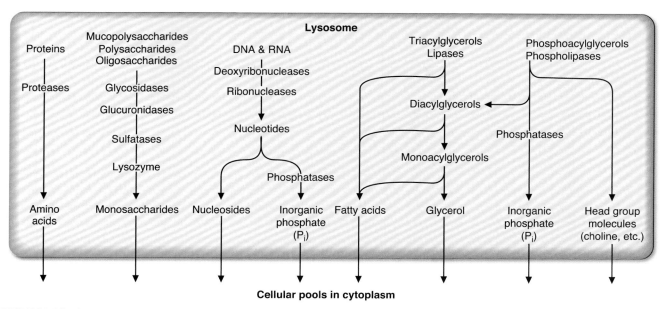

FIGURE 10.12 Lysosomal reactions. Most lysosomal enzymes are hydrolases, which cleave peptide, ester, and glycosidic bonds by adding the components of water across the bond. These enzymes are active at the acidic pH of the lysosome and inactive if accidentally released into the cytosol.

A. Lysosomal Hydrolases

The lysosomal digestive enzymes include *nucleases, phosphatases, glycosidases, esterases,* and *proteases* (Fig. 10.12). These enzymes are all hydrolases, enzymes that cleave amide, ester, and other bonds through the addition of water. Many of the products of lysosomal digestion, such as the amino acids, return to the cytosol. Lysosomes are therefore involved in recycling compounds. The proteases are classified as serine, cysteine, or aspartyl proteases, depending on the amino acid residue at the active site of the enzyme involved in the hydrolytic reaction. The cysteine proteases are also known as *cathepsins*.

Most of these lysosomal hydrolases have their highest activity near a pH of approximately 5.5 (the optimal pH for hydrolysis). The intralysosomal pH is maintained near 5.5 principally by v-ATPases (vesicular ATPases), which actively pump protons into the lysosome. The cytosol and other cellular compartments have a pH nearer 7.2 and are therefore protected from escaped lysosomal hydrolases.

B. Endocytosis, Phagocytosis, and Autophagy

Lysosomes are formed from digestive vesicles called *endosomes*, which are involved in receptor-mediated endocytosis. They also participate in digestion of foreign cells acquired through phagocytosis and the digestion of internal contents in the process of autophagocytosis.

1. Receptor-Mediated Endocytosis

Lysosomes are involved in the digestion of compounds brought into the cells in endocytotic clathrin-coated vesicles formed by the plasma membrane. These vesicles fuse to form multivesicular bodies called *early endosomes*. The early endosomes can either recycle back to the cell surface or mature into late endosomes as they recycle clathrin, lipids, and other membrane components back to the plasma membrane in vesicles called *recycling endosomes*. The late endosomes mature into lysosomes as they progressively accumulate newly synthesized acid hydrolases and vesicular proton pumps brought to them in clathrin-coated vesicles from the Golgi. Thus, lysosomes do not acquire their full digestive power until after sorting of membrane lipids and proteins for recycling.

Genetic defects in lysosomal enzymes, or in proteins such as the mannose 6-phosphate receptors required for targeting the enzymes to the lysosome, lead to an abnormal accumulation of undigested material in lysosomes that may be converted to residual bodies. The accumulation may be so extensive that normal cellular function is compromised, particularly in neuronal cells. Genetic diseases such as *Tay-Sachs* disease (an accumulation of partially digested gangliosides in lysosomes) and *Pompe* disease (an accumulation of glycogen particles in lysosomes) are caused by the absence or deficiency of specific lysosomal enzymes. Such diseases, in which a lysosomal function is compromised, are known as *lysosomal storage diseases*.

The elevated level of uric acid in **Lotta T.'s** blood led to the deposition of monosodium urate crystals in the joint space (synovial fluid) of her right great toe, resulting in podagra (painful great toe). Neutrophils, the mediators of the acute inflammation that followed, attempted to phagocytose the urate crystals. The engulfed urate crystals were deposited in the late endosomes and lysosomes of the neutrophil. Because urate crystals are particles that cannot be degraded by any of the lysosomal acid hydrolases, their accumulation caused lysis of the lysosomal membranes, followed by cell lysis and release of lysosomal enzymes into the joint space. The urate crystals also resulted in release of chemical mediators of inflammation that recruited other cells into the area. This further amplified the acute inflammatory reaction in the tissues of the joint capsule (synovitis), leading to the extremely painful swelling of acute gouty arthritis.

Within the Golgi, enzymes are targeted for endosomes (and eventually lysosomes) by addition of mannose 6-phosphate residues that bind to mannose 6-phosphate receptor proteins in the Golgi membrane. The mannose 6-phosphate receptors together with the associated bound acid hydrolases are incorporated into the clathrin-coated Golgi transport vesicles and the vesicles are released. The transport vesicles lose their clathrin coat and then fuse with the late endosomal membrane. The acidity of the endosome releases the acid hydrolases from the receptors into the vesicle lumen. The receptors are eventually recycled back to the Golgi.

2. Phagocytosis and Autophagy

One of the major roles of lysosomes is phagocytosis. Neutrophils and macrophages, the major phagocytic cells, devour pathogenic microorganisms and clean up wound debris and dead cells, thus aiding in repair. As bacteria or other particles are enclosed into clathrin-coated pits in the plasma membrane, these vesicles bud off to form intracellular phagosomes. The phagosomes fuse with lysosomes, where the acidity and digestive enzymes destroy the contents. Pinocytotic vesicles also may fuse with lysosomes.

In *autophagy* (self-eating), intracellular components such as organelles or glycogen particles are surrounded by a membrane derived from endoplasmic reticulum (ER) vesicles, forming an autophagosome. The autophagosome fuses with a lysosome, and lysosomal enzymes digest the contents of the phagolysosome. Organelles usually turn over much more rapidly than the cells in which they reside (e.g., approximately four mitochondria in each liver cell are degraded per hour). Cells that are damaged, but still viable, recover in part by using autophagy to eliminate damaged components.

If a significant amount of undigestible material remains within the lysosome after the digestion process is completed, the lysosome is called a *residual body*. Depending on the cell type, residual bodies may be expelled (exocytosis) or remain indefinitely in the cell as lipofuscin granules that accumulate with age.

IV. Mitochondria

Mitochondria contain most of the enzymes for the pathways of fuel oxidation and oxidative phosphorylation and thus generate most of the ATP required by mammalian cells. Each mitochondrion is surrounded by two membranes, an *outer membrane* and a highly impermeable *inner membrane*, separating the mitochondrial *matrix* from the cytosol (Fig. 10.13). The inner membrane forms invaginations known as *cristae* containing the electron-transport chain and ATP synthase. Most of the enzymes for the Krebs TCA cycle and other pathways for oxidation are located in the mitochondrial matrix, the compartment enclosed by the inner mitochondrial membrane. (The TCA cycle and the electron-transport chain are described in more detail in Chapters 23 and 24.)

The inner mitochondrial membrane is highly impermeable, and the proton gradient that is built up across this membrane during oxidative phosphorylation is essential for ATP generation from adenosine diphosphate (ADP) and phosphate. The transport of ions and other small molecules across the inner mitochondrial membrane occurs principally through facilitative transporters in a type of secondary active transport powered by the proton gradient established by the electron transport chain. The outer membrane contains pores made from proteins called *porins* and is permeable to molecules with a molecular weight up to about 1,000 Da.

Mitochondria can replicate by division; however, most of their proteins must be imported from the cytosol. Mitochondria contain a small amount of DNA, which encodes for only 13 different subunits of proteins involved in oxidative phosphorylation. Most of the enzymes and proteins in mitochondria are encoded by nuclear DNA and synthesized on cytoplasmic ribosomes. They are imported through membrane pores by a receptor-mediated process involving members of

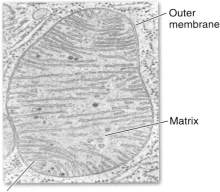

Inner membrane
folded into cristae

Outer
membrane

Matrix

|— 1 μm —|

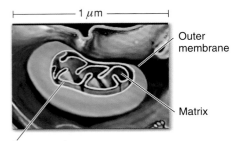

Inner membrane
folded into cristae

Outer
membrane

Matrix

FIGURE 10.13 Mitochondrion. Electron micrograph (**top**); three-dimensional drawing (**bottom**).

the heat-shock family of proteins (proteins whose synthesis is induced by an elevation of temperature or other indicators of stress). Mutations in mitochondrial DNA result in several genetic diseases that affect skeletal muscle, neuronal tissue, and renal tissue (known as *mitochondrial disorders*). Mitochondrial inheritance is maternal because the sperm do not contribute mitochondria to the fertilized egg. Spontaneous mutations within mitochondrial DNA have been implicated with the mechanism of aging.

V. Peroxisomes

Peroxisomes are cytoplasmic organelles, similar in size to lysosomes, that are involved in *oxidative reactions* using *molecular oxygen*. These reactions produce the toxic chemical *hydrogen peroxide* (H_2O_2), which is subsequently used or degraded within the peroxisome by catalase and other enzymes. Peroxisomes function in the oxidation of very-long-chain fatty acids (containing 20 or more carbons) to shorter-chain fatty acids, the conversion of cholesterol to bile acids, and the synthesis of *ether lipids* called *plasmalogens*. They are bounded by a single membrane.

Like mitochondria, peroxisomes can replicate by division. However, they are dependent on the import of proteins to function. They contain no DNA.

VI. Nucleus

The largest of the subcellular organelles of animal cells is the *nucleus* (Fig. 10.14). Most of the genetic material of the cell is located in the chromosomes of the nucleus, which are composed of DNA, an equal weight of small, positively charged proteins called *histones*, and a variable amount of other proteins. This nucleoprotein complex is called *chromatin*. The *nucleolus*, a substructure of the nucleus, is the site of *ribosomal RNA* (rRNA) transcription and processing and of *ribosome assembly*. Ribosomes are required for the synthesis of proteins. Replication, transcription, translation, and the regulation of these processes are the major focus of the molecular biology section of this text (see Section III).

The nucleus is separated from the rest of the cell (the cytoplasm) by the nuclear envelope, which consists of two membranes joined at *nuclear pores*. The outer nuclear membrane is continuous with the rough ER (RER). Transport through the pores is bidirectional, as illustrated by the following example. To convert the genetic code of the DNA into the primary sequence of a protein, DNA is transcribed into RNA, which is modified and edited into messenger RNA (mRNA). The mRNA travels through the nuclear pores into the cytoplasm, where it is translated into the primary sequence of a protein on ribosomes. Ribosomes, which are generated in the nucleolus, also must travel through nuclear pores to the cytoplasm. Conversely, proteins required for replication, transcription, and other processes enter into the nucleus through these pores. These proteins contain a specific sequence of amino acids known as a *nuclear localization signal*. Thus, the direction of transport through the pore is specific for the molecule or complex being transported across the membrane.

VII. Endoplasmic Reticulum

The ER is a network of membranous tubules within the cell consisting of *smooth endoplasmic reticulum* (SER), which lacks ribosomes, and RER, which is studded with ribosomes (Fig. 10.15). The SER has several functions. It contains enzymes for the synthesis of many lipids, such as triacylglycerols and phospholipids. It also contains the *cytochrome P450 oxidative enzymes* involved in metabolism of drugs and toxic chemicals like ethanol and the synthesis of hydrophobic molecules like steroid hormones. Glycogen is stored in regions of liver cells that are rich in SER.

 Pyruvate transfer across the inner mitochondrial membrane is dependent on the proton gradient, and the carrier for pyruvate transports both pyruvate and a proton into the matrix of the mitochondria. Such transport allows for the accumulation of pyruvate within the organelle at concentrations greater than in the cytosol. This is an example of which type of transport?

Several diseases are associated with peroxisomes. Peroxisomal diseases are caused by mutations that affect either the synthesis of functional peroxisomal enzymes or their incorporation into peroxisomes. For example, adrenoleukodystrophy involves a mutation that decreases the content of a fatty acid transporter in the peroxisomal membrane. Zellweger syndrome is caused by the failure to complete the synthesis of peroxisomes.

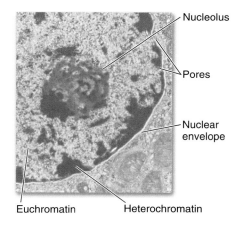

Nucleolus

Pores

Nuclear envelope

Euchromatin   Heterochromatin

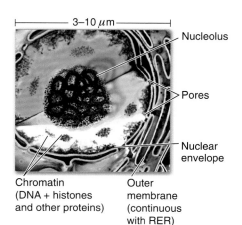

3–10 μm

Nucleolus

Pores

Nuclear envelope

Chromatin (DNA + histones and other proteins)   Outer membrane (continuous with RER)

FIGURE 10.14 Nucleus. Electron micrograph **(top)**; three-dimensional drawing **(bottom)**. *RER*, rough endoplasmic reticulum.

Cotransport of pyruvate and a proton, down the proton's electrochemical gradient, is an example of secondary active transport. Energy has been expended, during the transfer of electrons through the electron transfer chain, to generate the proton gradient across the inner mitochondrial membrane. The energy of the proton gradient is then used by the carrier to carry protons down their electrochemical gradient (favorable), bringing pyruvate along with the protons. This will allow pyruvate active transport, secondary to favorable proton entry into the mitochondrial matrix.

Chronic ingestion of ethanol has increased the content of MEOS, the microsomal ethanol oxidizing system, in **Al M.'s** liver. MEOS is a cytochrome P450 enzyme that catalyzes the conversion of ethanol, NADPH, and O_2 to acetaldehyde, $NADP^+$, and 2 H_2O (see Chapter 9). The adjective *microsomal* is a term derived from experimental cell biology that is sometimes used for processes that occur in the ER. When cells are lysed in the laboratory, the ER is fragmented into vesicles called *microsomes*, which can be isolated by centrifugation. Microsomes, as such, are not actually present in cells.

The monomeric G-protein Arf (a member of the Ras superfamily of regulatory proteins; see Section III.C.2 in Chapter 9) was named for its contribution to the pathogenesis of cholera and not for its normal function in the assembly of intracellular vesicles. In the case of cholera, it is required for the transport of *V. cholerae* A toxin subunit into the cell. The cholera toxin is endocytosed in caveolae vesicles that subsequently merge with lysosomes (or are transformed into lysosomes), where the acidic pH contributes to activation of the toxin. As the toxin is transported through the Golgi and ER, it is further processed and activated. Arf forms a complex with the A-subunit that promotes its travel between compartments. The A-subunit is actually an ADP-ribosylase (an enzyme that cleaves NAD and attaches the ADP portion to a protein) (see Chapter 6, Fig. 6.13), and hence, Arf became known as the *ADP-ribosylating factor*. The ADP-ribosylation of proteins regulating the CFTR chloride channel led to **Dennis V.'s** dehydration and diarrhea.

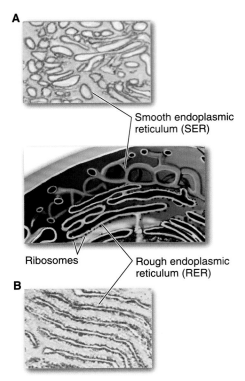

FIGURE 10.15 **A.** Smooth endoplasmic reticulum. **B.** Rough endoplasmic reticulum. **A** and **B** are electron micrographs. A three-dimensional drawing is in the **middle**.

The RER is involved in the synthesis of certain proteins. Ribosomes attached to the membranes of the RER give them their "rough" appearance. Proteins produced on these ribosomes enter the lumen of the RER, travel to another membrane system (the *Golgi complex*) in vesicles, and are subsequently either secreted from the cell, sequestered within membrane-enclosed organelles such as lysosomes, or embedded in the plasma membrane. *Posttranslational modifications* of these proteins, such as the initiation of *N*-linked glycosylation, the addition of lipid-based anchors, and disulfide formation, occur in the RER. In contrast, proteins encoded by the nucleus and found in the cytoplasm, peroxisomes, or mitochondria are synthesized on free ribosomes in the cytosol and are seldom modified by the attachment of oligosaccharides.

VIII. Golgi Complex

The *Golgi complex* is involved in modifying proteins produced in the RER and in *sorting and distributing* these proteins to the lysosomes, secretory vesicles, or the plasma membrane. It consists of a curved stack of flattened vesicles in the cytoplasm that is generally divided into three compartments: the *cis* Golgi network, which is often convex and faces the nucleus; the *medial* Golgi stacks; and the *trans* Golgi network, which often faces the plasma membrane. Vesicles transport material to and from the Golgi. The Golgi complex also participates in posttranslational modification of proteins, such as complex branched-chain oligosaccharide addition, sulfation, and phosphorylation.

IX. Cytoskeleton

The structure of the cell, the shape of the cell surface, and the arrangement of subcellular organelles are organized by three major protein components: *microtubules* composed of *tubulin*, which move and position organelles and vesicles; *thin filaments* composed of *actin*, which form a cytoskeleton; and *intermediate filaments* (IF) composed of different fibrous proteins. Actin and tubulin, which are also involved in cell movement, are dynamic structures composed of continuously associating and dissociating globular subunits. IFs, which play a structural role, are composed of stable fibrous proteins that turn over more slowly than do the components of microtubules and thin filaments.

A. Microtubules

Microtubules, cylindrical tubes composed of tubulin subunits, are present in all nucleated cells and the platelets in blood (Fig. 10.16). They are responsible for the positioning of organelles in the cell cytoplasm and the movement of vesicles, including phagocytic vesicles, exocytotic vesicles, and the transport vesicles between the ER, Golgi, and endosomes. They also form the spindle apparatus for cell division. The microtubule network (the minus end) begins in the nucleus at the centriole and extends outward to the plasma membrane (usually the plus end). Microtubule-associated proteins (MAPs) attach microtubules to other cellular components and can determine cell shape and polarity.

Motor proteins called *kinesins* and *cytoplasmic dyneins* use ATP energy to move cargo along the microtubules. Kinesins move molecules, vesicles, and organelles toward the plus end of the microtubule, usually toward the plasma membrane. Cytoplasmic dyneins are huge proteins that move vesicles and organelles to the minus end, generally toward the nucleus. They are also involved in the positioning of the Golgi complex and the movement of chromosomes during mitosis.

Microtubules consist of polymerized arrays of α- and β-tubulin dimers that form 13 protofilaments organized around a hollow core (see Fig. 10.16). Three different tubulin polypeptides (α, β, and γ) of similar amino acid composition are encoded by related genes; α- and β-dimers polymerize to form most microtubules, and γ-tubulin is found only in the centrosomes and spindle pole bodies. Two other forms of tubulin, δ and ε, have been found in centrioles. Tubulin dimers composed of one α-subunit and one β-subunit bind guanosine triphosphate (GTP), which creates a conformational change in the dimer that favors addition of dimers to the tubulin polymer. The dimers can add to and dissociate from both ends of the tubulin, but the end to which they add more rapidly (the plus end) has a net rate of growth, and the end to which they add more slowly (the minus end) has a net rate of loss. As GTP is hydrolyzed to guanosine diphosphate (GDP), the binding of tubulin subunits is weakened, resulting in their dissociation (dynamic instability). Thus, the net rate and direction of growth are dictated by the fastest growing end of the microtubule.

B. Actin Filaments

Actin filaments form a critical network that controls the shape of the cell and movement of the cell surface, thereby allowing cells to move, divide, engulf particles, and contract. Actin is present in all living cells. The actin polymer, called *F-actin*, is composed of a helical arrangement of globular G-actin subunits (Fig. 10.17). Within the polymer, each G-actin subunit contains a bound ATP or ADP that holds the actin fold into a closed conformation (see Chapter 7). The actin polymer is dynamic. New subunits of G-actin containing ATP continuously combine with the assembled F-actin polymer at the plus end. As F-actin elongates, bound ATP is hydrolyzed to ADP, so that most of the polymer contains G-actin–ADP subunits. The conformation of ADP-actin favors dissociation from the minus end of the polymer; thus, the polymer is capable of lengthening from the plus end. This directional growth can account for certain types of cell movement and shape changes: the formation of pseudopodia that surround other cells during phagocytosis, the migration of cells in the developing embryo, or the movement of white blood cells through tissues.

 Lotta T. was given colchicine, a drug that is frequently used to treat gout in its initial stages. One of colchicine's actions is to prevent phagocytic activity by binding to dimers of the α- and β-subunits of tubulin. When the tubulin dimer–colchicine complexes bind to microtubules, further polymerization of the microtubules is inhibited, depolymerization predominates, and the microtubules disassemble. Microtubules are necessary for vesicular movement of urate crystals during phagocytosis and release of mediators that activate the inflammatory response. Thus, colchicine diminishes the inflammatory response, swelling, and pain caused by formation of urate crystals.

 Colchicine, an initial drug used to treat **Lotta T.**, has a narrow therapeutic index (i.e., the amount of drug that produces the desirable therapeutic effect is not much lower than the amount that produces an adverse effect). Its therapeutic effect depends on inhibiting tubulin synthesis in neutrophils, but it can also prevent tubulin synthesis (and, thus, cell division and other cellular processes) in other cells. Fortunately, neutrophils concentrate colchicine, so they are affected at lower concentrations of colchicine than other cell types. Neutrophils lack the transport protein P-glycoprotein, a member of the ABC cassette family (which includes the CFTR channel). In most other cell types, P-glycoprotein exports chemicals such as colchicine, thus preventing their accumulation.

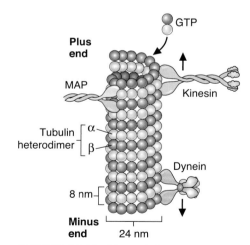

FIGURE 10.16 Microtubules composed of αβ-tubulin heterodimers. These proteins project outward to attach the microtubules to other cellular components. The microtubule grows by the addition of αβ-dimers containing bound guanosine triphosphate (GTP) to the plus end of the polymer. Kinesin and dyneins are motor proteins that transport cargo (e.g., vesicles) along the microtubule. *MAP*, microtubule-associated protein.

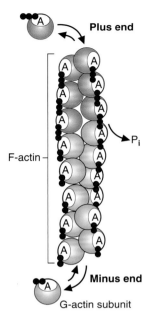

FIGURE 10.17 Actin filaments. The polymer F-actin is assembled from G-actin subunits containing bound adenosine triphosphate (ATP). While bound, the ATP is slowly hydrolyzed to adenosine diphosphate (ADP). The conformational change shifts the equilibrium so that dissociation of the G-actin subunits is favorable at the minus end of the polymer. Once they are dissociated, the actin subunits exchange ADP for ATP, which may again associate with the actin polymer. At the plus end of the molecule, association is favored over dissociation. P_i, inorganic phosphate.

Actin polymers form the thin filaments (also called *microfilaments*) in the cell that are organized into compact ordered bundles or loose network arrays by cross-linking proteins. Short actin filaments bind to the cross-linking protein spectrin to form the cortical actin skeleton network (see Fig. 10.5). In muscle cells, long actin filaments combine with thick filaments, composed of the protein myosin, to produce muscle contraction. The assembly of G-actin subunits into polymers, bundling of fibers, and attachments of actin to spectrin and to the plasma membrane proteins and organelles are mediated by several actin-binding proteins and G-proteins from the Rho family.

C. Intermediate Filaments

IFs are composed of fibrous protein polymers that provide structural support to membranes of the cells and scaffolding for attachment of other cellular components. Each IF subunit is composed of a long rodlike α-helical core containing globular spacing domains, and globular *N*- and *C*-terminal domains. The α-helical segments of two subunits coil around each other to form a coiled coil and then combine with another dimer coil to form a tetramer. Depending on the type of filament, the dimers may be either hetero- or homodimers. The tetramers join end to end to form protofilaments, and approximately eight protofilaments combine to form filaments (Fig. 10.18). Filament assembly is partially controlled through phosphorylation.

In contrast to actin thin filaments, the 50 or so different types of IFs are each composed of a different protein having the same general structure described previously. Some of the IFs, such as the nuclear lamins, are common to all cell types. These filaments provide a latticelike support network attached to the inner nuclear membrane. Other IFs are specific for types of cells (e.g., epithelial cells have cytokeratins, and neurons have neurofilaments). These provide an internal network that helps to support the shape and resilience of the cell.

CLINICAL COMMENTS

Al M. Al M. has been drinking for 5 years and has begun to exhibit mental and systemic effects of chronic alcohol consumption. In his brain, ethanol has altered the fluidity of neuronal lipids, causing changes in their response to neurotransmitters released from exocytotic vesicles. In his liver, increased levels of the MEOS (cytochrome P450-2E1) located in the SER have increased his rate of ethanol oxidation to acetaldehyde, a compound that is toxic to the cells. His liver also continues to oxidize ethanol to acetaldehyde through a cytosolic enzyme, liver alcohol dehydrogenase.

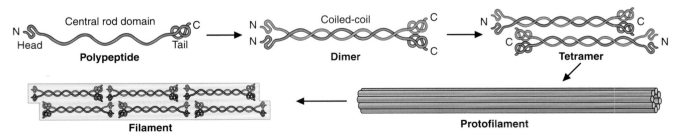

FIGURE 10.18 Formation of a cytokeratin filament. The central rod of the keratin monomer is principally an α-helical structure. A specific acidic keratin monomer combines with a specific basic keratin monomer to form a heterodimer coil (a coiled-coil structure). Two dimers combine in antiparallel fashion to form a tetramer, and the tetramers combine head to tail to form protofilaments. Approximately eight protofilaments combine to form a filament. The filament is thicker than actin filaments (called *thin filaments* or *microfilaments*) and thinner than microtubules (thick tubes) and is therefore called an *intermediate filament*.

One of the toxic effects of acetaldehyde is inhibition of tubulin polymerization. Tubulin is used in the liver for secretion of very low-density lipoprotein particles containing newly synthesized triacylglycerols. As a result, these triacylglycerols accumulate in the liver, and he has begun to develop a fatty liver. Acetaldehyde may also damage protein components of the inner mitochondrial membrane and affect its ability to pump protons to the cytosol.

Lotta T. Lotta T. had a rapid and gratifying clinical response to the hourly administration of colchicine. This drug diminishes phagocytosis and the subsequent release of the lysosomal enzymes that initiate the inflammatory response in synovial tissue.

The inflammatory response that causes the symptoms of an acute attack of gout begins when neutrophils and macrophages ingest urate crystals. In neutrophils, urate activates the conversion of the polyunsaturated fatty acid arachidonic acid (present in membrane phospholipids) to leukotriene B_4. The release of this messenger contributes to the pain. Colchicine, through its effect on tubulin, inhibits phagocytosis, leukotriene B_4 release, and recruitment and cell division of additional cells involved in inflammation. Colchicine also inhibits the tubulin-dependent release of histamine from mast cells. As a result, there was a rapid improvement in the pain and swelling in Lotta's great toe.

After the gout attack subsided, Ms. T. was placed on daily allopurinol, a drug that inhibits urate production (see Chapter 8). During the next 6 months of allopurinol therapy, Ms. T.'s blood urate levels decreased. She did not have another gout attack during this time.

Dennis V. Dennis V. was diagnosed with cholera. He was placed on intravenous rehydration therapy, followed by oral rehydration therapy with high glucose- and Na^+-containing fluids (to be continued in Chapter 11).

V. cholerae secrete a toxin consisting of one A- and multiple B-subunits. The B-subunits allowing binding to the intestinal epithelia, and the A-subunit is processed and transported into the cell, where it associates with the monomeric G-protein Arf (ADP-ribosylation factor). The cholera toxin A-subunit ADP-ribosylates the Gα-subunit of the heterotrimeric G-protein $G\alpha_s$ (a process discussed in Chapter 11). The net result is activation of protein kinase A, which then phosphorylates the CFTR chloride channel so that it remains permanently open. The subsequent efflux of chloride, sodium, and water into the bowel lumen is responsible for **Dennis V.'s** diarrhea and subsequent dehydration.

BIOCHEMICAL COMMENTS

Differences between Bacterial and Human Cells. Different species of bacteria have some common structural features that distinguish them from animal cells. They are single-cell organisms that are classified as prokaryotes ("before nucleus"). Their genetic material (DNA) is concentrated in the central region of the cell, called a *nucleoid* rather than a nucleus, because it is not separated from the rest of the cellular contents by a membrane. Likewise, bacteria contain no cytoplasmic organelles defined by membranes. They do have a plasma membrane that encloses the cytoplasm. External to the plasma membrane is a peptidoglycan cell wall composed of extensively cross-linked polysaccharides that form a protective shield on the surface of the cell.

Bacterial cells obtain nutrients from the medium on which they grow. Many of their metabolic pathways for fuel oxidation are similar to those in eukaryotes and generate nicotinamide adenine dinucleotide (NADH) and ATP; however, individual steps in these pathways may use different coenzymes or very different enzymes for catalysis than do human cells. Like human cells, bacteria use intermediates of glycolysis and other basic degradative pathways to serve as precursors for biosynthetic pathways, and energy acquired from catabolic pathways is used in anabolic pathways. Aerobic bacteria, such as *Escherichia coli*, contain enzymes of the TCA cycle and the components of the electron-transport chain, which are located in the cell membrane. However, many bacteria are anaerobes and can function in the absence of oxygen.

Many of the metabolic differences between human cells and bacteria are related to their interactions with their environment. Some bacteria, such as *E. coli*, can adapt to adverse or changing conditions (high vs. low O_2 tension, or a single supply of nutrients from which to synthesize all required components) by dramatic shifts in the genes that are transcribed. Other bacteria find a unique environmental niche where they do not have to compete with other bacteria for nutrients (e.g., *Lactobacilli* in yogurt are adapted to an acidic pH). In contrast, the human cells are adapted to interacting with blood and interstitial fluid, which provides a well-controlled pH, a constant nutrient supply, and a medium for communication between very distant cells. As a consequence of their constant environment, adult human cells seldom need to adapt (or can adapt) to widely fluctuating conditions through large variations in the genes transcribed. As a consequence of being organized into a multicellular organism, human cell types have been able to specialize in function, structure, and enzyme content.

KEY CONCEPTS

- The cell is the basic unit of living organisms.
- Unique features of each cell type define tissue specificity and function.
- Despite the variety of cell types, there are many common features that all cells share, such as the presence of a plasma membrane.
  - The plasma membrane is composed primarily of lipids and proteins (both integral and peripheral).
  - Specific transport proteins are required to allow compounds to cross membranes, either by facilitative diffusion, gated channels, or active transport.
  - Eukaryotes contain intracellular organelles, whereas prokaryotic cells do not.
- In eukaryotes, the intracellular organelles consist of lysosomes, the nucleus, ribosomes, the ER, the Golgi apparatus, mitochondria, peroxisomes, and the cytoplasm. Each organelle contributes a different function to the cell. Some cells may lack one or more of these internal organelles.
  - Lysosomes are the intracellular organelles of digestion.
  - The nucleus contains the genetic material of the cell and is the site of RNA synthesis.
  - Ribosomes are intracellular organelles on which protein synthesis occurs.
  - The ER contains enzymes for the synthesis of many lipids, for drug and toxic chemical metabolism, and for posttranslational modification of proteins.
  - The Golgi complex modifies proteins produced in the ER and sorts and distributes them to other organelles.
  - The mitochondria are the cells' power plants, synthesizing ATP.
  - The peroxisomes sequester various oxidative reactions that have the potential to generate dangerous radical species.
  - The cytoskeleton aids in defining the structure of the cell, the shape of the cell surface, and the arrangement of subcellular organelles within the cytoplasm.
- The diseases discussed in this chapter are summarized in Table 10.1.

TABLE 10.1 Diseases Discussed in Chapter 10		
DISORDER OR CONDITION	**GENETIC OR ENVIRONMENTAL**	**COMMENTS**
Cholera	Environmental	Watery diarrhea leading to dehydration and hypovolemic shock caused by cholera toxin ADP-ribosylating a class of G-proteins, altering their function and affecting water and salt transport across the intestinal mucosa. Treat with a glucose electrolyte solution to increase coupled glucose–sodium uptake into the intestinal epithelial cells, reversing the loss of water from these cells.
Gout	Both	Treat by inhibiting xanthine oxidase, thereby reducing the production of uric acid, using the analog allopurinol. Before allopurinol, the patient is treated with colchicine, which blocks microtubule formation and the migration of neutrophils to the affected area.
Gas gangrene	Environmental	Bacterial infection that secretes a toxin which is a phospholipase, leading to cell membrane destruction. This leads to capillary destruction and impaired blood flow to the affected area.
Alcoholism	Both	Ethanol poisoning caused by increased production of acetaldehyde resulting from the combined actions of alcohol dehydrogenase and the induction of the microsomal ethanol oxidizing system (MEOS). MEOS is induced because of the high levels of ethanol in the patient's diet.

REVIEW QUESTIONS—CHAPTER 10

1. Bacteria contain a cell wall and a plasma membrane. Antibiotics targeting the cell wall do not affect human cells because the human cells do not express a cell wall. However, antibiotics cannot target plasma membranes because both bacteria and humans express such membranes. Which one of the following is a characteristic of the eukaryotic plasma membrane?
   A. It is composed principally of triacylglycerols and cholesterol.
   B. It contains principally nonpolar lipids.
   C. It contains phospholipids with their acyl groups extending into the cytosol.
   D. It contains more phosphatidylserine in the inner than the outer leaflet.
   E. It contains oligosaccharides sandwiched between the inner and outer leaflets.

2. A marathon runner releases epinephrine before a race, which binds to a receptor with seven transmembrane domains. Such transmembrane proteins can be best described by which one of the following?
   A. They can usually be dissociated from membranes without disrupting the lipid bilayer.
   B. They are classified as peripheral membrane proteins.
   C. They contain hydrophobic amino acid residues at their carboxyl terminus.
   D. They contain hydrophilic amino acid residues extending into the lipid bilayer.
   E. They contain membrane-spanning regions that are α-helices.

3. A patient had a sudden heart attack caused by inadequate blood flow through the vessels of the heart. As a consequence, there was an inadequate supply of oxygen to generate ATP in his cardiomyocytes. The compartment of the cardiomyocyte most directly involved in ATP generation is which one of the following?
   A. Mitochondrion
   B. Peroxisome
   C. Lysosome
   D. Nucleus
   E. Golgi

4. One manner in which type 2 diabetes occurs is via a reduction in the release of insulin from the pancreas. The release of insulin from the β-cells of the pancreas requires Ca^{2+} influx through a channel that is activated by a change in the membrane potential across the plasma membrane. The movement of calcium across

the membrane is an example of which one of the following?

A. Voltage-gated channel
B. Passive diffusion
C. Active transport
D. Ligand-gated channel
E. Phosphorylation-gated channel

5. Lysosomes function to help fight infection and to degrade unwanted metabolites in the cell. ATP is required for the appropriate functioning of the lysosome because of which one of the following?

A. Maintaining an acidic environment in the lysosome
B. Maintaining a basic environment in the lysosome
C. Regulation of enzyme activity
D. Activation of lysosomal zymogens
E. As a cofactor for lysosomal hydrolases

6. Mature red blood cells are different from most other cells in the human body in that they do not contain a nucleus and must use anaerobic metabolism instead of aerobic metabolism. Anaerobic metabolism is required for these cells because of which one of the following?

A. Oxygen cannot enter red blood cells.
B. The red blood cells lack a plasma membrane.
C. The red blood cells lack mitochondria.
D. The red blood cells lack enzymes for glucose metabolism.
E. Oxygen cannot bind to any proteins in the red blood cell.

7. Normal or physiologic serum sodium (Na^+) levels are around 140 mEq/L, whereas potassium (K^+) levels are 3.5 to 5.0 mEq/L. Intracellular concentrations are reversed with a high K^+ level and much lower Na^+ level. This ion imbalance is accomplished by the Na^+,K^+-ATPase, which is a protein that can be best described by which one of the following?

A. It catalyzes simple diffusion.
B. It catalyzes primary active transport.
C. It exchanges two Na^+ ions for three K^+ ions.
D. It catalyzes the transport of glucose down its concentration gradient.
E. It catalyzes the efflux of urea from the cell.

8. A sweat chloride test is ordered on a patient with suspected cystic fibrosis. The defective protein in this patient, if the sweat test is positive, is best described by which one of the following?

A. It is a chloride channel that uses energy for diffusion.
B. It is a voltage-gated chloride channel.
C. It is a ligand-gated chloride channel.
D. It is an active transport system for sodium.
E. It is a passive diffusion system for sodium that does not require energy.

9. An inherited mutation in the dystrophin gene is responsible for Duchenne muscular dystrophy. Which one of the following statements accurately describes a property of dystrophin?

A. It is a spectrin-like lipid.
B. It is part of the inner membrane or cortical skeleton.
C. It is a spectrin-like carbohydrate.
D. It is a transmembrane protein.
E. It functions as a hormone or neurotransmitter finder.

10. A patient has peripheral vascular disease, an atherosclerotic narrowing of arteries and arterioles. One type of medication to treat this condition alters the fluidity of the red blood cell so it can "bend" past these obstructions and deliver oxygen to the tissues past the obstruction. Theoretically, which one of the following diets would work in the same manner?

A. High in saturated fats
B. Low in saturated fats
C. High in unsaturated fats
D. Low in unsaturated fats
E. Diet devoid of all fats

ANSWERS

1. **The answer is D.** Phosphatidylserine, the only lipid with a net negative charge at neutral pH, is located in the inner leaflet, where it contributes to the more negatively charged intracellular side of the membrane. The expression of phosphatidylserine in the outer leaflet of the plasma membrane is often associated with aging. The membrane is composed principally of phospholipids and cholesterol (thus, A is incorrect). Phospholipids are amphipathic (contain polar and nonpolar ends; see Chapter 5), with their polar head groups extending into the aqueous medium inside and outside of the cell. The fatty acyl groups of the two layers face each other on the inside of the bilayer, and the polar oligosaccharide groups of glycoproteins and glycolipids extend into the aqueous medium (thus, B, C, and E are incorrect).

2. **The answer is E.** The transmembrane regions are α-helices with hydrophobic amino acid side chains binding to membrane lipids. The hydrophobic interactions hinder their extraction (thus, A and D are incorrect). Because they are not easily extracted, they are classified as integral proteins (thus, B is incorrect). The carboxyl and amino terminals of transmembrane proteins extend into the aqueous intra- and extracellular medium and thus need to contain many hydrophilic residues (thus, C is incorrect).

3. **The answer is A.** Most of fuel oxidation and ATP generation occurs in the mitochondrion. Although some may also occur in the cytosol, the amount produced in the cytoplasm is much smaller than in the mitochondria in most cells.

4. **The answer is A.** Channels which open in response to a change in ion concentration across the membrane (which results in a change in membrane potential, or voltage, across the membrane) are known as *voltage-gated channels*. The calcium influx is not passive diffusion because a carrier is required (the channel). This is not an active transport process because calcium is flowing down its concentration gradient and the cell is not concentrating calcium within it. A ligand-gated channel opens when a particular ligand binds to it, not when the membrane potential changes. There is no phosphorylation event required in the opening of this calcium channel, so it is not an example of a phosphorylation-gated channel.

5. **The answer is A.** ATP is required by the vesicular ATPase, which uses the energy of ATP hydrolysis to concentrate protons within the lysosome, which generates the acidic environment required for enzyme activity. Answer B is, therefore, incorrect because lysosomes are acidic compared to the cytoplasm, not basic. ATP is not required to either activate or regulate, or act as a cofactor for, any lysosomal hydrolase.

6. **The answer is C.** Oxygen enters red blood cells via diffusion across its plasma membrane and binds to hemoglobin within the cell. Aerobic metabolism requires the presence of mitochondria, which are lacking in red blood cells. The red blood cell metabolizes glucose for energy, so the enzymes for glucose metabolism are present in the cell.

7. **The answer is B.** Energy is needed to create the ion imbalance across the membrane, so the protein does not catalyze simple diffusion. The Na^+,K^+-ATPase catalyzes the hydrolysis of ATP to create the ion gradient by exchanging three sodium ions (from the cytoplasm) for two potassium ions (from outside the cell). This results in the export of sodium, and uptake of potassium, in an electrogenic manner (charge imbalance across the membrane). This is an example of primary active transport. The Na^+ gradient then powers the transport of glucose into the cell against its concentration gradient (an example of secondary active transport). Urea leaving liver cells is not powered by a sodium gradient.

8. **The answer is C.** The CFTR is an example of a ligand-gated channel regulated through phosphorylation-gated channels. The CFTR allows chloride ions to cross the membrane but not sodium ions. It is considered simple diffusion even though ATP is involved. Energy is not required in simple diffusion as it is in an active transport system.

9. **The answer is B.** Dystrophin is a spectrin-like protein (not lipid) that is present in skeletal muscle cells. It binds with actin to form the inner membrane skeleton or the cortical skeleton. It is a peripheral membrane protein, not a transmembrane protein, and therefore does not bind hormones or neurotransmitters.

10. **The answer is C.** Unsaturated fatty acid chains form a pocket for cholesterol binding which prevents the hydrophobic chains from packing too closely together thereby maintaining fluidity of the membrane and allowing the red blood cells to "deform" through small spaces. The fluidity of the plasma membrane is also partially determined by the unsaturated fatty acid content of the diet, so a diet high in unsaturated fat would theoretically act like the medication. Saturated fats do not bind to cholesterol in this manner and also tend to decrease the fluidity of the membrane.

11 Cell Signaling by Chemical Messengers

Within a complex organism such as the human, the different organs, tissues, and cell types have developed specialized functions. Yet each cell must contribute in an integrated way as the body grows, differentiates, and adapts to changing conditions. Such integration requires communication that is carried out by chemical messengers traveling from one cell to another by direct contact of cells with the extracellular matrix or by direct contact of one cell with another. The eventual goal of such signals is to change actions carried out in target cells by intracellular proteins (metabolic enzymes, gene regulatory proteins, ion channels, or cytoskeletal proteins). In this chapter, we present a basic overview of signaling by chemical messengers.

Chemical Messengers. Chemical messengers (also called signaling molecules) transmit messages between cells. They are **secreted** from one cell in **response to a specific stimulus** and **travel to a target cell**, where they **bind to a specific receptor** and **elicit a response** (Fig. 11.1). In the nervous system, these chemical messengers are called **neurotransmitters**; in the **endocrine system**, they are **hormones**; and in **the immune system**, they are called **cytokines**. Additional chemical messengers include **retinoids**, **eicosanoids**, and **growth factors**. Depending on the distance between the secreting and target cells, chemical messengers can be classified as **endocrine** (travel in the blood), **paracrine** (travel between nearby cells), or **autocrine** (act on the same cell that produces the message).

Receptors and Signal Transduction. Receptors are proteins that contain a binding site specific for a single chemical messenger and another binding site involved in transmitting the message (see Fig. 11.1). The second binding site may interact with another protein or with DNA. They may be either **plasma membrane receptors** (which span the plasma membrane and contain an extracellular binding domain for the messenger) or **intracellular binding proteins** (for messengers able to diffuse into the cell) (see Fig. 11.1). Most plasma membrane receptors fall into the categories of **ion-channel receptors**, **tyrosine kinase receptors**, **tyrosine kinase–associated receptors**, **serine–threonine kinase receptors**, or **heptahelical receptors** (proteins with seven α-helices spanning the membrane). When a chemical messenger binds to a receptor, the signal it is carrying must be converted into an intracellular response. This conversion is called **signal transduction**.

Signal Transduction for Intracellular Receptors. Most intracellular receptors are **gene-specific transcription factors**, proteins that bind to DNA and regulate the transcription of certain genes. (Gene transcription is the process of copying the genetic code from DNA to RNA and is discussed further in Chapter 15.)

Signal Transduction for Plasma Membrane Receptors. Mechanisms of signal transduction that follow the binding of signaling molecules to plasma membrane receptors include phosphorylation of receptors at tyrosine residues (**receptor tyrosine kinase** activity), conformational changes in **signal transducer proteins** (e.g., proteins with Src homology 2 [**SH2**] domains, the **monomeric guanosine triphosphate [GTP]-binding proteins [G-proteins] like Ras, or heterotrimeric G-proteins**), or increases in the levels of **intracellular second messengers**. Second messengers are nonprotein molecules that are generated inside the cell in response

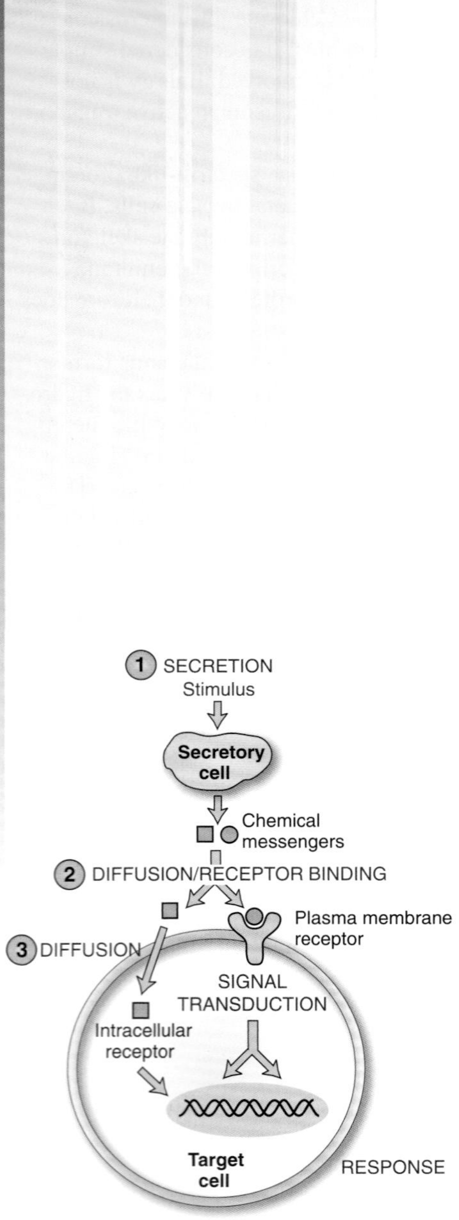

FIGURE 11.1 General features of chemical messengers. (*1*) Secretion of chemical message. (*2*) Binding of message to cell surface receptor. (*3*) Diffusion of a hydrophobic message across the plasma membrane and binding to an intracellular receptor.

to hormone binding and that continue transmission of the message. Examples include 3′,5′-cyclic adenosine monophosphate (**cAMP**), inositol trisphosphate (**IP₃**), and diacylglycerol (**DAG**).

Signaling often requires a rapid response and rapid termination of the message, which may be achieved by degradation of the receptor itself, by degradation of the messenger or second messenger, the conversion of GTP to guanosine diphosphate (GDP) on GTP-dependent signaling molecules, deactivation of signal transduction kinases by phosphatases, or other means.

THE WAITING ROOM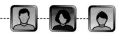

 Mia S. is a 37-year-old woman who complains of increasing muscle fatigue, which she notices mostly with eating: Halfway through a meal, she has trouble chewing her food. If she rests for 5 to 10 minutes, her strength returns to normal. She also notes that if she talks on the phone, her ability to form words gradually decreases because of fatigue of the muscles of speech. She also reports that by evening, her upper eyelids droop to the point that she has to pull her upper lids back in order to see normally. These symptoms are becoming increasingly severe. When Mia is asked to sustain an upward gaze, her upper eyelids eventually drift downward involuntarily. When she is asked to hold both arms straight out in front of her for as long as she is able, both arms begin to drift downward within minutes. Her physician suspects that Mia has myasthenia gravis and orders a test to determine whether she has antibodies in her blood directed against the acetylcholine (ACh) receptor.

 Ann R., who suffers from anorexia nervosa, has increased her weight to 102 lb from a low of 85 lb (see Chapter 9). On the advice of her physician, she has been eating more to prevent fatigue during her daily jogging regimen. She runs about 10 miles before breakfast every second day and forces herself to drink a high-energy supplement immediately afterward.

 Dennis V. was hospitalized for dehydration resulting from cholera toxin (see Chapter 10). In his intestinal mucosal cells, the cholera toxin A-subunit indirectly activated the cystic fibrosis transmembrane conductance regulator (CFTR) channel, resulting in secretion of chloride and sodium ions into his intestinal lumen. Ion secretion was followed by loss of water, resulting in vomiting and watery diarrhea. Dennis is being treated for hypovolemic shock by replacing his fluid loss with intravenous fluids.

I. General Features of Chemical Messengers

Certain universal characteristics of chemical messenger systems are illustrated in Figure 11.1. Signaling generally follows this sequence: (1) the chemical messenger is secreted from a specific cells in response to a stimulus; (2) the messenger diffuses or is transported through blood or other extracellular fluid to the target cell; (3) a molecule in the target cell, termed a *receptor* (a plasma membrane receptor or intracellular receptor), specifically binds the messenger; (4) binding of the messenger to the receptor elicits a response; (5) the signal ceases and is terminated. Chemical messengers elicit their response in the target cell without being metabolized by the cell.

An additional feature of chemical messenger systems is that the specificity of the response is dictated by the type of receptor and its location. Generally, each receptor binds only one specific chemical messenger, and each receptor initiates a characteristic signal transduction pathway that will ultimately activate or inhibit certain processes in the cell. Only certain cells, the target cells, carry receptors for that messenger and are capable of responding to its message.

 ACh is released by neurons and acts on ACh receptors at neuromuscular junctions to stimulate muscle contraction. Myasthenia gravis is an acquired autoimmune disease in which most patients have developed pathogenic antibodies against these receptors. **Mia S.'s** decreasing ability to form words as well as her other symptoms of muscle weakness are being caused by the inability of ACh to stimulate repeated muscle contraction when the numbers of effective ACh receptors at neuromuscular junctions are greatly reduced.

 Endocrine hormones enable **Ann R.** to mobilize fuels from her adipose tissue during her periods of fasting and during jogging. Although she fasts overnight, α-cells of her pancreas increase secretion of the polypeptide hormone glucagon. The stress of prolonged fasting and chronic exercise stimulates release of cortisol, a steroid hormone, from her adrenal cortex. The exercise of jogging also increases secretion of the hormones epinephrine and norepinephrine from the adrenal medulla. Each of these hormones is being released in response to a specific signal and causes a characteristic response in a target tissue, enabling her to exercise. However, each of these hormones binds to a different type of receptor and works in a different way.

Ann R.'s fasting is accompanied by high levels of the endocrine hormone glucagon, which is secreted in response to low blood glucose levels. It enters the blood and acts on the liver to stimulate several pathways, including the release of glucose from glycogen stores (glycogenolysis) (see Chapter 3). The specificity of its action is determined by the location of receptors. Although liver parenchymal cells have glucagon receptors, skeletal muscle and many other tissues do not. Therefore, glucagon cannot stimulate glycogenolysis in these tissues.

The means of signal termination is an exceedingly important aspect of cell signaling, and failure to terminate a signal contributes to several diseases such as cancer.

A. General Features of Chemical Messenger Systems Applied to the Nicotinic Acetylcholine Receptor

The individual steps involved in cell signaling by chemical messengers are illustrated with *acetylcholine* (ACh), a neurotransmitter that acts on *nicotinic acetylcholine receptors* on the plasma membrane of certain muscle cells. This system exhibits the classic features of chemical messenger release and specificity of response.

Neurotransmitters are secreted from neurons in response to an electrical stimulus called the *action potential* (a voltage difference across the plasma membrane caused by changes in Na^+ and K^+ gradients that is propagated along a nerve). The neurotransmitters diffuse across a synapse to another excitable cell, where they elicit a response (Fig. 11.2). ACh is the neurotransmitter at neuromuscular junctions, where it transmits a signal from a motor nerve to a muscle fiber that elicits contraction of the fiber. Prior to release, ACh is sequestered in vesicles clustered near an active zone in the *presynaptic membrane*. This membrane also has voltage-gated Ca^{2+} channels that open when the action potential reaches them, resulting in an influx of Ca^{2+}. The Ca^{2+} triggers fusion of the vesicles with the plasma membrane, and ACh is released into the synaptic cleft. Thus, the chemical messenger is released from a specific cell in response to a specific stimulus. The mechanism of vesicle fusion with the plasma membrane is common to the release of many second messengers.

ACh diffuses across the synaptic cleft to bind to the nicotinic ACh receptor on the plasma membrane of the muscle cells (Fig. 11.3). The subunits of the receptor are assembled around a channel, which has a funnel-shaped opening in the center. As ACh binds to one of the subunits of the receptor, a conformational change

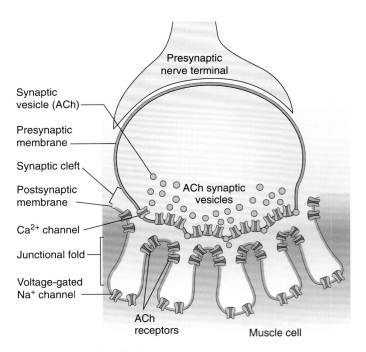

FIGURE 11.2 Acetylcholine (ACh) receptors at the neuromuscular junction. A motor nerve terminates in several branches; each branch terminates in a bulb-shaped structure called the *presynaptic bouton*. Each bouton synapses with a region of the muscle fiber that contains junctional folds. At the crest of each fold, there is a high concentration of ACh receptors, which are gated ion channels.

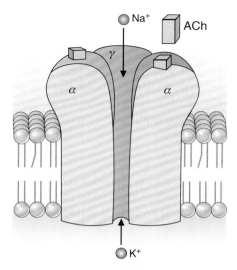

Na⁺   ACh

γ

α   α

K⁺

FIGURE 11.3   The nicotinic acetylcholine (ACh) receptor. Each receptor is composed of five subunits, and each subunit has four membrane-spanning helical regions. For clarity, only three subunits are shown in this figure. The two α-subunits are identical and contain binding sites for ACh. When two ACh molecules are bound, the subunits change their conformation so that the channel in the center of the receptor is open, allowing K^+ ions to diffuse out and Na^+ ions to diffuse in.

opens the narrow portion of the channel (the gate), allowing Na^+ to diffuse in and K^+ to diffuse out (a uniform property of all receptors is that signal transduction begins with conformational changes in the receptor). The change in ion concentration activates a sequence of events that eventually triggers the cellular response—contraction of the fiber.

Once ACh secretion stops, the message is rapidly terminated by *acetylcholinesterase*, an enzyme located on the postsynaptic membrane that cleaves ACh. It is also terminated by diffusion of ACh away from the synapse. Rapid termination of messages is a characteristic of systems that require a rapid response from the target cell.

B. Endocrine, Paracrine, and Autocrine Actions

The actions of chemical messengers are often classified as endocrine, paracrine, or autocrine (Fig. 11.4). Each endocrine hormone (e.g., insulin) is secreted by a specific cell type (generally in an endocrine gland), enters the blood, and exerts its actions on specific target cells, which may be some distance away. In contrast to endocrine hormones, paracrine actions are those carried out on nearby cells, and the location of the cells plays a role in the specificity of the response. Synaptic transmission by ACh and other neurotransmitters (sometimes called *neurocrine signaling*) is an example of paracrine signaling. ACh activates only those ACh receptors that are located across the synaptic cleft from the signaling nerve, not every muscle cell with ACh receptors. Paracrine actions are also very important in limiting the immune response to a specific location in the body, a feature that helps prevent the development of autoimmune disease. Autocrine actions involve a messenger that acts on the cell from which it is secreted or on nearby cells that are the same type as the secreting cells.

C. Types of Chemical Messengers

There are three types of major signaling systems in the body employing chemical messengers: the nervous system, the endocrine system, and the immune system. Some messengers are difficult to place in just one such category.

 Myasthenia gravis is a disease of autoimmunity, which in most cases is caused by the production of an antibody directed against the ACh receptor in skeletal muscle. In this disease, B- and T-lymphocytes cooperate in producing a variety of antibodies against the nicotinic ACh receptor. The antibodies then bind to various locations in the receptor and cross-link the receptors, forming a multireceptor antibody complex. The complex is endocytosed and incorporated into lysosomes, where it is degraded. **Mia S.**, therefore, has fewer functional receptors on the muscle cell membrane for ACh to activate.

 ACh acts on two different types of receptors; nicotinic and muscarinic. Nicotinic receptors (for which nicotine is an activator) are found at the neuromuscular junction of skeletal muscle cells, as well as in the parasympathetic nervous system. Muscarinic receptors (for which muscarine, a mushroom toxin, is an activator) are found at the neuromuscular junction of cardiac and smooth muscle cells, as well as in the sympathetic nervous system. Curare (a paralyzing agent) is an inhibitor of nicotinic ACh receptors, whereas atropine is an inhibitor of muscarinic ACh receptors. Atropine can be used under conditions in which acetylcholinesterase has been inactivated by various nerve gases or chemicals such that atropine will block the effects of the excess ACh present at the synapse.

 Mia S. could be tested with an inhibitor of acetylcholinesterase, edrophonium chloride, which is administered intravenously. After this drug inactivates acetylcholinesterase, ACh that is released from the nerve terminal accumulates in the synaptic cleft. Even though Mia expresses fewer ACh receptors on her muscle cells (owing to the autoantibody-induced degradation of receptors), by increasing the local concentration of ACh, these receptors have a higher probability of being occupied and activated. Therefore, acute intravenous administration of this short-acting drug briefly improves muscular weakness in patients with myasthenia gravis.

A. Endocrine

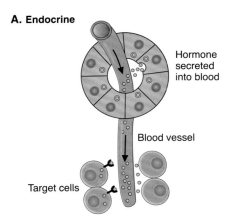

Hormone secreted into blood

Blood vessel

Target cells

B. Paracrine

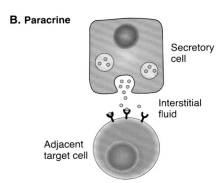

Secretory cell

Interstitial fluid

Adjacent target cell

C. Autocrine

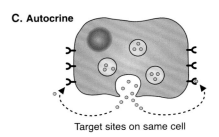

Target sites on same cell

Y Receptor　○ Hormone or other chemical messenger

FIGURE 11.4 Endocrine, autocrine, and paracrine actions of hormones and other chemical messengers.

The catecholamine hormone epinephrine (also called *adrenaline*) is the fright, fight, and flight hormone. Epinephrine and the structurally similar hormone norepinephrine are released from the adrenal medulla in response to a variety of immediate stresses, including pain, hemorrhage, exercise, hypoglycemia, and hypoxia. Thus, as **Ann R.** begins to jog, there is a rapid release of epinephrine and norepinephrine into her blood.

1. The Nervous System

The nervous system secretes two types of messengers: small-molecule neurotransmitters, often called *biogenic amines*, and neuropeptides. Small-molecule neurotransmitters are nitrogen-containing molecules, several of which are amino acids or derivatives of amino acids (e.g., ACh, epinephrine, and γ-aminobutyrate; Fig. 11.5). Neuropeptides are usually small peptides (between 4 and 35 amino acids), secreted by neurons, that act as neurotransmitters at synaptic junctions or are secreted into the blood to act as neurohormones.

2. The Endocrine System

Endocrine hormones are defined as compounds secreted from specific endocrine cells in endocrine glands, which reach their target cells following transport through the blood. Insulin, for example, is an endocrine hormone secreted from the β-cells of the pancreas. Classic hormones are generally divided into the structural categories of polypeptide hormones (e.g., insulin; see Fig. 6.12 for the structure of insulin), catecholamines such as epinephrine (which is also a neurotransmitter), steroid hormones (which are derived from cholesterol), and thyroid hormone (which is derived from tyrosine). Many of these endocrine hormones also exert paracrine or autocrine actions. The hormones that regulate metabolism are discussed throughout this chapter and in subsequent chapters of this text.

Some compounds that are normally considered hormones are more difficult to categorize. For example, retinoids, which are derivatives of vitamin A (also called *retinol*) and vitamin D (which is also derived from cholesterol) are usually classified as hormones, although they are not synthesized in endocrine cells.

3. The Immune System

The messengers of the immune system, called *cytokines*, are small proteins with a molecular weight of approximately 20,000 Da. Cytokines regulate a network of responses designed to kill invading microorganisms. The different classes of cytokines (interleukins, tumor necrosis factors, interferons, and colony-stimulating factors) are secreted by cells of the immune system and usually alter the behavior of other cells in the immune system by activating the transcription of genes for proteins involved in the immune response. *Chemokines* are chemotactic cytokines in that these molecules have the ability to induce movement in targeted cells toward the source of the chemokines.

4. The Eicosanoids

The *eicosanoids* (including prostaglandins [PG], thromboxanes, and leukotrienes) control cellular function in response to injury (Fig. 11.6). These compounds are all

$$H_3C-\overset{\overset{\displaystyle O}{\|}}{C}-O-CH_2-CH_2-\overset{+}{N}(CH_3)_3$$

Acetylcholine

$$^-OOC-CH_2-CH_2-CH_2-\overset{+}{N}H_3$$

γ-Aminobutyrate (GABA)

Epinephrine

FIGURE 11.5 Small-molecule neurotransmitters.

derived from arachidonic acid, a 20-carbon polyunsaturated fatty acid that is usually present in cells as part of the membrane lipid phosphatidylcholine (see Chapter 5, Fig. 5.19). Although almost every cell in the body produces an eicosanoid in response to tissue injury, different cells produce different eicosanoids. The eicosanoids act principally in paracrine and autocrine functions, affecting the cells that produce them or their neighboring cells. For example, vascular endothelial cells (cells that line the vessel wall) secrete the prostaglandin prostacyclin (PGI$_2$), which acts on nearby smooth muscle cells to cause vasodilation (expansion of blood vessels). The synthesis and metabolism of the eicosanoids are discussed further in Chapter 31.

5. Growth Factors

Growth factors are polypeptides that function through stimulation of cellular proliferation (hyperplasia) or cell size (hypertrophy). For example, platelets aggregating at the site of injury to a blood vessel secrete platelet-derived growth factor (PDGF). PDGF stimulates the proliferation of nearby smooth muscle cells, which eventually form a plaque covering the injured site. Some growth factors are considered hormones, and some have been called *cytokines*.

II. Intracellular Transcription Factor Receptors

A. Intracellular versus Plasma Membrane Receptors

The structural properties of a messenger determine, to some extent, the type of receptor it binds. Most receptors fall into two broad categories: *intracellular receptors* or *plasma membrane receptors* (Fig. 11.7). Messengers using intracellular receptors must be hydrophobic molecules able to diffuse through the plasma membrane into cells. In contrast, polar molecules such as peptide hormones, cytokines, and catecholamines cannot rapidly cross the plasma membrane and must bind to a plasma membrane receptor.

Most of the intracellular receptors for lipophilic messengers are *gene-specific transcription factors*. A transcription factor is a protein that binds to a specific site

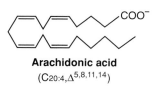

Arachidonic acid
(C$_{20:4}$, $\Delta^{5,8,11,14}$)

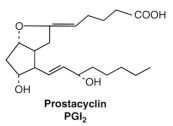

Prostacyclin
PGI$_2$

FIGURE 11.6 Eicosanoids are derived from arachidonic acid and retain its original 20 carbons (thus, the name *eicosanoids*). All prostaglandins, such as prostacyclin, also have an internal ring.

 Lotta T. suffered enormously painful gout attacks affecting her great toe (see "Clinical Comments," Chapter 8). The extreme pain was caused by the release of a leukotriene that stimulated pain receptors. The precipitated urate crystals in her big toe stimulated recruited inflammatory cells to release the leukotriene.

Cell-surface receptors

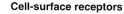
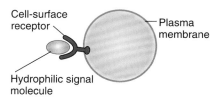

Cell-surface receptor

Plasma membrane

Hydrophilic signal molecule

Intracellular receptors

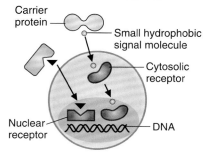

Carrier protein

Small hydrophobic signal molecule

Cytosolic receptor

Nuclear receptor

DNA

FIGURE 11.7 Intracellular versus plasma membrane receptors. Plasma membrane receptors have extracellular binding domains. Intracellular receptors bind steroid hormones or other messengers that are able to diffuse through the plasma membrane. Their receptors may reside in the cytoplasm and translocate to the nucleus, reside in the nucleus bound to DNA, or reside in the nucleus bound to other proteins.

on DNA and regulates the rate of transcription of a gene (i.e., synthesis of mRNA; see Chapter 16). External signaling molecules bind to transcription factors that bind to a specific sequence on DNA and regulate the expression of only certain genes; they are called *gene-specific* or *site-specific transcription factors*.

B. The Steroid Hormone/Thyroid Hormone Superfamily of Receptors

Lipophilic hormones that use intracellular gene-specific transcription factors include the steroid hormones (such as estrogen and cortisol), thyroid hormone, retinoic acid (the active form of vitamin A), and vitamin D (Fig. 11.8). Because these compounds are water-insoluble, they are transported in the blood bound to serum albumin, which has a hydrophobic binding pocket, or to more specific transport proteins such as steroid hormone-binding globulin (SHBG) or thyroid hormone-binding globulin (TBG). The intracellular receptors for these hormones are structurally similar and are referred to as the *steroid hormone/thyroid hormone superfamily of receptors*.

The steroid hormone/thyroid hormone superfamily of receptors reside primarily in the nucleus, although some members are also found in the cytoplasm. The glucocorticoid receptor, for example, exists as cytoplasmic multimeric complexes associated

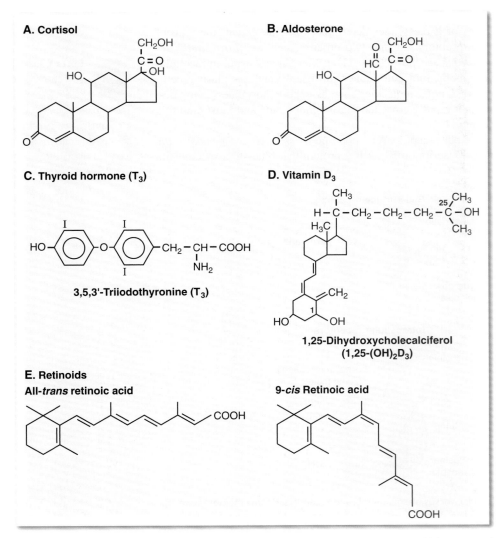

FIGURE 11.8 Steroid hormone–thyroid hormone superfamily. **A.** Cortisol (a glucocorticoid). **B.** Aldosterone (a mineralocorticoid). **C.** Thyroid hormone. **D.** Vitamin D$_3$. **E.** Retinoids.

with heat-shock proteins. When the hormone cortisol (a glucocorticoid) binds, the receptor undergoes a conformational change and dissociates from the heat-shock proteins, exposing a nuclear translocation signal (a signal specifying its transport to the nucleus). The receptors dimerize and the complex (including bound hormone) translocates to the nucleus where it binds to a portion of the DNA called the *hormone response element* (e.g., the glucocorticoid receptor binds to the glucocorticoid response element [GRE]). The majority of the intracellular receptors, however, reside principally in the nucleus, and some of these are constitutively bound to their response element in DNA (e.g., the thyroid hormone receptor). Binding of the hormone changes their activity and their ability to associate with, or disassociate from, DNA. Regulation of gene transcription by these receptors is described in more detail in Chapter 16.

As an example of the complexity that can occur with the steroid hormone superfamily of receptors, several nuclear receptors play important roles in intermediary metabolism and they have become the targets of lipid-lowering drugs. These include the peroxisome proliferator-activated receptors (PPAR α, β, and γ), the liver X-activated receptor (LXR), the farnesoid X-activated receptor (FXR), and the pregnane X receptor (PXR). These receptors form heterodimers with the 9-*cis*-retinoic acid receptor (RXR) and bind to their appropriate response elements in DNA in an inactive state. When the activating ligand binds to the receptor (fatty acids and their derivatives for the PPARs, oxysterols for LXR, bile salts for FXR, and secondary bile salts for PXR), the complex is activated and gene expression is altered. Unlike the cortisol receptor, these receptors reside in the nucleus and are activated once their ligands enter the nucleus and bind to them.

III. Plasma Membrane Receptors and Signal Transduction

All plasma membrane receptors are proteins with certain features in common: an extracellular domain that binds the chemical messenger, one or more membrane-spanning domains that are α-helices, and an intracellular domain that initiates signal transduction. As the ligand binds to the extracellular domain of its receptor, it causes a conformational change that is communicated to the intracellular domain through the rigid α-helix of the transmembrane domain. The activated intracellular domain initiates a characteristic signal transduction pathway that usually involves the binding of specific intracellular signal transduction proteins. Signal transduction pathways run in one direction. From a given point in a signal transduction pathway, events closer to the receptor are referred to as *upstream*, and events closer to the response are referred to as *downstream*.

The pathways of signal transduction for plasma membrane receptors have two major types of effects on the cell: (1) rapid and immediate effects on cellular ion levels or activation/inhibition of enzymes and/or (2) slower changes in the rate of gene expression for a specific set of proteins. Often, a signal transduction pathway will ultimately produce both kinds of effects.

A. Major Classes of Plasma Membrane Receptors

Individual plasma membrane receptors are grouped into three categories: *ion-channel receptors*, *receptors that are kinases or bind to and activate kinases*, and *receptors that work through second messengers*. This classification is based on the receptor's general structure and means of signal transduction.

1. Ion-Channel Receptors

The ion-channel receptors are similar in structure to the previously discussed nicotinic ACh receptor (see Fig. 11.3). Signal transduction consists of the conformational change when ligand binds. Most small-molecule neurotransmitters and some neuropeptides use ion-channel receptors.

The steroid hormone cortisol is synthesized and released from the adrenal cortex in response to the polypeptide hormone adrenal corticotrophic hormone (ACTH). Chronic stress (pain, hypoglycemia, hemorrhage, and exercise) signals are passed from the brain cortex to the hypothalamus to the anterior pituitary, which releases ACTH. Cortisol acts on tissues to change enzyme levels and redistribute nutrients in preparation for acute stress. For example, it increases transcription of the genes for regulatory enzymes in the pathway of gluconeogenesis (called *gene-specific activation of transcription*, or *induction of protein synthesis*). The net result of this activity is an increased cellular content of the enzymes. Induction of gluconeogenic enzymes prepares the liver to respond rapidly to hypoglycemia with increased synthesis of glucose. **Ann R.**, who has frequently been fasting and exercising, has an increased capacity for gluconeogenesis in her liver.

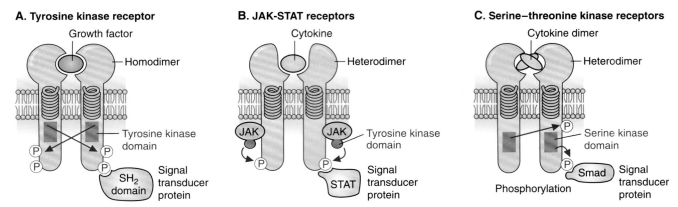

A. Tyrosine kinase receptor

Growth factor

Homodimer

Tyrosine kinase domain

SH₂ domain

Signal transducer protein

B. JAK-STAT receptors

Cytokine

Heterodimer

JAK JAK

Tyrosine kinase domain

STAT

Signal transducer protein

C. Serine–threonine kinase receptors

Cytokine dimer

Heterodimer

Serine kinase domain

Smad

Signal transducer protein

Phosphorylation

FIGURE 11.9 Receptors that are kinases or that bind kinases. The kinase domains are shown in *red*, and the phosphorylation sites are indicated with *red arrows*. **A.** Tyrosine kinase receptors. **B.** Janus kinase (JAK)-signal transducer and activator of transcription (STAT) receptors. STAT proteins are phosphorylated by the activated JAK kinase, which is associated with the cytokine receptor. **C.** Serine–threonine kinase receptors. Smad proteins are phosphorylated by the activated receptors.

Heptahelical receptors

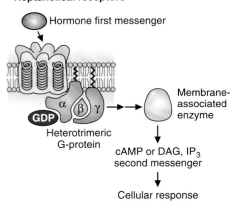

Hormone first messenger

Membrane-associated enzyme

α β γ

GDP

Heterotrimeric G-protein

cAMP or DAG, IP₃ second messenger

Cellular response

FIGURE 11.10 G-protein–coupled receptors and second messengers. The secreted chemical messenger (hormone, cytokine, or neurotransmitter) is the first messenger, which binds to a plasma membrane receptor such as the heptahelical receptors. The activated hormone–receptor complex activates a heterotrimeric G-protein (via an exchange of guanosine triphosphate for the bound guanosine diphosphate [GDP]; see Fig. 11.17) and, via stimulation of membrane-bound enzymes, different G-proteins lead to generation of one or more intracellular second messengers, such as 3′,5′-cyclic adenosine monophosphate (cAMP), diacylglycerol (DAG), or inositol trisphosphate (IP₃).

2. Receptors that Are Kinases or that Bind Kinases

There are several types of receptors that are kinases or bind kinases, as illustrated in Figure 11.9. Protein kinases transfer a phosphate group from adenosine triphosphate (ATP) to the hydroxyl group of a specific amino acid side chain in the target protein. Their common feature is that the intracellular kinase domain of the receptor (or the kinase domain of the associated protein) is activated when the messenger binds to the extracellular domain. The receptor kinase phosphorylates an amino acid residue (serine, threonine, tyrosine, or, rarely, histidine) on the receptor (autophosphorylation) and/or an associated protein. The message is propagated downstream through signal transducer proteins that bind to the activated messenger–receptor complex (e.g., *s*ignal *t*ransducer and *a*ctivator of *t*ranscription [STAT], Smad (named after the first two proteins identified, Sma in *Caenorhabditis elegans* and Mad in *Drosophila*), or an Src homology 2 [SH2] domain-containing protein such as growth factor receptor–bound protein 2 [Grb2]).

3. Heptahelical Receptors

Heptahelical receptors (also called *G-protein–coupled receptors* [GPCRs]) contain seven membrane-spanning α-helices and are the most common type of plasma membrane receptor (Fig. 11.10). They work through second messengers, which are small nonprotein compounds, such as cAMP, generated inside the cell in response to messenger binding to the receptor. They continue intracellular transmission of the message from the hormone/cytokine/neurotransmitter, which is the "first" messenger. Second messengers are present in low concentrations so that modulation of their level, and hence the message, can be rapidly initiated and terminated.

B. Signal Transduction through Tyrosine Kinase Receptors

The tyrosine kinase receptors are depicted in Figure 11.9A. They generally exist in the membrane as monomers with a single membrane-spanning helix. One molecule of the growth factor generally binds two molecules of the receptor and promotes their dimerization (Fig. 11.11). Once the receptor dimer has formed, the intracellular tyrosine kinase domains of the receptor phosphorylate each other on certain tyrosine residues (autophosphorylation). The phosphotyrosine residues form specific binding sites for signal transducer proteins.

1. Ras and the MAP Kinase Pathway

The Ras–mitogen-activated protein (MAP) kinase pathway demonstrates how receptor tyrosine kinases can activate signaling through the assembly of protein complexes,

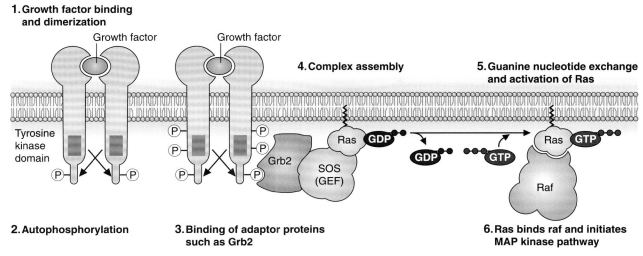

1. Growth factor binding and dimerization

Growth factor

Growth factor

4. Complex assembly

5. Guanine nucleotide exchange and activation of Ras

Tyrosine kinase domain

Ras GDP

GDP

GTP

Ras GTP

Grb2

SOS (GEF)

Raf

2. Autophosphorylation

3. Binding of adaptor proteins such as Grb2

6. Ras binds raf and initiates MAP kinase pathway

FIGURE 11.11 Signal transduction by tyrosine kinase receptors. (*1*) Binding and dimerization. (*2*) Autophosphorylation. (*3*) Binding of Grb2 and SOS. (*4*) SOS is a guanine nucleotide exchange factor (GEF) that binds Ras, a monomeric G-protein anchored to the plasma membrane. (*5*) GEF activates the exchange of guanosine triphosphate (GTP) for bound guanosine diphosphate (GDP) on Ras. (*6*) Activated Ras containing GTP binds the target enzyme Raf, thereby activating it and a series of downstream kinases known as the mitogen-activated protein (MAP) kinase pathway.

caused by protein–protein interactions. In this pathway, one of the domains of the receptor containing a phosphotyrosine residue forms a binding site for intracellular proteins with a specific three-dimensional structure known as the *SH2 domain* (the SH2 domain, named for the first protein in which it was found, the Src protein of the Rous sarcoma virus). The adaptor protein Grb2 is one of the proteins with an SH2 domain that binds to phosphotyrosine residues on growth factor receptors. Binding to the receptor causes a conformational change in Grb2 that activates another binding site called an *SH3 domain*. These activated SH3 domains bind the protein SOS (SOS is an acronym for "son of sevenless," a name that is not related to the function or structure of the compound). SOS is a guanine nucleotide exchange factor (GEF) for Ras, a monomeric G-protein located in the plasma membrane (see Chapter 9, Section III.C.2). SOS catalyzes exchange of GTP for guanosine diphosphate (GDP) on Ras, causing a conformational change in Ras that promotes binding of the protein Raf. Raf is a serine protein kinase that is also called *m*itogen-*a*ctivated *p*rotein *ki*nase *ki*nase *ki*nase (MAPKKK). Raf begins a sequence of successive phosphorylation steps called a *phosphorylation cascade*. When one of the kinases in a cascade is phosphorylated, it binds and phosphorylates the next enzyme downstream in the cascade. The MAP kinase cascade ultimately leads to an alteration of gene transcription factor activity, thereby either upregulating or downregulating transcription of many genes involved in cell survival and proliferation.

Although many different signal transducer proteins have SH2 domains, and many receptors have phosphotyrosine residues, a signal transducer protein may only be specific for one type of receptor. This specificity of binding results from the fact that each phosphotyrosine residue has a different amino acid sequence around it that forms the binding domain. Similarly, the SH2 domain of the transducer protein is only part of its binding domain. Conversely, however, several transducer proteins will bind to multiple receptors (such as Grb2).

Many tyrosine kinase receptors (as well as heptahelical receptors) also have additional signaling pathways involving intermediates such as phosphatidylinositol phosphates.

2. Phosphatidylinositol Phosphates in Signal Transduction

Phosphatidylinositol signaling molecules can be generated through either tyrosine kinase receptors or heptahelical receptors. Phosphatidylinositol phosphates serve two

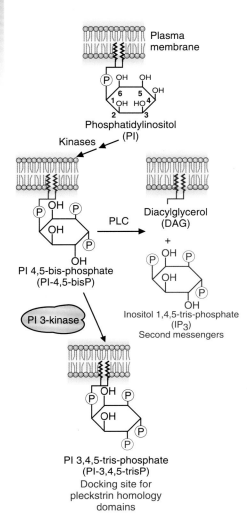

FIGURE 11.12 Major route for generation of the phosphatidyl inosilide signal molecules inositol 1′,4′,5′-trisphosphate (IP₃), and phosphatidylinositol 3′,4′,5′-trisphosphate (PI-3,4,5-trisP). Phosphatidylinositol 3′-kinase (PI 3-kinase) phosphorylates phosphatidylinositol 4′,5′-bisphosphate (PI-4,5-bisP) and phosphatidylinositol 4-phosphate (not shown) at the 3 position. Prime symbols are sometimes used in these names to denote the inositol ring. Diacylglycerol (DAG) is also a second messenger. *PLC*, phospholipase C.

different functions in signal transduction: (1) Phosphatidylinositol 4′,5′-bisphosphate (PI-4,5-bisP) can be cleaved to generate the two intracellular second messengers, DAG and IP₃; and (2) phosphatidylinositol 3′,4′,5′-trisphosphate (PI-3,4,5-trisP) can serve as a plasma-membrane docking site for signal transduction proteins.

Phosphatidylinositol, which is present in the inner leaflet of the plasma membrane, is converted to PI-4,5-bisP by kinases that phosphorylate the inositol ring at the 4′ and 5′ positions (Fig. 11.12). PI-4,5-bisP, which has three phosphate groups, is cleaved by a phospholipase C isozyme to generate IP₃ and DAG. The phospholipase isozyme Cγ (PLCγ) is activated by tyrosine kinase growth-factor receptors, and phospholipase Cβ is activated by a heptahelical receptor–G-protein signal transduction pathway.

PI-4,5-bisP can also be phosphorylated at the 3′ position of inositol by the enzyme phosphatidylinositol 3′-kinase (PI 3-kinase) to form PI-3,4,5-trisP (see Fig. 11.12). PI-3,4,5-trisP (and PI-3,4-bisP) form membrane docking sites for proteins that contain a certain sequence of amino acids called the *pleckstrin homology* (PH) domain. PI 3-kinase contains an SH2 domain and is activated by binding to a specific phosphotyrosine site on a tyrosine kinase receptor or receptor-associated protein. The protein *p*hosphatase and *ten*sin homolog (PTEN) catalyzes the dephosphorylation of PI-3,4,5-trisP to PI-4,5-bisP, thereby removing the primary signal from the pathway. Mutations within PTEN, or misexpression of PTEN, can lead to cancer (see Chapter 18).

3. The Insulin Receptor

The insulin receptor, a member of the tyrosine kinase family of receptors, provides a good example of divergence in the pathway of signal transduction. Unlike other growth-factor receptors, the insulin receptor exists in the membrane as a preformed dimer, with each half containing an α- and a β-subunit (Fig. 11.13). The β-subunits autophosphorylate each other when insulin binds, thereby activating the receptor. The activated phosphorylated receptor binds a protein called *i*nsulin *r*eceptor *s*ubstrate (*IRS*). The activated receptor kinase phosphorylates IRS at multiple sites, creating multiple binding sites for different proteins with SH2 domains. One of the sites binds the adapter protein Grb2, which leads to the activation of Ras and the MAP kinase pathway. At another phosphotyrosine site, PI 3-kinase binds and is activated.

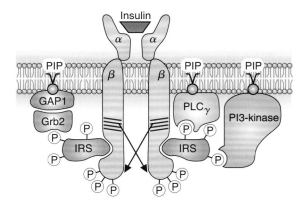

FIGURE 11.13 Insulin receptor signaling. The insulin receptor is a dimer of two membrane-spanning α–β pairs. The tyrosine kinase domains are shown in *red*, and *arrows* indicate autocross-phosphorylation. The activated receptor binds IRS molecules (insulin receptor substrates) and phosphorylates IRS at multiple sites, thereby forming binding sites for proteins with SH2 domains, examples being Grb2, phospholipase Cγ (PLCγ), and phosphatidylinositol (PI) 3-kinase. Both PLCγ and PI 3-kinase are associated with various phosphatidylinositol phosphates (all designated with *PIP*) in the plasma membrane and are an important part of second messenger production. Grb2 associates with a protein known as GAP1 (Grb2-associated protein), which has a pleckstrin homology domain that associates with phosphatidylinositol phosphates in the membrane.

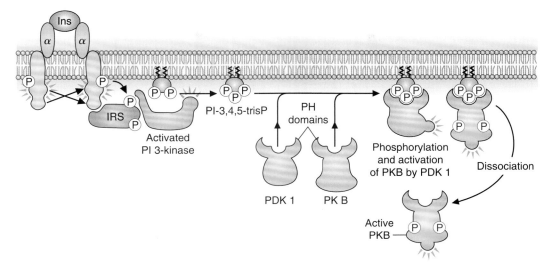

FIGURE 11.14 The insulin receptor–protein kinase B (Akt) signaling pathway. *Ins*, insulin; *IRS*, insulin receptor substrate; *PH* domains, pleckstrin homology domains; *PDK1*, phosphoinositide-dependent protein kinase-1; *PKB*, protein kinase B; *PI-3,4,5-trisP*, phosphatidylinositol 3′,4′,5′-trisphosphate; *PI 3-kinase*, phosphatidylinositol 3′-kinase.

This pathway will lead to the activation of protein kinase B (PKB). At a third site, PLC_γ binds and is activated. The insulin receptor can also transmit signals through direct docking with other signal transduction intermediates.

The signal pathway initiated by the insulin–receptor complex involving PI 3-kinase leads to activation of protein kinase B (also called *Akt*), a serine–threonine kinase that mediates many of the downstream effects of insulin (Fig. 11.14). PI 3-kinase binds to IRS and phosphorylates PI-4,5-bisP in the membrane to form PI-3,4,5-trisP. Protein kinase B and *p*hosphoinositide-*d*ependent *k*inase-*1* (PDK1) are recruited to the membrane by their PH domains, where PDK1 phosphorylates and activates protein kinase B. One of the signal transduction pathways for Akt leads to the effects of insulin on glucose metabolism. Other pathways result in the phosphorylation of a host of other proteins that affect cell growth and survival. In general, phosphorylation of these proteins by Akt promotes cell survival. The action of insulin is covered in more detail in Chapters 26, 36, and 43. It is important to note that other receptors' tyrosine kinase receptors will also lead to the activation of the Akt pathway through the direct binding of PI 3-kinase to activated receptors (see Section III.B.2 of this chapter).

 Insulin is a growth factor that is essential for cell viability and growth. It increases general protein synthesis, which strongly affects muscle mass through hypertrophy. However, it also regulates immediate nutrient availability and storage, including glucose transport into skeletal muscle and glycogen synthesis. Thus, **Dianne A.** and other patients with type 1 diabetes mellitus who lack insulin rapidly develop hyperglycemia once insulin levels drop too low. They also exhibit muscle "wasting." To mediate the diverse regulatory roles of insulin, the signal transduction pathway diverges after activation of the receptor and phosphorylation of IRS, which has multiple binding sites for different signal-mediator proteins.

C. Signal Transduction by Cytokine Receptors: Use of JAK-STAT Proteins

Tyrosine kinase–associated receptors in the cytokine receptor family transduce signals through *ja*nus *k*inase (JAK)/STAT proteins to regulate the proliferation of certain cells involved in the immune response (see Fig. 11.9B). The receptors themselves have no intrinsic kinase activity but bind (associate with) a tyrosine kinase of the JAK family. Their signal transducer proteins, called STATs, are themselves gene-specific transcription factors. Thus, cytokine receptors use a more direct route for propagation of the signal to the nucleus than tyrosine kinase receptors.

Each receptor monomer has an extracellular domain, a membrane-spanning region, and an intracellular domain. As the cytokine binds to these receptors, they form dimers or trimers (either between the same or distinct receptor molecules) and may cluster (Fig. 11.15). The activated receptor-associated tyrosine kinases phosphorylate each other on tyrosine residues and also phosphorylate tyrosine residues on the receptor, forming phosphotyrosine-binding sites for the SH2 domain of a STAT. STATs are inactive in the cytoplasm until they bind to the receptor complex, where they are also phosphorylated by the bound JAK. Phosphorylation changes the

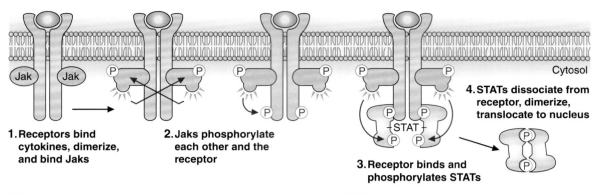

FIGURE 11.15 Steps in cytokine receptor signaling. *Jak*, janus kinase; *STAT*, signal transducer and activator of transcription.

conformation of the STAT, causing it to dissociate from the receptor and dimerize with another phosphorylated STAT, thereby forming an activated transcription factor. The STAT dimer translocates to the nucleus and binds to a response element on DNA, thereby regulating gene transcription.

There are many different STAT proteins, each with a slightly different amino acid sequence. Receptors for different cytokines bind different STATs, which then form heterodimers in various combinations. This microheterogeneity allows different cytokines to target different genes. STAT signaling is regulated in several ways. Two prominent types are a protein family known as *s*uppressors *of c*ytokine *s*ignaling (*SOCS*) and *p*rotein *i*nhibitors of *a*ctivated STAT (*PIAS*). Both SOCS and PIAS genes are induced by activated STAT in order to limit the duration of the second message.

D. Receptor Serine–Threonine Kinases

Proteins in the transforming growth factor superfamily use receptors that have serine–threonine kinase activity and associate with proteins from the Smad family, which are gene-specific transcription factors (see Fig. 11.9C). This superfamily includes (1) transforming growth factor β (TGF-β), a cytokine/hormone involved in tissue repair, immune regulation, and cell proliferation; and (2) bone morphogenetic proteins (BMPs), which control proliferation, differentiation, and cell death during development.

A simplified version of TGF-β binding to its receptor complex and activating Smads is illustrated in Figure 11.16. The TGF-β receptor complex is composed of two different single membrane-spanning receptor subunits (type I and type II), which have different functions even though they both have serine kinase domains.

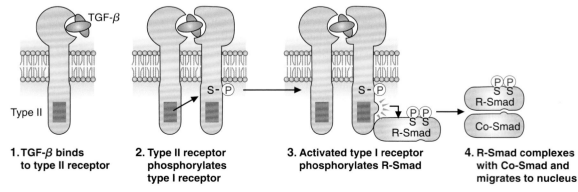

FIGURE 11.16 Serine–threonine receptors and Smad proteins. Transforming growth factor β (TGF-β), which is composed of two identical subunits, communicates through a receptor dimer of type I and type II subunits that have serine kinase domains. The type I receptor phosphorylates an R-Smad (receptor-specific Smad), which binds a Co-Smad (common Smad, also called Smad 4). The Smad dimer then translocates to the nucleus to activate or inhibit the expression of target genes.

TGF-β binds to a type II receptor. The activated type II receptor recruits a type I receptor, which it phosphorylates at a serine residue, forming an activated receptor complex. The type I receptor then binds a receptor-specific Smad protein (called an *R-Smad*), which it phosphorylates on serine residues. The phosphorylated R-Smad undergoes a conformational change and dissociates from the receptor. It then forms a complex with another member of the Smad family, Smad 4 (Smad 4 is known as the *common Smad, Co-Smad*, and is not phosphorylated). The Smad complex, which may contain several Smads, translocates to the nucleus, where it activates or inhibits the transcription of target genes. Receptors for distinct ligands bind different Smads, which bind to alternative sites on DNA and regulate the transcription of different sets of genes. There is also an inhibitory Smad that is activated which acts to regulate the extent of Smad activation (another example of signal termination).

E. Signal Transduction through Heptahelical Receptors

The heptahelical receptors are named for their seven membrane-spanning domains, which are α-helices (see Fig. 11.10; see also Fig. 7.9). Although hundreds of hormones and neurotransmitters work through heptahelical receptors, the extracellular binding domain of each receptor is specific for just one polypeptide hormone, catecholamine, or neurotransmitter (or a close structural analog). Heptahelical receptors have no intrinsic kinase activity but initiate signal transduction through heterotrimeric G-proteins composed of α-, β-, and γ-subunits. However, different types of heptahelical receptors bind different G-proteins, and different G-proteins exert different effects on their target proteins. The activation of the G-protein leads to second messenger production within the cells. Second messengers are present in low concentrations so that modulation of their level, and hence the message, can be rapidly initiated and terminated.

I. Heterotrimeric G-Proteins

The function of heterotrimeric G-proteins is illustrated in Figure 11.17 using a hormone that activates adenylyl cyclase (e.g., glucagon or epinephrine). While the α-subunit contains bound GDP, it remains associated with the β- and γ-subunits, either free in the membrane or bound to an unoccupied receptor (see Fig. 11.17, part 1). When the hormone binds, it causes a conformational change in the receptor that promotes GDP dissociation and GTP binding. The exchange of GTP for bound GDP causes dissociation of the α-subunit from the receptor and from the β- and γ-subunits (see Fig. 11.17, part 2). The α- and γ-subunits are tethered to the intracellular side of the plasma membrane through lipid anchors, but the subunits can still move laterally on the membrane surface. The GTP α-subunit binds its target enzyme in the membrane, thereby changing its activity. In this example, the α-subunit binds and activates adenylyl cyclase, thereby increasing synthesis of cAMP (see Fig. 11.17, part 3).

With time, the Gα-subunit inactivates itself by hydrolyzing its own bound GTP to GDP and inorganic phosphate (P_i) (an intrinsic GTPase activity). This action is unrelated to the number of cAMP molecules formed. Like the monomeric G-proteins, the α-subunit now containing GDP dissociates from its target protein, adenylyl cyclase (see Fig. 11.17, part 4). It reforms the trimeric G-protein complex, which may return to bind the empty hormone receptor. As a result of this GTPase "internal clock," sustained elevation of hormone levels is necessary for continued signal transduction and elevation of cAMP. G-proteins in which the internal clock has become defective (either through mutation or modification by toxins) can become permanently activated, thereby continuously stimulating their signal transduction pathway.

There are a large number of different heterotrimeric G-protein complexes which are generally categorized according to the activity of the α-subunit (Table 11.1). The 20 or so different isoforms of Gα fall into five broad categories: $G\alpha_s$, $G\alpha_{i/o}$, $G\alpha_t$, $G\alpha_{q/11}$, and $G\alpha_{12/13}$. $G\alpha_s$ refers to α-*subunits*, which, like the one in Figure 11.17, stimulate adenylyl cyclase (hence the *s*). Gα-subunits that inhibit adenylyl cyclase are called $G\alpha_i$. The β- and γ-subunits likewise exist as different isoforms, which also transmit messages. $G\alpha_{qs}$ subunits activate phospholipase C_β, which generates

ACh has two types of receptors: nicotinic ion-channel receptors (the receptors inhibited by antibodies in myasthenia gravis) and muscarinic receptors (which exist as a variety of subtypes). The M2 muscarinic receptors activate a $G\alpha_{i/o}$ heterotrimeric G-protein in which release of the βγ-subunit controls K^+ channels and pacemaker activity in the heart. Epinephrine has several types and subtypes of heptahelical receptors: β-Adrenergic receptors work through a $G\alpha_s$ and stimulate adenylyl cyclase, α_2-adrenergic receptors in other cells work through a $G\alpha_i$ protein and inhibit adenylyl cyclase, and α_1-adrenergic receptors work through $G\alpha_q$ subunits and activate phospholipase C_β. This variety in receptor types allows a messenger to have different actions in different cells.

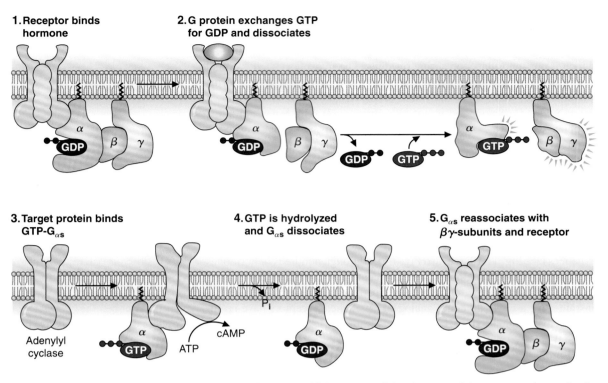

1. Receptor binds hormone

2. G protein exchanges GTP for GDP and dissociates

3. Target protein binds GTP-G$_{\alpha s}$

Adenylyl cyclase

ATP

cAMP

4. GTP is hydrolyzed and G$_{\alpha s}$ dissociates

P$_i$

5. G$_{\alpha s}$ reassociates with βγ-subunits and receptor

FIGURE 11.17 Serpentine receptors and heterotrimeric G-proteins. (*1*) The intracellular domains of the receptor form a binding site for a G-protein that contains guanosine diphosphate (GDP) bound to the α-subunit. (*2*) Hormone binding to the receptor promotes the exchange of guanosine triphosphate (GTP) for GDP. As a result, the complex disassembles, releasing the G-protein α-subunit from the β–γ complex. (*3*) The G$_s$ α-subunit binds to a target enzyme (in the example shown, the target is adenylyl cyclase), thereby changing its activity (for the "s" G-proteins, the activity is stimulated). The β–γ complex may simultaneously target another protein and change its activity. (*4*) Over time, bound GTP is hydrolyzed to GDP, causing dissociation of the α-subunit from the target protein, thereby reducing the activity of the target protein. (*5*) The GDP α-subunit reassociates with the βγ-subunit and the hormone receptor. *ATP*, adenosine triphosphate; *cAMP*, 3′,5′-cyclic adenosine monophosphate.

second messengers based on phosphatidylinositol. Gα$_t$ subunits activate cGMP phosphodiesterase. Gα$_{12/13}$ subunits activate a GEF, which activates the small GTP-binding protein Rho, which is involved in cytoskeletal alterations.

2. Adenylyl Cyclase and cAMP Phosphodiesterase

cAMP is referred to as a *second messenger* because changes in its concentration reflect changes in the concentration of the hormone (the first messenger). When a hormone binds and adenylyl cyclase is activated, it synthesizes cAMP from ATP.

TABLE 11.1 Subunits of Heterotrimeric G-Proteins

Gα-SUBUNIT	ACTION	SOME PHYSIOLOGIC USES
α$_s$; Gα(s)[a]	Stimulates adenylyl cyclase	Glucagon and epinephrine to regulate metabolic enzymes, regulatory polypeptide hormones to control steroid hormone and thyroid hormone synthesis, and by some neurotransmitters (e.g., dopamine) to control ion channels
α$_{i/o}$; Gα(i/o) (signal also flows through βγ-subunits)	Inhibits adenylyl cyclase	Epinephrine; many neurotransmitters, including acetylcholine, dopamine, serotonin
α$_t$; Gα(t)	Stimulates cGMP phosphodiesterase	Has a role in the transducin pathway, which mediates detection of light in the eye
α$_{q/11}$; Gα(q/11)	Activates phospholipase C$_\beta$	Epinephrine, acetylcholine, histamine, thyroid-stimulating hormone (TSH), interleukin-8, somatostatin, angiotensin
α$_{12/13}$; Gα(12/13)	Activate Rho-GEF (guanine nucleotide exchange factor)	Thromboxane A2, lysophosphatidic acid act as signals to alter cytoskeletal elements

cGMP, cyclic guanosine monophosphate.

[a] There is a growing tendency to designate the heterotrimeric G-protein subunits without using subscripts so that they are actually visible to the naked eye.

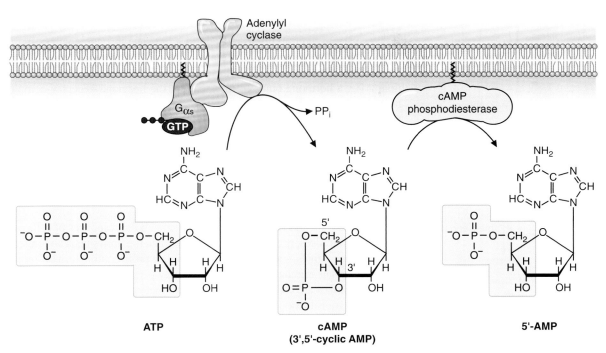

FIGURE 11.18 Formation and cleavage of the cyclic phosphodiester bond in 3′,5′-cyclic adenosine monophosphate (cAMP). When activated by Gα$_s$, adenylyl cyclase converts adenosine triphosphate (ATP) to cAMP + pyrophosphate (PP$_i$). cAMP phosphodiesterase hydrolyzes cAMP to 5′-AMP.

cAMP is hydrolyzed to AMP by cAMP phosphodiesterase, which also resides in the plasma membrane (Fig. 11.18). The concentration of cAMP and other second messengers is kept at very low levels in cells by balancing the activity of these two enzymes (the cyclase and the phosphodiesterase) so that cAMP levels can change rapidly when hormone levels change. Some hormones change the concentration of cAMP by targeting the phosphodiesterase enzyme rather than adenylyl cyclase. For example, insulin lowers cAMP levels by causing phosphodiesterase activation.

cAMP exerts diverse effects in cells. It is an allosteric activator of protein kinase A (PKA) (see Chapter 9, Section III.B.3), which is a serine–threonine protein kinase that phosphorylates a large number of metabolic enzymes, thereby providing a rapid response to hormones like glucagon and epinephrine. It is also the enzyme that phosphorylates the CFTR, activating the channel. PKA substrates also include, among many, phosphorylase kinase (regulation of glycogen degradation) and phospholamban (regulation of cardiac contractility). The catalytic subunits of PKA also enter the nucleus and phosphorylate a gene-specific transcription factor called *cyclic-AMP response element-binding protein* (CREB). Thus, cAMP also activates a slower response pathway, gene transcription. In other cell types, cAMP activates ligand-gated channels directly.

Some signaling pathways cross from the receptor tyrosine kinase pathway of MAP kinase activation to CREB activation, and the heterotrimeric G-protein pathways diverge to include a route to the MAP kinase pathway. These types of complex interconnections in signaling pathways are sometimes called *hormone cross-talk*.

3. Phosphatidylinositol Signaling by Heptahelical Receptors

Certain heptahelical receptors bind the q isoform of the Gα-subunit (Gα$_q$), which activates the target enzyme phospholipase C$_\beta$ (see Fig. 11.12). When it is activated, phospholipase C$_\beta$ hydrolyzes the membrane lipid PI-4,5-bisP into two second messengers, DAG and IP$_3$. IP$_3$ has a binding site in the sarcoplasmic reticulum and the endoplasmic reticulum that stimulates the release of Ca^{2+}. Ca^{2+} activates enzymes containing the calcium–calmodulin subunit, including a protein kinase. DAG, which remains in the membrane, activates protein kinase C, which then propagates the response by phosphorylating target proteins.

 Dennis V. was hospitalized for dehydration resulting from cholera toxin (see Chapter 10). The cholera toxin A-subunit was absorbed into the intestinal mucosal cells where it was processed and complexed with adenosine diphosphate [ADP]-ribosylation factor (Arf), a small G-protein that is normally involved in vesicular transport. Cholera A toxin is a nicotinamide adenine dinucleotide (NAD)-glycohydrolase, which cleaves NAD and transfers the ADP-ribose portion to other proteins. It ADP-ribosylates the Gα$_s$ subunit of heterotrimeric G-proteins, thereby inhibiting their GTPase activity. As a consequence, they remain actively bound to adenylyl cyclase, resulting in increased production of cAMP. The CFTR channel is activated, resulting in secretion of chloride ion and Na$^+$ ion into the intestinal lumen. The ion secretion is followed by loss of water, resulting in vomiting and watery diarrhea.

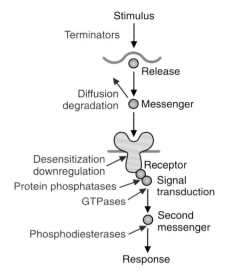

FIGURE 11.19 Sites of signal termination. Processes that terminate signals are shown in *red*.

F. Changes in Response to Signals

Tissues vary in their ability to respond to a message through changes in receptor activity or number. Many receptors contain intracellular phosphorylation sites that alter their ability to transmit signals. Receptor number is also varied through downregulation. After a hormone binds to the receptor, the hormone–receptor complex may be taken into the cell by the process of endocytosis in clathrin-coated pits (see Chapter 10, Section II.C) The receptors may be degraded or recycled back to the cell surface. This internalization of receptors decreases the number available on the surface under conditions of constant high hormone levels when hormones occupy more of the receptors and results in decreased synthesis of new receptors. Hence, it is called *downregulation*.

IV. Signal Termination

Some signals, such as those that modify the metabolic responses of cells or that transmit neural impulses, need to turn off rapidly when the hormone is no longer being produced. Other signals, such as those that stimulate proliferation, turn off more slowly. In contrast, signals regulating differentiation may persist throughout our lifetime. Many chronic diseases are caused by failure to terminate a response at the appropriate time.

Signal transduction pathways can be terminated by a variety of means (Fig. 11.19). The first level of termination is the chemical messenger itself. When the stimulus is no longer applied to the secreting cell, the messenger is no longer secreted and existing messenger is catabolized. For example, many polypeptide hormones such as insulin are taken up into the liver and degraded. Termination of the ACh signal by acetylcholinesterase has already been mentioned.

Within each pathway of signal transduction, the signal may be turned off at specific steps. For example, serpentine receptors can be desensitized to the messenger by phosphorylation, internalization, and degradation. G-proteins, both monomeric and heterotrimeric, automatically terminate messages as they hydrolyze GTP via their intrinsic GTPase activity. Although G-proteins do have intrinsic GTPase activity, this activity is relatively weak and can be accelerated through interaction with a class of proteins known as *GTPase-activating proteins* (GAPs). Termination also can be achieved through degradation of the second messenger (e.g., phosphodiesterase cleavage of cAMP). Each of these terminating processes is also highly regulated.

Another important pathway for reversing the message typically used by receptor kinase pathways is through protein phosphatases, enzymes that reverse the action of kinases by removing phosphate groups from proteins. These are specific tyrosine or serine–threonine phosphatases (enzymes that remove the phosphate group from specific proteins) for all of the sites that are phosphorylated by signal transduction kinases. There are even receptors that are protein phosphatases.

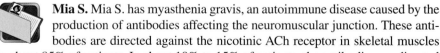

CLINICAL COMMENTS

Mia S. Mia S. has myasthenia gravis, an autoimmune disease caused by the production of antibodies affecting the neuromuscular junction. These antibodies are directed against the nicotinic ACh receptor in skeletal muscles in about 85% of patients. In about 10% to 15% of patients, the antibodies are directed against other proteins in the neuromuscular junction. The diagnosis is made by history (presence of typical muscular symptoms), physical examination (presence of inability to do specific repetitive muscular activity over time), and the presence of antibodies against ACh receptors. The diagnosis can be further confirmed by neurophysiologic testing, including a diagnostic procedure involving repetitive electrical nerve stimulation and an electromyogram (EMG) showing a partial blockade of ion flux across muscular membranes. The prognosis for this otherwise debilitating disease has improved dramatically with the advent of new therapies. Virtually all myasthenia patients can live full, productive lives with proper treatment. These therapies include anticholinesterase agents; immunosuppressive drugs, such as glucocorticoids, azathioprine, or mycophenolate; thymectomy (removal of the thymus gland, which offers long-term benefit that may eliminate the need for a continuing medical therapy by reducing immunoreactivity); intravenous immunoglobulin (IVIG; which decreases the effect the effect of autoantibodies); and plasmapheresis (which reduces anti-ACh receptor antibody levels). IVIG and plasmapheresis are reserved as a means of rapidly helping the patient through a period of serious myasthenia signs and symptoms.

Ann R. Anorexia nervosa presents as a distorted visual self-image often associated with compulsive exercise. Although Ann has been gaining weight, she is still relatively low on stored fuels needed to sustain the metabolic requirements of exercise. Her prolonged starvation has resulted in release of the steroid hormone cortisol and the polypeptide hormone glucagon, whereas levels of the polypeptide hormone insulin have decreased. Cortisol activates transcription of genes for some of the enzymes of gluconeogenesis (the synthesis of glucose from amino acids and other precursors; see Chapter 3). Glucagon binds to heptahelical receptors in liver and adipose tissue and, working through cAMP and PKA, activates many enzymes involved in fasting fuel metabolism. Insulin, which is released when Ann drinks her high-energy supplement, works through a specialized tyrosine kinase receptor to promote fuel storage. Epinephrine, a catecholamine released when she exercises, promotes fuel mobilization.

Dennis V. In the emergency department, Dennis received intravenous rehydration therapy (normal saline [0.9% NaCl]) and oral hydration therapy containing Na^+, K^+, and glucose or a digest of rice (which contains glucose and amino acids). Glucose is absorbed from the intestinal lumen via the sodium-dependent glucose cotransporters, which cotransport Na^+ into the cells together with glucose. Many amino acids are also absorbed by Na^+-dependent cotransport. With the return of Na^+ to the cytoplasm, water efflux from the cell into the intestinal lumen decreases. Dennis quickly recovered from his bout of cholera. Cholera is self-limiting, possibly because the bacteria remain in the intestine, where they are washed out of the system by the diffuse watery diarrhea. Antibiotics (tetracycline or doxycycline) can also be used, particularly in severe cases, to decrease the duration of the diarrhea and vibrio excretion. Over the past 3 years, **Percy V.** has persevered through the death of his wife and the subsequent calamities of his grandson Dennis V., including salicylate poisoning, suspected malathion poisoning, and now cholera. Mr. V. has decided to send his grandson home for the remainder of the summer.

BIOCHEMICAL COMMENTS

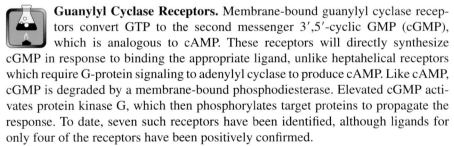

Guanylyl Cyclase Receptors. Membrane-bound guanylyl cyclase receptors convert GTP to the second messenger 3',5'-cyclic GMP (cGMP), which is analogous to cAMP. These receptors will directly synthesize cGMP in response to binding the appropriate ligand, unlike heptahelical receptors which require G-protein signaling to adenylyl cyclase to produce cAMP. Like cAMP, cGMP is degraded by a membrane-bound phosphodiesterase. Elevated cGMP activates protein kinase G, which then phosphorylates target proteins to propagate the response. To date, seven such receptors have been identified, although ligands for only four of the receptors have been positively confirmed.

A soluble form of guanylyl cyclase exists, located in the cytoplasm, and is a receptor for nitric oxide (NO), a neurotransmitter/neurohormone. NO is a lipophilic gas that is able to diffuse into the cell. This receptor thus is an exception to the rule that intracellular receptors are gene transcription factors. The membrane-bound receptors will bind atrial natriuretic peptide, brain natriuretic peptide, and C-type natriuretic peptide, as well as guanylin.

cGMP-elevating drugs have been used in humans to treat a variety of disorders such as angina pectoris (glycerol trinitrate decomposes to NO, which activates a guanylyl cyclase), heart failure (using nesiritide, which is synthetic β-natriuretic peptide, a ligand for activation of a guanylyl cyclase receptor), and erectile dysfunction (through drugs that inhibit a cGMP phosphodiesterase [designated PDE5], such as sildenafil).

A laboratory test to confirm the diagnosis of myasthenia gravis uses the patient's sera as a source of antibodies directed against the ACh receptor. Human cell lines, grown in the laboratory and producing the ACh receptor, are used as a source of soluble receptor (the cells are lysed and a solubilized membrane fraction, which contains the receptor, is obtained). The soluble receptor is incubated with radioactively labeled α-bungarotoxin, which binds very specifically and tightly to the ACh receptor. A sample of the patient's sera is incubated with the bungarotoxin–receptor complex, and the extent to which antibodies bind to the receptor complex is determined as a measurement of reduced bungarotoxin binding to the receptor. A positive result indicates the presence of anti-ACh receptor antibodies in the sera.

KEY CONCEPTS

- In order to integrate cellular function with the needs of the organism, cells communicate with each other via chemical messengers. Chemical messengers include neurotransmitters (for the nervous system), hormones (for the endocrine system), cytokines (for the immune system), retinoids, eicosanoids, and growth factors.
- Chemical messengers transmit their signals by binding to receptors on target cells. When a messenger binds to a receptor, a signal transduction pathway is activated which generates second messengers within the cell.
- Receptors can be either plasma membrane proteins or intracellular binding proteins.
- Intracellular receptors act primarily as transcription factors, which regulate gene expression in response to a signal being released.
- Plasma membrane receptors fall into different classes, such as ion-channel receptors, tyrosine kinase receptors, tyrosine kinase–associated receptors, serine–threonine kinase receptors, or G-protein–coupled receptors (GPCRs), also known as *serpentine receptors*.
  - Ion-channel receptors respond to a stimulus by allowing ion flux across the membrane.
  - Tyrosine kinase and tyrosine kinase–associated receptors respond to a stimulus through activation of a tyrosine kinase activity, which phosphorylates specific target proteins to elicit a cellular response.
  - Serine–threonine kinase receptors respond to a stimulus that activates a serine–threonine kinase, which then transmits signals through activation of Smad proteins, which are transcription factors.
  - GPCRs respond to a stimulus by activating a guanine nucleotide-binding protein (G-protein), which, in its activated GTP-binding state, activates a target protein. G-proteins contain intrinsic GTPase activity, thereby limiting the time for which they are active.
- Signal termination can occur via a variety of mechanisms such as destruction of the chemical messenger; inactivation of second messages, such as loss of cAMP; or removal of covalent bonds added as a result of the primary message (e.g., dephosphorylation).
- Diseases discussed in this chapter are summarized in Table 11.2.

TABLE 11.2   Diseases Discussed in Chapter 11

DISORDER OR CONDITION	GENETIC OR ENVIRONMENTAL	COMMENTS
Myasthenia gravis	Environmental	Autoantibodies to the acetylcholine receptor (and others at the neuromuscular junction), leading to neuromuscular dysfunction.
Cholera	Environmental	Watery diarrhea leading to dehydration and hypovolemic shock caused by cholera toxin ADP-ribosylating a class of G-proteins, altering their function and affecting water and salt transport across the intestinal mucosa. Main treatment is with a glucose–electrolyte solution to increase coupled glucose–sodium uptake into the intestinal epithelial cells, reversing the loss of water from these cells.
Anorexia nervosa	Both	Effects of inadequate nutrition on hormone release and response. Cortisol, glucagon, and epinephrine levels are all increased under these conditions.

ADP, adenosine diphosphate.

REVIEW QUESTIONS—CHAPTER 11

Questions 1 and 2 are based on the following patient.

1. A patient has severe weakness of a muscle group after repeatedly contracting that muscle group. After rest, the muscle appears to function normally unless repeatedly contracted again. The antibody causing this disease process would directly affect which one of the following?
   A. The number of ACh vesicles
   B. Voltage-gated Ca^{2+} channels
   C. Na^+ and K^+ gradients
   D. ACh receptors in smooth muscle
   E. ACh receptors in skeletal muscle

2. In the patient described in the previous question, ACh and other similar neurotransmitters use which one of the following modes of action to transmit their signal?
   A. Endocrine
   B. Paracrine
   C. Autocrine
   D. Neuropeptide
   E. Cytokine

Use the following information to answer Questions 3 and 4. You do not need to know more about parathyroid hormone or pseudohypoparathyroidism than the information given.

Pseudohypoparathyroidism is a heritable disorder caused by target-organ unresponsiveness to parathyroid hormone (a polypeptide hormone secreted by the parathyroid gland). One of the mutations that causes this disease occurs in the gene encoding $G\alpha_s$ in certain cells.

3. The receptor for parathyroid hormone is most likely which one of the following?
   A. An intracellular transcription factor
   B. A cytoplasmic guanylyl cyclase
   C. A receptor that must be endocytosed in clathrin-coated pits to transmit its signal
   D. A heptahelical receptor
   E. A tyrosine kinase receptor

4. This mutation most likely has which one of the following characteristics?
   A. It is a gain-of-function mutation.
   B. It decreases the GTPase activity of the $G\alpha_s$ subunit.
   C. It decreases synthesis of cAMP in response to parathyroid hormone.
   D. It decreases generation of IP_3 in response to parathyroid hormone.
   E. It decreases synthesis of PI-3,4,5-trisP in response to parathyroid hormone.

5. Techniques are available to allow one to introduce mutations in proteins at a selected amino acid residue (site-directed mutagenesis). Which step of the signal transduction pathway would be blocked if you created a tyrosine kinase receptor in which all of the tyrosine residues normally phosphorylated on the receptor were converted to phenylalanine residues?
   A. Grb2 binding to the receptor to propagate the response
   B. Binding of the growth factor to the receptor
   C. Induction of a conformational change in the receptor upon growth factor binding
   D. Activation of the receptor's intrinsic tyrosine kinase activity
   E. Dimerization of the receptors

6. A patient has been diagnosed with a glucagonoma, a pancreatic tumor that independently and episodically secretes glucagon. Which one of the following would be expected in this patient?
   A. Low serum glucose
   B. Increased glycogenolysis in the liver
   C. Increased glycogenolysis in muscle tissue
   D. Increased glycogenesis in the liver
   E. Increased glycogenesis in muscle tissue

7. Curare has been given as a paralyzing agent in patients undergoing surgical procedures, and its mode of action is best described by inhibiting the action of which one of the following?
   A. Atropine
   B. Muscarinic receptors
   C. Nicotinic receptors
   D. The formation of ACh
   E. The breakdown of ACh

8. A patient with allergies is taking a drug that blocks the actions of leukotrienes. The leukotrienes are derived from which one of the following molecules?
   A. Oleic acid
   B. Linolenic acid
   C. Stearic acid
   D. Arachidonic acid
   E. Palmitic acid

9. A pheochromocytoma is an adrenal tumor that episodically produces epinephrine and/or norepinephrine. Tissues that respond to these adrenal hormones must express which one of the following?
   A. A tyrosine kinase receptor
   B. An intracellular receptor
   C. A ligand-gated receptor
   D. The Smad transcription factor
   E. A heptahelical receptor

10. A male with chronic alcoholism and cirrhosis of the liver has low sexual desire, poor sexual functioning, a need to shave only every 3 days, and normal-sized testicles. Which one of the following best explains these symptoms?
   A. Increased MEOS (microsomal ethanol oxidizing system)
   B. Decreased MEOS (microsomal ethanol oxidizing system)
   C. Normal thyroid hormone
   D. Low serum albumin
   E. Low plasma membrane receptors

1. **The answer is E.** This patient has myasthenia gravis caused by the production of an antibody directed against ACh receptors in skeletal muscles (not smooth muscle), resulting in fewer functional receptors but not affecting the number of ACh vesicles, Na^+ and K^+ gradients, or voltage-gated Ca^{2+} channels.

2. **The answer is B.** Endocrine action is defined as a hormone secreted by a specific cell type with action on specific target cells usually some distance away. Paracrine actions are hormones secreted by a cell and binding to nearby cells. Autocrine action involves a messenger that acts on the cell from which it was secreted. ACh activates only those ACh receptors located across the synaptic cleft from the signaling nerve and not every cell that contains ACh receptors. ACh is a nitrogen-containing small-molecule neurotransmitter or biogenic amine, not a neuropeptide. Cytokines are messengers of the immune system.

3. **The answer is D.** Parathyroid hormone is a polypeptide hormone and thus must bind to a plasma membrane receptor instead of an intracellular receptor (thus, A and B are incorrect). Hormones that bind to plasma membrane receptors do not need to enter the cell to transmit their signals (thus, C is incorrect). Heptahelical receptors work through heterotrimeric G-proteins that have an α-subunit, and tyrosine kinase receptors work through monomeric G-proteins that have no subunits (thus, D is correct and E is incorrect).

4. **The answer is C.** $Gα_s$ normally activates adenylyl cyclase to generate cAMP in response to parathyroid hormone. Because the patient has end-organ unresponsiveness, he must have a deficiency in the signaling pathway (thus, A is incorrect) and cAMP will be decreased. Decreased GTPase activity will increase binding to adenylyl cyclase and increase responsiveness (thus, B is incorrect). Neither IP_3 nor PI-3,4,5-trisP is involved in signal transduction by the $Gα_s$ subunit.

5. **The answer is A.** Grb2 binding to the receptor requires phosphotyrosine residues on the receptor. Grb2 normally binds to the receptor through its SH2 domains, which recognize phosphotyrosine residues on the receptor. In the absence of these phosphotyrosine residues, Grb2 would not be able to bind to the receptor. Growth factor binding to the receptor does not require phosphotyrosine residues. It is the binding of the growth factor to the receptor, through a conformational change in the receptor that activates the intrinsic tyrosine kinase of the receptor, which then leads to autophosphorylation of the receptor. The lack of intracellular tyrosine residues on the receptor will not alter the events initiated by the

conformational change of the receptor. Dimerization of receptors occurs upon binding growth factor and is not dependent on the activation of the tyrosine kinase activity or on autophosphorylation of the receptor.

6. **The answer is B.** Glucagon increases blood/serum glucose by stimulating the release of glucose from liver glycogen stores. Liver parenchymal cells express glucagon receptors but muscle cells do not, so muscle cells do not respond to glucagon. Glucagon therefore stimulates liver glycogenolysis but has no effect on muscle cells. Glycogenesis, the synthesis of glycogen, is an effect of insulin but not glucagon.

7. **The answer is C.** Curare is an inhibitor of nicotinic (skeletal and parasympathetic) ACh receptors causing muscle paralysis, but curare does not affect the heart or the sympathetic nervous system (which express muscarinic ACh receptors). Curare inhibits only ACh receptors, not ACh production or elimination. Atropine blocks the effects of excess ACh and is a completely different medication than curare.

8. **The answer is D.** PG, thromboxanes, and leukotrienes are eicosanoids and are all derived from arachidonic acid, a 20-carbon fatty acid derived from linoleic acid (an essential fatty acid). Arachidonic acid cannot be derived from any of the other fatty acids listed as possible answers.

9. **The answer is E.** Catecholamines are polar molecules that are not hydrophobic and cannot rapidly cross the plasma membrane (they do not bind to an intracellular receptor). They must bind to a plasma membrane receptor, which in this case is a heptahelical receptor linked to a G-protein. Catecholamines do not directly activate tyrosine kinase receptors or ligand-gated receptors, nor do they lead to the activation of Smad (which is a function of TGF-β receptors).

10. **The answer is D.** The patient is manifesting a low functioning level of testosterone. Testosterone is a steroid hormone that is lipophilic (hydrophobic) and must be transported in blood bound to albumin. Alcoholics with cirrhosis produce less albumin than normal and are usually protein-malnourished, which further decreases serum albumin. The low serum albumin thus decreases functional or transported levels of testosterone. Normal-sized testicles imply normal production of testosterone. MEOS helps to metabolize alcohol but has nothing to do with testosterone. Being a hydrophobic molecule, testosterone diffuses through the plasma membrane and does not use a plasma membrane receptor; it binds to an intracellular transcription factor receptor. Expressing normal thyroid hormone would not produce any of these symptoms.

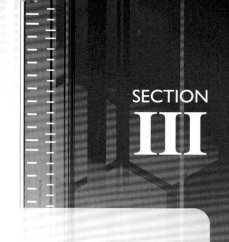

Gene Expression and the Synthesis of Proteins

In the middle of the 20th century, DNA was identified as the genetic material and its structure was determined. Using this knowledge, researchers then discovered the mechanisms by which genetic information is inherited and expressed. During the last quarter of the 20th century, our understanding of this critical area of science, known as *molecular biology*, grew at an increasingly rapid pace. We now have techniques to probe the human genome that will completely revolutionize the way medicine is practiced in the 21st century.

The genome of a cell consists of all its genetic information, encoded in DNA. In eukaryotes, DNA is located mainly in nuclei, but small amounts are also found in mitochondria. Nuclear genes are packaged in chromosomes that contain DNA and protein in tightly coiled structures (Chapter 12).

The molecular mechanism of inheritance involves a process known as *replication*, in which the strands of parental DNA serve as templates for the synthesis of DNA copies (Fig. III.1) (Chapter 13). After DNA replication, cells divide, and these DNA copies are passed to daughter cells. Alterations in genetic material occur by recombination (the exchange of genetic material between chromosomes) and by mutation (the result of chemical changes that alter DNA). DNA repair mechanisms correct much of this damage, but, nevertheless, many gene alterations are passed to daughter cells.

The expression of genes within cells requires two processes: transcription and translation (see Fig. III.1) (Chapters 14 and 15). DNA is transcribed to produce RNA. Three major types of RNA are transcribed from DNA and subsequently participate in the process of translation (the synthesis of proteins). Messenger RNA (mRNA) carries the genetic information from the nucleus to the cytoplasm, where translation occurs on ribosomes—structures that contain proteins complexed with ribosomal RNA (rRNA). Transfer RNA (tRNA) carries individual amino acids to the ribosomes, where they are joined in peptide linkage to form proteins. During translation, the sequence of nucleic acid bases in mRNA is read in sets of three (each set of three bases constitutes a codon). The sequence of codons in the mRNA dictates the sequence of amino acids in the protein. Proteins function in cell structure, signaling, and catalysis and, therefore, determine the appearance and behavior of cells and the organism as a whole. The regulation of gene expression (Chapter 16) determines which proteins are synthesized and the amount synthesized at any time, thus allowing cells to undergo development and differentiation and to respond to changing environmental conditions.

Research in molecular biology has produced a host of techniques, known collectively as *recombinant DNA technology*, *biotechnology*, or *genetic engineering*, that can be used for the diagnosis and treatment of disease (Chapter 17). These techniques can detect a number of genetic diseases that previously could only be diagnosed after symptoms appeared. Diagnosis of these diseases can now be made with considerable accuracy even before birth, and carriers of these diseases also can be identified.

 Many drugs used in medicine to treat bacterial infections are targeted to interfere with the bacteria's ability to synthesize RNA and proteins. Thus, medical students need to know the basics of bacterial DNA replication, RNA synthesis, and protein synthesis to understand the mechanism of action of these drugs.

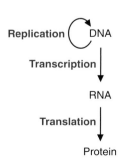

Replication DNA

Transcription

RNA

Translation

Protein

FIGURE III.1 Replication, transcription, and translation. Replication: DNA serves as a template for producing DNA copies. Transcription: DNA serves as a template for the synthesis of RNA. Translation: RNA provides the information for the synthesis of proteins.

Ethical dilemmas have come together with technological advances in molecular biology. Consider the case of a patient with a mild case of ornithine transcarbamoylase deficiency, a urea-cycle defect that, if untreated, leads to elevated ammonia levels and nervous system dysfunction. The patient was being treated effectively by dietary restriction of protein. However, in 1999, he was treated with a common virus carrying the normal gene for ornithine transcarbamoylase. The patient developed a severe immune response to the virus and died as a result of the treatment. This case history raises the issues of appropriate patient consent, appropriate criteria to be included in this type of study, and the types of diseases for which gene therapy is appropriate. These are issues that are still applicable over 15 years after this unfortunate incident, and that you, the student, will be facing as you enter your practice of medicine.

Tumors may be benign or malignant. A tumor is malignant if it invades locally or if cells break away from the tumor, enter the blood stream, and travel to other parts of the body where they establish new growths (a process called *metastasis*), resulting in destruction of the tissues they invade. Many of the drugs used to treat malignant tumors are directed toward inhibition of DNA replication. These chemotherapeutic drugs are more toxic to cancer cells than to normal cells because the cancer cells divide more rapidly. However, such drugs also may inhibit normal rapidly dividing cells, such as the cells of the bone marrow (causing a decrease in white blood cell count) or cells in the hair follicles (resulting in hair loss during chemotherapy).

With recent developments in the field of gene therapy, diseases that for centuries have been considered hopeless are now potentially curable. Much of the therapy for these diseases is currently experimental. However, during the 21st century, physicians may be using genetic engineering techniques routinely for both the diagnosis and treatment of their patients.

Replication and cell division are highly regulated processes in the human. *Cancer* is a group of diseases in which a cell in the body has been transformed and begins to grow and divide out of control (Chapter 18). It results from multiple mutations or changes in DNA structure in the genes that activate cell growth, called *proto-oncogenes*, and those that ensure that DNA replication and repair are normal, called *growth-suppressor* or *tumor-suppressor genes*. Mutations that activate proto-oncogenes to oncogenes disturb the regulation of the cell cycle and the rate of cell proliferation. Mutations that disrupt tumor-suppressor genes lead to an increased incidence of these proto-oncogene–activating mutations. Such mutations may be inherited, causing a predisposition to a type of cancer. They also may arise from DNA replication or copying errors that remain uncorrected, from chemicals or radiation that damages DNA, from translocation of pieces of chromosomes from one chromosome to another during replication, or from incorporation of viral-encoded DNA into the genome.

Structure of the Nucleic Acids

Nucleotides in DNA and RNA. Nucleotides are the monomeric units of the nucleic acids DNA and RNA. Each nucleotide consists of a heterocyclic **nitrogenous base**, a **sugar**, and **phosphate. DNA** contains the purine bases **adenine** (A) and **guanine** (G) and the pyrimidine bases **cytosine** (C) and **thymine** (T). **RNA** contains A, G, and C, but it has **uracil** (U) instead of thymine. In DNA, the sugar is **deoxyribose**, whereas in RNA, it is **ribose**.

Polynucleotides such as DNA and RNA are linear sequences of nucleotides linked by **3'- to 5'-phosphodiester bonds** between the sugars (Fig. 12.1). The bases of the nucleotides can interact with other bases or with proteins.

DNA Structure. Genetic information is encoded by the sequence of different nucleotide bases in DNA. **DNA** is **double-stranded**; it contains **two antiparallel polynucleotide strands.** The two strands are joined by hydrogen bonding between their bases to form **base pairs. Adenine** pairs with **thymine**, and **guanine** pairs with **cytosine.** The two DNA strands run in **opposite directions**. One strand runs in a 5'-to-3' direction, and the other strand runs in a 3'-to-5' direction. The two DNA strands wind around each other, forming a **double helix**.

Transcription of a gene generates a **single-stranded RNA** that is identical in nucleotide sequence to one of the strands of the duplex DNA. The three major types of RNA are **messenger RNA** (mRNA), **ribosomal RNA** (rRNA), and **transfer RNA** (tRNA).

RNA Structures. mRNAs contain the nucleotide sequence that is converted into the amino acid sequence of a protein in the process of translation. Eukaryotic mRNA has a structure known as a **cap** at the 5'-end, a sequence of adenine nucleotides (a **poly[A] tail**) at the 3'-end, and a **coding region** in between containing **codons** that dictate the sequence of amino acids in a protein or relay a signal. Each codon in the genetic code is a different sequence of three nucleotides.

rRNAs and tRNAs are part of the apparatus for protein synthesis, but they do not encode proteins. **rRNA** has **extensive internal base pairing** and complexes with proteins to form **ribonucleoprotein particles** called **ribosomes.** The ribosomes bind mRNA and tRNAs during translation. Each **tRNA** binds and **activates a specific amino acid** for insertion into the polypeptide chain and therefore has a somewhat different nucleotide sequence than other tRNAs. A unique trinucleotide sequence on each tRNA called an **anticodon** binds to a complementary codon on the mRNA, thereby ensuring insertion of the correct amino acid. In spite of their differences, all tRNAs contain several unusual nucleotides and assume a similar **cloverleaf** structure.

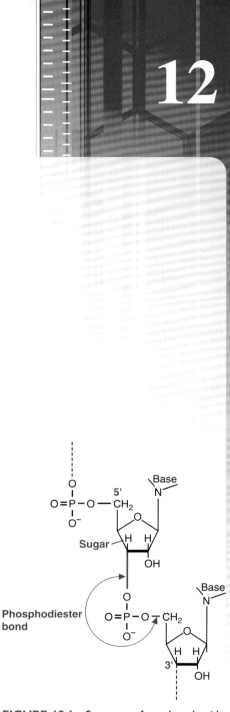

FIGURE 12.1 Structure of a polynucleotide. The 5'-carbon of the top sugar and the 3'-carbon of the bottom sugar are indicated. Because the sugar is ribose, this is an example of RNA.

An adenoma is a mass of rapidly proliferating cells called a *neoplasm* (neo = new; plasm = growth), which is formed from epithelial cells growing into a glandlike structure. The cells lining all the external and internal organs are epithelial cells, and most human tumors are adenocarcinomas. Adenomatous polyps are adenomas that grow into the lumen of the colon or rectum. The term *malignant* applied to a neoplasm refers to invasive, unregulated growth. **Clark T.** has an adenocarcinoma, which is a malignant adenoma that has started to grow through the wall of the colon into surrounding tissues. Cells from adeno-carcinomas can break away and spread through the blood or lymph to other parts of the body, where they form "colony" tumors. This process is called *metastasis*.

The Gram stain is a standard laboratory test that can be used to determine what type of bacteria is present in an infection. The test is based on the cell wall of the bacteria trapping a specific dye (crystal violet). Gram-positive bacteria, which trap the dye, have a thicker cell wall than gram-negative bacteria, which exclude the dye. Gram-positive and gram-negative bacteria have differences in the sugar and protein composition of their outer cell walls as well as the lipid components associated with the cell walls. Because of these dif-ferences in cell-wall structure, antibiotics will affect each class of bacteria differently. Typing the bacteria using the Gram stain should allow the appropri-ate treatment options for the patient to be better determined.

Isabel S. is a 26-year-old intravenous drug user who has used shared needles. She presented to the emergency department with an abscess on her right arm where she injects. She reported that a few months ago, she had a 3-week course of a flulike syndrome with fever, malaise, and muscle aches. She was offered an HIV test, which was positive, and a multidrug regimen was initiated.

Clark T. had a screening colonoscopy at age 50 years during which they removed several intestinal polyps whose pathology was consistent with adenomas. He did not return for a 3-year colonoscopic examination as instructed for surveillance. At age 59 years he reappeared, complaining of maroon-colored stools, an indication of intestinal bleeding. The source of the blood loss was an adenocarcinoma growing from a colonic polyp of the large intestine. At surgery, it was found that the tumor had invaded the gut wall and penetrated the visceral peritoneum, and several pericolic lymph nodes contained cancer cells. A computed tomography scan of the abdomen and pelvis showed several small nodules of meta-static cancer in the liver. Following resection of the tumor in both the colon and liver, the oncologist began treatment with 5-fluorouracil (5-FU) combined with other chemotherapeutic agents.

Paul T. complains to his physician of a 3-day history of worsening fever and cough. His cough produces thick yellow-brown sputum. He has crackles on pulmonary examination at the right base of his lungs. He is empirically started on azithromycin for community-acquired pneumonia. A stain of his sputum shows many gram-positive diplococci. A sputum culture confirms that he has a respiratory infection, in this case caused by *Streptococcus pneumoniae*.

I. DNA Structure

A. Location of DNA

DNA and *RNA* serve as the genetic material for prokaryotic and eukaryotic cells, for viruses, and for plasmids, each of which stores it in a different arrangement or location. In prokaryotes, DNA is not separated from the rest of the cellular contents. In eukaryotes, however, DNA is located in the nucleus, where it is separated from the rest of the cell by the nuclear envelope (see Fig. 10.14), and in the mitochondria. Eukaryotic nuclear DNA is bound to proteins, forming a complex called *chromatin*. During interphase (when cells are not dividing), some of the chromatin is diffuse (euchromatin) and some is dense (heterochromatin), but no distinct structures can be observed. However, before mitosis (when cells divide), the DNA is replicated, resulting in two identical chromosomes called *sister chromatids*. During metaphase (a period in mitosis), these condense into discrete, visible chromosomes.

DNA is a double-stranded molecule that forms base pairs (bp), via hydrogen bonding, between strands (see the following paragraph). The *base pair* designation is often used to indicate the size of a DNA molecule. For example, in a stretch of DNA 200 bp long, both strands are included, with 200 bases in each strand, for a total of 400 bases.

Less than 0.1% of the total DNA in a cell is present in mitochondria. The genetic information in a mitochondrion is encoded in <20,000 bp of DNA; the information in a human haploid nucleus (i.e., an egg or a sperm cell) is encoded in about 3×10^9 (3 billion) bp. The DNA and protein-synthesizing systems in mitochondria more closely resemble the systems in bacteria, which do not have membrane-enclosed organelles, than those in the eukaryotic nucleus and cytoplasm. It has been sug-gested that mitochondria were derived from ancient bacterial invaders of primordial eukaryotic cells.

Viruses are small infectious particles consisting of a DNA or RNA genome (but not both), proteins required for pathogenesis or replication, and a protein coat. They lack, however, complete systems for DNA replication, production of RNA (transcription), and synthesis of proteins (translation). Consequently, viruses must invade other cells and commandeer their DNA, RNA, and protein-synthesizing machinery to reproduce. Both eukaryotes and prokaryotes can be infected by viruses. Viruses that infect bacteria are known as *bacteriophages* (or more simply as *phages*).

Plasmids are small, circular DNA molecules that can enter bacteria and replicate autonomously; that is, outside the host genome. In contrast to viruses, plasmids are not infectious; they do not convert their host cells into factories devoted to plasmid production. Plasmids do, however, often carry genes, some of which confer resistance to antibiotics. Genetic engineers use plasmids as tools for transfer of foreign genes into bacteria because segments of DNA can readily be incorporated into plasmids.

B. Determination of the Structure of DNA

In 1865, Frederick Meischer first isolated DNA, obtaining it from pus scraped from surgical bandages. Initially, scientists speculated that DNA was a cellular storage form for inorganic phosphate, an important but unexciting function that did not spark widespread interest in determining its structure. In fact, the details of DNA structure were not fully determined until 1953, almost 90 years after it had first been isolated but only 9 years after it had been identified as the genetic material.

Early in the 20th century, the *bases* of DNA were identified as the purines adenine (A) and guanine (G) and the pyrimidines cytosine (C) and thymine (T) (Fig. 12.2). The sugar was found to be deoxyribose, a derivative of ribose, lacking a hydroxyl group on carbon 2 (see Fig. 12.2).

Nucleotides, composed of a base, a sugar, and phosphate, were found to be the monomeric units of the nucleic acids (Table 12.1). In nucleosides, the nitrogenous base is linked by an *N*-glycosidic bond to the anomeric carbon of the sugar, either ribose or deoxyribose. The atoms in the sugar are numbered using the prime symbol (′) to distinguish them from the numbering of the atoms in the nitrogenous base. A nucleotide is a nucleoside with an inorganic phosphate attached to a 5′-hydroxyl group of the sugar in ester linkage (Fig. 12.3). The names and abbreviations of nucleotides specify the base, the sugar, and the number of phosphates attached (*mono*phosphate [MP], *di*phosphate [DP], *tri*phosphate [TP]). In deoxynucleotides, the prefix "d" precedes the abbreviation. For example, GDP is guanosine diphosphate (the base guanine attached to a ribose that has two phosphate

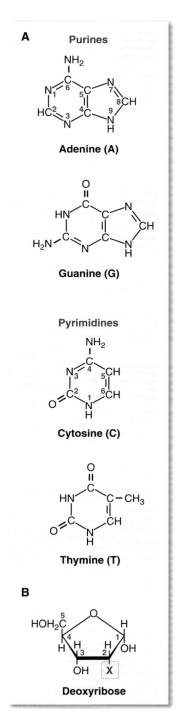

FIGURE 12.2   A. Purine and pyrimidine bases in DNA. **B.** Deoxyribose and ribose, the sugars of DNA and RNA, respectively. The carbon atoms are numbered from 1 to 5. When the sugar is attached to a base, the carbon atoms are numbered from 1′ to 5′ to distinguish it from the base. In deoxyribose, the X = H; in ribose, the X = OH.

TABLE 12.1	Names of Bases and Their Corresponding Nucleosides[a]
BASE	**NUCLEOSIDE**
Adenine (A)	Adenosine
Guanine (G)	Guanosine
Cytosine (C)	Cytidine
Thymine (T)	Thymidine
Uracil (U)	Uridine
Hypoxanthine (I)	Inosine[b]

[a]If the sugar is deoxyribose rather than ribose, the nucleoside has "deoxy" as a prefix (e.g., deoxyadenosine). Nucleotides are given the name of the nucleoside plus mono-, di-, or triphosphate (e.g., adenosine triphosphate, deoxyadenosine triphosphate).

[b]The base hypoxanthine is not found in DNA but is produced during degradation of the purine bases. It is found in certain tRNA molecules. Its nucleoside, inosine, is produced during synthesis of the purine nucleotides (see Chapter 39).

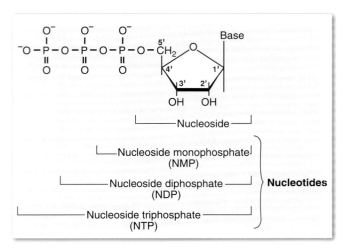

FIGURE 12.3 Nucleoside and nucleotide structures displayed with ribose as the sugar. The corresponding deoxyribonucleotides are abbreviated dNMP, dNDP, and dNTP. N = any base (A, G, C, U, or T). The hydrogen atoms (H) have been removed from the figure to improve clarity.

After **Isabel S.** was diagnosed with HIV, she was treated with a multidrug regimen. One of the first drugs used to treat HIV was zidovudine (ZDV), formerly called *AZT*. This is a nucleoside analog reverse transcriptase inhibitor drug and is an analog of the thymine nucleotide found in DNA (the modified group is shown in the *dashed box*). ZDV is phosphorylated in the body by the kinases that normally phosphorylate nucleosides and nucleotides. As the viral DNA chain is being synthesized in a human cell, ZDV is then added to the growing 3′-end by viral reverse transcriptase. However, ZDV lacks a 3′-OH group, and therefore, no additional nucleotides can be attached through a 5′→3′-bond. Thus, chain elongation of the DNA is terminated. Reverse transcriptase has a higher affinity for ZDV than do normal human cellular DNA polymerases, enabling the drug to target viral replication more specifically than cellular replication. Lamivudine (3TC, 2′,3′-dideoxy-3′-thiacytidine) is also a nucleoside analog reverse transcriptase inhibitor with an analog of cytidine and is used more commonly as a first-line agent.

ZDV,
an analog of deoxythymidine

groups) and dATP is deoxyadenosine triphosphate (the base adenine attached to a deoxyribose with three phosphate groups).

In 1944, after Oswald Avery's experiments establishing DNA as the genetic material were published, interest in determining the structure of DNA intensified. Digestion with enzymes of known specificity proved that inorganic phosphate joined the nucleotide monomers, forming a phosphodiester bond between the 3′-carbon of one sugar and the 5′-carbon of the next sugar along the polynucleotide chain (Fig. 12.4). Another key to DNA structure was provided by Erwin Chargaff. He analyzed the base composition of DNA from various sources and concluded that on a molar basis, the amount of adenine was always equal to the amount of thymine and the amount of guanine was equal to the amount of cytosine.

During this era, James Watson and Francis Crick joined forces and, using the X-ray diffraction data of Maurice Wilkins and Rosalind Franklin, incorporated the available information into a model for DNA structure. In 1953, they published a brief paper (~900 words), describing DNA as a double helix consisting of two polynucleotide strands joined by pairing between the bases (adenine with thymine and guanine with cytosine). The model of *base pairing* they proposed, and the implications of the model for understanding DNA replication, formed the basis of modern molecular biology.

C. Concept of Base Pairing

As proposed by Watson and Crick, each DNA molecule consists of two polynucleotide chains joined by hydrogen bonds between the bases. In each base pair, a purine on one strand forms hydrogen bonds with a pyrimidine on the other strand. In one type of base pair, adenine on one strand pairs with thymine on the other strand (Fig. 12.5). This base pair is stabilized by two hydrogen bonds. The other base pair, formed between guanine and cytosine, is stabilized by three hydrogen bonds. As a consequence of base pairing, the two strands of DNA are complementary; that is, adenine on one strand corresponds to thymine on the other strand, and guanine corresponds to cytosine.

The concept of base pairing proved to be essential for determining the mechanism of DNA replication (in which the copies of DNA are produced that are distributed to daughter cells) and the mechanisms of transcription and translation (in which mRNA is produced from genes and used to direct the process of protein synthesis). As Watson and Crick implied in their article, base pairing allows one strand of DNA

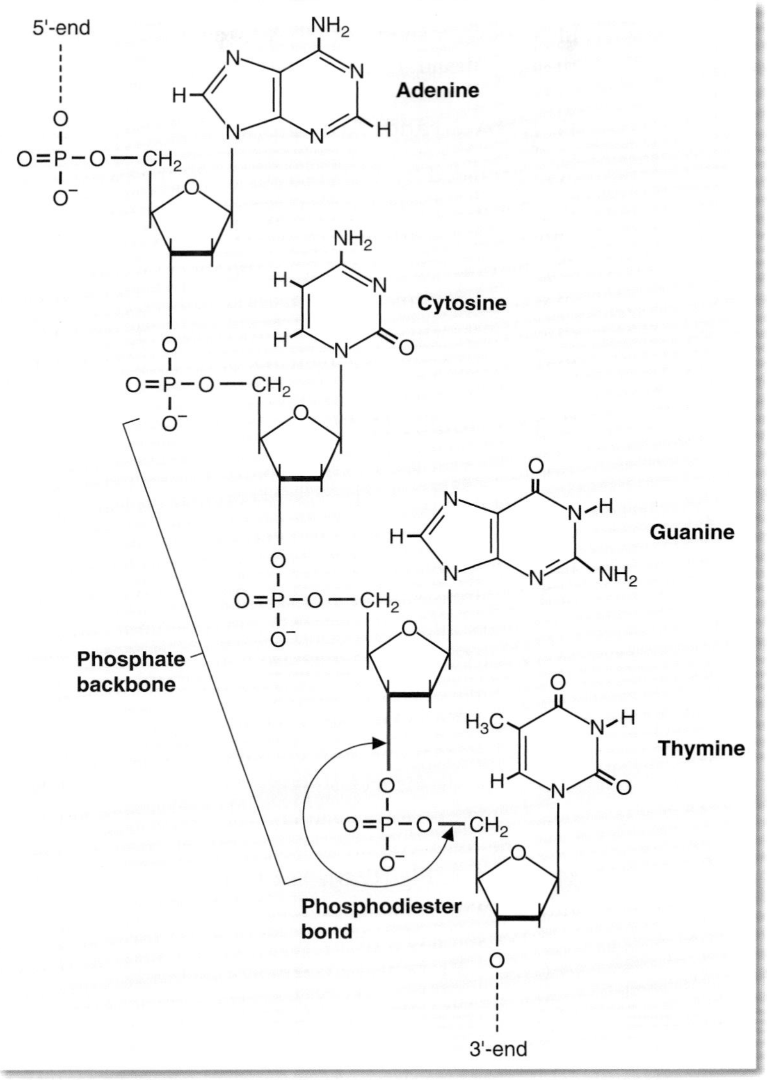

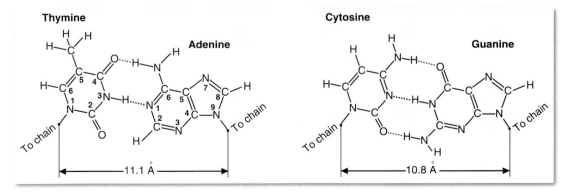

FIGURE 12.4   A segment of a polynucleotide chain of DNA. The *dashes* at the 5'- and 3'-ends indicate that the molecule contains more nucleotides than are shown. The hydrogen atoms (H) have been omitted from the sugar structures to increase the clarity of the figure.

FIGURE 12.5   Base pairs of DNA. Note that the purine bases are "flipped over" from the positions in which they are usually shown (see Fig. 12.4). The bases must be in this orientation to form base pairs. The *dotted lines* indicate hydrogen bonds between the bases. Although the hydrogen bonds participate in holding the bases and thus the two DNA strands together, they are weaker than covalent bonds and allow the DNA strands to separate during replication and transcription.

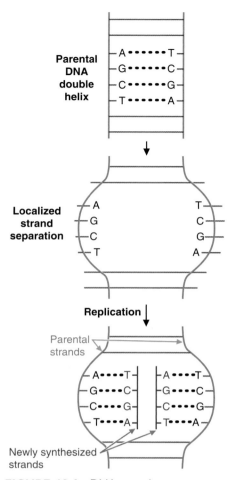

FIGURE 12.6 DNA strands serve as templates. During replication, the strands of the helix separate in a localized region. Each parental strand serves as a template for the synthesis of a new DNA strand.

to serve as a template for the synthesis of the other strand (Fig. 12.6). Base pairing also allows a strand of DNA to serve as a template for the synthesis of a complementary strand of RNA.

D. DNA Strands Are Antiparallel

As concluded by Watson and Crick, the two complementary strands of DNA run in opposite directions (antiparallel). On one strand, the 5′-carbon of the sugar is above the 3′-carbon (Fig. 12.7). This strand is said to run in a 5′-to-3′ direction. On the other strand, the 3′-carbon is above the 5′-carbon. This strand is said to run in a 3′-to-5′ direction. Thus, the strands are antiparallel (i.e., they run in opposite directions). This concept of directionality of nucleic acid strands is essential for understanding the mechanisms of replication and transcription.

E. The Double Helix

Because each base pair contains a purine bonded to a pyrimidine, the strands are equidistant from each other throughout. If two strands that are equidistant from each other are twisted at the top and the bottom, they form a double helix (Fig. 12.8). In the *double helix* of DNA, the base pairs that join the two strands are stacked like a spiral staircase along the central axis of the molecule. The electrons of the adjacent base pairs interact, generating hydrophobic stacking forces that, in addition to the hydrogen bonding of the base pairs, stabilize the helix.

The phosphate groups of the sugar–phosphate backbones are on the outside of the helix (see Fig. 12.8). Each phosphate has two oxygen atoms forming the phosphodiester bonds that link adjacent sugars. However, the third –OH group on the phosphate is free and dissociates a hydrogen ion at physiologic pH. Therefore, each DNA helix has negative charges coating its surface that facilitate the binding of specific proteins.

The helix contains grooves of alternating size, known as the *major* and *minor* *grooves* (see Fig. 12.8). The bases in these grooves are exposed and therefore can interact with proteins or other molecules.

Watson and Crick described the B form of DNA, a right-handed helix, with 3.4 Å (1 Å = 10^{-8} cm) between base pairs and 10.4 bp per turn. Although this form predominates in vivo, other forms also occur (Fig. 12.9). The A form, which predominates

Multidrug regimens used to treat cancers (e.g., lymphomas) sometimes include the drug doxorubicin (Adriamycin). It is a natural product with a complex multiring structure that intercalates or slips in between the stacked base pairs of DNA and inhibits replication and transcription. It will inhibit DNA synthesis in all cells but will preferentially affect rapidly growing cells (such as tumor cells as compared to normal cells).

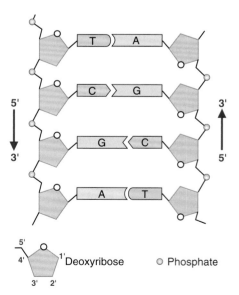

FIGURE 12.7 Antiparallel strands of DNA. For the strand on the left, the 5′-carbon of each sugar is above the 3′-carbon, so the 5′-to-3′ direction is from top to bottom. For the strand on the right, the 5′-carbon of each sugar is below the 3′-carbon, so the 5′-to-3′ direction is from bottom to top.

A

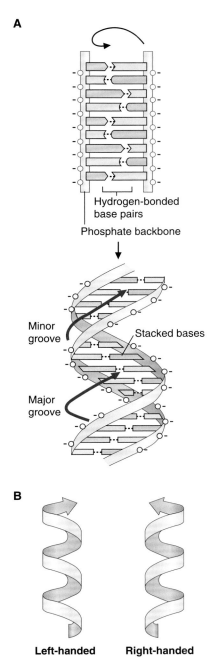

Hydrogen-bonded
base pairs

Phosphate backbone

Minor
groove

Stacked bases

Major
groove

B

Left-handed   Right-handed

FIGURE 12.8   A. Two DNA strands twist to form a double helix. The distance between the two phosphodiester backbones is about 11 Å. The hydrogen-bonded base pairs, shown bonded by *dotted lines*, create stacking forces with adjacent base pairs. Each phosphate group contains one negatively charged oxygen atom that provides the phosphodiester backbone with a negative charge. Because of the twisting of the helix, grooves are formed along the surface; the larger one is the major groove and the smaller one is the minor groove. **B.** If you look up through the bottom of a helix along the central axis and the helix spirals away from you in a clockwise direction (toward the *arrowhead* in the drawing), it is a right-handed helix. If it spirals away from you in a counterclockwise direction, it is a left-handed helix.

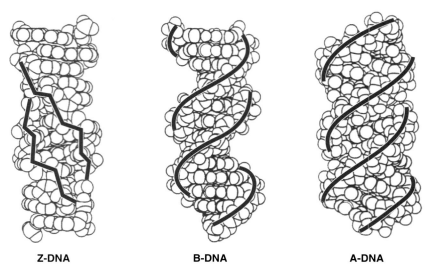

FIGURE 12.9 Z, B, and A forms of DNA. The *solid red lines* connect one phosphate group to the next. (Modified from Saenger W. *Principles of Nucleic Acid Structure.* New York, NY: Springer-Verlag; 1984:257–286.)

in DNA–RNA hybrids, is similar to the B form but is more compact (2.3 Å between base pairs and 11 bp per turn). In the Z form, the bases of the two DNA strands are positioned toward the periphery of a left-handed helix. There are 3.8 Å between base pairs and 12 bp per turn in Z-DNA. This form of the helix was designated "Z" because, in each strand, a line connecting the phosphates "zigs" and "zags" (see Fig. 12.9). Z-DNA is formed transiently in cells and can be stabilized by specific Z-DNA–binding proteins. Z-DNA formation has been linked to transcriptional initiation (the initiation of RNA synthesis from the DNA template); however, its physiologic significance is still elusive. For the rest of this text, we will focus only on B-DNA.

F. Characteristics of DNA

Both alkali and heat cause the two strands of the DNA helix to separate (denature). Many techniques used to study and analyze DNA or to produce recombinant DNA molecules make use of this property. Although alkali causes the two strands of DNA to separate, it does not break the phosphodiester bonds (Fig. 12.10). In contrast, the phosphodiester bonds of RNA are cleaved by alkali because of the hydroxyl group on the 2′-carbon losing its proton, allowing the negatively charged oxygen to attack, and break, the phosphodiester linkage. Therefore, alkali is used to remove RNA from DNA and to separate DNA strands before, or after, electrophoresis (separation by size in an electric field) on polyacrylamide or agarose gels.

Heat alone converts double-stranded DNA to single-stranded DNA. The separation of strands is called *melting*, and the temperature at which 50% of the DNA is separated is called the T_m. If the temperature is slowly decreased, complementary single strands can realign and base-pair, reforming a double helix that is essentially identical to the original DNA. This process is known as *renaturation, reannealing,* or *hybridization* (Fig. 12.11). Hybridization is used extensively in research and clinical testing (see Chapter 17).

II. Structure of Chromosomes

A. Size of DNA Molecules

A prokaryotic cell generally contains a single *chromosome* composed of double-stranded DNA that forms a circle. These circular DNA molecules are extremely large. The entire chromosome of the bacterium *Escherichia coli,* composed of a single

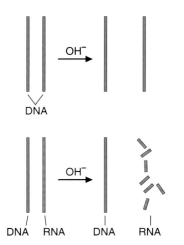

FIGURE 12.10 Effect of alkali on DNA and RNA. DNA strands stay intact but they separate. RNA strands are degraded to nucleotides.

circular double-stranded DNA molecule, contains $>4 \times 10^6$ bp. Its molecular weight is $>2{,}500 \times 10^6$ g/mol (compared to the molecular weight for a glucose molecule of 180 g/mol). If this molecule were linear, its length would measure almost 2 mm. DNA from eukaryotic cells is approximately 1,000 times larger than that from bacterial cells. In eukaryotes, each chromosome contains one continuous linear DNA helix. The DNA of the longest human chromosome is >7 cm in length. In fact, if the DNA from all 46 chromosomes in a diploid human cell were placed end to end, our total DNA would span a distance of about 2 m (>6 ft). Our total DNA contains about 6×10^9 bp.

B. Packaging of DNA

DNA molecules require special packaging to enable them to reside within cells because the molecules are so large. In *E. coli,* the circular DNA is supercoiled and attached to an RNA–protein core. Recall that DNA consists of a double helix, with the two strands of DNA wrapping around each other to form a helical structure. In order to compact, the DNA molecule coils about itself to form a structure called a *supercoil*. A telephone cord, which connects the handpiece to the phone, displays supercoiling when the coiled cord wraps about itself. When the strands of a DNA molecule separate and unwind over a small local region (which occurs during DNA replication), supercoils are introduced into the remaining portion of the molecule, thereby increasing stress on this portion of the molecule. Enzymes known as *topoisomerases* relieve this stress so that unwinding of the DNA strands can occur. This will be discussed in greater detail in Chapter 13.

Packaging of eukaryotic DNA is much more complex than that of prokaryotic DNA because eukaryotic DNA is larger and must be contained within the nucleus of the cell. Eukaryotic DNA binds to an equal weight of *histones*, which are small basic proteins containing large amounts of arginine and lysine. The complex of DNA and proteins is called *chromatin*. The organization of eukaryotic DNA into chromatin is essential for controlling transcription as well as for packaging. When chromatin is extracted from cells, it has the appearance of beads on a string (Fig. 12.12). The beads with DNA protruding from each end are known as *nucleosomes*, and the beads themselves are known as *nucleosome cores* (Fig. 12.13). Two molecules of each of four histone classes (histones H2A, H2B, H3, and H4) form the center of the core around which approximately 140 bp of double-stranded DNA are wound. The DNA wrapped around the nucleosome core is continuous and joins one nucleosome core to the next. The DNA joining the cores is complexed with the fifth type of histone, H1. Further compaction of chromatin occurs as the strings of nucleosomes wind into helical tubular coils called *solenoid* structures.

Although complexes of DNA and histones form the nucleosomal substructures of chromatin, other types of proteins are also associated with DNA in the nucleus. These proteins were given the unimaginative name of *nonhistone chromosomal proteins.* The cells of different tissues contain different amounts and types of these proteins, which include enzymes that act on DNA and factors that regulate transcription.

C. The Human Genome

The *genome*, or total genetic content, of a human *haploid* cell (a sperm or an egg) is distributed in 23 chromosomes. Haploid cells contain one copy of each chromosome. The haploid *egg* and haploid sperm cells combine to form the *diploid* zygote, which continues to divide to form our other cells (mitosis), also diploid. In diploid cells, there are thus 22 pairs of *autosomal chromosomes*, with each pair composed of two *homologous chromosomes* containing a similar series of genes (Fig. 12.14). In addition to the autosomal chromosomes, each diploid cell has two *sex chromosomes*, designated X and Y. A female has two X chromosomes, and a male has one X and one Y chromosome. The total number of chromosomes per diploid cell is 46.

Genes are arranged linearly along each chromosome. A *gene*, in genetic terms, is the fundamental unit of heredity. In structural terms, a gene encompasses the DNA sequence that encodes the structural components of the gene product (whether it be

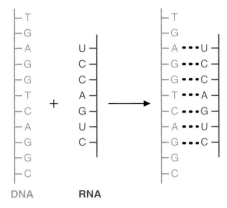

FIGURE 12.11 Hybridization of DNA and complementary RNA.

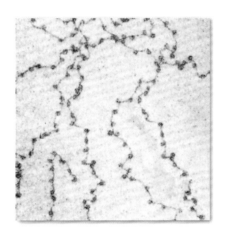

FIGURE 12.12 Chromatin showing "beads on a string" structure.

 If histones contain large amounts of arginine and lysine, will their net charge be positive or negative?

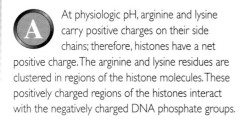 At physiologic pH, arginine and lysine carry positive charges on their side chains; therefore, histones have a net positive charge. The arginine and lysine residues are clustered in regions of the histone molecules. These positively charged regions of the histones interact with the negatively charged DNA phosphate groups.

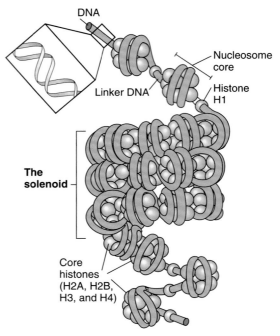

FIGURE 12.13 A polynucleosome, indicating the histone cores and linker DNA. The DNA is depicted in *blue*, whereas the histones are depicted as *light brown spheres*.

a polypeptide chain or an RNA molecule) along with the DNA sequences adjacent to the 5′-end of the gene that regulates its expression. A *genetic locus* is a specific position or location on a chromosome. Each gene on a chromosome in a diploid cell is matched by an alternate version of the gene at the same genetic locus on the homologous chromosome (Fig. 12.15). These alternate versions of a gene are called *alleles*. We thus have two alleles of each gene, one from our mother and one from our father. If the alleles are identical in base sequence, we are homozygous for this gene.

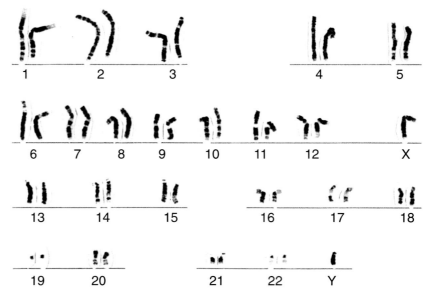

FIGURE 12.14 Human chromosomes from a male diploid cell. Each diploid cell contains 22 pairs of autosomes (numbered chromosomes 1 through 22) plus one X and one Y. Each female diploid cell contains two X chromosomes. Each haploid cell contains chromosomes 1 through 22 plus either an X or a Y. (From Gelehrter TD, Collins FS, Ginsburg D. *Principles of Medical Genetics.* 2nd ed. Baltimore, MD: Williams & Wilkins; 1998:18.)

If the alleles differ, we are heterozygous for this gene and may produce two versions of the encoded protein that differ somewhat in primary structure.

The genomes of prokaryotic and eukaryotic cells differ in size. The genome of the bacterium *E. coli* contains approximately 3,000 genes. All of this bacterial DNA has a function; it either codes for proteins, rRNA, and tRNA, or it serves to regulate the synthesis of these gene products. In contrast, the genome of the human haploid cell contains between 20,000 and 25,000 genes, about seven to eight times the number in *E. coli*. The function of most of this extra DNA has not been determined (an issue considered in more detail in Chapter 15).

III. Structure of RNA

A. General Features of RNA

RNA is similar to DNA. Like DNA, it is composed of nucleotides joined by 3'- to 5'-phosphodiester bonds, the purine bases adenine and guanine, and the pyrimidine base cytosine. However, its other pyrimidine base is uracil rather than thymine. Uracil and thymine are identical bases except that thymine has a methyl group at position 5 of the ring (Fig. 12.16). In RNA, the sugar is ribose, which contains a hydroxyl group on the 2'-carbon (see Fig. 12.3; the prime refers to the position on the ribose ring). As indicated previously, the presence of the 2'-hydroxyl is what renders RNA susceptible to alkaline hydrolysis.

RNA chains are usually single-stranded and lack the continuous helical structure of double-stranded DNA. However, RNA still has considerable secondary and tertiary structure because base pairs can form in regions where the strand loops back on itself. As in DNA, pairing between the bases is complementary and antiparallel. But in RNA, adenine pairs with uracil rather than thymine (see Fig. 12.16B). Base pairing in RNA can be extensive, and the irregular looped structures that are generated are important for the binding of molecules, such as enzymes, that interact with specific regions of the RNA.

The three major types of RNA (mRNA, rRNA, and tRNA) participate directly in the process of protein synthesis. Other, less abundant RNAs are involved in replication

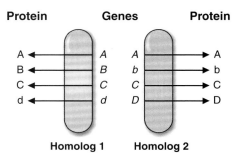

FIGURE 12.15 Homologous chromosomes and their protein products. A set of homologous chromosomes is shown diagrammatically. (Of course, during interphase, when they are producing their protein products, they cannot be visualized as discrete entities.) Four genes are shown as examples on each homolog. The genes of the homologs are alleles (e.g., *AA, Bb, CC, dD*). They may be identical (e.g., *AA, CC*) or they may differ (e.g., *Bb, dD*) in DNA sequence. Thus, the corresponding protein products may be identical, or they may differ in amino acid sequence.

Will S. has sickle cell anemia (see Chapters 6 and 7). He has two alleles for the β-globin gene that both generate the mutated form of hemoglobin, HbS. His younger sister Amanda, a carrier for sickle cell trait, has one normal allele (which produces HbA) and one that produces HbS. A carrier would theoretically be expected to produce HbA:HbS in a 50:50 ratio. However, what is generally seen in electrophoresis is a 60:40 ratio of HbA:HbS. Dramatic deviations from this ratio imply the occurrence of an additional hemoglobin mutation (e.g., thalassemia).

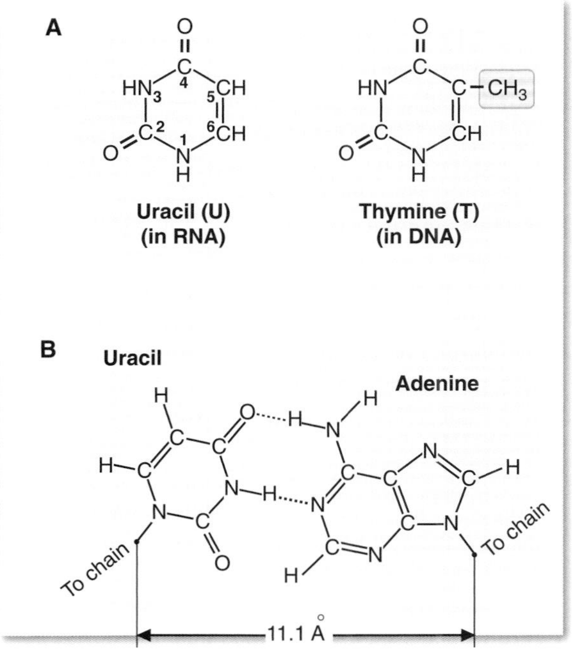

FIGURE 12.16 **A.** Comparison of the structures of uracil and thymine. They differ in structure only by a methyl group, shown in the *yellow box*. **B.** A uracil–adenine base pair in RNA.

Clark T.'s original benign adenomatous polyp was located in the ascending colon. Because Mr. T.'s father died of a cancer of the colon, his physician had warned him that his risk for developing colon cancer was two to three times higher than for the general population. Unfortunately, Mr. T. neglected to have a repeat colonoscopic examination after 3 years as recommended, and he developed an adenocarcinoma that metastasized.

Mr. T. is being treated with several chemotherapy agents, including 5-FU, a pyrimidine base similar to uracil and thymine. 5-FU inhibits the synthesis of the thymine nucleotides required for DNA replication. Thymine is normally produced by a reaction catalyzed by thymidylate synthase, an enzyme that converts deoxyuridine monophosphate (dUMP) to deoxythymidine monophosphate (dTMP). 5-FU is converted in the body to 5-FdUMP, which binds tightly to thymidylate synthase in a transition-state complex and inhibits the reaction (recall that thymine is 5-methyluracil). Thus, thymine nucleotides cannot be generated for DNA synthesis, and the rate of cell proliferation decreases.

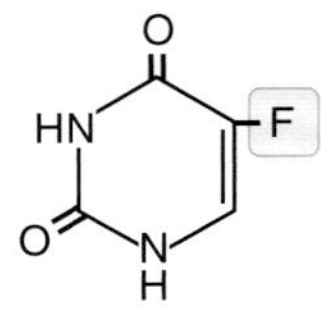

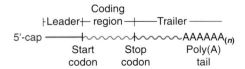

**5-Fluorouracil (5-FU),
an analogue of uracil or thymine**

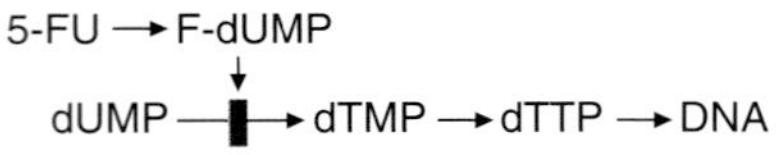

5-FU → F-dUMP

dUMP ⟶╫⟶ dTMP → dTTP → DNA

Coding

├Leader┤─ region ─┼──Trailer ───

5'-cap ────────┼〰〰〰〰〰AAAAAA(n)

Start   Stop   Poly(A)
codon   codon   tail

FIGURE 12.17 The regions of eukaryotic mRNA. The *wavy line* indicates the polynucleotide chain of the mRNA and the *As* comprise the poly(A) tail. The 5'-cap consists of a guanosine residue linked at its 5'-hydroxyl group to three phosphates, which are linked to the 5'-hydroxyl group of the next nucleotide in the RNA chain (a 5'–5' triphosphate linkage). The start and stop codons represent where protein synthesis is initiated and terminated from this mRNA.

or in the processing of RNA; that is, in the conversion of RNA precursors to their mature forms or destruction of existing RNA molecules (see Chapter 17). Other forms of RNA are involved in gene regulation (e.g., microRNA; see Chapter 16).

Some RNA molecules are capable of catalyzing reactions. Thus, RNA, as well as protein, can have enzymatic activity. Certain rRNA precursors can remove internal segments of themselves, splicing the remaining fragments together. Because this RNA is changed by the reaction that it catalyzes, it is not truly an enzyme and therefore has been termed a *ribozyme*. Other RNAs act as true catalysts, serving as ribonucleases that cleave other RNA molecules or as a peptidyl transferase, the enzyme in protein synthesis that catalyzes the formation of peptide bonds.

B. Structure of mRNA

Each mRNA molecule contains a nucleotide sequence that is converted into the amino acid sequence of a polypeptide chain in the process of translation. In eukaryotes, mRNA is transcribed from protein-coding genes as a long primary transcript that is processed in the nucleus to form mRNA. The various processing intermediates, which are mRNA precursors, are called *pre-mRNA* or *h*eterogenous *n*uclear RNA (*hnRNA*). mRNA travels through nuclear pores to the cytoplasm, where it binds to ribosomes and tRNAs and directs the sequential insertion of the appropriate amino acids into a polypeptide chain.

Eukaryotic mRNA consists of a leader sequence at the 5'-end, a coding region, and a trailer sequence at the 3'-end (Fig. 12.17). The leader sequence begins with a guanosine cap structure at its 5'-end. The coding region begins with a trinucleotide start codon that signals the beginning of translation, followed by the trinucleotide codons for amino acids, and ends at a termination signal. The trailer sequence terminates at its 3'-end with a poly(A) tail that may be up to 200 nucleotides long. Most of the leader sequence, all of the coding region, and most of the trailer are formed by transcription of the complementary nucleotide sequence in DNA. However, the terminal guanosine in the cap structure and the poly(A) tail do not have complementary sequences; they are added after transcription has been completed (posttranscriptionally).

C. Structure of rRNA

Ribosomes are subcellular ribonucleoprotein complexes on which protein synthesis occurs. Different types of ribosomes are found in prokaryotes and in the cytoplasm and mitochondria of eukaryotic cells (Fig. 12.18). Prokaryotic ribosomes contain three types of rRNA molecules with sedimentation coefficients of 16S, 23S, and 5S. A sedimentation coefficient is a measure of the rate of sedimentation of a macromolecule in a high-speed centrifuge (ultracentrifuge). The units of sedimentation are expressed in Svedberg units (S). The 30S ribosomal subunit contains the 16S rRNA complexed with proteins, and the 50S ribosomal subunit contains the 23S and 5S rRNAs complexed with proteins. The 30S and 50S ribosomal subunits join to form the 70S ribosome, which participates in protein synthesis. Although larger macromolecules generally have higher sedimentation coefficients than do smaller macromolecules, sedimentation coefficients are not additive. Because frictional forces acting on the surface of a macromolecule slow its migration through the solvent, the rate of sedimentation depends not only on the density of the macromolecule but also on its shape.

Cytoplasmic ribosomes in eukaryotes contain four types of rRNA molecules of 18S, 28S, 5S, and 5.8S. The 40S ribosomal subunit contains the 18S rRNA complexed with proteins, and the 60S ribosomal subunit contains the 28S, 5S, and 5.8S rRNAs complexed with proteins. In the cytoplasm, the 40S and 60S ribosomal subunits combine to form the 80S ribosomes that participate in protein synthesis.

Mitochondrial ribosomes, with a sedimentation coefficient of 55S, are smaller than cytoplasmic ribosomes. Their properties are similar to those of the 70S ribosomes of bacteria.

rRNAs contain many loops and exhibit extensive base pairing in the regions between the loops. The sequences of the rRNAs of the smaller ribosomal subunits exhibit secondary structures that are common to many different species.

D. Structure of tRNA

During protein synthesis, *tRNA* molecules carry amino acids to ribosomes and ensure that they are incorporated into the appropriate positions in the growing polypeptide chain. This is done through base pairing in an antiparallel manner of three bases of the tRNA (the *anticodon*) with the three base codons within the coding region of the mRNA. Therefore, cells contain at least 20 different tRNA molecules that differ somewhat in nucleotide sequence, one for each of the amino acids found in proteins. Many amino acids have more than one tRNA.

tRNA molecules contain not only the usual nucleotides but also derivatives of these nucleotides that are produced by posttranscriptional modifications. In eukaryotic cells, 10% to 20% of the nucleotides of tRNA are modified. Most tRNA molecules contain ribothymidine (rT), in which a methyl group is added to uridine to form ribothymidine. They also contain dihydrouridine (D), in which one of the double bonds of the base is reduced, and pseudouridine (ψ), in which uracil is attached to ribose by a carbon–carbon bond rather than a nitrogen–carbon bond (see Chapter 14). The base at the 5′-end of the anticodon of tRNA is also frequently modified.

tRNA molecules are small compared with both mRNA and the large rRNA molecules. On average, tRNA molecules contain about 80 nucleotides and have a sedimentation coefficient of 4S. Because of their small size and high content of modified nucleotides, tRNAs were the first nucleic acids to be sequenced. Since 1965, when Robert Holley deduced the structure of the first tRNA, the nucleotide sequences of many different tRNAs have been determined. Although their primary sequences differ, all tRNA molecules can form a structure resembling a cloverleaf (discussed in more detail in Chapter 14).

E. Other Types of RNA

In addition to the three major types of RNA described previously, other RNAs are present in cells. These RNAs include the *oligonucleotides* that serve as primers for DNA replication and the RNAs in the *small nuclear ribonucleoproteins* (snRNPs or snurps) that are involved in the splicing and modification reactions that occur during the maturation of RNA precursors (see Chapter 14). Also included are *microRNAs*, which participate in the regulation of gene expression (see Chapters 16 and 18).

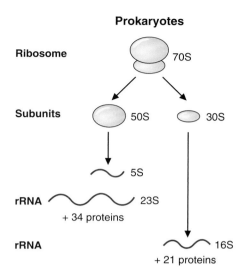

Prokaryotes

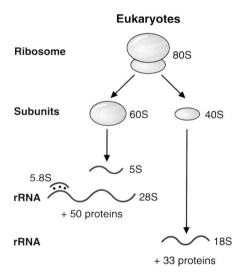

Eukaryotes

FIGURE 12.18 Comparison of prokaryotic and eukaryotic ribosomes. The cytoplasmic ribosomes of eukaryotes are shown. Mitochondrial ribosomes are similar to prokaryotic ribosomes, but they are smaller (55S rather than 70S).

CLINICAL COMMENTS

Isabel S. Isabel S.'s infection with HIV was from needles contaminated with HIV. Without treatment, her HIV will progress and will result in the development of AIDS. The progressive immunologic deterioration that accompanies this disease ultimately results in life-threatening opportunistic infections with fungi (e.g., *Candida, Cryptococcus, Pneumocystis jirovecii* [formerly known as *Pneumocystis carinii*]), other viruses (e.g., cytomegalovirus, herpes simplex), and bacteria (e.g., *Mycobacterium, Salmonella*). The immunologic incompetence also frequently results in the development of certain neoplasms (e.g., Kaposi sarcoma, non-Hodgkin lymphoma) as well as meningitis, neuropathies, and neuropsychiatric disorders causing cognitive dysfunction. Although recent advances in drug therapy can slow or stop the course of the disease, no cure is yet available.

Clark T. Clark T.'s original benign adenomatous polyp was located on the right side of the colon, which is less common than the left side but is increasing in incidence. Because Mr. T.'s father died from a cancer of

 Azithromycin, the antibiotic used to treat **Paul T.**, inhibits protein synthesis on prokaryotic ribosomes but not on eukaryotic ribosomes. It binds to the 50S ribosomal subunit, which is absent in eukaryotes. Therefore, it will selectively inhibit bacterial growth. However, because mitochondrial ribosomes are similar to those of bacteria, mitochondrial protein synthesis can also be inhibited. This fact is important in understanding some of the side effects of antibiotics that work by inhibiting bacterial protein synthesis.

Clark T. completed his first course of intravenous chemotherapy in the hospital. He tolerated the therapy with only mild anorexia and diarrhea and with only a mild leukopenia (a decreased white blood cell count; *leuko* = white). Thirty days after the completion of the initial course, these symptoms abated and he started his second course of chemotherapy, including 5-FU as an outpatient.

Because 5-FU inhibits synthesis of thymine, DNA synthesis is affected in all cells in the human body that are rapidly dividing, such as the cells in the bone marrow that produce leukocytes and the mucosal cells lining the intestines. Inhibition of DNA synthesis in rapidly dividing cells contributes to the side effects of 5-FU and many other chemotherapeutic drugs.

the colon, his physician had warned him that his risk for developing colon cancer was two to three times higher than for the general population. Unfortunately, Mr. T. neglected to have his annual colonoscopic examinations as prescribed, and he developed an adenocarcinoma that metastasized.

The most malignant characteristic of neoplasms is their ability to metastasize; that is, form a new neoplasm at a noncontiguous site. The initial site of metastases for a tumor is usually at the first capillary bed encountered by the malignant cells once they are released. Thus, cells from tumors of the gastrointestinal tract often pass through the portal vein to the liver, which is **Clark T.'s** site of metastasis. Because his adenocarcinoma has metastasized, there is little hope of eradicating it, and his therapy with 5-FU and other chemotherapy agents is palliative (directed toward reducing the severity of the disease and alleviating the symptoms without actually curing the disease). Although if the metastatic disease in the liver responds to the chemotherapy, those lesions may then be able to be resected, resulting in improved survival.

Paul T. Paul T.'s infection was treated with azithromycin, a macrolide antibiotic. Because this agent can inhibit mitochondrial protein synthesis in eukaryotic cells, it has the potential to alter host-cell function, leading to such side effects as epigastric distress, diarrhea, and, infrequently, cholestatic jaundice.

BIOCHEMICAL COMMENTS

Retroviruses. RNA also serves as the genome for certain types of viruses, including retroviruses. HIV is an example of a retrovirus (Fig. 12.19). Because they are not capable of reproducing independently, viruses must invade host cells to reproduce. Some viruses that are pathogenic to humans contain DNA as their genetic material; others contain RNA as their genetic material. HIV invades cells of the immune system and prevents the affected individual from mounting an adequate immune response to combat infections.

According to the "central dogma" proposed by Francis Crick, information flows from DNA to RNA to proteins. For the most part, this concept holds true. However, retroviruses provide one violation of this rule. When retroviruses invade cells, their RNA genome is transcribed to produce a DNA copy. The enzyme that catalyzes this process is encoded in the viral RNA and is known as *reverse transcriptase*. This DNA copy integrates into the genome of the infected cell, and enzymes of the host cell are used to produce many copies of the viral RNA, as well as viral proteins, which can be packaged into new viral particles.

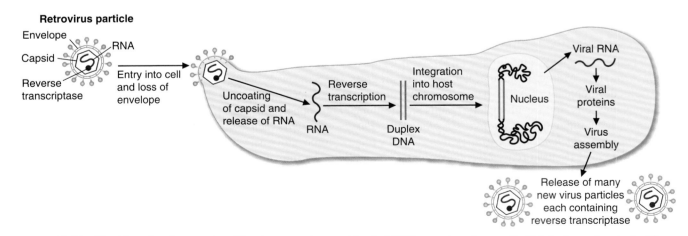

FIGURE 12.19 The life cycle of a retrovirus. The virus contains two identical RNA strands, only one of which is shown for clarity. After penetrating the plasma membrane, the single-stranded viral RNA genome is reverse-transcribed to a double-stranded DNA form. The viral DNA migrates to the nucleus and integrates into the chromosomal DNA, where it is transcribed to form a viral RNA transcript. The viral transcript can form the viral RNA genome for progeny viruses, or it can be translated to generate viral structural proteins.

KEY CONCEPTS

- The central dogma of molecular biology is that DNA is transcribed to RNA, which is translated to protein.
- Nucleotides, consisting of a nitrogenous base, a five-carbon sugar, and phosphate, are the monomeric units of the nucleic acids DNA and RNA (see Chapter 5).
- DNA contains the sugar 2'-deoxyribose; RNA contains ribose.
- DNA and RNA contain the purine bases adenine (A) and guanine (G).
- DNA contains the pyrimidine bases cytosine (C) and thymine (T), whereas RNA contains C and uracil (U).
- DNA and RNA are linear sequences of nucleotides linked by phosphodiester bonds between the 3'-sugar of one nucleotide and the 5'-sugar of the next nucleotide.
- Genetic information is encoded by the sequence of the nucleotide bases in DNA.
- DNA is double stranded; one strand runs in the 5'-to-3' direction, whereas the other is antiparallel and runs in the 3'-to-5' direction.
- The two strands of DNA wrap about each other to form a double helix and are held together by hydrogen bonding between bases in each strand and by hydrophobic interactions between the stacked bases in the core of the molecule.
- The base adenine hydrogen-bonds to thymine, whereas cytosine hydrogen-bonds to guanine.
- Transcription of a gene generates a single-stranded RNA; the three major types of RNA are messenger RNA (mRNA), ribosomal RNA (rRNA), and transfer RNA (tRNA).
- Eukaryotic mRNA is modified at both the 5'- and 3'-ends. In between, it contains a coding region for the synthesis of a protein.
- Codons within the coding region dictate the sequence of amino acids in a protein. Each codon is three nucleotides long.
- rRNA and tRNA are required for protein synthesis.
  - rRNA is complexed with proteins to form ribonucleoprotein particles called *ribosomes*, which bind mRNA and tRNAs during translation.
  - tRNA contains an anticodon that binds to a complementary codon on mRNA, ensuring insertion of the correct amino acid into the protein being synthesized.
- The diseases discussed in this chapter are summarized in Table 12.2.

TABLE 12.2   Diseases Discussed in Chapter 12

DISORDER OR CONDITION	GENETIC OR ENVIRONMENTAL	COMMENTS
AIDS	Environmental	AIDS is due to infection by the HIV, a retrovirus containing an RNA genome. Through its growth in immune cells, active infection by the virus leads to an immunocompromised state. Nucleoside analogs are one class of drugs used to treat people with HIV infections.
Adenocarcinoma	Both	Use of nucleotide analogs as chemotherapeutic agents. Specifically, 5-fluorouracil is used to inhibit deoxythymidine monophosphate (dTMP) synthesis by the enzyme thymidylate synthase, which leads to the death of rapidly proliferating cells.
Pneumonia	Environmental	A bacteria-induced illness in the lungs, leading to fever and cough. Treated with antibiotics. Certain antibiotics target bacterial protein synthesis but may also inhibit mitochondrial protein synthesis.

REVIEW QUESTIONS—CHAPTER 12

Directions: For each question below, select the single best answer.

1. Viruses cause many human infections such as hepatitis, encephalitis, and the "common cold." Which one of the following is a common trait of all these viruses?
   A. They are small, circular DNA molecules that enter bacteria and replicate outside the host genome.
   B. Upon infecting eukaryotic cells, they are called *phages*.
   C. All the common cold viruses contain both DNA and RNA genomes.
   D. In order to reproduce, they must use the infected cell's DNA, RNA, and protein-synthesizing machinery.
   E. Upon becoming infectious, they are called *plasmids*.

2. Many drugs used to treat cancers inhibit DNA replication, whereas some will inhibit the pathways required to synthesize proteins from certain genes. Which one of the following accurately describes a step leading from DNA replication to the synthesis of a protein?
   A. Translation of a gene generates a single-stranded RNA that is complementary to both strands of the DNA.
   B. Transcription of a gene generates a single-stranded RNA that is complementary to one of the DNA strands.
   C. tRNA encodes the proteins during translation.
   D. mRNA encodes the proteins during transcription.
   E. rRNA encodes the proteins during transcription.

3. Gout is caused by the deposition of urate crystals in the joints and kidney. Purines are metabolized to uric acid, whereas pyrimidines, when metabolized, do not generate uric acid. Which one of the following should be restricted in the diet of a patient with gout?
   A. Cytosine
   B. Guanine
   C. Thymine
   D. Uracil
   E. Deoxyribose

4. A patient has a microcytic, hypochromic anemia. In order to ascertain the cause of the anemia, the patient's hemoglobin was isolated, and it was determined that there was much more β-chain present than α-chain, indicating an α-thalassemia. To determine the genetic basis of the thalassemia, nucleic acids were isolated from the blood of the patient. During the procedure of isolating the nucleic acids, both heat and alkali treatment were required. The alkali and heat were included owing to which ONE of the following?
   A. Alkali causes the two strands of DNA and RNA to separate.
   B. Heat causes the two strands of DNA and RNA to separate.
   C. Alkali cleaves the phosphodiester bonds of DNA and RNA, degrading them to nucleotides.
   D. Alkali separates the strands of DNA and degrades RNA to nucleotides.
   E. Alkali separates the strands of RNA and degrades DNA to nucleotides.

5. Targeting certain structural features of eukaryotic mRNA can result in an inhibition of protein synthesis. Which one of the following describes a unique aspect of eukaryotic mRNA?
   A. A polyguanosine tail is found at the 3'-end.
   B. The 5'-end begins with a leader sequence that contains an adenine cap.
   C. The cap and tail of the mRNA are added posttranscriptionally.
   D. The leader sequence contains a guanosine cap at the 3'-end of the mRNA.
   E. The poly(A) tail is found at the 3'-end of the mRNA.

6. Some chemotherapeutic drugs alter the ability of DNA polymerase to faithfully replicate. For the DNA sequence 5'–ATCGATCGATCGATCG–3', which one of the following represents the sequence and polarity of the complementary strand?
   A. 5'–ATCTATCGATCGATCG–3'
   B. 3'–ATCGATCGATCGATCG–5'
   C. 5'–CGAUCGAUCAUCGAU–3'
   D. 5'–CGATCGATCGATCGAT–3'
   E. 3'–CGATCGATCGATCGAT–5'

7. Certain drugs inhibit bacterial RNA synthesis. If the DNA strand 5'–GCTATGCATCGTGATC GAATTGCGT–3' serves as a template for the synthesis of RNA, which one of the following choices gives the sequence and polarity of the newly synthesized RNA?
   A. 5'–ACGCAATTCGATCACGATGCATAGC–3'
   B. 5'–UGCGUUAAGCUAGUGCUACGUAUCG–3'
   C. 5'–ACGCAAUUCGAUCACGAUGCAUAGC–3'
   D. 5'–CGAUACGUAGCACUAGCUUAACGCA–3'
   E. 5'–GCTATGCATCGTGATCGAATTGCGT–3'

8. Understanding the structure of DNA, and the process of replication, enabled various drugs to be developed that interfered with DNA replication. In DNA, the bond between the deoxyribose sugar and the phosphate is best described by which one of the following?
   A. A polar bond
   B. An ionic bond
   C. A hydrogen bond
   D. A covalent bond
   E. A van der Waals bond

9. Certain drugs can intercalate between DNA bases and alter the backbone of the DNA. The backbone of a DNA strand is composed of which of the following? Choose the one best answer.
   A. Phosphates and sugars
   B. Bases and phosphates
   C. Nucleotides and sugars
   D. Phosphates and nucleosides
   E. Sugars and bases

10. Analysis of one strand of a double-stranded piece of DNA displayed 20 mol % A, 25 mol % T, 30 mol % G, and 25 mol % C. Which one of the following accurately represents the composition of the complementary strand?
    A. A is 25 mol %, T is 20 mol %, G is 25 mol %, and C is 30 mol %.
    B. [A] is 30 mol %, [T] is 25 mol %, [G] is 20 mol %, and [C] is 25 mol %.

C. [U] is 25 mol %, [T] is 20 mol %, [G] is 25 mol %, and [C] is 30 mol %.
D. [A] is 25 mol %, [T] is 25 mol %, [G] is 25 mol %, and [C] is 25 mol %.
E. The composition of the complementary strand cannot be determined from the data given.

ANSWERS

1. **The answer is D.** Viruses consist of either a DNA or RNA genome but not both. All the viruses that cause the common cold are RNA viruses. When viruses infect bacteria (prokaryotes), they are called *bacteriophages* or *phages*. Plasmids are not viruses and are not infectious. Plasmids are small, circular DNA molecules that can replicate autonomously, whereas viruses cannot and must use the host cell's DNA, RNA, and protein-synthesizing machinery.

2. **The answer is B.** rRNA and tRNA are part of the apparatus for protein synthesis, but the sequences of rRNA and tRNA do not encode proteins. mRNA carries the genetic information that is converted into the amino acid sequence of a protein, but that is used in the process of translation. Transcription of a gene from DNA generates RNA that is complementary to only one strand of DNA.

3. **The answer is B.** Adenine and guanine are purines, which form urate during their metabolism. Cytosine, thymine, and uracil are pyrimidines that follow different metabolic pathways and do not form uric acid. Deoxyribose is a component of DNA, but it is a sugar and not a purine base, and it is not converted to uric acid.

4. **The answer is D.** Both alkali and heat cause the two strands of DNA to separate. Alkali does not break the phosphodiester bonds of DNA but does cleave the phosphodiester bonds of RNA, degrading RNA to nucleotides. RNA is single stranded, not double stranded. In the analysis of DNA, many techniques call for its separation from RNA (the alkali treatment) and its denaturation (separation of the double strands).

5. **The answer is E.** The leader sequence begins with an N^7-methylguanosine cap at the 5′-end of the mRNA. The coding region of the mRNA then follows. The 3′-end of the mRNA contains a polyadenine tail, which aids in the stability of the mRNA. Only the tail of the mRNA is added after transcription of the mRNA.

6. **The answer is D.** The complementary strand must run in the opposite direction, so the 5′-end must base-pair with the G at the 3′-end of the given strand. Therefore, the 5′-end of the complementary strand must be C. G would then base-pair to C, A to T, and T to A. Answer B is incorrect because the bases do not base-pair with each other with the sequences indicated, C is incorrect because U is not found in DNA, and E is incorrect because it has the wrong polarity (the 5′-T in answer E would not base-pair with the 3′-G in the given sequence).

7. **The answer is C.** The RNA strand must be complementary to the DNA strand, and A in DNA base-pairs with U in RNA, whereas T in DNA base-pairs with A in RNA, G in DNA base-pairs with C in RNA, and C in DNA base-pairs with G in RNA. Answers A and E are incorrect because they contain T, which is found in DNA, not RNA. Answer B is incorrect because the base-pairing rules are broken when the strands are aligned in antiparallel fashion. Answers D is incorrect because the polarity of the strand is incorrect (if one were to switch the 5′- and 3′-ends, the answer would be correct).

8. **The answer is D.** The phosphate is in an ester bond between two deoxyribose groups, generating the phosphodiester bond in the DNA backbone (these are covalent bonds). None of the other types of bonds is correct.

9. **The answer is A.** The DNA backbone is composed of the phosphates and deoxyribose in phosphodiester linkages. The bases are internal to the backbone, base-paired to bases in the complementary strand, and form stacking interactions within the double helix.

10. **The answer is A.** The base pairs in double-stranded DNA require that [A] = [T], and [C] = [G]. Therefore, if the concentration of A in one strand is 20 mol %, the concentration of T in the complementary strand must also be 20 mol %. For the example given, then, [A] would be 25 mol %, [T] would be 20 mol %, [G] would be 25 mol %, and [C] would be 30 mol %.

13

Synthesis of DNA

DNA synthesis occurs by the process of **replication**. During replication, each of the two parental strands of DNA serves as a **template** for the synthesis of a complementary strand. Thus, each DNA molecule generated by the replication process contains one intact parental strand and one newly synthesized strand (Fig. 13.1). In eukaryotes, **DNA replication** occurs during the **S phase** of the **cell cycle**, which is followed by the G_2 phase. The cell **divides** during the next phase **(M)**, and each daughter cell receives an exact copy of the DNA of the parent cell.

The Replication Fork. In both prokaryotes and eukaryotes, the site at which replication is occurring at any given moment is called the **replication fork**. As replication proceeds, the two parental strands separate in front of the fork. Behind the fork, each newly synthesized strand of DNA base-pairs with its complementary parental template strand. A complex of proteins is involved in replication. **Helicases and topoisomerases** unwind the parental strands, and **single-strand binding proteins** prevent them from reannealing.

The major enzyme involved in replication is a **DNA polymerase** that copies each parental template strand in the 3'-to-5' direction, producing new strands in a 5'-to-3' direction. **Deoxyribonucleoside triphosphates** serve as the precursors. One strand of newly synthesized DNA grows continuously, whereas the other strand is synthesized discontinuously in short segments known as **Okazaki fragments**. These fragments are subsequently joined by **DNA ligase**.

Initiation. DNA polymerase cannot initiate the synthesis of new strands. Therefore, a short **primer** is produced which contains ribonucleotides (RNA). DNA polymerase can add deoxyribonucleotides to the 3'-end of this primer. This RNA primer is subsequently removed and replaced by deoxyribonucleotides.

Telomeres. The ends of linear chromosomes are called **telomeres**. The enzyme **telomerase**, an RNA-dependent DNA polymerase that carries its own RNA template, is required for their replication.

Errors and Repair. Errors that occur **during replication** can lead to deleterious **mutations**. However, many errors are corrected by enzyme activities associated with the complex at the replication fork. The **error rate** is thus kept at a very low level.

Damage to DNA molecules also causes mutations. **Repair mechanisms** correct DNA damage, usually by removing and replacing the damaged region. The intact, undamaged strand serves as a template for the DNA polymerase involved in the repair process.

Recombination. Although cells have mechanisms to correct replication errors and to repair DNA damage, some genetic change is desirable. It produces new proteins or variations of proteins that may increase the survival rate of the species. Genetic change is produced by unrepaired mutations and by a mechanism known as **recombination**, in which portions of chromosomes are exchanged.

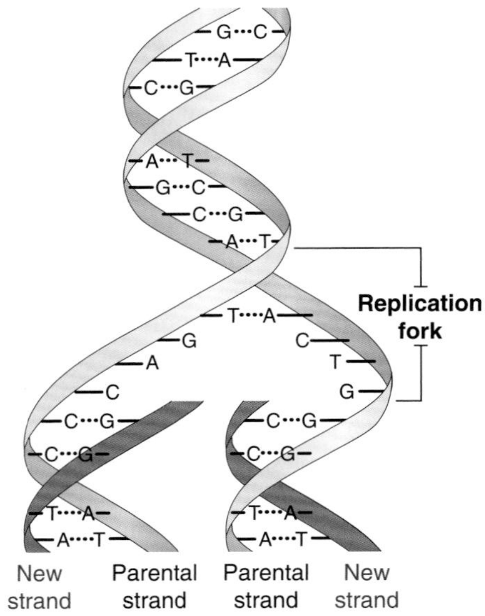

FIGURE 13.1 A replicating DNA helix. The parental strands separate at the replication fork. Each parental strand serves as a template for the synthesis of a new strand.

THE WAITING ROOM

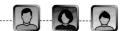

Isabel S. is having difficulty complying with her multidrug regimen. She often forgets to take her pills. When she returns for a checkup, she asks if it is that important to take her pills every day for treatment of HIV.

Dianne A. responded to treatment for her diabetes mellitus but subsequently developed a low-grade fever, an increase in urinary urgency and frequency, and burning at the urethral opening with urination (dysuria). A urinalysis showed a large number of white blood cells and many gram-negative bacilli. A urine culture indicated many colonies of *Escherichia coli,* which is sensitive to several antibiotics, including the quinolone ciprofloxacin.

Calvin A. is a 46-year-old man who noted a superficial, brownish-black, 5-mm nodule with irregular borders in the skin on his chest. He was scheduled for outpatient surgery, at which time a wide excision biopsy was performed such that the complete mole was removed and biopsied. Examination of the nodule revealed histologic changes characteristic of a malignant melanoma reaching a thickness of only 0.7 mm (Stage I).

Michael T. is a 62-year-old electrician who has smoked two packs of cigarettes per day for 40 years. He recently noted that his chronic cough had gotten worse. His physician ordered a chest X-ray, which showed a 2-cm nodule in the upper lobe of the right lung. A computed tomography (CT) scan was performed and confirmed a 2-cm nodule very concerning for malignancy. The patient was taken for surgery and the nodule excised. The pathology showed a poorly differentiated adenocarcinoma of the lung. Malignant neoplasms (new growth, a tumor) of epithelial cell origin (including the intestinal lining, cells of the skin, and cells lining the airways of the lungs) are called *carcinomas*. If the cancer grows in a gland-like pattern, it is an *adenocarcinoma*.

Collection of a patient's urine allows many variables to be examined, including sugar (glucose) levels, creatinine (kidney function) levels, ketone bodies (significant fatty acid oxidation), and crystal or bacterial infiltration. In the case of bacteria, the finding of any bacteria in the urine is unusual because normal urine is sterile. If large numbers of organisms are seen microscopically and they are accompanied by white blood cells, a urinary tract infection is the diagnosis. In **Dianne A.'s** case, the bacteria were demonstrated to be gram-negative (see Chapter 12)—specifically, *E. coli.* Typing the bacteria will allow the appropriate antibiotic to be given to cure the infection.

I. DNA Synthesis in Prokaryotes

The basic features of the mechanism of DNA replication are illustrated by the processes occurring in the bacterium *E. coli*. This bacillus grows symbiotically in the human colon. It has been extensively studied and serves as a model for the more complex, and consequently less well understood, processes that occur in eukaryotic cells.

A. Bidirectional Replication

Replication of the circular double-stranded DNA of the chromosome of *E. coli* begins with the binding of approximately 30 molecules of the protein DnaA at a single point of origin (known as the *origin of replication*), designated *oriC*, where the DNA coils around the DnaA core (Fig. 13.2). With the assistance of other proteins (e.g., a helicase, gyrase, and single-stranded binding protein), the two parental strands separate within this region, and both strands are copied simultaneously. Synthesis begins at the origin and occurs at two *replication forks* that move away from the origin bidirectionally (in both directions at the same time). Replication ends on the other side of the chromosome at a termination point. One round of synthesis, involving the incorporation of over 4 million nucleotides in each new strand of DNA, is completed in approximately 40 minutes. However, a second round of synthesis can begin at the origin before the first round is finished. These multiple initiations of replication allow bacterial multiplication to occur much more quickly than the time it takes to complete a single round of replication.

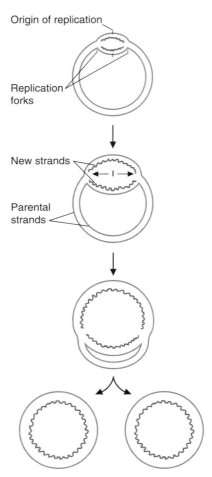

FIGURE 13.2 Bidirectional replication of a circular chromosome. Replication begins at the point of origin (*oriC*) and proceeds in both directions at the same time. Parental strands are shown in *blue*; newly synthesized strands are shown in *red*.

B. Semiconservative Replication

Each daughter chromosome contains one of the parental DNA strands and one newly synthesized complementary strand. Therefore, replication is said to be *semiconservative*; that is, the parental strands are conserved but are no longer together. Each one is paired with a newly synthesized strand (see Figs. 13.1 and 13.2).

C. DNA Unwinding

Replication requires separation of the parental DNA strands and unwinding of the helix ahead of the replication fork. *Helicases* (an example of which is the protein DnaB) separate the DNA strands and unwind the parental duplex. Single-strand binding proteins prevent the strands from reassociating and protect them from enzymes that cleave single-stranded DNA (Fig. 13.3). *Topoisomerases*, enzymes that can break phosphodiester bonds and rejoin them, relieve the supercoiling of the parental duplex caused by unwinding. DNA gyrase is a major topoisomerase in bacterial cells.

D. DNA Polymerase Action

Enzymes that catalyze the synthesis of DNA are known as *DNA polymerases*. E. coli has three DNA polymerases: Pol I, Pol II, and Pol III. *Pol III* is the major replicative enzyme (Table 13.1). All DNA polymerases that have been studied copy a DNA

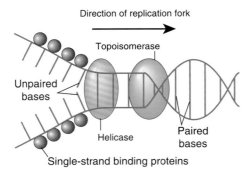

FIGURE 13.3 Proteins involved in separating and unwinding parental DNA strands at the replication fork in prokaryotes.

TABLE 13.1 Functions of Bacterial DNA Polymerases		
POLYMERASES	**FUNCTIONS***ᵃ*	**EXONUCLEASE ACTIVITY***ᵇ*
Pol I	Filling of gap after removal of RNA primer DNA repair Removal of RNA primer in conjunction with RNase H	5'-to-3' and 3'-to-5'
Pol II	DNA repair	3'-to-5'
Pol III	Replication; synthesis of DNA	3'-to-5'

*ᵃ*Synthesis of new DNA strands always occurs in a 5'-to-3' direction.
*ᵇ*Exonucleases remove nucleotides from the ends of DNA strands, acting either at the 5'-end (cleaving 5'-to-3') or at the 3'-end (cleaving 3'-to-5'). Endonucleases cleave bonds within polynucleotide chains.

template strand in its 3'-to-5' direction, producing a new strand in the 5'-to-3' direction (Fig. 13.4). Deoxyribonucleoside triphosphates (dATP, dGTP, dCTP, and dTTP) serve as substrates for the addition of nucleotides to the growing chain.

The incoming nucleotide forms a base pair with its complementary nucleotide on the template strand. Then, an ester bond is formed between the first (or α) 5'-phosphate of the incoming nucleotide and the free 3'-hydroxyl group at the end of the growing chain. Pyrophosphate is released. The release of pyrophosphate (formed from the β- and γ-phosphates of the nucleotide) and its subsequent cleavage by a pyrophosphatase provide the energy that drives the polymerization reaction.

DNA polymerases that catalyze the synthesis of new strands during replication exhibit a feature called *processivity*. They remain bound to the parental template strand while continuing to "process" down the chain rather than dissociating and reassociating as each nucleotide is added. Consequently, synthesis is much more rapid than it would be with an enzyme that was not processive.

 Dianne A.'s urinary tract infection was treated with ciprofloxacin, a fluorinated member of the quinolone family. This group of drugs inhibits bacterial DNA gyrase, a topoisomerase that unwinds the closed circular bacterial DNA helix ahead of the replication fork and thus inhibits bacterial DNA synthesis. Because eukaryotic cells use a different protein as a topoisomerase and do not contain DNA gyrase, they are not affected by quinolones.

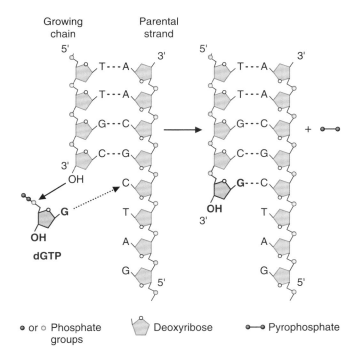

FIGURE 13.4 Action of DNA polymerase. Deoxyribonucleoside triphosphates serve as precursors (substrates) used by DNA polymerase to lengthen the DNA chain. DNA polymerase copies the DNA template strand in the 3'-to-5' direction. The new strand grows in the 5'-to-3' direction. *dGTP,* deoxyguanosine triphosphate.

One of the drugs used to treat **Isabel S.** was lamivudine, a nucleotide reverse transcriptase inhibitor (NRTI). It is a dideoxynucleoside, an example of which is shown in the following figure. For an early-generation NRTI, didanosine, the base in the drug is hypoxanthine. For lamivudine, the base is cytosine.

HOCH$_2$ O Base

H H
H H

A dideoxynucleoside

The dideoxynucleosides do not have a hydroxyl group on either the 2'- or 3'-carbon. They can be converted to dideoxynucleoside triphosphates in cells and, like zidovudine (ZDV), terminate chain growth when incorporated into DNA. In the case of the dideoxynucleosides, chain termination results from the absence of a hydroxyl group on the 3'-carbon. The HIV mutates very rapidly (mostly because reverse transcriptase lacks 3'-to-5' exonuclease activity, which is the proofreading activity) and frequently develops resistance to one or more of these drugs. Therefore, it is recommended that patients with AIDS take several drugs, including two NRTIs.

RNase H is a ribonuclease that specifically degrades RNA from an RNA–DNA hybrid. The HIV (see Chapter 12) converts an RNA genome to a double-stranded DNA copy using the enzyme reverse transcriptase. An intermediate in the conversion of the single-stranded RNA genome to double-stranded DNA is an RNA–DNA hybrid. To remove the RNA so a double-stranded DNA molecule can be made, reverse transcriptase also contains RNase H activity. Because reverse transcriptase lacks error-checking capabilities, the HIV genome can mutate at a rapid rate. **Isabel S.** takes many drugs because of the need to block HIV replication at multiple steps in order to "keep ahead" of the high mutation rate of the virus. The RNase H activity of reverse transcriptase has proven to be a difficult target for drug development to block HIV genome replication, although research in this area is still quite active.

E. Base-Pairing Errors

In *E. coli,* the replicative enzyme Pol III also performs a proofreading or editing function. This enzyme has 3'-to-5' exonuclease activity in addition to its polymerase activity (see Table 13.1). If the nucleotide at the end of the growing chain is incorrectly base-paired with the template strand, Pol III removes this nucleotide before continuing to lengthen the growing chain. This proofreading activity eliminates most base-pairing errors as they occur. Only about one base pair in a million is mismatched in the final DNA product; the error rate is about 10^{-6}. If this proofreading activity is experimentally removed from the enzyme, the error rate increases to about 10^{-3}.

After replication, other mechanisms replace mismatched bases that escaped proofreading so that the fidelity of DNA replication is very high. The two processes of proofreading and postreplication mismatch repair result in an overall error rate of about 10^{-10}; that is, less than one mismatched base pair in 10 billion.

F. RNA Primer Requirement

DNA polymerase cannot initiate the synthesis of new strands; it requires the presence of a free 3'-OH group to function. Therefore, a *primer* is required to supply the free 3'-OH group. This primer is an RNA oligonucleotide. It is synthesized in a 5'-to-3' direction by an RNA polymerase (*primase*) that copies the DNA template strand. DNA polymerase initially adds a deoxyribonucleotide to the 3'-hydroxyl group of the primer and then continues adding deoxyribonucleotides to the 3'-end of the growing strand (Fig. 13.5).

G. The Replication Fork

Both parental strands are copied at the same time in the direction of the replication fork, an observation that is difficult to reconcile with the known activity of DNA polymerase, which can produce chains only in a 5'-to-3' direction. Because the parental strands run in opposite directions relative to each other, synthesis should occur in a 5'-to-3' direction *toward* the fork on one template strand and in a 5'-to-3' direction *away* from the fork on the other template strand.

Okazaki resolved this dilemma by showing that synthesis on one strand, called the *leading strand*, is continuous in the 5'-to-3' direction toward the fork. The other strand, called the *lagging strand*, is synthesized discontinuously in short fragments (see Fig. 13.5). These fragments, named for Okazaki, are produced in a 5'-to-3' direction (away from the fork) but then are joined together so that, overall, synthesis proceeds toward the replication fork.

H. DNA Ligase

As replication progresses, the RNA primers are removed from Okazaki fragments, probably by the combined action of DNA polymerase I (Pol I, using its 5'-to-3' exonuclease activity) and *RNase H*, an enzyme that removes RNA from DNA–RNA hybrids. Pol I fills in the gaps produced by removal of the primers. Because DNA polymerases cannot join two polynucleotide chains together, an additional enzyme, *DNA ligase*, is required to perform this function. The 3'-hydroxyl group at the end of one fragment is ligated to the phosphate group at the 5'-end of the next fragment (Fig. 13.6).

II. DNA Synthesis in Eukaryotes

The process of replication in eukaryotes is similar to that in prokaryotes. Differences in the processes are related mainly to the vastly larger amount of DNA in eukaryotic cells (>1,000 times the amount in *E. coli*) and the association of eukaryotic DNA with histones in nucleosomes. Enzymes with DNA polymerase, primase, ligase,

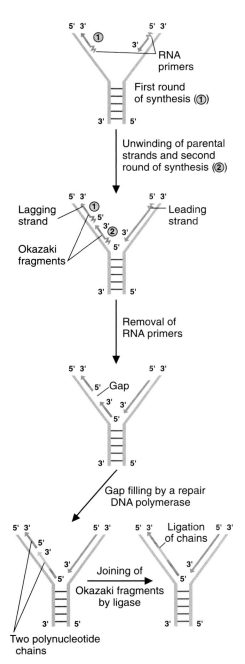

FIGURE 13.5 Synthesis of DNA at the replication fork. (See Fig. 13.6 for the ligation reaction.)

helicase, and topoisomerase activity are all present in eukaryotes, although these enzymes differ in some respects from those of prokaryotes.

A. Eukaryotic Cell Cycle

The *cell cycle* of eukaryotes consists of four phases (Fig. 13.7). The first three phases (G_1, S, and G_2) constitute *interphase*. Cells spend most of their time in these three phases, carrying out their normal metabolic activities. The fourth phase is *mitosis*, the process of cell division. This phase is very brief.

The first phase of the cell cycle, G_1 (the first "gap" phase), is the most variable in length. Late in G_1, the cells prepare to duplicate their chromosomes (e.g., by producing nucleotide precursors). In the second (S) phase, DNA replicates.

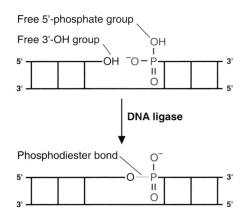

FIGURE 13.6 Action of DNA ligase. Two polynucleotide chains, one with a free 3'-OH group and one with a free 5'-phosphate group, are joined by DNA ligase, which forms a phosphodiester bond.

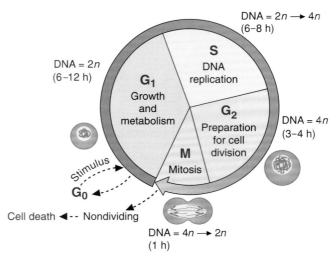

FIGURE 13.7 Eukaryotic cell cycle. The times given for the length of each phase are for cells growing in culture. DNA content is expressed as 2N (diploid) and, after DNA replication, as 4N (tetraploid).

Although Prometheus was chained to a rock as punishment for his theft of fire from the gods, and a vulture pecked at his liver each day, he survived. Can you guess why?

In the human body, many cells cycle frequently—for example, hair follicles, skin cells, and cells of the duodenal crypts. Other cells, such as the precursors of red blood cells, divide several times and then lose their nuclei and leave the cell cycle to form mature red blood cells. These cells transport oxygen and carbon dioxide among the lungs and other tissues for about 120 days and then die. Other cells are normally quiescent (in G_0). However, they can be stimulated to divide. In many instances, the stimuli are growth factors or hormones (e.g., mammary alveolar cells, uterine cells). In the case of liver cells, the stimulus is produced by death of some of the cells.

Nucleosomes disassemble as the replication forks advance. Throughout S phase, the synthesis of histones and other proteins associated with DNA is markedly increased. The amount of DNA and histones both double and chromosomes are duplicated. Histones complex with DNA, and nucleosomes are formed very rapidly behind the advancing replication forks.

During the third phase of the cell cycle, G_2 (the second "gap" phase), the cells prepare to divide and synthesize tubulin for construction of the microtubules of the spindle apparatus. Finally, division occurs in the brief mitotic or *M phase*.

Following mitosis, some cells reenter G_1, repeatedly going through the phases of the cell cycle and dividing. Other cells arrest in the cycle after mitosis, never to divide again, or they enter an extended G_1 phase (sometimes called G_0), in which they remain quiescent but metabolically active for long periods of time. Upon the appropriate signal, cells in G_0 are stimulated to reenter the cycle and divide.

B. Points of Origin for Replication

In contrast to bacterial chromosomes (see Section I.A of this chapter), eukaryotic chromosomes have multiple points of origin at which replication begins. "Bubbles" appear at these points on the chromosomes. At each end of a bubble, a replication fork forms; thus, each bubble has two forks. DNA synthesis occurs at each of these forks, as illustrated in Figure 13.8. As the bubbles enlarge, they eventually merge and replication is completed. Because eukaryotic chromosomes contain multiple points of origin of replication (and, thus, multiple replicons, or units of replication), duplication of such large chromosomes can occur within a few hours.

C. Eukaryotic DNA Polymerases

Fifteen different DNA polymerases have been identified in eukaryotic cells. Examples of some of these polymerases, and their properties, are shown in Table 13.2. Polymerases δ (Pol δ) and ε (Pol ε) are the major replicative enzymes. Polymerase α is also involved in replication. Polymerases δ and ε, as well as Pol α, appear to be involved in DNA repair. Polymerase γ is located in mitochondria and replicates the DNA of this organelle. Polymerases ζ, κ, η, and ι, which lack 5′ exonuclease activity, are used when DNA is damaged and are known as *bypass polymerases* because they can "bypass" the damaged area of DNA and continue replication.

TABLE 13.2 Functions of Some Eukaryotic DNA Polymerases

POLYMERASE	FUNCTIONS[a]	EXONUCLEASE ACTIVITY
Pol α	Replication (in a complex with primase and aids in starting the primer) DNA repair	None
Pol β	DNA repair exclusively	None
Pol γ	DNA replication in mitochondria	3'-to-5'
Pol δ	Replication (processive DNA synthesis on lagging strand) DNA repair	3'-to-5'
Pol ε	Replication (processive DNA synthesis on leading strand) DNA repair	3'-to-5'
Pol κ	DNA repair (bypass polymerase)[b]	None
Pol η	DNA repair (bypass polymerase)	None
Pol ζ	DNA repair (bypass polymerase)	None
Pol ι	DNA repair (bypass polymerase)	None

[a]Synthesis of new DNA strands always occurs in a 5'-to-3' direction.
[b]Bypass polymerases are able to "bypass" areas of DNA damage and continue DNA replication. Some enzymes are error-free and insert the correct bases; other enzymes are error-prone and sometimes insert incorrect bases.

D. The Eukaryotic Replication Complex

Many proteins bind at or near the replication fork and participate in the process of duplicating DNA (Fig. 13.9 and Table 13.3). Polymerases δ and ε are the major replicative enzymes. However, before the DNA polymerases can act, a primase associated with Pol α produces an RNA primer (~10 nucleotides in length).

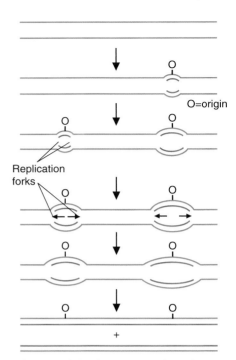

FIGURE 13.8 Replication of a eukaryotic chromosome. Synthesis is bidirectional from each point of origin (O) and semiconservative. Each daughter DNA helix contains one intact parental strand (*blue line*) and one newly synthesized strand (*red line*).

A Liver cells are in G_0. Up to 90% of the human liver can be removed. The remaining liver cells are stimulated to reenter the cell cycle and divide, regenerating a mass equivalent to the original mass of the liver within a few weeks. The myth of Prometheus indicates that the capacity of the liver to regenerate was recognized even in ancient times.

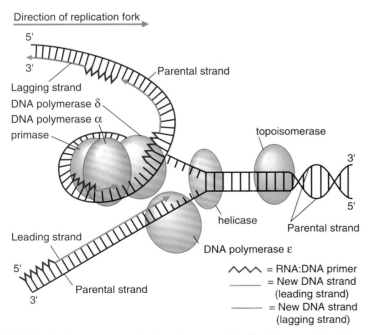

FIGURE 13.9 Replication complex in eukaryotes. The lagging strand is shown looped around the replication complex to demonstrate that all DNA synthesis is in the 5'-to-3' direction. Single-strand binding proteins (not shown) are bound to the unpaired single-stranded DNA. Other proteins also participate in this complex (see text).

TABLE 13.3	Major Proteins Involved in Replication
DNA polymerases	Add nucleotides to a strand growing in a 5'-to-3' direction, copying a DNA template in a 3'-to-5' direction
Primase	Synthesizes RNA primers
Helicases	Separate parental DNA strands; that is, unwind the double helix
Single-strand binding proteins	Prevent single strands of DNA from reassociating
Topoisomerases	Relieve torsional strain on parental duplex caused by unwinding
Enzymes that remove primers	RNase H hydrolyzes RNA of DNA–RNA hybrids Flap endonuclease 1 (FEN1) recognizes "flap" (Unannealed portion of RNA) near 5'-end of primer and cleaves downstream in DNA region of primer; the flap is created by polymerase δ displacing the primer as the Okazaki fragment is synthesized
DNA ligase	Joins, by forming a phosphodiester bond, two adjacent DNA strands that are bound to the same template
PCNA	Enhances processivity of the DNA polymerases; binds to many proteins present at the replication fork

PCNA, proliferating cell nuclear antigen.

Then, Pol α adds about 20 deoxyribonucleotides to this RNA and dissociates from the template because of the low processivity of Pol α. Pol α also lacks proofreading activity (3'-to-5' exonuclease activity). On the leading strand, Pol ε adds deoxyribonucleotides to this RNA–DNA primer, continuously producing this strand. Pol ε is a highly processive enzyme.

The lagging strand is produced from a series of Okazaki fragments (see Fig. 13.5). Synthesis of each Okazaki fragment is initiated by Pol α and its associated primase, as described previously. After Pol α dissociates, Pol δ adds deoxyribonucleotides to the primer, producing an Okazaki fragment. Pol δ stops synthesizing one fragment when it reaches the start of the previously synthesized Okazaki fragment (see Fig. 13.5). The primer of the previously synthesized Okazaki fragment is removed by flap endonuclease 1 (FEN1) and RNase H. The gap left by the primer is filled by Pol δ using the parental DNA strand as its template and the newly synthesized Okazaki fragment as its primer. DNA ligase subsequently joins the Okazaki fragments together (see Fig. 13.6). Okazaki fragments are much smaller in eukaryotes than in prokaryotes (~200 nucleotides vs. 1,000 to 2,000 nucleotides). Because the size of eukaryotic Okazaki fragments is equivalent to the size of the DNA found in nucleosomes, it seems likely that one nucleosome at a time may release its DNA for replication.

Obviously, eukaryotic replication requires many proteins. The complexity of the fork and the fact that it is not completely understood limits the detail shown in Figure 13.9. One protein that is not shown in Figure 13.9 is proliferating cell nuclear antigen (PCNA), which is involved in organizing and orchestrating the replication process on both the leading and lagging strands. PCNA is often used clinically as a diagnostic marker for proliferating cells.

Additional activities that occur during replication include proofreading and DNA repair. Pols δ and ε, which are part of the replication complex, exhibit the 3'-to-5' exonuclease activity required for proofreading. Enzymes that catalyze repair of mismatched bases are also present (see Section III.B.3). Consequently, eukaryotic replication occurs with high fidelity; approximately one mispairing occurs for every 10^9 to 10^{12} nucleotides incorporated into growing DNA chains.

E. Replication at the Ends of Chromosomes

Eukaryotic chromosomes are linear and the ends of the chromosomes are called *telomeres*. As DNA replication approaches the end of the chromosome, a problem develops in the lagging strand (Fig. 13.10). Either primase cannot lay down a primer

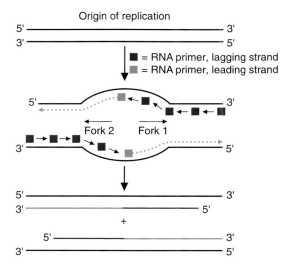

Origin of replication

■ = RNA primer, lagging strand
■ = RNA primer, leading strand

Fork 2   Fork 1

FIGURE 13.10 The end-replication problem in linear chromosomes. After replication and removal of the RNA primers, the telomeres have 3′ overhangs. When these molecules are replicated, chromosome shortening will result. The figure depicts a linear chromosome with one origin of replication. At the origin, two replication forks are generated, moving in opposite directions, labeled as *Fork 1* and *Fork 2*. As *Fork 1* moves to the right, the bottom strand is read in the 3′-to-5′ direction, which means it is the template for the leading strand. The newly synthesized DNA complementary to the upper strand at *Fork 1* will be the lagging strand. Now consider *Fork 2*. As this replication fork moves to the left, the upper strand is read in the 3′-to-5′ direction, so the newly synthesized DNA complementary to this strand will be the leading strand. For this fork, the newly synthesized DNA complementary to the bottom strand will be the lagging strand. The overhangs result from degradation of the RNA primers at the 5′-ends of the lagging strand, resulting in a 3′ overhang.

at the very end of the chromosome, or, after DNA replication is complete, the RNA at the end of the chromosome is degraded. Consequently, the newly synthesized strand is shorter at the 5′-end, and there is a 3′ overhang in the DNA strand being replicated. If the chromosome became shorter with each successive replication, genes would be lost. How is this problem solved?

The 3′ overhang is lengthened by the addition of nucleotides so that primase can bind and synthesize a primer for the complementary strand. Telomeres consist of a repeating sequence of bases (TTAGGG for humans), which may be repeated thousands of times. The enzyme telomerase contains both proteins and RNA and acts as an RNA-dependent DNA polymerase (just like reverse transcriptase). The RNA within telomerase contains the complementary copy of the repeating sequence in the telomeres and can base-pair with the existing 3′ overhang (Fig. 13.11). The polymerase activity of telomerase then uses the existing 3′-hydroxyl group of the overhang as a primer and its own RNA as a template and

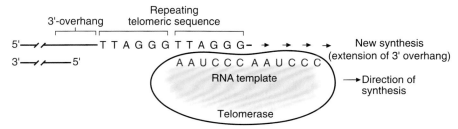

FIGURE 13.11 Telomerase action. The RNA present in telomerase base-pairs with the overhanging 3′-end of telomeres and extends it by acting as both a template and a reverse transcriptase. After copying a small number of repeats, the complex moves down to the 3′-end of the overhang and repeats the process.

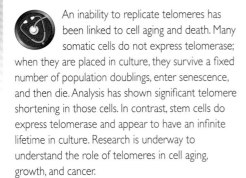

An inability to replicate telomeres has been linked to cell aging and death. Many somatic cells do not express telomerase; when they are placed in culture, they survive a fixed number of population doublings, enter senescence, and then die. Analysis has shown significant telomere shortening in those cells. In contrast, stem cells do express telomerase and appear to have an infinite lifetime in culture. Research is underway to understand the role of telomeres in cell aging, growth, and cancer.

Michael T. has been smoking for 40 years because of the highly addictive nature of nicotine in tobacco and in spite of the warnings on cigarette packs that this habit can be dangerous and even deadly. The burning of tobacco, and, for that matter, the burning of any organic material, produces many different carcinogens such as benzo[*a*]pyrene. These carcinogens coat the airways and lungs. They can cross cell membranes and interact with DNA, causing damage to bases that interferes with normal base pairing. If these DNA lesions cannot be repaired or if they are not repaired rapidly enough, a permanent mutation can be produced when the cells replicate. Some mutations are silent, whereas other mutations can lead to abnormal cell growth, and cancer results.

Melanomas develop from exposure of the skin to the UV rays of the sun. The UV radiation causes pyrimidine dimers to form in DNA. Mutations may result from nonrepair of the dimers that produce melanomas, which appear as dark brown growths on the skin.

Fortunately, **Calvin A.'s** malignant skin lesion was discovered at an early stage. Because there was no evidence of cancer in the margins of the resected mass, full recovery was expected. However, lifelong surveillance for return of the melanoma was recommended.

synthesizes new DNA that lengthens the 3′-end of the DNA strand. The telomerase moves down the DNA toward the new 3′-end and repeats the process many times. When the 3′-overhang is sufficiently long, primase binds and synthesis of the complementary strand is initiated. Even after this lengthening process, there is still a 3′ overhang that forms a complicated structure with telomere-binding proteins to protect the ends of the chromosomes from damage and nuclease attack once they have been lengthened.

III. DNA Repair

A. Actions of Mutagens

Despite proofreading and mismatch repair (see the following) during replication, some mismatched bases do persist. Additional problems may arise from DNA damaged by *mutagens*, chemicals produced in cells, inhaled, or absorbed from the environment which cause mutations. Mutagens that cause normal cells to become cancer cells are known as *carcinogens*. Unfortunately, mismatching of bases and DNA damage produce thousands of potentially mutagenic lesions in each cell every day. Without repair mechanisms, we could not survive these assaults on our genes.

DNA damage can be caused by radiation and by chemicals (Fig. 13.12). These agents can directly affect the DNA or they can act indirectly. For example, X-rays, a type of ionizing radiation, act indirectly to damage DNA by exciting water in the cell and generating the hydroxyl radical, which reacts with DNA, thereby altering the structure of the bases or cleaving the DNA strands.

Although exposure to X-rays is infrequent, it is more difficult to avoid exposure to cigarette smoke and virtually impossible to avoid exposure to sunlight. Cigarette smoke contains carcinogens such as the aromatic polycyclic hydrocarbon benzo[*a*]pyrene (see Fig. 13.12). When this compound is oxidized by cellular enzymes, which normally act to make foreign compounds more water-soluble and easy to excrete, it becomes capable of forming bulky adducts with guanine residues in DNA. Ultraviolet (UV) rays from the sun, which also produce distortions in the DNA helix, excite adjacent pyrimidine bases on DNA strands, causing them to form covalent dimers, usually in the form of thymine dimers (Fig. 13.13).

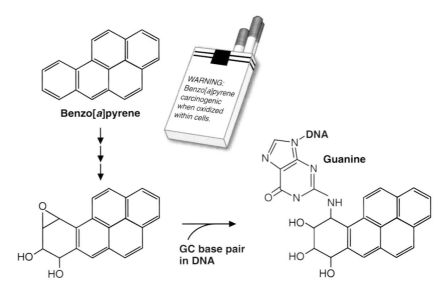

FIGURE 13.12   Oxidation of benzo[*a*]pyrene and covalent binding to DNA. Benzo[*a*] pyrene is not carcinogenic until it is oxidized within cells. Then, it can bind covalently to guanine residues in DNA, interrupting hydrogen bonding in G–C base pairs and producing distortions of the helix, interfering with replication of the DNA at this site.

B. Repair Mechanisms

The mechanisms used for the repair of DNA have many similarities (Fig. 13.14). First, a distortion in the DNA helix is recognized, and the region containing the distortion is removed. The gap in the damaged strand is replaced by the action of a DNA polymerase that uses the intact, undamaged strand as a template, and synthesizes DNA in the 5'-to-3' direction. Finally, a ligase seals the nick in the strand that has undergone repair. The one exception to this scheme occurs in bacteria. Bacteria can remove thymine dimers by photoactivating enzymes that cleave the bonds between the bases using energy from visible light. In this process, nucleotides are not released from the damaged DNA.

1. Nucleotide Excision Repair

Nucleotide excision repair (NER) involves local distortions of the DNA helix, such as mismatched bases or bulky adducts (e.g., oxidized benzo[a]pyrene) (Fig. 13.15; see also Fig. 13.14). Specific repair endonucleases cleave the abnormal chain and remove the distorted region. The gap is then filled by a DNA polymerase that adds deoxyribonucleotides, one at a time, to the 3'-end of the cleaved DNA, using the intact complementary DNA strand as a template. The newly synthesized segment is joined to the 5'-end of the remainder of the original DNA strand by a DNA ligase.

2. Base Excision Repair

DNA glycosylases recognize small distortions in DNA involving lesions caused by damage to a single base. A glycosylase cleaves the *N*-glycosidic bond that joins the damaged base to deoxyribose (see Fig. 13.15). The sugar–phosphate backbone of the DNA now lacks a base at this site (known as an *apurinic* or *apyrimidinic site*, or an *AP site*). Then, an apurinic/apyrimidinic (AP) endonuclease cleaves

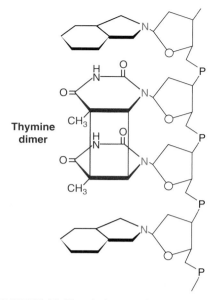

FIGURE 13.13 A thymine dimer in a DNA strand. Ultraviolet light can cause two adjacent pyrimidines to form a covalent dimer.

Pyrimidine dimers occur frequently in the skin. Usually, repair mechanisms correct this damage and cancer rarely occurs. However, in individuals with XP, cancers are extremely common. These individuals have defects in their DNA repair systems. The first defect to be identified was a deficiency of the endonuclease involved in removal of pyrimidine dimers from DNA. Because of the inability to repair DNA, the frequency of mutation increases. A cancer develops once proto-oncogenes or tumor suppressor genes mutate (see Chapter 18). By scrupulously avoiding sunlight, these individuals can reduce the number of skin cancers that develop.

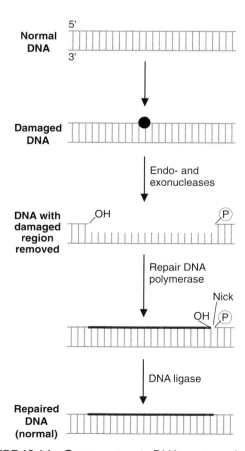

FIGURE 13.14 Common steps in DNA repair mechanisms.

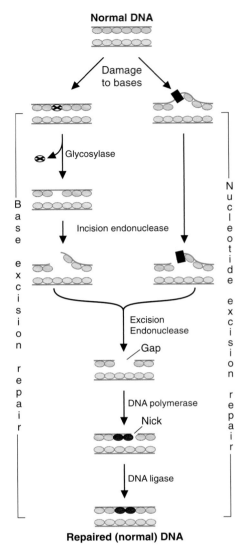

FIGURE 13.15 Types of damage and various repair mechanisms. In base excision repair, the glycosylase cleaves the glycosidic bond between the altered base (shown with an *X*) and ribose. In nucleotide excision repair, the entire nucleotide is removed at once. The gap formed by the incision (cut) and excision (removal) endonucleases is usually several nucleotides wider than that shown.

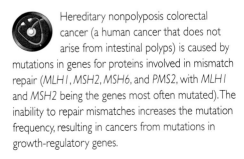

Q Spontaneous deamination occurs frequently in human DNA, and cytosine is a base that is often deaminated. How will cytosine deamination, if not repaired, lead to a mutation in the DNA?

Hereditary nonpolyposis colorectal cancer (a human cancer that does not arise from intestinal polyps) is caused by mutations in genes for proteins involved in mismatch repair (*MLH1*, *MSH2*, *MSH6*, and *PMS2*, with *MLH1* and *MSH2* being the genes most often mutated). The inability to repair mismatches increases the mutation frequency, resulting in cancers from mutations in growth-regulatory genes.

the sugar–phosphate strand at this site. Subsequently, the same types of enzymes involved in other types of repair mechanisms restore this region to normal.

3. Mismatch Repair

Mismatched bases (bases that do not form normal Watson–Crick base pairs) are recognized by enzymes of the mismatch repair system. Because neither of the bases in a mismatch is damaged, these repair enzymes must be able to determine which base of the mismatched pair to correct.

The mismatch–repair enzyme complex acts during replication when an incorrect but normal base (i.e., A, G, C, or T) is incorporated into the growing chain (Fig. 13.16). In bacteria, parental DNA strands contain methyl groups on adenine bases in specific sequences. During replication, the newly synthesized strands are not immediately methylated. Before methylation occurs, the proteins involved in mismatch repair can distinguish parental from newly synthesized strands. A region of the new, unmethylated strand, containing the mismatched base, is removed and replaced.

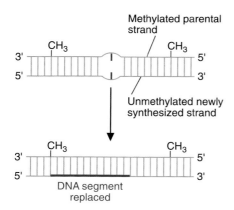

Methylated parental strand

Unmethylated newly synthesized strand

DNA segment replaced

FIGURE 13.16 Mismatch repair. Normal, undamaged, but mismatched bases bind proteins of the mismatch repair system. In bacteria, these proteins recognize the older, parental strand because it is methylated and replace a segment of newly synthesized (and unmethylated) DNA containing the mismatched base. The mechanism for distinguishing between parental and newly synthesized strands in humans is not as well understood.

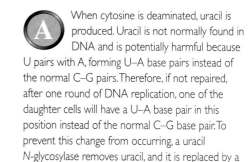

When cytosine is deaminated, uracil is produced. Uracil is not normally found in DNA and is potentially harmful because U pairs with A, forming U–A base pairs instead of the normal C–G pairs. Therefore, if not repaired, after one round of DNA replication, one of the daughter cells will have a U–A base pair in this position instead of the normal C–G base pair. To prevent this change from occurring, a uracil N-glycosylase removes uracil, and it is replaced by a cytosine via base excision repair.

Human enzymes also can distinguish parental from newly synthesized strands and repair mismatches. However, the mechanism for strand recognition has not yet been as clearly defined as those in bacteria. Otherwise, the process in bacteria and eukaryotes is very similar.

4. Transcription-Coupled Repair

Genes that are actively transcribed to produce messenger RNA (mRNA) are preferentially repaired. The RNA polymerase that is transcribing a gene (see Chapter 14 for a description of the process) stalls when it encounters a damaged region of the DNA template. Excision-repair proteins are attracted to this site and repair the damaged region, similar to the process of NER. Subsequently, RNA polymerase can resume transcription.

IV. Genetic Rearrangements

The exchange of segments between DNA molecules occurs quite frequently and is responsible for genetic alterations that can have beneficial or devastating consequences for affected individuals and, in some instances, for their offspring. The DNA segments that are exchanged may be homologous (i.e., of very similar sequence) or they may be totally unrelated. The size of these segments can range from a few nucleotides to tens of thousands of nucleotides and can include many different genes or portions of genes. Many of the enzymes involved in these exchanges are the same as or similar to those used for replication and repair and include endonucleases, exonucleases, unwinding enzymes, topoisomerases, DNA polymerases, and ligases.

One type of genetic rearrangement that has been observed for many years is "crossing over" between homologous chromosomes during meiosis. Another type occurs in stem cells as they differentiate into lymphocytes. Segments of the genes of stem cells are rearranged so that the mature cell is capable of producing only a single type of antibody (see Figs. 16.10 and 7.19). Other types of genetic exchanges involve transposable elements (transposons) that can move from one site in the genome to another or produce copies that can be inserted into new sites. Translocations occur when chromosomes break and portions randomly become joined to other chromosomes, producing gross changes that can be observed under the light microscope. Genetic exchanges can even occur between species—for example, when foreign DNA is inserted into the human genome as a result of viral infection.

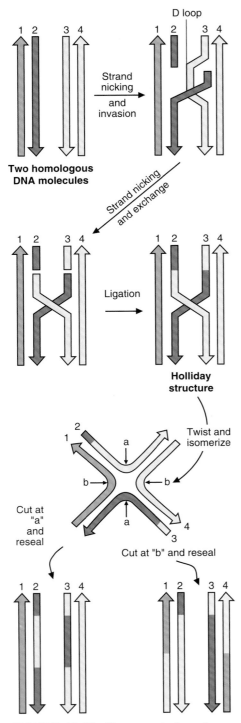

FIGURE 13.17 Key steps in homologous recombination. *D loop*, displacement loop.

A. General or Homologous Recombination

Various models, supported by experimental evidence, have been proposed for the mechanism of recombination between homologous DNA sequences. Although these mechanisms are complex, a simplified scheme for one type of recombination is presented in Figure 13.17.

Initially, two homologous chromosomes or segments of double-helical (duplex) DNA that have very similar, but not necessarily identical, sequences become aligned (see Fig. 13.17). One strand of one duplex is nicked by an enzyme and invades the other DNA duplex, base-pairing with a region of complementary sequence. The match between the sequences does not have to be perfect, but a significant number of bases must pair so that the strand displaced from its partner can form a displacement loop (D loop). This D loop is nicked, and the displaced strand now base-pairs with the former partner of the invading strand. Ligation occurs, and a Holliday structure is generated (see Fig. 13.17). The branch point of the Holliday structure can migrate and may move many thousands of nucleotides from its original position. The Holliday structure, named for the scientist who discovered it, is finally cleaved and then re-ligated, forming two chromosomes that have exchanged segments. In addition to enzymes similar to those used in DNA replication, enzymes for strand invasion, branch migration, and cleavage of the Holliday structure are required. Homologous recombination also is an important component of repairing double-strand breaks in DNA.

B. Translocations

Breaks in chromosomes, caused by agents such as X-rays or chemical carcinogens, can result in gross chromosomal rearrangements (Fig. 13.18). If the free ends of the DNA at the break point reseal with the free ends of a different broken chromosome, a translocation is produced. These exchanges of large portions of chromosomes can have deleterious effects and are observed frequently in cancer cells.

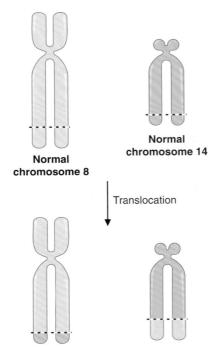

FIGURE 13.18 A chromosomal translocation. A portion of the long arm of chromosome 8 is exchanged for a portion of the long arm of chromosome 14. This chromosomal translocation occurs in Burkitt lymphoma.

C. Transposable Elements

Movable (or transposable) genetic elements, "jumping genes," were first observed by Barbara McClintock in the 1940s. Her work, initially greeted with skepticism, was ultimately accepted, and she was awarded the Nobel Prize in 1983.

Transposons are segments of DNA that can move from their original position in the genome to a new location (Fig. 13.19). They are found in all organisms. Transposons contain the gene for an enzyme called a *transposase*, which is involved in cleaving the transposon from the genome and moving it from one location to another.

Retroposons are similar to transposons except that they involve an RNA molecule. Reverse transcriptase (see below) makes a single-stranded DNA copy of the RNA which is converted to a double-stranded DNA. The double-stranded DNA is then inserted into the genome at multiple locations, forming a repetitive element in the DNA.

V. Reverse Transcriptase

Reverse transcriptase is an enzyme that uses a single-stranded RNA template and makes a DNA copy (Fig. 13.20). The RNA template can be transcribed from DNA by RNA polymerase or obtained from another source such as an RNA virus. The DNA copy of the RNA produced by reverse transcriptase is known as *complementary DNA* (because it is complementary to the RNA template) or *cDNA*. Retroviruses (RNA viruses) contain a reverse transcriptase, which copies the viral RNA genome. A double-stranded cDNA is produced, which can become integrated into the human genome (see Fig. 12.19). After integration, the viral genes may be inactive, or they may be transcribed, sometimes causing diseases such as AIDS or cancer (see Chapter 18). The integration event may also disrupt an adjacent cellular gene, which also may lead to disease (see Chapter 18).

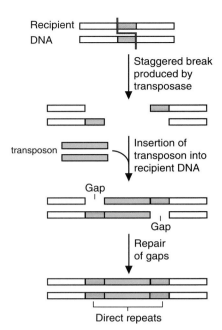

FIGURE 13.19 Transposons. The steps involved in transposition are shown. Direct repeats (the areas in *blue*) are regions of DNA that have the same base sequence in the 5′-to-3′ direction. They are created after the transposon integrates into the chromosome.

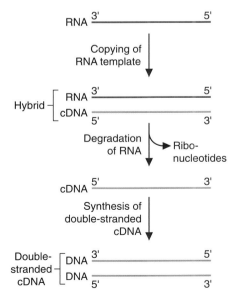

FIGURE 13.20 Action of reverse transcriptase. This enzyme catalyzes the production of a DNA copy (cDNA) from an RNA template. The RNA of a DNA–RNA hybrid is degraded by an associated activity of reverse transcriptase (designated as *RNase H*), and the single DNA strand is used as a template to make double-stranded DNA. This figure is a simplified version of a more complex process.

CLINICAL COMMENTS

Isabel S. Isabel S. contracted HIV when she used needles contaminated with HIV to inject drugs intravenously. Intravenous drug users account for about 10% of newly diagnosed HIV cases in the United States. HIV mutates rapidly, and therefore, current treatment involves a combination of drugs that affect different aspects of its life cycle (designated *HAART*, for *h*ighly *a*ctive *a*ntiretroviral *t*herapy). This multidrug therapy lowers the viral titer (the number of viral particles found in a given volume of blood), sometimes to undetectable levels. However, if treatment is not followed carefully (i.e., if the patient is not "compliant"), the titer increases rapidly. Therefore, Isabel's physician emphasized that she must carefully follow her drug regimen and worked with her to ensure that she was able to take all her medications.

Dianne A. Dianne A.'s poorly controlled diabetes mellitus predisposed her to a urinary tract infection because glucose in the urine serves as a "culture medium" for bacterial growth. The kidney glomerulotubular unit reabsorbs filtered glucose so that, normally, the urine is glucose-free. However, when serum blood glucose levels exceed 175 to 185 mg/dL (the tubular threshold for glucose), the capacity for reabsorption is exceeded. In Ms. A.'s case, blood glucose levels frequently exceed this threshold.

Calvin A. The average person has about 30 moles on the body surface, yet only about 20 people out of every 100,000 develop a malignant melanoma. The incidence of malignant melanoma, however, is rising rapidly. Because about 10% of patients with malignant melanoma die as a result of this cancer, the physician's decision to biopsy a pigmented mole with an irregular border and variation of color probably saved Calvin's life.

Michael T. Lung cancer currently accounts for about 15% of all cancers in men and women. The overall 5-year survival rate is approximately 15%. Thankfully, cigarette smoking has declined in the United States. Whereas 50% of men and 32% of women smoked in 1965, these figures have, in 2014, fallen to 18.8% and 14.8%, respectively.

BIOCHEMICAL COMMENTS

DNA Repair and Disease. DNA serves a unique role within a cell in that it produces the blueprint for gene expression throughout the lifetime of the cell. However, DNA is present in limited copies within cells (unlike RNA and proteins), and various agents often compromise its structural integrity. The DNA, then, must be continually monitored for damage; when damage is found, repair mechanisms are required to restore the DNA to its original structure. If the integrity of the DNA cannot be maintained, deleterious mutations may accumulate in the genome, ultimately having a negative impact on the person as a whole. Failures in DNA repair mechanisms will lead to disease, as indicated by the examples below.

DNA can undergo various types of damage within the cells aqueous environment. DNA undergoes spontaneous hydrolysis of the *N*-glycosidic bonds, generating apurinic or apyrimidinic sites within the DNA. Failure to repair these sites (via base excision repair) will lead to changes in nucleotide sequence of the DNA. DNA, when exposed to UV light rapidly forms thymine dimers, which will interfere with DNA replication unless repaired. DNA exposure to X-rays or ionizing radiation will lead to single-strand or double-strand breaks within the DNA. Failure to repair these breaks will lead to replicative errors. The DNA is also exposed to environmental toxins, leading to chemically modified bases, which need to be repaired before DNA replication occurs; otherwise, the risk of inappropriate base-pairing during replication is greatly increased.

DNA repair disorders, caused by mutations in single genes, often give rise to a cell that actively accumulates mutations and can eventually turn into a cancer cell (see Chapter 18). A common theme in DNA repair enzyme mutations is the clinical display of cancer. It is important to note that the mutations themselves do not directly lead to cancer; rather, successive cell generations, each with accumulated mutations caused by DNA repair defects, will eventually acquire a mutation that leads to growth advantages and cancer. Distinct examples of such diseases are described in the following paragraph.

The first example is the mutations that give rise to XP. XP is primarily a defect in NER (see Fig. 13.15). There are at least 13 genes responsible for XP and its variants, all of which are involved in NER and/or transcription-coupled repair. The disorder is seen clinically as sun hypersensitivity resulting in skin abnormalities. It leads to a significantly greater risk of developing skin cancer, in particular at a younger age than in the general population. This results from an inability to remove UV-induced thymine dimers in the DNA, leading to mismatches being created during DNA replication through the thymine dimer.

Mutations in proteins specifically responsible for transcription-coupled repair lead to Cockayne syndrome, which presents clinically as premature aging. Cells with these mutations cannot transcribe damaged genes. If the DNA cannot be repaired because of the defect in transcription-coupled repair, premature cell death can result from the reduction of gene expression. There are also specific mutations within the XP constellation of genes that give rise to a phenotype that reflects traits of both XP and Cockayne syndrome, indicating that there are commonalities in symptoms when either NER or transcription-coupled repair is defective.

Hereditary nonpolyposis colon cancer (HNPCC) is caused by mutations in enzymes present in intestinal epithelial cells that are responsible for mismatch repair. The inability to repair mismatches will eventually lead to a series of mutations within the cells, leading to colon cancer (most commonly right-sided). This disorder is inherited, and the affected individuals have an increased risk of several cancers, with colorectal cancer being the most common. In addition, they have an early age of onset of the cancers as compared to the general population.

Hereditary breast cancer (*BRCA1* and *BRCA2*) results from the inheritance of mutations in proteins responsible for the DNA repair of single-strand and double-strand breaks. Inheritance of mutations in these genes will predispose the patients to an earlier age of onset of the disorder. The roles of *BRCA1* and *BRCA2* will be discussed further in Chapter 18.

KEY CONCEPTS

- Replication of the genome requires DNA synthesis.
- During replication, each of the two parental strands of DNA serves as a template for the synthesis of a complementary strand.
- The site at which replication is occurring is called the *replication fork*.
- Helicases and topoisomerases are required to unwind the DNA helix of the parental strands.
- DNA polymerase is the major enzyme involved in replication.
- DNA polymerase copies each parental template strand in the 3′-to-5′ direction, producing new strands in a 5′-to-3′ direction.
- The precursors for replication are deoxyribonucleotide triphosphates.
- As DNA synthesis proceeds in the 5′-to-3′ direction, one parental strand is synthesized continuously, whereas the other exhibits discontinuous synthesis, creating small fragments named Okazaki fragments which are subsequently joined. This is necessary because DNA polymerase can only synthesize DNA in the 5′-to-3′ direction.

- DNA polymerase requires a free 3'-hydroxyl group of a nucleotide primer in order to replicate DNA. The primer is synthesized by the enzyme primase, which provides an RNA primer.
- The enzyme telomerase synthesizes the replication of the ends of linear chromosomes (telomeres).
- Errors during replication can lead to mutations, so error checking and repair systems function to maintain the integrity of the genome.
- Table 13.4 summarizes the diseases discussed in this chapter.

TABLE 13.4	Diseases Discussed in Chapter 13	
DISORDER OR CONDITION	**GENETIC OR ENVIRONMENTAL**	**COMMENTS**
HIV/AIDS	Environmental	The rationale for multidrug regime for AIDS patients is explained.
Urinary tract infection	Environmental	Antibiotics to treat such infections can target prokaryotic specific enzymes involved in DNA synthesis.
Melanoma	Both	Drugs used to treat cancer can inhibit DNA replication by a variety of mechanisms.
Lung cancer	Both	Drugs used to treat cancer can inhibit DNA replication.
Hereditary nonpolyposis colon cancer	Genetic	Mutations in enzymes required for DNA mismatch repair can lead to mutations in genes regulating cell proliferation.
Cockayne syndrome	Genetic	Mutations in enzymes required for transcription-coupled DNA repair lead to premature cell death and a premature aging phenotype.
Xeroderma pigmentosum	Genetic	Mutations involved in nucleotide excision repair lead to a greatly elevated risk for the development of skin cancer.
Hereditary breast cancer	Genetic	Mutations in the genes *BRCA1* and *BRCA2* lead to defects in the repair of single-strand and double-strand breaks in DNA.

REVIEW QUESTIONS—CHAPTER 13

1. A variety of drugs can alter DNA replication in eukaryotic cells. Which one of the following steps could be a target for such a drug? Choose the one best answer.
   A. The enzyme family of DNA polymerases, which unwinds parental strands
   B. The enzyme family of topoisomerases, which copy each parental strand in the 3'-to-5' direction
   C. The enzyme family of helicases, which copy each parental strand in the 5'-to-3' direction
   D. The finding that both strands of newly synthesized DNA always grow continuously
   E. The enzyme DNA ligase, which joins Okazaki fragments

2. There are a variety of DNA polymerases in both bacterial and eukaryotic cells. Targeting which one of the following properties of DNA polymerases would result in inhibiting DNA synthesis?
   A. The initiation de novo of the synthesis of new DNA strands
   B. The formation of phosphodiester bonds through hydrogen bonding
   C. The cleavage of released pyrophosphate that provides the energy for the polymerization reaction
   D. The dissociation and reassociation of the enzyme with DNA as each nucleotide is added to an existing DNA chain
   E. The process of copying a template strand in its 3'-to-5' direction, producing a new strand in the 5'-to-3' direction

3. An antibiotic that inhibits bacterial DNA polymerases can damage human mitochondria owing to which one of the following eukaryotic DNA polymerases being most similar to a prokaryotic DNA polymerase?
   - A. α
   - B. β
   - C. γ
   - D. δ
   - E. ε

4. A drug that inhibits DNA replication, but is inactivated by chromosomes containing telomeres, would prove to be a very useful antibiotic. Telomeres can be best described by which one of the following?
   - A. Telomeres are only present in circular chromosomes.
   - B. Before telomerase action, and after DNA replication, there is a 3′ overhang of the newly synthesized strand.
   - C. Before telomerase action, and after DNA replication, there is a 5′ overhang of the strand being replicated.
   - D. In human DNA, telomeres consist of repeating sequences of TTAGGT.
   - E. Somatic eukaryotic cells do not contain telomeres.

5. Diseases caused by defects in DNA repair systems put the patient at risk for developing cancers. DNA repair mechanisms can be best described by which one of the following?
   - A. Proofreading works as the bases are paired and eliminates all base-pairing errors.
   - B. After replication, no further repairs are possible.
   - C. Genes that produce mRNA have a unique repair system.
   - D. Genes that produce transfer RNA (tRNA) have a unique repair system.
   - E. DNA glycosylases recognize distortion of the DNA helix owing to bulky adducts being present on a base within the DNA.

6. Translocations cause some of the most recognized genetic syndromes in human offspring. A translocation can be best described by which one of the following?
   - A. They always produce cancer.
   - B. They always produce mental retardation.
   - C. They have to involve the exchange of an entire chromosome.
   - D. They can only occur in the presence of reverse transcriptase.
   - E. They can occur in somatic or stem cells.

7. The retroviruses, including HIV, use an RNA genome. In order to generate DNA from the genomic RNA, the enzyme reverse transcriptase is required. Reverse transcriptase differs specifically from DNA Pol δ by which one of the following?
   - A. Synthesizing DNA in the 5′-to-3′ direction
   - B. Expressing 3′-to-5′ exonuclease activity
   - C. Using Watson–Crick base-pair rules during DNA synthesis
   - D. Synthesizing DNA in the 3′-to-5′ direction
   - E. Inserting inosine into a growing DNA chain

8. The large DNA molecules in human chromosomes take more time to replicate than the smaller, circular bacterial chromosomes. If a 1,000-kilobase (kb) fragment of DNA has 10 evenly spaced and symmetric replication origins, and DNA polymerase moves at 1 kb per second, how many seconds will it take to produce two daughter molecules? (Ignore potential problems at the ends of this linear piece of DNA.) Assume that the 10 origins are evenly spaced from each other but not from the ends of the chromosome.
   - A. 20
   - B. 30
   - C. 40
   - D. 50
   - E. 100

9. DNA replication is a different process than DNA repair. Mutations in DNA repair enzymes can lead to disease—especially certain forms of cancer. Primase is not required during DNA repair processes because of which one of the following?
   - A. All of the primase is associated with replication origins.
   - B. RNA would be highly mutagenic at a repair site.
   - C. Repair DNA polymerases do not require a primer.
   - D. Replicative DNA polymerases do not require a primer.
   - E. DNA polymerases (both repair and replicative) can use any 3′-OH for elongation.

10. The key mechanistic failure in patients with XP involves which one of the following?
    - A. Mutation in the primase gene
    - B. Inability to excise a section of the UV-damaged DNA
    - C. Mutation of one of the mismatch repair components
    - D. Inability to synthesize DNA across the damaged region
    - E. Loss of proofreading capacity

ANSWERS

1. **The answer is E.** Helicases and topoisomerases unwind the parental strands. DNA polymerases copy each parental template in the 3'-to-5' direction, producing new strands in a 5'-to-3' direction. One strand of newly synthesized DNA grows continuously, but the other strand is synthesized discontinuously in short segments knows as Okazaki fragments. These fragments are subsequently joined by DNA ligase. Targeting a single enzyme with a drug is more likely to succeed than inhibiting an entire family of enzymes.

2. **The answer is E.** DNA polymerases catalyze the synthesis of DNA but cannot initiate the synthesis of new strands de novo, because a short primer first must be synthesized by DNA primase (a DNA-dependent RNA polymerase). Phosphodiester bonds, which link the backbone, are covalent bonds and are not formed from hydrogen bonds. During the course of adding a nucleotide to an existing DNA chain, pyrophosphate is released, and its subsequent hydrolysis (pyrophosphate contains a high-energy bond) by the enzyme pyrophosphatase (not DNA polymerase) provides the energy that drives the polymerization reactions. DNA polymerases exhibit processivity, in which the enzyme remains bound to the parental template strand as the enzyme creates new phosphodiester bonds while reading the template. The enzyme does not dissociate and reassociate after each nucleotide is added to the existing DNA strand. DNA polymerases copy a template in the 3'-to-5' direction, producing new strands in a 5'-to-3' direction.

3. **The answer is C.** Mitochondria in human cells are very similar to bacteria and are theorized to have arisen from bacteria that developed a symbiotic relationship with the host cell. Polymerase γ is located in mitochondria and replicates the DNA of this organelle. Polymerases δ and ε are the major replicative enzymes in the eukaryotic nucleus. Polymerase α is involved in DNA repair. Polymerase β participates in base excision repair.

4. **The answer is B.** Eukaryotic chromosomes are linear, and the ends of the chromosomes are called *telomeres*. Bacteria have circular DNA and therefore have no telomeres. Telomeres in humans consist of a repeating sequence of TTAGGG. The newly synthesized DNA strand, before telomerase action, is shorter at the 5'-end so that the strand being replicated has an overhang at the 3'-end. Somatic cells have telomeres, but as they age, their expression of telomerase decreases, so the cells only survive for a fixed number of population doublings.

5. **The answer is C.** Proofreading, an inherent property of most DNA polymerase owing to its 3' exonuclease activity, eliminates base-pairing errors as they occur during replication, but proofreading does not eliminate all errors made by DNA polymerase. Postreplication error repair systems replace mismatched bases that are missed by proofreading. Genes that produce mRNA contain a unique transcription-coupled repair system (repair occurs as the genes are transcribed). Nucleotide excision repair involves local distortion of the DNA helix, such as in bulky adducts, whereas DNA glycosylases recognize damage to a single base.

6. **The answer is E.** Translocations can occur in both somatic and stem cells. Translocations occur frequently and can be either beneficial or devastating. Some translocations can lead to developmental delay, and some can lead to a higher risk of developing cancer, but they also can be beneficial or have no discernable effect. Translocation consists of a portion of one chromosome being exchanged for a portion of another chromosome. Reverse transcriptase is found in RNA viruses and has no role in human translocation.

7. **The answer is B.** A DNA polymerase's 3'-to-5' exonuclease activity is required for proofreading (check the base just inserted, and if it is incorrect, remove it), and reverse transcriptase does not have this activity, whereas Pol δ does. Both reverse transcriptase and Pol δ synthesize DNA in the 5'-to-3' directions (all DNA polymerases do this), and both follow standard Watson–Crick base-pairing rules (A with T or U, G with C). Neither polymerase can synthesize DNA in the wrong direction (3'-to-5') or insert inosine into a growing DNA chain. Thus, the only difference between the two polymerases is answer B. Pol δ is used primarily for lagging-strand synthesis during DNA replication, although it also has repair functions.

8. **The answer is D.** In 50 seconds, each replication origin will have synthesized 100 kb of DNA (50 in each direction). Because there are 10 origins, 10 × 100 will yield the 1,000 kb needed to replicate the DNA. The first origin will be 50 kb from one end, and the remaining 9 origins will each be 100 kb apart.

9. **The answer is E.** The role of the primer is to provide a free 3'-OH group for DNA polymerase to add the next nucleotide and form a phosphodiester bond. When DNA repair occurs, one of the remaining bases in the DNA will have a free 3'-OH, which repair DNA polymerases (such as DNA pol I in bacteria) will use to begin extension of the DNA.

10. **The answer is B.** XP is a set of diseases all related to an inability to repair thymine dimers, leading to an inability to excise UV-damaged DNA. It does not affect bypass polymerases, which can synthesize across the damaged region, sometimes making mutations in its path. The primase gene, or mismatch repair, is not involved in excising thymine dimers. Proofreading ability of DNA polymerases is likewise not involved in this process.

Transcription: Synthesis of RNA

Synthesis of RNA from a **DNA template** is called **transcription**. Genes are transcribed by enzymes called **RNA polymerases** that generate a **single-stranded RNA** identical in sequence (with the exception of U in place of T) to one of the strands of the double-stranded DNA. The DNA strand that directs the sequence of nucleotides in the RNA by **complementary base pairing** is the template strand. The RNA strand that is initially generated is the **primary transcript**. The DNA **template is copied** in the **3′-to-5′ direction**, and the **RNA transcript** is **synthesized** in the **5′-to-3′ direction**. RNA polymerases differ from DNA polymerases in that they can **initiate** the **synthesis** of new strands in the absence of a primer.

In addition to catalyzing the polymerization of **ribonucleotides**, RNA polymerases must be able to recognize the appropriate gene to transcribe, the appropriate strand of the double-stranded DNA to copy, and the **start point** of transcription (Fig. 14.1). Specific sequences on DNA, called **promoters**, determine where the RNA polymerase binds and how frequently it initiates transcription. Other regulatory sequences, such as **promoter-proximal elements** and **enhancers**, also affect the frequency of transcription.

In **bacteria**, a **single RNA polymerase** produces the primary transcript precursors for all three major classes of RNA: messenger RNA (mRNA), ribosomal RNA (rRNA), and transfer RNA (tRNA). Because bacteria do not contain nuclei, ribosomes bind to mRNA as it is being transcribed, and protein synthesis occurs simultaneously with transcription.

Eukaryotic genes are transcribed in the nucleus by **three different RNA polymerases**, each principally responsible for one of the major classes of RNA. The primary transcripts are **modified** and **trimmed** to produce the mature RNAs. The precursors of **mRNA** (called **pre-mRNA**) have a **guanosine** "cap" added at the 5′-end and a **poly(A) "tail"** at the 3′-end. **Exons**, which contain the coding sequences for the proteins, are separated in **pre-mRNA** by **introns**, regions that have no coding function. During **splicing reactions**, introns are removed and the exons connected to form the mature mRNA. In eukaryotes, tRNA and rRNA precursors are also modified and trimmed, although not as extensively as pre-mRNA.

FIGURE 14.1 Regions of a gene. A gene is a segment of DNA that functions as a unit to generate an RNA product or, through the processes of transcription and translation, a polypeptide chain. The transcribed region of a gene contains the template for synthesis of an RNA, which begins at the start point. A gene also includes regions of DNA that regulate production of the encoded product, such as a promoter region. In a structural gene, the transcribed region contains the coding sequences that dictate the amino acid sequence of a polypeptide chain.

The thalassemias are a heterogenous group of hereditary anemias that constitute the most common gene disorder in the world, with a carrier rate of almost 7%. The disease was first discovered in countries around the Mediterranean Sea and was named for the Greek word *thalassa*, meaning "sea." However, it is also present in areas extending into India and China that are near the equator.

The thalassemia syndromes are caused by mutations that decrease or abolish the synthesis of the α- or β-chains in the adult hemoglobin A tetramer. Individual syndromes are named according to the chain whose synthesis is affected and the severity of the deficiency. Thus, in β^0-thalassemia, the superscript 0 denotes that none of the β-chain is present; in β^+-thalassemia, the plus sign denotes a partial reduction in the synthesis of the β-chain. More than 170 different mutations have been identified that cause β-thalassemia; most of these interfere with the transcription of β-globin mRNA or its processing or translation.

The measurement of hemoglobin levels in blood is important for the appropriate diagnosis of many diseases such as anemia. Laboratories measure hemoglobin content by first exposing the sample (usually lysed blood cells to release the hemoglobin from the red blood cells) to an oxidizing agent, which converts the ferrous iron in hemoglobin to its ferric state. The level of ferric iron is then determined with a second reagent (either a cyanide or azide derivative), which reacts with the ferric iron and generates a colored product whose concentration can be determined spectrophotometrically.

THE WAITING ROOM

 Lisa N. is a 4-year-old girl of Mediterranean ancestry whose height and body weight are below the 20th percentile for girls of her age. She tires easily and complains of loss of appetite and shortness of breath on exertion. A dull pain has been present in her right upper quadrant for the last 3 months and she appears pale. Initial laboratory studies indicate a severe anemia (decreased red blood cell count) with a hemoglobin of 7.0 g/dL (reference range = 12 to 16 g/dL). A battery of additional hematologic tests reveals that Lisa has β^+-thalassemia, intermediate type.

 Isabel S., a patient with HIV (see Chapters 12 and 13), has developed a cough that produces a gray, slightly blood-tinged sputum. A chest X-ray indicates a cavitary infiltrate in the right upper lung field. A stain of sputum shows the presence of acid-fast bacilli, suggesting a diagnosis of pulmonary tuberculosis caused by *Mycobacterium tuberculosis*.

 Catherine T. picked mushrooms in a wooded area near her home. A few hours after eating one small mushroom, she experienced mild nausea and diarrhea. She brought a mushroom with her to the hospital emergency department. A poison expert identified it as *Amanita phalloides* (the "death cap"). These mushrooms contain the toxin α-amanitin.

 Sarah L., a 28-year-old computer programmer, notes increasing fatigue, pleuritic chest pain, and a nonproductive cough. In addition, she complains of joint pains, especially in her hands. A rash on both cheeks and the bridge of her nose ("butterfly rash") has been present for the last 6 months. Initial laboratory studies reveal a subnormal white blood cell count and a mild reduction in hemoglobin. Tests result in a diagnosis of systemic lupus erythematosus (SLE) (frequently called *lupus*).

I. Action of RNA Polymerase

Transcription, the synthesis of RNA from a DNA template, is carried out by *RNA polymerases* (Fig. 14.2). Like DNA polymerases, RNA polymerases catalyze the formation of ester bonds between nucleotides that base-pair with the complementary nucleotides on the DNA template. Unlike DNA polymerases, RNA polymerases can initiate the synthesis of new chains in the absence of primers. They also lack the 3'-to-5' exonuclease activity found in DNA polymerases, although they do perform rudimentary error-checking through a different mechanism. A strand of DNA serves as the template for RNA synthesis and is copied in the 3'-to-5' direction. Synthesis of the new RNA molecule occurs in the 5'-to-3' direction. The ribonucleoside triphosphates adenosine triphosphate (ATP), guanosine triphosphate (GTP), cytidine triphosphate (CTP), and uridine triphosphate (UTP) serve as the precursors. Each nucleotide base sequentially pairs with the complementary deoxyribonucleotide base on the DNA template (A, G, C, and U pair with T, C, G, and A, respectively). The polymerase forms an ester bond between the α-phosphate on the ribose 5'-hydroxyl of the nucleotide precursor and the ribose 3'-hydroxyl at the end of the growing RNA chain. The cleavage of a high-energy phosphate bond in the nucleotide triphosphate and release of pyrophosphate (from the β- and γ-phosphates) provide the energy for this polymerization reaction. Subsequent cleavage of the pyrophosphate by a pyrophosphatase also helps to drive the polymerization reaction forward by removing a product. The overall error rate of RNA polymerase is 1 in 100,000 bases.

RNA polymerases must be able to recognize the start point for transcription of each gene and the appropriate strand of DNA to use as a template. They also must be sensitive to signals that reflect the need for the gene product and control the frequency of transcription. A region of regulatory sequences called the *promoter*

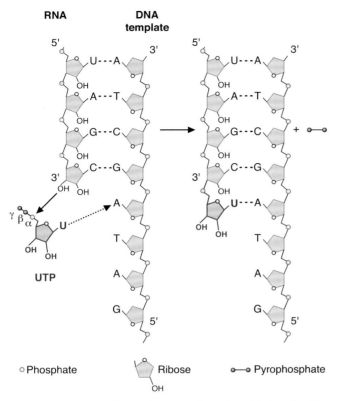

Phosphate   Ribose   Pyrophosphate

FIGURE 14.2 RNA synthesis. The α-phosphate from the added nucleotide connects the ribosyl groups.

Patients with AIDS frequently develop tuberculosis. After **Isabel S.'s** sputum stain suggested that she had tuberculosis, a multidrug antituberculous regimen, which includes an antibiotic of the rifamycin family (rifampin), was begun. A culture of her sputum was done to confirm the diagnosis.

Rifampin inhibits bacterial RNA polymerase, selectively killing the bacteria that cause the infection. The nuclear RNA polymerase from eukaryotic cells is not affected. Although rifampin can inhibit the synthesis of mitochondrial RNA, the concentration required is considerably higher than that used for treatment of tuberculosis.

(often composed of smaller sequences called *boxes* or *elements*), usually contiguous with the transcribed region, controls the binding of RNA polymerase to DNA and identifies the start point (see Fig. 14.1). The frequency of transcription is controlled by regulatory sequences within the promoter and nearby the promoter (promoter-proximal elements) and by other regulatory sequences, such as enhancers (also called *distal-promoter elements*), that may be located at considerable distances—sometimes thousands of nucleotides—from the start point. Both the promoter-proximal elements and the enhancers interact with proteins that stabilize RNA polymerase binding to the promoter.

II. Types of RNA Polymerases

Bacterial cells have a single RNA polymerase that transcribes DNA to generate all of the different types of RNA (mRNA, rRNAs, and tRNA. The RNA polymerase of *Escherichia coli* contains five subunits (2α, β, β', and ω), which form the core enzyme. Another protein called a σ *(sigma) factor* binds the core enzyme and directs binding of RNA polymerase to specific promoter regions of the DNA template. The σ factor dissociates shortly after transcription begins. *E. coli* has several different σ factors that recognize the promoter regions of different groups of genes. The major σ factor is σ^{70}, a designation related to its molecular weight of 70,000 Da.

In contrast to prokaryotes, eukaryotic cells have three RNA polymerases (Table 14.1). Polymerase I produces most of the rRNAs, polymerase II produces mRNA and microRNAs (microRNAs regulate gene expression and are discussed in more detail in Chapter 16), and polymerase III produces small RNAs, such as tRNA and 5S rRNA. All of these RNA polymerases have the same mechanism of action. However, they recognize different types of promoters.

The mushrooms picked by **Catherine T.** contained α-amanitin, an inhibitor of eukaryotic RNA polymerases:

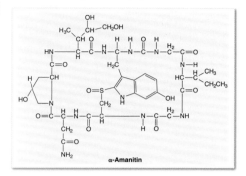

α-Amanitin

It is particularly effective at blocking the action of RNA polymerase II. This toxin initially causes gastrointestinal disturbances, then electrolyte imbalance and fever, followed by liver and kidney dysfunction. Around 10% to 20% of individuals who ingest α-amanitin die within 10 days.

TABLE 14.1	**Products of Eukaryotic RNA Polymerases**	
POLYMERASE	**PRODUCT**	
RNA polymerase I	Ribosomal RNA (rRNA)	
RNA polymerase II	Messenger RNA (mRNA) + microRNA (miRNA)	
RNA polymerase III	Transfer RNA (tRNA) + other small RNAs	

A. Sequences of Genes

Double-stranded DNA consists of a *coding strand* and a *template strand* (Fig. 14.3). The DNA template strand is the strand that is used by RNA polymerase during the process of transcription. It is complementary and antiparallel both to the coding (nontemplate) strand of the DNA and to the RNA transcript produced from the template. Thus, the coding strand of the DNA is identical in base sequence and direction to the RNA transcript except, of course, that wherever this DNA strand contains a T, the RNA transcript contains a U. By convention, the nucleotide sequence of a gene is represented by the letters of the nitrogenous bases of the coding strand of the DNA duplex. It is written from left to right in the 5′-to-3′ direction.

During translation, mRNA is read 5′-to-3′ in sets of three bases, called *codons*, that determine the amino acid sequence of the protein (see Fig. 14.3) Thus, the base sequence of the coding strand of the DNA can be used to determine the amino acid sequence of the protein. For this reason, when gene sequences are given, they refer to the coding strand.

A gene consists of the transcribed region and the regions that regulate transcription of the gene (e.g., promoter and enhancer regions) (Fig. 14.4). The base in the coding strand of the gene serving as the start point for transcription is numbered +1. This nucleotide corresponds to the first nucleotide incorporated into the RNA at the 5′-end of the transcript. Subsequent nucleotides within the transcribed region of the gene are numbered +2, +3, and so on, toward the 3′-end of the gene. Untranscribed sequences to the left of the start point, known as the *5′-flanking* region of the gene, are numbered −1, −2, −3, and so on, starting with the nucleotide (−1) immediately to the left of the start point (+1) and moving from right to left. By analogy to a river, the sequences to the left of the start point are said to be *upstream* from the start point and those to the right are said to be *downstream*.

B. Recognition of Genes by RNA Polymerase

For genes to be expressed, RNA polymerase must recognize the appropriate point at which to start transcription and the strand of the DNA to transcribe (the template strand). RNA polymerase also must recognize which genes to transcribe because transcribed genes are only a small fraction of the total DNA. The genes that are

Q Why is it important for RNA polymerase to distinguish between the two DNA strands at the promoter?

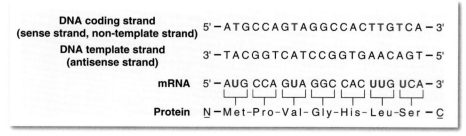

FIGURE 14.3 Relationship between the coding strand of DNA (also known as the *sense strand*, or the *nontemplate strand*), the DNA template strand (also known as the *antisense strand*), the messenger RNA (mRNA) transcript, and the protein produced from the gene. The bases in mRNA are used in sets of three (called *codons*) to specify the order of the amino acids inserted into the growing polypeptide chain during the process of translation (see Chapter 15).

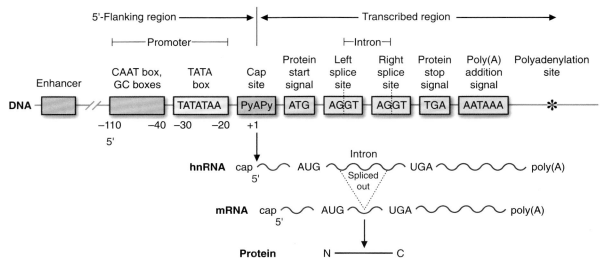

FIGURE 14.4 A schematic view of a eukaryotic gene, and steps required to produce a protein product. The gene consists of promoter and transcribed regions. The transcribed region contains introns, which do not contain coding sequences for proteins, and exons, which do carry coding sequences for proteins. The first RNA form produced is heterogeneous nuclear RNA (hnRNA), which contains both intronic and exonic sequences. The hnRNA is modified such that a cap is added at the 5′-end (cap site) and a poly(A) tail is added to the 3′-end. The introns are removed (a process called splicing) to produce the mature messenger RNA (mRNA), which leaves the nucleus to direct protein synthesis in the cytoplasm. Py is pyrimidine (C or T). Although the TATA box is still included in this figure for historical reasons, only 12.5% of eukaryotic promoters contain this sequence.

transcribed differ from one type of cell to another and change with alterations in physiologic conditions. These signals in DNA that RNA polymerase recognizes are called *promoters*. Promoters are sequences in DNA (often composed of smaller sequences called *boxes* or *elements*) that determine the start point and the frequency of transcription. Because they are located on the same molecule of DNA and near the gene they regulate, they are said to be *cis*-acting (i.e., *cis* refers to acting on the same side). Proteins that bind to these DNA sequences and facilitate or prevent the binding of RNA polymerase are said to be *trans*-acting.

 The two strands of DNA are antiparallel, with complementary nucleotides at each position. Because RNA synthesis always occurs in the 5′-to-3′ direction, each strand would produce a different mRNA, resulting in different codons for amino acids and a different protein product. Therefore, it is critical that RNA polymerase transcribe the correct strand.

C. Promoter Regions of Genes for mRNA

The binding of RNA polymerase and the subsequent initiation of gene transcription involves several *consensus sequences* in the promoter regions of the gene (Fig. 14.5). A consensus sequence is the sequence that is most commonly found in a given region when many genes are examined. In prokaryotes, an adenine- and thymine-rich consensus sequence in the promoter determines the start point of transcription by binding proteins that facilitate the binding of RNA polymerase. In the prokaryote *E. coli,* this consensus sequence is TATAAT, which is known as the *TATA* or *Pribnow box.* It is centered about -10 and is recognized by the sigma factor σ^{70}. A similar sequence in the -25 region of about 12.5% of eukaryotic genes has a consensus sequence of TATA(A/T)A. (The [A/T] in the fifth position indicates that either A or T occurs with equal frequency.) This eukaryotic sequence is also known as a *TATA box,* but it is sometimes named the Hogness or Hogness–Goldberg box after its discoverers. Other consensus sequences involved in binding of RNA polymerase are found farther upstream in the promoter region (see Fig. 14.5) or downstream after the transcriptional start signal. Bacterial promoters contain a sequence of TTGACA in the -35 region. Eukaryotes frequently have disparate sequences, such as the TF$_{II}$B-recognition element (a GC-rich sequence, abbreviated as BRE), the initiator element, the downstream promoter element (DPE), and the motif ten element (MTE). The DPE and MTE are found downstream from the transcription start site. Eukaryotic genes also contain promoter-proximal elements (in the region of -100 to -200), which are sites that bind other gene regulatory proteins. Genes vary

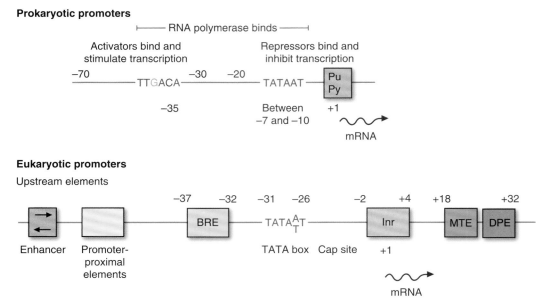

FIGURE 14.5 Prokaryotic and eukaryotic promoters. The promoter-proximal region contains binding sites for transcription factors that can accelerate the rate at which RNA polymerase binds to the promoter. *BRE*, TF$_{II}$B recognition element; *MTE*, motif ten element; *DPE*, downstream promoter element; *Pu*, purine; *Py*, pyrimidine.

Lisa N. has a β^+-thalassemia classified clinically as β-thalassemia intermedia. She produces an intermediate amount of functional β-globin chains (her hemoglobin is 7.0 g/dL; normal is 12 to 16 g/dL). β-Thalassemia intermedia is usually the result of two different mutations (one that mildly affects the rate of synthesis of β-globin and one severely affecting its rate of synthesis); or, less frequently, homozygosity for a mild mutation in the rate of synthesis; or a complex combination of mutations. For example, mutations within the promoter region of the β-globin gene could result in a significantly decreased rate of β-globin synthesis in an individual who is homozygous for the allele, without completely abolishing synthesis of the protein.

Two of the point mutations that result in a β^+-phenotype are within the TATA box (A → G or A → C in the −28 to −31 region) for the β-globin gene. These mutations reduce the accuracy of the start point of transcription so that only 20% to 25% of the normal amount of β-globin is synthesized. Other mutations that also reduce the frequency of β-globin transcription have been observed farther upstream in the promoter region (−87 C → G and −88 C → T).

in the number of such sequences present. An analysis of nearly 10,000 promoter sequences indicated that the initiator element was the most common element in these promoters (~50%), whereas BRE and DPE were present in about 15% of the promoters, and TATA, the least abundant, at 12.5% of the promoters.

In bacteria, several protein-producing genes may be linked together and controlled by a single promoter. This genetic unit is called an *operon* (Fig. 14.6). One mRNA is produced that contains the coding information for all of the proteins encoded by the operon. Proteins bind to the promoter and either inhibit or facilitate transcription of the operon. *Repressors* are proteins that bind to a region in the promoter known as the *operator* and inhibit transcription by preventing the binding of RNA polymerase to DNA. *Activators* are proteins that stimulate transcription by binding within the −35 region or upstream from it, facilitating the binding of RNA polymerase. (Operons are described in more detail in Chapter 16.)

Q What property of an AT-rich region of a DNA double helix makes it suitable to serve as a recognition site for the start point of transcription?

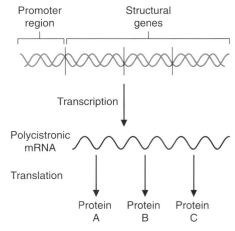

FIGURE 14.6 Bacterial operon. A cistron encodes a single polypeptide chain. In bacteria, a single promoter may control transcription of an operon containing many cistrons. A single polycistronic messenger RNA (mRNA) is transcribed. Its translation produces several polypeptide chains.

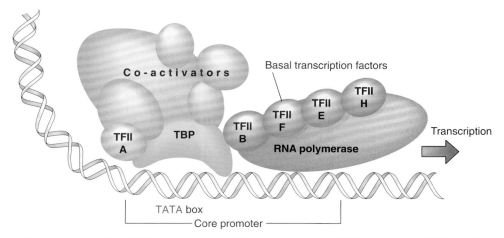

FIGURE 14.7 Transcription apparatus. The TATA-binding protein (TBP), a component of TF$_{II}$D, binds to the TATA box. Transcription factors TF$_{II}$A and -B bind to TBP. RNA polymerase binds, and then TF$_{II}$E, -F, and -H bind. This complex can transcribe at a basal level. Some coactivator proteins are present as a component of TF$_{II}$D, and these can bind to other regulatory DNA-binding proteins (called *specific transcription factors* or *transcriptional activators*). TF$_{II}$D also recognizes the initiator element and the downstream promoter element in the case of TATA-less promoters (see Fig. 14.5).

In eukaryotes, proteins known as *general transcription factors* (or basal factors) bind to the TATA box (or other promoter elements, in the case of TATA-less promoters) and facilitate the binding of RNA polymerase II, the polymerase that transcribes mRNA (Fig. 14.7). This binding process involves at least six basal transcription factors (labeled as TF$_{II}$s, transcription factors for RNA polymerase II). The TATA-binding protein (TBP), which is a component of TF$_{II}$D, initially binds to the TATA box. TF$_{II}$D consists of both the TBP and several transcriptional coactivators. Components of TF$_{II}$D will also recognize initiator and DPE boxes in the absence of a TATA box. TF$_{II}$A and TF$_{II}$B interact with TBP. RNA polymerase II binds to the complex of transcription factors and to DNA and is aligned at the start point for transcription. TF$_{II}$E, TF$_{II}$F, and TF$_{II}$H subsequently bind, cleaving ATP, and transcription of the gene is initiated.

With only these transcription (or basal) factors and RNA polymerase II attached (the basal transcription complex), the gene is transcribed at a low or basal rate. TF$_{II}$H plays several roles in both transcription and DNA repair. In both processes, it acts as an ATP-dependent DNA helicase, unwinding DNA for either transcription or repair to occur. Two of the forms of xeroderma pigmentosum (XPB and XPD; see Chapter 13) arise from mutations within two different helicase subunits of TF$_{II}$H. TF$_{II}$H also contains a kinase activity, and RNA polymerase II is phosphorylated by this factor during certain phases of transcription.

The rate of transcription can be further increased by binding of other regulatory DNA-binding proteins to additional gene regulatory sequences (such as the promoter-proximal or enhancer regions). These regulatory DNA-binding proteins are called *gene-specific transcription factors* (or transactivators) because they are specific to the gene involved (see Chapter 16). They interact with coactivators in the basal transcription complex. These are depicted in Figure 14.7 under the general term *coactivators*. Coactivators consist of transcription-associated factors (TAFs) that interact with transcription factors through an activation domain on the transcription factor (which is bound to DNA). The TAFs interact with other factors (described as the mediator proteins), which in turn interact with the RNA polymerase complex. These interactions are further discussed in Chapter 16.

(A) In regions where DNA is being transcribed, the two strands of the DNA must be separated. AT base pairs in DNA are joined by only two hydrogen bonds, whereas GC pairs have three hydrogen bonds. Therefore, in AT-rich regions of DNA, the two strands can be separated more readily than in regions that contain GC base pairs.

III. Transcription of Bacterial Genes

In bacteria, binding of RNA polymerase with a σ factor to the promoter region of DNA causes the two DNA strands to unwind and separate within a region

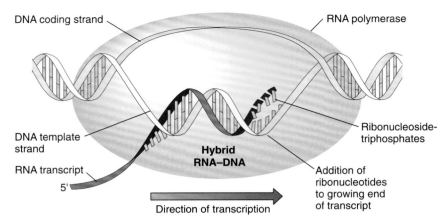

FIGURE 14.8 An overview of transcription at the site of RNA synthesis.

approximately 10 to 20 nucleotides in length. As the polymerase transcribes the DNA, the untranscribed region of the helix continues to separate, whereas the transcribed region of the DNA template rejoins its DNA partner (Fig. 14.8). The σ factor is released when the growing RNA chain is approximately 10 nucleotides long. The elongation reactions continue until the RNA polymerase encounters a transcription termination signal. One type of termination signal involves the formation of a hairpin loop in the transcript, preceding several U residues. The second type of mechanism for termination involves the binding of a protein, the rho factor, which causes release of the RNA transcript from the template in an energy-requiring mechanism. The signal for both termination processes is the sequence of bases in the newly synthesized RNA.

A *cistron* is a region of DNA that encodes a single polypeptide chain. In bacteria, mRNA is usually generated from an operon as a *polycistronic transcript* (one that contains the information to produce several different proteins). Because bacteria do not contain a nucleus, the polycistronic transcript is translated as it is being transcribed. This process is known as *coupled transcription translation*. This transcript is not modified and trimmed, and it does not contain introns (regions within the coding sequence of a transcript that are removed before translation occurs). Several different proteins are produced during translation of the polycistronic transcript, one from each cistron (see Fig. 14.6).

In prokaryotes, rRNA is produced as a single long transcript that is cleaved to produce the 16S, 23S, and 5S rRNAs. tRNA is also cleaved from larger transcripts (Fig. 14.9). One of the cleavage enzymes, RNase P, is a protein containing an RNA molecule. This RNA actually catalyzes the cleavage reaction.

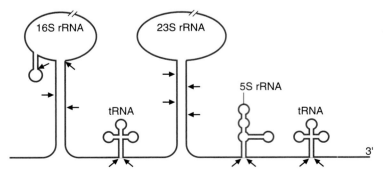

FIGURE 14.9 Bacterial ribosomal RNA (rRNA) and transfer RNA (tRNA) transcripts. One large precursor is cleaved (at *arrows*) to produce 16S, 23S, and 5S rRNA and some tRNAs.

IV. Transcription of Eukaryotic Genes

The process of transcription in eukaryotes is similar to that in prokaryotes. RNA polymerase binds to the transcription factor complex in the promoter region and to the DNA, the helix unwinds within a region near the start point of transcription, DNA strand separation occurs, synthesis of the RNA transcript is initiated, and the RNA transcript is elongated, copying the DNA template. The DNA strands separate as the polymerase approaches and rejoin as the polymerase passes.

One of the major differences between eukaryotes and prokaryotes is that eukaryotes have more elaborate mechanisms for processing the transcripts, particularly the precursors of mRNA (pre-mRNA). Eukaryotes also have three polymerases rather than just the one present in prokaryotes. Other differences include the facts that (1) eukaryotic mRNA usually contains the coding information for only one polypeptide chain and (2) eukaryotic RNA is transcribed in the nucleus and migrates to the cytoplasm where translation occurs. Thus, coupled transcription translation does not occur in eukaryotes.

A. Synthesis of Eukaryotic mRNA

In eukaryotes, extensive processing of the primary transcript occurs before the mature mRNA is formed and can migrate to the cytosol where it is translated into a protein product. RNA polymerase II synthesizes a large primary transcript from the template strand that is capped at the 5′-end as it is transcribed (Fig. 14.10). The transcript also rapidly acquires a poly(A) tail at the 3′-end. Pre-mRNAs thus contain untranslated regions at both the 5′- and 3′-ends (the leader and trailing sequences, respectively). These untranslated regions are retained in the mature mRNA. The coding region of the pre-mRNA, which begins with the start codon for protein synthesis and ends with the stop codon, contains both exons and introns. *Exons* consist of the nucleotide codons that dictate the amino acid sequence of the eventual protein product. Between the exons, interspersing regions called *introns* contain nucleotide sequences that are removed by splicing reactions to form the mature RNA. The mature RNA thus contains a leader sequence (that includes the cap), a coding region comprising exons, and a trailing sequence that includes the poly(A) tail.

There are three different types of methyl caps, shown in *red*:

$$CH_3 (N^7)$$
$$G - 5' - P\ P\ P - 5' - N_1\ N_2\ N_3 - - - - CAP\ 0$$

$\boxed{CAP\ 0}$

(CH_3)-SAM

$\boxed{CAP\ 1}$

$$CH_3 (N^7) \qquad CH_3$$
$$G - 5' - P\ P\ P - 5' - N_1 - N_2\ N_3 - - - - CAP\ 1$$

(CH_3)-SAM

$\boxed{CAP\ 2}$

$$CH_3 (N^7) \qquad CH_3\ CH_3$$
$$G - 5' - P\ P\ P - 5' - N_1 - N_2 - N_3 - - - - CAP\ 2$$

CAP 0 refers to the methylated guanosine (on the nitrogen at the seven position, N^7) added in the 5′-to-5′ linkage to the mRNA; *CAP 1* refers to CAP 0 with the addition of a methyl group to the 2′-carbon of ribose on the nucleotide (N_1) at the 5′-end of the chain; and *CAP 2* refers to CAP 1 with the addition of another 2′-methyl group to the next nucleotide (N_2). The methyl groups are donated by S-adenosylmethionine (*SAM*).

Once SAM donates its methyl group, it must be regenerated by reactions that require the vitamins folate and B_{12}. Thus, formation of mRNA is also one of the processes affected by a deficiency of these vitamins.

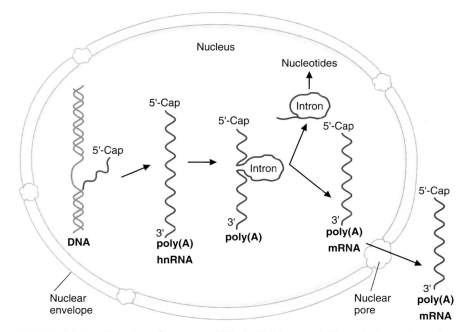

FIGURE 14.10 Overview of messenger RNA (mRNA) synthesis. Transcription produces heterogeneous nuclear RNA (hnRNA, also known as pre-mRNA) from the DNA template. hnRNA processing involves addition of a 5′-cap and a poly(A) tail and splicing to join exons and remove introns. The product, mRNA, migrates to the cytoplasm, where it will direct protein synthesis.

Within about 4 weeks of initiation of treatment for tuberculosis, culture results of **Isabel S.'s** sputum confirmed the diagnosis of pulmonary tuberculosis caused by *M. tuberculosis*. Therefore, the multidrug therapy, which included the antibiotic rifampin, was continued. Rifampin binds to the RNA polymerases of several bacteria. *M. tuberculosis* rapidly develops resistance to rifampin through mutations that result in an RNA polymerase that cannot bind the complex structure. Simultaneous treatment with drugs that work through different mechanisms decreases the selective advantage of the mutation and the rate at which resistance develops.

This mature mRNA complexes with the poly(A)-binding protein and other proteins. It travels through pores in the nuclear envelope into the cytoplasm. There it combines with ribosomes and directs the incorporation of amino acids into proteins.

1. Transcription and Capping of mRNA

Capping of the primary transcript synthesized by RNA polymerase II occurs at its 5′-end as it is being transcribed (Fig. 14.11). The 5′-terminal, the initial nucleotide of the transcript, is a pyrimidine with three phosphate groups attached to the 5′-hydroxyl of the ribose. To form the cap, the terminal triphosphate loses one phosphate, forming a 5′-diphosphate. The β-phosphate of the diphosphate then attacks the α-phosphate of GTP, liberating pyrophosphate and forming an unusual 5′-to-5′ triphosphate linkage. A methyl group is transferred from SAM, a universal methyl donor, to position 7 of the added guanine ring. Methylation also occurs on the ribose 2′-hydroxyl group in the terminal nucleotide to which the cap is attached and sometimes on the 2′-hydroxyl group of the adjacent nucleotide ribose. This cap seals the 5′-end of the primary transcript and decreases the rate of degradation. It also serves as a recognition site for the binding of the mature mRNA to a ribosome at the initiation of protein synthesis.

2. Addition of a Poly(A) Tail

After the RNA polymerase transcribes the stop codon for protein translation, it passes a sequence called the *polyadenylation signal* (AAUAAA) (Fig. 14.12). It continues past the polyadenylation signal until it reaches an unknown, and possibly nonspecific, termination signal many nucleotides later. However, as the primary transcript is released from the RNA polymerase elongation complex, an enzyme complex binds to the polyadenylation signal and cleaves the primary transcript approximately 10 to 20 nucleotides downstream, thereby forming the 3′-end. Following this cleavage, a poly(A) tail that can be >200 nucleotides in length is added to the 3′-end. Thus, there is no poly(dT) sequence in the DNA template that corresponds to this tail; it is added after transcription is completed. ATP serves as

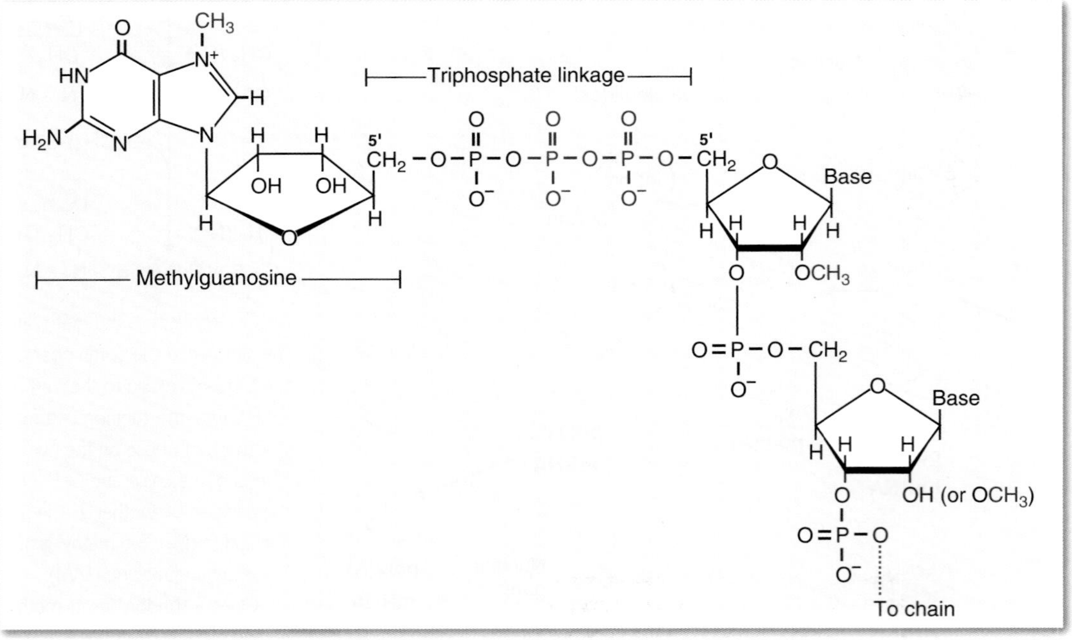

FIGURE 14.11   The cap structure in eukaryotic mRNA. The phosphates in *red* originated from the original RNA transcript; the phosphate in *black* comes from guanosine triphosphate (GTP). S-Adenosylmethionine (SAM) donates the methyl groups (shown in *red*) required for cap synthesis. A CAP 1 structure is shown.

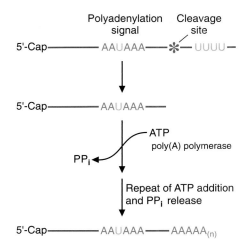

FIGURE 14.12 Synthesis of the poly(A) tail. As RNA polymerase continues to transcribe the DNA, enzymes cleave the transcript (heterogeneous nuclear RNA [hnRNA]) at a point 10 to 20 nucleotides beyond an AAUAAA sequence, just before a run of Us (or Gs). Approximately 250 adenine nucleotides are then added to the 3′-end of the hnRNA, one at a time, by poly(A) polymerase. *ATP*, adenosine triphosphate; *PP_i*, pyrophosphate.

the precursor for the sequential addition of the adenine nucleotides. They are added one at a time, with poly(A) polymerase catalyzing each addition. The poly(A) tail is a protein-binding site that protects the mRNA from degradation.

3. Removal of Introns

Eukaryotic pre-mRNA transcripts contain regions known as *exons* and *introns*. Exons appear in the mature mRNA; introns are removed from the transcript and are not found in the mature mRNA (see Fig. 14.10). Therefore, introns do not contribute to the amino acid sequence of the protein. Some genes contain 50 or more introns. These introns are carefully removed from the pre-mRNA transcript, and the exons are spliced together so that the appropriate protein is produced from the gene.

The consensus sequences at the intron/exon boundaries of the pre-mRNA are AGGU (AGGT in the DNA). The sequences vary to some extent on the exon side of the boundaries, but almost all introns begin with a 5′-GU and end with a 3′-AG (Fig. 14.13). These intron sequences at the left splice site and the right splice site are therefore invariant. Because every 5′-GU and 3′-AG combination does not result in a functional splice site, clearly other features (still to be determined) within the exon or intron help to define the appropriate splice sites.

A complex structure known as a *spliceosome* ensures that exons are spliced together with great accuracy (Fig. 14.14). *Small nuclear ribonucleoproteins* (snRNPs), called "snurps," are involved in formation of the spliceosome. Because snurps are rich in uracil, they are identified by numbers preceded by a U.

Exons frequently code for separate functional or structural domains of proteins. Proteins with similar functional regions (e.g., ATP- or nicotinamide adenine dinucleotide [NAD]-binding regions) frequently have similar domains, although their overall structure and amino acid sequence is quite different. A process known as *exon shuffling* has probably occurred throughout evolution, allowing new proteins to develop with functions similar to those of other proteins.

B. Synthesis of Eukaryotic rRNA

rRNAs form the ribonucleoprotein complexes on which protein synthesis occurs. In eukaryotes, the rRNA gene exists as many copies in the nucleolar organizer region of the nucleus (Fig. 14.15, circle 1). Each gene produces a large, 45S transcript (synthesized by RNA polymerase I) that is cleaved to produce the 18S, 28S, and

 Lisa N. has β^+-thalassemia (enough of the β-chain is produced to maintain blood hemoglobin levels >6.0 g/dL). One mutation resulting in β^+-thalassemia is a point mutation (AATAAA → AACAAA) that changes the sequence in hnRNA at the polyadenylation signal site from AAUAAA to AACAAA. Homozygous individuals with this mutation produce only one-tenth the amount of normal β-globin mRNA.

 Some types of β^0-thalassemia (little or none of the hemoglobin β-chain produced) are caused by homozygous mutations in the splice-junction sequences at intron/exon boundaries. In some individuals, an AT replaces a GT in the gene at the 5′-end of the first or second intron. Mutations also occur within the splice-junction sequences at the 3′-ends of introns (which are normally GT at the donor-site 5′-end and AG at the acceptor-site 3′-end). Mutations at either site totally abolish normal splicing and result in β^0-thalassemia.

├─Exon─┼──Intron──┼─Exon─┤

hnRNA 5′-cap ──── AG GU ──── AG G(U) ── 3′

FIGURE 14.13 Splice junctions in heterogeneous nuclear RNA (hnRNA). The intron sequences shown in the *boxes* are invariant. They always appear at this position in introns. The sequences on the exon side of the splice sites are more variable.

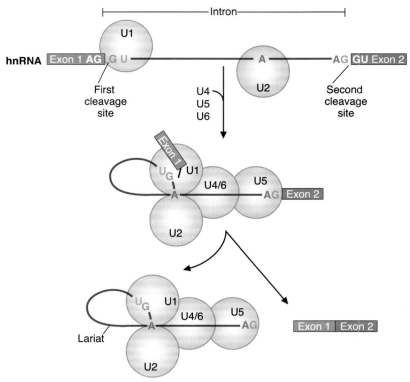

FIGURE 14.14   Splicing process. Nuclear ribonucleoproteins (snurps U1 to U6) bind to the intron, causing it to form a loop. The complex is called a spliceosome. The U1 snurp binds near the first exon/intron junction, and U2 binds within the intron in a region containing an adenine nucleotide residue. Another group of snurps, U4, U5, and U6, binds to the complex, and the loop is formed. The phosphate attached to the G residue at the 5′-end of the intron forms a 2′–5′ linkage with the 2′-hydroxyl group of the adenine nucleotide residue. Cleavage occurs at the end of the first exon, between the AG residues at the 3′-end of the exon and the GU residues at the 5′-end of the intron. The complex continues to be held in place by the spliceosome. A second cleavage occurs at the 3′-end of the intron after the AG sequence. The exons are joined together. The intron, shaped like a lariat, is released and degraded to nucleotides.

SLE is an autoimmune disease characterized by a particular spectrum of autoantibodies against many cellular components, including chromatin, ribonucleoprotein, and cell membrane phospholipids. In this disorder, the body makes these antibodies against its own components. snRNPs are one of the targets of these antibodies. In fact, snRNPs were discovered as a result of studies using antibodies obtained from patients with SLE.

Tests were performed on **Sarah L.'s** blood to detect levels of antibodies including antibodies to nuclear antigens (ANA), antibodies to double-stranded DNA (anti-dsDNA), and antibodies to ribonucleoproteins (these were historically known as *Smith proteins*, for the first patient in which they were discovered. It has since been shown that the snRNPs correspond to the Smith antigens). The tests were strongly positive and, in conjunction with her symptoms, led to a diagnosis of SLE.

5.8S rRNAs. Approximately 1,000 copies of this gene are present in the human genome. The genes are linked in tandem, separated by spacer regions that contain the termination signal for one gene and the promoter for the next. Promoters for rRNA genes are located in the 5′-flanking region of the genes and extend into the region surrounding the start point. rRNA genes caught in the act of transcription by electron micrographs show that many RNA polymerase I molecules can be attached to a gene at any given time, all moving toward the 3′-end as the 45S rRNA precursors are synthesized.

As the 45S rRNA precursors are released from the DNA, they complex with proteins, forming ribonucleoprotein particles that generate the granular regions of the nucleolus (see Fig. 14.15, circle 2). Processing of the transcript occurs in the granular regions. 5S rRNA, produced by RNA polymerase III from genes located outside the nucleolus in the nucleoplasm, migrates into the nucleolus and joins the ribonucleoprotein particles.

One to two percent of the nucleotides of the 45S precursor become methylated, primarily on the 2′-hydroxyl groups of ribose moieties (see Fig. 14.15, circle 3). These methyl groups may serve as markers for cleavage of the 45S precursors and are conserved in the mature rRNA. A series of cleavages in the 45S transcripts occur to produce the mature rRNAs (Fig. 14.16).

In the production of cytoplasmic ribosomes in human cells, one portion of the 45S rRNA precursor becomes the 18S rRNA that, complexed with proteins, forms

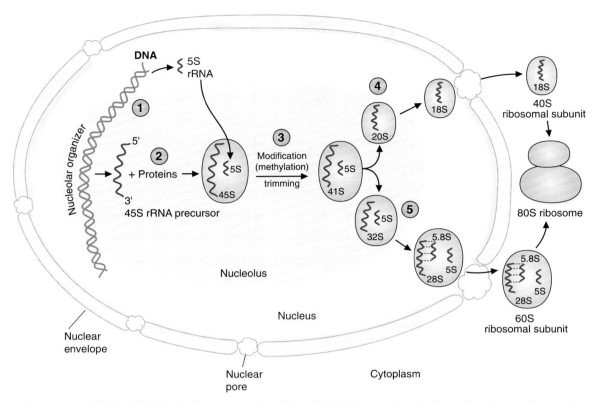

FIGURE 14.15 Ribosomal RNA (rRNA) and ribosome synthesis. The 5S rRNA is transcribed in the nucleoplasm and moves into the nucleolus. The other rRNAs are transcribed from DNA and mature in the nucleolus, forming the 40S and 60S ribosomal subunits, which migrate to the cytoplasm. See the text for a detailed explanation.

the small 40S ribosomal subunit (Fig. 14.15, circle 4). Another segment of the precursor folds back on itself and is cleaved, forming 28S rRNA, hydrogen-bonded to the 5.8S rRNA. The 5S rRNA, transcribed from nonnucleolar genes, and several proteins complex with the 28S and 5.8S rRNAs to form the 60S ribosomal subunit (Fig. 14.15, circle 5). The ribosomal subunits migrate through the nuclear pores. In the cytoplasm, the 40S and 60S ribosomal subunits interact with mRNA, forming the 80S ribosomes on which protein synthesis occurs.

C. Synthesis of Eukaryotic tRNA

A tRNA has one binding site for a specific sequence of three nucleotides in mRNA (the anticodon site) and another binding site for the encoded amino acid. Thus, tRNAs ensure that the genetic code is translated into the correct sequence of amino acids. At least 20 types of tRNAs occur in cells, one for every amino acid that is incorporated into growing polypeptide chains during the synthesis of proteins. tRNAs have a cloverleaf structure that folds into a three-dimensional L shape and contain several bases that are modified posttranscriptionally (Fig. 14.17). The loop closest to the 5′-end is known as the *D-loop* because it contains dihydrouridine (D). The second, or *anticodon loop*, contains the trinucleotide anticodon that base-pairs with the codon on mRNA. The third loop (the *TΨC loop*) contains both ribothymidine (T) and pseudouridine (Ψ). A fourth loop, known as the *variable loop* because it varies in size, is frequently found between the anticodon and TΨC loops. Base pairing occurs in the stem regions of tRNA, and a three-nucleotide sequence (e.g., CCA) at the 3′-end is the attachment site for the specific amino acid carried by each tRNA. Different tRNAs bind different amino acids. The three-dimensional structure of tRNA has been determined and is shown in Figure 14.18. tRNA is produced by RNA polymerase III, which recognizes, along with promoter-proximal elements,

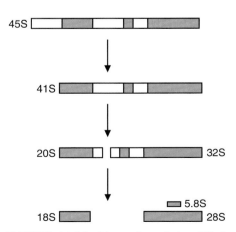

FIGURE 14.16 Maturation of the 45S ribosomal RNA (rRNA) precursor. The *clear regions* are removed, and the *red regions* become the mature rRNAs. (The 5S rRNA is not produced from this precursor.)

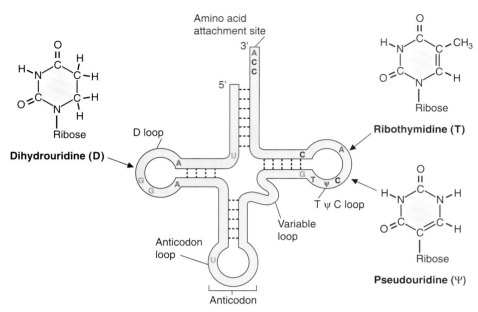

FIGURE 14.17 The transfer RNA (tRNA) cloverleaf. Bases that commonly occur in a particular position are indicated by *letters*. Base pairing in stem regions is indicated by *dotted lines* between the strands. The locations of the modified bases dihydrouridine (D), ribothymidine (T), and pseudouridine (Ψ) are indicated. *D loop*, contains dihydrouridine.

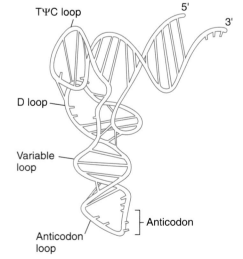

FIGURE 14.18 The three-dimensional folding of transfer RNA (tRNA). *D loop*, contains dihydrouridine. (Reprinted with permission from Kim SH, Suddath FL, Quigley GJ, et al. *Science*. 1974;185:436. Copyright © 1974 American Association for the Advancement of Science.)

a split promoter within the transcribed region of the gene (Fig. 14.19). One segment of the promoter is located between +8 and +19. A second segment is 30 to 60 base pairs (bp) downstream from the first.

tRNA precursors of approximately 100 nucleotides in length are generated. (Fig. 14.20, circle 1). The pre-tRNA assumes a cloverleaf shape and is subsequently cleaved at the 5′- and 3′-ends (see Fig. 14.20, circle 2). The enzyme that acts at the 5′-end is RNase P, similar to the RNase P of bacteria. Both enzymes contain a small RNA (M1) that has catalytic activity and serves as an endonuclease. Some tRNA precursors contain introns that are removed by endonucleases. To close the opening, a 2′- or 3′-phosphate group from one end is ligated to a 5′-hydroxyl on the other end by an RNA ligase.

The bases are modified at the same time the endonucleolytic cleavage reactions are occurring (see Fig. 14.20, circle 3). Three modifications occur in most tRNAs: (1) Uracil is methylated by SAM to form thymine; (2) one of the double bonds of uracil is reduced to form dihydrouracil; and (3) a uracil residue (attached to ribose by an *N*-glycosidic bond) is rotated to form pseudouridine, which contains uracil linked to ribose by a carbon–carbon bond (see Fig. 14.17). Other, less common but more complex modifications also occur and involve bases other than uracil. Of particular note is the deamination of adenine in the nucleoside adenosine to form the base hypoxanthine and the nucleoside inosine.

The final step in forming the mature tRNA is the addition of a CCA sequence at its 3′-end (see Fig. 14.20, circle 4). These nucleotides are added one at a time

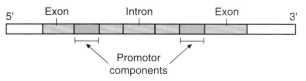

FIGURE 14.19 Promoter for transfer RNA (tRNA) transcription. The segments of the genes from which the mature tRNA is produced are indicated in *purple*. The two regions of the promoter lie within these segments and are indicated in *green*.

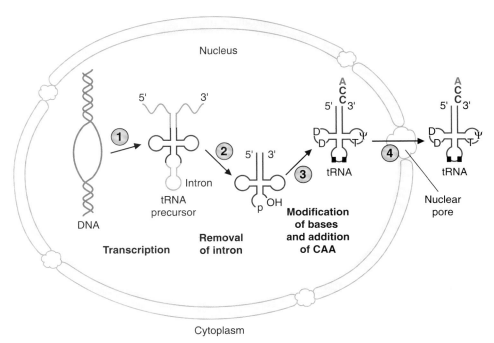

FIGURE 14.20   Overview of transfer RNA (tRNA) synthesis. D, T, Ψ, and ■ indicate modified bases. *D*, dihydrouracil; *T*, ribothymidine; Ψ, pseudouridine; ■, other modified bases.

by nucleotidyltransferase. The tRNA then migrates to the cytoplasm. The terminal adenosine at the 3′-end is the site at which the specific amino acid for each tRNA is bound and activated for incorporation into a protein.

V. Differences in Size between Eukaryotic and Prokaryotic DNA

A. Diploid versus Haploid

Except for the germ cells, most normal human cells are diploid. Therefore, they contain two copies of each chromosome, and each chromosome contains genes that are alleles of the genes on the homologous chromosome. Because one chromosome in each set of homologous chromosomes is obtained from each parent, the alleles can be identical, containing the same DNA sequence, or they can differ. A diploid human cell contains 2,000 times more DNA than the genome of the bacterium in the haploid *E. coli* cell (~4 × 10⁶ bp).

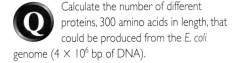

Calculate the number of different proteins, 300 amino acids in length, that could be produced from the *E. coli* genome (4 × 10⁶ bp of DNA).

B. Introns

Eukaryotic introns contribute to the DNA size difference between bacteria and human cells. In eukaryotic genes, introns (noncoding regions) occur within sequences that code for proteins. Consequently, the primary transcript (heterogeneous nuclear RNA [hnRNA]) averages roughly 10 times longer than the mature mRNA produced by removal of the introns. In contrast, bacterial genes do not contain introns.

C. Repetitive Sequences in Eukaryotic DNA

Although being diploid and containing introns account for some of the difference between the DNA content of humans and bacteria, a large difference remains that is related to the greater complexity of the human organism. Bacterial cells have a single copy of each gene, called *unique DNA*, and they contain very little DNA

Four million base pairs contain $(4 \times 10^6)/3$ or 1.33 million codons. If each protein contained approximately 300 amino acids, *E. coli* could produce about 4,000 different proteins [$(1.33 \times 10^6)/300$].

Alu sequences in DNA were named for the enzyme Alu (obtained from *Arthrobacter luteus*), which is able to cleave them. Alu sequences make up 6% to 8% of the human genome. In some cases of familial hypercholesterolemia, homologous recombination is believed to have occurred between two Alu repeats, resulting in a large deletion in the low-density lipoprotein (LDL)–receptor gene. The LDL receptor mediates uptake of the cholesterol-containing LDL particle into many cell types, and, in the absence of functional LDL receptors, blood cholesterol levels are elevated. Patients who are homozygous for this mutation may die from cardiac disease as early as in their second or third decade of life.

that does not produce functional products. Eukaryotic cells contain substantial amounts of DNA that does not code for functional products (i.e., proteins or rRNA and tRNA). In addition, some genes that encode functional products are present in multiple copies, called *highly repetitive* or *moderately repetitive* DNA. About 64% of the DNA in the human genome is unique, consisting of DNA sequences present in one or a very few copies in the genome (Fig. 14.21). Some of the unique DNA sequences are transcribed to generate mRNA, which is translated to produce proteins.

Highly repetitive DNA consists of sequences approximately 6 to 100 bp in length that are present in hundreds of thousands to millions of copies, clustered within a few locations in the genome (see Fig. 14.21). It occurs in centromeres (which join sister chromatids during mitosis) and in telomeres (the ends of chromosomes). This DNA represents approximately 10% of the human genome. It is not transcribed.

Moderately repetitive DNA is present in a few to tens of thousands of copies in the genome (see Fig. 14.21). This fraction constitutes approximately 25% of the human genome. It contains DNA that is functional and transcribed to produce rRNA, tRNA, and also some mRNA. The histone genes, present in a few hundred copies in the genome, belong to this class. Moderately repetitive DNA also includes some gene sequences that are functional but not transcribed. Promoters and enhancers (which are involved in regulating gene expression) are examples of gene sequences in this category. Other groups of moderately repetitive gene sequences that have been found in the human are called the *Alu sequences* (~300 bp in length). Alu sequences are also examples of *short interspersed elements* (SINEs). The *long*

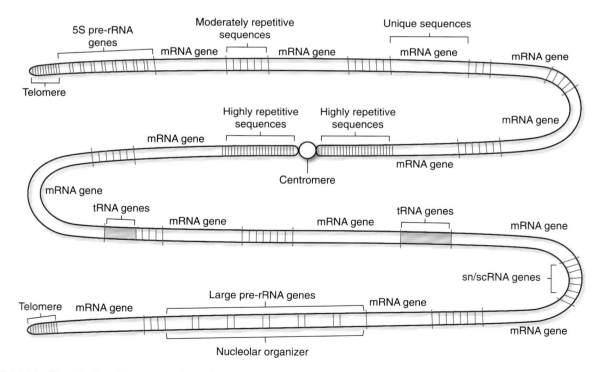

FIGURE 14.21 Distribution of unique, moderately repetitive, and highly repetitive sequences in a hypothetical human chromosome. Unique genes encode messenger RNA (mRNA). These genes occur in single copies. The genes for the large ribosomal RNA (rRNA) and the transfer RNA (tRNA) precursors occur in multiple copies that are clustered in the genome. The large rRNA genes form the nucleolar organizer. Moderately repetitive sequences are dispersed throughout the genome, and highly repetitive sequences are clustered around the centromere and at the ends of the chromosome (the telomeres). Small nuclear RNA (snRNA) and small cytoplasmic RNA (scRNA) are usually found in ribonuclear protein particles. *sn/sc RNA*, small nuclear, small cytoplasmic RNAs, usually found in ribonucleoprotein particles. (From Wolfe SL. *Mol and Cell Biol.* 1993:761.)

*inter*spersed *e*lements (LINEs) are 6,000 to 7,000 bp in length. The functions of the Alu and LINE sequences have not been determined.

D. Summary of the Differences between Eukaryotic and Prokaryotic DNA and RNA

Several differences between eukaryotes and prokaryotes affect the processes of replication, transcription, and translation, in addition to the content of their DNA. Eukaryotic DNA is complexed with histones, and prokaryotic DNA is not. In eukaryotic cells, the process of transcription, which occurs in the nucleus, is separated by the nuclear envelope from the process of translation (protein synthesis from the mRNA template), which occurs in the cytoplasm. Because prokaryotes lack nuclei, the processes of transcription and translation occur simultaneously. Transcription of bacterial DNA requires only one promoter per operon. In contrast, human DNA requires one promoter for each gene.

Complexity may explain some of the differences between the DNA content of bacteria and humans. But an extension of this line of reasoning would lead to the conclusion that frogs are more complex than humans because frogs have 8 ft of DNA per diploid nucleus, compared to the 6 ft in a human cell. Logic, or perhaps vanity, suggests that the amount of DNA per cell does not necessarily reflect the complexity of the organism. One of the features of frog DNA that may explain its length is that frogs have more repetitive DNA than humans. More than 75% of the frog genome is in the moderately and highly repetitive category, whereas only about 35% of the human genome is repetitive.

Major differences between prokaryotic and eukaryotic DNA and RNA are summarized in Table 14.2. LINEs make up about 5% of the human genome. In some patients with hemophilia (a disease in which blood does not clot normally), a LINE sequence has been inserted into exon 14 of the gene for factor VIII, a protein of the blood-clotting system. The insertion of the LINE sequence leads to the production of a nonfunctional protein.

 The mutations that cause the thalassemias affect the synthesis of either the α- or the β-chains of adult hemoglobin, causing an anemia. They are classified by the chain affected (α- or β-) and by the amount of chain synthesized (0 for no synthesis and + for synthesis of some functional chains). They are also classified as major, intermediate, or minor, according to the severity of the clinical disorder. β-Thalassemia major (also called *homozygous β-thalassemia*) is a clinically severe disorder requiring frequent blood transfusions. It is caused by the inheritance of two alleles for a severe mutation. In β-thalassemia intermedia, the patient exhibits a less severe clinical phenotype and is able to maintain hemoglobin levels >6 to 7 g/dL. It is usually the result of two different mild mutations or homozygosity for a mild mutation. β-Thalassemia minor (also known as *β-thalassemia trait*) is a heterozygous disorder involving a single mutation that is often clinically asymptomatic.

During embryonic and fetal life, the β-chain is replaced by the ε- and γ-chains, respectively. As a result, patients with severe mutations in the α-chain tend to die in utero, whereas those with mutations in the β-chains exhibit symptoms postnatally, because hemoglobin F ($\alpha_2\gamma_2$) is normally replaced with adult hemoglobin A ($\alpha_2\beta_2$) after birth.

TABLE 14.2	Differences between Eukaryotes and Prokaryotes	
	EUKARYOTES (HUMAN)	**PROKARYOTES** (*Escherichia coli*)
Nucleus	Yes	No
Chromosomes		
Number	23 per haploid cell	1 per haploid cell
DNA	Linear	Circular
Histones	Yes	No
Genome		
Diploid	Somatic cells	No
Haploid	Germ cells	All cells
Size	3×10^9 bp per haploid cell	4×10^6 bp
Genes		
Unique	64%	100%
Repetitive		
Moderately	25%	None
Highly	10%	None
Operons	No	Yes
mRNA		
Polycistronic	No	Yes
Introns (hnRNA)	Yes	No
Translation	Separate from transcription	Coupled with transcription

bp, base pairs; mRNA, messenger RNA; hnRNA, heterogeneous nuclear RNA.

CLINICAL COMMENTS

Lisa N. Patients with β^+-thalassemia who maintain their hemoglobin levels >6.0 to 7.0 g/dL are usually classified as having thalassemia intermedia. In the β-thalassemias, the α-chains of adult hemoglobin A ($\alpha_2\beta_2$) continue to be synthesized at a normal rate. These chains accumulate in the bone marrow in which the red blood cells are synthesized during the process of erythropoiesis (generation of red blood cells). The accumulation of α-chains diminishes erythropoiesis, resulting in an anemia. Individuals who are homozygous for a severe mutation require constant transfusions.

Individuals with thalassemia intermedia, such as **Lisa N.**, could have inherited two different defective alleles, one from each parent. One parent may be a "silent" carrier, with one normal allele and one mildly affected allele. This parent produces enough functional β-globin so few or no clinical symptoms of thalassemia appear. (However, they generally have a somewhat decreased amount of hemoglobin, resulting in microcytic hypochromic red blood cells.) When this parent contributes the mildly defective allele and the other heterozygous parent contributes a more severely defective allele, thalassemia intermedia occurs in the child. The child is thus heterozygous for two different defective alleles.

Isabel S. Isabel S. was treated with a multidrug regimen for tuberculosis because the microbes that cause the disease frequently become resistant to the individual drugs. The current approach in patients with *M. tuberculosis* is to initiate antimycobacterial therapy with four agents because the mycobacteria frequently become resistant to one or more of the individual antitubercular drugs. The same approach is taken for patients with HIV, with careful attention given to drug interactions. Isabel was started on isoniazid (INH), rifampin, pyrazinamide, and ethambutol. Isoniazid inhibits the biosynthesis of mycolic acids, which are important constituents of the mycobacterial cell wall. Isoniazid is often prescribed with vitamin B$_6$ (pyridoxine) because isoniazid can interfere with the activation of this vitamin (to pyridoxal phosphate), which can lead to an alteration in normal cellular metabolism and result in a clinical neuropathy. Rifampin binds to and inhibits bacterial RNA polymerase, which selectively kills the bacteria that cause the infection. Pyrazinamide, a synthetic analog of nicotinamide, targets the mycobacterial fatty acid synthase I gene involved in mycolic acid biosynthesis in *M. tuberculosis*. Ethambutol blocks arabinosyl transferases that are involved in cell wall biosynthesis.

Just as bacteria can become resistant to drugs, so can HIV. Because of this concern, patients with HIV are treated with multidrug regimens. Multidrug regimens usually include two nucleoside reverse transcriptase inhibitors (NRTIs), such as lamivudine (3TC, Epivir) and abacavir, as well as a third agent. The third agent is usually either a nonnucleoside reverse transcriptase inhibitor (NNRTI), an example of which is efavirenz; a protease inhibitor (PI), an example of which is indinavir; or an integrase inhibitor. PIs prevent the HIV polyprotein from being cleaved into its mature products (see "Biochemical Comments"). The drugs are often combined into one pill to make it easier to take. **Isabel S.** was started on efavirenz as her third drug and was counseled on not getting pregnant because this drug is teratogenic.

Catherine T. The toxin α-amanitin is capable of causing irreversible hepatocellular and renal dysfunction through inhibition of mammalian RNA polymerases. α-Amanitin is particularly effective at blocking the action of RNA polymerase II. Fortunately, **Catherine T.'s** toxicity proved mild. She developed only gastrointestinal symptoms and slight changes in her hepatic and renal function, which returned to normal within a few weeks. Treatment was primarily supportive, with fluid and electrolyte replacement for that lost through the gastrointestinal tract. No effective antidote is available for the *Amanita phalloides* toxin.

Sarah L. SLE is a multisystem disease characterized by inflammation related to the presence of autoantibodies in the blood. These autoantibodies react with antigens normally found in the nucleus, cytoplasm, and plasma membrane of the cell. Such "self" antigen–antibody (autoimmune) interactions initiate an inflammatory cascade that produces the broad symptom profile of multiorgan dysfunction found in **Sarah L.**

Pharmacologic therapy for SLE involves anti-inflammatory drugs and immunosuppressive agents. It can include nonsteroidal anti-inflammatory drugs (NSAIDs), corticosteroids, antimalarials, or immunosuppressive drugs. Plaquenil is an antimalarial drug used to treat skin and joint symptoms in SLE, although its exact mechanism of action in these patients is not fully understood. Sarah was placed on such a drug regimen.

BIOCHEMICAL COMMENTS

Production of the Virus that Causes AIDS. AIDS is caused by the HIV. Two forms of the virus have been discovered, HIV-1, which is prevalent in industrialized countries, and HIV-2, which is prevalent in certain regions of Africa. Eight to 10 years or more can elapse between the initial infection and development of the full-blown syndrome.

Proteins in the viral coat bind to membrane protein receptors (named CD4) of helper T-lymphocytes, a class of cells involved in the immune response. Subsequently, conformational changes occur that allow the viral-coat proteins to bind to a chemokine coreceptor in the cell membrane. The lipid in the viral coat then fuses with the cell membrane, and the viral core enters the cell, releasing its RNA and enzymes (including the reverse transcriptase) by a process called *uncoating*. Reverse transcriptase uses the viral RNA as a template to produce a single-stranded DNA copy, which then serves as a template for synthesis of a double-stranded DNA. An integrase enzyme, also carried by the virus, enables this DNA to integrate into the host cell genome as a provirus (Fig. 14.22).

In the initial stage of transcription of the provirus, the transcript is spliced, and three proteins—Nef, Tat, and Rev—are produced. Tat stimulates transcription of the viral genes. As Rev accumulates, it allows unspliced viral RNA to leave the nucleus and to produce proteins of the viral envelope and viral core, including reverse transcriptase. Two of the envelope glycoproteins (gp41 and gp120, which are derived from the *env* gene product) form a complex that embeds in the cell membrane. The other proteins, which are translated as a polyprotein and cleaved by the viral protease (one of the targets of anti-HIV drugs), combine with the full-length viral RNA to form core viral particles, which bud from the cell membrane. Thus, the virus obtains its lipid coat from the host cell membrane, and the coat contains the viral proteins gp41 and gp120. These surface proteins of the virus bind to CD4 receptors on other human helper T-lymphocytes, and the infection spreads.

In an uninfected person, helper T-lymphocytes usually number approximately 1,000/mL. Infection with HIV causes the number of these cells to decrease, which results in a deficiency of the immune system. When the number of T-lymphocytes drops to <200/mL, the disease is in an advanced stage, and opportunistic infections, such as tuberculosis, occur. Although macrophages and dendritic cells lack CD4 receptors, they can also become infected with HIV and can carry the virus to the central nervous system.

The most effective means of combating HIV infection involves the use of drugs that inhibit the viral reverse transcriptase or the viral protease. However, these drugs only hold the infection at bay; they do not effect a cure.

 Studies have indicated that a failure to dispose properly of cellular debris, a normal by-product of cell death, may lead to the induction of autoantibodies directed against chromatin in patients with SLE. Normal cells have a finite lifetime and are programmed to die (apoptosis) through a distinct biochemical mechanism. One of the steps in this mechanism is the stepwise degradation of cellular DNA (and other cellular components). If the normal intracellular components are exposed to the immune system, autoantibodies against them may be generated. The enzyme in cells that degrades DNA is deoxyribonuclease I (DNase I), and individuals with SLE have reduced serum activity levels of DNase I compared with individuals who do not have the disease. Through an understanding of the molecular mechanism whereby autoantibodies are generated, it may be possible to develop therapies to combat this disorder.

 Drugs currently used to treat HIV act on the viral reverse transcriptase or the protease (see Fig. 14.22). The nonnucleoside drugs (e.g., efavirenz) bind to reverse transcriptase and inhibit its action. The nucleoside analogs (e.g., lamivudine) add to the 3'-end of the growing DNA transcript produced by reverse transcriptase and prevent further elongation. The PI (e.g., indinavir) bind to the protease and prevent it from cleaving the polyprotein.

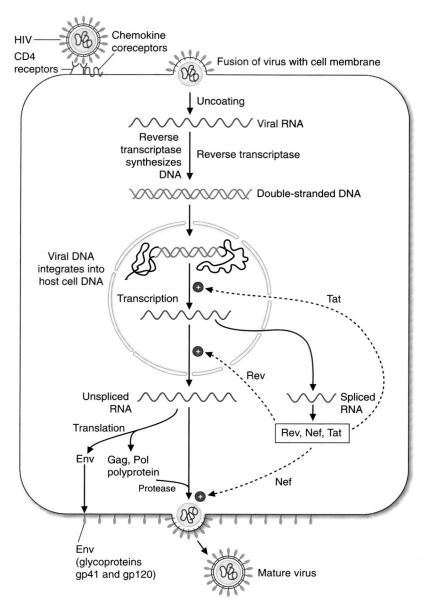

FIGURE 14.22 Infection of a host cell by HIV. The HIV particle binds to the CD4 receptor and a chemokine coreceptor in the host cell membrane. The virus enters the cell and uncoats, releasing its RNA and proteins. The viral enzyme reverse transcriptase produces a double-stranded DNA copy that is integrated into the host cell genome. HIV is now a provirus. Transcripts of the viral DNA are spliced and translated to produce the proteins Tat, Rev, and Nef. Tat stimulates transcription of the viral DNA, and Rev causes the viral RNA transcripts to leave the nucleus unspliced. The unspliced RNA serves as the viral genome and also codes for the proteins of the viral core and envelope. The envelope proteins (gp41 and gp120, which are derived from the Env protein) enter the cell membrane. The viral core proteins are synthesized as a polyprotein, which is cleaved by a protease as the viral particles form and bud from the cell membrane. The particles carry membrane lipid as a coat that contains gp41 and gp120. Nef indirectly aids in the assembly of viral particles. *Pol* is the reverse transcriptase produced from the viral RNA. ⊕, stimulates.

KEY CONCEPTS

- Transcription is the synthesis of RNA from a DNA template.
- The enzyme RNA polymerase transcribes genes into a single-stranded RNA.
- The RNA produced is complementary to one of the strands of DNA, which is known as the *template strand*. The other DNA strand is the coding, or sense, strand.
- Bacteria contain a single RNA polymerase; eukaryotic cells use three different RNA polymerases.
- The DNA template is copied in the 3′-to-5′ direction and the RNA transcript is synthesized in the 5′-to-3′ direction.
- In contrast to DNA polymerases, RNA polymerases do not require a primer to initiate transcription, nor do they contain extensive error-checking capabilities.
- Promoter regions, specific sequences in DNA, determine where on the DNA template RNA polymerase binds to initiate transcription.
- Transcription initiation requires several protein factors to allow for efficient RNA polymerase binding to the promoter.
- Other DNA sequences, such as promoter-proximal elements and enhancers, affect the rate of transcription initiation through the interactions of DNA-binding proteins with RNA polymerase and other initiation factors.
- Eukaryotic genes contain exons and introns. Exons specify the coding region of proteins, whereas introns have no coding function.
- The primary transcript of eukaryotic genes is modified to remove the introns (splicing) before a final, mature mRNA is produced.
- Table 14.3 summarizes the diseases discussed in this chapter.

TABLE 14.3 Diseases Discussed in Chapter 14

DISORDER OR CONDITION	GENETIC OR ENVIRONMENTAL	COMMENTS
β-Thalassemia	Genetic	An anemia caused by an imbalance in β- and α-globin chain synthesis. For a β-thalassemia, more α-chain is synthesized than functional β-chain.
Tuberculosis	Environmental	The drug rifampin, among others, is used to treat tuberculosis via inhibition of bacterial RNA polymerase.
Mushroom poisoning (α-amanitin poisoning)	Environmental	Inhibition of RNA polymerase II by α-amanitin. There is no effective antidote for this poison.
Systemic lupus erythematosus (SLE)	Both	The development of autoantibodies directed against various cellular proteins, including those involved in RNA processing (such as complexes involved in RNA splicing, the snurps).

REVIEW QUESTIONS—CHAPTER 14

1. A gene would need to contain which one of the following templates to generate the short transcript AUCCGUACG (note that all sequences are written from 5′ to 3′)?
   A. ATCCGTACG
   B. CGTACGGAT
   C. AUCCGUACG
   D. TAGGCATGC
   E. GCATGCCTA

2. Given that the LD$_{50}$ (the dose at which 50% of the recipients die) of amanitin is 0.1 mg/kg of body weight, and that the average mushroom contains 7 mg of amanitin, how many mushrooms must be consumed by **Catherine T.** (50 kg of body weight) to be above the LD$_{50}$?
   A. 1
   B. 2
   C. 3
   D. 4
   E. 5

3. Mutations in DNA large distances from a structural gene can lead to over- or underexpression of that gene. Which one of the following eukaryotic DNA control sequences does not need to be in a fixed location and is most responsible for high rates of transcription of particular genes?
   A. Promoter
   B. Promoter-proximal element
   C. Enhancer
   D. Operator
   E. Splice donor site

4. Which one of the following is true of both eukaryotic and prokaryotic gene expression and would therefore not be an effective target for drug development?
   A. After transcription, a 3′-poly(A) tail and a 5′-cap are added to mRNA.
   B. Translation of mRNA can begin before transcription is complete.
   C. mRNA is synthesized in the 3′-to-5′ direction.
   D. RNA polymerase binds at a promoter region upstream of the gene.
   E. Mature mRNA is always precisely collinear to the gene from which it was transcribed.

5. A family has two children, both of whom have a form of β-thalassemia. One child is almost nonsymptomatic, whereas the other requires frequent blood transfusions for his disease. The α-globin to β-globin ratio in the more severely affected child is most likely to be which one of the following?
   A. 5:1
   B. 2:1
   C. 1:1
   D. 1:2
   E. 1:5

6. Certain drugs can be used as antibiotics because they affect bacterial RNA polymerases but not eukaryotic RNA polymerases. RNA polymerase is a key enzyme in the process of transcription, which can be best described by which one of the following?
   A. The single-stranded RNA produced is identical to one of the strands of double-stranded DNA.
   B. The single-stranded RNA produced is identical to both of the strands of double-stranded DNA.
   C. Eukaryotic genes are transcribed in the cytosol by three different RNA polymerases.
   D. RNA polymerase cannot initiate new strand synthesis and must have a primer.
   E. Eukaryotic genes are transcribed in the nucleus by three different DNA polymerases.

7. Eukaryotic cells contain multiple RNA polymerases, which makes it difficult to block all RNA synthesis with one drug targeted to a specific polymerase. Which one of the following best describes properties of eukaryotic RNA polymerases?
   A. Polymerase I produces most of the rRNA.
   B. Polymerase II produces most of the tRNA.

C. Polymerase III produces most of the mRNA.
D. All three RNA polymerases have the same mechanism of action and bind to the same promotor sequences on DNA.
E. Enhancers identify the start point for transcription for all three polymerases.

8. The production of mRNA in eukaryotic cells requires a large number of steps, and drugs targeted to any of these steps could block mRNA production. Which one of the following accurately describes a part of the process of producing mRNA from a eukaryotic gene?
   A. The sense strand of DNA is the strand used by RNA polymerase during transcription.
   B. The antisense DNA strand is identical to the RNA transcript except that the DNA strand contains thymine and the RNA strand contains uracil.
   C. The first RNA form produced contains both intron and exon sequences.
   D. Mature mRNA contains a cap at the 5′-end, a poly(A) tail at the 3′ end, introns, and exons.
   E. During processing in the nucleus of a precursor mRNA, introns and exons are shuffled in sequence to produce the mature mRNA.

9. Genetic abnormalities in DNA are transcribed into mRNA. This error then causes tRNA to use an incorrectly coded amino acid to produce a protein, which may then malfunction because of the alteration in primary structure of the synthesized protein. The tRNAs used for protein synthesis can be best described by which one of the following?
   A. A specific tRNA can code for multiple different amino acids.
   B. tRNA contains a codon site that binds with an anticodon of mRNA.
   C. tRNA contains one specific binding site for both the sequence of three nucleotides in mRNA and the encoded amino acid.
   D. One of the loops of tRNA contains the anticodon.
   E. The D loop contains the anticodon.

10. A researcher wants to develop an antibiotic that targets histones and introns in bacteria, and she has applied for a grant. Why would the grant's physician/biochemist advisor advise against funding this grant application?
    A. The proposed antibiotic would have no effect on bacteria but could harm human cells.
    B. The proposed antibiotic would negatively affect both bacteria and human cells.
    C. The proposed antibiotic would have no effect on either bacteria or human cells.
    D. Bacteria have histones but do not have introns.
    E. Bacteria have introns but do not have histones.

ANSWERS

1. **The answer is B.** The transcript that is produced is copied from the DNA template strand, which must be of the opposite orientation from the transcript. So the 5′-end of the template strand should base-pair with the 3′-end of the transcript, or the G. Thus, CGTACGGAT would base-pair with the transcript and would represent the template strand.

2. **The answer is A. Catherine T.** weighs 50 kg, and if 0.1 mg/kg of body weight is the LD_{50}, then for Amanda, 5 mg of toxin would bring her to the LD_{50}. Because one mushroom contains 7 mg of the toxin, ingesting just one mushroom could be fatal.

3. **The answer is C.** Enhancer sequences can be thousands of bases away from the basal promoter and still stimulate transcription of the gene. This is accomplished by looping of the DNA so that the proteins binding to the enhancer sequence (transactivators) can also bind to proteins bound to the promoter (coactivators). A promoter-proximal element is a DNA sequence near to the promoter that can bind transcription factors that aid in recruiting RNA polymerase to the promoter region.

4. **The answer is D.** Both prokaryotes and eukaryotes require RNA polymerase binding to an upstream promoter element. Answer A applies only to eukaryotes; prokaryote mRNA is not capped, nor does it contain a poly(A) tail. Prokaryotes have no nucleus; therefore, the 5′-end of an mRNA is immediately available for ribosome binding and initiation of translation (thus, B is incorrect). Answer C is incorrect overall; RNA synthesis, like DNA synthesis, is always in the 5′-to-3′ direction. Answer E is incorrect because introns are present only in eukaryotic genes.

5. **The answer is A.** A β-thalassemia refers to a condition in which the α-chain of globin is produced in excess of the β-chain. The greater the ratio of α- to β-chain, the more severe the disease. Patients are usually asymptomatic at a ratio of 2:1, but once the ratio is greater than 2:1, symptoms will become evident. The reduction in β-globin synthesis can come about because of splicing mutations, promoter mutations, or point mutations within the coding regions of the β-globin gene.

6. **The answer is A.** The single-stranded RNA produced by transcription is identical in sequence to one (not both) of the DNA strands except that the RNA strand contains the base uracil in locations where the DNA strand contains thymine. Eukaryotic genes are transcribed in the nucleus (not cytosol) by three different RNA polymerases (not DNA polymerases). RNA polymerase does not require a primer to initiate transcription, unlike DNA polymerase, which does require a primer to initiate DNA replication.

7. **The answer is A.** The promotor region on the DNA identifies the start point of transcription for each gene. Enhancers are distal promoter elements that stabilize RNA polymerase binding to the promoter, but enhancers do not identify the initiation point for transcription. All of the RNA polymerases have the same mechanism of action but differ in which promoters they recognize (the sequence of promoters differs for each polymerase) owing to the use of different accessory factors in forming the initiation complex. Polymerase I produces rRNA; polymerase II, mRNA; and polymerase III, tRNA in eukaryotic cells.

8. **The answer is C.** The sense (or coding) strand of DNA is identical to the mRNA produced, with the exception of the DNA containing thymine and the RNA containing uracil. The template (or antisense) strand of DNA is the strand that is used by RNA polymerase to produce a complementary RNA sequence to the template strand (thus, the antisense strand is complementary to the mRNA produced and is not identical to it). The first RNA form produced by RNA polymerase is hnRNA, which contains both intron (noncoding) and exon (coding sequences) sequences. hnRNA is modified by the addition of a cap to the 5′-end, a poly(A) tail added to the 3′-end, and all introns removed. During processing, the intron sequences are removed from the hnRNA to produce the mature mRNA.

9. **The answer is D.** tRNA contains a three-base sequence known as the *anticodon*, which binds to a corresponding complementary codon on the mRNA. The amino acid is covalently linked to the tRNA at its 3′-end, which is distinct from the anticodon site. A particular tRNA only links to one amino acid, not multiple amino acids. In the cloverleaf structure of tRNA, one of the loops contains the anticodon that is distinct from the D loop, which frequently contains dihydrouridine as an unusual base.

10. **The answer is A.** Bacteria do not have histones or introns, but humans have both. The proposed antibiotic would have no effect on bacteria but could have a deleterious effect on human cells.

15

Translation: Synthesis of Proteins

Proteins are produced by the process of **translation**, which occurs on **ribosomes** and is directed by **messenger RNA (mRNA)**. The genetic message encoded in DNA is first transcribed into mRNA, and the **nucleotide sequence** in the coding region of the mRNA is then translated into the **amino acid sequence** of the protein.

Translation of the Code. The portion of mRNA that specifies the amino acid sequence of the protein is read in **codons**, which are **sets of three nucleotides** that specify individual amino acids (Fig 15.1). The codons on mRNA are read sequentially in the 5'-to-3' direction, starting with the **5'-AUG** (or "start" codon) that specifies **methionine** and sets the **reading frame** and ending with a **3'-termination** (or "stop") codon (**UAG**, **UGA**, or **UAA**). The protein is synthesized from its **N terminus** to its **C terminus**.

Each amino acid is carried to the ribosome by an **aminoacyl–transfer RNA (tRNA)** (i.e., a tRNA with an amino acid covalently attached). **Base pairing** between the **anticodon** of the tRNA and the **codon** on the mRNA ensures that each amino acid is inserted into the growing polypeptide at the appropriate position.

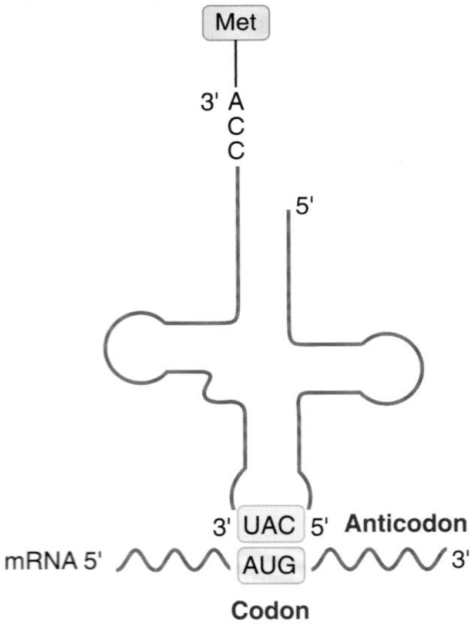

Synthesis of the Protein. Initiation involves formation of a complex containing the initial **methionyl-tRNA** bound to the AUG "start" codon of the **mRNA** and to the "P" site of the **ribosome**. It requires guanosine triphosphate (**GTP**) and proteins known as **eukaryotic initiation factors** (eIFs).

Elongation of the polypeptide involves **three steps:** (1) **binding** of an **aminoacyl-tRNA** to the "A" site on the ribosome, where it base-pairs with the second codon on the mRNA; (2) **formation** of a **peptide bond** between the first and second amino acids; and (3) **translocation**, movement of the mRNA relative to the ribosome, so that the third mRNA codon moves into the "A" site. These three **elongation steps** are **repeated** until a **termination** codon aligns with the site on the ribosome where the next aminoacyl-tRNA would normally bind. **Release factors** bind instead, causing the completed protein to be released from the ribosome.

After one ribosome binds and moves along the mRNA, translating the polypeptide, another ribosome can bind and begin translation. The complex of a single mRNA with multiple ribosomes is known as a **polysome**.

Folding and Modification and Targeting of the Protein. Folding of the polypeptide into its three-dimensional configuration occurs as the polypeptide is being translated. This process involves proteins called **chaperones**. **Modification** of amino acid residues in a protein occurs during or after translation. Proteins synthesized on **cytosolic ribosomes** are released into the cytosol or transported into mitochondria, peroxisomes, and the nucleus. Proteins synthesized on ribosomes attached to the **rough endoplasmic reticulum** (RER) are destined for lysosomes, cell membranes, or secretion from the cell. These proteins are transferred to the **Golgi complex**, where they are modified and **targeted** to their ultimate locations.

FIGURE 15.1 Binding of transfer RNA (tRNA) to a codon on messenger RNA (mRNA). The tRNA contains an amino acid at its 3'-end that corresponds to the codon on mRNA with which the anticodon of the tRNA can base-pair. Note that the codon–anticodon pairing is complementary and antiparallel.

THE WAITING ROOM

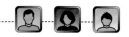

 Lisa N., a 4-year-old patient with β⁺-thalassemia intermedia (see Chapter 14), showed no improvement in her symptoms at her second visit. Her hemoglobin level was 7.3 g/dL (reference range for females = 12 to 16 g/dL).

 Jay S. is a 9-month-old male infant of Ashkenazi Jewish parentage. His growth and development were normal until age 5 months, when he began to exhibit mild, generalized muscle weakness. By 7 months, he had poor head control and slowed development of motor skills, and he was increasingly inattentive to his surroundings. His parents also noted unusual eye movements and staring episodes. On careful examination of his retinae, his pediatrician observed a "cherry red" spot within a pale macula. The physician suspected Tay–Sachs disease and sent samples of his whole blood to the molecular biology–genetics laboratory.

 Paul T. returned to his physician's office after 5 days of azithromycin therapy (see Chapter 12) feeling significantly better. The sputum sample from his previous visit had been cultured. The results confirmed that his respiratory infection was caused by *Streptococcus pneumoniae* and that the organism was sensitive to penicillin, macrolides (e.g., erythromycin, clarithromycin), tetracycline, and other antibiotics.

 Edna R., a 25-year-old junior medical student, brings her healthy 4-month-old daughter, **Beverly**, to the pediatrician for her second diphtheria, tetanus, and pertussis (DTaP, acellular pertussis) immunization, along with the following immunizations: pneumococcal, inactivated polio, *Haemophilus* influenza, and rotavirus. Edna tells the doctor that her great-great aunt had died of diphtheria during an epidemic many years ago.

 The results of tests performed in the molecular biology laboratory show that **Jay S.** has an insertion in exon 11 of the α-chain of the hexosaminidase A gene, the most common mutation found in patients of Ashkenazi Jewish background who have Tay–Sachs disease. Hexosaminidase A, the enzyme activity that is lacking in **Jay S.**, can be assayed using a serum sample and a substrate that releases a fluorescent dye upon being hydrolyzed. When measuring enzyme activity, one needs to be careful to distinguish between hexosaminidase A activity and a closely related activity from hexosaminidase B. This is accomplished by differential heat inactivation of the sample (exposure of the sample to 50°C will inactivate hexosaminidase A activity but not hexosaminidase B activity). For prenatal screening, molecular techniques are the preferred method because of their sensitivity and the limited amount of sample available (see Chapter 17).

I. The Genetic Code

Transcription, the transfer of the genetic message from DNA to RNA, and *translation*, the transfer of the genetic message from the nucleotide language of nucleic acids to the amino acid language of proteins, both depend on base pairing. In the late 1950s and early 1960s, molecular biologists attempting to decipher the process of translation recognized two problems. The first involved decoding the relationship between the language of the nucleic acids and the language of the proteins, and the second involved determining the molecular mechanism by which translation between these two languages occurs.

Twenty different amino acids are commonly incorporated into proteins, and therefore, the protein alphabet has 20 characters. The nucleic acid alphabet, however, has only four characters, corresponding to the four nucleotides of mRNA (A, G, C, and U). If two nucleotides constituted the code for an amino acid, then only 4^2 (or 16) amino acids could be specified. Therefore, the number of nucleotides that code for an amino acid has to be at least three, providing 4^3 (or 64) possible combinations or *codons*—more than required, but not excessive.

Scientists set out to determine the specific codons for each amino acid. In 1961, Marshall Nirenberg produced the first crack in the genetic code (the collection of codons that specifies all the amino acids found in proteins). He showed that poly(U), a polynucleotide in which all the bases are uracil, produced polyphenylalanine in a cell-free protein-synthesizing system. Thus, UUU must be the codon for phenylalanine. As a result of experiments using synthetic polynucleotides in place of mRNA, other codons were identified.

The pioneering molecular biologists recognized that, because amino acids cannot bind directly to the sets of three nucleotides that form their codons, adapters are required. The adapters were found to be transfer RNA (tRNA) molecules. Each tRNA molecule contains an *anticodon* and covalently binds a specific amino acid at its 3′-end (see Chapters 12 and 14). The anticodon of a tRNA molecule is a set of three nucleotides that can interact with a codon on mRNA (see Fig. 15.1). In order to interact, the codon and anticodon must be complementary (i.e., they must be able to form base pairs in an antiparallel orientation). Thus, the anticodon of a tRNA serves as the link between an mRNA codon and the amino acid that the codon specifies.

Obviously, each codon present within mRNA must correspond to a specific amino acid. Nirenberg found that trinucleotides of known base sequence could bind to ribosomes and induce the binding of specific aminoacyl-tRNAs (i.e., tRNAs with amino acids attached covalently). As a result of these and the earlier experiments, the relationship between all 64 codons and the amino acids they specify (the entire genetic code) was determined by the mid-1960s (Table 15.1).

Three of the 64 possible codons (UGA, UAG, and UAA) terminate protein synthesis and are known as stop or *nonsense codons*. The remaining 61 codons specify amino acids. Two amino acids each have only one codon (AUG for methionine; UGG for tryptophan). The remaining amino acids have multiple codons.

A. The Code Is Degenerate Yet Unambiguous

Because many amino acids are specified by more than one codon, the genetic code is described as *degenerate*, which means that an amino acid may have more than one codon. However, each codon specifies only one amino acid, and the genetic code is thus unambiguous.

Inspection of a codon table shows that in most instances of multiple codons for a single amino acid, the variation occurs in the third base of the codon (see Table 15.1). Crick noted that the pairing between the 3′-base of the codon and the 5′-base of the anticodon does not always follow the strict base-pairing rules that he and Watson had previously discovered (i.e., A pairs with U, and G with C). This observation resulted in the *wobble hypothesis*.

At the third base of the codon (the 3′-position of the codon and the 5′-position of the anticodon), the base pairs can wobble. For example, G can pair with U, and A, C, or U can pair with the unusual base hypoxanthine (I) found in tRNA. Thus, three of the four codons for alanine (GCU, GCC, and GCA) can pair with a single tRNA that contains the anticodon 5′-IGC-3′ (Fig. 15.2). If each of the 61 codons for amino acids required a distinct tRNA, cells would contain 61 tRNAs. However, because of wobble between the codon and anticodon, fewer than 61 tRNAs are required to translate the genetic code.

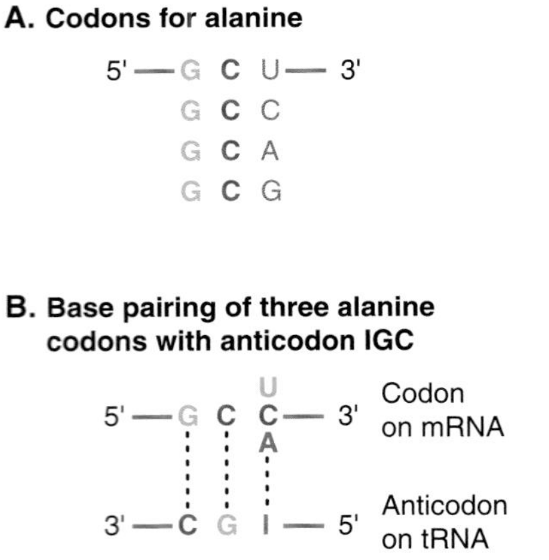

A. Codons for alanine

```
5' — G  C  U — 3'
     G  C  C
     G  C  A
     G  C  G
```

B. Base pairing of three alanine codons with anticodon IGC

```
              U
5' — G  C  C — 3'   Codon
     :  :  :  A      on mRNA
     :  :  :
3' — C  G  I — 5'   Anticodon
                     on tRNA
```

FIGURE 15.2 Base pairing of codons for alanine with 5′-IGC-3′. **A.** The variation is in the third base. **B.** The first three of these codons can pair with a transfer RNA (tRNA) that contains the anticodon 5′-IGC-3′. Hypoxanthine (I) is an unusual base found in tRNA that can form base pairs with U, C, or A. It is formed by the deamination of adenine. Hypoxanthine is the base attached to ribose in the nucleoside inosine. The single-letter abbreviation for hypoxanthine is I, referring to the nucleoside inosine. *mRNA,* messenger RNA.

TABLE 15.1 The Genetic Code

FIRST BASE	SECOND BASE				THIRD BASE
(5′)	**U**	**C**	**A**	**G**	**(3′)**
U	Phe	Ser	Tyr	Cys	U
	Phe	Ser	Tyr	Cys	C
	Leu	Ser	Stop	Stop	A
	Leu	Ser	Stop	Trp	G
C	Leu	Pro	His	Arg	U
	Leu	Pro	His	Arg	C
	Leu	Pro	Gln	Arg	A
	Leu	Pro	Gln	Arg	G
A	Ile	Thr	Asn	Ser	U
	Ile	Thr	Asn	Ser	C
	Ile	Thr	Lys	Arg	A
	Met	Thr	Lys	Arg	G
G	Val	Ala	Asp	Gly	U
	Val	Ala	Asp	Gly	C
	Val	Ala	Glu	Gly	A
	Val	Ala	Glu	Gly	G

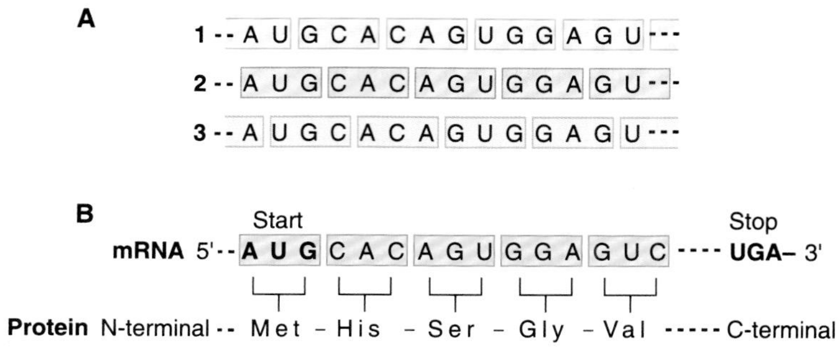

A

```
1 -- A U G C A C A G U G G A G U ---

2 -- A U G C A C A G U G G A G U ---

3 -- A U G C A C A G U G G A G U ---
```

B

```
              Start                              Stop
mRNA 5'-- A U G C A C A G U G G A G U C ---- UGA- 3'
          └┬┘ └┬┘ └┬┘ └┬┘ └┬┘
Protein N-terminal -- Met – His – Ser – Gly – Val ----- C-terminal
```

FIGURE 15.3 Reading frame of messenger RNA (mRNA). **A.** For any given mRNA sequence, there are three possible reading frames (*1, 2,* and *3*). **B.** An AUG near the 5'-end of the mRNA (the start codon) sets the reading frame for translation of a protein from the mRNA. The codons are read in linear order, starting with this AUG. (The other potential reading frames are not used. They would give proteins with different amino acid sequences.)

All organisms studied so far use the same genetic code, with some rare exceptions. One exception occurs in human mitochondrial mRNA, in which UGA codes for tryptophan instead of serving as a stop codon, AUA codes for methionine instead of isoleucine, and CUA codes for threonine instead of leucine.

B. The Code Is Nonoverlapping

mRNA does not contain extra nucleotides, or punctuation, to separate one codon from the next, and the codons do not overlap. Each nucleotide is read only once. Beginning with a start codon (AUG) near the 5'-end of the mRNA, the codons are read sequentially, ending with a stop codon (UGA, UAG, or UAA) near the 3'-end of the mRNA.

C. Relationship between mRNA and the Protein Product

The start codon (AUG) sets the reading frame—the order in which the sequence of bases in the mRNA is sorted into codons (Fig. 15.3). The order of the codons in the mRNA determines the sequence in which amino acids are added to the growing polypeptide chain. Thus, the order of the codons in the mRNA determines the linear sequence of amino acids in the protein.

II. Effects of Mutations

Mutations that result from damage to the nucleotides of DNA molecules or from unrepaired errors during replication (see Chapter 13) can be transcribed into mRNA and therefore can result in the translation of a protein with an abnormal amino acid sequence. Various types of mutations can occur which have different effects on the encoded protein (Table 15.2).

TABLE 15.2	Types of Mutations	
TYPE	**DESCRIPTION**	**EXAMPLE**
Point	A single base change	
Silent	A change that specifies the same amino acid	CGA → CGG
		Arg → Arg
Missense	A change that specifies a different amino acid	CGA → CCA
		Arg → Pro
Nonsense	A change that produces a stop codon	CGA → UGA
		Arg → Stop
Insertion	An addition of one or more bases	
Deletion	A loss of one or more bases	

Silent point mutations can also lead to disease if they create a new splice site during mRNA processing. Hutchinson–Gilford progeria syndrome (HGPS), a premature aging disorder, can result from a mutation in the lamin A gene (*LMNA* gene) in which the base at position 1,824 in the gene is altered from a cytosine to a thymine. This single nucleotide change does not alter the amino acid sequence (the codon indicated a glycine before the change and indicates a glycine after the change), but it does create a cryptic splice site in exon 11, which gives rise to a prelamin A that is missing 50 amino acids. The loss of these amino acids interferes with posttranslational processing of the protein as well as disruption of the nuclear membrane, telomere dysfunction, chromatin-remodeling defects, and epigenetic alterations.

 Sickle cell anemia is caused by a missense mutation. In each of the alleles for β-globin, **Will S.'s** DNA has a single base change (see Chapter 6). In the sickle cell gene, G*T*G replaces the normal GAG. Thus, in the mRNA, the codon GUG replaces GAG and a valine residue replaces a glutamate residue in the protein. The amino acid change is indicated as *E6V*; the normal glutamate (E) at position 6 of the β-chain has been replaced by a valine (V).

 One type of thalassemia is caused by a nonsense mutation. Codon 17 of the β-globin chain is changed from UGG to UGA. This change results in the conversion of a codon for a tryptophan residue to a stop codon. Other types of thalassemia are caused by deletions in the globin genes. Patients have been studied who have large deletions in either the 5'- or the 3'-coding region of the β-globin gene, removing almost one-third of the DNA sequence.

Is it possible that **Lisa N.** has either a nonsense mutation in codon 17 or a large deletion of the β-globin gene?

A. Point Mutations

Point mutations occur when only one base in DNA is altered, producing a change in a single base of an mRNA codon. There are three basic types of point mutations: silent mutations, missense mutations, and nonsense mutations. Point mutations are said to be "silent" when they do not affect the amino acid sequence of the protein. For example, a codon change from CG*A* to CG*G* does not affect the protein because both of these codons specify arginine (see Table 15.1). In *missense mutations*, one amino acid in the protein is replaced by a different amino acid. For example, a change from C*G*A to C*C*A causes arginine to be replaced by proline. A nonsense mutation causes the premature termination of a polypeptide chain. For example, a codon change from *C*GA to *U*GA causes a codon for arginine to be replaced by a stop codon, so synthesis of the mutant protein terminates at this point.

B. Insertions, Deletions, and Frameshift Mutations

An *insertion* occurs when one or more nucleotides are added to DNA. If the insertion does not generate a stop codon, a protein with more amino acids than normal could be produced.

When one or more nucleotides are removed from DNA, the mutation is known as a *deletion*. If the deletion does not affect the normal start and stop codons, a protein with fewer than the normal number of amino acids could be produced.

A *frameshift mutation* occurs when the number of inserted or deleted nucleotides is not a multiple of three (Fig. 15.4). The reading frame shifts at the point where the insertion or deletion begins. Beyond that point, the amino acid sequence of the protein translated from the mRNA differs from the normal protein.

III. Formation of Aminoacyl-tRNA

A tRNA that contains an amino acid attached covalently to its 3'-end is called an *aminoacyl-tRNA* and is considered to be charged. Aminoacyl-tRNAs are named both for the amino acid and the tRNA that carries the amino acid. For example, the tRNA for alanine (tRNA^{Ala}) acquires alanine to become alanyl-tRNA^{Ala}. A particular tRNA recognizes only the AUG start codon that initiates protein synthesis and not other AUG codons that specify insertion of methionine within the polypeptide chain. This initiator methionyl-tRNA^{Met} is denoted by the subscript "i" in methionyl-tRNA$_i^{Met}$.

Amino acids are attached to their tRNAs by highly specific enzymes known as *aminoacyl-tRNA synthetases*. Twenty different synthetases exist; one for each amino acid. Each synthetase recognizes a particular amino acid and all of the tRNAs that carry that amino acid.

The formation of the ester bond that links the amino acid to the tRNA by an aminoacyl-tRNA synthetase is an energy-requiring process that occurs in two steps.

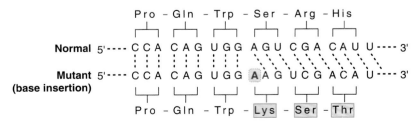

FIGURE 15.4 A frameshift mutation. The insertion of a single nucleotide (the A in the *dotted red box*) causes the reading frame to shift so that the amino acid sequence of the protein translated from the mRNA is different after the point of insertion. A similar effect can result from the insertion or deletion of nucleotides if the number inserted or deleted is not a multiple of three.

The amino acid is activated in the first step when its carboxyl group reacts with adenosine triphosphate (ATP) to form an enzyme-aminoacyl–adenosine monophosphate (AMP) complex and pyrophosphate (Fig. 15.5). The cleavage of a high-energy bond of ATP in this reaction provides energy, and the subsequent cleavage of pyrophosphate by a pyrophosphatase helps to drive the reaction by removing one of the products. In the second step, the activated amino acid is transferred to the 2′- or 3′-hydroxyl group (depending on the type of aminoacyl-tRNA synthetase that catalyzes the reaction) of the ribose connected to the 3′-terminal A residue of the tRNA, and AMP is released (recall that all tRNAs have a CCA added to their 3′-end post-transcriptionally). The energy in the aminoacyl-tRNA ester bond is subsequently used in the formation of a peptide bond during the process of protein synthesis. The aminoacyl-tRNA synthetase provides the first error-checking step in preserving the fidelity of translation. The enzymes check their work, and if the incorrect amino acid has been linked to a particular tRNA, the enzyme will remove the amino acid from the tRNA and try again using the correct amino acid.

Some aminoacyl-tRNA synthetases use the anticodon of the tRNA as a recognition site as they attach the amino acid to the hydroxyl group at the 3′-end of the tRNA (Fig. 15.6). However, other synthetases do not use the anticodon but recognize only bases located at other positions in the tRNA. Nevertheless, insertion of the amino acid into a growing polypeptide chain depends solely on the bases of the anticodon, through complementary base pairing with the mRNA codon.

IV. Process of Translation

Translation of a protein involves three steps: *initiation, elongation,* and *termination.* It begins with the formation of the initiation complex. Subsequently, synthesis of the polypeptide occurs by a series of elongation steps that are repeated as each amino acid is added to the growing chain (Fig. 15.7). Termination occurs where the mRNA contains an in-frame stop codon, and the completed polypeptide chain is released.

A. Initiation of Translation

In eukaryotes, initiation of translation involves formation of an *initiation complex* composed of methionyl-tRNA$_i^{Met}$, mRNA, and a ribosome (Fig. 15.8). Methionyl-tRNA$_i^{Met}$ (also known as *Met-tRNA$_i^{Met}$*) initially forms a complex with the protein

A nonsense mutation at codon 17 would cause premature termination of translation. A nonfunctional peptide containing only 16 amino acids would result, producing a β⁰-thalassemia if the mutation occurred in both alleles. A large deletion in the coding region of the gene could also produce a truncated protein. If **Lisa N.** has a nonsense mutation or a large deletion, it could be in only one allele. The mutation in the other allele must be milder because she produces some normal β-globin. Her hemoglobin is 7.3 g/dL, typical of thalassemia intermedia (a β⁺-thalassemia).

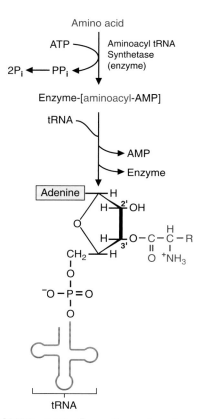

FIGURE 15.5 Formation of aminoacyl-transfer RNA (tRNA). The amino acid is first activated by reacting with adenosine triphosphate (ATP). The amino acid is then transferred from the aminoacyl-AMP to tRNA. *AMP,* adenosine monophosphate; *P$_i$,* inorganic phosphate; *PP$_i$,* pyrophosphate.

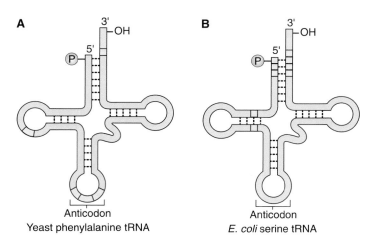

FIGURE 15.6 Some aminoacyl-transfer RNA (tRNA) synthetase recognition sites on tRNA. Each aminoacyl-tRNA synthetase is specific for certain tRNAs, which it "recognizes" by binding the sequences of nucleotides called *recognition sites,* shown in *green.* In some cases, the anticodon is a recognition site; in others, it is not. This is true for human tRNAs as well as for those shown here. *E. coli, Escherichia coli.*

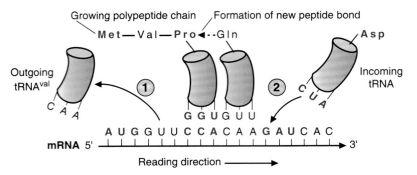

FIGURE 15.7 Overview of the process of translation. (*1*) Once a transfer RNA (tRNA) has donated its amino acid to the growing polypeptide chain (which itself is still linked to a tRNA), it is released from the mRNA. (*2*) A new aminoacyl-tRNA binds to the correct codon in the mRNA to donate its amino acid to the growing polypeptide chain.

eukaryotic initiation factor 2 (eIF2), which binds GTP. This complex then binds to the small (40S) ribosomal subunit with the participation of eukaryotic initiation factor 3 (eIF3). eIF3 also participates in preventing premature association of the 60S ribosomal subunit with the pre-initiation complex. The cap at the 5′-end of the mRNA binds to components of the eIF4 complex, eIF4F, known as the *cap-binding complex*. eIF4F is a complex comprising eIF4E, eIF4A, and eIF4G. The mRNA, in association with the cap-binding complex, then binds to the eIFs-Met-tRNA$_i^{Met}$–40S ribosome complex. In a reaction that requires hydrolysis of ATP (because of the helicase activity of an eIF subunit), this complex unwinds a hairpin loop in the mRNA and scans the mRNA until it locates the AUG start codon (usually the first AUG in the mRNA). GTP is hydrolyzed, the initiation factors (IFs) are released, and the large ribosomal (60S) subunit binds. The ribosome is now complete. It contains one small and one large subunit, and it has three binding sites for tRNA, known as the *P* (*peptidyl*), *A* (*aminoacyl*), and *E* (*ejection*) sites. During initiation,

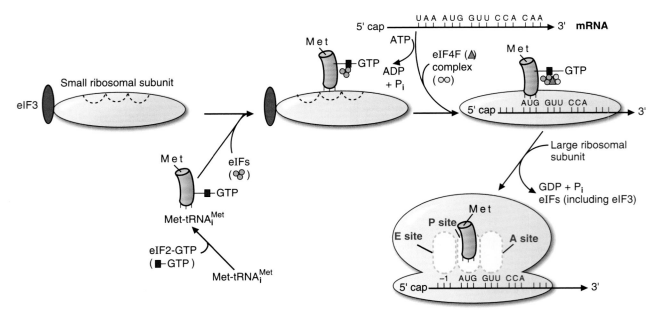

FIGURE 15.8 Initiation of protein synthesis. *P site*, peptidyl site on the ribosome; *A site*, aminoacyl site on the ribosome; *E site*, free transfer RNA (tRNA) ejection site (the A, P, and E sites or portions of them are indicated by *dashed lines*); *eIF*, eukaryotic initiation factor; *mRNA*, messenger RNA; *ADP*, adenosine diphosphate; *ATP*, adenosine triphosphate; *GDP*, guanosine diphosphate; *GTP*, guanosine triphosphate; *P$_i$*, inorganic phosphate; *Met*, methionyl. This is a simplified version of translational initiation; many more initiation factors and steps are required.

TABLE 15.3   Differences between Eukaryotes and Prokaryotes in the Initiation of Protein Synthesis

	EUKARYOTES	PROKARYOTES
Binding of mRNA to small ribosomal subunit	Cap at 5′-end of mRNA binds eIFs and 40S ribosomal subunit containing tRNA$_i^{Met}$. mRNA is scanned for AUG start codon within the Kozak consensus sequence.	Shine–Dalgarno sequence upstream of initiating AUG binds to complementary sequence in 16S rRNA.
First amino acid	Methionine	Formyl-methionine
Initiation factors	eIFs (12 or more)	IFs (3)
Ribosomes	80S	70S
	(40S and 60S subunits)	(30S and 50S subunits)

mRNA, messenger RNA; rRNA, ribosomal RNA; tRNA, transfer RNA; IF, initiation factor; eIFs, eukaryotic initiation factor.

Met-tRNA$_i^{Met}$ binds to the ribosome at the P site, which is located initially at the start codon for translation. Eukaryotes also contain a Kozak consensus sequence which is recognized by the ribosome as the translational start site (the sequence is A or G – CC*AUG*G, where the purine base is three bases upstream of the AUG start codon). The Kozak sequence aids in defining the initial AUG codon for translation. Loss of this sequence reduces the efficiency of translational initiation.

The initiation process differs for prokaryotes and eukaryotes (Table 15.3). In bacteria, the initiating methionyl-tRNA is formylated, producing a formyl-methionyl-tRNA$_f^{Met}$ that participates in formation of the initiation complex (Fig. 15.9). Only three IFs are required to generate this complex in prokaryotes compared with the dozen or more required by eukaryotes. The ribosomes also differ in size. Prokaryotes have 70S ribosomes, composed of 30S and 50S subunits; eukaryotes have 80S ribosomes, composed of 40S and 60S subunits. Unlike eukaryotic mRNA, bacterial mRNA is not capped. Identification of the initiating AUG triplet in prokaryotes occurs when a sequence in the mRNA (known as the *Shine–Dalgarno sequence*) binds to a complementary sequence near the 3′-end of the 16S ribosomal RNA (rRNA) of the small ribosomal subunit.

Initiation of translation is also regulated at the level of the IFs. For example, insulin, an anabolic hormone, stimulates general protein synthesis by activating eIF4E. Normally, eIF4E is bound to an inhibitor protein, designated 4E-binding protein (4E-BP). When insulin binds to its cell surface receptor, it initiates an intracellular sequence of events resulting in phosphorylation of 4E-BP. Phosphorylated 4E-BP no longer binds to eIF4E, and eIF4E is now free to participate in the initiation of protein synthesis.

Similarly, eIF2 is a regulator of the initiation step in protein synthesis. When it is phosphorylated, it is inactive and protein synthesis cannot begin. Conditions such as starvation, heat shock, and viral infection result in phosphorylation of eIF2 by a specific kinase.

The regulation of globin synthesis by heme in reticulocytes illustrates the role of eIF2 in the regulation of translation. Reticulocytes, which are the precursors of red blood cells, synthesize the oxygen-carrying hemoglobin molecules from the globin polypeptide chains and the Fe-binding pigment heme. In the absence of heme, the rate of initiation of globin synthesis decreases. Heme acts by inhibiting the phosphorylation of eIF2. Thus, eIF2 is active in the presence of heme and globin synthesis is initiated.

And finally, both eIF2 and elongation factor 1 (EF1) are types of heterotrimeric G-proteins (see Chapter 11). They dramatically change their conformation and actively form complexes when they bind GTP but become inactive and dissociate when they hydrolyze this GTP to guanosine diphosphate (GDP). GTP can then displace the bound GDP to reactivate eIF2 or EF1.

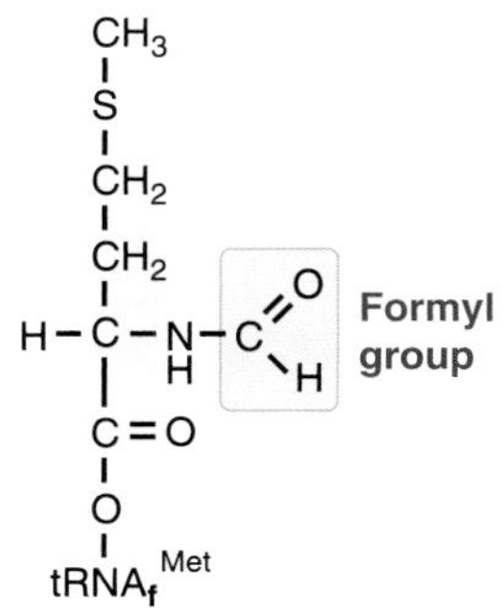

FIGURE 15.9 Bacterial tRNA containing formyl-methionine. The initial methionine is not formylated in eukaryotic protein synthesis.

Many antibiotics that are used to combat bacterial infections in humans take advantage of the differences between the mechanisms for protein synthesis in prokaryotes and eukaryotes. For example, streptomycin binds to the 30S ribosomal subunit of prokaryotes. It interferes with initiation of protein synthesis and causes misreading of mRNA. Streptomycin, however, was not used to treat **Paul T.** because it can cause permanent hearing loss. Its use is therefore confined mainly to the treatment of tuberculosis or other infections that do not respond adequately to other antibiotics. Another example is tetracycline, which binds to the 30S ribosomal subunit of prokaryotes and inhibits binding of aminoacyl-tRNA to the A site of the ribosome.

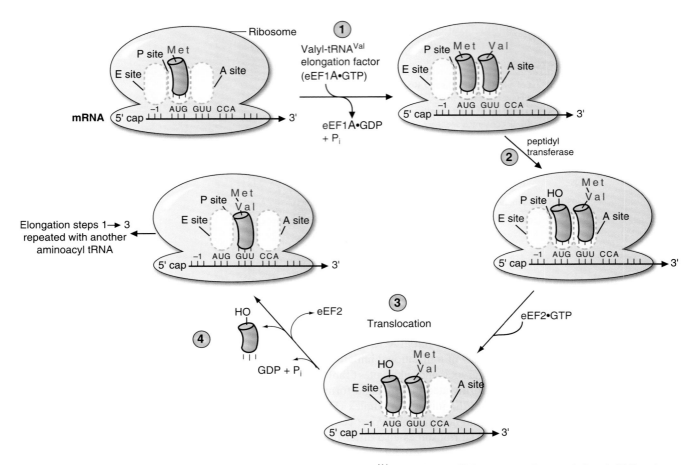

FIGURE 15.10 Elongation of a polypeptide chain. (*1*) Binding of valyl-tRNA^{Val} to the A site. (*2*) Formation of a peptide bond. (*3*) Translocation. (*4*) Ejection of the free tRNA. After step 4, step 1 is repeated using the aminoacyl-tRNA for the new codon in the A site. Steps 2, 3, and 4 follow. These four steps keep repeating until termination occurs. *EF*, elongation factor; *P$_i$*, inorganic phosphate; *GDP*, guanosine diphosphate; *GTP*, guanosine triphosphate; *mRNA*, messenger RNA; *tRNA*, transfer RNA; *P site*, peptidyl site; *A site*, aminoacyl site; *E site*, free tRNA ejection site.

B. Elongation of Polypeptide Chains

After the initiation complex is formed, addition of each amino acid to the growing polypeptide chain involves binding of an aminoacyl-tRNA to the A site on the ribosome, formation of a peptide bond, and translocation of the peptidyl-tRNA to the P site (Fig. 15.10). The peptidyl-tRNA contains the growing polypeptide chain.

1. Binding of Aminoacyl-tRNA to the A Site

When Met-tRNA$_i$ (or a peptidyl-tRNA) is bound to the P site, the mRNA codon in the A site determines which aminoacyl-tRNA will bind to that site. An aminoacyl-tRNA binds when its anticodon is antiparallel and complementary to the mRNA codon. In eukaryotes, the incoming aminoacyl-tRNA first combines with eEF1A containing bound GTP before binding to the mRNA–ribosome complex. eEF1A is similar to the α-subunit of a heterotrimeric G-protein in that it contains GTPase activity (see Chapter 11). When the aminoacyl-tRNA–eEF1A–GTP complex binds to the A site, GTP is hydrolyzed to GDP as the ribosome activates the GTPase activity of eEF1A. This prompts dissociation of eEF1A–GDP from the aminoacyl-tRNA ribosomal complex, thereby allowing protein synthesis to continue. The binding of the appropriate aminoacyl-tRNA to the A site comprises the second error-checking step in protein synthesis. If an improper aminoacyl-tRNA is brought to the A site, the ribosomal activation of the GTPase of eEF1A does not occur and the complex will leave the binding site along with the aminoacyl-tRNA. Only when the GTP is hydrolyzed can eEF1A release the aminoacyl-tRNA and dissociate from the complex.

The antibiotic levofloxacin (a quinolone) inhibits two bacterial enzymes: DNA gyrase and topoisomerase IV. The bacterium causing **Paul T.'s** infection was found to be sensitive to levofloxacin, and this could have been used in place of azithromycin.

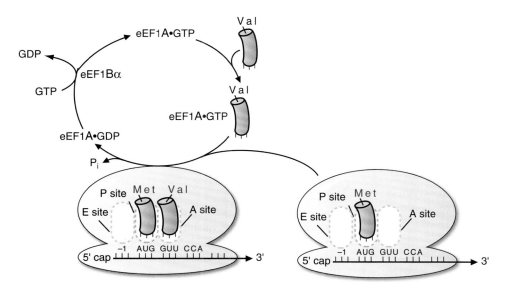

FIGURE 15.11 Recycling of eEF1A in eukaryotes. eEF1A contains a GTPase activity, which is activated upon binding to the ribosome. Guanosine triphosphate (GTP) is hydrolyzed, and eEF1A is released from the ribosome, binding to eEFIBα. eEFIBα is a guanine nucleotide exchange factor and accelerates the substitution of GTP for the guanosine diphosphate (GDP) on eEF1A. Once this occurs, eEF1A is ready for another round of translation. In prokaryotes, eEF1A corresponds to EF-Tu, and the protein corresponding to eEFIBα is EF-Ts. *EF*, elongation factor; P_i, inorganic phosphate; *P site*, peptidyl site; *A site*, aminoacyl site; *E site*, free tRNA ejection site.

Once released, the free eEF1A-GDP binds with the eEFB1α, which accelerates the replacement of bound GDP with GTP (Figure 15.11). Thus, eEF1A–GTP is ready to bind another aminoacyl-tRNA molecule and continue protein synthesis.

The process of elongation is very similar in prokaryotes, except that the corresponding factor for eEF1A is named *EF-Tu* and the associating elongation factors are called *EF-Ts* instead of eEFB1α.

2. Formation of a Peptide Bond

In the first round of elongation, the amino acid on the tRNA in the A site forms a peptide bond with the methionine on the tRNA in the P site. In subsequent rounds of elongation, the amino acid on the tRNA in the A site forms a peptide bond with the peptide on the tRNA in the P site (see Fig. 15.10). Peptidyltransferase, which is not a protein but the rRNA of the large ribosomal subunit, catalyzes the formation of the peptide bond. The tRNA in the A site now contains the growing polypeptide chain, and the tRNA in the P site is uncharged (i.e., it no longer contains an amino acid or a peptide).

3. Translocation

Translocation in eukaryotes involves another G-protein, elongation factor eEF2 (EF-G in prokaryotes), that complexes with GTP and binds to the ribosome, causing a conformational change that moves the mRNA and its base-paired tRNAs with respect to the ribosome. The uncharged tRNA moves from the P site to the E site. It is released from the ribosome when the next charged tRNA enters the A site. The peptidyl-tRNA moves into the P site, and the next codon of the mRNA occupies the A site. During translocation, GTP is hydrolyzed to GDP, which is released from the ribosome along with the elongation factor (see Fig. 15.10).

C. Termination of Translation

The three elongation steps are repeated until a termination (stop) codon moves into the A site on the ribosome. Because no tRNAs with anticodons that can pair with stop codons normally exist in cells, release factors bind to the ribosome instead, causing peptidyltransferase to hydrolyze the bond between the peptide chain and tRNA. The newly synthesized polypeptide is released from the ribosome, which dissociates into its individual subunits, releasing the mRNA.

 The macrolide antibiotics (e.g., erythromycin, clarithromycin, azithromycin) bind to the 50S ribosomal subunit of bacteria and inhibit translocation. Azithromycin was used to treat **Paul T.** because he had taken it previously without difficulty. It has less-serious side effects than many other antibiotics and can be used as an alternative drug in patients who are allergic to penicillin, like Mr. T. After 2 weeks of therapy, Mr. T. recovered from his infection.

 Chloramphenicol is an antibiotic that interferes with the peptidyltransferase activity of the 50S ribosomal subunit of bacteria. It was not used to treat **Paul T.** because it is very toxic to humans, partly because of its effect on mitochondrial protein synthesis.

Diphtheria is a highly contagious disease caused by a toxin secreted by the bacterium *Corynebacterium diphtheriae*. Although the toxin is a protein, it is not produced by a bacterial gene but by a gene brought into the bacterial cell by an infecting bacteriophage.

Diphtheria toxin is composed of two protein subunits. The B-subunit binds to a cell surface receptor, facilitating the entry of the A-subunit into the cell. In the cell, the A-subunit catalyzes a reaction in which the ADP-ribose (ADPR) portion of NAD is transferred to eEF2 (ADP-ribosylation). In this reaction, the ADPR is attached covalently to a posttranslationally modified histidine residue known as *diphthamide*. ADP-ribosylation of eEF2 inhibits protein synthesis, leading to cell death. Children, including **Edna R.'s** daughter, should be immunized against this often-fatal disease at an early age, unless there is a contraindication.

Currently, owing to misperceptions of vaccine side effects, some parents are not having their children immunized. The decrease in the incidence of infectious disease in the United States has led to complacency. Anyone who remembers the summertime fear of poliomyelitis in the 1940s and 1950s realizes that immunizations are a blessing that should be available to all children. This has been reinforced by several outbreaks, including the measles outbreak in Anaheim, California, at Disneyland in December 2015.

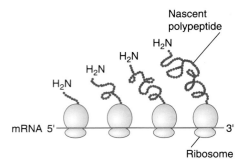

FIGURE 15.12 A polysome. The complex of messenger RNA (mRNA) and multiple ribosomes, each of which is producing a polypeptide chain, is called a *polysome*.

Protein synthesis requires a considerable amount of energy. Formation of each aminoacyl-tRNA requires the equivalent of two high-energy phosphate bonds because ATP is converted to AMP and pyrophosphate, which is cleaved to form two inorganic phosphates. As each amino acid is added to the growing peptide chain, two GTPs are hydrolyzed, one at the step involving eEF1A and the second at the translocation step. Thus, four high-energy bonds are cleaved for each amino acid of the polypeptide. In addition, energy is required for initiation of synthesis of a polypeptide chain and for synthesis from nucleoside triphosphate precursors of the mRNA, tRNA, and rRNA involved in translation.

V. Polysomes

As one ribosome moves along the mRNA, producing a polypeptide chain, a second ribosome can bind to the vacant 5′-end of the mRNA. Many ribosomes can simultaneously translate a single mRNA, forming a complex known as a *polysome* or *polyribosome* (Fig. 15.12). A single ribosome covers approximately 80 nucleotides of mRNA. Therefore, ribosomes are positioned on mRNA at intervals of approximately 100 nucleotides. The growing polypeptide chains attached to the ribosomes become longer as each ribosome moves from the 5′-end toward the 3′-end of the mRNA.

VI. Processing of Proteins

Nascent polypeptide chains (i.e., polypeptides that are in the process of being synthesized) are processed. As they are being produced, they travel through a tunnel in the ribosome, which can hold roughly 30 amino acid residues. As polymerization of the chain progresses, the amino acid residues at the *N*-terminal end begin to emerge from this protected region within the ribosome and to fold and refold into the three-dimensional conformation of the polypeptide. Proteins bind to the nascent polypeptide and mediate the folding process. These mediators are called *chaperones* (they are members of the heat-shock family of proteins; see Chapter 7) because they prevent improper interactions from occurring. Disulfide-bond formation between cysteine residues is catalyzed by protein disulfide isomerases and may also be involved in producing the three-dimensional structure of the polypeptide.

VII. Posttranslational Modifications

After proteins emerge from the ribosome, they may undergo *posttranslational modifications*. The initial methionine is removed by specific proteases; methionine is not the *N*-terminal amino acid of all mature proteins. Subsequently, other specific cleavages also may occur that convert proteins to more active forms (e.g., the conversion of proinsulin to insulin). In addition, amino acid residues within the peptide chain can be modified enzymatically to alter the activity or stability of the protein, direct the protein to a subcellular compartment, or prepare it for secretion from the cell.

Amino acid residues are modified enzymatically by the addition of various types of functional groups (Table 15.4). For example, the *N*-terminal amino acid is sometimes *acetylated*, and methyl groups can be added to lysine residues (*methylation*). These changes alter the charge on the protein. Proline and lysine residues can be modified by *hydroxylation*. In collagen, hydroxylation leads to stabilization of the protein. *Carboxylations* are important especially for the function of proteins involved in blood coagulation. Formation of γ-carboxyglutamate allows these proteins to chelate Ca^{2+}, a step in clot formation. Fatty acids or other hydrophobic groups (e.g., prenyl groups) anchor the protein in membranes (*fatty acylation and prenylation*). An adenosine diphosphate (ADP)-ribose group can be transferred from nicotinamide adenine dinucleotide (NAD^+) to certain proteins (*ADP-ribosylation*). The addition and removal of phosphate groups (which bind covalently to serine, threonine, or tyrosine residues) serve to regulate the activity of many proteins

TABLE 15.4	Posttranslational Modifications of Proteins
Acetylation	
ADP-ribosylation	
Carboxylation	
Fatty acylation	
Glycosylation	
Hydroxylation	
Methylation	
Phosphorylation	
Prenylation	

(e.g., the enzymes of glycogen degradation and regulators of gene transcription) (*phosphorylation*). *Glycosylation*, the addition of carbohydrate groups, is a common modification that occurs mainly on proteins that are destined to be secreted or incorporated into lysosomes or cellular membranes.

VIII. Targeting of Proteins to Subcellular and Extracellular Locations

Many proteins are synthesized on polysomes in the cytosol. After they are released from ribosomes, they remain in the cytosol, where they carry out their functions. Other proteins synthesized on cytosolic ribosomes enter organelles such as mitochondria or nuclei. These proteins contain amino acid sequences called *targeting sequences* or *signal sequences* that facilitate their transport into a certain organelle. Another group of proteins are synthesized on ribosomes bound to the RER. These proteins are destined for secretion or for incorporation into various subcellular organelles (e.g., lysosomes, endoplasmic reticulum [ER], Golgi complex) or cellular membranes, including the plasma membrane.

Proteins that enter the RER as they are being synthesized have signal peptides near their *N* termini that do not have a common amino acid sequence. However, they do contain several hydrophobic residues and are 15 to 30 amino acids in length (Fig. 15.13). A *signal-recognition particle* (*SRP*) binds to the ribosome and to the

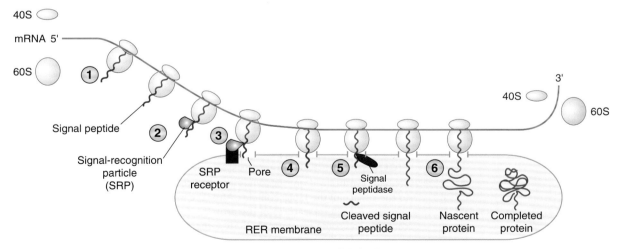

FIGURE 15.13 Synthesis of proteins on the rough endoplasmic reticulum (RER). (*1*) Translation of the protein begins in the cytosol. (*2*) As the signal peptide emerges from the ribosome, a signal-recognition particle (SRP) binds to it and to the ribosome and inhibits further synthesis of the protein. (*3*) The SRP binds to the SRP receptor in the RER membrane, docking the ribosome on the RER. (*4*) The SRP is released and protein synthesis resumes. (*5*) As the signal peptide moves through a pore into the RER, a signal peptidase removes the signal peptide. (*6*) Synthesis of the nascent protein continues, and the completed protein is released into the lumen of the RER. *mRNA*, messenger RNA.

signal peptide as the nascent polypeptide emerges from the tunnel in the ribosome and translation ceases. When the SRP subsequently binds to an SRP receptor (docking protein) on the RER, translation resumes and the polypeptide begins to enter the lumen of the RER. The signal peptide is removed by the signal peptidase, and the remainder of the newly synthesized protein enters the lumen of the RER. These proteins are transferred in small vesicles to the Golgi complex.

The Golgi complex serves to process the proteins it receives from the RER and to sort them so that they are delivered to their appropriate destinations (Fig. 15.14). Processing, which can be initiated in the ER, involves glycosylation, the addition of carbohydrate groups, and modification of existing carbohydrate chains. Sorting signals permit delivery of proteins to their target locations. For example, glycosylation of enzymes destined to become lysosomal enzymes results in the presence of a mannose 6-phosphate residue on an oligosaccharide attached to the enzyme. This residue is recognized by the mannose 6-phosphate receptor protein, which incorporates the enzyme into a clathrin-coated vesicle. The vesicle travels to endosomes and

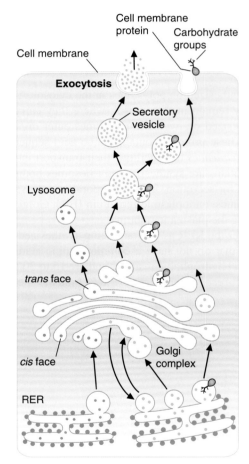

FIGURE 15.14 Fate of proteins synthesized on the rough endoplasmic reticulum (RER). Proteins synthesized on ribosomes attached to the endoplasmic reticulum travel in vesicles to the *cis* face of the Golgi complex. After the membranes fuse, the proteins enter the Golgi complex. Structural features of the proteins determine their fate. Some remain in the Golgi complex, and some return to the RER. Others bud from the *trans* face of the Golgi complex in vesicles. These vesicles can become lysosomes or secretory vesicles, depending on their contents. Secretory proteins are released from the cell when secretory vesicles fuse with the cell membrane (exocytosis). Proteins with hydrophobic regions embedded in the membrane of secretory vesicles become cell membrane proteins. See Chapter 10 for descriptions of the endoplasmic reticulum, Golgi complex, lysosomes, and the cell membrane, and also for an explanation of the process of exocytosis.

is eventually incorporated into lysosomes. Other proteins containing a Lys–Asp–Glu–Leu (KDEL) sequence at their carboxyl terminus are returned to the ER from the Golgi. Proteins with hydrophobic regions can embed in various membranes. Some proteins, whose sorting signals have not yet been determined, enter secretory vesicles and travel to the cell membrane where they are secreted by the process of exocytosis.

CLINICAL COMMENTS

 Lisa N. Lisa N. has a β^+-thalassemia classified clinically as β-thalassemia intermedia. She produces an intermediate amount of functional β-globin chains (her hemoglobin is 7.3 g/dL; normal is 12 to 16 g/dL). In β^0-thalassemia, little or none of the hemoglobin β-chain is produced. β-Thalassemia intermedia is usually the result of two different mutations (one that mildly affects the rate of synthesis of β-globin and one that severely affects its rate of synthesis); or, less frequently, homozygosity for a mild mutation in the rate of synthesis; or a complex combination of mutations. The mutations that cause the thalassemias have been studied extensively, and some are summarized in Table 15.5. For each of these mutations, the student should now be able to explain why the mutation results in a β^+- or β^0-thalassemia.

Jay S. The molecular biology–genetics laboratory's report on **Jay S.'s** white blood cells indicated that he had a deficiency of hexosaminidase A caused by a defect in the gene encoding the α-subunit of this enzyme (variant B, Tay–Sachs disease). Hexosaminidases are lysosomal enzymes that are necessary for the normal degradation of glycosphingolipids such as the gangliosides. Gangliosides are found in high concentrations in neural ganglia, although they are produced in many areas of the nervous system. When the activity of these degradative enzymes is absent or subnormal, partially degraded gangliosides accumulate in lysosomes in various cells of the central nervous system, causing a wide array of neurologic disorders known collectively as *gangliosidoses*. When the enzyme deficiency is severe, symptoms appear within the first 3 to 5 months of life. Eventually, symptoms include upper and lower motor neuron deficits, visual difficulties that can progress to blindness, seizures, and increasing cognitive dysfunction. By the second year of life, the patient may regress to a completely vegetative state, often succumbing to bronchopneumonia caused by aspiration or an inability to cough.

Edna R. With the availability of diphtheria toxoid as part of the almost universal diphtheria, tetanus, and pertussis (DTaP) immunization practiced in the United States, fatalities caused by infection by the gram-positive bacillus *C. diphtheriae* are rare. Most children, as is the case with **Edna R.'s** daughter Beverly, are immunized. In unimmunized individuals, however, symptoms are caused by a bacterial exotoxin encoded by a phage that infects the bacterial cells. The toxin enters human cells, inhibiting protein synthesis and, ultimately, causing cell death. Complications related to cardiac and nervous system involvement are the major causes of morbidity and mortality. Patients for whom a definitive diagnosis of diphtheria is established are treated with equine diphtheria antitoxin and antibiotics.

Paul T. Paul's use of the antibiotic azithromycin effectively cleared up his pneumonia caused by *S. pneumoniae*. His physician released Paul with no further follow up appointments necessary.

BIOCHEMICAL COMMENTS

 Antibiotics that Inhibit Protein Synthesis. The processes of translation on bacterial ribosomes and on the cytoplasmic ribosomes of eukaryotic cells have many similarities, but there are several subtle differences. Antibiotics

 I-cell disease (mucolipidosis II) is an inherited disorder of protein targeting. Lysosomal proteins are not sorted properly from the Golgi to the lysosomes, and lysosomal enzymes end up being secreted from the cell. This is because of a mutation in the enzyme N-acetylglucosamine phosphotransferase, which is a required first step for attaching the lysosomal targeting signal, mannose 6-phosphate, to lysosomal proteins. Thus, lysosomal proteins cannot be targeted to the lysosomes, and these organelles become clogged with materials that cannot be digested, destroying overall lysosomal function. This leads to a lysosomal storage disease of severe consequence, with death before the age of 8 years.

TABLE 15.5 **Some Examples of Mutations in β-Thalassemia**		
TYPE OF MUTATION	**PHENOTYPE**	**ORIGIN**
Nonsense		
Codon 17 (A → T)	β^0	Chinese
Codon 39 (C → T)	β^0	Mediterranean
Codon 121 (A → T)	β^0	Polish
Frameshift		
Codon 6 (−1 bp)	β^0	Mediterranean
Codon 16 (−1 bp)	β^0	Asian Indian
Codon 41/42 (−4 bp)	β^0	Asian Indian, Chinese
Codon 71/72 (+1 bp)	β^0	Chinese
Promoter		
Position −88 (C → T)	β^+	African American
Position −31 (A → G)	β^+	Japanese
Position −28 (A → C)	β^+	Kurdish
Cap site		
Position +1 (A → C)	β^+	Asian Indian
Splice junction		
Intron 1, position 1 (G → A)	β^0	Mediterranean
Intron 1, 3'-end (−25 bp)	β^0	Asian Indian
Intron 2, position 1 (G → A)	β^0	Mediterranean
Intron 2, 3'-end (A → G)	β^0	African American
Intron, internal		
Intron 1, position 5 (G → T)	β^+	Mediterranean
Intron 1, position 6 (T → C)	β^+	Mediterranean
Intron 2, position 110 (G → A)	β^+	Mediterranean
Intron 2, position 654 (C → T)	β^0	Chinese
Intron 2, position 745 (C → G)	β^+	Mediterranean
Exon, internal		
Codon 24 (T → A)	β^+	African American
Codon 26 (G → A)	β^E	Southeast Asian
Codon 27 (G → T)	$\beta^{Knossos}$	Mediterranean
RNA		
Cleavage/polyadenylation		
AATAAA to AACAAA	β^+	African American

bp, base pair(s).
Data from Scriver CR, Beaudet AL, Sly WS, et al. *The Metabolic and Molecular Basis of Inherited Diseases.* Vol. 3. New York, NY: McGraw-Hill; 1995:3456–3457.

act at steps at which these differences occur, and different antibiotics target each of the major steps of protein synthesis (Table 15.6). Therefore, these compounds can be used selectively to prevent bacterial protein synthesis and inhibit bacterial proliferation while having little or no effect on human cells. Caution must be exercised in their use, however, because some of the antibiotics affect human mitochondria, which have a protein-synthesizing system similar to that of bacteria. Another problem with these drugs is that bacteria can become resistant to their action. Mutations in genes that encode the proteins or RNA of bacterial ribosomes can cause resistance. Resistance also

TABLE 15.6	Inhibitors of Protein Synthesis in Prokaryotes
ANTIBIOTIC	**MODE OF ACTION**
Streptomycin	Binds to the 30S ribosomal subunit of prokaryotes, thereby preventing formation of the initiation complex. It also causes misreading of mRNA.
Tetracycline	Binds to the 30S ribosomal subunit and inhibits binding of aminoacyl-tRNA to the A site.
Chloramphenicol	Binds to the 50S ribosomal subunit and inhibits peptidyltransferase.
Erythromycin	Binds to the 50S ribosomal subunit and prevents translocation.

mRNA, messenger RNA; tRNA, transfer RNA; A site, aminoacyl site.

results when bacteria take up plasmids that carry genes for inactivation of the antibiotic. Because of the widespread and often indiscriminate use of antibiotics, strains of bacteria are rapidly developing that are resistant to all known antibiotics.

 Streptomycin. Streptomycin inhibits translation initiation by binding to three proteins and probably the 16S rRNA of the 30S ribosomal subunit of bacteria. Abnormal initiation complexes, known as *streptomycin monosomes*, accumulate. Streptomycin can also cause misreading of mRNA, resulting in premature termination of translation or in the incorporation of incorrect amino acids into polypeptide chains that have already been initiated. The use of this antibiotic is limited because it causes ototoxicity that can result in loss of hearing.

 Tetracycline. Tetracycline binds to the 30S ribosomal subunit of bacteria and prevents an aminoacyl-tRNA from binding to the A site on the ribosome. This effect of the drug is reversible; thus, when the drug is removed, bacteria resume protein synthesis and growth, resulting in a rekindling of the infection. Furthermore, tetracycline is not absorbed well from the intestine, and its concentration can become elevated in the contents of the gut, leading to changes in the intestinal flora. Because it has been used to treat human infections and has been added to animal feed to prevent animal infections, humans have had extensive exposure to tetracycline. As a result, resistant strains of bacteria have developed.

 Chloramphenicol. Chloramphenicol binds to the 50S ribosomal subunit of bacteria and prevents binding of the amino acid portion of the aminoacyl-tRNA, effectively inhibiting peptidyltransferase action. This antibiotic is used only for certain extremely serious infections such as meningitis and typhoid fever. Chloramphenicol readily enters human mitochondria, where it inhibits protein synthesis. Cells of the bone marrow often fail to develop in patients treated with chloramphenicol, and use of this antibiotic has been linked to fatal blood dyscrasias, including an aplastic anemia.

 Erythromycin. Erythromycin and the other macrolide antibiotics bind to the 50S ribosomal subunit of bacteria near the binding site for chloramphenicol. They prevent the translocation step, the movement of the peptidyl-tRNA from the A site to the P site on the ribosome. Because the side effects are less severe and more readily reversible than those of many other antibiotics, the macrolides are often used to treat infections in persons who are allergic to penicillin, an antibiotic that inhibits bacterial cell-wall synthesis. However, bacterial resistance to erythromycin is increasing. Therefore, its close relative, azithromycin, is often used.

KEY CONCEPTS

- Translation is the process of translating the sequence of nucleotides in mRNA to an amino acid sequence of a protein.
- Translation proceeds from the amino to the carboxyl terminus, reading the mRNA in the 5′-to-3′ direction.

- Protein synthesis occurs on ribosomes.
- The mRNA is read in codons, sets of three nucleotides that specify individual amino acids.
- AUG, which specifies methionine, is the start codon for all protein synthesis.
- Specific stop codons (UAG, UGA, and UAA) signal when the translation of the mRNA is to end.
- Amino acids are linked covalently to tRNA by the enzyme aminoacyl-tRNA synthetase, creating charged tRNA.
- Charged tRNAs base-pair with the codon via the anticodon region of the tRNA.
- Protein synthesis is divided into three stages: initiation, elongation, and termination.
- Multiprotein factors are required for each stage of protein synthesis.
- Proteins fold as they are synthesized.
- Specific amino acid side chains may be modified after translation by a process known as *posttranslational modification*.
- Mechanisms within eukaryotic cells specifically target newly synthesized proteins to different compartments in the cell.
- Table 15.7 summarizes the diseases discussed in this chapter.

TABLE 15.7 Diseases Discussed in Chapter 15		
DISORDER OR CONDITION	**GENETIC OR ENVIRONMENTAL**	**COMMENTS**
β-Thalassemia	Genetic	Lisa N. has β-thalassemia intermedia, indicating that the β-globin gene product is produced at reduced levels as compared to the α-globin gene product. This can happen because of a variety of mutations.
Tay–Sachs disease	Genetic	Mutation in a gene encoding a lysosomal enzyme, leading to loss of lysosomal function and death at an early age for the patient
Pneumonia	Environmental	Although rifampin was used to treat the bacterial infection previously (acting on bacterial RNA polymerase), the mechanism of other antibiotics that target prokaryotic protein synthesis are also discussed.
Diphtheria, pertussis	Environmental	Diphtheria toxin catalyzes the ADP-ribosylation of eEF2, a necessary factor for eukaryotic protein synthesis. This results in cell death. Vaccination against pertussis antigens will prevent infection.
I-cell disease (mucolipidosis II)	Genetic	Mutation in posttranslational processing that leads to mistargeting of enzymes destined for the lysosomes. Disease leads to lysosomal dysfunction and early death.
Hutchinson–Gilford progeria syndrome	Genetic	An example of a silent mutation in terms of amino acid substitution, but the single-nucleotide change creates an alternative splice site which leads to a loss of 50 amino acids from the precursor lamin A protein. This leads to altered posttranslational processing and the symptoms of a premature aging disease.

ADP, adenosine diphosphate; eEF2, eukaryotic elongation factor 2.

REVIEW QUESTIONS—CHAPTER 15

1. Antibiotics can target differences in processing of the genetic code between bacteria and humans. In the readout of the genetic code in prokaryotes, which one of the following processes acts before any of the others?
   A. tRNA$_i$ alignment with mRNA
   B. Termination of transcription
   C. Movement of the ribosome from one codon to the next
   D. Recruitment of termination factors to the A site
   E. Export of mRNA from the nucleus

2. Genetic mutations can be simulated in laboratory situations. tRNA charged with cysteine can be chemically treated so that the amino acid changes its identity to alanine. If some of this charged tRNA is added to a protein-synthesizing extract that contains *all* the normal components required for translation, which of the following statements represents the most likely outcome after adding an mRNA that has both Cys and Ala codons in the normal reading frame?
   A. Cysteine would be added each time the alanine codon was translated.
   B. Alanine would be added each time the cysteine codon was translated.
   C. The protein would have a deficiency of cysteine residues.
   D. The protein would have a deficiency of alanine residues.
   E. The protein would be entirely normal.

3. Human and bacterial DNA differ in the organization of genetic information. A series of eukaryotic gene sequences (coding sequences) is given below. Based on this portion of the sequence, which gene could produce a protein that contains 300 amino acids and has a phenylalanine residue near its *N* terminus? The phenylalanine codons (5′-to-3′) are UUU and UUC.
   A. 5′-CCATGCCATTTGCATCA -3′
   B. 5′-CCATGCCATTTGCATGA-3′
   C. 5′-CCATGCCAATTTGCATC-3′
   D. 5′-CCATCCCATTTGCATGA-3′
   E. 5′-CCATCCCATTTGCATCA-3′

4. A drug is being designed to block eukaryotic translation. Which of the following would be an appropriate target for the drug? Choose the one best answer.

5. A gene has undergone a mutation in which a certain codon has been altered, through a single nucleotide change, into a Phe codon. Which one of the following amino acids could the original codon code for?
   A. Pro
   B. Leu
   C. Gly
   D. Asn
   E. Arg
   F. Trp

6. A mutation in a gene has led to the generation of a nonsense codon in the corresponding protein. If this is caused by a single nucleotide change, the original codon may have coded for which one of the following amino acids?
   A. Gly
   B. Pro
   C. Phe
   D. Asn
   E. Trp

7. Which type of mutation leads to sickle cell anemia? Choose the one best answer.
   A. Silent
   B. Nonsense
   C. Insertion
   D. Deletion
   E. Missense

8. The creation of a stop codon in DNA often leads to a deleterious condition. If a mutation in DNA caused a stop codon TAG to be created on the coding strand between the TATA box and the transcription initiation site, what would be the most likely outcome?
   A. No effect
   B. Loss of transcription
   C. Loss of translation
   D. A shorter protein
   E. A mistake in splicing

9. A temperature-sensitive variant of *Escherichia coli* was discovered which had a complete loss of protein synthetic ability after about five generations of growth at the nonpermissive temperature. Analysis of the components required for protein synthesis indicated that mRNA

	N-Formyl-methionine Linked to tRNA	The Nuclear mRNA Ribosomal Complex	Enzymes Necessary for Splicing	The Initiator tRNA for Methionine	An Enzyme Involved in 5′-Cap Formation
A	Yes	Yes	No	No	Yes
B	Yes	No	Yes	No	No
C	Yes	Yes	Yes	No	Yes
D	No	No	No	Yes	No
E	No	Yes	Yes	Yes	No
F	No	No	No	Yes	Yes

synthesis (transcription) still occurred at the nonpermissive temperature, and the mRNA produced had normal half-lives. The transcription of rRNA and tRNA was also normal as was ribosome structure. A potential protein in which loss of activity at the nonpermissive temperature would lead to these findings is which one of the following?

A. A spliceosome protein
B. A tRNA-modifying enzyme
C. The capping protein
D. Poly(A) polymerase
E. A nuclear mRNA export protein

10. A new patient, recently admitted to the hospital, has contracted diphtheria. A family history indicates that the patient had never been vaccinated against this pathogen. Protein synthesis in the patient's cells is inhibited owing to which one of the following?

A. An inhibition of RNA polymerase II activity
B. An inhibition of peptidyltransferase activity
C. An inhibition of the assembly of the translation-initiation complex
D. An inhibition of the translocation step of protein synthesis
E. An inhibition of the termination of protein synthesis.

ANSWERS

1. **The answer is A.** It is important to note that the question is asking about prokaryotic mechanisms. In prokaryotes, there is no nucleus (thus, E cannot be correct), and translation begins before transcription is terminated (coupled translation–transcription, thus B is incorrect). Therefore, before the ribosome can move from one codon to the next (translocation), or the protein synthesis machinery terminates (via termination factors), the initiating tRNA must bind and align with the mRNA to initiate translation, indicating that answer A is the first step of the choices listed that must occur.

2. **The answer is C.** Because the extract contains all normal components, the Cys-tRNA charged with alanine will compete with Cys-tRNA charged with cysteine for binding to the cysteine codons. Thus, the protein will have some alanines put in the place of cysteine, leading to a deficiency of cysteine residues. Answer A is incorrect because the tRNA recognizes the cysteine codon, not the alanine codon. Answer B is incorrect because of the competition mentioned previously.

3. **The answer is A.** In order to answer this question, one first needs to find the start codon: AUG in mRNA and ATG in DNA. Bases 3 to 5 in the sequence contain this element. Next, the sequence needs to specify a phenylalanine residue near the amino terminus, which is UUU or UUC in mRNA, or TTT or TTG in DNA, but these sequences need to be in frame with the initiating methionine codon. The last element to look for is the absence of a premature stop codon because this protein is 300 amino acids long. There is no stop sequence in the remaining bases of this piece of DNA. For answer B, the last three bases of this sequence are TGA, which in mRNA would be UGA, and this is an in-frame stop signal. This sequence would not give rise to a protein that contained 300 amino acids. For answer C, the TTT in that sequence (bases 10 to 12) are not in frame with the initiating methionine, indicating that there is not a phenylalanine near the amino terminus in the protein encoded by this sequence. For answers D and E, there are no ATG sequences, indicating that the initiating

methionine is absent and that this stretch of DNA cannot code for the amino-terminal end of a protein.

4. **The answer is F.** *N*-Formyl-methionine is used for the initiation of prokaryotic protein synthesis but not eukaryotic protein synthesis. In eukaryotes, the mRNA is processed within the nucleus and then exported into the cytoplasm before ribosomes can bind to it, so there is no nuclear mRNA–ribosome complex formed. Splicing occurs in the nucleus, but splicing errors will not alter translation. Eukaryotic translation requires an initiator tRNA for methionine, so if that tRNA were unavailable, there would be no eukaryotic translation occurring. The cap on eukaryotic mRNA is necessary for appropriate IF binding to allow the charged initiator tRNA and ribosomes to bind to the mRNA. In the absence of cap formation, eukaryotic translation would be inhibited.

5. **The answer is B.** The codons for Phe are UUC and UUU. Leucine has six codons, and single nucleotide changes in four of those codons would result in a Phe codon. This is not the case for Pro, Gly, Asn, or Arg codons; in order to convert those codons to a Phe codon, two nucleotide changes are required. Answering this question required consultation with the genetic code.

6. **The answer is E.** A nonsense codon is the conversion of a codon to a stop codon. The stop codons are UGA, UAG, and UAA. The codon for Trp is UGG, which can be converted to UGA or UAG with a single nucleotide change. None of the other amino acid codons, with a single nucleotide change, can be converted into a stop codon.

7. **The answer is E.** A single mutation of one amino acid (valine for glutamate) causes sickle cell anemia. This change specifies a different amino acid (missense). A silent mutation specifies the same amino acid and has no consequence. A nonsense mutation is a change to a stop codon. An insertion is an addition of at least one base within the DNA. A deletion is a loss of at least one base in the DNA sequence. Sickle cell anemia could also be considered a point mutation since only a single base is changed which codes for a different amino acid.

8. **The answer is A.** There is no coding sequence between the TATA box (the promoter region where RNA polymerase binds) and the transcription initiation site, so the presence of a TAG in the DNA will not affect protein synthesis. In fact, the RNA corresponding to this sequence (UAG) will not even be synthesized because the transcription initiation site occurs after this sequence in the DNA. The introns and exons are not affected by this mutation, and splicing will occur normally. Thus, the mRNA produced would be of normal size and would produce a normal-sized protein.

9. **The answer is B.** All tRNA molecules have the nucleotides CCA added to the 3′-end of the tRNA after it has been transcribed. The ribose on the 3′-terminal adenine is the one that accepts amino acids to form aminoacyl-tRNA. The absence of this A residue would prevent the charging of the tRNA molecules, which would lead to cessation of all protein synthesis. It would require several generations of growth such that any functional enzyme produced would have been degraded after that many generations. Spliceosomes are eukaryotic-specific because bacterial genes do not contain introns that need to be spliced from the initial transcript. There are multiple aminoacyl-tRNA synthetases, and lacking one would lead to incomplete protein synthesis (protein synthesis would stop when this particular charged tRNA needed to be brought to the ribosome), but some protein synthesis would occur. Prokaryotic RNA is not capped; nor are poly(A) tails added to each mRNA, as in eukaryotic cells. Prokaryotes do not contain a nucleus.

10. **The answer is D.** Diphtheria toxin catalyzes the ADP-ribosylation of eEF2, thereby inhibiting the activity of this factor, which is required for the translocation step of protein synthesis. The toxin does not affect RNA polymerase II, the peptidyltransferase activity of the large ribosomal subunit, the initiation complex required for ribosome assembly, or the termination steps of protein synthesis.

16

Regulation of Gene Expression

Gene expression, the generation of a protein or RNA product from a particular gene, is controlled by complex mechanisms. Normally, only a fraction of the genes in a cell are expressed at any time. Gene expression is regulated differently in prokaryotes and eukaryotes.

Regulation of Gene Expression in Prokaryotes. In **prokaryotes**, gene expression is regulated mainly by controlling the **initiation of gene transcription**. Sets of genes that encode proteins with related functions are organized into **operons**, and each operon is under the control of **a single promoter** (or regulatory region). Regulatory proteins called **repressors** bind to the promoter and inhibit the binding of RNA polymerase (**negative control**), whereas **activator proteins** facilitate RNA polymerase binding (**positive control**). Repressors are controlled by nutrients or their metabolites, classified as **inducers** or corepressors. Regulation also may occur through **attenuation of transcription**.

Eukaryotes: Regulation of Gene Expression at the Level of DNA. In eukaryotes, activation of a gene requires changes in the state of chromatin (**chromatin remodeling**) that are facilitated by **acetylation of histones and methylation of bases**. These changes in DNA determine which genes are available for transcription.

Regulation of Eukaryotic Gene Transcription. Transcription of specific genes is regulated by proteins (called **specific transcription factors** or **transactivators**) that bind to **gene regulatory sequences** (called **promoter-proximal elements**, **response elements**, or **enhancers**) that activate or inhibit assembly of the basal transcription complex and RNA polymerase at a TATA box or similar regulatory element. These specific transcription factors, which may bind to DNA sequences some distance from the promoter, interact with coactivators or corepressors that bind to components of the basal transcription complex. These protein factors are said to work in "**trans**"; the DNA sequences to which they bind are said to work in "**cis**."

Other Sites for Regulation of Eukaryotic Gene Expression. Regulation also occurs during the **processing** of RNA, during RNA **transport** from the nucleus to the cytoplasm, and at the level of **translation** in the cytoplasm. Regulation can occur simultaneously at multiple levels for a specific gene, and many factors act in concert to stimulate or inhibit expression of a gene.

THE WAITING ROOM

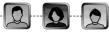

Charles F., a 68-year-old man, complained of fatigue, loss of appetite, and a low-grade fever. An open biopsy of a lymph node indicated the presence of non-Hodgkin lymphoma, follicular type. Computed tomography and other noninvasive procedures showed a diffuse process with bone marrow involvement. He is receiving multidrug chemotherapy with R-CHOP (rituximab, cyclophosphamide, doxorubicin, vincristine, and prednisone).

Mannie W. is a 56-year-old man who complains of weight loss related to a decreased appetite and increased fatigue. He notes discomfort in the left upper quadrant of his abdomen. On physical examination, he is noted to be pale and to have ecchymoses (bruises) on his arms and legs. His spleen is markedly enlarged.

Initial laboratory studies show a hemoglobin of 10.4 g/dL (normal = 13.5 to 17.5 g/dL) and a leukocyte (white blood cell) count of 106,000 cells/mm³ (normal = 4,500 to 11,000 cells/mm³). The majority of the leukocytes are granulocytes (white blood cells arising from the myeloid lineage), some of which have an "immature" appearance. The percentage of lymphocytes in the peripheral blood is decreased. A bone marrow aspiration and biopsy show the presence of an abnormal chromosome (the Philadelphia chromosome) in dividing marrow cells.

Ann R., who has anorexia nervosa, has continued on an almost meat-free diet (see Chapters 1, 3, 9, and 11). She now appears emaciated and pale. Her hemoglobin is 9.7 g/dL (normal = 12 to 16 g/dL), her hematocrit (volume of packed red cells) is 31% (reference range for women = 36% to 46%), and her mean corpuscular volume (the average volume of a red cell) is 70 femtoliters (fL; 1 fL is 10^{-15} L) (reference range = 80 to 100 fL). These values indicate an anemia that is microcytic (small red cells) and hypochromic (light in color, indicating a reduced amount of hemoglobin per red cell). Her serum ferritin (the cellular storage form of iron) was also subnormal. Her plasma level of transferrin (the iron transport protein in plasma) is higher than normal, but its percentage saturation with iron is below normal. This laboratory profile is consistent with changes that occur in an iron deficiency state.

I. Gene Expression Is Regulated for Adaptation and Differentiation

Virtually all cells of an organism contain identical sets of genes. However, at any given time, only a small number of the total genes in each cell are expressed (i.e., generate a protein or RNA product). The remaining genes are inactive. Organisms gain several advantages by regulating the activity of their genes. For example, both prokaryotic and eukaryotic cells adapt to changes in their environment by turning the expression of genes on and off. Because the processes of RNA transcription and protein synthesis consume a considerable amount of energy, cells conserve fuel by making proteins only when they are needed.

In addition to regulating gene expression to adapt to environmental changes, eukaryotic organisms alter expression of their genes during development. As a fertilized egg becomes a multicellular organism, different kinds of proteins are synthesized in varying quantities. In humans, as the child progresses through adolescence and then into adulthood, physical and physiologic changes result from variations in gene expression and, therefore, of protein synthesis. Even after an organism has reached the adult stage, regulation of gene expression enables certain cells to undergo differentiation to assume new functions.

Many of the drugs used by **Charles F.** inhibit the proliferation of cancer cells in various ways. Doxorubicin (Adriamycin) is a large nonpolar molecule synthesized by fungi that intercalates between DNA bases, inhibiting replication and transcription and forming DNA with single- and double-strand breaks. Vincristine binds to tubulin and inhibits formation of the mitotic spindle, thereby preventing cell division. Cyclophosphamide is an alkylating agent that damages DNA by covalently attaching alkyl groups to DNA bases. Rituximab is an anti-CD20 antibody which specifically targets B-cells (including the tumor cells) for destruction (a form of immunotherapy). Prednisone is a steroid hormone; its effect on cancer cells is not exactly understood, but it is given to help manage the side effects of the other agents.

The measurement of iron in the blood needs to account for iron associated with hemoglobin, free iron, and iron bound to its carrier protein, transferrin. When a physician orders a determination of serum iron, the order refers to ferric iron (Fe^{3+}) bound to transferrin and not to the ferrous iron (Fe^{2+}) bound to circulating hemoglobin (which may be present in the plasma as a result of occasional red-cell lysis). Measurement of ferric iron has been adapted to automated spectrophotometric analysis. In most cases, the samples are acidified to remove the ferric ion from transferrin. The iron is then reduced to the ferrous state by a reducing agent (such as ascorbic acid), and the level of iron is determined by its binding to a dye that changes color when ferrous ion binds to it.

The total iron-binding capacity (TIBC) is determined by adding ferric ion to the sample to saturate all transferrin-binding sites in the sample. Excess iron (free iron, not bound to transferrin) is precipitated by treatment with $MgCO_3$, and the precipitate is removed by centrifugation. The resulting soluble sample is then analyzed for Fe^{3+}, as described previously. By comparing the levels of Fe^{3+} bound both before and after saturation, one can determine what percentage of transferrin contained bound iron. For a woman between the ages of 16 and 40 years, the percentage saturation should be in the range of 20% to 50%. **Ann R.'s** iron saturation is below this normal range, indicating an iron deficiency.

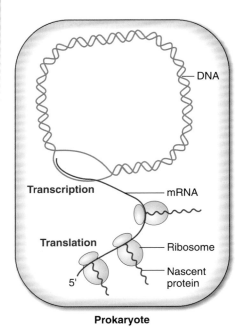

Prokaryote

FIGURE 16.1 *Escherichia coli* cell. In prokaryotes, DNA is not separated from the rest of the cellular contents by a nuclear envelope; therefore, simultaneous transcription and translation occur in bacteria. Once a small piece of messenger RNA (mRNA) is synthesized, ribosomes bind to the mRNA and translation begins.

II. Regulation of Gene Expression in Prokaryotes

Prokaryotes are single-celled organisms and therefore require less complex regulatory mechanisms than the multicellular eukaryotes (Fig. 16.1). The most extensively studied prokaryote is the bacterium *Escherichia coli*, an organism that thrives in the human colon, usually enjoying a symbiotic relationship with its host. Based on the size of its genome (4×10^6 base pairs), *E. coli* should be capable of making several thousand proteins. However, under normal growth conditions *E. coli* synthesizes only about 600 to 800 different proteins. Thus, many genes are inactive and *E. coli* will only synthesize those genes that generate the proteins required for growth in that particular environment.

All *E. coli* cells of the same strain are morphologically similar and contain an identical circular chromosome (see Fig. 16.1). As in other prokaryotes, DNA is not complexed with histones, no nuclear envelope separates the genes from the contents of the cytoplasm, and gene transcripts do not contain introns. In fact, as messenger RNA (mRNA) is being synthesized, ribosomes bind and begin to produce proteins, so that transcription and translation occur simultaneously (known as *coupled transcription–translation*). The mRNA molecules in *E. coli* have a very short half-life and are degraded within a few minutes. mRNA molecules must be constantly generated from transcription to maintain synthesis of its proteins. Thus, regulation of transcription, principally at the level of initiation, is sufficient to regulate the level of proteins within the cell.

A. Operons

The genes encoding proteins are called *structural genes*. In the bacterial genome, the structural genes for proteins involved in performing a related function (such as the enzymes of a biosynthetic pathway) are often grouped sequentially into units called *operons* (Fig. 16.2, and see Fig. 14.6). The genes in an operon are coordinately expressed; that is, they are either all turned on or all turned off. When an operon is expressed, all of its genes are transcribed (refer to Chapter 14, Section III). A single polycistronic mRNA is produced that codes for all of the proteins of the operon. This polycistronic mRNA contains multiple sets of start and stop codons that allow several different proteins to be produced from this single transcript at the translational level. Transcription of the genes in an operon is regulated by the *promoter*, which is located in the operon at the 5′-end, upstream from the structural genes.

B. Regulation of RNA Polymerase Binding by Repressors

In bacteria, the principal means of regulating gene transcription is through repressors, which are regulatory proteins that prevent the binding of RNA polymerase

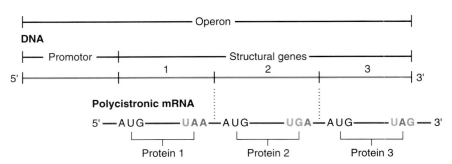

FIGURE 16.2 An operon. The structural genes of an operon are transcribed as one long polycistronic messenger RNA (mRNA). During translation, different start (AUG) and stop (UAA, UGA or UAG) codons lead to several distinct proteins being produced from this single mRNA.

to the promoter and thus act on initiation of transcription (Fig. 16.3). In general, regulatory mechanisms such as repressors, which work through inhibition of gene transcription, are referred to as *negative control*, and mechanisms that work through stimulation of gene transcription are called *positive control*.

The repressor is encoded by a regulatory gene (see Fig. 16.3). Although this gene is considered part of the operon, it is not always located near the remainder of the operon. Its product, the *repressor protein*, diffuses to the promoter and binds to a region of the operon called the *operator*. The operator is located within the promoter or near its 3'-end, just upstream from the transcription start point. When a repressor is bound to the operator, the operon is not transcribed because the repressor protein either physically blocks the binding of RNA polymerase to the promoter or prevents the RNA polymerase from initiating transcription. Two regulatory mechanisms work through controlling repressors: induction (an inducer inactivates the repressor) and repression (a corepressor is required to activate the repressor).

1. Inducers

Induction involves a small molecule, known as an *inducer*, which stimulates expression of the operon by binding to the repressor and changing its conformation so that it can no longer bind to the operator (Fig. 16.4). The inducer is either a nutrient or a metabolite of the nutrient. In the presence of the inducer, RNA polymerase can therefore bind to the promoter and transcribe the operon. The key to this mechanism is that in the absence of the inducer, the repressor is active, transcription is repressed, and the genes of the operon are not expressed.

Consider, for example, induction of the *lac* operon of *E. coli* by lactose (Fig. 16.5). The enzymes for metabolizing glucose by glycolysis are produced constitutively; that is, they are constantly being made. If the milk sugar lactose is available, the cells adapt and begin to produce the three additional enzymes required for lactose metabolism, which are encoded by the *lac* operon. A metabolite of lactose (allolactose) serves as an inducer, binding to the repressor and inactivating it. Because the inactive repressor no longer binds to the operator, RNA polymerase can bind to the promoter and transcribe the structural genes of the *lac* operon, producing a polycistronic mRNA that encodes for the three additional proteins. However, the presence of glucose can prevent activation of the *lac* operon (see "Stimulation of RNA Polymerase Binding" in Section II.C). It is important to realize that the *lac* operon is expressed at very low levels (basal levels) even in the absence of repressor. Thus, even in the absence of lactose, a small amount of permease is present in the cellular membrane. Therefore, when lactose does become available in the environment, a few molecules of lactose are able to enter the cell and can be metabolized to allolactose. The few molecules of allolactose produced are sufficient to induce the operon. As the amount of permease increases, more lactose can be transported into the cell to be used as an energy source.

2. Corepressors

In a regulatory model called *repression*, the repressor is inactive until a small molecule called a *corepressor* (a nutrient or its metabolite) binds to the repressor, activating it (Fig. 16.6). The repressor–corepressor complex then binds to the operator, preventing binding of RNA polymerase and gene transcription. Consider, for example, the *trp* operon, which encodes the five enzymes required for the synthesis of the amino acid tryptophan. When tryptophan is available, *E. coli* cells save energy by no longer making these enzymes. Tryptophan is a corepressor that binds to the inactive repressor, causing it to change conformation and bind to the operator, thereby inhibiting transcription of the operon. Thus, in the repression model, the repressor is inactive without a corepressor; in the induction model, the repressor is active unless an inducer is present.

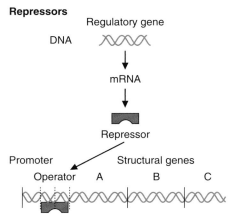

Repressors

FIGURE 16.3 Regulation of operons by repressors. When the repressor protein is bound to the operator (a DNA sequence adjacent to, or within, the promoter), RNA polymerase cannot bind, and transcription therefore does not occur. *mRNA*, messenger RNA.

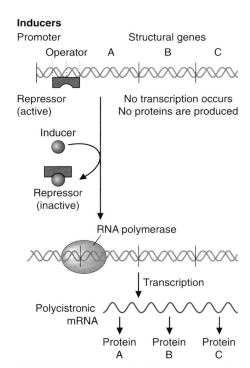

Inducers

FIGURE 16.4 An inducible operon. In the absence of an inducer, the repressor binds to the operator, preventing the binding of RNA polymerase. When the inducer is present, the inducer binds to the repressor, inactivating it. The inactive repressor no longer binds to the operator. Therefore, RNA polymerase can bind to the promoter region and transcribe the structural genes. *mRNA*, messenger RNA.

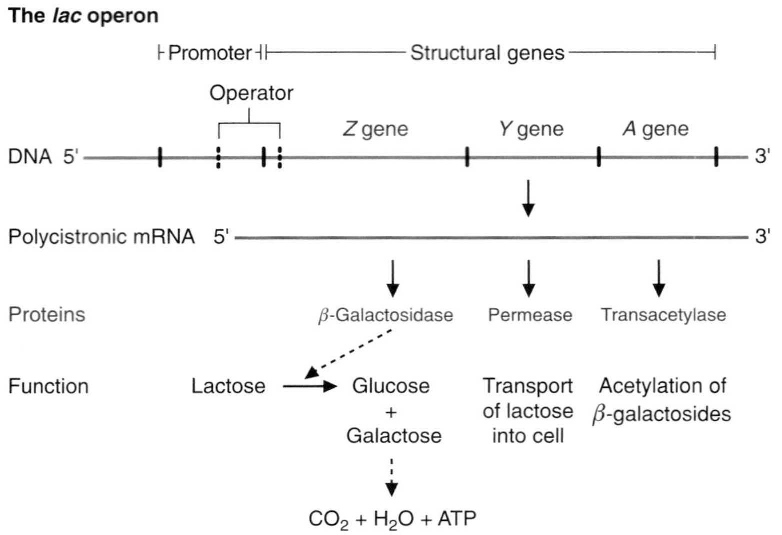

The *lac* operon

Promoter ─┤├──────── Structural genes ────────┤

Operator

Z gene   *Y* gene   *A* gene

DNA 5' ────────────────────────────── 3'

↓

Polycistronic mRNA 5' ────────────────── 3'

↓   ↓   ↓

Proteins   β-Galactosidase   Permease   Transacetylase

Function   Lactose ⟶ Glucose   Transport   Acetylation of
                              +   of lactose   β-galactosides
                           Galactose   into cell

↓

$CO_2 + H_2O$ + ATP

FIGURE 16.5   The protein products of the *lac* operon. Lactose is a disaccharide that is hydrolyzed to glucose and galactose by β-galactosidase (the *Z* gene). Both glucose and galactose can be oxidized by the cell for energy. The permease (*Y* gene) enables the cell to take up lactose more readily. The *A* gene produces a transacetylase that acetylates β-galactosides. The function of this acetylation is not clear. The promoter binds RNA polymerase and the operator binds a repressor protein. Lactose is converted to allolactose, an inducer that binds the repressor protein and prevents it from binding to the operator. Transcription of the *lac* operon also requires activator proteins that are inactive when glucose levels are high. ATP, adenosine triphosphate; *mRNA*, messenger RNA.

C. Stimulation of RNA Polymerase Binding

In addition to regulating transcription by means of repressors that inhibit RNA polymerase binding to promoters (negative control), bacteria regulate transcription by means of activating proteins that bind to the promoter and stimulate the binding of RNA polymerase (positive control). Transcription of the *lac* operon, for example, can be induced by allolactose only if glucose is absent. The presence or absence of glucose is communicated to the promoter by a regulatory protein named the *cyclic adenosine monophosphate* (cAMP) *receptor protein* (CRP) (Fig. 16.7). This regulatory protein is also called a *catabolite activator protein* (CAP). A decrease in glucose levels increases levels of the intracellular second messenger cAMP by a

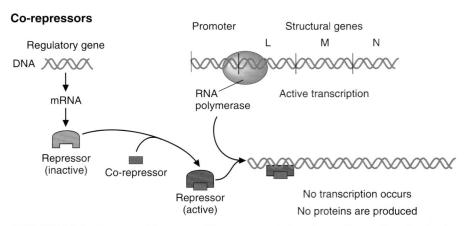

FIGURE 16.6   A repressible operon. The repressor is inactive until a small molecule, the corepressor, binds to it. The repressor–corepressor complex binds to the operator and prevents transcription. *mRNA*, messenger RNA.

A. In the presence of lactose and glucose

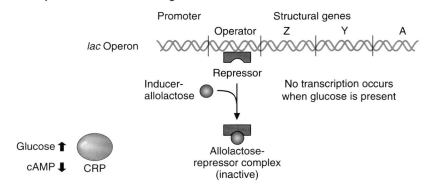

B. In the presence of lactose and absence of glucose

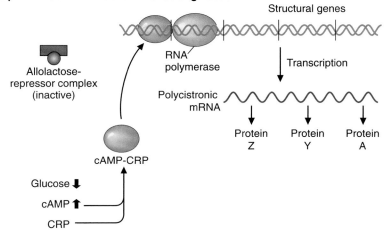

FIGURE 16.7 Catabolite repression of stimulatory proteins. The *lac* operon is used as an example. **A.** The inducer allolactose (a metabolite of lactose) inactivates the repressor. However, because of the absence of the required coactivator, cAMP–CRP, no transcription occurs unless glucose is absent. **B.** In the absence of glucose, cAMP levels rise. cAMP forms a complex with the cAMP receptor protein (CRP). The binding of the cAMP–CRP complex to a regulatory region of the operon permits the binding of RNA polymerase to the promoter. Now, the operon is transcribed, and the proteins are produced. *cAMP*, cyclic adenosine mo-nophosphate; *mRNA*, messenger RNA.

mechanism that involves glucose transport into the bacteria. cAMP binds to CRP and the cAMP–CRP complex binds to a regulatory region of the operon, stimulating binding of RNA polymerase to the promoter and transcription. When glucose is present, cAMP levels decrease, CRP assumes an inactive conformation that does not bind to the operon, and the recruitment of RNA polymerase to the promoter is reduced, resulting in inhibition of transcription. Thus, the enzymes encoded by the *lac* operon are not produced if cells have an adequate supply of glucose, even if lactose is present at very high levels.

D. Regulation of RNA Polymerase Binding by Sigma Factors

E. coli has only one RNA polymerase. Sigma factors bind to this RNA polymerase, stimulating its binding to certain sets of promoters, thus simultaneously activating transcription of several operons. The standard sigma factor in *E. coli* is σ^{70}, a protein with a molecular weight of 70,000 Da (see Chapter 14). Other sigma factors also exist. For example, σ^{32} helps RNA polymerase recognize promoters for the different operons that encode the heat-shock proteins. Thus, increased transcription of the genes for heat-shock proteins, which prevent protein denaturation at high temperatures, occurs in response to elevated temperatures.

E. Attenuation of Transcription

Some operons are regulated by a process that interrupts (attenuates) transcription after it has been initiated (Fig. 16.8). For example, high levels of tryptophan attenuate transcription of the *E. coli trp* operon as well as repress its transcription. As mRNA is being transcribed from the *trp* operon, ribosomes bind and rapidly begin to translate the transcript. Near the 5'-end of the transcript are several codons for tryptophan. Initially, high levels of tryptophan in the cell result in high levels of Trp-tRNA^{Trp} and rapid translation of the transcript. However, rapid translation generates a hairpin loop in the mRNA that serves as a termination signal for RNA polymerase, and transcription terminates. Conversely, when tryptophan levels are low, levels of Trp-tRNA^{Trp} are low, and ribosomes stall at codons for tryptophan. A different hairpin loop forms in the mRNA that does not terminate transcription, and the complete mRNA is transcribed. Attenuation requires coupled transcription and translation, so this mechanism is not applicable to eukaryotic systems.

The tryptophan, histidine, leucine, phenylalanine, and threonine operons are regulated, in part, by attenuation. Repressors and activators also act on the promoters of some of these operons, allowing the levels of these amino acids to be very carefully and rapidly regulated.

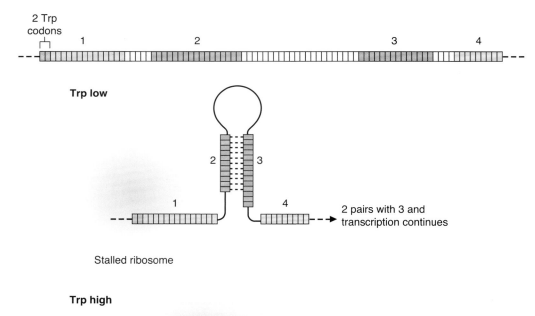

FIGURE 16.8 Attenuation of the *trp* operon. Sequences 2, 3, and 4 in the messenger RNA (mRNA) transcript can form base pairs (2 with 3 or 3 with 4) that generate hairpin loops. When tryptophan levels are low, the ribosome stalls at the adjacent Trp codons in sequence 1, the 2–3 loop forms, and transcription continues. When tryptophan levels are high, translation is rapid and the ribosome blocks formation of the 2–3 loop. Under these conditions, the 3–4 loop forms and terminates transcription.

III. Regulation of Gene Expression in Eukaryotes

Multicellular eukaryotes are much more complex than single-celled prokaryotes. As the human embryo develops into a multicellular organism, different sets of genes are turned on and different groups of proteins are produced, resulting in differentiation into morphologically distinct cell types that are able to perform different functions. Even beyond development, certain cells within the organism continue to differentiate, such as those that produce antibodies in response to an infection, renew the population of red blood cells, and replace digestive cells that have been sloughed into the intestinal lumen. All of these physiologic changes are dictated by complex alterations in gene expression.

A. Regulation at Multiple Levels

Differences between eukaryotic and prokaryotic cells result in different mechanisms for regulating gene expression. DNA in eukaryotes is organized into the nucleosomes of chromatin, and genes must be in an active structure to be expressed in a cell. Furthermore, operons are not present in eukaryotes, and the genes that encode proteins that function together are usually located on different chromosomes. For example, the gene for α-globin is on chromosome 16, whereas the gene for β-globin is on chromosome 11. Thus, each gene needs its own promoter. In addition, the processes of transcription and translation are separated in eukaryotes by intracellular compartmentation (nucleus and cytosol, or endoplasmic reticulum [ER]) and by time (eukaryotic heterogeneous nuclear RNA [hnRNA, also known as *pre-RNA*] must be processed and translocated out of the nucleus before it is translated). Thus, regulation of eukaryotic gene expression occurs at multiple levels:

- DNA and the chromosome, including chromosome remodeling and gene rearrangement
- Transcription, primarily through transcription factors that affect binding of RNA polymerase to the promoter
- Processing of transcripts
- Initiation of translation and stability of mRNA

Once a gene is activated through chromatin remodeling, the major mechanism of regulating expression affects initiation of transcription at the promoter.

B. Regulation of Availability of Genes for Transcription

Once a haploid sperm and egg combine to form a diploid cell, the number of genes in human cells remains approximately the same. As cells differentiate, different genes are available for transcription. A typical nucleus contains chromatin that is condensed (heterochromatin) and chromatin that is diffuse (euchromatin) (see Chapter 12). The genes in heterochromatin are inactive, whereas those in euchromatin produce mRNA. Long-term changes in the activity of genes occur during development as chromatin goes from a diffuse to a condensed state or vice versa.

The cellular genome is packaged together with histones into nucleosomes, and initiation of transcription is prevented if the promoter region is part of a nucleosome. Thus, activation of a gene for transcription requires changes in the state of the chromatin, called *chromatin remodeling*. The availability of genes for transcription also can be affected in certain cells, or under certain circumstances, by *gene rearrangements*, *amplification*, or *deletion*. For example, during lymphocyte maturation, genes are rearranged to produce a variety of different antibodies. The term *epigenetics* is used to refer to changes in gene expression without altering the sequence of the DNA. Chromatin remodeling and DNA methylation are such changes that can be inherited and that contribute to the regulation of gene expression.

I. Chromatin Remodeling

The remodeling of chromatin generally refers to displacement of the nucleosome from specific DNA sequences so that transcription of the genes in that sequence can

Alteration of gene expression is a common finding in cancer cells. Alterations in HAT or HDAC activity may contribute to dysregulation of cellular proliferation in certain tumors. These alterations in HAT or HDAC activity are usually caused by mutations in transcription factors or coactivators, which have either enhanced, or reduced, their ability to recruit HATs or HDACs to a preinitiation complex at the promoter. HDACs have been shown to be excellent therapeutic targets for drugs that inhibit their activity. Some of these inhibitors display antiproliferative activity on a variety of human cancer cell lines and are currently in clinical trials.

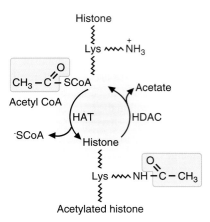

FIGURE 16.9   Histone acetylation. *CoA*, coenzyme A; *HAT*, histone acetyltransferase; *HDAC*, histone deacetylase.

be initiated. This occurs through two different mechanisms. The first mechanism is by an adenosine triphosphate (ATP)–driven chromatin remodeling complex, which uses energy from ATP hydrolysis to unwind certain sections of DNA from the nucleosome core. The second mechanism is by covalent modification of the histone tails through acetylation (Fig. 16.9). Histone acetyltransferases (HATs) transfer an acetyl group from acetyl coenzyme A (acetyl-CoA) to lysine residues in the histone tails (the amino-terminal ends of histones H2A, H2B, H3, and H4) of the histone octamer. This reaction removes a positive charge from the ε-amino group of the lysine, thereby reducing the electrostatic interactions between the histones and the negatively charged DNA, making it easier for DNA to unwind from the histones. The acetyl groups can be removed by histone deacetylases (HDAC). Each histone has several lysine residues that may be acetylated and, through a complex mixing of acetylated and nonacetylated sites, different segments of DNA can be freed from the nucleosome. Several transcription factors and coactivators contain HAT activity, which facilitates the binding of these factors to the DNA and also facilitates simultaneous activation of the gene and initiation of its transcription.

2. Methylation of DNA

Cytosine residues in DNA can be methylated to produce 5-methylcytosine. The methylated cytosines are located in CG-rich sequences (called *CG* or *CpG islands*), which are often near or in the promoter region of a gene. In certain instances, genes that are methylated are less readily transcribed than those that are not methylated. For example, globin genes are more extensively methylated in nonerythroid cells (cells that are not a part of the erythroid, or red blood cell, lineage) than in cells in which these genes are expressed (e.g., erythroblasts and reticulocytes). Methylation is a mechanism for regulating gene expression during differentiation, particularly in fetal development.

3. Gene Rearrangement

Segments of DNA can move from one location to another in the genome, associating with each other in various ways so that different proteins are produced (Fig. 16.10). The most thoroughly studied example of gene rearrangement occurs in cells that produce antibodies. Antibodies contain two light chains and two heavy chains, each of which contains both a variable region and a constant region (see Chapter 7, Section VIII, Fig. 7.19). Cells called *B-cells* make antibodies. In the precursors of B-cells, hundreds of V_H sequences, approximately 20 D_H sequences and approximately 6 J_H sequences, are located in clusters within a long region of the chromosome (see Fig. 16.10). During the production of the immature B-cells, a series of recombinational events occurs that joins one V_H, one D_H, and one J_H sequence into a single exon.

Methylation has been implicated in genomic imprinting, a process that occurs during the formation of the eggs or sperm that blocks the expression of the gene in the fertilized egg. Males methylate a different set of genes than females. This sex-dependent differential methylation has been studied most extensively in two human disorders, Prader-Willi syndrome and Angelman syndrome. Both syndromes, which have very different symptoms, result from deletions of the same region of chromosome 15 (a microdeletion of <5 megabases in size). If the deletion is inherited from the father, Prader-Willi syndrome is seen in the child. If the deletion is inherited from the mother, Angelman syndrome is observed. A disease occurs when a gene that is in the deleted region of one chromosome is methylated on the other chromosome. The mother methylates different genes than the father, so different genes are expressed depending on which parent transmitted the intact chromosome. For example, for Prader-Willi syndrome, if genes 1, 2, and 3 are deleted in the paternal chromosome and gene 2 is methylated (Me) in the maternal chromosome, only genes 1 and 3 will be expressed. For Angelman syndrome, genes 1, 2, and 3 are deleted on the maternal chromosome and gene 1 is methylated on the paternal chromosome, so only genes 2 and 3 are expressed.

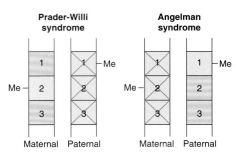

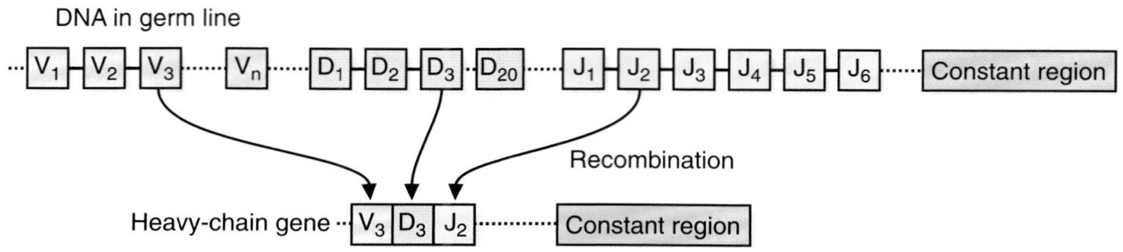

DNA in germ line

...V_1 V_2 V_3 ... V_n ...... D_1 D_2 D_3 ... D_{20} ...... J_1 J_2 J_3 J_4 J_5 J_6 ...... Constant region

Recombination

Heavy-chain gene ... V_3 D_3 J_2 .... Constant region

FIGURE 16.10 Rearrangement of DNA. The heavy-chain gene from which lymphocytes produce immunoglobulins is generated by combining specific segments from among a large number of potential sequences in the DNA of precursor cells. The variable and constant regions of immunoglobulins (antibodies) are described in Chapter 7.

This exon now encodes the variable region of the heavy chain of the antibody. Given the large number of immature B-cells that are produced, virtually every recombinational possibility occurs, so that all VDJ combinations are represented within this cell population. Later in development, during differentiation of mature B-cells, recombinational events join a VDJ sequence to one of the nine heavy-chain elements. When the immune system encounters an antigen, the one immature B-cell that can bind to that antigen (because of its unique manner of forming the VDJ exon) is stimulated to proliferate (clonal expansion) and to produce antibodies against the antigen.

4. Gene Amplification

Gene amplification is not the usual physiologic means of regulating gene expression in normal cells, but it does occur in response to certain stimuli if the cell can obtain a growth advantage by producing large amounts of a protein. In gene amplification, certain regions of a chromosome undergo repeated cycles of DNA replication. The newly synthesized DNA is excised and forms small, unstable chromosomes called *double minutes*. The double minutes integrate into other chromosomes throughout the genome, thereby amplifying the gene in the process. Normally, gene amplification occurs through errors during DNA replication and cell division, and, if the environmental conditions are appropriate, cells containing amplified genes may have a growth advantage over those without the amplification.

5. Gene Deletions

With a few exceptions, the deletion of genetic material is likewise not a normal means of controlling transcription, although such deletions do result in disease. Gene deletions can occur through errors in DNA replication and cell division and are usually noticed only if a disease results. For example, various types of cancers result from the loss of a good copy of a tumor-suppressor gene, leaving the cell with a mutated copy of the gene (see Chapter 18).

C. Regulation at the Level of Transcription

The transcription of active genes is regulated by controlling assembly of the basal transcription complex containing RNA polymerase and its binding to distinct elements of the promoter, such as the TATA or Inr box (see Chapter 14). The basal transcription complex contains $TF_{II}D$ (which binds to elements within the promoter, such as the TATA or Inr box), and other proteins called *general (basal) transcription factors* (such as $TF_{II}A$) that form a complex with RNA polymerase II. Additional transcription factors that are ubiquitous to all promoters bind upstream at various sites in the promoter region. They increase the frequency of transcription and are required for a promoter to function at an adequate level. Genes that are regulated solely by these consensus elements in the promoter region are said to be constitutively expressed.

The control region of a gene also contains DNA regulatory sequences that are specific for that gene and may increase its transcription 1,000-fold or more (Fig. 16.11). Gene-specific transcription factors (also called *transactivators* or *activators*) bind to these regulatory sequences and interact with mediator proteins such

Although rearrangements of short DNA sequences are difficult to detect, microscopists have observed major rearrangements for many years. Such major rearrangements, known as *translocations*, can be observed in metaphase chromosomes under the microscope. **Mannie W.** has such a translocation, known as the *Philadelphia chromosome* because it was first observed in that city. The Philadelphia chromosome is produced by a balanced exchange between chromosomes 9 and 22. In this translocation, most of a gene from chromosome 9, the *c-abl* gene, is transferred to the *BCR* gene on chromosome 22. This creates a fused *BCR-abl* gene. The *c-abl* gene is a tyrosine kinase (see Chapter 11), and its regulation by the BCR promoter results in uncontrolled growth stimulation rather than differentiation in cells containing this translocation.

Historically, non-Hodgkin lymphoma was treated with methotrexate, and this drug is still used in certain cases of lymphoma. It inhibits cell proliferation by inhibiting dihydrofolate reductase. Dihydrofolate reductase reduces dihydrofolate to tetrahydrofolate, a cofactor required for synthesis of thymine and purine nucleotides. Methotrexate resistance, however, was frequently observed in patients. Sometimes, rapidly dividing cancer cells treated with methotrexate amplify the gene for dihydrofolate reductase, producing hundreds of copies in the genome. These cells generate large amounts of dihydrofolate reductase, and normal doses of methotrexate are no longer adequate. Gene amplification is one of the mechanisms by which patients become resistant to a drug. Methotrexate is no longer used for the treatment of non-Hodgkin lymphoma, having been supplanted by specific immunotherapy.

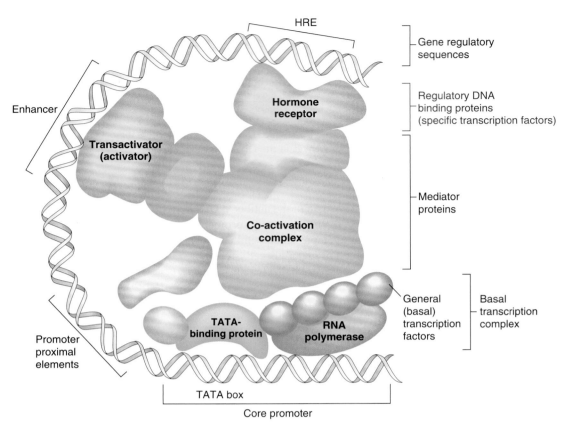

FIGURE 16.11 The gene regulatory control region consists of the promoter region and additional gene regulatory sequences, including enhancers and hormone response elements (HRE). In this case, a promoter containing a TATA box is shown. Gene regulatory proteins that bind directly to DNA (regulatory DNA-binding proteins) are usually called *specific transcription factors* or *transactivators*; they may be either activators or repressors of the transcription of specific genes. The specific transcription factors bind mediator proteins (coactivators or corepressors) that interact with the general transcription factors of the basal transcription complex. The basal transcription complex contains RNA polymerase and associated general transcription factors (TF$_{II}$ factors) and binds, in this case, to the TATA box of the promoter, initiating gene transcription.

 In fragile X syndrome, a GCC triplet is amplified on the 5'-side of a gene (fragile X mental retardation 1 [FMR-1]) associated with the disease. This gene is located on the X chromosome. The disease is named for the finding that when cells containing this triplet repeat expansion are cultured in the absence of folic acid (which impairs nucleotide production and hence the replication of DNA), the X chromosome develops single- and double-strand breaks in its DNA. These were termed *fragile sites*. It was subsequently determined that the *FMR-1* gene was located in one of these fragile sites. A normal person has about 30 copies of the GCC triplet, but in affected individuals, thousands of copies can be present. This syndrome, which is a common form of inherited intellectual developmental disorder, affects about 1 in 3,500 males and 1 in 4,000 to 1 in 6,000 females worldwide.

as coactivators. By forming a loop in the DNA, coactivators interact with the basal transcription complex and can activate its assembly at the initiation site on the promoter. These DNA regulatory sequences may be some distance from the promoter and may be either upstream or downstream of the initiation site.

Depending on the system, the terminology used to describe components of gene-specific regulation varies somewhat. For example, in the original terminology, DNA regulatory sequences called *enhancers* bound transactivators, which bound coactivators. Similarly, silencers bound corepressors. Hormones bound to hormone receptors, which bound to hormone response elements in DNA. Although these terms are still used, they are often replaced by more general terms such as *DNA regulatory sequences* and *specific transcription factors*, in recognition of the fact that many transcription factors activate one gene while inhibiting another or that a specific transcription factor may be changed from a repressor to an activator by phosphorylation.

1. Gene-Specific Regulatory Proteins

The regulatory proteins that bind directly to DNA sequences are most often called *transcription factors* or *gene-specific transcription factors* (if it is necessary to distinguish them from the general transcription factors of the basal transcription complex). They also can be called *activators* (or *transactivators*), *inducers*, *repressors*, or *nuclear receptors*. In addition to their DNA-binding domain, these proteins usually have a domain that binds to mediator proteins (coactivators, corepressors, or TATA-binding protein–associated factors [TAFs]). Coactivators, corepressors, and other mediator proteins do not bind directly to DNA but generally bind to components of the basal transcription complex and mediate its assembly at the promoter. They can be specific for a given gene transcription factor or general and bind many different gene-specific transcription factors. Certain coactivators have HAT activity, and certain corepressors have histone deacetylase activity. When the appropriate interactions among the transactivators, coactivators, and the basal transcription complex occur, the rate of transcription of the gene is increased (induction).

Some regulatory DNA-binding proteins inhibit (repress) transcription and may be called *repressors*. Repression can occur in several ways. A repressor bound to its specific DNA sequence may inhibit binding of an activator to its regulatory sequence. Alternatively, the repressor may bind a corepressor that inhibits binding of a coactivator to the basal transcription complex. The repressor may bind a component of the basal transcription complex directly. Some steroid hormone receptors that are transcription factors bind either coactivators or corepressors, depending on whether the receptor contains bound hormone. Furthermore, a particular transcription factor may induce transcription when it is bound to the regulatory sequence of one gene and may repress transcription when it is bound to the regulatory sequence of another gene.

2. Transcription Factors that Are Steroid Hormone/Thyroid Hormone Receptors

In humans, steroid hormones and other lipophilic hormones activate or inhibit transcription of specific genes through binding to nuclear receptors that are gene-specific transcription factors (Fig. 16.12A). The nuclear receptors bind to DNA regulatory sequences called *hormone response elements* and induce or repress transcription of

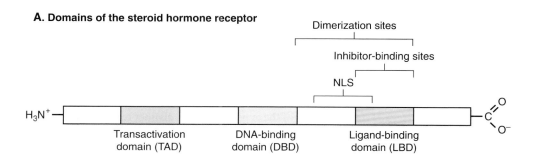

A. Domains of the steroid hormone receptor

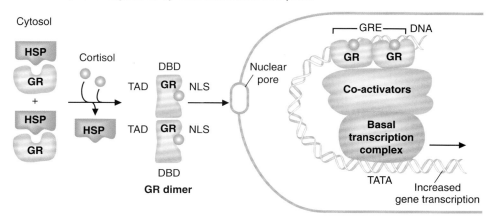

B. Transcriptional regulation by steroid hormone receptors

FIGURE 16.12   Steroid hormone receptors. **A.** Domains of the steroid hormone receptor. The transactivation domain (TAD) binds coactivators; DNA-binding domain (DBD) binds to the hormone response element in DNA; ligand-binding domain (LBD) binds hormone; NLS is the nuclear localization signal; the dimerization sites are the portions of the protein involved in forming a dimer. The inhibitor-binding site binds heat-shock proteins and masks the nuclear localization signal. **B.** Transcriptional regulation by steroid hormone receptors. *HSP*, heat-shock protein; *GRE*, glucocorticoid response element; *GR*, glucocorticoid receptor.

In a condition known as *androgen insensitivity*, patients produce androgens (the male sex steroids), but target cells fail to respond to these steroid hormones because they lack the appropriate intracellular transcription factor receptors (androgen receptors). Therefore, the transcription of the genes responsible for masculinization is not activated. A patient with this condition has an XY (male) karyotype (set of chromosomes) but has external characteristics of a female. External male genitalia do not develop, but testes are present, usually in the inguinal region or abdomen.

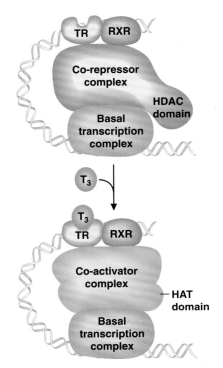

FIGURE 16.13 Activity of the thyroid hormone receptor–retinoid receptor dimer (TR-RXR) in the presence and absence of thyroid hormone (T₃). *HAT*, histone acetyltransferase; *HDAC*, histone deacetylase.

target genes. The receptors contain a hormone (ligand)-binding domain, a DNA-binding domain, and a dimerization domain that permits two receptor molecules to bind to each other, forming characteristic homodimers or heterodimers. A transactivation domain binds the coactivator proteins that interact with the basal transcription complex. The receptors also contain a nuclear localization signal domain that directs them to the nucleus at various times after they are synthesized.

Various members of the steroid hormone/thyroid hormone receptor family work in different ways. The *glucocorticoid receptor*, which binds the steroid hormone cortisol, resides principally in the cytosol bound to heat-shock proteins. As cortisol binds, the receptor dissociates from the heat-shock proteins, exposing the nuclear localization signal (see Fig. 16.12B). The receptors form homodimers that are translocated to the nucleus, where they bind to the hormone response elements (glucocorticoid response elements [GRE]) in the DNA control region of certain genes. The transactivation domains of the receptor dimers bind mediator proteins, thereby activating transcription of specific genes and inhibiting transcription of others.

Other members of the steroid hormone/thyroid hormone family of receptors are also gene-specific transactivation factors but generally form heterodimers that bind constitutively to a DNA regulatory sequence in the absence of their hormone ligand and repress gene transcription (Fig. 16.13). For example, the *thyroid hormone receptor* forms a heterodimer with the retinoid X receptor (RXR) that binds to thyroid hormone response elements and to corepressors (including one with histone deacetylase activity), thereby inhibiting expression of certain genes. When thyroid hormone binds, the receptor dimer changes conformation and the transactivation domain binds coactivators, thereby initiating transcription of the genes.

The RXR, which binds the retinoid 9-*cis*-retinoic acid, can form heterodimers with at least eight other nuclear receptors. Each heterodimer has a different DNA binding specificity. This allows the RXR to participate in the regulation of a wide variety of genes and to regulate gene expression differently, depending on the availability of other active receptors.

3. Structure of DNA-Binding Proteins

Several unique structural motifs have been characterized for specific transcription factors. Each of these proteins has a distinct recognition site (DNA-binding domain) that binds to the bases of a specific sequence of nucleotides in DNA. Four of the best-characterized structural motifs are zinc fingers, b-zip proteins (including leucine zippers), helix-turn-helix, and helix-loop-helix.

Zinc-finger motifs (commonly found in the DNA-binding domain of steroid hormone receptors) contain a bound zinc chelated at four positions with either histidine or cysteine in a sequence of approximately 20 amino acids (Fig. 16.14). The result is a relatively small, tight, autonomously folded domain. The zinc is required

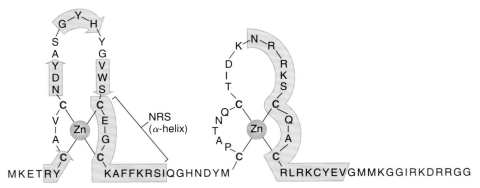

FIGURE 16.14 Zinc fingers of the estrogen receptor. In each of the two zinc fingers, one zinc ion is coordinated with four cysteine residues, shown in *red*. The region labeled *α-helix* with *NRS* forms an α-helix that contains a nucleotide recognition signal (NRS). This signal consists of a sequence of amino acid residues that bind to a specific base sequence in the major groove of DNA. Regions enclosed in *boxed arrows* participate in rigid helices.

A. Zinc fingers   **B. Leucine zipper**   **C. Helix-turn-helix**   **D. Helix-loop-helix**

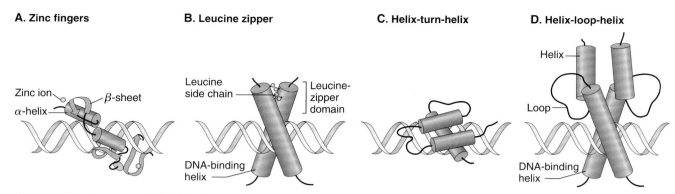

FIGURE 16.15 Interaction of DNA-binding proteins with DNA. **A.** Zinc-finger motifs consist of an α-helix and a β-sheet in which four cysteine and/or histidine residues coordinately bind a zinc ion. The nucleotide recognition signal (contained within the α-helix) of at least one zinc finger binds to a specific sequence of bases in the major groove of DNA. **B.** Leucine-zipper motifs form from two distinct polypeptide chains. Each polypeptide contains a helical region in which leucine residues are exposed on one side. These leucines form hydrophobic interactions with each other, causing dimerization. The remaining helices interact with DNA. **C.** Helix-turn-helix motifs contain three (or sometimes four) helical regions, one of which binds to DNA, whereas the others lie on top and stabilize the interaction. **D.** Helix-loop-helix motifs contain helical regions that bind to DNA like leucine zippers. However, their dimerization domains consist of two helices, each of which is connected to its DNA-binding helix by a loop.

to maintain the tertiary structure of this domain. Eukaryotic transcription factors generally have two to six zinc-finger motifs that function independently. At least one of the zinc fingers forms an α-helix containing a nucleotide recognition signal, a sequence of amino acids that fits specifically into the major groove of DNA (Fig. 16.15A).

As an example of zinc-finger transcription factors, two estrogen receptors combine to form a dimer that binds to a palindrome in the promoter region of certain genes (see Figs. 16.11 and 16.12). A palindrome is a sequence of bases that is identical on both the parallel and the antiparallel strand, and which could base pair together. For example, the sequence 5′-ATCGCGAT-3′ base-pairs to form the sequence 3′-TAGCGCTA-5′, which, when written in the 5′-to-3′ direction, is ATCGCGAT. Each estrogen receptor is approximately 73 amino acids long and contains two zinc fingers. Each zinc is chelated to two cysteines in an α-helix and two cysteines in a β-sheet region. The position of the nucleotide recognition sequence in an α-helix keeps the sequence in a relatively rigid conformation as it fits into the major groove of DNA. The zinc finger that lies closest to the carboxyl terminus is involved in dimerization with the second estrogen receptor, thus inverting the nucleotide recognition sequence to match the other half of the palindrome. The dimer-palindrome requirement enormously enhances the specificity of binding, and, consequently, only those genes with the appropriate DNA sequences are affected. A wide variety of transcription factors contain the zinc-finger motif, including the steroid hormone receptors such as the estrogen and the glucocorticoid receptors. Other transcription factors that contain zinc-finger motifs include Sp1 and polymerase III transcription factor TF$_{III}$A (part of the basal transcription complex), which has nine zinc-finger motifs.

Leucine zippers also function as dimers to regulate gene transcription (see Fig. 16.15B). The leucine-zipper motif is an α-helix of 30 to 40 amino acid residues that contains a leucine every seven amino acids, positioned so that they align on the same side of the helix. Two helices dimerize so that the leucines of one helix align with the other helix through hydrophobic interactions to form a coiled coil. The dimers can be either homodimers or heterodimers (e.g., the transcription factor AP1 is a heterodimer whose subunits are coded by the *fos* and *jun* genes). The portions of the dimer adjacent to the zipper "grip" the DNA through basic amino acid residues (arginine and lysine) that bind to the negatively charged phosphate groups. This DNA-binding portion of the molecule also contains a nucleotide recognition signal.

In the *helix-turn-helix* motif, one helix fits into the major groove of DNA, making most of the DNA-binding contacts (see Fig. 16.15C). It is joined to a segment containing two additional helices that lie across the DNA-binding helix at right angles. Thus, a very stable structure is obtained without dimerization. An example of helix-turn-helix transcriptions factors is the homeodomain proteins (proteins that play critical roles in the regulation of gene expression during development).

Helix-loop-helix transcription factors are a fourth structural type of DNA-binding protein (see Fig. 16.15D). They also function as dimers that fit around and grip DNA in a manner geometrically similar to leucine-zipper proteins. The dimerization region consists of a portion of the DNA-gripping helix and a loop to another helix. Like leucine zippers, helix-loop-helix factors can function as either hetero- or homodimers. These factors also contain regions of basic amino acids near the amino terminus and are also called *basic helix-loop-helix* (bHLH) proteins. Many of the transcription factors containing the helix-loop-helix motif are involved in cellular differentiation (such as myogenin in skeletal muscle, neurogenin in neurogenesis, and SCL/tal-1 in hematopoiesis and blood cell development).

4. Regulation of Transcription Factors

The activity of gene-specific transcription factors is regulated in several different ways. Because transcription factors must interact with a variety of coactivators to stimulate transcription, the availability of coactivators or other mediator proteins is critical for transcription factor function. If a cell upregulates or downregulates its synthesis of coactivators, the rate of transcription can also be increased or decreased. Transcription factor activity can be modulated by changes in the amount of transcription factor synthesized (see Section III.C.5), by binding a stimulatory or inhibitory ligand (e.g., steroid hormone binding to the steroid hormone receptors) and by stimulation of nuclear entry (illustrated by the glucocorticoid receptor). The ability of a transcription factor to influence the transcription of a gene is also augmented or antagonized by the presence of other transcription factors. For example, the thyroid hormone receptor is critically dependent on the concentration of the retinoid receptor to provide a dimer partner. Another example is provided by the phosphoenolpyruvate (PEP) carboxykinase gene, which is induced or repressed by a variety of hormone-activated transcription factors (see Section III.C.5). Frequently, transcription factor activity is regulated through phosphorylation.

Growth factors, cytokines, polypeptide hormones, and several other signal molecules regulate gene transcription through phosphorylation of specific transcription factors by receptor kinases. Examples include STAT proteins, which are transcription factors phosphorylated by cytokine receptors, and Smad proteins, which are transcription factors phosphorylated by serine/threonine kinase receptors such as the transforming growth factor β (TGF-β) receptor (see Chapter 11).

Nonreceptor kinases, such as protein kinase A, also regulate transcription factors through phosphorylation. Many hormones generate the second messenger cAMP, which activates protein kinase A. Activated protein kinase A enters the nucleus and phosphorylates the transcription factor CREB (*c*AMP *r*esponse *e*lement–*b*inding protein). CREB is constitutively bound to the DNA response element CRE (*c*AMP *r*esponse *e*lement) and is activated by phosphorylation. Other hormone signaling pathways, such as the mitogen-activated protein (MAP) kinase pathway, also lead to the phosphorylation of CREB (as well as many other transcription factors).

5. Multiple Regulators of Promoters

The same transcription factor inducer can activate transcription of many different genes if the genes each contain a common response element. Furthermore, a single inducer can activate sets of genes in an orderly, programmed manner (Fig. 16.16). The inducer initially activates one set of genes. One of the protein products of this

Before the advent of specifically targeted monoclonal antibody therapy, the cytokine interferon was used to treat tumors of blood cell origin. Interferons, cytokines produced by cells that have been infected with a virus, bind to the cytokine family of cell surface receptors. When an interferon binds, JAK (*janus kinase*, a receptor-associated tyrosine kinase) phosphorylates a STAT transcription factor (see Chapter 11). The phosphorylated STAT proteins are released from the JAK–receptor complex, dimerize, enter the nucleus, and bind to specific gene regulatory sequences. Different combinations of phosphorylated STAT proteins bind to different sequences and activate transcription of a different set of genes. One of the genes activated by interferon produces the oligonucleotide 2′-5′-oligo(A), which is an activator of a ribonuclease. This RNase degrades mRNA, thus inhibiting synthesis of the viral proteins required for its replication. In addition to stimulating degradation of mRNA, interferon also leads to the phosphorylation of eIF2α (a necessary factor for protein synthesis), which inactivates the eIF2α complex. This enables interferon to prevent the synthesis of viral proteins.

In addition to antiviral effects, interferons were shown to have antitumor effects. The mechanisms of the antitumor effects are not well understood but are probably likewise related to stimulation of specific gene expression by STAT proteins. Interferon-α, produced by recombinant DNA technology, had been used in the past to treat patients such as **Charles F.** who have certain types of nodular lymphomas, and patients such as **Mannie W.** who have chronic myelogenous leukemia. As targeted therapy became available to reduce the side effects of treatments, interferon therapy was reduced in scope.

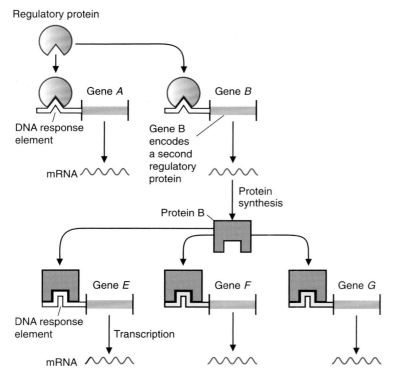

FIGURE 16.16 Activation of sets of genes by a single inducer. Each gene in a set has a common DNA regulatory element so that one regulatory protein can activate all the genes in the set. In the example shown, the first regulatory protein stimulates the transcription of genes A and B, which have a common DNA regulatory sequence in their control regions. The protein product of gene B is itself a transcriptional activator, which in turn stimulates the transcription of genes E, F, and G, which likewise contain common response elements. *mRNA*, messenger RNA.

 The enzyme PEP carboxykinase (PEPCK) is required for the liver to produce glucose from amino acids and lactate. **Ann R.**, who has an eating disorder, needs to maintain a certain blood glucose level to keep her brain functioning normally. When her blood glucose levels drop, cortisol (a glucocorticoid) and glucagon (a polypeptide hormone) are released. In the liver, glucagon increases intracellular cAMP levels, resulting in activation of protein kinase A and subsequent phosphorylation of CREB. Phosphorylated CREB binds to its response element in DNA, as does the cortisol receptor. Both transcription factors enhance transcription of the *PEPCK* gene (see Fig. 16.17). Insulin, which is released when blood glucose levels rise after a meal, can inhibit expression of this gene, in part by leading to the dephosphorylation of CREB.

set of genes can then act as a specific transcription factor for another set of genes. If this process is repeated, the net result is that one inducer can set off a series of events that results in the activation of many different sets of genes.

An example of a transcriptional cascade of gene activation is observed during adipocyte (fat cell) differentiation. Fibroblast-like cells can be induced to form adipocytes by the addition of dexamethasone (a steroid hormone), cAMP-elevating agents, and insulin to the cells. These factors induce the transient expression of two similar transcription factors named C/EPB-β and C/EPB-δ. The names stand for *CCAAT enhancer–binding protein*, and β and δ are two forms of these factors that recognize CCAAT sequences in DNA. The C/EPB transcription factors then induce the synthesis of yet another transcription factor, named the *peroxisome proliferator-activated receptor γ* (PPAR-γ), which forms heterodimers with RXR to regulate the expression of yet another transcription factor, C/EPB-α. The combination of PPAR-γ and C/EPB-α then leads to the expression of adipocyte-specific genes.

An individual gene contains many different response elements and enhancers, and genes that encode different protein products contain different combinations of response elements and enhancers. Thus, each gene does not have a single unique protein that regulates its transcription. Rather, as different proteins are stimulated to bind to their specific response elements and enhancers in a given gene, they act cooperatively to regulate expression of that gene (Fig. 16.17). Overall, a relatively small number of response elements and enhancers and a relatively small number of regulatory proteins generate a wide variety of responses from different genes.

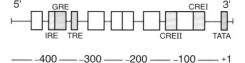

FIGURE 16.17 A simplified view of the regulatory region of the *PEPCK* gene. *Boxes* represent various response elements in the 5′-flanking region of the gene. Not all elements are labeled. Regulatory proteins bind to these DNA elements and stimulate or inhibit the transcription of the gene. This gene encodes the enzyme phosphoenolpyruvate carboxykinase (PEPCK), which catalyzes a reaction of gluconeogenesis (the pathway for production of glucose) in the liver. Synthesis of the enzyme is stimulated by glucagon (by a cyclic adenosine monophosphate [cAMP]-mediated process), by glucocorticoids, and by thyroid hormone. Synthesis of PEPCK is inhibited by insulin. *CRE*, cAMP response element; *TRE*, thyroid hormone response element; *GRE*, glucocorticoid response element; *IRE*, insulin response element.

D. Posttranscriptional Processing of RNA

After the gene is transcribed (i.e., posttranscription), regulation can occur during processing of the RNA transcript (hnRNA) into the mature mRNA. The use of alternative splice sites or sites for addition of the poly(A) tail (polyadenylation sites) can result in the production of different mRNAs from a single hnRNA and, consequently, in the production of different proteins from a single gene.

1. Alternative Splicing and Polyadenylation Sites

Processing of the primary transcript involves the addition of a cap to the 5'-end, removal of introns, and polyadenylation (the addition of a poly(A) tail to the 3'-end) to produce the mature mRNA (see Chapter 14). In certain instances, the use of alternative splicing and polyadenylation sites causes different proteins to be produced from the same gene. For example, genes that code for antibodies are regulated by alterations in the splicing and polyadenylation sites, in addition to undergoing gene rearrangement (Fig. 16.18). At an early stage of maturation, pre–B-lymphocytes produce immunoglobulin M (IgM) antibodies that are bound to the cell membrane. Later, a shorter protein (immunoglobulin D [IgD]) is produced that no longer binds to the cell membrane but is secreted from the cell.

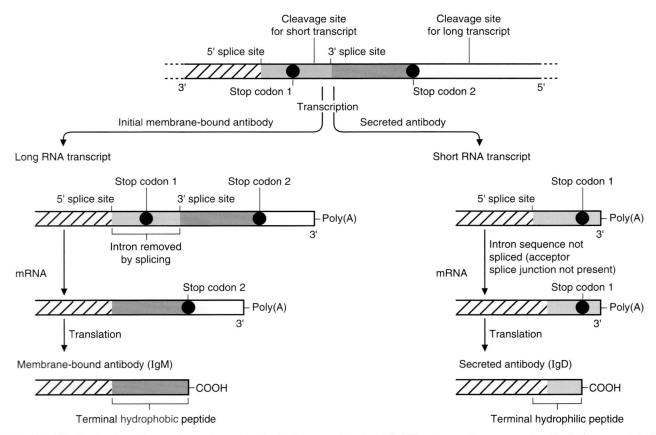

FIGURE 16.18 Production of a membrane-bound antibody (immunoglobulin M [IgM]) and a smaller secreted antibody (immunoglobulin D [IgD]) from the same gene. Initially, the lymphocytes produce a long transcript that is cleaved and polyadenylated after the second stop codon. The intron that contains the first stop codon is removed by splicing between the 5'- and 3'-splice sites. Therefore, translation ends at the second stop codon, and the protein contains a hydrophobic exon at its C-terminal end that becomes embedded in the cell membrane. After antigen stimulation, the cells produce a shorter transcript by using a different cleavage and polyadenylation site. This transcript lacks the 3'-splice site for the intron, so the intron is not removed. In this case, translation ends at the first stop codon. The IgD antibody does not contain the hydrophobic region at its C terminus, so it is secreted from the cell. *mRNA*, messenger RNA.

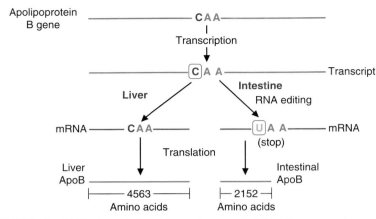

FIGURE 16.19 RNA editing. In liver, the apolipoprotein B (*ApoB*) gene produces a protein that contains 4,563 amino acids. In intestinal cells, the same gene produces a protein that contains only 2,152 amino acids. Conversion of a C to a U (through deamination) in the RNA transcript generates a stop codon in the intestinal messenger RNA (mRNA). Thus, the protein produced in the intestine (named apoB-48) is only 48% of the length of the protein produced in the liver (named apoB-100).

2. RNA Editing

In some instances, RNA is "edited" after transcription. Although the sequence of the gene and the primary transcript (hnRNA) are the same, bases are altered or nucleotides are added or deleted after the transcript is synthesized, so the mature mRNA differs in different tissues (Fig. 16.19). This leads to the synthesis of proteins with different activities in those tissues.

E. Regulation at the Level of Translation and the Stability of mRNA

Although the regulation of expression of most genes occurs at the level of transcription initiation, some genes are regulated at the level of initiation of translation, whereas others are regulated by altering the stability of the mRNA transcript.

1. Initiation of Translation

In eukaryotes, regulation of gene expression at the level of translation usually involves the initiation of protein synthesis by eukaryotic initiation factors (eIFs), which are regulated through mechanisms that involve phosphorylation (see Chapter 15, Section IV). For example, heme regulates translation of globin mRNA in reticulocytes by controlling the phosphorylation of eIF2α (Fig. 16.20). In reticulocytes (red blood cell precursors), globin is produced when heme levels in the cell are high but not when they are low. Because reticulocytes lack nuclei, globin synthesis must be regulated at the level of translation rather than at transcription. Heme acts by preventing phosphorylation of eIF2α by a specific kinase (heme-regulated inhibitor kinase) that is inactive when heme is bound. Thus, when heme levels are high, eIF2α is not phosphorylated and is active, resulting in globin synthesis. Similarly, in other cells, conditions such as starvation, heat shock, or viral infections may result in activation of a specific kinase that phosphorylates eIF2α to an inactive form. Another example is provided by insulin, which stimulates general protein synthesis by inducing the phosphorylation of 4E-BP, a binding protein for eIF4E. When 4E-BP, in its nonphosphorylated state, binds eIF4E, the initiating protein is sequestered from participating in protein synthesis. When 4E-BP is phosphorylated, as in response to insulin binding to its receptor on the cell surface, the 4E-BP dissociates from eIF4E, leaving eIF4E in the active form, and protein synthesis is initiated.

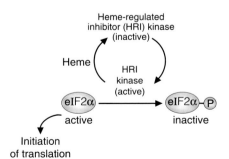

FIGURE 16.20 Heme prevents inactivation of eIF2α. When eIF2α is phosphorylated by heme-regulated inhibitor kinase, it is inactive and protein synthesis cannot be initiated. Heme inactivates the heme-regulated inhibitor kinase, thereby preventing phosphorylation of eIF2α and activating translation of the globin messenger RNA (mRNA). *IF*, initiation factor.

Ferritin synthesis

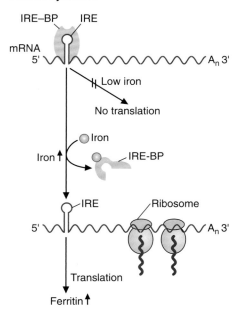

FIGURE 16.21 Translational regulation of ferritin synthesis. The messenger RNA (mRNA) for ferritin has an iron response element (IRE). When the iron response element–binding protein (IRE-BP) does not contain bound iron, it binds to IRE, preventing translation. When IRE-BP binds iron, it dissociates and the mRNA is translated.

A different mechanism for regulation of translation is illustrated by iron regulation of ferritin synthesis (Fig. 16.21). Ferritin, the protein involved in the storage of iron within cells, is synthesized when iron levels increase. The mRNA for ferritin has an iron response element (IRE), consisting of a hairpin loop near its 5′-end, which can bind a regulatory protein called the *iron response element–binding protein* (IRE-BP). When IRE-BP does not contain bound iron, it binds to the IRE and prevents initiation of translation. When iron levels increase and IRE-BP binds iron, it changes to a conformation that can no longer bind to the IRE on the ferritin mRNA. Therefore, the mRNA is translated and ferritin is produced.

2. microRNAs

microRNAs (miRNAs) are small RNA molecules that regulate protein expression at a posttranscriptional level. An miRNA can either induce the degradation of a target mRNA or block translation of the target mRNA. In either event, the end result is reduced expression of the target mRNA.

miRNAs were first discovered in nematodes and have since been shown to be present in plant and animal cells. There are believed to be approximately 1,000 miRNA genes in the human genome, some of which are located within the introns of the genes they regulate. Other miRNA genes are organized into operons, such that certain miRNA families are produced at the same time. It is also evident that one miRNA can regulate multiple mRNA targets and that a particular mRNA may be regulated by more than one miRNA.

The biogenesis of miRNA is shown in Figure 16.22. miRNA is transcribed by RNA polymerase II and is capped and polyadenylated in the same manner as mRNA. The initial RNA product is designated the primary miRNA (pri-miRNA). The pri-miRNA is modified in the nucleus by an RNA-specific endonuclease named *Drosha*, in concert with a double-stranded RNA-binding protein, *DGCR8/Pasha*. The action of Drosha is to create a stem-loop RNA structure of about 70 to 80 nucleotides in length, which is the precursor miRNA (pre-miRNA). The pre-miRNA is exported form the nucleus to the cytoplasm (via the protein exportin 5), where it interacts with another RNA endonuclease named *Dicer* and Dicer's binding partner *t*ransactivation *r*esponse RNA-*b*inding *p*rotein (TRBP). Dicer cleaves the pre-miRNA to mature miRNA (a double-stranded RNA with a two-nucleotide overhang at the ends). One of the strands of the miRNA (known as the *guide strand*) is incorporated into the

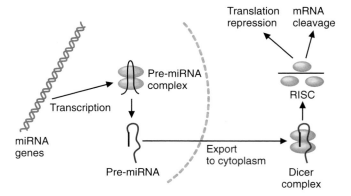

FIGURE 16.22 MicroRNA (miRNA) synthesis and action. *miRNA* genes are transcribed in the nucleus by RNA polymerase II, generating the primary miRNA, processed to a precursor miRNA (pre-miRNA), and then exported to the cytoplasm. In the cytoplasm, the pre-miRNA is further processed by a ribonuclease (Dicer), and the resulting double-stranded miRNA is strand-selected, with the guide strand (designated in *black*) entering the RNA-induced silencing complex (RISC). The guide strand of RISC targets the complex to the 3′-untranslated region of the target messenger RNA (mRNA), leading to either degradation of the mRNA or an inhibition of translation.

RNA-induced silencing complex (RISC), while the other RNA strand (the passenger strand) is degraded. The major protein in RISC is known as *argonaute*. It is the RISC that will block translation of the target mRNA.

The guide strand leads the RISC to the target mRNA, as the guide strand forms base pairs within a section of the 3′-untranslated region of the mRNA. If there is a high homology in base pairing, then argonaute, a ribonuclease, will degrade the mRNA. However, if the homology between the guide strand and the target mRNA is poor (owing to mismatches), then translation of the mRNA will be blocked.

The net result of miRNA expression is the loss of target mRNA translation. As miRNAs have multiple targets, and these targets will vary from tissue to tissue, an alteration in miRNA expression will have profound effects on gene expression within cells. As will be discussed in Chapter 18, tumors can result from the loss, or overexpression, of miRNA genes.

F. Transport and Stability of mRNA

Stability of an mRNA also plays a role in regulating gene expression because mRNAs with long half-lives can generate more protein than can those with shorter half-lives. The mRNA of eukaryotes is relatively stable (with half-lives measured in hours to days), although it can be degraded by nucleases in the nucleus or cytoplasm before it is translated. To prevent degradation during transport from the nucleus to the cytoplasm, mRNA is bound to proteins that help to prevent its degradation. Sequences at the 3′-end of the mRNA appear to be involved in determining its half-life and binding proteins that prevent degradation. One of these is the poly(A) tail, which protects the mRNA from attack by nucleases. As mRNA ages, its poly(A) tail becomes shorter.

An example of the role of mRNA degradation in control of translation is provided by the transferrin receptor mRNA (Fig. 16.23). The transferrin receptor is a protein located in cell membranes that permits cells to take up transferrin, the protein that transports iron in the blood. The rate of synthesis of the transferrin receptor increases when intracellular iron levels are low, enabling cells to take up more iron. Synthesis of the transferrin receptor, like that of the ferritin receptor, is regulated by the binding of the IRE-BP to the IREs. However, in the case of the transferrin receptor mRNA, the IREs are hairpin loops located at the 3′-end of the mRNA and not at the 5′-end where translation is initiated. When the IRE-BP does not contain bound iron, it has a high affinity for the IRE hairpin loops. Consequently, IRE-BP prevents degradation of the mRNA when iron levels are low, thus permitting synthesis of more transferrin receptor so that the cell can take up more iron. Conversely, when iron levels are elevated, IRE-BP binds iron and has a low affinity for the IRE hairpin loops of the mRNA. Without bound IRE-BP at its 3′-end, the mRNA is rapidly degraded and the transferrin receptor is not synthesized.

CLINICAL COMMENTS

Charles F. Follicular lymphomas are one of the most common subsets of non-Hodgkin lymphoma (~30% of cases). Patients with a more aggressive course, as seen in **Charles F.**, die within 3 to 5 years after diagnosis if left untreated. In patients treated with multidrug chemotherapy (in this case, R-CHOP), a positive response rate of 96% has been reported, with a 5-year overall survival of approximately 80%.

Mannie W. Mannie W. has chronic myelogenous leukemia (CML), a hematologic disorder in which the proliferating leukemic cells are believed to originate from a single line of primitive myeloid cells. It is classified as one of the myeloproliferative disorders, and CML is distinguished by the presence of a specific cytogenetic abnormality of the dividing marrow cells known as the

 Follicular lymphoma is one type of non-Hodgkin lymphoma. The most frequent form of non-Hodgkin lymphoma is diffuse large B-cell lymphoma. A recent study has shown that miRNA expression is different between these two different types of tumors and is different from normal B-cells. miRNA "signatures" are being developed for different tumor types, with the ultimate goal being individualized therapy based on the miRNA expression profile in a particular tumor. For example, in follicular lymphoma (which is the disorder displayed by **Charles F.**), the majority of misexpressed miRNAs are overexpressed, whereas in diffuse large B-cell lymphoma, these genes exhibit reduced expression. Therapeutic treatments are being developed to downregulate expression of the altered miRNAs in follicular lymphoma, which should alter overall gene expression in the tumor cells and perhaps halt their runaway proliferation. Such approaches show promise as molecular medicine becomes an important tool in the physician's arsenal for treating disease.

Transferrin receptor synthesis

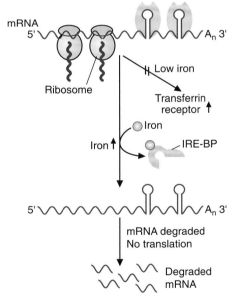

FIGURE 16.23 Regulation of degradation of the messenger RNA (mRNA) for the transferrin receptor (TfR). Degradation of the TfR mRNA is prevented by binding of the iron response element–binding protein (IRE-BP) to IREs, which are hairpin loops located at the 3′-end of the transferrin receptor mRNA. When iron levels are high, IRE-BP binds iron and is not bound to the TfR mRNA. The TfR mRNA is rapidly degraded, preventing synthesis of the transferrin receptor.

Omnipotent stem cells in the bone marrow normally differentiate and mature in a highly selective and regulated manner, becoming red blood cells, white blood cells, or platelets. Cytokines stimulate differentiation of the stem cells into the lymphoid and myeloid lineages. The lymphoid lineage gives rise to B- and T-lymphocytes, which are white blood cells that work together to generate antibodies for the immune response. The myeloid lineage gives rise to three types of progenitor cells: erythroid, granulocytic–monocytic, and megakaryocytic. The erythroid progenitor cells differentiate into red blood cells (erythrocytes), and the other myeloid progenitors give rise to nonlymphoid white blood cells and platelets. Various medical problems can affect this process. In **Mannie W.**, who has CML, a single line of primitive myeloid cells undergo the event which leads to the Philadelphia chromosome being generated. This produces leukemic cells that proliferate abnormally, causing a large increase in the number of white blood cells in the circulation. The Philadelphia chromosome is a somatic translocation not found in the germ line. In **Lisa N.**, who has a deficiency of red blood cells caused by her β^+-thalassemia (see Chapter 15), differentiation of precursor cells into mature red blood cells is stimulated to compensate for the anemia.

Ann R. has a hypochromic anemia, which means that her red blood cells are pale because they contain low levels of hemoglobin. Because of her iron deficiency, her reticulocytes do not have sufficient iron to produce heme, the required prosthetic group of hemoglobin. Consequently, eIF2α is phosphorylated in her reticulocytes and cannot activate initiation of globin translation.

Philadelphia chromosome, found in >90% of cases. In most instances, the cause of CML is unknown, but the disease occurs with an incidence of around 1.5 per 100,000 population in Western societies.

Ann R. Ann R.'s iron stores are depleted. Normally, about 16% to 18% of total body iron is contained in ferritin, which contains a spherical protein (apoferritin) that is capable of storing as many as 4,000 atoms of iron in its center. When an iron deficiency exists, serum and tissue ferritin levels fall. Conversely, the levels of transferrin (the blood protein that transports iron) and the levels of the transferrin receptor (the cell surface receptor for transferrin) increase.

BIOCHEMICAL COMMENTS

Regulation of Transcription by Iron. A cell's ability to acquire and store iron is a carefully controlled process. Iron obtained from the diet is absorbed in the intestine and released into the circulation, where it is bound by transferrin, the iron transport protein in plasma. When a cell requires iron, the plasma iron–transferrin complex binds to the transferrin receptor in the cell membrane and is internalized into the cell. Once the iron is freed from transferrin, it then binds to ferritin, which is the cellular storage protein for iron. Ferritin has the capacity to store up to 4,000 molecules of iron per ferritin molecule. Both transcriptional and translational controls work to maintain intracellular levels of iron (see Figs. 16.21 and 16.23). When iron levels are low, the IRE-BP binds to specific hairpin structures on both the ferritin and transferrin receptor mRNAs. This binding event stabilizes the transferrin receptor mRNA so that it can be translated and the number of transferrin receptors in the cell membrane increased. Consequently, cells will take up more iron, even when plasma transferrin/iron levels are low. The binding of IRE-BP to the ferritin mRNA, however, blocks translation of the mRNA. With low levels of intracellular iron, there is little iron to store and less need for intracellular ferritin. Thus, the IRE-BP can stabilize one mRNA and block translation from a different mRNA.

What happens when iron levels rise? Iron will bind to the IRE-BP, thereby decreasing its affinity for mRNA. When the IRE-BP dissociates from the transferrin receptor mRNA, the mRNA becomes destabilized and is degraded, leading to less receptor being synthesized. Conversely, dissociation of the IRE-BP from the ferritin mRNA allows that mRNA to be translated, thereby increasing intracellular levels of ferritin and increasing the capacity of the cell for iron storage.

Why does an anemia result from iron deficiency? When an individual is deficient in iron, the reticulocytes do not have sufficient iron to produce heme, the required prosthetic group of hemoglobin. When heme levels are low, eIF2α (see Fig. 16.20) is phosphorylated and becomes inactive. Thus, globin mRNA cannot be translated because of the lack of heme. This results in red blood cells with inadequate levels of hemoglobin for oxygen delivery, and in an anemia.

KEY CONCEPTS

- Prokaryotic gene expression is primarily regulated at the level of initiation of gene transcription. In general, there is one protein per gene.
  - Sets of genes that encode proteins with related functions are organized into operons.
  - Each operon is under the control of a single promoter.
  - Repressors bind to the promoter to inhibit RNA polymerase binding.
  - Activators facilitate RNA polymerase binding to the repressor.

- Eukaryotic gene regulation occurs at several levels.
  - At the DNA structural level, chromatin must be remodeled to allow access for RNA polymerase, which is accomplished, in part, by proteins with histone acetyltransferase activity.
  - Transcription is regulated by transcription factors that either enhance or restrict RNA polymerase access to the promoter.
  - Transcription factors can bind to promoter-proximal elements, certain response elements, or enhancer regions which are a great distance from the promoter.
  - Coactivators (mediator proteins) bind to the transactivation domains of transcription factors to enhance assembly of the basal transcription complex.
  - RNA processing (including alternative splicing), transport from the nucleus to the cytoplasm, and translation are also regulated in eukaryotes.
  - MicroRNA expression alters translation of expressed mRNAs.
- Diseases discussed in this chapter are found in Table 16.1.

TABLE 16.1   Diseases Discussed in Chapter 16

DISORDER OR CONDITION	GENETIC OR ENVIRONMENTAL	COMMENTS
Non-Hodgkin lymphoma, follicular type	Both	Treatment with multiple drugs, all targeted to inhibiting cell proliferation, but through different mechanisms. DNA synthesis is targeted, as is tubulin action (to block cell division). DNA damage is induced, and thymidine synthesis is also blocked to inhibit further DNA replication.
Chronic myelogenous leukemia (CML)	Both	More than 80% of CML arises owing to the generation of the Philadelphia chromosome, which is created by an exchange of genetic material between chromosomes 9 and 22. This translocation creates a unique fusion protein (BCR-abl), which facilitates uncontrolled proliferation of cells that express this fusion protein.
Anorexia nervosa	Both	The patient's poor diet has led to a hypochromic anemia caused by low iron levels. This leads to a reduction of expression of serum and tissue ferritin but an increase of expression of the transferrin protein and the transferrin receptor.
Angelman and Prader-Willi syndromes	Genetic	The use of base methylation, within promoter regions, to regulate gene expression. The methylation of key bases within the promoter leads to nonexpression of the gene and forms the basis for imprinting. This is an example of epigenetic modification of gene expression.
Fragile X disease	Genetic	A significant number of triplet repeat expansions within a gene may lead to dysfunction of the protein product, resulting in disease. In fragile X, impairment of cognitive function is the primary symptom, owing to expansions in the *FMR-1* gene on the X chromosome.
Androgen insensitivity	Genetic	Lack of androgen receptors, leading to default female sex characteristics. The patient produces androgens but cannot respond to them. These patients have an XY genotype but female sex characteristics.

REVIEW QUESTIONS—CHAPTER 16

1. Bacteria can coordinately express several genes simultaneously. Which one of the following explains why several different proteins can be synthesized from a typical prokaryotic mRNA?
   - A. Any of the three reading frames can be used.
   - B. There is redundancy in the choice of codon/tRNA interactions.
   - C. The gene contains several operator sequences from which to initiate translation.
   - D. Alternative splicing events are commonly found.
   - E. Many RNAs are organized in a series of consecutive translational cistrons.

2. *E. coli* will only express genes for lactose metabolism when lactose is present in the growth medium. In *E. coli*, under high-lactose, high-glucose conditions, which one of the following could lead to maximal transcription activation of the *lac* operon?
   - A. A mutation in the *lac I* gene (which encodes the repressor)
   - B. A mutation in the CRP-binding site leading to enhanced binding
   - C. A mutation in the operator sequence
   - D. A mutation leading to enhanced cAMP levels
   - E. A mutation leading to lower binding of repressor

3. Expression of the lactose operon in *E. coli* can be quite complex. A mutation in the *lac I* (repressor) gene of a "noninducible" strain of *E. coli* resulted in an inability to synthesize any of the proteins of the *lac* operon. Which one of the following provides a rational explanation?
   - A. The repressor has lost its affinity for the inducer.
   - B. The repressor has lost its affinity for the operator.
   - C. A *trans*-acting factor can no longer bind to the promoter.
   - D. The CAP protein is no longer being made.
   - E. Lactose feedback inhibition becomes constitutive.

4. Many transcription factors, which act as dimers, bind to palindromic sequences in their target DNA. Which one of the following double-stranded DNA sequences shows perfect dyad symmetry (the same sequence of bases on both strands)?
   - A. GAACTGCTAGTCGC
   - B. GGCATCGCGATGCC
   - C. TAATCGGAACCAAT
   - D. GCAGATTTTAGACG
   - E. TGACCGGTGACCGG

5. Transcription factors can be activated in several ways as well as inhibited under certain conditions. Which one of the following describes a common theme in the structure of DNA-binding proteins?
   - A. The presence of a specific helix that lies across the major or minor groove of DNA
   - B. The ability to recognize RNA molecules with the same sequence
   - C. The ability to form multiple hydrogen bonds between the protein peptide backbone and the DNA phosphodiester backbone
   - D. The presence of zinc
   - E. The ability to form dimers with disulfide linkages

6. Altered eukaryotic DNA can lead to mutations; however, the alteration in DNA does not necessarily have to be within an exon. Which one of the following best represents an epigenetic alteration in DNA which could lead to altered gene regulation?
   - A. Deamination of C to U in DNA
   - B. Deamination of A to I in DNA
   - C. Methylation of C residues in DNA
   - D. Substitution of an A for a G in DNA
   - E. A simple base deletion in the DNA

7. An altered response to hormones can occur if the receptor contains a mutation. A nuclear receptor has a mutation in its transactivation domain, such that it can no longer bind to other transcription factors. Which one of the following is most likely to occur when this receptor binds its cognate ligand?
   - A. Inability to bind to DNA
   - B. Enhanced ability to bind to DNA
   - C. Enhanced transcription of hormone-responsive genes
   - D. Enhanced dimerization of hormone receptors
   - E. Reduced transcription of hormone-responsive genes

8. A patient presents with a β-thalassemia. Such a disorder could result from a mutation located in which of the following? Choose the one best answer.

	An intron of the β-globin gene	An exon of the β-globin gene	An intron of the α-globin gene	The promoter region of the β-globin gene	The promoter region of the α-globin gene
A	No	No	Yes	No	Yes
B	Yes	Yes	No	Yes	Yes
C	No	No	Yes	No	Yes
D	Yes	Yes	No	Yes	No
E	No	No	Yes	No	No
F	Yes	Yes	No	Yes	No

9. In response to foreign organisms, humans produce a variety of antibodies that can bind to the organism. In the production of human antibodies, which one of the following can cause the production of different proteins from a single gene?
   A. Pretranscription processing of hnRNA
   B. Removal of introns from hnRNA
   C. Addition of a cap to the 5′-end of hnRNA
   D. Addition of a cap to the 3′-end of hnRNA
   E. Alternative sites for synthesizing the poly(A) tail

10. A eukaryotic cell line grows normally at 30°C, but at 42°C, its growth rate is reduced owing to iron toxicity. At the elevated temperature, the cell displays elevated free intracellular iron levels, coupled with high levels of transferrin receptor. Ferritin levels within the cell are extremely low at the elevated temperature. These results can be explained by a single-nucleotide mutation in which one of the following proteins?
    A. Transferrin
    B. Ferritin
    C. Transferrin receptor
    D. IRE-BP
    E. RNA polymerase

ANSWERS

1. **The answer is E.** Many prokaryotic genes are organized into operons, in which one polycistronic mRNA contains the translational start and stop sites for several related genes. Although each gene within the mRNA can be read from a different reading frame, the reading frame is always consistent within each gene (thus, A is incorrect). Redundancy in codon/tRNA interactions has nothing to do with multiple cistrons within an mRNA (thus, B is incorrect). Operator sequences are in DNA and initiate transcription, not translation (thus, C is incorrect). Alternative splicing occurs only in eukaryotes (which have introns), not in prokaryotes (thus, D is incorrect).

2. **The answer is D.** In order to transcribe the *lac* operon, the repressor protein (*lac I* gene product) must bind allolactose and leave the operator region, and the cAMP–CRP complex must bind to the promoter in order for RNA polymerase to bind. Of the choices offered, only raising cAMP levels can allow transcription of the operon when both lactose and glucose are high. Raising cAMP, even though glucose is present, will allow the cAMP–CRP complex to bind and recruit RNA polymerase. Answers that call for mutations in the repressor (answers A and E) will not affect binding of cAMP–CRP. Mutations in the DNA (answers B and C) do not allow CRP binding in the absence of cAMP.

3. **The answer is A.** The repressor will bind to the operator and block transcription of all genes in the operon unless prevented by the inducer allolactose. If the repressor has lost its affinity for the inducer, it cannot dissociate from the operator and the genes in the operon will not be expressed (thus, E is incorrect). If the repressor has lost its affinity for the operator (answer B), then the operon would be expressed constitutively. Because the question states that there is a mutation in the *I* (repressor) gene, answer D is incorrect, and mutations in the *I* gene do not affect *trans*-acting factors from binding to the promoter, although the only other one for the *lac* operon is the CRP.

4. **The answer is B.** The sequence, if read in the 5′-to-3′ direction, is identical to the complementary sequence read 5′-to-3′. None of the other sequences fits this pattern.

5. **The answer is A.** All DNA-binding proteins contain an α-helix that binds to the major or minor groove in DNA. These proteins do not recognize RNA molecules (thus, B is incorrect), nor do they form bonds between the peptide backbone and the DNA backbone (thus, C is incorrect; if this were correct, how could there be any specificity in protein binding to DNA?). Only zinc fingers contain zinc, and dimers are formed by hydrogen bonding—not by disulfide linkages.

6. **The answer is C.** Epigenetic events include histone acetylation and DNA methylation—alterations to the DNA which do not involve altering the base-pairing characteristics of the DNA (or causing insertions or deletions within the DNA). Deamination of C or A residues (to U or I, respectively) will lead to altered base pairing when the DNA is replicated (methylation of C does not alter the base-pairing properties of the C). Substitution of one base for another also leads to an alteration in base-pairing properties.

7. **The answer is E.** The transactivation domain of the receptor is required to recruit other positive acting factors to the promoter region of the gene in order to enhance transcription. Lack of this domain, and reduced recruitment of coactivators, would lead to reduced transcription. The receptor would still be able to bind to DNA (i.e., through a different site on the receptor, the DNA-binding domain), although its affinity for DNA is not enhanced by lack of the transactivation domain. The transactivation domain is not related to the dimerization domain of hormone receptors.

8. **The answer is B.** A β-thalassemia refers to a disorder in which the number of α-globin chains exceeds that of the β-globin genes. This can occur because of a stop codon being introduced into an exon of the β-globin

gene, or loss of a splice site in the β-globin gene (which could occur in an intron or exon). An imbalance in chain synthesis could also occur because of a mutation in the β-globin gene promoter, or in the α-globin gene promoter that enhanced α-globin synthesis relative to β-globin gene synthesis. A mutation in an intron of the α-globin gene would not lead to more α-globin protein than β-globin protein.

9. **The answer is E.** After the gene is transcribed (post-transcription), the use of alternative splice sites or sites for addition of the poly(A) tail can result in different mRNAs (and therefore different proteins) from a single hnRNA. Introns are inert (noncoding) and would have no effect. Alternative splicing would remove exons, but all introns are removed from the hnRNA. The cap (on the 5′-end) is required for translation but would not alter the reading frame of the protein.

10. **The answer is D.** Ferritin is the cellular storage protein for iron. Transferrin is the transport protein for iron in plasma. The transferrin receptor binds the iron–transferrin complex for transport of iron into the cell.

The synthesis of both the transferrin receptor and ferritin are controlled by the IRE-BP. At the low temperature, the IRE-BP binds to the 3′-end of the transferrin receptor mRNA, stabilizing the mRNA so that it can be translated to produced transferrin receptor proteins. When intracellular iron levels increase, the iron binds to IRE-BP, displacing the protein from the mRNA, which leads to degradation of the mRNA and reduced synthesis of the transferrin receptor. In a similar fashion, the IRE-BP binds to the 5′-end of the ferritin mRNA, blocking ferritin synthesis. When intracellular iron levels increase, the IRE-BP falls off the mRNA, and ferritin is synthesized to bind the intracellular iron and prevent free iron toxicity in the cell. In this cell line, the IRE-BP is mutated such that at the elevated temperature it cannot bind iron, meaning that the IRE-BP remains bound to the transferrin receptor and ferritin mRNA molecules. This leads to a lack of ferritin and to overexpression of transferrin receptor in the membrane. The cell will accumulate iron but will not have adequate ferritin for the iron to bind to, leading to elevated free iron levels in the cell.

Use of Recombinant DNA Techniques in Medicine

17

The rapid development of techniques in molecular biology is revolutionizing the practice of medicine. The potential uses of these techniques for the diagnosis and treatment of disease are vast.

Clinical Applications. Polymorphisms, inherited differences in DNA base sequences, are abundant in the human population, and many alterations in DNA sequences are associated with diseases. Tests for DNA sequence variations are more sensitive than many other techniques (such as enzyme assays) and permit recognition of diseases at earlier, and therefore potentially more treatable, stages. These tests also can identify carriers of inherited diseases so they can receive appropriate counseling. Because genetic variations are so distinctive, **DNA fingerprinting** (analysis of DNA sequence differences) can be used to determine family relationships or to help identify the perpetrators of a crime.

Techniques of molecular biology are used in the **prevention** and **treatment** of disease. For example, recombinant DNA techniques provide human insulin for the treatment of diabetes, factor VIII for the treatment of hemophilia, and vaccines for the prevention of hepatitis. Although treatment of disease by gene therapy is in the experimental phase of development, the possibilities are limited only by the human imagination and, of course, by ethical considerations. The ability to rapidly analyze the genome and **proteome** (all expressed proteins) of a cell enables different variants of a particular disease to be identified and treated appropriately.

Techniques. To recognize normal or pathologic genetic variations, DNA must be isolated from the appropriate source, and adequate amounts must be available for study. Techniques for **isolating** and **amplifying** genes and studying and **manipulating** DNA sequences involve the use of **restriction enzymes**, **cloning vectors**, **polymerase chain reaction (PCR)**, **gel electrophoresis**, **blotting onto nitrocellulose paper**, and the preparation of **labeled probes that hybridize** to the appropriate target DNA sequences. Techniques to analyze all expressed genes within a cell require **gene chip** assays, which can lead to a genetic profile of normal versus diseased cells. **Gene therapy** involves isolating normal genes and inserting them into diseased cells so that the normal genes are expressed, permitting the diseased cells to return to a normal state. Ablation of gene expression is possible using techniques based on **small interfering RNA** (siRNA). Students should have a general understanding of recombinant DNA techniques to appreciate their current use and the promise they hold for the future. Rapid sequencing of DNA and complementary DNA (cDNA; next-generation sequencing) allows for rapid determination of mutations in the genome and changes in gene expression.

Cystic fibrosis is a disease caused by an inherited deficiency in the cystic fibrosis transmembrane conductance regulator (CFTR) protein, which is a chloride channel (see Chapter 10, Fig. 10.9). In the absence of chloride secretion, thick mucus blocks the pancreatic duct, resulting in decreased secretion of digestive enzymes into the intestinal lumen. The resulting malabsorption of fat and other foodstuffs decreases growth and may lead to varying degrees of small-bowel obstruction. Liver and gallbladder secretions may be similarly affected. Eventually, atrophy of the secretory organs or ducts may occur. Thick mucus also blocks the airways, markedly diminishing air exchange and predisposing the patient to stasis of secretions, diminished immune defenses, and increased secondary infections. Defects in the CFTR chloride channel also affect sweat composition, increasing the sodium and chloride content of the sweat, thereby providing a diagnostic tool.

THE WAITING ROOM

 Edna R., a third-year medical student, has started working in the hospital blood bank two nights a week (see Chapter 15 for an introduction to Edna R. and her daughter, Beverly). Because she will be handling human blood products, she must have a series of hepatitis B vaccinations. She has reservations about having these vaccinations and inquires about the efficacy and safety of the vaccines currently in use.

 Susan F. is a 3-year-old Caucasian girl who has been diagnosed with cystic fibrosis (CF). Her growth rate has been in the 30th percentile over the last year. Since birth, she has had occasional episodes of spontaneously reversible and minor small-bowel obstruction. These episodes are superimposed on gastrointestinal symptoms that suggest a degree of dietary fat malabsorption, such as bulky, glistening, foul-smelling stools two or three times per day. She has experienced recurrent flare-ups of bacterial bronchitis/bronchiolitis in the last 10 months, each time caused by *Pseudomonas aeruginosa*. A quantitative sweat test was unequivocally positive (excessive sodium and chloride were found in her sweat on two occasions). Based on these findings, the pediatrician informed Susan's parents that Susan probably has CF. A sample of her blood was sent to a DNA testing laboratory to confirm the diagnosis and to determine specifically which one of the many potential genetic mutations known to cause CF was present in her cells.

 Carrie S., Will S.'s 19-year-old sister, is considering marriage. Her growth and development have been normal, and she is free of symptoms of sickle cell anemia. Because a younger sister, Amanda, was tested and found to have sickle trait (expressing one normal β-globin gene and one sickle β-globin gene), and because of Will's repeated sickle crises, Carrie wants to know whether she also has sickle trait (see Chapters 6 and 7 for **Will S.'s** history). A hemoglobin electrophoresis is performed that shows the composition of her hemoglobin to be 58% HbA, 39% HbS, 1% HbF, and 2% HbA$_2$, a pattern consistent with the presence of sickle cell trait. The hematologist who saw her in the clinic on her first visit is studying the genetic mutations of sickle cell trait and asks Carrie for permission to draw additional blood for more sophisticated analysis of the genetic disturbance that causes her to produce HbS. Carrie informed her fiancé that she has sickle cell trait and that she wants to delay their marriage until he is tested.

 Victoria T. was a 21-year-old woman who was the victim of a rape and murder. Her parents told police that she left her home and drove to the local convenience store. When she had not returned home an hour later, her father went to the store to look for Victoria. He found her car still parked in front of the store and called the police. They searched the area around the store and found **Victoria T.'s** body in a wooded area behind the building. She had been sexually assaulted and strangled. Medical technologists from the police laboratory collected a semen sample from vaginal fluid and took samples of dried blood from under the victim's fingernails. Witnesses identified three men who spoke to Victoria while she was at the convenience store. DNA samples were obtained from these suspects to determine whether any of them was the perpetrator of the crime.

 Isabel S.'s cough is slightly improved on a multidrug regimen for pulmonary tuberculosis, but she continues to have night sweats. She is tolerating her current HIV therapy well but complains of weakness and fatigue. The man with whom she had shared "dirty" needles to inject drugs accompanies Isabel to the clinic and requests that he be tested for the presence of HIV.

I. Recombinant DNA Techniques

Techniques for joining DNA sequences into new combinations (*recombinant DNA*) were originally developed as research tools to explore and manipulate genes and to produce the gene products (protein). Now, they are also being used to identify mutated genes associated with disease and to correct genetic defects. These techniques will soon replace many current clinical testing procedures. A basic appreciation of recombinant DNA techniques is required to understand how genetic variations among individuals are determined and how these differences can be used to diagnose disease. The first steps in determining individual variations in genes involve isolating the genes (or fragments of DNA) that contain variable sequences and obtaining adequate quantities for study. The Human Genome Project has succeeded in sequencing the 3 billion bases of the human genome and can now be used as a template to discover and understand the molecular basis of disease.

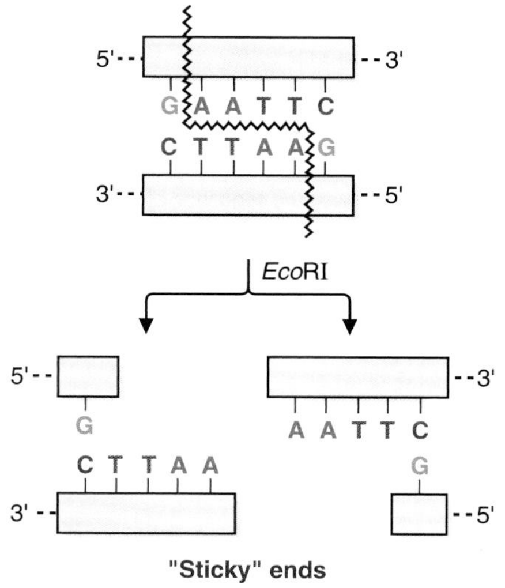

A. Strategies for Obtaining Fragments of DNA and Copies of Genes

I. Restriction Fragments

Enzymes called *restriction endonucleases* enable molecular biologists to cleave segments of DNA from the genome of various types of cells or to fragment DNA obtained from other sources. A *restriction enzyme* is an endonuclease that specifically recognizes a short sequence of DNA, usually 4 to 6 base pairs (bp) in length, and cleaves a phosphodiester bond in both DNA strands within this sequence (Fig. 17.1). A key feature of restriction enzymes is their specificity. A restriction enzyme always cleaves at the same DNA sequence and cleaves only at that particular sequence. Most of the DNA sequences recognized by restriction enzymes are palindromes, that is, both strands of DNA have the same base sequence when read in a 5'-to-3' direction. The cuts made by these enzymes are usually "sticky" (i.e., the products are single-stranded at the ends, with one strand overhanging the other, so they anneal with complementary sequences to the overhang). However, sometimes they are blunt (the products are double-stranded at the ends, with no overhangs). Hundreds of restriction enzymes with different specificities have been isolated (Table 17.1).

FIGURE 17.1 Action of restriction enzymes. Note that the DNA sequence shown is a palindrome: each strand of the DNA, when read in a 5'-to-3' direction, has the same sequence. Cleavage of this sequence by *Eco*RI produces single-stranded (or "sticky") ends or tails. Not shown is an example of an enzyme that generates blunt ends (see Table 17.1).

TABLE 17.1	Sequences Cleaved by Selected Restriction Enzymes[a]	
RESTRICTION ENZYME	**SOURCE**	**CLEAVAGE SITE**
*Alu*I (blunt ends)	*Arthrobacter luteus*	5'–AG CT–3' 3'–TC GA–5'
*Bam*HI	*Bacillus amyloliquefaciens* H	5'–G GATCC–3' 3'–CCTAG G–5'
*Eco*RI	*Escherichia coli* RY13	5'–G AATTC–3' 3'–CTTAA G–5'
*Hae*III (blunt ends)	*Haemophilus aegyptius*	5'–GG CC–3' 3'–CC GG–5'
*Hind*III	*Haemophilus influenzae* R_d	5'–A AGCTT–3' 3'–TTCGA A–5'
*Msp*I	*Moraxella* species	5'–C CGG–3' 3'–GGC C–5'
*Mst*II	*Microcoleus*	5'–CC TNAGG–3' 3'–GGANT CC–5'
*Not*I	*Nocardia otitidis*	5'–GC GGCCGC–3' 3'–CGCCGG CG–5'
*Pst*I	*Providencia stuartii* 164	5'–CTGCA G–3' 3'–G ACGTC–5'
*Sma*I (blunt ends)	*Serratia marcescens* S_b	5'–CCC GGG–3' 3'–GGG CCC–5'

[a]Restriction enzymes are named for the bacterium from which they were isolated (e.g., *Eco* is from *Escherichia coli.*). Unless otherwise indicated, they all create "sticky" overhanging ends. N stands for any base.

Q Which one of the following sequences is most likely to be a restriction enzyme recognition sequence? All of the sequences are written in standard notation, with the top strand going in the 5'-to-3' direction, left to right.

(A) GT CCT G
CA GGA C

(B) TA CGAT
AT GCTA

(C) CT GA G
GA CTC

(D) AT CCTA
TA GGAT

The answer is C. C follows the palindromic sequence CTNAG, where N can be any base. None of the other sequences is this close to a palindrome. Although most restriction enzymes recognize a "perfect" palindrome, in which the sequence of bases in each strand are the same, others may have intervening bases between the regions of identity, as in this example. Note also the specificity of the enzyme *MstII* in Table 17.1.

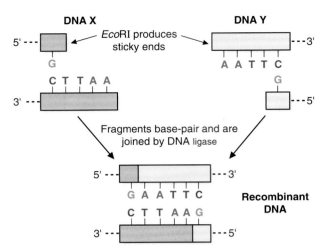

FIGURE 17.2 Production of recombinant DNA molecules with restriction enzymes and DNA ligase. The *dashes* at the 5′- and 3′-ends indicate that this sequence is part of a longer DNA molecule.

In sickle cell anemia, the point mutation that converts a glutamate residue to a valine residue (GAG to GTG) occurs in a site that is cleaved by the restriction enzyme *MstII* (recognition sequence CCTNAGG, where N can be any base) within the normal β-globin gene. The sickle cell mutation causes the β-globin gene to lose this *MstII* restriction site. Therefore, because **Will S.** is homozygous for the sickle cell gene, neither of the two alleles of his β-globin gene will be cleaved at this site.

Restriction endonucleases were discovered in bacteria in the late 1960s and 1970s. These enzymes were named for the fact that bacteria use them to "restrict" the growth of viruses (bacteriophage) that infect the bacterial cells. They cleave the phage DNA into smaller pieces so the phage cannot reproduce in the bacterial cells. However, they do not cleave the bacterial DNA, because its bases are methylated at the restriction sites by DNA methylases. Restriction enzymes also restrict uptake of DNA from the environment, and they restrict mating with nonhomologous species.

Restriction fragments of DNA can be used to identify variations in base sequence in a gene. However, they also can be used to synthesize a *recombinant DNA* (also called *chimeric DNA*), which is composed of molecules of DNA from different sources that have been recombined in vitro (outside the organism; e.g., in a test tube). The sticky ends of two unrelated DNA fragments can be joined to each other if they have sticky ends that are complementary. Complementary ends are obtained by cleaving the unrelated DNAs with the same restriction enzyme (Fig. 17.2). After the sticky ends of the fragments base-pair with each other, the fragments can be attached covalently by the action of DNA ligase.

2. DNA Produced by Reverse Transcriptase

If messenger RNA (mRNA) transcribed from a gene is isolated, this mRNA can be used as a template by the enzyme reverse transcriptase (see Chapter 12, "Biochemical Comments"), which produces a DNA copy (cDNA) of the RNA. In contrast to DNA fragments cleaved from the genome by restriction enzymes, DNA produced by reverse transcriptase does not contain introns because mRNA, which has no introns, is used as a template. cDNA also lacks the regulatory regions of a gene because those sequences (promoter, promoter-proximal elements, and enhancers) are not transcribed into mRNA.

3. Chemical Synthesis of DNA

Automated machines can synthesize oligonucleotides (short molecules of single-stranded DNA) up to 150 nucleotides in length. These machines can be programmed to produce oligonucleotides with a specified base sequence. Although entire genes cannot yet be synthesized in one piece, appropriate overlapping pieces of genes can be made and then ligated together to produce a fully synthetic gene. In addition, oligonucleotides can be prepared that will base-pair with segments of genes. These oligonucleotides can be used in the process of identifying, isolating, and amplifying genes.

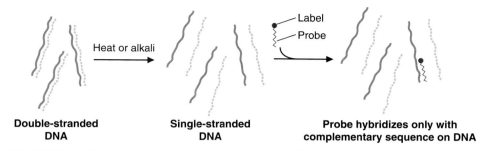

FIGURE 17.3   Use of probes to identify DNA sequences. The probe can be either DNA or RNA.

B. Techniques for Identifying DNA Sequences

1. Probes

A probe is a single-strand polynucleotide of DNA or RNA that is used to identify a complementary sequence on a larger single-stranded DNA or RNA molecule (Fig. 17.3). Formation of base pairs with a complementary strand is called *annealing* or *hybridization*. Probes can be composed of cDNA (produced from mRNA by reverse transcriptase), fragments of genomic DNA (cleaved by restriction enzymes from the genome), chemically synthesized oligonucleotides, or, occasionally, RNA.

The conditions of hybridization can be manipulated to provide different degrees of stringency. *Stringency* refers to how exact a match the probe must have to the DNA to which it is hybridizing in order for significant hybridization to occur. Low-stringency conditions allow several mismatches between the two nucleic acid strands to be tolerated (nonstandard base pairs); high stringency requires an exact match of the complementary sequences before hybridization can take place. Stringency can be manipulated by raising or lowering the temperature (increased temperature increases stringency) and raising or lowering the salt concentration in the hybridization reaction (high salt concentration reduces the stringency because it negates the electrostatic repulsion between the phosphates in the DNA backbone of two mismatched DNA strands). Thus, a high-stringency hybridization (looking for an exact match) will be performed at high temperature and low salt concentrations.

To identify the target sequence, the probe must carry a *label* (see Fig. 17.3). If the probe has a radioactive label such as ^{32}P, it can be detected by autoradiography. An autoradiogram is produced by covering the material containing the probe with a sheet of X-ray film. Electrons (β-particles) emitted by disintegration of the radioactive atoms expose the film in the region directly over the probe. Several techniques can be used to introduce labels into these probes. Not all probes are radioactive. Some are chemical adducts (compounds that bind covalently to DNA) that can be identified by, for example, fluorescence microscopy.

2. Gel Electrophoresis

Gel electrophoresis is a technique that uses an electrical field to separate molecules on the basis of size. Because DNA contains negatively charged phosphate groups, it will migrate in an electrical field toward the positive electrode (Fig. 17.4). Shorter molecules migrate more rapidly through the pores of a gel than do longer molecules, so separation is based on length. Gels composed of polyacrylamide, which can separate DNA molecules that differ in length by only one nucleotide, are used to determine the base sequence of DNA. Agarose gels are used to separate longer DNA fragments that have larger size differences.

The bands of DNA in the gel can be visualized by various techniques. Staining with dyes such as ethidium bromide allows direct visualization of DNA bands under ultraviolet light. Specific sequences are generally detected by means of a labeled probe.

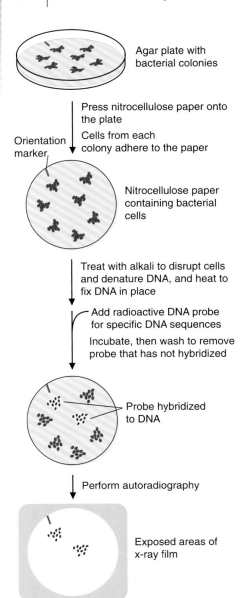

FIGURE 17.5 Identification of bacterial colonies containing specific DNA sequences. The autoradiogram can be used to identify bacterial colonies on the original agar plate that contain the desired DNA sequence. Note that an orientation marker is placed on the nitrocellulose and the agar plate so the results of the autoradiogram can be properly aligned with the original plate of bacteria.

Western blots are one of the tests for the AIDS virus. Antibodies to HIV proteins in the blood are detected by using the blood to probe a nitrocellulose filter that has HIV proteins on it. A positive result would show that the blood contains antibodies to HIV proteins, indicating that the individual has been infected with HIV. Tests performed on **Isabel S.'s** friend showed that he was HIV-positive.

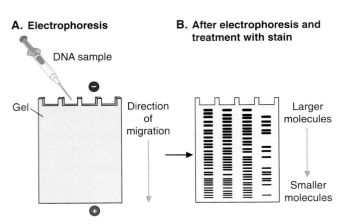

FIGURE 17.4 Gel electrophoresis of DNA. **A.** DNA samples are placed into depressions ("wells") at one end of a gel, and an electrical field is applied. The DNA migrates toward the positive electrode at a rate that depends on the size of the DNA molecules. As the gel acts as a sieve, shorter molecules migrate more rapidly than longer molecules. **B.** The gel is removed from the apparatus. The bands are not visible until techniques are performed to visualize them (see Fig. 17.6).

3. Detection of Specific DNA Sequences

To detect specific sequences, DNA is usually transferred to a solid support, such as a sheet of nitrocellulose paper. For example, if bacteria are growing on an agar plate, cells from each colony will adhere to a nitrocellulose sheet pressed against the agar, and an exact replica of the bacterial colonies can be transferred to the nitrocellulose paper (Fig. 17.5). A similar technique is used to transfer bands of DNA from electrophoretic gels to nitrocellulose sheets. After bacterial colonies or bands of DNA are transferred to nitrocellulose paper, the paper is treated with an alkaline solution and then heated. Alkaline solutions denature DNA (i.e., separate the two strands of each double helix), and the heating fixes the DNA on the filter paper such that it will not move from its position during the rest of the blotting procedure. The single-stranded DNA is then hybridized with a probe, and the regions on the nitrocellulose blot containing DNA that base-pairs with the probe are identified.

E. M. Southern developed the technique, which bears his name, for identifying DNA sequences on gels. *Southern blots* are produced when DNA on a nitrocellulose blot of an electrophoretic gel is hybridized with a DNA probe. Molecular biologists decided to continue with this geographic theme as they named two additional techniques. *Northern blots* are produced when RNA on a nitrocellulose blot is hybridized with a DNA probe. A slightly different but related technique, known as a *Western blot*, involves separating proteins by gel electrophoresis and probing with labeled antibodies for specific proteins (Fig. 17.6).

4. DNA Sequencing

The most common procedure for determining the sequence of nucleotides in a DNA strand was developed by Frederick Sanger and involves the use of dideoxynucleotides. Dideoxynucleotides (see Chapter 13) lack a 3'-hydroxyl group (in addition to lacking the 2'-hydroxyl group that is normally absent from DNA deoxynucleotides). Thus, once they are incorporated into a replicating DNA chain, the next nucleotide cannot add, and polymerization is terminated. In this procedure, only one of the four dideoxynucleotides (dideoxyadenosine triphosphate [ddATP], dideoxythymidine triphosphate [ddTTP], dideoxyguanosine triphosphate [ddGTP], or dideoxycytidine triphosphate [ddCTP]) is added to a tube containing all four normal deoxynucleotides, DNA polymerase, a primer, and the template strand for the DNA that is being sequenced (Fig. 17.7). As DNA polymerase catalyzes the sequential addition of complementary bases to the 3'-end, the dideoxynucleotide competes with its corresponding normal nucleotide for insertion. Whenever the dideoxynucleotide is incorporated,

A. Terminates with ddATP

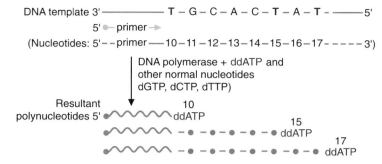

B. If synthesis is terminated with:

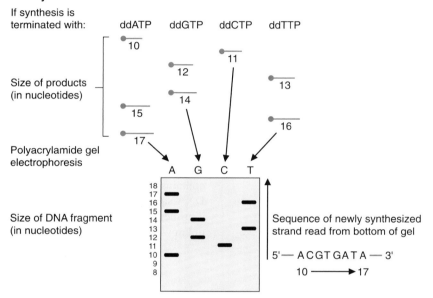

FIGURE 17.6 Southern, Northern, and Western blots. For Southern blots, DNA molecules are separated by electrophoresis, denatured, transferred to nitrocellulose paper (by "blotting"), and hybridized with a DNA probe. For Northern blots, RNA is electrophoresed and treated similarly except that alkali is not used (first, because alkali hydrolyzes RNA, and second, because RNA is already single-stranded). For Western blots, proteins are electrophoresed, transferred to nitrocellulose, and probed with a specific antibody.

FIGURE 17.7 The Sanger method of DNA sequencing. **A.** A reaction mixtures contain one of the dideoxynucleotides, such as ddATP, and some of the normal nucleotide, dATP, which compete for incorporation into the growing polynucleotide chain. When a T is encountered on the template strand (position 10), some of the molecules will incorporate a ddATP and the chain will be terminated. Those that incorporate a normal dATP will continue growing until position 15 is reached, where they will incorporate either a ddATP or the normal dATP. Only those that incorporate a dATP will continue growing to position 17. Thus, strands of different length from the 5'-end are produced, corresponding to the position of a T in the template strand. **B.** DNA sequencing by the dideoxynucleotide method. Four tubes are used. Each one contains DNA polymerase, a DNA template hybridized to a primer, plus dATP, dGTP, dCTP, and dTTP. Either the primer or the nucleotides must have a radioactive label, so bands can be visualized on the gel by autoradiography. Only one of the four dideoxyribonucleotides (ddNTPs) is added to each tube. Termination of synthesis occurs where the ddNTP is incorporated into the growing chain. The template is complementary to the sequence of the newly synthesized strand. Automated DNA sequencers use fluorescent-labeled ddNTPs and a column to separate the oligonucleotides by size. As samples leave the column, their fluorescence is analyzed to determine which base has terminated synthesis of that fragment. *dATP*, deoxyadenosine triphosphate; *dTTP*, deoxythymidine triphosphate; *dGTP*, deoxyguanosine triphosphate; *dCTP*, deoxycytidine triphosphate; *ddATP*, dideoxyadenosine triphosphate; *ddTTP*, dideoxythymidine triphosphate; *ddGTP*, dideoxyguanosine triphosphate; *ddCTP*, dideoxycytidine triphosphate.

One of the drugs used to treat HIV is didanosine, a nucleotide reverse transcriptase inhibitor (NRTI). This drug is a purine nucleoside composed of the base hypoxanthine linked to dideoxyribose. In cells, didanosine is phosphorylated to form a nucleotide that adds to growing DNA strands. Because dideoxynucleotides lack both 2'- and 3'-hydroxyl groups, DNA synthesis is terminated. Reverse transcriptase has a higher affinity for the dideoxynucleotides than does the cellular DNA polymerase, so the use of this drug will affect reverse transcriptase to a greater extent than the cellular enzyme.

further polymerization of the strand cannot occur, and synthesis is terminated. Some of the chains will terminate at each of the locations in the template strand that is complementary to the dideoxynucleotide. Consider, for example, a growing polynucleotide strand in which adenine (A) should add at positions 10, 15, and 17. Competition between ddATP and dATP for each position results in some chains terminating at position 10, some at 15, and some at 17. Thus, DNA strands of varying lengths are produced from a template. The shortest strands are closest to the 5'-end of the growing DNA strand because the strand is synthesized in a 5'-to-3' direction.

Four separate reactions are performed, each with only one of the dideoxynucleotides present (ddATP, ddTTP, ddGTP, ddCTP), plus a complete mixture of normal nucleotides (see Fig. 17.7B). In each tube, some strands are terminated whenever the complementary base for that dideoxynucleotide is encountered. If these strands are subjected to gel electrophoresis, the sequence 5' → 3' of the DNA strand complementary to the template can be determined by "reading" from the bottom to the top of the gel; that is, by noting the lanes (A, G, C, or T) in which bands appear, starting at the bottom of the gel and moving sequentially toward the top.

5. Next-Generation DNA Sequencing

The original limitation in the traditional Sanger method of sequencing DNA was speed; it took an extended period of time to generate significant amounts of sequence data. Improvements in the speed of sequencing have led to next-generation sequencing, which allow for sequencing of an entire genome in less than 1 day.

This technique involves mechanical fractionation of the genome, followed by the addition of known sequences of DNA to the ends of the unknown DNA (Fig. 17.8). The fractionated DNA, with known ends, is added to a glass slide which contains bound DNA complementary to the added ends of the unknown DNA. The DNA samples are amplified (see Section I.C.3 on PCR) and then sequenced using a primer that is complementary to the known sequence of DNA on the ends of the unknown DNA. Many thousands of pieces of DNA are sequenced simultaneously

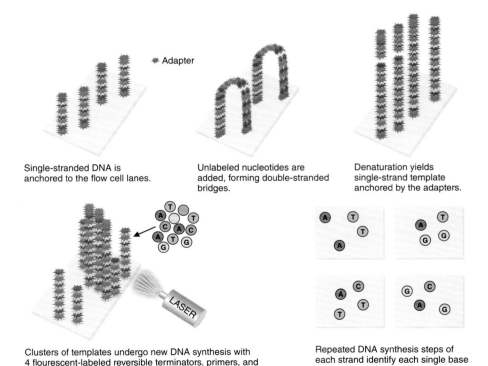

Single-stranded DNA is anchored to the flow cell lanes.

Unlabeled nucleotides are added, forming double-stranded bridges.

Denaturation yields single-strand template anchored by the adapters.

Clusters of templates undergo new DNA synthesis with 4 flourescent-labeled reversible terminators, primers, and DNA polymerase to identify the first base of each cluster after laser excitation and imaging.

Repeated DNA synthesis steps of each strand identify each single base in order, one at a time.

FIGURE 17.8 A simplified depiction of next-generation sequencing. See text for details. (From Ross JS, Cronin M. Whole cancer genome sequencing by next-generation methods. *Am J Clin Path.* 2011;136[4]:527–539.)

on the slide. In this case, one sequences the unknown fragments one nucleotide at a time. Each deoxynucleotide in the reaction mixture is linked to a different fluorophore as well as to a chemical blocking agent at the 3′-hydroxyl group on the ribose. After the first nucleotide has been added to the primer, a computer analyzes the fluorescence of all the DNA sequences on the slide and stores the data. Chemicals are then added to remove both the blocking groups from the 3′-hydroxyl groups and the fluorophores from the nucleotides already incorporated into the DNA. DNA synthesis is then initiated to add the next base to the primer, and the process is repeated. This continues for up to 100 bases, such that 100-base-long sequences are stored in the computer for each piece of unknown DNA on the slide. The computer then analyzes these sequences, looks for overlaps in sequence, and can generate an entire sequence of the DNA being analyzed. Multiple variations of this procedure have been developed and have begun to revolutionize clinical testing.

 Noninvasive prenatal testing is based on next-generation sequencing and is used to determine, early in a pregnancy, if certain chromosomal abnormalities are present (trisomies or monosomies) as well as the sex of the fetus. Fetal DNA can be found in the mother's blood, and through analysis of the DNA, and determining chromosome ratios by sequencing, it can be determined if multiple copies of a particular chromosome are present in the fetus. This is currently used only as a screening procedure; positive results require confirmation by an invasive technique such as amniocentesis.

C. Techniques for Amplifying DNA Sequences

To study genes or other DNA sequences, adequate quantities of material must be obtained. It is often difficult to isolate significant quantities of DNA from the original source. For example, an individual cannot usually afford to part with enough tissue to provide the amount of DNA required for clinical testing. Therefore, the available quantity of DNA has to be amplified.

1. Cloning of DNA

The first technique developed for amplifying the quantity of DNA is known as *cloning* (Fig. 17.9). The DNA that you want amplified (the "foreign" DNA) is attached to a *vector* (a carrier DNA), which is introduced into a host cell that makes multiple copies of the DNA. The foreign DNA and the vector DNA are usually cleaved with the same restriction enzyme, which produces complementary sticky ends in both DNAs. The foreign DNA is then added to the vector. Base pairs form between the complementary single-stranded regions, and DNA ligase joins the molecules to produce a chimera, or recombinant DNA. As the host cells divide, they replicate their own DNA, and they also replicate the DNA of the vector, which includes the foreign DNA.

If the host cells are bacteria, commonly used vectors are *bacteriophage* (viruses that infect bacteria), *plasmids* (extrachromosomal pieces of circular DNA that are taken up by bacteria), or *cosmids* (plasmids that contain DNA sequences from the lambda bacteriophage). When eukaryotic cells are used as the host, the vectors are often retroviruses, adenoviruses, free DNA, or DNA coated with a lipid layer (liposomes). The foreign DNA sometimes integrates into the host-cell genome, or it exists as episomes (extrachromosomal fragments of DNA) (see Section III.E).

Host cells that contain recombinant DNA are called *transformed cells* if they are bacteria or *transfected* (or *transduced*, if the vector is a virus) cells if they are eukaryotes. Markers in the vector DNA are used to identify cells that have been transformed, and probes for the foreign DNA can be used to determine that the host cells actually contain the foreign DNA. If the host cells containing the foreign DNA are incubated under conditions in which they replicate rapidly, large quantities of the foreign DNA can be isolated from the cells. With the appropriate vector and growth conditions that permit expression of the foreign DNA, large quantities of the protein produced from this DNA can be isolated.

2. Libraries

Specific collections of DNA fragments are known as *libraries*. A *genomic library* is a set of host cells (or phage) that collectively contain all of the DNA sequences from the genome of another organism. Thus, a genomic library contains promoter and intron sequences of every gene. A *cDNA library* is a set of host cells that collectively contain all the DNA sequences produced by reverse transcriptase from the mRNA obtained from cells (or tissue) of a particular type. Therefore, a cDNA library contains complementary DNA for all the genes expressed in that cell type,

Q In the early studies on CF, DNA sequencing was used to determine the type of defect in patients. Buccal cells were obtained from washes of the mucous membranes of the mouth, DNA isolated from these cells was amplified by PCR, and DNA sequencing of the CF gene was performed. A sequencing gel for the region in which the normal gene differs from the mutant gene is shown here. What is the difference between the normal and the mutant CF gene sequence shown on the gel, and what effect would this difference have on the protein produced from this gene?

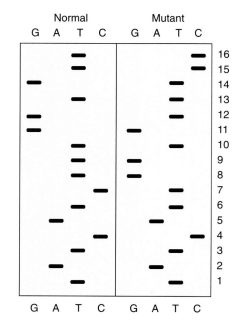

In individuals of northern European descent, 70% of the cases of CF are caused by a deletion of three bases in the CF gene. In the region of the gene shown on the gels, the base sequence (read from the bottom to the top of the gel) is the same for the normal and mutant gene for the first 6 positions, and the bases in positions 10 through 16 of the normal gene are the same as the bases in positions 7 through 13 of the mutant gene. Therefore, a three-base deletion in the mutant gene corresponds to bases 7 through 9 of the normal gene.

	Ile	Ile	Phe	Gly

Normal sequence: **T A T C A T C T T T G G T**

CF sequence: **T A T C A T - - - T G G T**

	Ile		Ile		Gly	

Loss of 3 bp (indicated by the *dashes*) maintains the reading frame, so only the single amino acid phenylalanine (F) is lost. Phenylalanine would normally appear as residue 508 in the protein. Therefore, the deletion is referred to as ΔF_{508}. The rest of the amino acid sequence of the normal and the mutant proteins is identical.

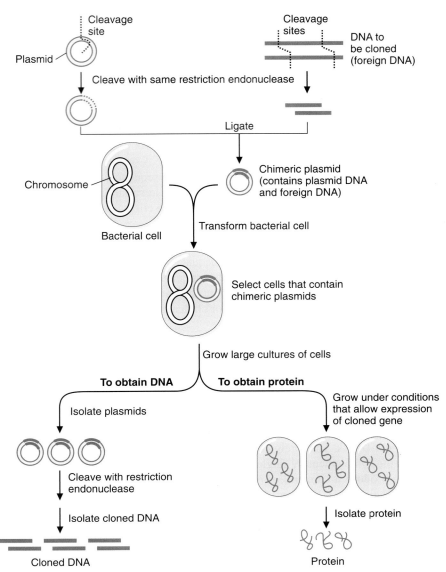

FIGURE 17.9 Simplified scheme for cloning of DNA in bacteria. A plasmid is a specific type of vector, or carrier, which can contain inserts of foreign DNA of up to 2.0 kilobase pairs in size. For clarity, the sizes of the pieces of DNA are not drawn to scale (e.g., the bacterial chromosomal DNA should be much larger than the plasmid DNA).

corresponding to the particular stage of differentiation of the cell when the mRNA was isolated. Because cDNA libraries are generated by reverse transcription of mRNA, promoter and intron sequences of genes are not present in those libraries.

The DNA fragments that are used to construct genomic libraries are much larger than those needed to construct cDNA libraries (for humans, a genomic library would need to represent all 3 billion bp in the haploid genome; the average mRNA is about 2,500 bases in size). Thus, different vectors are used to construct genomic libraries compared to cDNA libraries. Bacteriophage, which can handle up to 20 kilobase pairs [kb] of foreign DNA; bacterial artificial chromosomes (BACs), which can handle up to 150 kb of foreign DNA; and yeast artificial chromosomes (YACs), which can handle up to 1,000 kb of foreign DNA are often used in construction of genomic libraries. For cDNA libraries, plasmids (which can accept up to 2 kb of foreign DNA) are usually the vector of choice.

To clone a gene, a suitable probe must be developed (derived from either an amino acid sequence within a protein or from a similar DNA sequence obtained from another species); the library is then screened with the probe (using techniques described previously) to find host cells that harbor DNA sequences complementary to the probe. Obtaining sufficient clones enable the complete cDNA, or gene, to be obtained and sequenced.

3. Polymerase Chain Reaction

The *polymerase chain reaction* (PCR) is an in vitro method that can be used for rapid production of very large amounts of specific segments of DNA. It is particularly suited for amplifying regions of DNA for clinical or forensic testing procedures because only a very small sample of DNA is required as the starting material. Regions of DNA can be amplified by PCR from a single strand of hair or a single drop of blood or semen.

First, a sample of DNA containing the segment to be amplified must be isolated. Large quantities of primers, the four deoxyribonucleoside triphosphates, and a heat-stable DNA polymerase are added to a solution in which the DNA is heated to separate the strands (Fig. 17.10). The primers are two synthetic oligonucleotides; one oligonucleotide is complementary to a short sequence in one strand of the DNA to be amplified, and the other is complementary to a sequence in the other DNA strand. As the solution is cooled, the oligonucleotides form base pairs with the DNA and serve as primers for the synthesis of DNA strands by a heat-stable DNA polymerase (this polymerase is isolated from *Thermus aquaticus*, a bacterium that grows in hot springs). The process of heating, cooling, and new DNA synthesis is repeated many times until a large number of copies of the DNA is obtained. The process is automated, so each round of replication takes only a few minutes, and in 20 heating and cooling cycles the DNA is amplified more than a million-fold.

 Although only small amounts of semen were obtained from **Victoria T.'s** body, the quantity of DNA in these specimens was able to be amplified by PCR. This technique provided sufficient amounts of DNA for comparison with DNA samples from the three suspects.

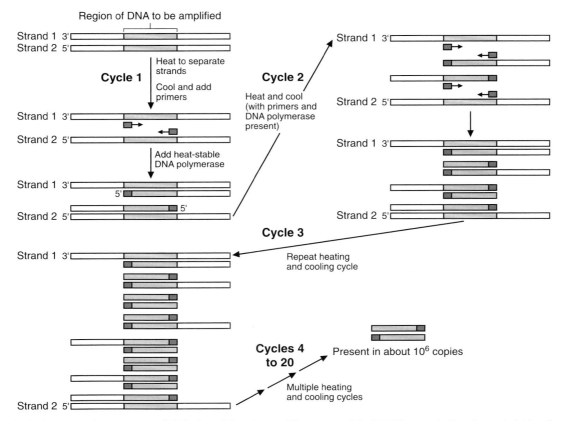

FIGURE 17.10 Polymerase chain reaction (PCR). *Strand 1* and *strand 2* are the original DNA strands. The short *dark blue fragments* are the primers. After multiple heating and cooling cycles, the original strands remain, but most of the DNA consists of amplified copies of the segment (shown in *lighter blue*) synthesized by the heat-stable DNA polymerase.

The mutation that causes sickle cell anemia abolishes a restriction site for the enzyme *Mst*II in the β-globin gene. The consequence of this mutation is that the restriction fragment produced by *Mst*II that includes the 5'-end of the β-globin gene is larger (1.3 kb) for individuals with sickle cell anemia than for normal individuals (1.1 kb). Analysis of restriction fragments provides a direct test for the mutation. In **Will S.'s** case, both alleles for β-globin lack the *Mst*II site and produce 1.3-kb restriction fragments; thus, only one band is seen in a Southern blot.

A

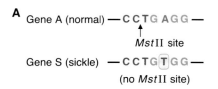

Gene A (normal) — C C T G A G G —

*Mst*II site

Gene S (sickle) — C C T G T G G —

(no *Mst*II site)

B

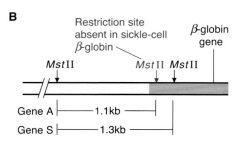

Restriction site absent in sickle-cell β-globin

β-globin gene

*Mst*II   *Mst*II *Mst*II

Gene A |————— 1.1kb ————|

Gene S |————— 1.3kb —————|

C

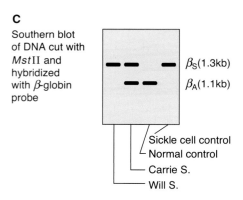

Southern blot of DNA cut with *Mst*II and hybridized with β-globin probe

β_S (1.3kb)
β_A (1.1kb)

Sickle cell control
Normal control
Carrie S.
Will S.

Carriers of sickle cell trait have both a normal and a mutant allele. Therefore, their DNA will produce both the larger and the smaller *Mst*II restriction fragments. When **Will S.'s** sister, **Carrie S.**, was tested, she was found to have both the small and the large restriction fragments, and her status as a carrier of sickle cell anemia, initially made on the basis of protein electrophoresis, was confirmed.

II. Use of Recombinant DNA Techniques for Diagnosis of Disease

A. DNA Polymorphisms

Polymorphisms are variations among individuals of a species in DNA sequences of the genome. They serve as the basis for using recombinant DNA techniques in the diagnosis of disease. The human genome probably contains millions of different polymorphisms. Some polymorphisms involve *point mutations*, the substitution of one base for another. *Deletions* and *insertions* are also responsible for variations in DNA sequences. Some polymorphisms occur within the coding region of genes. Others are found in noncoding regions that are closely linked to genes involved in the cause of inherited disease, in which case they can be used as a marker for the disease. Because only about 1.5% of the human genome codes for genes, most polymorphisms are present in noncoding regions of the genome.

B. Detection of Polymorphisms

1. Restriction Fragment Length Polymorphisms

Occasionally, a point mutation occurs in a recognition site for one of the restriction enzymes. The restriction enzyme, therefore, can cut at this restriction site in DNA from most individuals but not in DNA from individuals with this mutation. Consequently, the restriction fragment that binds a probe for this region of the genome will be larger for a person with the mutation than for most members of the population. Mutations also can create restriction sites that are not normally present. In this case, the restriction fragment from this region of the genome will be smaller for a person with the mutation than for most individuals. These variations in the length of restriction fragments are known as *restriction fragment length polymorphisms* (RFLPs).

In some cases, the mutation that causes a disease affects a restriction site within the coding region of a gene. In many cases, however, the mutation does not alter a restriction site within the gene of interest. In some cases, an RFLP close to the gene may be discovered (tightly linked; i.e., physically close on the DNA molecule). This RFLP can still serve as a biologic marker for the disease. Both types of RFLPs can be used for genetic testing to determine whether an individual has the disease.

2. Detection of Mutations by Allele-Specific Oligonucleotide Probes

Other techniques have been developed to detect mutations because many mutations associated with genetic diseases do not occur within restriction enzyme recognition sites or cause detectable restriction fragment length differences when digested with restriction enzymes. For example, oligonucleotide probes (containing 15 to 20 nucleotides) can be synthesized that are complementary to a DNA sequence that includes a mutation. Different probes are produced for alleles that contain mutations and for those that have a normal DNA sequence. The region of the genome that contains the abnormal gene is amplified by PCR, and the samples of DNA are placed in narrow bands on nitrocellulose paper ("slot blotting"). The paper is then treated with the radioactive probe for either the normal or the mutant sequence. Appropriate manipulation of the hybridization conditions (e.g., high temperature and low salt concentration) will allow probes with only a one-base difference to distinguish between normal and mutant alleles, making this test a very sensitive technique. Autoradiograms indicate whether the normal or mutant probe has preferentially base-paired (hybridized) with the DNA—that is, whether the alleles are normal or mutated. Carriers, of course, have two different alleles: one that binds to the normal probe and one that binds to the mutant probe.

3. Testing for Mutations by Polymerase Chain Reaction

If an oligonucleotide that is complementary to a DNA sequence containing a mutation is used as a primer for PCR, the DNA sample used as the template will be amplified only if it contains the mutation. If the DNA is normal (does not contain the mutation), the primer will not hybridize because of the one-base difference, and the DNA will not be amplified. This concept is extremely useful for clinical testing. In fact, several oligonucleotides, each specific for a different mutation and each containing a different label, can be used as primers in a single PCR reaction. This procedure results in rapid and relatively inexpensive testing for multiple mutations.

4. Detection of Polymorphisms Caused by Repetitive DNA

Human DNA contains many sequences that are repeated in tandem a variable number of times at certain loci in the genome. These regions are called *highly variable regions* because they contain a *variable number of tandem repeats* (VNTR). Digestion with restriction enzymes that recognize sites that flank the VNTR region produces fragments containing these loci, which differ in size from one individual to another, depending on the number of repeats that are present. Probes used to identify these restriction fragments bind to or near the sequence that is repeated (Fig. 17.11).

The restriction fragment patterns produced from these loci can be used to identify individuals as accurately as the traditional fingerprint. In fact, this restriction fragment technique has been called *DNA fingerprinting* and is gaining widespread use in forensic analysis. Family relationships can be determined by this method, and it can be used to help acquit or convict suspects in criminal cases.

Individuals who are closely related genetically will have restriction fragment patterns (DNA fingerprints) that are more similar than those who are more distantly related. Only monozygotic twins will have identical patterns.

How does one determine the DNA sequence of a gene that contains a mutation to develop specific probes to that mutation? First, the gene that causes the disease must be identified. This is done by a process known as *positional cloning*, which involves linking polymorphic markers to the disease. Individuals who express the disease will exhibit a specific subset of polymorphic markers, whereas individuals who do not express the disease will not express the same subset of polymorphic markers. Once such polymorphic markers are identified, identification of the disease gene can occur using these markers, in either of two ways. The first way is to use the polymorphic markers as probes to screen a human genomic library. This will identify pieces of human DNA that contain the polymorphic marker. These pieces of DNA can then be used as probes to expand the region of the genome surrounding this marker (chromosome walking). Potential genes within this region are identified (using data available from the sequencing of the human genome), and the sequence of bases within each gene is compared with the sequence of bases in the genes of individuals who have the disease. The one gene that shows an altered sequence in disease-carrying individuals compared with normal individuals is the tentative disease gene. The second method to identify the disease gene is to screen the already sequenced human genome via database searching for genes near the identified polymorphic markers. Once identified, such genes would need to be sequenced in normal and afflicted individuals to identify the disease gene. Through the sequencing of genes from many people afflicted with the disease, the types of mutations that lead to this disease can be characterized and specific tests developed to determine whether individuals express these particular mutations.

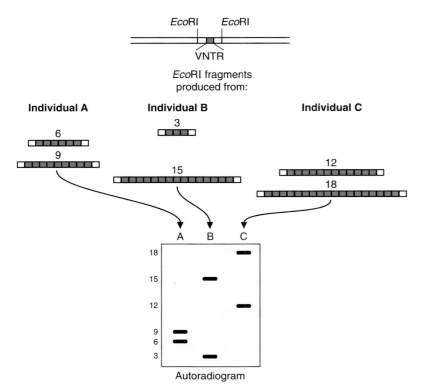

FIGURE 17.11 Restriction fragments produced from a gene with a variable number of tandem repeats (VNTR). Each individual has two homologs of every somatic chromosome and thus two genes each containing this region with a VNTR. Cleavage of each individual's genomic DNA with a restriction enzyme produces two fragments containing this region. The length of the fragments depends on the number of repeats they contain. Electrophoresis separates the fragments, and a labeled probe that binds to the fragments allows them to be visualized. Each *short blue block* represents one repeat.

Q Testing for CF by DNA sequencing is time-consuming and expensive. Therefore, another technique that uses allele-specific oligonucleotide probes has been developed. **Susan F.** and her family were tested using this method. Oligonucleotide probes, complementary to the region where the three-base deletion is located, have been synthesized. One probe binds to the mutant (ΔF_{508}) gene and the other to the normal gene.

DNA was isolated from Susan, her parents, and two siblings and was amplified by PCR. Samples of the DNA were spotted on nitrocellulose paper and treated with the oligonucleotide probes, and the following results were obtained. (*Dark spots* indicate binding of the probe.)

Autoradiogram

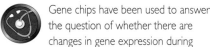

Normal probe

ΔF_{508} probe

Father
Child 1
Child 2
Susan F.
Mother

Which members of Susan's family have CF, which are normal, and which are carriers?

Gene chips have been used to answer the question of whether there are changes in gene expression during dieting. Gene chips containing approximately 47,000 unique genes were used, and the probes were cDNA prepared from adipose tissue of control and calorie-restricted overweight women. Upon caloric restriction, 334 transcripts were upregulated, whereas 342 transcripts were reduced in expression, as compared to the control group. As expected, many of the genes corresponded to those involved in metabolism and metabolic regulation. Increased use of these techniques will, in the future, enable development of pharmaceutic agents that specifically target transcripts involved in weight regulation, with the goal being the development and implementation of new and improved weight loss drugs.

5. DNA Chips (Microarrays)

Over the past 15 years, a technique has been developed that permits screening many genes simultaneously to determine which alleles of these genes are present in samples obtained from patients. The surface of a small chip is dotted with thousands of pieces of single-stranded DNA, each representing a different gene or segment of a gene. The chip is then incubated with a sample of a patient's DNA, and the pattern of hybridization is determined by computer analysis. The results of the hybridization analysis can be used, for example, to determine which one of the many known mutations for a particular genetic disease is the specific defect underlying a patient's problem. An individual's gene chip also may be used to determine which alleles of drug-metabolizing enzymes are present and, therefore, the likelihood of that individual having an adverse reaction to a particular drug.

Another use for a DNA chip is to determine which genes are being expressed in cells. If the mRNA from a tissue specimen is used to produce cDNA by reverse transcriptase, the cDNA will hybridize with only those genes being expressed in that tissue. In the case of a cancer patient, this technique could be used to determine the classification of the cancer much more rapidly and more accurately than the methods traditionally used by pathologists. The treatment then could be tailored more specifically to the individual patient. This technique also can be used to identify the genes required for tissue specificity (e.g., the difference between a muscle cell and a liver cell) and differentiation (the conversion of precursor cells into the different cell types). Experiments using gene chips are helping us to understand differentiation and may open the opportunity to artificially induce differentiation and tissue regeneration in the treatment of disease.

The advent of next-generation sequencing has led to a technique known as *RNA-SEQ*, which enables an investigator to determine which mRNA is being expressed in a particular tissue and also how much mRNA is present in the cell. As an overview, mRNA is isolated from a cell and converted to cDNA, and the cDNA molecules are sequenced using next-generation techniques. The intensity of the fluorescent signals during sequencing can quantitate the amount of starting cDNA, and comparing sequences obtained with genomic databases can identify the genes that have produced the mRNA under analysis. RNA-SEQ avoids using gene chips and does not restrict the results to only those genes that are represented on the gene chip.

As another example of the myriad uses of gene chips, a gene chip has been developed for the diagnosis of infectious disease. This gene chip contains 29,445 distinct oligonucleotides (60 bases long) that correspond to vertebrate viruses, bacteria, fungi, and parasites. Patient samples (nose aspirates, urine, blood, or tissue samples) are used as a source of RNA, which is converted to cDNA. Specific regions of the cDNA are amplified by PCR (the products of the PCR are fluorescent because of the incorporation of fluorescent primers in the procedure). Hybridization of the fluorescent probe with the chip allows identification of the infectious agent. The possibilities for gene chip applications in the future are virtually limitless.

The huge amount of information now available from the sequencing of the human genome, and the results available from gene chip experiments, has greatly expanded the field of bioinformatics. Bioinformatics can be defined as the gathering, processing, data storage, data analysis, information extraction, and visualization of biologic data. Bioinformatics also provides scientists with the capability to organize vast amounts of data in a manageable form that allows easy access and retrieval. Powerful computers are required to perform these analyses. As an example of an experiment that requires these tools, suppose you want to compare the effects of two different immunosuppressant drugs on gene expression in lymphocytes. Lymphocytes would be treated with either nothing (the control) or with the drugs individually (experimental samples). RNA would be isolated from the cells during drug treatment and the RNA converted to fluorescent cDNA using the enzyme reverse transcriptase and a fluorescent nucleotide analog. The cDNA produced from your three samples would be used as probes for a gene chip containing DNA fragments from more than 5,000 human genes. The samples would be allowed to hybridize to the chips, and you would then have 15,000 results to interpret (the extent of hybridization of each cDNA sample with each of the 5,000 genes on the chip). Computers are used to analyze the fluorescent spots on the chips and to compare the levels of fluorescent intensity from one chip to another. In this way, you could group genes showing similar levels of stimulation or inhibition in the presence of the drugs and compare the two drugs with respect to which genes have had their levels of expression altered by drug treatment.

(A) Individuals to which both probes hybridize are carriers (because they contain one normal allele and one mutant allele). Thus, the father and mother are both carriers of the defective allele, as is one of the two siblings (child 2). Susan has the disease (expressing only the mutant allele), and the other sibling (child 1) is not a carrier for the disease (expressing only the normal allele).

III. Use of Recombinant DNA Techniques for the Prevention and Treatment of Disease

A. Vaccines

Before the advent of recombinant DNA technology, vaccines were made exclusively from infectious agents that had been either killed or attenuated (altered so that they can no longer multiply in an inoculated individual). Both types of vaccines were potentially dangerous because they could be contaminated with the live infectious agent. In fact, in a small number of instances, disease has actually been caused by vaccination. For the vaccine to be successful in preventing future infections, the human immune system must respond to the antigenic proteins on the surface of an infectious agent. The immune system is then prepared if the body is exposed to the infectious agent in the future. By recombinant DNA techniques, these antigenic proteins can be solely produced in large quantities, completely free of the infectious agent, and used in a vaccine. Thus, any risk of infection by the vaccine is eliminated. The first successful recombinant DNA vaccine to be produced was for the hepatitis B virus (HBV).

More recently, DNA vaccines have been used to achieve similar results. The theory behind DNA vaccines is to allow DNA to enter cells within a tissue, which then transcribe and translate the protein product encoded by the gene. This protein is an antigen from the organism against which antibody production is desired. The host then generates an immune response to the antigen, generating protection for the host. Although this therapy has been successful in rats, it has not yet evolved to the point of being successful in humans, perhaps as a result of insufficient cells accepting and expressing the DNA vaccine. Ongoing research is geared toward increasing the number of cells that receive the DNA, thereby enhancing immunogenicity.

B. Production of Therapeutic Proteins

1. Insulin and Growth Hormone

Recombinant DNA techniques are used to produce proteins that have therapeutic properties. One of the first such proteins to be produced was human *insulin*. Recombinant DNA corresponding to the A-chain of human insulin was prepared and inserted into plasmids that were used to transform *Escherichia coli* cells. The bacteria then synthesized the insulin chain, which was purified. A similar process was used to obtain B-chains. The A- and B-chains were then mixed and allowed to fold and form disulfide bonds, producing active insulin molecules (Fig. 17.12). Insulin is not glycosylated, so there was no problem with differences in glycosyltransferase activity between *E. coli* and human cell types.

Human growth hormone has also been produced in *E. coli* and is used to treat children with growth-hormone deficiencies. Before production of recombinant growth hormone, growth hormone isolated from cadaver pituitary tissue was used, which was in short supply.

(M) A current method for forensic analysis of DNA samples is to take advantage of the presence of short tandem repeat (STR) sequences in the DNA. The number of repeats differs among alleles, so an analysis of 8 to 16 STRs is usually sufficient for a statistically valid match. The DNA to be analyzed is amplified in a PCR reaction with all of the primers (for all 8 to 16 STR regions) simultaneously (a process known as multiplexing). The primers are labeled with a fluorescent nucleotide, and they have been designed such that each STR amplification will yield a different-sized amplification product. After the PCR has been completed, the fluorescent DNA samples are analyzed by size via capillary electrophoresis and a fluorescent detector. The sizes of the fragments are determined using time of elution from the column (and comparison to known size standards). If the multiplex PCR analyzed 8 STR regions, it is possible for 16 different-sized bands (two alleles for each STR) to be generated from each individual donating DNA. These products are compared to the products obtained from the unknown sample, and matches (or nonmatches) can be determined. These procedures are now automated and are very precise.

DNA samples were obtained from each of the three suspects in **Victoria T.'s** rape and murder case, and these samples were compared with the victim's DNA by using DNA fingerprinting. Because **Victoria T.'s** sample size was small, PCR was used to amplify the regions containing the VNTRs. The results, using a probe for one of the repeated sequences in human DNA, are shown in the accompanying figure to illustrate the process. For more positive identification, several different restriction enzymes and probes were used. The DNA from suspect 2 produced the same VNTR pattern as the DNA from the semen obtained from the victim. If the other restriction enzymes and probes corroborate this finding, suspect 2 can be identified by DNA fingerprinting as the rapist/murderer.

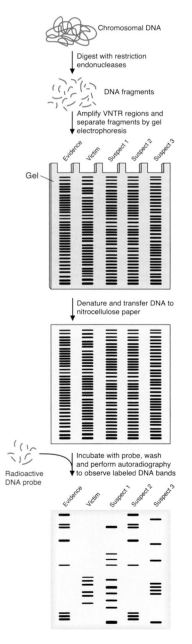

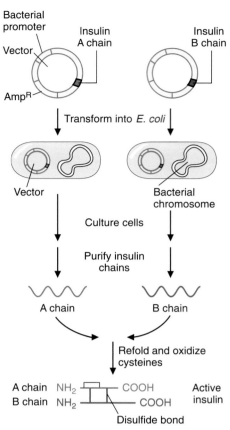

FIGURE 17.12 Production of human insulin in *Escherichia coli*. Amp^R is the gene for ampicillin resistance. The presence of Amp^R allows bacterial cells that contain the vector to grow in the presence of ampicillin. Cells that lack the Amp^R gene die in the presence of ampicillin. Because *E. coli* cannot process preproinsulin, a synthetic scheme was developed whereby each individual chain of insulin was expressed, produced, and purified, and then the two chains were linked together in a test tube.

2. Complex Human Proteins

More complex proteins have been produced in mammalian cell culture using recombinant DNA techniques. The gene for *factor VIII*, a protein involved in blood clotting, is defective in individuals with hemophilia. Before genetically engineered factor VIII became available, several patients with hemophilia died of AIDS or hepatitis that they contracted from transfusions of contaminated blood or from factor VIII isolated from contaminated blood.

Tissue plasminogen activator (TPA) is a protease in blood that converts plasminogen to plasmin. Plasmin is a protease that cleaves fibrin (a major component of blood clots), so administered TPA dissolves blood clots. Recombinant TPA, produced in mammalian cell cultures, can be administered during or immediately after a heart attack to dissolve the thrombi that occlude coronary arteries and prevent oxygen from reaching the heart muscle. It can also be used to treat other serious conditions caused by blood clots, including stroke and pulmonary embolism.

Hematopoietic growth factors also have been produced in mammalian cell cultures by recombinant DNA techniques. Erythropoietin can be used in certain types of anemias to stimulate the production of red blood cells. Colony-stimulating factors (CSFs) and interleukins (ILs) can be used after bone marrow transplants and after chemotherapy to stimulate white blood cell production and decrease the risk of infection. Recombinant β-interferon is the first drug known to decrease the frequency and severity of episodes resulting from the effects of demyelination in patients with multiple sclerosis.

A method for producing human proteins that has proven to be successful involves transgenic animals. These animals (usually goat or sheep) have been genetically engineered to produce human proteins in the mammary gland and secrete them into milk. The gene of interest is engineered to contain a promoter that is only active in the mammary glands under lactating conditions. The vector containing the gene and promoter is inserted into the nucleus of a freshly fertilized egg, which is then implanted into a foster mother. The female animal progeny are tested for the presence of this transgene, and milk from the positive animals is collected. Large quantities of the protein of interest can then be isolated from the relatively small number of proteins present in milk.

C. Small Interfering RNA

In several disorders, it would be advantageous to reduce the expression of a particular gene. This has, in the past, been very difficult to do, but a recently discovered series of reactions will allow this to occur, and the technique is already showing promise as a therapeutic tool. One way to reduce expression of a particular protein is to reduce the level of mRNA within the cell that codes for the protein. This can occur by either specifically degrading this mRNA or by blocking translation from the mRNA of interest. It turns out that eukaryotic cells have a built-in system to silence gene expression via reduction of mRNA levels, a process known as *gene silencing*. Gene silencing comes about via the transcription of genes known as *microRNAs* (miRNA; see Chapter 16). The miRNAs are processed to form a small (21 to 24 bp) double-stranded RNA molecule. The double-stranded RNA is separated into single strands, and the strand that is complementary to a specific mRNA is guided to the mRNA, which is either degraded or inhibited from participation in translation, depending on the miRNA. If the miRNA pairing is exact with its target, mRNA degradation is initiated. If the miRNA pairing with the target is inexact, inhibition of translation results (see Fig. 16.21).

Since this expression-ablation pathway was first discovered, it has been shown that the introduction of chemically synthesized double-stranded RNA molecules into cells will generate small interfering RNAs (siRNAs) to inhibit production of a cellular protein. Although this technique holds great promise for antiviral and anticancer therapies, a great deal of work still needs to be done to optimize delivery of the double-stranded RNA to the target tissue and to optimize the stability of the agent. Alternative approaches include the induction, or inhibition, of certain miRNA genes.

D. Genetic Counseling

One means of preventing disease is to avoid passing defective genes to offspring. If individuals are tested for genetic diseases, particularly members of families that are known to carry a defective gene, genetic counselors can inform the individuals of their risks and options. With this information, people can decide in advance whether to have children.

Screening tests based on the recombinant DNA techniques outlined in this chapter have been developed for many inherited diseases. Although these tests are currently expensive, particularly if entire families have to be screened, the cost may be trivial compared with the burden of raising children with severe disabilities. Obviously, cost and ethical considerations must be taken into account, but recombinant DNA technology has provided individuals with the ability to make choices.

Screening can be performed on the prospective parents before conception. If they decide to conceive, the fetus can be tested for the genetic defect. In some cases, if the fetus has the defect, treatment can be instituted at an early stage, even in utero. For certain diseases, early therapy leads to a more positive outcome.

When **Edna R.** began working with patients, she received the hepatitis B vaccine. The HBV infects the liver, causing severe damage. The virus contains a surface antigen (HBsAg) or coat protein for which the gene has been isolated. However, because the protein is glycosylated, it could not be produced in *E. coli*. (Bacteria, because they lack subcellular organelles, cannot produce glycosylated proteins.) Therefore, a yeast (eukaryotic) expression system was used that produced a glycosylated form of the protein. The viral protein, separated from the small amount of contaminating yeast protein, is used as a vaccine for immunization against HBV infection.

Dianne A. is using a recombinant human insulin called lispro (Humalog) (see Chapter 6, Fig. 6.12). Lispro was genetically engineered so that lysine is at position 28 and proline is at position 29 of the B-chain (the reverse of their positions in normal human insulin). Dianne injects lispro right before each meal to help keep her blood sugars controlled. The switch of position of the two amino acids leads to a faster acting insulin homolog. The lispro is absorbed from the site of injection much more quickly than other forms of insulin, and it acts to lower blood glucose levels much more rapidly than the other insulin forms.

Carrie S.'s fiancé decided to be tested for the sickle cell gene. He was found to have both the 1.3-kb and the 1.1-kb *Mst*II restriction fragments that include a portion of the β-globin gene. Therefore, like Carrie, he also is a carrier for the sickle cell gene.

A defect in the adenosine deaminase (ADA) gene causes severe combined immunodeficiency syndrome (SCID). When ADA is defective, deoxyadenosine and dATP accumulate in rapidly dividing cells, such as lymphocytes, and prove toxic to these cells. Cells of the immune system cannot proliferate at a normal rate. When an appropriate donor is available, bone marrow transplantation can be performed in the first 3 months of life with a reasonable degree of success. Without this, children with SCID usually die at an early age because they cannot combat infections. To survive, they must be confined to a sterile environmental "bubble."

In 1990, a 4-year-old girl, for whom no donor was available, was treated with infusions of her own lymphocytes that had been treated with a retrovirus containing a normal ADA gene. Although she had not responded to previous therapy, she improved significantly after this attempt at gene therapy. This disease is still being treated with gene therapy in combination with replacement enzyme infusion.

E. Gene Therapy

The ultimate cure for genetic diseases is to introduce normal genes into individuals who have defective genes. Currently, gene therapy is being attempted in animals, cell cultures, and human subjects. It is not possible at present to replace a defective gene with a normal gene at its usual location in the genome of the appropriate cells. However, as long as the gene is expressed at the appropriate time and produces adequate amounts of the protein to return the person to a normal state, the gene does not have to integrate into the precise place in the genome. Sometimes, the gene does not even have to be in the cells that normally contain it.

Retroviruses were the first vectors used to introduce genes into human cells. Normally, retroviruses enter target cells, their RNA genome is copied by reverse transcriptase, and the double-stranded DNA copy is integrated into the host-cell genome (see Fig. 14.22). If the retroviral genes (e.g., *gag, pol,* and *env*) are first removed and replaced with the therapeutic gene, the retroviral genes integrated into the host-cell genome will produce the therapeutic protein rather than the viral proteins (Fig. 17.13).

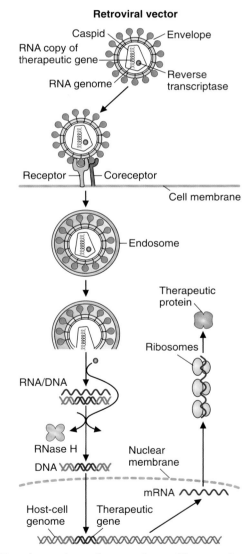

FIGURE 17.13 Use of retroviruses for gene therapy. The retrovirus carries an RNA copy of the therapeutic gene into the cell. The endosome that contains the virus dissolves, and the RNA and viral reverse transcriptase are released. This enzyme copies the RNA, making a double-stranded DNA that integrates into the host-cell genome. Transcription and translation of this DNA (the therapeutic gene) produces the therapeutic protein. (The virus does not multiply because its genes were removed and replaced by the RNA copy of the therapeutic gene.)

This process works only when the human host cells are undergoing division, so it has limited applicability. Other problems with this technique are that it can only be used with small genes (≤8 kb), and it may disrupt other genes because the insertion point is random, thereby possibly resulting in cancer.

Adenoviruses, which are natural human pathogens, can also be used as vectors. As in retroviral gene therapy, the normal viral genes required for synthesis of viral particles are replaced with the therapeutic genes. The advantages to using an adenovirus are that the introduced gene can be quite large (~36 kb), and infection does not require division of host cells. The disadvantage is that genes carried by the adenovirus do not integrate stably into the host genome, resulting in only transient expression of the therapeutic proteins (but preventing disruption of host genes and the complications that may arise from it). Thus, the treatment must be repeated periodically. Another problem with adenoviral gene therapy is that the host can mount an immune response to the pathogenic adenovirus, causing complications, including death.

To avoid the problems associated with viral vectors, researchers are employing treatment with DNA alone or with DNA coated with a layer of lipid (i.e., in liposomes). Adding a ligand for a receptor located on the target cells could aid delivery of the liposomes to the appropriate host cells. Many problems still plague the field of gene therapy. In many instances, the therapeutic genes must be targeted to the cells where they normally function—a difficult task at present. Deficiencies in dominant genes are more difficult to treat than those in recessive genes, and the expression of the therapeutic genes often needs to be carefully regulated. Although the field is moving forward, progress is slow. As mentioned previously, current research is exploring the use of siRNA to block expression of oncogenes in tumor cells, although significant clinical impact is most likely years away.

F. Transgenic Animals

The introduction of normal genes into somatic cells with defective genes corrects the defect only in the treated individuals, not in their offspring. To eliminate the defect for future generations, the normal genes must be introduced into the germ cell line (the cells that produce sperm in males or eggs in females). Experiments with animals indicate that gene therapy in germ cells is feasible. Genes can be introduced into fertilized eggs from which transgenic animals develop, and these transgenic animals can produce apparently normal offspring.

In fact, if the nucleus isolated from the cell of one animal is injected into the enucleated egg from another animal of the same species and the egg is implanted in a foster mother, the resulting offspring is a "clone" of the animal from which the nucleus was derived. Clones of sheep and pigs have been produced, and similar techniques could be used to clone humans. Obviously, these experiments raise many ethical questions that will be difficult to answer.

IV. Proteomics

The techniques described previously have concentrated on nucleic acid identification, but there have also been rapid advances in analyzing all proteins expressed by a cell at a particular stage of development. The techniques are sophisticated enough to allow comparisons between two different samples, such as normal cells and cancer cells from the same tissue. An abbreviated view of this technique is shown in Figure 17.14. Proteins from the two different cell types (A and B) are isolated and labeled with different fluorescent dyes. The proteins are then separated by two-dimensional gel electrophoresis (the first dimension, or separation, is by charge, and the second dimension is by size), which generates a large number of spots that can be viewed under a fluorescent imaging device; each of these spots corresponds to an individual protein. A computer aligns the spots from the two samples and can determine, by the level of fluorescence expressed at each protein spot, if a protein

Another form of SCID is X-linked and is known as X-SCID. This disease results from mutations in a common subunit protein of multiple cytokine receptors. The cDNA corresponding to this subunit was delivered to patient lymphocytes using a retroviral vector, and the success rate of reconstituting the immune system was high for patients who received this gene therapy. The enthusiasm concerning the treatment was tempered, however, by the development of leukemia in three of the patients who were part of the initial trial. Retroviruses randomly insert their DNA copy of their genome into the host chromosome. In the patients who developed leukemia, it has been determined that the vector inserted near the *LMO2* gene, a known proto-oncogene (see Chapter 18). The insertional event triggered activation (or overexpression) of *LMO2*, leading to uncontrolled cell proliferation. Current research is now directed to attempt to target areas of insertion for vectors used in gene therapy.

Adenoviral vectors have been used in an aerosol spray to deliver normal copies of the *CFTR* gene to cells of the lung in patients with CF. Some cells took up this gene, and the patients experienced moderate improvement. However, stable integration of the gene into the genome did not occur, and cells affected by the disease other than those in the lung (e.g., pancreatic cells) did not benefit. Nevertheless, this approach marked a significant forward step in the development of gene therapy. Adenoviral vectors were also used in an attempt to treat ornithine transcarbamoylase deficiency (a disorder of nitrogen metabolism). In this trial, a volunteer died following a severe immune response to the adenoviral vector. This unfortunate result has led to a reevaluation of the safety of viral vectors for gene therapy.

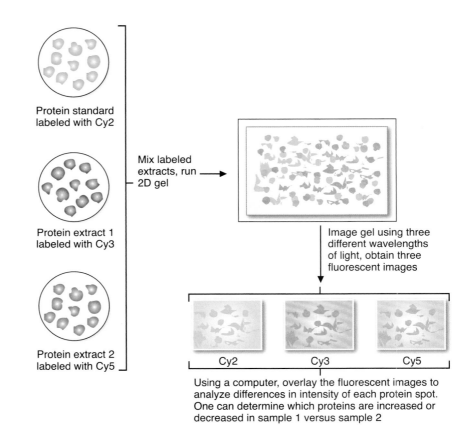

FIGURE 17.14 Using proteomics to determine if a protein is up- or downregulated. See text for more details. *2D*, two-dimensional.

has been up- or downregulated in one sample compared to the other. Proteins whose expression levels change can then be identified by sensitive techniques involving protein mass spectrometry.

The proteomics approach holds great promise in molecularly fingerprinting particular tumors and for discovering novel targets for drug development that are only expressed in the cancerous state. A physician's knowledge of the markers expressed by a particular tumor should allow for specific drug regimens to be used; no longer will one treatment be the norm for a particular tumor. Depending on a patient's proteome, treatments for the patient's specific tumor can be devised and prescribed.

 The most common CF mutation is a 3-bp deletion that causes the loss of phenylalanine at position 508 (Δ508; the Δ indicates deletion). This mutation is present in the CFTR protein in >70% of patients with CF. The defective protein is synthesized in the endoplasmic reticulum but is misfolded. It is, therefore, not transported to the Golgi but is degraded by a proteolytic enzyme complex called the proteasome. Other mutations responsible for CF generate an incomplete mRNA because of premature stop signals, frame shifts, or abnormal splice sites, or the mutations create a CFTR channel in the membrane that does not function properly.

CLINICAL COMMENTS

Edna R. In reading about development of the hepatitis B vaccine, **Edna R.** learned that the first vaccine available for HBV, marketed in 1982, was a purified and "inactivated" vaccine containing HBV virus that had been chemically killed. The virus was derived from the blood of known HBV carriers. Later, "attenuated" vaccines were used, in which the virus remained live but was altered so that it no longer multiplied in the inoculated host. Both the inactivated and the attenuated vaccines are potentially dangerous because they can be contaminated with live infectious HBV.

The modern "subunit" vaccines, first marketed in 1987, were made by recombinant DNA techniques described earlier in this chapter. Because this vaccine consists solely of the viral surface protein or antigen to which the immune system responds, there is no risk for infection with HBV.

Susan F. CF is a genetically determined autosomal-recessive disease that can be caused by a variety of mutations within the CF gene located on chromosome 7. **Susan F.** was found to have a 3-bp deletion at residue 508 of the CF gene (the mutation present in ~85% of white patients with CF in the United States). This mutation is generally associated with a more severe clinical course than many other mutations that cause the disease. However, other genes and environmental factors may modify the clinical course of the disease, so it is not currently possible to counsel patients accurately about prognosis based on their genotype.

CF is a relatively common genetic disorder in the United States, with a carrier rate of approximately 5% in Caucasians. The disease occurs in 1/3,000 Caucasian births in the country (1/17,000 in African Americans and 1/31,000 in Asians).

 Carrie S. After learning the results of their tests for the sickle cell gene, **Carrie S.** and her fiancé consulted a genetic counselor. The counselor informed them that, because they were both carriers of the sickle cell gene, their chance of having a child with sickle cell anemia was fairly high (~1 in 4). She told them that prenatal testing was available with fetal DNA obtained from cells by amniocentesis or chorionic villus sampling. If these tests indicated that the fetus had sickle cell disease, abortion was a possibility. Carrie, because of her religious background, was not sure that abortion was an option for her. Nonetheless, having witnessed her brother's sickle cell crises for many years, she also was not sure that she wanted to risk having a child with the disease. Her fiancé also felt that, at 25 years of age, he was not ready to deal with such difficult problems. They mutually agreed to cancel their marriage plans.

 Victoria T. DNA fingerprinting represents an important advance in forensic medicine. Before development of this technique, identification of criminals was far less scientific. The suspect in the rape and murder of **Victoria T.** was arrested and convicted, mainly on the basis of the results of DNA fingerprint analysis.

This technique has been challenged in some courts on the basis of technical problems in statistical interpretation of the data and sample collection. It is absolutely necessary for all of the appropriate controls to be run, including samples from the victim's DNA as well as the suspect's DNA. Another challenge to the fingerprinting procedure has been raised because PCR is such a powerful technique that it can amplify minute amounts of contaminating DNA from a source unrelated to the case.

 What are the statistical issues relating to DNA fingerprinting? Through the analysis of a large number of individuals of different ethnicities, one can determine the frequency of a particular DNA polymorphism within that distinct population. By matching 8 to 16 polymorphisms (using multiplexed PCR for polymorphic STRs) from DNA at the crime scene with DNA from a suspect, one can determine the odds of that match happening by chance. For example, let us assume that a suspect's DNA was compared with DNA found at the crime scene for four unique polymorphisms within the suspect's ethnic group. The frequency of polymorphism A in that population is 1 in 20; of polymorphism B, 1 in 30; of polymorphism C, 1 in 50; and of polymorphism D, 1 in 100. The odds of the suspect's DNA matching the DNA found at the crime scene for all four polymorphisms would be the product of each individual probability, or $(1/20) \times (1/30) \times (1/50) \times (1/100)$. This comes out to a 1 in 3 million chance that an individual would have the same polymorphisms in his or her DNA as that found at the crime scene. The question left to the courts is whether the 1 in 3 million match is sufficient to convict the suspect of the crime. Given that there may be 30 million individuals in the United States within the same ethnic group as the suspect, there would then be 30 people within the country who would match the DNA polymorphisms found at the scene of the crime. Can the court be sure that the suspect is the correct individual? Clearly, the use of DNA fingerprinting is much clearer when a match is not made, for that immediately indicates that the suspect was not at the scene of the crime.

BIOCHEMICAL COMMENTS

 Mapping of the Human Genome. The Human Genome Project began in 1990, and by the summer of 2000, the entire human genome had been mapped. This feat was accomplished in far less than the expected time as a result of both cooperative and competitive interactions of laboratories in the private as well as public sectors.

The human genome contains $>3 \times 10^9$ (3 billion) bp. A large percentage of this genome (<95%) does not code for the amino acid sequences of proteins or for functional RNA (such as ribosomal RNA [rRNA] or transfer RNA [tRNA]) but is composed of repetitive sequences, introns, and other noncoding elements of unknown function. The human genome is estimated to contain only about 20,000 to 25,000 genes; however, significantly more proteins are produced than there are genes. This arises from alternative splicing and various posttranslational modifications. Further analysis of the proteome may prove to be more informative than the genome.

Analysis of the genome has led to the identification of a large number of single nucleotide polymorphisms (SNPs), which refer to a single nucleotide change within a given DNA sequence as compared between individuals. For such a change to be considered an SNP (as opposed to a random mutation), the polymorphism must be

Over the past few years, a revolutionary new technique, based on a rudimentary immune system found in microbes and archaea, has enabled scientists to knock out, or insert, targeted genes in cells. The technique is known as CRISPR/Cas, for clustered *regulatory interspaced short palindromic repeats* (CRISPR)–*associated system* (Cas represents nucleases and helicases). Within the clustered repeats of these regions of the bacterial genome were found DNA sequences from bacteriophage. If a similar phage were to infect the bacteria, the host cell would use a defense mechanism that would recognize the invading DNA and degrade it using the *Cas* genes. Scientists have used the specificity of this system to successfully alter genes in cultured cells, either by knocking them out (destroying their ability to code for a functional protein) or by replacing the gene with a modified one. This technique has matured enough to enable a strain of mosquitoes to be created which would render females unable to breed, and this would have the potential to eliminate certain strains of mosquitoes (e.g., those that carry the malaria parasite) from existence. Scientists in China have successfully altered the β-globin gene in human embryos as a test to see if thalassemia can be treated with CRISPR/Cas technology. These early experiments have demonstrated that there are still technical issues concerning nonspecific gene integration to work out, but the potential for this technique is enormous. There also are significant ethical issues associated with this technique, including the ability to remove a species from existence and altering the human genome before birth. The medical implications for this technique are endless, but it is not clear that the ethical issues will be resolved as easily as the scientific technique.

present within 1% of the population. SNPs are plentiful in the human genome, occurring every 100 to 300 bp; therefore, SNPs are useful tools for mapping disease genes within the chromosome. SNPs are also being used in place of STR sequences in forensic DNA analysis.

When identification of a wayward gene is announced on the morning news, the average citizen may expect a cure for the genetic disease to be available that evening. Although knowledge of the chromosomal location and the sequence of genes will result in the rapid development of tests to determine whether an individual carries a defective gene, the development of a treatment for the genetic disease caused by the defective gene is not that easy or that rapid. As outlined in the section on gene therapy, many technical problems need to be solved before gene therapy becomes common. In addition to solving the molecular puzzles involved in gene therapy, we also will have to deal with many difficult ethical as well as technical questions.

Is it appropriate to replace defective genes in somatic cells to relieve human suffering? Many people may agree with this goal. But there is a related question: Is it appropriate to replace defective genes *in the germ cell line* to relieve human suffering? Fewer people may agree with this goal. Genetic manipulation of somatic cells affects only one generation; these cells die with the individual. Germ cells, however, live on, producing each successive generation.

The techniques developed to explore the human genome could be used for many purposes. What are the limits for the application of the knowledge gained by advances in molecular biology? Who should decide what the limits are, and who should serve as the "genetic police"? If we permit experiments that involve genetic manipulation of the human germ cell line, however nobly conceived, could we, in our efforts to "improve" ourselves, genetically engineer the human race into extinction?

KEY CONCEPTS

- Techniques for isolating and amplifying genes and studying and manipulating DNA sequences are currently being used in the diagnosis, prevention, and treatment of disease.
- These techniques require an understanding of the following tools and processes:
    - Restriction enzymes
    - Cloning vectors
    - Polymerase chain reaction
    - Dideoxy DNA sequencing
    - Gel electrophoresis
    - Nucleic acid hybridization
    - Expression vectors
- Recombinant DNA molecules produced by these techniques can be used as diagnostic probes, in gene therapy, or for the large-scale production of proteins for the treatment of disease.
- Identified genetic polymorphisms, inherited differences in DNA base sequences between individuals, can be used for both diagnosis of disease and the generation of an individual's molecular fingerprint.
- Genetic treatment of disease is possible, using either gene therapy or gene-ablation techniques. Technical difficulties currently restrict the widespread use of these treatments.
- Proteomics is the study of proteins expressed by a cell. Differences in protein expression between normal and cancer cells can be used to identify potential targets for future therapy.
- Diseases discussed in this chapter are summarized in Table 17.2.

TABLE 17.2 Diseases Discussed in Chapter 17

DISORDER OR CONDITION	GENETIC OR ENVIRONMENTAL	COMMENTS
Cystic fibrosis	Genetic	Cystic fibrosis is caused by a mutation in the cystic fibrosis transmembrane conductance regulator (CFTR) protein, which is a chloride channel. The most common mutation in the *CFTR* gene is Δ508, a triplet deletion that removes codon 508 from the primary sequence. The disease leads to pancreatic duct blockage as well as clogged airways.
Hepatitis B	Environmental	Vaccine development for hepatitis B using molecular genetic techniques to produce recombinant virus proteins
Sickle cell disease	Genetic	The development of genetic testing for sickle cell disease based on understanding the base change in DNA which leads to the disease

REVIEW QUESTIONS—CHAPTER 17

1. Many molecular techniques use electrophoresis of DNA fragments. Electrophoresis resolves double-stranded DNA fragments based on which one of the following?
   A. Sequence
   B. Molecular weight
   C. Isoelectric point
   D. Frequency of CTG repeats
   E. Secondary structure

2. Restriction enzymes can recognize, for the most part, a four-base sequence, a six-base sequence, or an eight-base sequence. If a restriction enzyme recognizes a six-base sequence, how frequently, on average, will this enzyme cut a large piece of DNA?
   A. Once every 16 bases
   B. Once every 64 bases
   C. Once every 256 bases
   D. Once every 1,024 bases
   E. Once every 4,096 bases

3. A forensic scientist is preparing to sequence some DNA found on a victim's clothing. Which one of the following sets of reagents will the technician require in order to carry out the Sanger technique for DNA sequencing? (The lists are not meant to be all-inclusive.)
   A. Deoxyribonucleotides, Taq polymerase, DNA primer
   B. Dideoxyribonucleotides, deoxyribonucleotides, template DNA
   C. Dideoxyribonucleotides, DNA primer, reverse transcriptase
   D. Two DNA primers, template DNA, Taq polymerase
   E. mRNA, dideoxynucleotides, reverse transcriptase

4. Certain diseases, such as fragile X syndrome, are caused by an expansion of triplet repeats within the gene. Which of the following sets of techniques would best enable a rapid determination if such a repeat were present within a gene? Choose the one best answer.
   A. PCR, RFLP analysis, but not SNP analysis
   B. PCR, RFLP analysis, and SNP analysis

   C. RFLP analysis, but not PCR or SNP analysis
   D. PCR, but not RFLP analysis or SNP analysis
   E. SNP analysis, but not PCR or RFLP analysis

5. The best method to determine whether albumin is transcribed in the liver of a mouse model of hepatocarcinoma is which one of the following?
   A. Genomic library screening
   B. Genomic Southern blot
   C. Tissue Northern blot
   D. Tissue Western blot
   E. VNTR analysis

6. Individuals metabolize drugs at different rates, owing to polymorphisms within the drug metabolizing genes. Which one of the following would be sufficient for testing the presence of such a polymorphism?
   A. Southern blots, PCR, SNP determinations, but not Northern blots
   B. Southern blot, PCR, SNP determinations, and Northern blots
   C. Southern blot, SNP determinations, Northern blot, but not PCR
   D. Southern blot, Northern blot, PCR, but not SNP determinations
   E. SNP determinations, but not Northern blot, Southern blot, or PCR

7. A scientist has cloned the cDNA for a particular gene and wants to analyze tissue expression of the gene by Northern blot analysis. She is surprised to see three positive bands in liver samples but only one band in all other tissues examined. A potential explanation for this finding is which one of the following?
   A. Liver contains three genes for this particular protein.
   B. RNA editing
   C. Posttranslational modifications
   D. Loss of a restriction endonuclease recognition site in the liver gene
   E. Alternative splicing

8. A scientist is attempting to understand the difference in gene expression between a prostate cancer cell and a non-cancer prostate cell. A gene chip experiment has identified 245 potential genes as being upregulated in the cancer cell line as compared to the noncancer cell line. Confirmation of this result can be obtained using which one of the following techniques?
   A. Southern blot
   B. Northern blot
   C. SNP analysis
   D. RFLP analysis
   E. PCR

9. When an individual has a test to determine whether he or she has been infected with HIV (the virus that causes AIDS), a Western blot is often used for confirmation purposes. For the Western blot test, which one of the following samples is run through the polyacrylamide gel, the contents of which will be transferred to filter paper for the blotting technique?
   A. Patient DNA cut with restriction enzymes
   B. A sample of the patient's blood
   C. Patient RNA prepared from DNA extracted from red blood cells
   D. Antibodies against HIV proteins
   E. Purified HIV proteins

10. The isolation and use of restriction endonucleases has allowed for a proliferation of techniques to generate recombinant DNA. Which of the following can describe recombinant DNA? Choose the one best answer.

	Recombinant DNA always refers to one DNA molecule derived from two or more different species.	Recombinant DNA techniques can be used to generate therapeutic proteins.	Bacteriophages were the source of the first restriction enzymes isolated.	Recombinant DNA has allowed for different types of insulin to be produced; some fast acting, some slow acting.	The use of gene therapy requires the production of recombinant DNA molecules.
A	Yes	No	Yes	No	Yes
B	Yes	No	No	No	No
C	Yes	No	Yes	Yes	Yes
D	No	Yes	No	Yes	No
E	No	Yes	No	Yes	Yes
F	No	Yes	Yes	No	No

ANSWERS

1. **The answer is B.** All DNA fragments are negatively charged and will migrate toward the positive electrode. The only difference between the fragments is their size, and the smaller fragments will move faster than the larger fragments because of their ability to squeeze through the gel at a faster rate.

2. **The answer is E.** The enzyme recognizes six bases, and the probability that the correct base is in each position is 1 in 4, so the overall probability is $(\frac{1}{4})^6$, or 1 in 4,096 bases.

3. **The answer is B.** The Sanger technique requires both deoxyribonucleotides and dideoxyribonucleotides and a template DNA. It does not use Taq polymerase (which is for PCR), nor does it need reverse transcriptase (which is required for producing DNA from RNA).

4. **The answer is A.** PCR experiments, using primers that flank the repeat area, can determine the number of repeats in a gene as compared to a gene with no or few repeats (the PCR product would be larger for a region containing multiple repeats as compared to a region with few repeats). Similarly, using restriction endonuclease recognition sites that flank the repeat, one

will see RFLPs, the length of the restriction fragment being dependent on the number of repeats in the gene. SNP analysis, however, examines SNPs, not multiple triplet repeats, and would not be a suitable method for determining a region of the genome that contained multiple triplet nucleotide repeats. Most individuals will have a certain number of repeats, and PCR and RFLP will enable expanded repeat regions to be distinguished from small repeat regions relatively easily.

5. **The answer is C.** A Northern blot allows one to determine which genes are being transcribed in a tissue at the time of mRNA isolation. The mRNA is run on a gel, transferred to filter paper, and then analyzed with a probe. If albumin is being transcribed, then a probe for albumin should give a positive result in the Northern blot. A library screening will not indicate if a particular gene is being transcribed, nor will a Southern blot. Those techniques will only allow one to determine that the gene is present in the genome. A Western blot analyzes protein content, not mRNA content. Analysis of VNTRs does not provide information about whether a gene is transcribed.

6. **The answer is A.** A polymorphism in the DNA may lead to altered restriction sites, which would be detected by Southern blots. The polymorphism, if it involved expansion of repeat sequences, would be detectable by Southern blots or PCR across the expanded region. Polymorphisms may be as small as a single nucleotide difference, which would be detectable by SNP analysis. Northern blots examine the transcript from the genes and would be the least likely technique to provide information concerning the polymorphism. The polymorphism may not be expressed within the exons of the genes, so a Northern blot would not show an extended, or truncated, mRNA. SNPs would also not be evident in Northern blots.

7. **The answer is E.** Certain primary transcripts have the capability to be spliced in alternative fashion, depending on the composition of the spliceosome in the tissues. In this case, the liver can splice in three ways, creating three different-sized transcripts, whereas all other tissues only splice in one way, creating just a single size of transcript. Because the genome is constant for all tissues, if the liver contained three genes for this transcript, the other tissues would as well. RNA editing will alter one base in a transcript but does not alter the overall size of the transcript. Posttranslational modifications occur to proteins after they are synthesized but not to RNA molecules (that would be posttranscriptional modifications). The loss of a restriction endonuclease recognition site within the liver gene would not alter the overall size of the transcript because this would be a mutation in the DNA. It is possible that this change created one alternative splicing event but not the three that are observed via the Northern blot.

8. **The answer is B.** If 245 genes are being upregulated in the cancer cells as compared to the normal cells, the mRNA levels for those 245 genes should be increased in the cancer cells as compared to the nontumor cells. One can therefore perform Northern blots, using cDNA corresponding to the genes as probes, of RNA from nontumor and tumor cells to determine if mRNA levels

actually do increase after transformation. A Southern blot will not show expression of genes just that the gene is present in the cells. SNP analysis will determine polymorphisms in DNA but cannot determine gene expression levels. Similarly, RFLP looks at differences in DNA structure but not at gene expression levels. PCR analyzes DNA as well, not gene expression. (RT-PCR, however, in which the mRNA is converted to DNA by reverse transcriptase, can determine mRNA levels between two different samples.)

9. **The answer is E.** The Western blot is used to determine if a patient's blood contains antibodies against HIV proteins (which would mean that the patient is infected with the HIV virus). In order to make this determination, purified HIV proteins are run through a polyacrylamide gel and transferred to filter paper, and the filter paper is blotted with a sample of the patient's blood. If the patient's blood has antibodies to the HIV proteins, these antibodies will bind to the filter and can be detected by second antibodies that recognize human antibodies and contain a fluorescent tag for detection. This test does not use DNA or RNA in the gel (a Western blot is the running of proteins through a gel), nor is the patient's blood run through a gel or antibodies to HIV proteins.

10. **The answer is E.** Restriction endonucleases were discovered in bacteria, and they are used to protect the bacteria from invasion by foreign DNA. Recombinant DNA refers to the generation of a piece of DNA from two other pieces of DNA in a test tube, and the DNA can be from the same or different species. Recombinant DNA techniques have been used to generate therapeutic proteins (such as factor VIII, growth hormone, and insulin). The use of recombinant DNA techniques has also allowed variants of therapeutic proteins to be synthesized (such as long- and short-acting variants of insulin). Gene therapy requires the use of recombinant DNA techniques to generate a gene, with appropriate promoter regions, to deliver to cells with an inability to produce the protein encoded by the recombinant DNA.

18

The Molecular Biology of Cancer

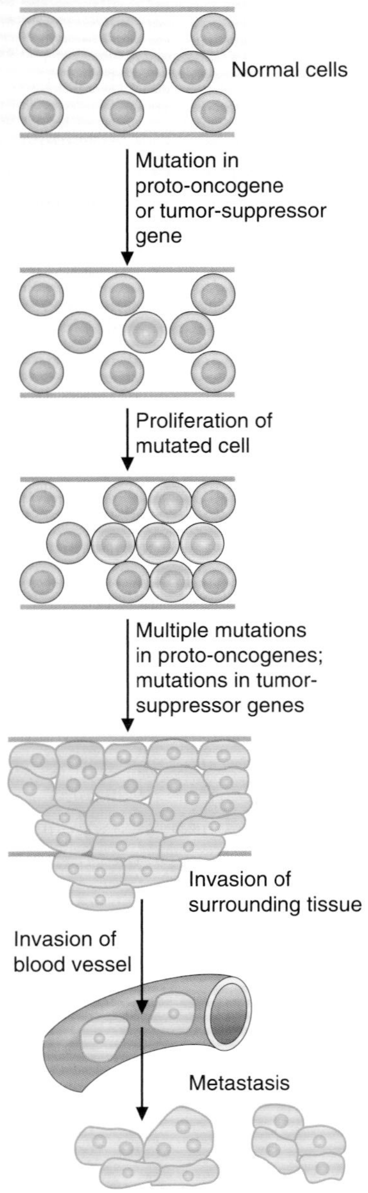

FIGURE 18.1 Development of cancer. Accumulation of mutations in a number of genes results in transformation. Cancer cells change morphologically, proliferate, invade other tissues, and metastasize.

The term **cancer** applies to a group of diseases in which **cells grow abnormally** and form a **malignant tumor**. Malignant cells can invade nearby tissues and **metastasize** (i.e., travel to other sites in the body, where they establish secondary areas of growth). This aberrant growth pattern results from **mutations in genes that regulate proliferation, differentiation, and survival of cells** in a multicellular organism. Because of these genetic changes, cancer cells no longer respond to the signals that govern growth of normal cells (Fig. 18.1.)

Oncogenes and Tumor-Suppressor Genes. The genes involved in the development of cancer are classified as **oncogenes** or **tumor-suppressor genes**. **Oncogenes** are mutated derivatives of normal genes (**proto-oncogenes**) whose function is to promote proliferation or cell survival. These genes can code for **growth factors, growth-factor receptors, signal transduction proteins, intracellular kinases, and transcription factors**. The process of transformation into a malignant cell may begin with a **gain-of-function** mutation in only one copy of a proto-oncogene. As the mutated cell proliferates, additional mutations can occur. **Tumor-suppressor genes** (normal growth–suppressor genes) encode proteins that **inhibit proliferation, promote cell death**, or **repair DNA**; both alleles need to be inactivated for transformation (**a loss of function**). Growth-suppressor genes have been called the guardians of the cell.

Cell Cycle Suppression and Apoptosis. Normal cell growth depends on a balanced regulation of **cell-cycle** progression and **apoptosis** (programmed cell death) by proto-oncogenes and growth-suppressor genes. At **checkpoints** in the **cell cycle**, products of **tumor-suppressor genes** slow growth in response to signals from the cell's environment, including external growth-inhibitory factors, or to allow time for repair of damaged DNA, or in response to other adverse circumstances in cells. Alternatively, cells with damaged DNA are targeted for **apoptosis** so that they will not proliferate. Many growth-stimulatory pathways involving proto-oncogenes, and growth-inhibitory controls involving a variety of tumor-suppressor genes, converge to regulate the activity of some key protein kinases, the **cyclin-dependent kinases**. These kinases act to control progression at specific points in the cell growth cycle. Apoptosis is initiated by either **death-receptor activation** or intracellular signals leading to release of the **mitochondrial protein cytochrome c**.

Mutations. Mutations in DNA that give rise to cancer may be **inherited** or may be caused by **chemical carcinogens, radiation, viruses**, and by **replication errors** that are not repaired. A cell population must accumulate **multiple mutations** for transformation to malignancy.

THE WAITING ROOM

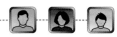

 Mannie W. has chronic myelogenous leukemia (CML), a disease in which a single line of myeloid cells in the bone marrow proliferates abnormally, causing a large increase in the number of nonlymphoid white blood cells (see Chapter 16). His myeloid cells contain the abnormal Philadelphia chromosome, which increases their proliferation. He has recently complained of pain and tenderness in various areas of his skeleton, possibly stemming from the expanding mass of myeloid cells within his bone marrow. He also reports a variety of hemorrhagic signs, including bruises (ecchymoses), bleeding gums, and the appearance of small red spots (petechiae caused by release of red cells into the skin).

 Michael T. was diagnosed with a poorly differentiated adenocarcinoma of the lung (see Chapter 13) after resection of a concerning nodule seen on a computed tomography (CT) scan of his chest. He survived the surgery and was recovering uneventfully until 6 months later, when he complained of an increasingly severe right temporal headache. A CT scan of his brain was performed. Results indicated that the cancer, which had originated in his lungs, had metastasized to his brain.

 Clark T. has had an intestinal adenocarcinoma resected, as well as several small metastatic nodules in his liver (see Chapters 12). He completed his second course of chemotherapy with 5-fluorouracil (5-FU) and oxaliplatin and had no serious side effects. He assured his physician at his most recent checkup that, this time, he intended to comply with any instructions his physicians gave him. He ruefully commented that he wished he had returned for regular examinations after his first colonoscopy.

 Calvin A. returned to his physician after observing a brownish-black irregular mole on his forearm (see Chapter 13). His physician thought the mole looked suspiciously like a malignant melanoma and referred him to a dermatologist who performed an excision biopsy (surgical removal for cytological analysis).

I. Causes of Cancer

The term *cancer* applies to a group of diseases in which cells grow abnormally and form a malignant tumor. Malignant cells can invade nearby tissues and metastasize (i.e., travel to other sites in the body where they establish secondary areas of growth). This aberrant growth pattern results from mutations in genes that regulate proliferation, differentiation, and survival of cells in a multicellular organism. Because of these genetic changes, cancer cells no longer respond to the signals that govern growth of normal cells.

Normal cells in the body respond to signals, such as cell–cell contact (contact inhibition), that direct them to stop proliferating. Cancer cells do not require growth-stimulatory signals, and they are resistant to growth-inhibitory signals. They are also resistant to *apoptosis*, the programmed cell death process whereby unwanted or irreparably damaged cells self-destruct. They have an infinite proliferative capacity and do not become senescent (i.e., they are immortalized). Furthermore, they can grow independent of structural support, such as the extracellular matrix (loss of anchorage dependence).

The study of cells in culture was, and continues to be, a great impetus for the study of cancer. Tumor development in animals can take months, and it was difficult to conduct experiments with tumor growth in animals. Once cells could be removed from an animal and propagated in a tissue culture dish, the onset of transformation (the normal cell becoming a cancer cell) could be seen in days.

Once cells were available to study, it was important to determine the criteria that distinguish transformed cells from normal cells in culture. Three criteria

 Determination of abnormal chromosome structures is done by karyotype analysis (see Fig. 12.14). Karyotypes are created by arresting cells in mitotic metaphase, a stage at which the chromosomes are condensed and visible under the light microscope. Nuclei are isolated and placed on a microscope slide, and the chromosomes are stained. Pictures of the chromosomes are obtained through the microscope, and the homologous chromosomes are paired. Through this type of analysis, translocations between chromosomes can be determined, as can trisomies and monosomies. As seen in the figure, this karyotype indicates a translocation between chromosomes 9 and 22 (a piece of chromosome 22 is now attached to chromosome 9; note the *arrows* in the figure). This is known as the *Philadelphia chromosome*, and it gives rise to CML, the disease exhibited by **Mannie W.**

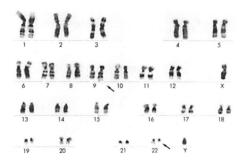

 Patients with leukemia can experience a variety of hemorrhagic (bleeding) manifestations caused by a decreased number of platelets. Platelets are small cells that initiate clot formation at the site of endothelial injury. Because of the uncontrolled proliferation of white cells within the limited space of the marrow, the normal platelet precursor cells (the megakaryocytes) in the marrow are "squeezed" or crowded and fail to develop into mature platelets. Consequently, the number of mature platelets (thrombocytes) in the circulation falls, and a thrombocytopenia develops. Because there are fewer platelets to contribute to clot formation, bleeding problems are common.

Malignant neoplasms (new growth, a tumor) of epithelial cell origin (including the intestinal lining, cells of the skin, and cells lining the airways of the lungs) are called *carcinomas*. If the cancer grows in a glandlike pattern, it is an adenocarcinoma. Thus, **Michael T.** and **Clark T.** have adenocarcinomas. **Calvin A.** had a carcinoma arising from melanocytes, which is technically a melanocarcinoma but is usually referred to as a *melanoma*.

Moles (also called *nevi*) are tumors of the skin. They are formed by melanocytes that have been transformed from highly dendritic single cells interspersed among other skin cells to round oval cells that grow in aggregates or "nests." Melanocytes produce the dark pigment melanin, which protects against sunlight by absorbing UV light. Additional mutations may transform the mole into a malignant melanoma.

The first experiments to show that oncogenes were mutant forms of proto-oncogenes in human tumors involved cells cultured from a human bladder carcinoma. The DNA sequence of the *ras* oncogene cloned from these cells differed from the normal *c-ras* proto-oncogene. Similar mutations were subsequently found in the *ras* gene of lung and colon tumors. **Clark T.'s** malignant polyp had a mutation in the *ras* proto-oncogene.

were established. The first is the requirement for serum in the cell culture medium to stimulate cell growth. *Serum* is the liquid fraction of clotted blood, and it contains many factors that stimulate cell proliferation. Transformed cells have, in general, a reduced requirement for serum: approximately 10% of that required for normal cells to grow. The second criterion is the ability to grow without attachment to a supporting matrix (anchorage dependence). Normal cells (such as fibroblasts or smooth muscle cells) require adherence to a substratum (in this case, the bottom of the plastic dish) and will not grow if suspended in a soft agar mixture. Transformed cells, however, have lost this anchorage dependence. The third and most stringent criterion used to demonstrate that cells are truly transformed is the ability of cells to form tumors when they are injected into mice that lack an immune system. Transformed cells will do so, whereas normal cells will not.

Drs. Michael Bishop and Harold Varmus demonstrated that cancer is not caused by unusual and novel genes but rather by mutation within existing cellular genes, and that for every gene that causes cancer (an *oncogene*), there is a corresponding cellular gene, called the *proto-oncogene*. Although this concept seems straightforward today, it was a significant finding when it was first announced and, in 1989, Drs. Bishop and Varmus were awarded the Nobel Prize in Medicine.

A single cell that divides abnormally eventually forms a mass called a *tumor*. A tumor can be benign and harmless; the common wart is a benign tumor formed from a slowly expanding mass of cells. In contrast, a malignant neoplasm (malignant tumor) is a proliferation of rapidly growing cells that progressively infiltrate, invade, and destroy surrounding tissue. Tumors develop angiogenic potential, which is the capacity to form new blood vessels and capillaries. Thus, tumors can generate their own blood supply to bring in oxygen and nutrients. Cancer cells also can metastasize, separating from the growing mass of the tumor and traveling through the blood or lymph to unrelated organs, where they establish new growths of cancer cells.

The transformation of a normal cell to a cancer cell begins with damage to DNA (base changes or strand breaks) caused by chemical carcinogens, ultraviolet (UV) light, viruses, or replication errors (see Chapter 13). Mutations result from the damaged DNA if it is not repaired properly or if it is not repaired before replication occurs. A mutation that can lead to transformation also may be inherited. When a cell with one mutation proliferates, this clonal expansion (proliferation of cells arising from a single cell) results in a substantial population of cells containing this one mutation, from which one cell may acquire a second mutation relevant to control of cell growth or death. With each clonal expansion, the probability of another transforming mutation increases. As mutations accumulate in genes that control proliferation, subsequent mutations occur even more rapidly, until the cells acquire the multiple mutations (in the range of four to seven) necessary for full transformation.

The transforming mutations occur in genes that regulate cellular proliferation and differentiation (proto-oncogenes), suppress growth (tumor-suppressor genes), target irreparably damaged cells for apoptosis, or repair damaged DNA. The genes that regulate cellular growth are called *proto-oncogenes*, and their mutated forms are called *oncogenes*. The term *oncogene* is derived from the Greek word *onkos*, meaning bulk or tumor. A transforming mutation in a proto-oncogene increases the activity or amount of the gene product (a gain-of-function mutation). Tumor-suppressor genes (normal growth–suppressor genes) and repair enzymes protect against uncontrolled cell proliferation. A transforming mutation in these protective genes results in a loss of activity or a decreased amount of the gene product.

In summary, cancer is caused by the accumulation of mutations in the genes involved in normal cellular growth and differentiation. These mutations give rise to cancer cells that are capable of unregulated, autonomous, and infinite proliferation. As these cancer cells proliferate, they impinge upon normal cellular functions, leading to the symptoms exhibited by individuals with the tumors.

II. Damage to DNA Leading to Mutations

A. Chemical and Physical Alterations in DNA

An alteration in the chemical structure of DNA, or of the sequence of bases in a gene, is an absolute requirement for the development of cancer. The function of DNA depends on the presence of various polar chemical groups in DNA bases, which are capable of forming hydrogen bonds between DNA strands or other chemical reactions. The oxygen and nitrogen atoms in DNA bases are targets for a variety of electrophiles (electron-seeking chemical groups). A typical sequence of events leading to a mutation is shown for dimethylnitrosamine in Figure 18.2. Chemical carcinogens (compounds that can cause transforming mutations) found in the environment and ingested in foods are generally stable lipophilic compounds that, like dimethylnitrosamine, must be activated by metabolism in the body to react with DNA (see also benzo[*a*]pyrene; Chapter 13, Section III.A and Fig. 13.12). Many chemotherapeutic agents, which are designed to kill proliferating cells by interacting with DNA, may also act as carcinogens and cause new mutations and tumors while eradicating the old. Structural alterations in DNA also occur through radiation and through UV light, which causes the formation of pyrimidine dimers. More than 90% of skin cancers occur in sunlight-exposed areas. UV rays derived from the sun induce an increased incidence of all skin cancers, including squamous cell carcinoma, basal cell carcinoma, and malignant melanoma of the skin. The wavelength of UV light that is most associated with skin cancer is UVB (280 to 320 nm), which forms pyrimidine dimers in DNA. This type of DNA damage is repaired by nucleotide excision repair pathways that require products of at least 20 genes. With excessive exposure to the sun, the nucleotide excision repair pathway is overwhelmed, and some damage remains unrepaired.

Each chemical carcinogen or reactant creates a characteristic modification in a DNA base. The DNA damage, if not repaired, introduces a mutation into the next generation when the cell proliferates.

B. Gain-of-Function Mutations in Proto-oncogenes

Proto-oncogenes are converted to oncogenes by mutations in the DNA that cause a gain in function; that is, the protein can now function better in the absence of the normal activating events. Several mechanisms that lead to the conversion of proto-oncogenes to oncogenes are known:

- Radiation and chemical carcinogens act (1) by causing a mutation in the regulatory region of a gene, increasing the rate of production of the proto-oncogene protein; or (2) by producing a mutation in the coding portion of the oncogene that results in the synthesis of a protein of slightly different amino acid composition capable of transforming the cell (Fig. 18.3A).
- The entire proto-oncogene or a portion of it may be transposed or translocated; that is, moved from one position in the genome to another (see Fig. 18.3B). In its new location, the proto-oncogene may be under the control of a promoter that is regulated in a manner different from the promoter that normally regulates this gene. This may allow the gene to be expressed in a tissue where it is not normally expressed or at higher-than-normal levels of expression. If only a portion of the proto-oncogene is translocated, it may be expressed as a truncated protein with altered properties, or it may fuse with another gene and produce a fusion protein containing portions of what are normally two separate proteins. The truncated or fusion protein may be hyperactive and cause inappropriate cell growth.
- The proto-oncogene may be amplified (see Fig. 18.3C), so that multiple copies of the gene are produced in a single cell. If more genes are active, more proto-oncogene protein will be produced, increasing the growth rate of the cells. As examples, the oncogene N-*myc* (a cell proliferation transcription

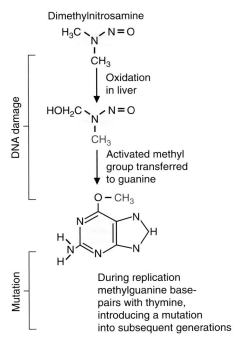

FIGURE 18.2 Mutations in DNA caused by nitrosamines. Nitrosamines are consumed in many natural products and are produced in the stomach from nitrites used as preservatives and secondary amines found in foods such as fish. They are believed to be responsible for the high incidence of gastric cancer in Japan and Iceland, where salt-preserved fish is a major dietary item. Nitrosamine metabolites methylate guanine (the transferred methyl group is shown in *red*).

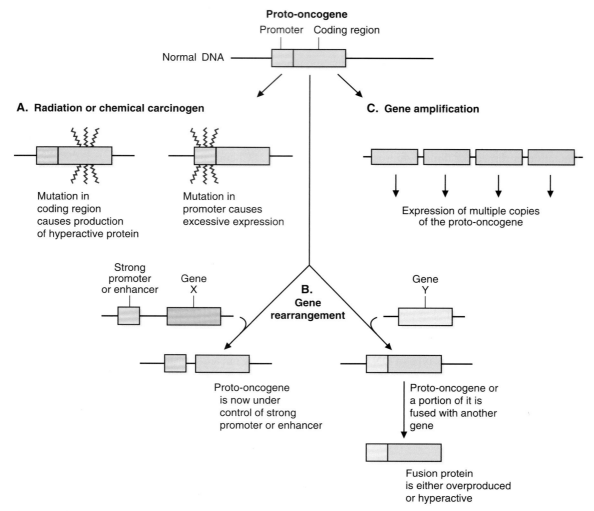

FIGURE 18.3 Transforming mutations in proto-oncogenes. **A.** Effect of radiation or chemical carcinogens on proto-oncogenes or their promoters. The mutations may be point mutations, deletions, or insertions. **B.** Gene rearrangements as caused by transposition or translocation of a proto-oncogene or proto-oncogene fragment. **C.** Amplification of a proto-oncogene allows more protein to be produced.

Burkitt lymphoma is a B-cell malignancy which usually results from a translocation between chromosomes 8 and 14. The translocation of genetic material moves the proto-oncogene transcription factor *c-myc* (normally found on chromosome 8) to another chromosome, usually chromosome 14. The translocated gene is now under the control of the promoter region for the immunoglobulin heavy-chain gene, which leads to inappropriate and overexpression of *c-myc*. The result may be uncontrolled cell proliferation and tumor development. All subtypes of Burkitt lymphoma contain this translocation. Epstein–Barr virus (EBV) infection of B-cells is also associated with certain types of Burkitt lymphoma.

factor, related to *c-myc*) is amplified in some neuroblastomas, and amplification of the *erb*-b2 oncogene (a growth-factor receptor) is associated with several breast carcinomas.

- If an oncogenic virus infects a cell, its oncogene may integrate into the host-cell genome, permitting production of the abnormal oncogene protein. The cell may be transformed and exhibit an abnormal pattern of growth. Rather than inserting an oncogene, a virus may simply insert a strong promoter into the host-cell genome. This promoter may cause increased or untimely expression of a normal proto-oncogene.

The important point to remember is that transformation results from abnormalities in the normal growth-regulatory program caused by gain-of-function mutations in proto-oncogenes. However, loss-of-function mutations also occur in the tumor-suppressor genes, repair enzymes, or activators of apoptosis, and a combination of both types of mutations is usually required for full transformation to a cancer cell.

C. Mutations in Repair Enzymes

Repair enzymes are the first line of defense preventing conversion of chemical damage in DNA to a mutation (see Chapter 13, Section III.B). DNA repair enzymes are tumor-suppressor genes in the sense that errors repaired before replication do not become mutagenic. DNA damage is constantly occurring from exposure to sunlight, background radiation, toxins, and replication errors. If DNA repair enzymes are absent, mutations accumulate much more rapidly, and once a mutation develops in a growth-regulatory gene, a cancer may arise. As an example, inherited mutations in the tumor-suppressor genes *brca1* and *brca2* predispose women to the development of breast cancer (see "Biochemical Comments" at the end of this chapter). The protein products of these genes play roles in DNA repair, recombination, and regulation of transcription. A second example, *hereditary nonpolyposis colorectal cancer* (HNPCC), was introduced in Chapter 13. It results from inherited mutations in enzymes involved in the DNA mismatch repair system.

III. Oncogenes

Proto-oncogenes control normal cell growth and division. These genes encode proteins that are growth factors, growth-factor receptors, signal transduction proteins, transcription factors, cell-cycle regulators, and regulators of apoptosis (Table 18.1). (The name representing the gene of an oncogene is referred to in lowercase letters and italics [e.g., *myc*], but the name of the protein product is capitalized and italics are not used [e.g., Myc]). The mutations in oncogenes that give rise to transformation are usually gain-of-function mutations; either a more active protein is produced or an increased amount of the normal protein is synthesized.

MicroRNAs (miRNAs) can also behave as oncogenes. If an miRNA is overexpressed (increased function), it can act as an oncogene if its target (which would exhibit reduced expression under these conditions) is a protein that is involved in inhibiting, or antagonizing, cell proliferation.

A. Oncogenes and Signal Transduction Cascades

All of the proteins in growth-factor signal transduction cascades are coded for by proto-oncogenes (Fig. 18.4).

1. Growth Factors and Growth-Factor Receptors

The genes for both growth factors and growth-factor receptors are proto-oncogenes.

Growth factors generally regulate growth by serving as ligands that bind to cellular receptors located on the plasma membrane (cell-surface receptors) (see Chapter 11). Binding of ligands to these receptors stimulates a signal transduction pathway in the cell that activates the transcription of certain genes. If too much of a growth factor or a growth-factor receptor is produced, the target cells may respond by proliferating inappropriately. Growth-factor receptors may also become oncogenic through translocation or point mutations in domains that affect binding of the growth factor, dimerization, kinase activity, or some other aspect of their signal transmission. In such cases, the receptor transmits a proliferative signal even though the growth factor normally required to activate the receptor is absent. In other words, the receptor is stuck in the "on" position.

2. Signal Transduction Proteins

The genes that encode proteins involved in growth-factor signal transduction cascades may also be proto-oncogenes. Consider, for example, the monomeric G-protein Ras. Binding of growth factor leads to the activation of Ras (see Fig. 11.11). When Ras binds guanosine triphosphate (GTP), it is active, but Ras slowly inactivates itself by hydrolyzing its bound GTP to guanosine diphosphate (GDP) and inorganic phosphate (P_i). This controls the length of time that Ras is active. Ras is converted to an oncogenic form by point mutations that decrease the activity of the GTPase domain of Ras, thereby increasing the length of time it remains in the active form.

Ras, when it is active, activates the serine–threonine kinase Raf (a mitogen-activated protein [MAP] kinase kinase kinase), which activates MEK (a MAP kinase

Mannie W.'s bone marrow cells contain the Philadelphia chromosome, typical of CML. The Philadelphia chromosome results from a reciprocal translocation between the long arms of chromosome 9 and 22. As a consequence, a fusion protein is produced that contains the N-terminal region of the Bcr protein from chromosome 22 and the C-terminal region of the Abl protein from chromosome 9. *Abl* is a proto-oncogene, and the resulting fusion protein (Bcr-Abl) has lost its regulatory region and is constitutively active, resulting in deregulated tyrosine kinase activity. When it is active, Abl stimulates the Ras pathway of signal transduction, leading to cell proliferation.

The gene for the human epidermal growth-factor receptor (*HER2*, *c-erb*-b2) is overexpressed in about 20% of breast cancer cases. Several drugs have been developed that recognize and blocks the receptor's action. The drug most studied, trastuzumab (Herceptin), has been shown to have survival benefits when used in combination with other chemotherapy. However, some tumors that overexpress *HER2* show resistance to Herceptin. Thus, it appears that a complete genotyping of breast cancer cells may be necessary (using the microarray or RNA-SEQ techniques described in Chapter 17) to develop an effective therapy for each patient with the disease, leading to individualized therapy.

TABLE 18.1 Classes of Oncogenes, Mechanism of Activation, and Associated Human Tumors

CLASS	PROTO-ONCOGENE	ACTIVATION MECHANISM	LOCATION	DISEASE
Growth Factors				
Platelet-derived growth-factor β-chain	sis	Overexpression	Secreted	Glioma Fibrosarcoma
Fibroblast growth factors	int-2	Amplification	Secreted	Breast cancer Bladder cancer Melanoma
	hst	Overexpression	Secreted	Stomach carcinoma
Growth-Factor Receptors				
Epidermal growth-factor receptor family	erb-b1	Overexpression	Cell membrane	Squamous cell carcinoma of the lung
	erb-b2	Amplification	Cell membrane	Breast, ovarian, lung, stomach cancers
Platelet-derived growth-factor receptor	PDGFR	Translocation	Cell membrane	Chronic myelomonocytic leukemia
Hedgehog receptor	SMO	Point mutation	Cell membrane	Basal cell carcinoma
Signal Transduction Proteins				
G-proteins	ras	Point mutation	Cytoplasm	Multiple cancers, including lung, colon, thyroid, pancreas, many leukemias
Serine–threonine kinase	akt2	Amplification	Cytoplasm	Ovarian carcinoma
	raf	Overexpression	Cytoplasm	Myeloid leukemia
Tyrosine kinase	abl	Translocation	Cytoplasm	Chronic myeloid leukemia Acute lymphoblastic leukemia
	src	Overexpression	Cytoplasm	Colon carcinoma
Hormone Receptors				
Retinoid receptor	RARα	Translocation	Nucleus	Acute promyelocytic leukemia
Transcription Factors				
	Hox11	Translocation	Nucleus	Acute T-cell leukemia
	Myc	Translocation	Nucleus	Burkitt lymphoma
		Amplification	Nucleus	Neuroblastoma, small-cell carcinoma of the lung
	fos, jun	Phosphorylation	Nucleus	Osteosarcoma, sarcoma
Apoptosis Regulators				
	Bcl-2	Translocation	Mitochondria	Follicular B-cell lymphoma
Cell-Cycle Regulators				
Cyclins	Cyclin D	Translocation	Nucleus	Lymphoma
		Amplification	Nucleus	Breast, liver, esophageal cancers
Cyclin-dependent kinase	CDK4	Amplification	Nucleus	Glioblastoma, sarcoma
		Point mutation	Nucleus	Melanoma

The table is not meant to be all-inclusive; only examples of each class of gene are presented.

kinase), which activates MAP kinase (Fig. 18.5). Activation of MAP kinase results in the phosphorylation of cytoplasmic and nuclear proteins, followed by increased transcription of the transcription-factor proto-oncogenes *myc* and *fos* (see the next section). Note that mutations in the genes for any of the proteins that regulate MAP kinase activity, as well as those proteins induced by MAP kinase activation, can lead to uncontrolled cell proliferation.

3. Transcription Factors

Many transcription factors, such as Myc and Fos, are proto-oncoproteins (the products of proto-oncogenes). MAP kinase, in addition to inducing *myc* and *fos,* also directly activates the AP-1 transcription factor through phosphorylation (see Fig. 18.5).

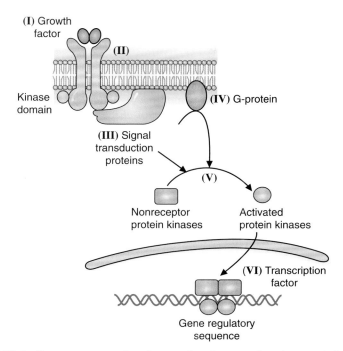

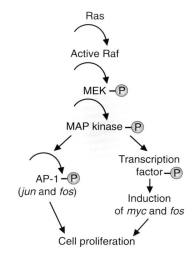

FIGURE 18.4 Proto-oncogene sites for transforming mutations in growth-factor signaling pathways. *(I)* The amount of growth factor. *(II)* The receptor, which normally must bind the growth factor to dimerize and activate a kinase domain. *(III)* Signal transduction proteins. Some, such as PI-3 kinase, form second messengers. *(IV)* G-proteins, and their regulators, which are also signal transduction proteins. *(V)* Nonreceptor protein kinase cascades, which lead to phosphorylation of transcription factors. *(VI)* Nuclear transcription factors that are normally activated through phosphorylation or binding of a ligand.

FIGURE 18.5 Phosphorylation cascade leading to activation of proto-oncogene transcription factors *myc*, *fos*, and *jun*. *MAP*, mitogen-activated protein; *MEK*, MAP kinase kinase.

AP-1 is a heterodimer formed by the protein products of the *fos* and *jun* families of proto-oncogenes. The targets of AP-1 activation are genes involved in cellular proliferation and progression through the cell cycle, as are the targets of the *myc* transcription factor. The synthesis of the transcription factor *c-myc* is tightly regulated in normal cells, and it is expressed only during the S phase of the cell cycle. In a large number of tumor types, this regulated expression is lost, and *c-myc* becomes inappropriately expressed or overexpressed throughout the cell cycle, driving cells continuously to proliferate.

The net result of alterations in the expression of transcription factors is the increased production of the proteins that carry out the processes required for proliferation.

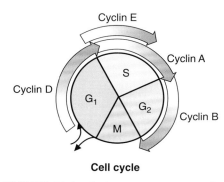

FIGURE 18.6 Cyclin synthesis during different phases of the cell cycle.

B. Oncogenes and the Cell Cycle

Growth factors, hormones, and other messengers activate the growth of human cells, involving DNA replication and cell division in the cell cycle. These activators work through cyclins and cyclin-dependent kinases (CDKs) that control progression from one phase of the cycle to another (Fig. 18.6). For quiescent cells to proliferate, they must leave G_0 and enter the G_1 phase of the cell cycle (see Chapter 13, Fig. 13.7). If the proper sequence of events occurs during G_1, the cells enter the S phase and are committed to DNA replication and cell division. Similarly, during G_2, cells make a commitment to mitotic division. CDKs are made constantly throughout the cell cycle but require binding of a specific cyclin to be active. Different cyclins made at different times in the cell cycle control each of the transitions (G_1/S, S/G_2, G_2/M).

The activity of the cyclin–CDK complex is further regulated through phosphorylation and through inhibitory proteins called *cyclin-dependent kinase inhibitors* (CKIs) (Fig. 18.7). CKIs slow cell-cycle progression by binding and inhibiting

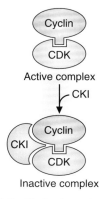

FIGURE 18.7 Cyclin-dependent kinase inhibitor (CKI) inhibition of cyclin/cyclin-dependent kinase (CDK) activity.

the CDK–cyclin complexes. CDKs are also controlled through activating phosphorylation by cyclin-activating kinases (CAKs) and inhibitory hyperphosphorylation kinases.

To illustrate the role of these proteins, consider some of the events that occur at the G$_1$/S checkpoint (Fig. 18.8). Because the cell is committed to DNA replication and division once it enters the S phase, multiple regulatory proteins are involved in determining whether the cell is ready to pass this checkpoint. These regulatory proteins include Cdk4 and Cdk6 (which are constitutively produced throughout the cell cycle), cyclin D (whose synthesis is induced only after growth-factor stimulation of a quiescent cell), the retinoblastoma gene product (Rb), and a class of transcription factors known collectively as *E2F*. In quiescent cells, Rb is complexed with E2F, resulting in inhibition of these transcription factors. Upon growth-factor stimulation, the cyclin Ds are induced (there are three types of cyclin D: D1, D2, and D3). They bind to Cdk4 and Cdk6, converting them to active protein kinases. One of the targets of cyclin/CDK phosphorylation is the Rb protein. Phosphorylation of Rb releases it from E2F, and E2F is then free to activate the transcription of genes required for entry into S phase. The Rb protein is a tumor-suppressor gene (more to follow).

The proteins induced by E2F include cyclin E, cyclin A, cdc25A (an activating protein phosphatase), and proteins required to bind at origins of replication to initiate DNA synthesis. The synthesis of cyclin E allows it to complex with Cdk2, forming another active cyclin complex that retains activity into S phase (see Fig. 18.6). One of the major functions of the cyclin E1–Cdk2 complex is hyperphosphorylation of the Rb protein, thereby keeping Rb in its inactive state. Cyclin A also complexes with Cdk2, and it phosphorylates, and inactivates, the E2F family of transcription factors. This ensures that the signals are not present for extended periods of time. Thus, each phase of the cell cycle activates the next through cyclin synthesis. The cyclins are removed by regulated proteolysis.

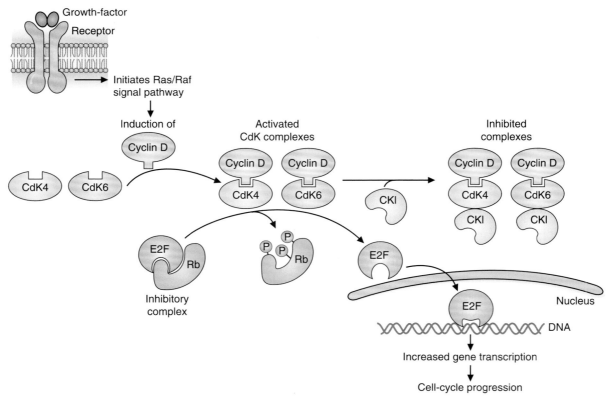

FIGURE 18.8 Control of the G$_1$/S transition in the cell cycle. The genes that encode cyclins and CDKs are oncogenes, and the gene that encodes the retinoblastoma protein (Rb) is a tumor-suppressor gene. *CDK*, cyclin-dependent kinase; *CKI*, cyclin-dependent kinase inhibitor.

Progression through the cell cycle is opposed by the CKIs (see Fig. 18.8). The CKIs regulating cyclin/CDK expression in the G₁ phase of the cell cycle fall into two categories: the Cip/Kip family and the INK4 (*inhibitors of cyclin-dependent kinase-4*) family. The Cip/Kip family members (p21, p27, and p57) have a broad specificity and inhibit all cyclin–CDK complexes. The INK4 family, which consists of p15, p16, p18, and p19, are specific for the cyclin D–Cdk4/6 family of complexes. The regulation of synthesis of different CKIs is complex, but some are induced by DNA damage to the cell and halt cell-cycle progression until the damage can be repaired. For example, the CKI p21 (a protein of 21,000 Da) is a key member of this group that responds to specific signals to block cell proliferation. If the damage cannot be repaired, an apoptotic pathway is selected and the cell dies.

In addition to sunlight and a preexisting nevus, hereditary factors also play a role in the development of malignant melanoma. Ten percent of melanomas tend to run in families. Some of the suspected melanoma-associated genes include the tumor-suppressor gene *p16* (an inhibitor of Cdk4) and *cdk4*. **Calvin A.** was the single child of parents who died in a car accident in their 50s, and thus, a familial tendency could not be assessed.

IV. Tumor-Suppressor Genes

Like the oncogenes, the tumor-suppressor genes encode molecules involved in the regulation of cell proliferation. Table 18.2 provides several examples. The normal function of tumor-suppressor proteins is generally to inhibit proliferation in response to certain signals such as DNA damage. The signal is removed when the cell is fully equipped to proliferate; the effect of the elimination of tumor-suppressor genes is to remove the brakes on cell growth. They affect cell-cycle regulation, signal transduction, transcription, and cell adhesion. The products of tumor-suppressor genes frequently modulate pathways that are activated by the products of proto-oncogenes.

Tumor-suppressor genes contribute to the development of cancer when both copies of the gene are inactivated. This is different from the case of proto-oncogene mutations because only one allele of a proto-oncogene needs to be converted to an oncogene to initiate transformation. As with the oncogenes, this is also applicable to miRNAs. If the expression of a particular miRNA is lost, the messenger RNA (mRNA) it regulates would be overexpressed, which could lead to enhanced cellular proliferation. Thus, miRNAs can be classified as either oncogenes (overexpression) or tumor suppressors (loss of function), depending on the genes that they regulate.

A. Tumor-Suppressor Genes that Regulate the Cell Cycle Directly

The two best-understood cell-cycle regulators that are also tumor suppressors are the retinoblastoma (*Rb*) and *p53* genes.

TABLE 18.2	Examples of Tumor Suppressors		
CLASS	**PROTEIN**	**LOCATION**	**ASSOCIATED DISEASES**
Adhesion protein receptor	E-cadherin	Cell membrane	Stomach cancer
	Patched	Cell membrane	Basal cell carcinoma
	TGF-β receptor	Cell membrane	Colon cancer
Signal transduction	NF-1	Under cell membrane	Neurofibrosarcoma
	Smad4/DPC	Cytoplasm/ nucleus	Pancreatic and colorectal cancers
Transcription factor cell-cycle regulator	WT-1	Nucleus	Wilms tumor
	p16(INK4)	Nucleus	Melanoma, lung, pancreatic cancers
	Retinoblastoma	Nucleus	Retinoblastoma, sarcomas
Cell cycle/apoptosis	p53	Nucleus	Most cancers
DNA repair	BRCA1	Nucleus	Breast cancer

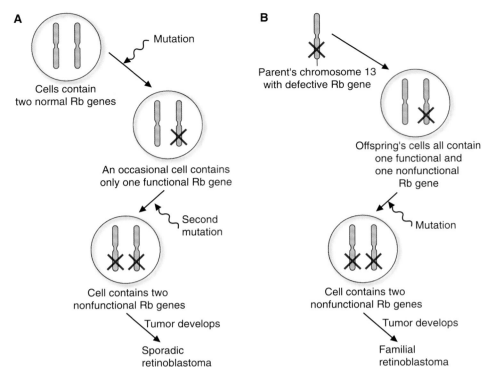

FIGURE 18.9 Mutations in the retinoblastoma (*Rb*) gene. **A.** Sporadic retinoblastoma. **B.** Familial retinoblastoma.

1. The Retinoblastoma Gene

As discussed previously, the retinoblastoma gene product, Rb, functions in the transition from G_1 to S phase and regulates the activation of members of the E2F family of transcription factors (see Fig. 18.8). If an individual inherits a mutated copy of the Rb allele, there is a 100% chance of that individual developing retinoblastoma because of the high probability that the second allele of Rb will gain a mutation (Fig.18.9). This is considered familial retinoblastoma. Individuals who do not inherit mutations in Rb, but who develop retinoblastoma, are said to have sporadic retinoblastoma and acquire two specific mutations, one in each Rb allele of the retinoblast, during their lifetime.

2. p53, The Guardian of the Genome

The p53 protein is a transcription factor that regulates the cell cycle and apoptosis, which is programmed cell death. Loss of both *p53* alleles is found in >50% of human tumors. p53 acts as the "guardian of the genome" by halting replication in cells that have suffered DNA damage and targeting unrepaired cells to apoptosis.

In response to DNA-damaging mutagens, ionizing radiation, or UV light, the level of p53 rises (Fig. 18.10, circle 1). p53, acting as a transcription factor, stimulates transcription of *p21* (a member of the Cip/Kip family of CKIs), as shown in Figure 18.10, circle 2. The p21 gene product inhibits the cyclin–CDK complexes, which prevents the phosphorylation of Rb and release of E2F proteins. The cell is thus prevented from entering S phase. p53 also stimulates the transcription of a number of DNA repair enzymes (including growth *a*rrest and *D*NA *d*amage [GADD45]) (Fig. 18.10, circle 3). If the DNA is successfully repaired, p53 induces its own downregulation through the activation of the *mdm2* gene. If the DNA repair was not successful, p53 activates several genes involved in apoptosis, including *bax* (discussed in the next section) and *insulinlike growth factor–binding protein 3* (IGF-BP3) (Fig. 18.10, circle 4). The IGF-BP3 protein product binds the receptor for insulinlike growth factor, which presumably induces apoptosis by blocking the

Inheritance of a mutation in *p53* leads to Li-Fraumeni syndrome, which is characterized by multiple types of tumors. Mutations in *p53* are present in >50% of human tumors. These are secondary mutations within the cell, and if *p53* is mutated, the overall rate of cellular mutation will increase because there is no p53 to check for DNA damage, to initiate the repair of the damaged DNA, or to initiate apoptosis if the damage is not repaired. Thus, damaged DNA is replicated, and the frequency of additional mutations within the same cell increases remarkably.

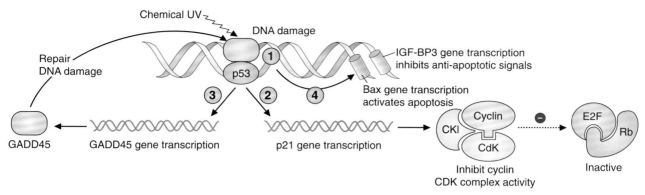

FIGURE 18.10 p53 and cell-cycle arrest. Mechanisms that recognize DNA damage stop p53 degradation and modify the p53 protein (*circle 1*). p53 stimulates the transcription of p21 (*circle 2*) and GADD45 (*circle 3*). p21 blocks the cyclin/CDK phosphorylation of Rb, which continues to inhibit the E2F family of transcription factors, thereby blocking cell progression through the cell cycle. GADD45 allows the DNA damage to be repaired. If the damage is not repaired, apoptotic genes are activated (*circle 4*). CDK, cyclin-dependent kinase; *Rb*, retinoblastoma; *UV*, ultraviolet.

antiapoptotic signaling by growth factors, and the cell enters a growth factor deprivation mode.

B. Tumor-Suppressor Genes that Affect Receptors and Signal Transduction

Tumor-suppressor genes may encode receptors, components of the signaling transduction pathway, or transcription factors.

1. Regulators of Ras

The Ras family of proteins is involved in signal transduction for many hormones and growth factors (see Section III.A.2) and is therefore oncogenic. The activity of these pathways is interrupted by *G*TPase-*a*ctivating *p*roteins [GAPs]; see Chapter 10, (Section III.E.1), which vary among cell types. Neurofibromin, the product of the tumor-suppressor gene *NF-1,* is a nervous system–specific GAP that regulates the activity of Ras in neuronal tissues. The growth signal is transmitted so long as the Ras protein binds GTP. Binding of NF-1 to Ras activates the GTPase domain of Ras, which hydrolyzes GTP to GDP, thereby inactivating Ras. Without a functional neurofibromin molecule, Ras is perpetually active.

2. Patched and Smoothened

A good example of tumor suppressors and oncogenes working together is provided by the coreceptor genes *patched* and *smoothened*, which encode the receptor for the hedgehog class of signaling peptides. (The strange names of some of the tumor-suppressor genes arose because they were first discovered in *Drosophila* [fruit fly], and the names of *Drosophila* mutations are often based on the appearance of a fly that expresses the mutation. Once the human homolog is found, it is given the same name as the *Drosophila* gene.) These coreceptors normally function to control growth during embryogenesis and illustrate the importance of maintaining a balance between oncogenes and tumor-suppressor genes. The Patched receptor protein inhibits Smoothened, its coreceptor protein. Binding of a hedgehog ligand to Patched releases the inhibition of Smoothened, which then transmits an activating signal to the nucleus, stimulating new gene transcription (Fig. 18.11). *Smoothened* is a proto-oncogene, and *patched* is a tumor-suppressor gene. If *patched* loses its function (definition of a tumor suppressor), then Smoothened can signal the cell to proliferate, even in the absence of a hedgehog signal. Conversely, if *smoothened* undergoes a gain-of-function mutation (definition of an oncogene), it can signal in the absence of the hedgehog signal, even in the presence of Patched. Inherited mutations in either *smoothened* or *patched* will lead to an increased incidence of basal cell carcinoma.

An inherited mutation in *NF-1* can lead to neurofibromatosis, a disease primarily of numerous benign, but painful, tumors of the nervous system. The movie *Elephant Man* was based on an individual who was believed to have had this disease. Recent analysis of the patient's remains, however, indicates that he may have suffered from the rare Proteus syndrome, not neurofibromatosis.

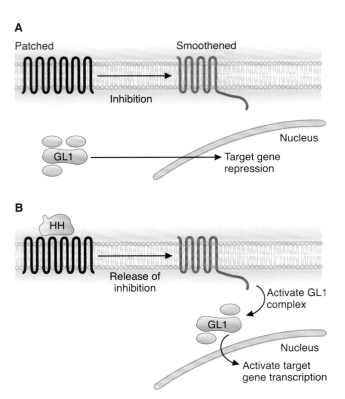

FIGURE 18.11 The Patched/Smoothened signaling system. **A.** In the absence of a hedge-hog (HH) signal, Smoothened is inactive owing to inhibition by the HH receptor Patched, and the GLI transcription factor complex acts as a repressor of transcription. **B.** When a ligand binds to the Patched receptor, the inhibition of Smoothened is repressed, leading to an activation of the GLI complex and active transcription of the target genes.

C. Tumor-Suppressor Genes that Affect Cell Adhesion

The cadherin family of glycoproteins mediates calcium-dependent cell–cell adhesion. Cadherins form intercellular complexes that bind cells together (Fig. 18.12A). They are anchored intracellularly by catenins, which bind to actin filaments. Loss of E-cadherin expression may contribute to the ability of cancer cells to detach and migrate in metastasis. Individuals who inherit a mutation in E-cadherin (this mutation is designated *CDH1*) are sharply predisposed to developing diffuse-type gastric cancer.

The catenin proteins have two functions: In addition to anchoring cadherins to the cytoskeleton, they act as transcription factors (see Fig. 18.12B). β-Catenin also binds to a complex that contains the regulatory protein *a*denomatous *pol*yposis *coli* (APC), which targets it for degradation. When the appropriate signal inactivates APC, β-catenin levels increase and it travels to the nucleus, where it activates *myc* and *cyclin D1* transcription, leading to cell proliferation. APC is a tumor-suppressor gene. If it is inactivated, it cannot bind β-catenin and inhibit cell proliferation. Mutations in APC or proteins that interact with it are found in the vast majority of sporadic human colon cancer. Inherited mutations in APC lead to one of the most common form of hereditary colon cancer, familial adenomatous polyposis (FAP).

V. Cancer and Apoptosis

In the body, superfluous or unwanted cells are destroyed by a pathway called *apoptosis*, or programmed cell death. Apoptosis is a regulated energy-dependent sequence of events by which a cell self-destructs. In this suicidal process, the

A. Catenins and cadherins in cell attachment

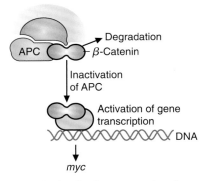

B. β-Catenin and APC in gene transcription

FIGURE 18.12 **A.** Catenins and cadherins. E-cadherin molecules form intercellular, calcium-dependent homodimers with cadherins from another cell, resulting in cell–cell adhesion. The cytoplasmic portion of E-cadherin is complexed to a variety of catenins, which anchor the cadherin to the actin cytoskeleton. **B.** β-Catenin and APC in transcription. The APC complex activates β-catenin for proteolytic degradation. If APC is inactivated, β-catenin levels increase. It acts as a transcription factor that increases synthesis of *myc* and other genes that regulate cell cycle progression.

cell shrinks, the chromatin condenses, and the nucleus fragments. The cell membrane forms blebs (outpouches), and the cell breaks up into membrane-enclosed apoptotic vesicles (apoptotic bodies) containing varying amounts of cytoplasm, organelles, and DNA fragments. Phosphatidylserine, a lipid on the inner leaflet of the cell membrane, is exposed on the external surface of these apoptotic vesicles. It is one of the phagocytic markers recognized by macrophages and other nearby phagocytic cells that engulf the apoptotic bodies.

Apoptosis is a normal part of multiple processes in complex organisms: embryogenesis, the maintenance of proper cell number in tissues, the removal of infected or otherwise injured cells, the maintenance of the immune system, and aging. It can be initiated by injury, radiation, free radicals or other toxins, withdrawal of growth factors or hormones, binding of proapoptotic cytokines, or interactions with cytotoxic T-cells in the immune system. Apoptosis can protect organisms from the negative effects of mutations by destroying cells with irreparably damaged DNA before they proliferate. Just as an excess of a growth signal can produce an excess of unwanted cells, the failure of apoptosis to remove excess or damaged cells can contribute to the development of cancer.

A. Normal Pathways to Apoptosis

Apoptosis can be divided into three general phases: an initiation phase, a signal integration phase, and an execution phase. Apoptosis can be initiated by external signals that work through death receptors such as tumor necrosis factor (TNF), or deprivation of growth hormones (Fig. 18.13). It can also be initiated by intracellular events that affect mitochondrial integrity (e.g., oxygen deprivation, radiation) and irreparably damaged DNA. In the signal integration phase, these proapoptotic signals are balanced against antiapoptotic cell survival signals by several pathways, including members of the Bcl-2 family of proteins. The execution phase is carried out by proteolytic enzymes called *caspases*.

1. Caspases

Caspases are cysteine proteases that cleave peptide bonds next to an aspartate residue. They are present in the cell as procaspases, zymogen-type enzyme precursors that are activated by proteolytic cleavage of the inhibitory portion of their polypeptide chain. The different caspases are generally divided into two groups according to their function: initiator caspases, which specifically cleave other procaspases; and execution caspases, which cleave other cellular proteins involved in maintaining cellular integrity (see Fig. 18.13). The initiator caspases are activated through two major signaling pathways: the death receptor pathway and the mitochondrial integrity pathway. They activate the execution caspases, which cleave protein kinases involved in cell adhesion, lamins that form the inner lining of the nuclear envelope, actin and other proteins required for cell structure, and DNA repair enzymes. They also cleave an inhibitor protein of the endonuclease *c*aspase-*a*ctivated *D*Nase (CAD), thereby activating CAD to initiate the degradation of cellular DNA. With destruction of the nuclear envelope, additional endonucleases (Ca^{2+}- and Mg^{2+}-dependent) also become activated.

2. The Death Receptor Pathway to Apoptosis

The death receptors are a subset of TNF-1 receptors, which includes Fas/CD95, TNF-receptor 1 (TNF-R1), and death receptor 3 (DR3). These receptors form a trimer that binds TNF-1 or another death ligand on its external domain and binds adaptor proteins to its intracellular domain (Fig.18.14). The activated TNF–receptor complex forms the scaffold for binding two molecules of procaspase 8 (or procaspase 10), which autocatalytically cleave each other to form active caspase 8 (or caspase 10). Caspases 8 and 10 are initiator caspases that activate execution caspases 3, 6, and 7. Caspase 3 also cleaves a Bcl-2 protein, Bid, to a form that activates the mitochondrial integrity pathway to apoptosis.

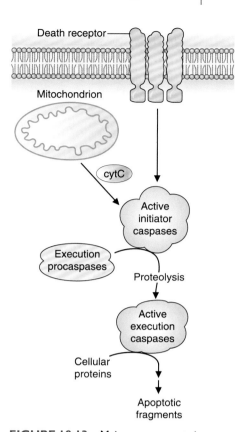

FIGURE 18.13   Major components in apoptosis. The release of cytochrome c (cytC) from mitochondria, or activation of death receptors, can lead to the initiation of apoptosis.

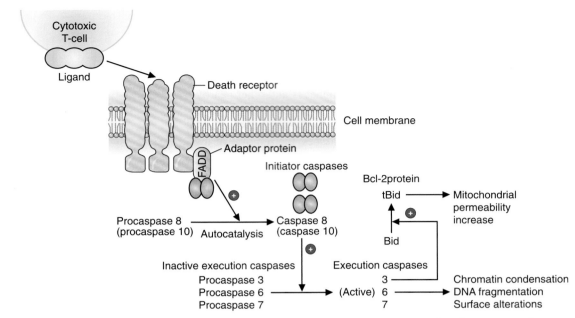

FIGURE 18.14 The death-receptor pathway to apoptosis. The ligand (either a free ligand or a cell surface-associated protein from another cell) binds to the death receptor, which makes a scaffold for autocatalytic activation of caspase 8 (and sometimes 10). Active caspase 8 (and sometimes 10) cleave apoptotic execution caspases directly. However, the pathway also activates Bid, which acts on mitochondrial membrane integrity. *FADD*, Fas-associated protein with death domain; *tBid*, truncated Bid.

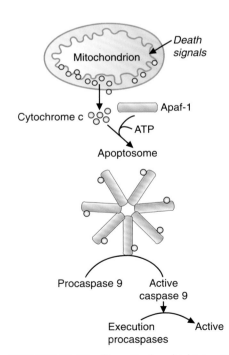

FIGURE 18.15 The mitochondrial integrity pathway releases cytochrome c, which binds to Apaf and forms a multimeric complex called the apoptosome. The apoptosome converts procaspase 9 to active caspase 9, an initiator caspase, which is released by the apoptosome into the cytosol. *ATP*, adenosine triphosphate.

3. The Mitochondrial Integrity Pathway to Apoptosis

Apoptosis is also induced by intracellular signals indicating that cell death should occur. Examples of these signals include growth-factor withdrawal, cell injury, the release of certain steroids, and an inability to maintain low levels of intracellular calcium. All of these treatments, or changes, lead to release of cytochrome c from the mitochondria (Fig. 18.15). Cytochrome c is a necessary protein component of the mitochondrial electron-transport chain that is loosely bound to the outside of the inner mitochondrial membrane. Its release initiates apoptosis.

In the cytosol, cytochrome c binds pro*a*poptotic *p*rotease-*a*ctivating *f*actor (Apaf). The Apaf/cytochrome c complex binds caspase 9, an initiator caspase, to form an active complex called the *apoptosome*. The apoptosome, in turn, activates execution caspases (3, 6, and 7) by zymogen cleavage.

4. Integration of Pro- and Antiapoptotic Signals by the Bcl-2 Family of Proteins

The Bcl-2 family members are decision makers that integrate pro-death and anti-death signals to determine whether the cell should commit suicide. Both proapoptotic and antiapoptotic members of the *Bcl-2* family exist (Table 18.3). Bcl-2 family members contain regions of homology, known as *Bcl-2 homology (BH) domains*. There are four such domains. The antiapoptotic factors contain all four domains (BH1 to BH4). The channel forming proapoptotic factors contain just three domains (BH1 to BH3), whereas the proapoptotic BH3 only family members contain just one BH domain, BH3.

The antiapoptotic *Bcl-2*–type proteins (including Bcl-2, Bcl-L, and Bcl-w) have at least two ways of antagonizing death signals. They insert into the outer mitochondrial membrane to antagonize channel-forming proapoptotic factors, thereby decreasing cytochrome c release. They may also bind cytoplasmic Apaf so that it cannot form the apoptosome complex (Fig. 18.16).

These antiapoptotic Bcl-2 proteins are opposed by proapoptotic family members that fall into two categories: ion-channel–forming members and BH3-only members.

TABLE 18.3	Examples of Bcl-2 Family Members

Antiapoptotic
  Bcl-2
  Bcl-x
  Bcl-w
Proapoptotic (Channel-forming)
  Bax
  Bak
  Bok
Proapoptotic (BH3-only)
  Bad
  Bid
  Bim

Roughly 30 Bcl-2 family members are currently known. These proteins play tissue-specific as well as signal pathway–specific roles in regulating apoptosis. The tissue specificity is overlapping. For example, Bcl-2 is expressed in hair follicles, kidney, small intestines, neurons, and the lymphoid system, whereas Bcl-x is expressed in the nervous system and hematopoietic cells.

The pro-death, ion-channel–forming members, such as Bax, are very similar to the antiapoptotic family members, except that they do not contain the binding domain for Apaf. They have the other structural domains, however, and when they dimerize with proapoptotic BH3-only members in the outer mitochondrial membrane, they form an ion channel that promotes cytochrome c release rather than inhibiting it (see Fig. 18.16). The pro-death BH3-only proteins (e.g., Bim and Bid) contain only the structural domain that allows them to bind to other Bcl-2 family members (the BH3 domain), and not the domains for binding to the membrane, forming ion channels, or binding to Apaf. Their binding activates the pro-death family members and inactivates the antiapoptotic members. When the cell receives a signal from a pro-death agonist, a BH3 protein like Bid is activated (see Fig. 18.16). The BH3 protein activates Bax (an ion-channel–forming proapoptotic channel member), which stimulates release of cytochrome c. Normally, Bcl-2 acts as a death antagonist by binding Apaf and keeping it in an inactive state. However, at the same time that Bid is activating Bax, Bid also binds to Bcl-2, thereby disrupting the Bcl-2–Apaf complex and freeing Apaf to bind to released cytochrome c to form the apoptosome.

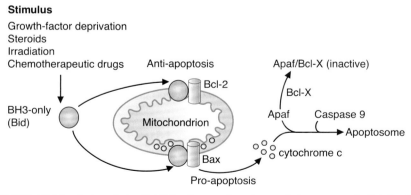

FIGURE 18.16 Roles of the Bcl-2 family members in regulating apoptosis. Bcl-2, which is antiapoptotic, binds Bid (or truncated Bid [tBid]) and blocks formation of channels that allow cytochrome c release from the mitochondria. Death signals result in activation of a BH3-only protein such as Bid, which can lead to mitochondrial pore formation, swelling, and release of cytochrome c. Bid binds to and activates the membrane ion-channel proapoptotic protein Bax, activating cytochrome c release, which binds to Apaf and leads to formation of the apoptosome.

When *Bcl-2* is mutated and oncogenic, it is usually overexpressed; for example, in follicular lymphoma and CML. Overexpression of *Bcl-2* disrupts the normal regulation of pro- and antiapoptotic factors and tips the balance to an antiapoptotic stand. This leads to an inability to destroy cells with damaged DNA, such that mutations can accumulate within the cell. Bcl-2 is also a multidrug-resistant transport protein, and if it is overexpressed, it will block the induction of apoptosis by antitumor agents by rapidly removing them from the cell. Thus, strategies are being developed to reduce Bcl-2 levels in tumors that overexpress it before initiating drug or radiation treatment.

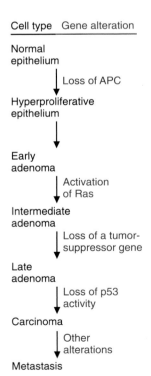

FIGURE 18.17 Possible steps in the development of colon cancer. The changes do not always occur in this order, but the most benign tumors have the lowest frequency of mutations, and the most malignant have the highest frequency.

B. Cancer Cells Bypass Apoptosis

Apoptosis should be triggered by several stimuli such as withdrawal of growth factors, elevation of p53 in response to DNA damage, monitoring of DNA damage by repair enzymes, or release of TNF or other immune factors. However, mutations in oncogenes can create apoptosis-resistant cells.

One of the ways this occurs is through activation of growth-factor–dependent signaling pathways that inhibit apoptosis, such as the PDGF/Akt/BAD pathway. Nonphosphorylated BAD acts like Bid in promoting apoptosis (see Fig. 18.16). Binding of the platelet-derived growth factor to its receptor activates PI-3 kinase, which phosphorylates and activates the serine–threonine kinase Akt (protein kinase B; see Chapter 11, Section III.B.3). Activation of Akt results in the phosphorylation of the proapoptotic BH3-only protein BAD, which inactivates it. The PDGF/Akt/BAD pathway illustrates the requirement of normal cells for growth-factor stimulation to prevent cell death. One of the features of neoplastic transformation is the loss of growth-factor dependence for survival. The MAP kinase pathway is also involved in regulating apoptosis and sends cell-survival signals. MAP kinase kinase phosphorylates and activates another protein kinase known as *RSK*. Like Akt, RSK phosphorylates BAD and inhibits its activity. Thus, BAD acts as a site of convergence for the PI-3 kinase/Akt and MAP kinase pathways in signaling cell survival. Gain-of-function mutations in the genes that control these pathways, such as *ras*, create apoptosis-resistant cells.

C. MicroRNAs and Apoptosis

Recent work has identified a number of miRNAs which regulate apoptotic factors. Bcl-2, for example, is regulated by at least two miRNAs, designated as miR-15 and miR-16. Expression of these miRNAs will control Bcl-2 (an antiapoptotic factor) levels in the cell. If, for any reason, the expression of these miRNAs is altered, Bcl-2 levels will also be altered, promoting either apoptosis (if Bcl-2 levels decrease) or cell proliferation (if Bcl-2 levels increase). Loss of both of these miRNAs is found in 68% of chronic lymphocytic leukemia (CLL) cells, most often caused by a deletion on chromosome 13q14. Loss of miR-15 and -16 expression would lead to an increase in Bcl-2 levels, favoring increased cell proliferation.

Other miRNA species have been identified which regulate factors involved in apoptosis. miR-21 regulates the expression of the programmed cell death 4 gene (PDCD4). PDCD4 is upregulated during apoptosis and functions to block translation. Loss of miR-21 activity would lead to cell death because PDCD4 would be overexpressed. However, overexpression of miR-21 would be antiapoptotic because PDCD4 expression would be ablated.

The miR-17 cluster regulates the protein kinase B/Akt pathway by modulating the levels of PTEN (the enzyme that converts phosphatidylinositol trisphosphate [PIP$_3$] to phosphatidylinositol bisphosphate [PIP$_2$]), as well as the levels of the E2F family of transcription factors. An upregulation of miR-17, acting as an oncogene, would decrease PTEN levels such that cellular proliferation is favored over apoptosis, resulting from the constant activation of the Akt pathway.

VI. Cancer Requires Multiple Mutations

Cancer takes a long time to develop in humans because multiple genetic alterations are required to transform normal cells into malignant cells (see Fig. 18.1). A single change in one oncogene or tumor-suppressor gene in an individual cell is not adequate for transformation. For example, if cells derived from biopsy specimens of normal cells are not already "immortalized"—that is, able to grow in culture indefinitely—addition of the *ras* oncogene to the cells is not sufficient for transformation. However, additional mutations in a combination of oncogenes—for example, *ras* and *myc*—can result in transformation (Fig. 18.17). Epidemiologists have estimated that four to seven mutations are required for normal cells to be transformed.

Cells accumulate multiple mutations through clonal expansion. When DNA damage occurs in a normally proliferative cell, a population of cells with that mutation is produced. Expansion of the mutated population enormously increases the probability of a second mutation in a cell containing the first mutation. After one or more mutations in proto-oncogenes or tumor-suppressor genes, a cell may proliferate more rapidly in the presence of growth stimuli and with further mutations grow autonomously; that is, independent of normal growth controls. Enhanced growth increases the probability of further mutations. Some families have a strong predisposition to cancer. Individuals in these families have inherited a mutation or deletion of one allele of a tumor-suppressor gene, and as progeny of that cell proliferate, mutations can occur in the second allele, leading to a loss of control of cellular proliferation. These familial cancers include familial retinoblastoma, FAPs of the colon, and multiple endocrine neoplasia (MEN), one form of which involves tumors of the thyroid, parathyroid, and adrenal medulla (MEN type II).

Studies of benign and malignant polyps of the colon show that these tumors have a number of different genetic abnormalities. The incidence of these mutations increases with the level of malignancy. In the early stages, normal cells of the intestinal epithelium proliferate, develop mutations in the *APC* gene, and polyps develop (see Fig. 18.17). This change is associated with a mutation in the *ras* proto-oncogene that converts it to an active oncogene. Progression to the next stage is associated with a deletion or alteration of a tumor-suppressor gene on chromosome 5. Subsequently, mutations occur in chromosome 18, inactivating a gene that may be involved in cell adhesion, and in chromosome 17, inactivating the *p53* tumor-suppressor gene. The cells become malignant, and further mutations result in growth that is more aggressive and metastatic. This sequence of mutations is not always followed precisely, but an accumulation of mutations in these genes is found in a large percentage of colon carcinomas.

 Michael T. had been smoking for 40 years before he developed lung cancer. The fact that cancer takes so long to develop has made it difficult to prove that the carcinogens in cigarette smoke cause lung cancer. Studies in England and Wales show that cigarette consumption by men began to increase in the early 1900s. After a 20-year lag, the incidence in lung cancer in men also began to rise. Women began smoking later, in the 1920s. Again, the incidence of lung cancer began to increase after a 20-year lag.

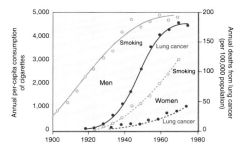

VII. At the Molecular Level, Cancer Is Many Different Diseases

More than 20% of the deaths in the United States each year are caused by cancer, with tumors of the lung, large intestine, and breast being the most common (Fig. 18.18). Different cell types typically use different mechanisms through which they lose the ability to control their own growth. An examination of the genes involved in the

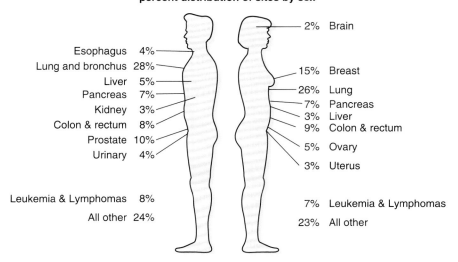

2014 Estimated cancer deaths, United States percent distribution of sites by sex

Esophagus 4%
Lung and bronchus 28%
Liver 5%
Pancreas 7%
Kidney 3%
Colon & rectum 8%
Prostate 10%
Urinary 4%

Leukemia & Lymphomas 8%
All other 24%

2% Brain
15% Breast
26% Lung
7% Pancreas
3% Liver
9% Colon & rectum
5% Ovary
3% Uterus

7% Leukemia & Lymphomas
23% All other

FIGURE 18.18 Estimated cancer deaths by site and sex. (Data from the American Cancer Society, Inc. *Cancer Facts and Figures, 2014.* www.cancer.org/research/cancerfactsstatistics /cancerfactsfigures2014/.).

A treatment for CML based on rational drug design has been developed. The fusion protein Bcr-Abl is found only in transformed cells that express the Philadelphia chromosome and not in normal cells. Once the structure of Bcr-Abl was determined, the drug imatinib (Gleevec) was designed to specifically bind to and inhibit only the active site of the fusion protein and not the normal protein. Imatinib was successful in blocking Bcr-Abl function, thereby stopping cell proliferation, and in some cells inducing apoptosis, so the cells would die. Because normal cells do not express the hybrid protein, they were not affected by the drug. The problem with this treatment is that some patients suffered relapses, and when their Bcr-Abl proteins were studied it was found that in some patients, the fusion protein had a single amino acid substitution near the active site that prevented imatinib from binding to the protein. Other patients had an amplification of the Bcr-Abl gene product. Other TKIs (such as dasatinib and nilotnib) can also be used in treating CML if a resistance to imatinib (Gleevec) is encountered.

development of cancer shows that a particular type of cancer can arise in multiple ways. For example, Patched and Smoothened are the receptor and coreceptor for the signaling peptide sonic hedgehog. Either mutation of *smoothened*, an oncogene, or inactivation of *patched*, a tumor-suppressor gene, can give rise to basal cell carcinoma. Similarly, TGF-β and its signal transduction proteins Smad4/DPC are part of the same growth-inhibiting pathway, and either may be absent in colon cancer. Thus, treatments that are successful for one patient with colon cancer may not be successful in a second patient with colon cancer because of the differences in the molecular basis of each individual's disease (this now appears to be the case with breast cancer as well). Medical practice in the future will require identifying the molecular lesions involved in a particular disease and developing appropriate treatments accordingly. The use of proteomics, RNA-SEQ, and gene chip technology (see Chapter 17) to genotype tumor tissues, and to understand which proteins they express, will aid greatly in allowing patient-specific treatments to be developed.

VIII. Viruses and Human Cancer

Three RNA retroviruses are associated with the development of cancer in humans: human T-lymphotrophic virus type 1 (HTLV-1), HIV, and hepatitis C. There are also DNA viruses associated with cancer, such as hepatitis B, EBV, human papillomavirus (HPV), and herpesvirus (HHV-8).

HTLV-1 causes adult T-cell leukemia. The HTLV-1 genome encodes a protein, Tax, which is a transcriptional coactivator. The cellular proto-oncogenes *c-sis* and *c-fos* are activated by Tax, thereby altering the normal controls on cellular proliferation and leading to malignancy. Thus, *tax* is a viral oncogene without a counterpart in the host-cell genome.

Infection with HIV, the virus that causes AIDS, leads to the development of neoplastic disease through several mechanisms. HIV infection leads to immunosuppression and, consequently, loss of immune-mediated tumor surveillance. HIV-infected individuals are predisposed to non-Hodgkin lymphoma, which results from an overproduction of T-cell lymphocytes. The HIV genome encodes a protein, Tat, a transcription factor that activates transcription of the *interleukin-6* (IL-6) and *interleukin-10* (IL-10) genes in infected T-cells. IL-6 and IL-10 are growth factors that promote proliferation of T-cells, and thus, their increased production may contribute to the development of non-Hodgkin lymphoma. Tat can also be released from infected cells and act as an angiogenic (blood vessel–forming) growth factor. This property is thought to contribute to the development of Kaposi sarcoma.

DNA viruses also cause human cancer, but by different mechanisms. Chronic hepatitis B infections will lead to hepatocellular carcinoma. A vaccine currently is available to prevent hepatitis B infections. EBV is associated with B- and T-cell lymphomas, Hodgkin disease, and other tumors. The EBV encodes a Bcl-2 protein that restricts apoptosis of the infected cell. HHV-8 has been associated with Kaposi sarcoma. Certain strains of papillomavirus are the major cause of cervical cancer, and a vaccine has been developed against those specific papillomavirus strains.

CLINICAL COMMENTS

Mannie W. The treatment of a symptomatic patient with CML whose white blood cell count is in excess of 50,000 cells/mL is initiated with a tyrosine kinase inhibitor (TKI). If one type is not tolerated or successful, another one is tried. In addition, both γ- and β-interferon have shown promise in increasing survival in these patients if they are intolerant to the TKI. Interestingly, the interferons have been associated with the disappearance of the Philadelphia chromosome in dividing marrow cells of some patients treated in this way. Hematopoietic stem cell transplantation can also be an option for treatment.

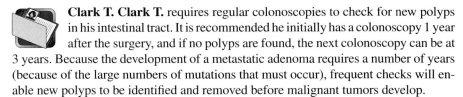 **Michael T.** Surgical resection of the lung nodule with an attempt at cure was justified in **Michael T.**, who had a good prognosis with a T_1,N_0,M_0 staging classification preoperatively. Because of his history and the characteristics of the nodule, there was a high probability it was a malignant nodule and a preoperative positron emission tomography (PET) scan did not show obvious signs of metastasis.

Unfortunately, Michael developed a metastatic lesion in the right temporal cortex of his brain 6 months later. Because metastases were almost certainly present in other organs, Michael's brain tumor was not treated surgically. In spite of palliative radiation therapy to the brain, **Michael T.** succumbed to his disease just 9 months after its discovery, an unusually virulent course for this malignancy. On postmortem examination, it was found that his body was riddled with metastatic disease.

 The TNM system is a cancer staging system that standardizes the classification of tumors. The T stands for the size and extent of the primary tumor (the higher number stands for a larger and more extensive tumor), the N stands for the amount of regional lymph nodes that are affected by the tumor (again, the higher the number, the worse the prognosis), and M stands for the presence of metastasis (0 for none, 1 for the presence of metastatic cells).

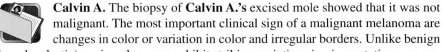 **Clark T. Clark T.** requires regular colonoscopies to check for new polyps in his intestinal tract. It is recommended he initially has a colonoscopy 1 year after the surgery, and if no polyps are found, the next colonoscopy can be at 3 years. Because the development of a metastatic adenoma requires a number of years (because of the large numbers of mutations that must occur), frequent checks will enable new polyps to be identified and removed before malignant tumors develop.

 Calvin A. The biopsy of **Calvin A.'s** excised mole showed that it was not malignant. The most important clinical sign of a malignant melanoma are changes in color or variation in color and irregular borders. Unlike benign (nondysplastic) nevi, melanomas exhibit striking variations in pigmentation, appearing in shades of black, brown, red, dark blue, and gray. Additional clinical warning signs of a melanoma are enlargement of a preexisting mole, itching or pain in a preexisting mole, or development of a new pigmented lesion during adult life. **Calvin A.** was advised to conduct a monthly self-examination, to have a clinical skin examination once or twice yearly, to avoid sunlight, and to use appropriate sunscreens.

Mutations associated with malignant melanomas include ras (gain of function in growth signal-transduction oncogene), p53 (loss of function of tumor-suppressor gene), p16 (loss of function in *cdk* inhibitor tumor-suppressor gene), cdk4 (gain of function in a cell-cycle progression oncogene), and cadherin/β-catenin regulation (loss of regulation that requires attachment).

BIOCHEMICAL COMMENTS

HNPCC and hereditary breast cancer both result from inherited mutations in genes involved in DNA repair.

HNPCC is estimated to account for between 2% and 3% of all colon cancer cases. These syndromes are heterogeneous, most likely owing to the finding that mutations in any of five genes could lead to colon cancer. The disease genes include *hMSH2*, *hMLH1*, *hPMS1*, *hPMS2*, and *hMSH6*. These genes all play a role in DNA mismatch repair, and all act as tumor suppressors (a loss of function is required for the tumor to develop).

It is important to understand that the lack of a DNA mismatch repair enzyme actually does not directly lead to cancer (such as an activating mutation in *myc* would do, for example). However, the lack of a functional mismatch repair system increases the frequency at which new mutations are introduced into somatic cells (particularly rapidly proliferating cells such as the colonic epithelium), such that eventually a mutation will result in a gene necessary for proper growth control. Once that mutation occurs, tumors can begin to develop.

Five percent to 10% of all breast cancer cases have been traced to inherited mutations in either one of two genes, *BRCA1* and *BRCA2*. *BRCA1* maps to chromosome 17 and acts as a tumor suppressor. The biochemical function of *BRCA1* is to participate in the response to DNA damage. *BRCA1* is phosphorylated by a variety of kinases, each of which is activated by a different form of DNA damage. *BRCA1* is primarily involved in repairing double-strand breaks in DNA, and in transcription-coupled repair. Once *BRCA1* is phosphorylated, it will signal for cell cycle arrest in order to allow the DNA damage to be repaired.

Women who carry a *BRCA1* mutation have a 55% to 65% risk of developing breast cancer, and about a 40% risk of ovarian cancer, by the age of 70 years. Men who carry *BRCA1* mutations have been shown to have a slight increase in breast cancer and prostate cancer.

The other gene involved in hereditary breast cancer is *BRCA2*, located on chromosome 13. *BRCA2* is required for DNA double-strand break repair, which is usually caused by ionizing radiation. As such, loss of *BRCA2* activity is required for cancer to develop, classifying *BRCA2* as a tumor suppressor. *BRCA2* is also required for homologous recombination between sister chromatids during meiosis and mitosis. *BRCA2* mutations have also been liked to increased incidence of breast and ovarian cancer in women, and breast cancer and prostate cancer in men. *BRCA1* and *BRCA2* mutations account for about 20% to 25% of all hereditary breast cancer cases.

An understanding of the roles of *BRCA1* and *BRCA2* in repairing double-strand breaks in DNA has led to the development of poly(ADP-ribose) polymerase 1 (PARP-1) inhibitors for the treatment of *BRCA1*- or *BRCA2*-induced breast cancers. Double-strand break repair occurs either by homologous recombination (requiring the activities of *BRCA1* and *BRCA2* proteins) or through nonhomologous end joining (NHEJ), which is an error-prone process, owing to trimming of the DNA ends before ligation.

Single-strand breaks in DNA are more common than double-strand breaks. The cellular mechanism for repairing single-strand breaks is dependent on PARP-1. PARP-1 produces large branched chains of poly(ADP-ribose), derived from NAD^+, at the site of damage, which acts as a docking station for proteins involved in repairing the single-strand break. Inhibiting PARP-1 would lead to an accumulation of single-strand breaks in the DNA.

PARP-1 inhibitors are effective in killing *BRCA1* or *BRCA2* mutated cells in that when single-strand breaks are not repaired, they often are converted to double-strand breaks when the replisome tries to replicate through the break. In a cell lacking *BRCA1* or *BRCA2* activity, the only way the DNA can be repaired is by NHEJ, which is an error-prone process. This leads to the cells accumulating a large number of mutations, eventually leading to cell death. Cells with functional *BRCA1* or *BRCA2* activity will not undergo that fate. Drugs which inhibit PARP-1 activity in cell culture are now in clinical trials, with very promising results.

KEY CONCEPTS

- *Cancer* is the term applied to a group of diseases in which cells no longer respond to normal constraints on growth.
- Cancer arises owing to mutations in the genome (either inherited or formed in somatic cells).
- The mutations that lead to cancer occur in certain classes of genes, including:
  - Those that regulate cellular proliferation and differentiation
  - Those that suppress growth
  - Those that target cells for apoptosis
  - Those that repair damaged DNA
- Mutations that lead to cancer can be either gain-of-function mutations or loss of activity within a protein.
  - Gain-of-function mutations occur in proto-oncogenes, resulting in oncogenes.
  - Loss-of-function mutations occur in tumor-suppressor genes.
- Examples of proto-oncogenes are those involved in signal transduction and cell cycle progression:
  - Growth factors and growth-factor receptors
  - Ras (a GTP-binding protein)
  - Transcription factors
  - Cyclins and proteins that regulate them
  - microRNAs which regulate growth-inhibitory proteins
- Examples of tumor-suppressor genes include the following:
  - Retinoblastoma (Rb) gene product, which regulates the G_1-to-S phase of the cell cycle
  - p53, which monitors DNA damage and arrests cell-cycle progression until the damage has been repaired

- Regulators of *ras*
- microRNAs that regulate growth-promoting signals
- Apoptosis (programmed cell death) leads to the destruction of damaged cells that cannot be repaired, and it consists of three phases:
  - Initiation phase (external signals or mitochondrial release of cytochrome c)
  - Signal integration phase
  - Execution phase
- Apoptosis is regulated by a group of proteins of the Bcl-2 family, which consists of both pro- and antiapoptotic factors.
- Cancer cells have developed mechanisms to avoid apoptosis.
- Multiple mutations are required for a tumor to develop in a patient, acquired over a number of years.
- Both RNA and DNA viruses can cause a normal cell to become transformed.
- Exploitation of DNA repair mechanisms may provide a novel means for regulating tumor cell growth.
- The diseases discussed in this chapter are summarized in Table 18.4.

TABLE 18.4   Diseases Discussed in Chapter 18

DISEASE OR DISORDER	ENVIRONMENTAL OR GENETIC	COMMENTS
Chronic myelogenous leukemia	Environmental	Chromosomal translocation leading to the novel Bcr-Abl protein being produced, leading to uncontrolled cell growth. Rational drug design has led to Bcr-Abl targeted agents, such as imatinib, which have a high rate of initial success in controlling tumor cell proliferation.
Lung adenocarcinoma	Environmental	Lung tumor caused by inhalation of mutagenic compounds over a number of years. Longitudinal data indicates a 20-year lag from the initiation of smoking and a rise in cancer incidence in such individuals.
Intestinal adenocarcinoma	Both	Colon tumors may result from environmental insult, leading to mutations, or an inherited mutation in a tumor-suppressor gene such as *APC*. Hereditary nonpolyposis colon cancer (HNPCC) is caused by inherited mutations in proteins involved in DNA mismatch repair.
Melanoma	Environmental	Tumor of the melanocyte, leading to uncontrolled cell growth. Mutations associated with malignant melanomas include *ras*, *p53*, *p16* (a regulator of Cdk4), *cdk4*, and cadherin/β-catenin regulation.
Burkitt lymphoma	Environmental	Disorder caused by a chromosomal translocation, in this case chromosomes 8 and 14, leading to the transcription factor *myc* being moved from chromosome 8 to 14. This leads to inappropriate and over expression of *c-myc*, leading to uncontrolled cell proliferation.
Li-Fraumeni syndrome	Genetic	An inherited mutation in the protein p53, which is responsible for protecting the genome against environmental damage. Lose of p53 activity will lead to an increased mutation rate, eventually leading to a mutation in a gene that regulates cell proliferation.
Neurofibromatosis	Genetic	A mutation in a protein (neurofibromin-1 [NF-1]) that regulates the GTPase activity of *ras*, which leads to numerous benign tumors of the nervous system.

1. The *ras* oncogene in **Clark T.'s** malignant polyp differs from the *c-ras* proto-oncogene only in the region that encodes the *N* terminus of the protein. This portion of the normal and mutant sequences is as follows:

```
              10            20            30
Normal  ATGACGGAATATAAGCTGGTGGTGGTGGGCGCCGGCGGT
Mutant  ATGACGGAATATAAGCTGGTGGTGGTGGGCGCCGTCGGT
```

This mutation is similar to the mutation found in the *ras* oncogene in various tumors. What type of mutation converts the *ras* proto-oncogene to an oncogene?
   A. An insertion that disrupts the reading frame of the protein
   B. A deletion that disrupts the reading frame of the protein
   C. A missense mutation that changes one amino acid within the protein
   D. A silent mutation that produces no change in the amino acid sequence of the protein
   E. An early termination that creates a stop codon in the reading frame of the protein

2. The mechanism through which Ras becomes an oncogenic protein is which one of the following?
   A. Ras remains bound to GAP.
   B. Ras can no longer bind cAMP.
   C. Ras has lost its GTPase activity.
   D. Ras can no longer bind GTP.
   E. Ras can no longer be phosphorylated by MAP kinase.

3. The ability of a normal cell to become a cancer cell can occur via a variety of mechanisms. Which one of the following best describes such a mechanism?
   A. Tumors arise via the acquisition of the ability to metabolize glucose at a faster rate than noncancer cells.
   B. Clonal expansion allows for a cell with a single mutation to become a cancer cell.
   C. Mutations in proto-oncogenes can lead to uncontrolled cell growth.
   D. Virtually all tumors arise via recombination events, leading to the formation of unusual and novel genes.
   E. Normal cellular oncogenes are mutated to proto-oncogenes, which leads to uncontrolled cellular proliferation.

4. Loss of both p53 protein alleles is found in >50% of human tumors. Which one of the following is a function of the p53 protein?
   A. Halting replication in cells that have suffered DNA damage
   B. Targeting repaired cells to undergo apoptosis
   C. Stimulating cyclin production
   D. Stimulating CDK production
   E. Stimulating phosphorylation of Rb

5. A tumor-suppressor gene is best described by which one of the following?
   A. A gain-of-function mutation leads to uncontrolled proliferation.
   B. A loss-of-function mutation leads to uncontrolled proliferation.
   C. When it is expressed, the gene suppresses viral genes from being expressed.
   D. When it is expressed, the gene specifically blocks the G_1/S checkpoint.
   E. When it is expressed, the gene induces tumor formation.

6. A tumor cell, owing to accumulated mutations, constitutively expresses the Akt pathway. Such cells bypass apoptosis because of which one of the following?
   A. Increased expression of cytochrome c
   B. Phosphorylation of BH3-only domain-containing proteins
   C. Phosphorylation of Bcl-2
   D. Increased expression of Apaf
   E. Decreased expression of caspases
   F. Phosphorylation of caspases

7. Inheriting a mutation in an enzyme necessary for DNA mismatch repair requires which one of the following to occur before a cell loses its ability to regulate its own proliferation?
   A. A mutation in *BRCA1* or *BRCA2*
   B. A mutation in the PDGF receptor
   C. A mutation on one *p53* gene
   D. A mutation in the *ras* gene
   E. A mutation in the corresponding normal allele

8. A tumor was found in which altered expression of a miRNA led to uncontrolled cellular proliferation. If the target of this miRNA was the Myc protein, how best would this miRNA be characterized?
   A. As an oncogene
   B. As a dominant-negative effector
   C. As a tumor suppressor
   D. As a factor that upregulates its target
   E. As a regulatory factor for an enzyme important in DNA repair

9. A 3-year-old girl is seen by a pediatric ophthalmologist because of reduced vision within her left eye. The doctor soon detects a mass growing within the eye, which is blocking her vision. Analysis of DNA from the girl's blood cells indicates a mutation in a tumor-suppressor gene which, when mutated, most often leads to tumor formation within the eyes. Which one of the following is a description of how this tumor-suppressor gene regulates the cell cycle?
   A. It encodes for a cyclin.
   B. In encodes for a CDK.

C. It encodes for a CKI.

D. It encodes a protein that regulates the transition from G_0 to G_1 phase in the cell cycle.

E. It encodes a protein that regulates the transition from G_1 to S phase in the cell cycle.

10. An individual has been diagnosed with hereditary diffuse type stomach cancer, in which rather than being located in one area of the stomach, the tumor is located in many areas of the stomach. A mutation in which one of the following proteins would lead to such a disorder?

A. p53 protein

B. NF-1

C. *Rb* gene

D. Cadherins

E. Caspases

ANSWERS

1. **The answer is C.** The *ras* oncogene has a point mutation in codon 12 (position 35 of the DNA chain) in which T replaces G. This changes the codon from one that specifies glycine to one that specifies valine. Thus, there is a single amino acid change in the proto-oncogene (a valine for a glycine) that changes *ras* to an oncogene.

2. **The answer is C.** Ras, when it is oncogenic, has lost its GTPase activity and thus remains active for a longer time. Answer A is incorrect because GAP proteins activate the GTPase activity of Ras and this mutation would make Ras less active. cAMP does not interact directly with Ras (thus, B is incorrect), and if Ras could no longer bind GTP, it would not be active (hence, D is also incorrect). Ras is not phosphorylated by the MAP kinase (thus, E is incorrect).

3. **The answer is C.** Cancers develop from mutations in normal cellular genes (the proto-oncogenes) that convert the genes to oncogenes. The oncogenes then alter cellular proliferation because they are not regulated in the same way as their corresponding proto-oncogene. Whereas a small number of tumors use recombination events to create a novel gene, this is not the usual mechanism for most tumors to develop. The proto-oncogenes need multiple mutations (4 to 7) for full transformation into oncogenes (clonal expansion of just a single mutation is usually not sufficient to form a tumor in vivo).

4. **The answer is A.** The p53 protein is a transcription factor that regulates the cell cycle and apoptosis. It has been named the "guardian of the genome" because it halts DNA replication in cells that have suffered DNA damage and, if the damage is too difficult to repair, targets such cells for apoptosis. Repaired cells are not targeted for apoptosis by p53. The p53 protein stimulates production of proteins that inhibit cyclin–CDK complexes, which prevents the phosphorylation of Rb and stops cells from further replicating their DNA.

5. **The answer is B.** Tumor-suppressor genes balance cell growth and quiescence. When they are not expressed (via loss-of-function mutations), the balance shifts to cell proliferation and tumorigenesis (thus, A is incorrect). Answer C is incorrect because tumor-suppressor genes do not act on viral genes, answer D is incorrect because tumor-suppressor genes are not specifically targeted to just one aspect of the cell cycle, and answer E is incorrect because a loss of expression of tumor-suppressor genes leads to tumor formation, not expression of these genes.

6. **The answer is B.** Growth factor deprivation can lead to apoptosis owing to the action of BH3-only domain members of the Bcl-2 family of proteins. The BH3-only domain proteins dimerize with channel-forming proteins in the outer mitochondrial membrane, allowing cytochrome c to leave the mitochondria and bind to Apaf, to form the apoptosome to initiate the apoptotic pathway. Growth factors, via activation of the Akt/protein kinase B pathway, lead to the phosphorylation of the BH3-only domain proteins and inactivate them, such that apoptosis is blocked. Because the cell in question is always expressing active Akt, the cell will be in a constant antiapoptotic state. Increased expression of cytochrome c will not lead to apoptosis or cell growth; it will not affect cellular proliferation. Bcl-2 is an antiapoptotic factor, but it is not phosphorylated by the Akt pathway. Increased expression of Apaf might lead to apoptosis if cytochrome c were released; its increased expression would not lead to uncontrolled cellular proliferation. Decreased expression of caspases would hinder apoptosis, but the Akt pathway does not alter the expression level of these proteases. Caspases are also not phosphorylated by Akt.

7. **The answer is E.** In order for a mutation in a DNA mismatch repair enzyme to be fully manifest, both alleles that code for this protein must be mutated; otherwise, 50% of the protein made would be functional, and that is often sufficient to allow for normal DNA repair. Mutating the corresponding normal allele would reduce the functional enzyme level to zero, and the lack of mismatch repair would eventually lead to mutations in genes involved in growth regulation, resulting in uncontrolled cellular proliferation. Mutations in *BRCA1* or *BRCA2* involve DNA repair of double-strand breaks, not mismatches. A mutation in the PDGF receptor may lead to transformation as a dominant oncogene, but it does not affect mismatch repair. A mutation in a *p53* gene would have no effect because *p53* is also a tumor

suppressor, and both copies of *p53* would need to be mutated for a tumor to develop. A mutation in *p53* would not, in combination with one mutation in a mismatch repair gene, lead to uncontrolled proliferation. A mutation in the *ras* gene, by itself, would lead to uncontrolled cellular proliferation because *ras* is a dominant oncogene, but the mechanism would not be by inability to repair DNA mismatches.

8. **The answer is C.** If *myc*, a proto-oncogene, is overexpressed, increased cell proliferation would result. One way *myc* could be overexpressed is if the miRNA regulating its expression were no longer expressed. In that case, *myc* mRNA levels would increase, and *myc* would be inappropriately expressed in the cell. For this to occur, the miRNA would have a loss of function, which is what defines a tumor-suppressor gene. The miRNA is downregulating, not upregulating, the expression of *myc*. A gain of function (such as overexpression of the miRNA) would define an oncogene. The miRNA is not acting as a dominant-negative effector, which is when one mutated copy of a protein (or RNA) interferes with the functioning of a functional protein produced by a normal allele. Myc is a transcription factor and not an enzyme needed for DNA repair.

9. **The answer is E.** The girl has retinoblastoma, which is caused by a mutation in the *Rb* gene, which is a tumor suppressor. The normal Rb protein binds to the E2F family of transcription factors, and when it does, transcription is inhibited. Phosphorylation of the Rb protein by cyclin–CDK complexes at the G_1/S interface of the cell cycle inactivates Rb, it dissociates from E2F, and transcription is now initiated, allowing cells to enter the S phase of the cycle. Because the mutation is in a tumor-suppressor gene, a loss of function is leading to tumor growth. Loss of Rb function leads to constant E2F activity, and the cell is always stimulated to proliferate (the checks and balances at the G_1/S boundary are lost). Loss of function of a cyclin, or a CDK, would stop cell growth (mutations in those genes would need to be gain-of-function mutations in order for a tumor to form). The CKIs are inhibitors, and loss of their function could lead to tumor growth, but such mutations would not be specific for retinoblastoma, as are mutations in the Rb protein.

10. **The answer is D.** Cadherins are membrane-bound glycoproteins involved in intracellular adhesion. Loss of function of a specific cadherin (E-cadherin) allows cell migration within the stomach, owing to the loss of intracellular adhesion. This allows tumor cells to leave their site of origin and move to other areas within the stomach (giving rise to the diffuse type of cancer found). p53 proteins and the Rb protein help regulate cell-cycle completion and cell reproduction, but these proteins do not regulate the ability of tumor cells to migrate. The protein produced by the *NF-1* gene (neurofibromin) binds to Ras and activates its GTPase activity, thereby reducing the amount of time that Ras is in its active state. Caspases are cysteine proteases involved in the apoptotic response.

Carbohydrate Metabolism, Fuel Oxidation, and the Generation of Adenosine Triphosphate

Glucose is central to all of metabolism. It is the universal fuel for human cells and the source of carbon for the synthesis of most other compounds. Every human cell type uses glucose to obtain energy. The release of insulin and glucagon by the pancreas aids in the body's use and storage of glucose. Other dietary sugars (mainly fructose and galactose) are converted to glucose or to intermediates of glucose metabolism.

Glucose is the precursor for the synthesis of an array of other sugars that are required for the production of specialized compounds such as lactose, cell surface antigens, nucleotides, or glycosaminoglycans. Glucose is also the fundamental precursor of noncarbohydrate compounds; it can be converted to lipids (including fatty acids, cholesterol, and steroid hormones), amino acids, and nucleic acids. Only those compounds that are synthesized from vitamins, essential amino acids, and essential fatty acids cannot be synthesized from glucose in humans.

All physiologic processes in living cells require energy transformation. Cells convert the chemical bond energy in foods into other forms, such as an electrochemical gradient across the plasma membrane, or the movement of muscle fibers in an arm, or assembly of complex molecules such as DNA. These energy transformations can be divided into three principal phases: (1) oxidation of fuels (fat, carbohydrate, and protein), (2) conversion of energy from fuel oxidation into the high-energy phosphate bonds of adenosine triphosphate (ATP), and (3) use of ATP phosphate bond energy to drive energy-requiring processes.

More than 40% of the calories in the typical diet in the United States are obtained from starch, sucrose, and lactose. These dietary carbohydrates are converted to glucose, galactose, and fructose in the digestive tract (Fig. IV.1). Monosaccharides are absorbed from the intestine, enter the blood, and travel to the tissues, where they are metabolized.

After glucose is transported into cells, it is phosphorylated by a hexokinase to form glucose 6-phosphate. Glucose 6-phosphate can then enter a number of metabolic pathways. The three that are common to all cell types are glycolysis, the pentose phosphate pathway, and glycogen synthesis (Fig. IV.2). In tissues, fructose and galactose are converted to intermediates of glucose metabolism. Thus, the fate of these sugars parallels that of glucose (Fig. IV.3).

The major fate of glucose 6-phosphate is oxidation via the pathway of glycolysis (see Chapter 22), which provides a source of ATP (the major energy currency of the cell) for all cell types. Cells that lack mitochondria cannot oxidize other fuels. They produce ATP from anaerobic glycolysis (the conversion of glucose to lactic acid). Cells that contain mitochondria oxidize glucose to CO_2 and H_2O via glycolysis and the tricarboxylic acid (TCA) cycle (Fig. IV.4). Some tissues, such as the brain, depend on the oxidation of glucose to CO_2 and H_2O for energy because they have a limited capacity to use other fuels. The oxidation of fuels to generate

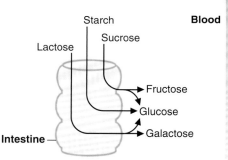

FIGURE IV.1 Overview of carbohydrate digestion. The major carbohydrates of the diet (starch, lactose, and sucrose) are digested to produce monosaccharides (glucose, fructose, and galactose), which enter the blood.

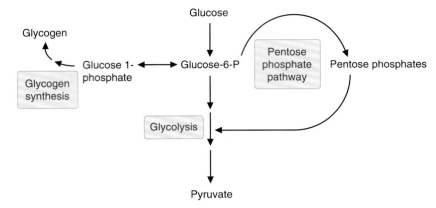

FIGURE IV.2   Major pathways of glucose metabolism.

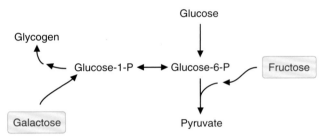

FIGURE IV.3   Overview of fructose and galactose metabolism. Fructose and galactose are converted to intermediates of glucose metabolism.

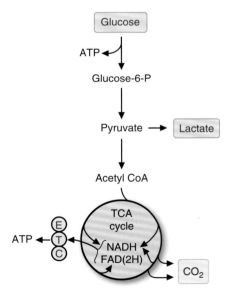

FIGURE IV.4   Conversion of glucose to lactate or to CO_2. *Acetyl CoA*, acetyl coenzyme A; *ETC*, electron-transport chain; *FAD(2H)*, reduced flavin adenine dinucleotide; *NADH*, reduced nicotinamide adenine dinucleotide; *TCA*, tricarboxylic acid.

ATP requires electron transfer through components of the inner mitochondrial membrane known as the *electron-transport chain* (ETC).

Glucose produces the intermediates of glycolysis and the TCA cycle that are used for the synthesis of amino acids and both the glycerol and fatty acid moieties of triacylglycerols (Fig. IV.5).

Another important fate of glucose 6-phosphate is oxidation via the pentose phosphate pathway, which generates nicotinamide adenine dinucleotide phosphate (NADPH). The reducing equivalents of NADPH are used for biosynthetic reactions and for the prevention of oxidative damage to cells (see Chapter 25). In this pathway, glucose undergoes oxidation and decarboxylation to five-carbon sugars (pentoses), which may reenter the glycolytic pathway. They also may be used for nucleotide synthesis (Fig. IV.6). There are also nonoxidative reactions, which can interconvert six- and five-carbon sugars.

Glucose 6-phosphate is also converted to UDP-glucose, which has many functions in the cell (Fig. IV.7). The major fate of UDP-glucose is the synthesis of glycogen, the storage polymer of glucose. Although most cells have glycogen to provide emergency supplies of glucose, the largest stores are in muscle and liver. Muscle glycogen is used to generate ATP during muscle contraction. Liver glycogen is used to maintain blood glucose during fasting and during exercise or periods of enhanced need. UDP-glucose is also used for the formation of other sugars, and galactose and glucose are interconverted while attached to UDP. UDP-galactose is used for lactose synthesis in the mammary gland. In the liver, UDP-glucose is oxidized to UDP-glucuronate, which is used to convert bilirubin and other toxic compounds to glucuronides for excretion (see Fig. IV.7).

Nucleotide sugars are also used for the synthesis of proteoglycans, glycoproteins, and glycolipids (see Fig. IV.7). Proteoglycans are major carbohydrate components of the extracellular matrix, cartilage, and extracellular fluids (such as the synovial fluid of joints), and they are discussed in more detail in Chapter 47.

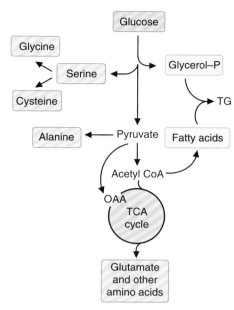

FIGURE IV.5 Conversion of glucose to amino acids and to the glycerol and fatty acid (FA) moieties of triacylglycerols (TG). *Acetyl CoA*, acetyl coenzyme A; *Glycerol-P*, glycerol 3-phosphate; *OAA*, oxaloacetate; *TCA*, tricarboxylic acid.

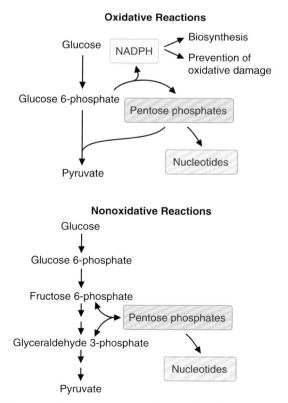

FIGURE IV.6 Overview of the pentose phosphate pathway. The oxidative reactions generate both reduced nicotinamide adenine dinucleotide phosphate (NADPH) and pentose phosphates. The nonoxidative reactions generate only pentose phosphates.

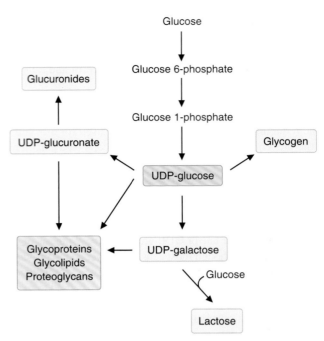

FIGURE IV.7 Products derived from uridine diphosphate (UDP)-glucose.

Most extracellular proteins are glycoproteins; that is, they contain covalently attached carbohydrates. For cell membrane glycoproteins and for glycolipids, the carbohydrate portion extends into the extracellular space.

All cells are continuously supplied with glucose under normal circumstances; the body maintains a relatively narrow range of glucose concentration in the blood (~70 to 100 mg/dL) in spite of the changes in dietary supply and tissue demand as we sleep and exercise. This process is called glucose homeostasis. Low blood glucose levels (hypoglycemia) are prevented by a release of glucose from the large glycogen stores in the liver (glycogenolysis); by synthesis of glucose from lactate, glycerol, and amino acids in liver (gluconeogenesis) (Fig. IV.8); and to a limited extent by a release of fatty acids from adipose tissue stores (lipolysis) to provide an alternate fuel when glucose is in short supply. High blood glucose levels (hyperglycemia) are prevented both by the conversion of glucose to glycogen and by its conversion to triacylglycerols in liver and adipose tissue. Thus, the pathways for glucose use as a fuel cannot be considered as totally separate from pathways involving amino acid and fatty acid metabolism (Fig. IV.9).

Intertissue balance in the use and storage of glucose during fasting and feeding is accomplished principally by the actions of the hormones of metabolic homeostasis—insulin and glucagon (Fig. IV.10). However, cortisol, epinephrine, norepinephrine, and other hormones are also involved in intertissue adjustments of supply and demand in response to changes of physiologic state.

The oxidation of our food is an energy-generating process. The first two phases of energy transformation are part of *cellular respiration*, the overall process of using O_2 and energy derived from oxidizing fuels to generate ATP. We need to breathe principally because our cells require O_2 to generate adequate amounts of ATP from the oxidation of fuels to CO_2. Cellular respiration uses >90% of the O_2 we inhale.

In phase 1 of respiration, energy is conserved from fuel oxidation by enzymes that transfer electrons from the fuels to the electron-accepting coenzymes nicotinamide adenine dinucleotide (NAD^+) and flavin adenine dinucleotide (FAD), which are reduced to NADH and FAD(2H), respectively (Fig. IV.11). The pathways for the oxidation of most fuels (glucose, fatty acids, ketone bodies, and many amino acids) converge in the generation of the activated 2-carbon acetyl group in acetyl

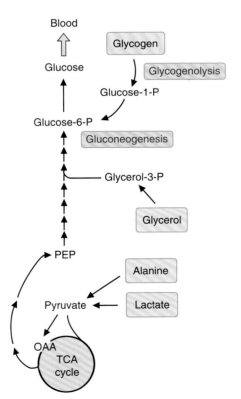

FIGURE IV.8 Production of blood glucose from glycogen (by glycogenolysis) and from alanine, lactate, and glycerol (by gluconeogenesis). *PEP*, phosphoenolpyruvate; *OAA*, oxaloacetate; *TCA*, tricarboxylic acid.

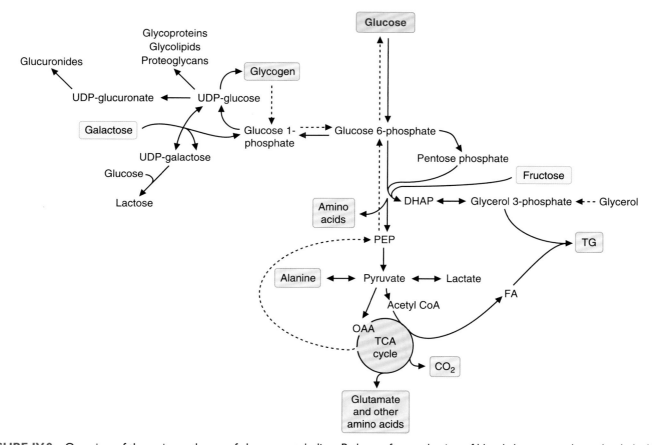

FIGURE IV.9   Overview of the major pathways of glucose metabolism. Pathways for production of blood glucose are shown by *dashed lines.* *Acetyl CoA,* acetyl coenzyme A; *DHAP,* dihydroxyacetone phosphate; *FA,* fatty acids; *OAA,* oxaloacetate; *PEP,* phosphoenolpyruvate; *TCA,* tricarboxylic acid; *TG,* triacylglycerols; *UDP,* uridine diphosphate.

coenzyme A (acetyl-CoA). The complete oxidation of the acetyl group to CO_2 occurs in the TCA cycle, which collects the energy mostly as NADH and FAD(2H).

In phase 2 of cellular respiration, the energy derived from fuel oxidation is converted to the high-energy phosphate bonds of ATP by the process of oxidative phosphorylation (see Fig. IV.11). Electrons are transferred from NADH and FAD(2H) to O_2 by the ETC, a series of electron-transfer proteins that are located in the inner mitochondrial membrane. Oxidation of NADH and FAD(2H) by O_2 generates an electrochemical potential across the inner mitochondrial membrane in the form of a transmembrane proton gradient (Δp). This electrochemical potential drives the synthesis of ATP from adenosine diphosphate (ADP) and inorganic phosphate (P_i) by a transmembrane enzyme called *ATP synthase* (or F_0F_1ATPase).

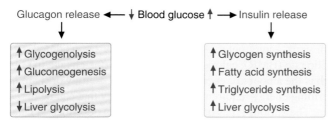

FIGURE IV.10   Pathways regulated by the release of glucagon (in response to a lowering of blood glucose levels) and insulin (released in response to an elevation of blood glucose levels). Tissue-specific differences occur in the response to these hormones, as detailed in the chapters of this section.

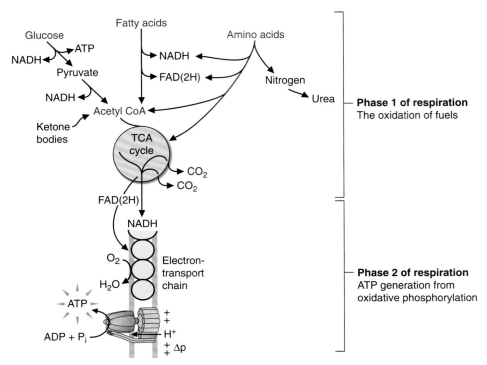

FIGURE IV.11 Cellular respiration. Δp, proton gradient; *Acetyl CoA*, acetyl coenzyme A; *ADP*, adenosine diphosphate; *ATP*, adenosine triphosphate; *FAD(2H)*, reduced flavin adenine dinucleotide; *NADH*, reduced nicotinamide adenine dinucleotide; P_i, inorganic phosphate; *TCA*, tricarboxylic acid.

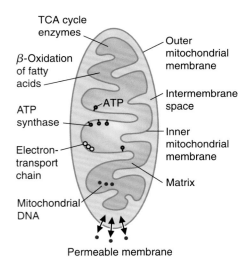

FIGURE IV.12 Oxidative metabolism in mitochondria. The inner mitochondrial membrane forms infoldings, called cristae, which enclose the mitochondrial matrix. Most of the enzymes for the tricarboxylic acid (TCA) cycle, the β-oxidation of fatty acids, and for mitochondrial DNA synthesis are found in the matrix. Adenosine triphosphate (ATP) synthase and the protein complexes of the electron-transport chain are embedded in the inner mitochondrial membrane. The outer mitochondrial membrane is permeable to small ions, but the inner mitochondrial membrane is impermeable to almost all molecules.

In phase 3 of cellular respiration, the high-energy phosphate bonds of ATP are used for processes such as muscle contraction (mechanical work), maintaining low intracellular Na^+ concentrations (transport work), synthesis of larger molecules such as DNA in anabolic pathways (biosynthetic work), or detoxification (biochemical work). As a consequence of these processes, ATP is either directly or indirectly hydrolyzed to ADP and P_i, or to AMP and pyrophosphate (PP_i).

Cellular respiration occurs in mitochondria (Fig. IV.12). The mitochondrial matrix, which is the compartment enclosed by the inner mitochondrial membrane, contains almost all of the enzymes for the TCA cycle and oxidation of fatty acids, ketone bodies, and most amino acids. The inner mitochondrial membrane contains the protein complexes of the ETC and ATP synthase, the enzyme complex that generates ATP from ADP and P_i. Some of the subunits of these complexes are encoded by mitochondrial DNA, which resides in the matrix. ATP is generated in the matrix, but most of the energy-using processes in the cell occur outside of the mitochondrion. As a consequence, newly generated ATP must be continuously transported to the cytosol by protein transporters in the impermeable inner mitochondrial membrane and by diffusion through pores in the more permeable outer mitochondrial membrane.

The rates of fuel oxidation and ATP use are tightly coordinated through feedback regulation of the ETC and the pathways of fuel oxidation. Thus, if less energy is required for work, more fuel is stored as glycogen or fat in adipose tissue. The basal metabolic rate (BMR), caloric balance, and ΔG (the change in Gibbs free energy, which is the amount of energy available to do useful work) are quantitative ways of describing energy requirements and the energy that can be derived from fuel oxidation. The various types of enzyme regulation described in Chapter 9 are all used to regulate the rate of oxidation of different fuels to meet energy requirements.

Fatty acids are a major fuel in the body. After eating, we store excess fatty acids and carbohydrates that are not oxidized as fat (triacylglycerols) in adipose tissue. Between meals, these fatty acids are released and circulate in blood bound to albumin. In muscle, liver, and other tissues, fatty acids are oxidized to acetyl-CoA in the pathway of β-oxidation. NADH and FAD(2H) generated from β-oxidation are reoxidized by O_2 in the ECT, thereby generating ATP (see Fig. IV.11). Small amounts of certain fatty acids are oxidized through other pathways that convert them to either oxidizable fuels or urinary excretion products (e.g., peroxisomal β-oxidation).

Not all acetyl-CoA generated from β-oxidation enters the TCA cycle. In the liver, acetyl-CoA generated from β-oxidation of fatty acids can also be converted to the ketone bodies acetoacetate and β-hydroxybutyrate. Ketone bodies are taken up by muscle and other tissues, which convert them back to acetyl-CoA for oxidation in the TCA cycle. They become a major fuel for the brain during prolonged fasting. The discussion of fatty acid oxidation and ketone body production occurs in Section V of this text.

Amino acids derived from dietary or body proteins are also potential fuels that can be oxidized to acetyl-CoA or converted to glucose and then oxidized (see Fig. IV.11). These oxidation pathways, like those of fatty acids, generate NADH or FAD(2H). Ammonia, which can be formed during amino acid oxidation, is toxic. It is therefore converted to urea in the liver and excreted in the urine. There are more than 20 different amino acids, each with a somewhat different pathway for oxidation of the carbon skeleton and conversion of its nitrogen to urea. Because of the complexity of amino acid metabolism, use of amino acids as fuels is considered separately in Section VII, Tissue Metabolism.

Glucose is a universal fuel used to generate ATP in every cell type in the body (Fig. IV.13). In glycolysis, 1 mole of glucose is converted to 2 moles of pyruvate and 2 moles of NADH by cytosolic enzymes. Small amounts of ATP are generated when high-energy pathway intermediates transfer phosphate to ADP in a process termed *substrate-level phosphorylation*. In aerobic glycolysis, the NADH produced from glycolysis is reoxidized by O_2 via the ETC, and pyruvate enters the TCA cycle. In anaerobic glycolysis, the NADH is reoxidized by conversion of pyruvate to lactate, which enters the blood. Although anaerobic glycolysis has a low ATP yield, it is important for tissues with a low oxygen supply and few mitochondria (e.g., the kidney medulla) or for tissues that are experiencing diminished blood flow (ischemia).

All cells continuously use ATP and require a constant supply of fuels to provide energy for the generation of ATP. Chapters 1 through 3 of this text outlined the basic patterns of fuel use in humans and provided information about dietary components.

The pathologic consequences of metabolic problems in fuel oxidation can be grouped into one of two categories: (1) lack of a required product or (2) excess of a substrate or pathway intermediate. The product of fuel oxidation is ATP, and an inadequate rate of ATP production occurs under a wide variety of medical conditions. Extreme conditions that interfere with ATP generation from oxidative phosphorylation, such as complete oxygen deprivation (anoxia) or cyanide poisoning, are fatal. A myocardial infarction is caused by a lack of adequate blood flow to regions of the heart (ischemia), thereby depriving cardiomyocytes of oxygen and fuel. Hyperthyroidism is associated with excessive heat generation from fuel oxidation, and in hypothyroidism, ATP generation can decrease to a fatal level. Conditions such as malnutrition, anorexia nervosa, or excessive alcohol consumption may decrease availability of thiamin, Fe^{2+}, and other vitamins and minerals required by the enzymes of fuel oxidation. Mutations in mitochondrial DNA or nuclear DNA result in deficient ATP generation from oxidative metabolism.

In contrast, problems arising from an excess of substrate or fuel are seen in diabetes mellitus, which may result in a potentially fatal ketoacidosis. Lactic acidosis occurs with a reduction in oxidative metabolism.

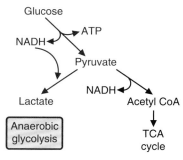

FIGURE IV.13   Glycolysis. In glycolysis, glucose is converted to pyruvate. If the pyruvate is reduced to lactate, the pathway does not require O_2 and is called anaerobic glycolysis (in *red*). If this pyruvate is converted instead to acetyl coenzyme A (acetyl-CoA) and oxidized in the tricarboxylic acid (TCA) cycle, glycolysis requires O_2 and is aerobic (in *black*). ATP, adenosine triphosphate; *NADH*, reduced nicotinamide adenine dinucleotide.

Definitions of prefixes and suffixes used in describing clinical conditions:

an-	Without
-emia	Blood
hyper-	Excessive, above normal
hypo-	Deficient, below normal
-osis	Abnormal or diseased state
-uria	Urine

Basic Concepts in the Regulation of Fuel Metabolism by Insulin, Glucagon, and Other Hormones

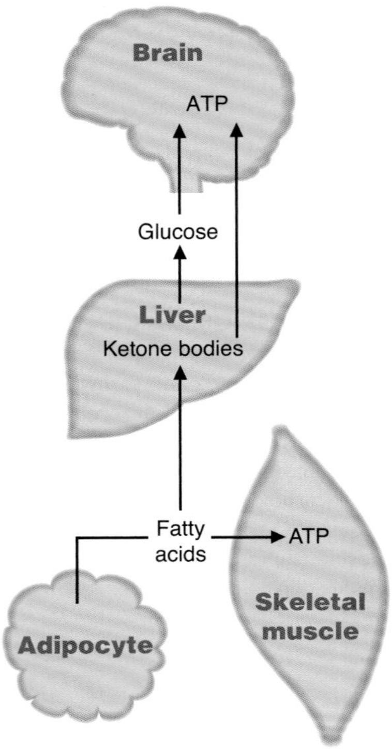

FIGURE 19.1 Maintenance of fuel supplies to tissues. Glucagon release activates the pathways shown. *ATP*, adenosine triphosphate.

All cells use adenosine triphosphate (ATP) continuously and require a constant supply of fuels to provide energy for ATP generation. **Insulin** and **glucagon** are the two major hormones that regulate fuel mobilization and storage. Their function is to ensure that cells have a constant source of glucose, fatty acids, and amino acids for ATP generation and for cellular maintenance (Fig. 19.1).

Because most tissues are partially or totally dependent on glucose for generation of ATP and for production of precursors of other pathways, insulin and glucagon **maintain blood glucose** levels near 80 to 100 mg/dL (90 mg/dL is the same as 5 mM) despite the fact that carbohydrate intake varies considerably over the course of a day. The maintenance of constant blood glucose levels (**glucose homeostasis**) requires these two hormones to regulate **carbohydrate**, **lipid**, and **amino acid metabolism** in accordance with the needs and capacities of individual tissues. Basically, the dietary intake of all fuels in excess of immediate need is stored, and the appropriate fuel is mobilized when a demand occurs. For example, when dietary glucose is not available to cells in sufficient quantities, fatty acids are mobilized and used by skeletal muscle as a fuel (see Chapters 2 and 30). Under these circumstances, the liver can also convert fatty acids to ketone bodies that can be used by the brain. The fatty acids that are mobilized under these conditions spare glucose for use by the brain and other glucose-dependent tissues (such as red blood cells).

Insulin and glucagon are important for the regulation of fuel storage and fuel mobilization (Fig. 19.2). Insulin, released from the β-cells of the pancreas in response to carbohydrate ingestion, promotes glucose use as a fuel and glucose storage as fat and glycogen. **Insulin, therefore, is a major anabolic hormone**. In addition to its storage function, insulin increases protein synthesis and cell growth. Blood insulin levels decrease as glucose is taken up by tissues and used. Glucagon, the major insulin **counterregulatory hormone**, is decreased in response to a carbohydrate meal and elevated during fasting. Its concentration in the blood increases as circulating levels of glucose fall, a response that promotes glucose production via **glycogenolysis** (glycogen degradation) and **gluconeogenesis** (glucose synthesis from amino acids and other noncarbohydrate precursors). Increased levels of circulating glucagon relative to insulin also stimulate the **mobilization of fatty acids** from adipose tissue. **Epinephrine** (the fight-or-flight hormone) and **cortisol** (a glucocorticoid released from the adrenal cortex in response to fasting and chronic stress) have effects on fuel metabolism that oppose those of insulin. Therefore, epinephrine and cortisol are considered to be insulin counterregulatory hormones.

Insulin and glucagon are polypeptide hormones synthesized as **prohormones** in the pancreatic β- and α-cells, respectively. **Proinsulin** is cleaved into mature insulin and a connection peptide (**C-peptide**) in storage vesicles and precipitated with Zn^{2+}. Insulin secretion is regulated principally by changes in blood glucose levels. Glucagon is also synthesized as a prohormone and cleaved into mature glucagon within storage vesicles. Its release is regulated principally through changes in the level of glucose and insulin bathing the α-cells located in the pancreatic islets of Langerhans.

Glucagon exerts its effects on cells by binding to a receptor located on the plasma membrane of target cells for this hormone. The binding to these specific receptors by glucagon stimulates the synthesis of the intracellular second messenger, cyclic adenosine monophosphate (**cAMP**) (Fig. 19.3). cAMP activates **protein kinase A (PKA)**, which phosphorylates key regulatory enzymes, thereby activating some while inhibiting others. Insulin, on the other hand, promotes the dephosphorylation of these key enzymes, leading to their activation or deactivation, depending on the enzyme. Changes of cAMP levels also induce or repress the synthesis of several enzymes.

Insulin binds to a receptor on the cell surface of insulin-sensitive tissues and initiates a cascade of intracellular events that differs from those stimulated by glucagon. Insulin binding activates both autophosphorylation of the receptor and the phosphorylation of other enzymes by the receptor's **tyrosine kinase** domain (see Chapter 11, Section III.B.3). The complete routes for **signal transduction** between this point and the final effects of insulin on the regulatory enzymes of fuel metabolism have not yet been fully established.

THE WAITING ROOM

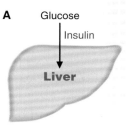

Deborah S. returned to her physician for her monthly office visit. She has been seeing her physician for more than a year because of obesity and elevated blood glucose levels. She still weighed 198 lb, despite trying to adhere to her diet. Her blood glucose level at the time of the visit, 2 hours after lunch, was 221 mg/dL (reference range = 80 to 140 mg/dL). Deborah suffers from type 2 diabetes, an impaired response to insulin. Understanding the actions of insulin and glucagon are critical for understanding this disorder.

Connie C. is a 46-year-old woman who 6 months earlier began noting episodes of fatigue and confusion in the morning before eating and sometimes after jogging. These episodes were occasionally accompanied by blurred vision and an unusually urgent sense of hunger. The ingestion of food relieved all of her symptoms within 25 to 30 minutes. In the last month, these attacks have occurred more frequently throughout the day, and she has learned to diminish their occurrence by eating between meals. As a result, she has recently gained 8 lb.

A random serum glucose level done at 4:30 P.M. during her first office visit was subnormal at 67 mg/dL. Her physician, suspecting she was having episodes of hypoglycemia, ordered a series of fasting serum glucose, insulin, and C-peptide levels. In addition, he asked Connie to keep a careful diary of all of the symptoms that she experienced when her attacks were most severe.

I. Metabolic Homeostasis

Living cells require a constant source of fuels from which to derive ATP for the maintenance of normal cell function and growth. Therefore, a balance must be achieved among carbohydrate, fat, and protein intake; their rates of oxidation; and their rates of storage when they are present in excess of immediate need. Alternatively, when the demand for these substrates increases, the rate of mobilization from storage sites and the rate of their de novo synthesis also require balanced regulation. The control of the balance between substrate need and substrate availability is referred to as *metabolic homeostasis* (Fig. 19.4). The intertissue integration required for metabolic homeostasis is achieved in three principal ways:

- The concentration of nutrients or metabolites in the blood affects the rate at which they are used or stored in different tissues.
- Hormones carry messages to their individual tissues about the physiologic state of the body and the nutrient supply or demand.
- The central nervous system uses neural signals to control tissue metabolism, either directly or through the release of hormones.

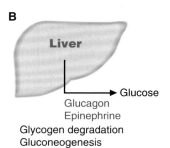

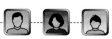

A Glucose

Triglyceride synthesis
Glycogen synthesis
Active glycolysis

B

Glucose

Glucagon
Epinephrine
Glycogen degradation
Gluconeogenesis

FIGURE 19.2 Insulin and the insulin counterregulatory hormones. **A.** Insulin promotes glucose storage as triglyceride or glycogen. **B.** Glucagon and epinephrine promote glucose release from the liver, activating glycogenolysis and gluconeogenesis. Cortisol will stimulate both glycogen synthesis and gluconeogenesis.

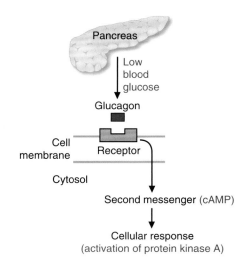

FIGURE 19.3 Cellular response to glucagon, which is released from the pancreas in response to a decrease in blood glucose levels. *cAMP,* cyclic adenosine monophosphate.

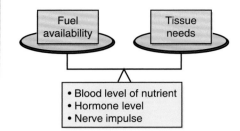

FIGURE 19.4 Metabolic homeostasis. The balance between fuel availability and the needs of tissues for different fuels is achieved by three types of messages: the level of the fuel or nutrients in the blood, the level of one of the hormones of metabolic homeostasis, or nerve impulses that affect tissue metabolism or the release of hormones.

Fatty acids provide an example of the influence that the level of a compound in the blood has on its own rate of metabolism. The concentration of fatty acids in the blood is the major factor determining whether skeletal muscles will use fatty acids or glucose as a fuel (see Chapter 30). In contrast, hormones are (by definition) intravascular carriers of messages between their sites of synthesis and their target tissues. Epinephrine, for example, is a flight-or-fight hormone that in times of stress signals an immediate need for increased fuel availability. Its level is regulated principally through the activation of the sympathetic nervous system.

Insulin and glucagon, however, are the two major hormones that regulate fuel storage and mobilization (see Fig. 19.2). Insulin is the major anabolic hormone of the body. It promotes the storage of fuels and the use of fuels for growth. Glucagon is the major hormone of fuel mobilization (Fig. 19.5). Other hormones, such as epinephrine, are released as a response of the central nervous system to hypoglycemia, exercise, or other types of physiologic stress. Epinephrine and other stress hormones also increase the availability of fuels (see Fig. 19.5). The major hormones of fuel homeostasis, insulin and glucagon, fluctuate continuously in response to our daily eating pattern.

Glucose has a special role in metabolic homeostasis. Many tissues (e.g., the brain, red blood cells, kidney medulla, exercising skeletal muscle) are dependent on glycolysis for all or a part of their energy needs. As a consequence, these tissues require uninterrupted access to glucose to meet their rapid rate of ATP use. In the adult, a minimum of 190 g glucose is required per day—approximately 150 g for the brain and 40 g for other tissues. Significant decreases of blood glucose <60 mg/dL limit glucose metabolism in the brain and may elicit hypoglycemic symptoms (as experienced by **Connie C.**), presumably because the overall process of glucose flux through the blood–brain barrier, into the interstitial fluid, and subsequently into the neuronal cells is slow at low blood glucose levels because of the K_m values of the glucose transporters required for this to occur (see Chapter 21).

The continuous efflux of fuels from their storage depots—during exercise, for example—is necessitated by the high amounts of fuel required to meet the need for ATP under these conditions. Disastrous results would occur if even a day's

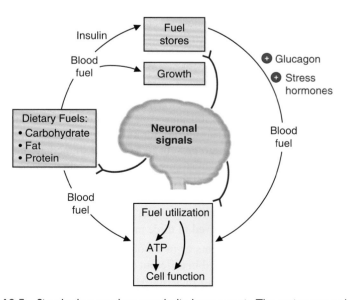

FIGURE 19.5 Signals that regulate metabolic homeostasis. The major stress hormones are epinephrine and cortisol. *ATP*, adenosine triphosphate.

supply of glucose, amino acids, and fatty acids could not enter cells normally and were instead left circulating in the blood. Glucose and amino acids would be at such high concentrations in the circulation that the hyperosmolar effect would cause progressively severe neurologic deficits and even coma. The concentration of glucose and amino acids would rise above the renal tubular threshold for these substances (the maximal concentration in the blood at which the kidney can completely resorb metabolites), and some of these compounds would be wasted as they spilled over into the urine. Nonenzymatic glycosylation of proteins would increase at higher blood glucose levels, altering the function of tissues in which these proteins reside. Triacylglycerols, present primarily in chylomicrons and very-low-density lipoproteins (VLDL), would rise in the blood, increasing the likelihood of atherosclerotic vascular disease. These potential metabolic derangements emphasize the need to maintain a normal balance between fuel storage and fuel use.

II. Major Hormones of Metabolic Homeostasis

The hormones that contribute to metabolic homeostasis respond to changes in the circulating levels of fuels that, in part, are determined by the timing and composition of our diet. Insulin and glucagon are considered the major hormone of metabolic homeostasis because they continuously fluctuate in response to our daily eating pattern. They provide good examples of the basic concept of hormonal regulation. Certain features of the release and action of other insulin counterregulatory hormones, such as epinephrine, norepinephrine, and cortisol, will be described and compared with insulin and glucagon.

Insulin is the major anabolic hormone that promotes the storage of nutrients: glucose storage as glycogen in liver and muscle, conversion of glucose to triacylglycerols in liver and their storage in adipose tissue, and amino acid uptake and protein synthesis in skeletal muscle (Fig. 19.6). It also increases the synthesis of albumin and other proteins by the liver. Insulin promotes the use of glucose as a fuel by facilitating its transport into muscle and adipose tissue. At the same time, insulin acts to inhibit fuel mobilization.

 Hyperglycemia may cause a constellation of symptoms such as polyuria and subsequent polydipsia (increased thirst). The inability to move glucose into cells necessitates the oxidation of lipids as an alternative fuel. As a result, adipose stores are used, and a patient with poorly controlled diabetes mellitus loses weight in spite of a good appetite. Extremely high levels of serum glucose can cause a hyperosmolar hyperglycemic state in patients with type 2 diabetes mellitus. Such patients usually have sufficient insulin responsiveness to block fatty acid release and ketone-body formation, but they are unable to significantly stimulate glucose entry into peripheral tissues. The severely elevated levels of glucose in the blood compared with those inside the cell leads to an osmotic effect that causes water to leave the cells and enter the blood. Because of the osmotic diuretic effect of hyperglycemia, the kidney produces more urine, leading to dehydration, which, in turn, may lead to even higher levels of blood glucose. If dehydration becomes severe, further cerebral dysfunction occurs and the patient may become comatose. Chronic hyperglycemia also produces pathologic effects through the nonenzymatic glycosylation of a variety of proteins. Hemoglobin A (HbA), one of the proteins that becomes glycosylated, forms HbA$_{1c}$ (see Chapter 7). **Deborah S.'s** high levels of HbA$_{1c}$ (9.5% of the total HbA, compared with the reference range of 4.7% to 6.4%) indicate that her blood glucose has been significantly elevated over the last 12 to 14 weeks, the half-life of hemoglobin in the bloodstream.

All membrane and serum proteins exposed to high levels of glucose in the blood or interstitial fluid are candidates for nonenzymatic glycosylation. This process distorts protein structure and slows protein degradation, which leads to an accumulation of these products in various organs, thereby adversely affecting organ function. These events contribute to the long-term microvascular and macrovascular complications of diabetes mellitus, which include diabetic retinopathy, nephropathy, and neuropathy (microvascular), in addition to coronary artery, cerebral artery, and peripheral artery disease and atherosclerosis (macrovascular).

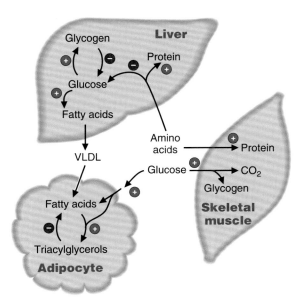

FIGURE 19.6 Major sites of insulin action on fuel metabolism. *VLDL*, very-low-density lipoprotein; ⊕, stimulated by insulin; ⊖, inhibited by insulin.

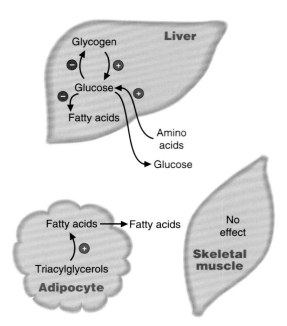

FIGURE 19.7 Major sites of glucagon action in fuel metabolism. $\oplus$, pathways stimulated by glucagon; $\ominus$, pathways inhibited by glucagon.

Glucagon acts to maintain fuel availability in the absence of dietary glucose by stimulating the release of glucose from liver glycogen (see Chapter 26); by stimulating gluconeogenesis from lactate, glycerol, and amino acids (see Chapter 28); and, in conjunction with decreased insulin, by mobilizing fatty acids from adipose triacylglycerols to provide an alternate source of fuel (see Chapter 30 and Fig. 19.7). Its sites of action are principally the liver and adipose tissue; it has no influence on skeletal muscle metabolism because muscle cells lack glucagon receptors. The message carried by glucagon is that "glucose is gone"; that is, the current supply of glucose is inadequate to meet the immediate fuel requirements of the body.

The release of insulin from the β-cells of the pancreas is dictated primarily by the level of glucose in the blood bathing the β-cells in the islets of Langerhans. The highest levels of insulin occur approximately 30 to 45 minutes after a high-carbohydrate meal (Fig. 19.8). They return to basal levels as the blood glucose concentration falls, approximately 2 hours after the meal. The release of glucagon from the α-cells of the pancreas, conversely, is controlled principally through a reduction of glucose and/or a rise in the concentration of insulin in the blood bathing the α-cells in the pancreas. Therefore, the lowest levels of glucagon occur after a high-carbohydrate meal. Because all of the effects of glucagon are opposed by insulin, the simultaneous stimulation of insulin release and suppression of glucagon secretion by a high-carbohydrate meal provides integrated control of carbohydrate, fat, and protein metabolism.

Insulin and glucagon are not the only regulators of fuel metabolism. The inter-tissue balance between the use and storage of glucose, fat, and protein is also accomplished by the circulating levels of metabolites in the blood, by neuronal signals, and by the other hormones of metabolic homeostasis (epinephrine, norepinephrine, cortisol, and others) (Table 19.1). These hormones oppose the actions of insulin by mobilizing fuels. Like glucagon, they are insulin counterregulatory hormones (Fig. 19.9). Of all these hormones, only insulin and glucagon are synthesized and released in direct response to changing levels of fuels in the blood. The release of cortisol, epinephrine, and norepinephrine is mediated by neuronal signals. Rising levels of the insulin counterregulatory hormones in the blood reflect, for the most part, a current increase in the demand for fuel.

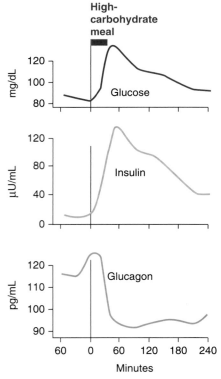

FIGURE 19.8 Blood glucose, insulin, and glucagon levels after a high-carbohydrate meal.

TABLE 19.1	Physiologic Actions of Insulin and Insulin Counterregulatory Hormones	
HORMONE	**FUNCTION**	**MAJOR METABOLIC PATHWAYS AFFECTED**
Insulin	Promotes fuel storage after a meal. Promotes growth	Stimulates glucose storage as glycogen (muscle and liver). Stimulates fatty acid synthesis and storage after a high-carbohydrate meal. Stimulates amino acid uptake and protein synthesis
Glucagon	Mobilizes fuels. Maintains blood glucose levels during fasting	Activates gluconeogenesis and glycogenolysis (liver) during fasting. Activates fatty acid release from adipose tissue
Epinephrine	Mobilizes fuels during acute stress	Stimulates glucose production from glycogen (muscle and liver). Stimulates fatty acid release from adipose issue
Cortisol	Provides for changing requirements during stress	Stimulates amino acid mobilization from muscle protein. Stimulates gluconeogenesis in order to produce glucose for liver glycogen synthesis. Stimulates fatty acid release from adipose issue

III. Synthesis and Release of Insulin and Glucagon

A. Endocrine Pancreas

Insulin and glucagon are synthesized in different cell types of the endocrine pancreas, which consists of microscopic clusters of small glands, the islets of Langerhans, scattered among the cells of the exocrine pancreas. The α-cells secrete glucagon and the β-cells secrete insulin into the hepatic portal vein via the pancreatic veins.

Connie C.'s studies confirmed that her fasting serum glucose levels were below normal, with an inappropriately high insulin level. She continued to experience the fatigue, confusion, and blurred vision she had described on her first office visit. These symptoms are referred to as the *neuroglycopenic manifestations of severe hypoglycemia* (neurologic symptoms resulting from an inadequate supply of glucose to the brain for the generation of ATP).

Connie also noted the symptoms that are part of the adrenergic response to hypoglycemic stress. Stimulation of the sympathetic nervous system (because of the low levels of glucose reaching the brain) results in the release of epinephrine, a stress hormone, from the adrenal medulla. Elevated epinephrine levels cause tachycardia (rapid heartbeat), palpitations, anxiety, tremulousness, pallor, and sweating.

In addition to the symptoms described by **Connie C.**, individuals may experience confusion, light-headedness, headache, aberrant behavior, blurred vision, loss of consciousness, or seizures. When severe and prolonged, death may occur.

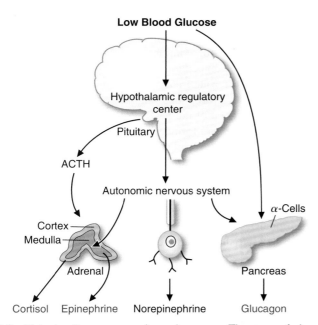

FIGURE 19.9 Major insulin counterregulatory hormones. The stress of a low blood glucose level mediates the release of the major insulin counterregulatory hormones through neuronal signals. Hypoglycemia is one of the stress signals that stimulates the release of cortisol, epinephrine, and norepinephrine. Adrenocorticotropic hormone (ACTH) is released from the pituitary and stimulates the release of cortisol (a glucocorticoid) from the adrenal cortex. Neuronal signals stimulate the release of epinephrine from the adrenal medulla and norepinephrine from nerve endings. Neuronal signals also play a minor role in the release of glucagon. Although norepinephrine has counterregulatory actions, it is not a major counterregulatory hormone.

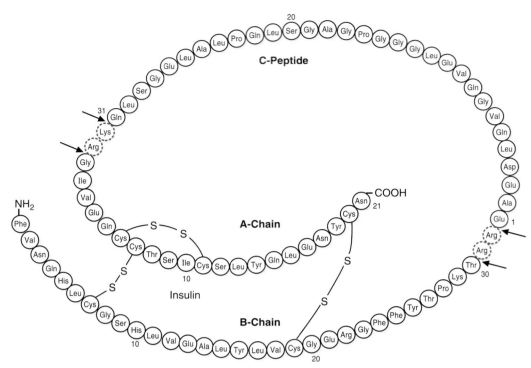

FIGURE 19.10 Cleavage of proinsulin to insulin. Proinsulin is converted to insulin by proteolytic cleavage, which removes the C-peptide and a few additional amino acid residues. Cleavage occurs at the *arrows*. (From Murray RK, Granner DK, Mayes PA, et al. *Harper's Biochemistry.* 23rd ed. Stanford, CT: Appleton & Lange; 1993:560.)

B. Synthesis and Secretion of Insulin

Insulin is a polypeptide hormone. The active form of insulin is composed of two polypeptide chains (the A-chain and the B-chain) linked by two interchain disulfide bonds. The A-chain has an additional intrachain disulfide bond (Fig. 19.10).

Insulin, like many other polypeptide hormones, is synthesized as a preprohormone that is converted in the rough endoplasmic reticulum (RER) to proinsulin. The "pre" sequence, a short hydrophobic signal sequence at the N-terminal end, is cleaved as it enters the lumen of the RER. Proinsulin folds into the proper conformation, and disulfide bonds are formed between the cysteine residues. It is then transported in microvesicles to the Golgi complex. It leaves the Golgi complex in storage vesicles, where a protease removes the biologically inactive "connecting peptide" (C-peptide) and a few small remnants, resulting in the formation of biologically active insulin (see Fig. 19.10). Zinc ions are also transported in these storage vesicles. Cleavage of the C-peptide decreases the solubility of the resulting insulin, which then coprecipitates with zinc. Exocytosis of the insulin storage vesicles from the cytosol of the β-cell into the blood is stimulated by rising levels of glucose in the blood bathing the β-cells.

Glucose enters the β-cell via specific glucose transporter proteins known as *GLUT 2* (see Chapter 21). Glucose is phosphorylated through the action of glucokinase to form glucose 6-phosphate, which is metabolized through glycolysis, the tricarboxylic acid (TCA) cycle, and oxidative phosphorylation. These reactions result in an increase in ATP levels within the β-cell (circle 1 in Fig. 19.11). As the β-cell ATP/adenosine diphosphate (ADP) ratio increases, the activity of a membrane-bound, ATP-dependent K^+ channel (K^+_{ATP}) is inhibited (i.e., the channel is closed) (circle 2 in Fig. 19.11). The closing of this channel leads to a membrane depolarization (because the membrane is normally hyperpolarized; see circle 3 in Fig. 19.11), which activates a voltage-gated Ca^{2+} channel that allows Ca^{2+} to enter the β-cell such that intracellular Ca^{2+} levels increase significantly

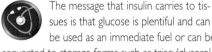

The message that insulin carries to tissues is that glucose is plentiful and can be used as an immediate fuel or can be converted to storage forms such as triacylglycerol in adipocytes or glycogen in liver and muscle.

Because insulin stimulates the uptake of glucose into tissues where it may be immediately oxidized or stored for later oxidation, this regulatory hormone lowers blood glucose levels. Therefore, one of the possible causes of **Connie C.'s** hypoglycemia is an insulinoma, a tumor that produces excessive insulin.

Whenever an endocrine gland continues to release its hormone in spite of the presence of signals that normally would suppress its secretion, this persistent inappropriate release is said to be "autonomous." Secretory neoplasms of endocrine glands generally produce their hormonal product autonomously in a chronic fashion.

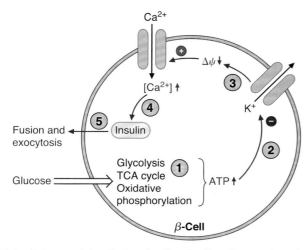

FIGURE 19.11 Release of insulin by the β-cells. Details are given in the text. *ATP*, adenosine triphosphate; *TCA*, tricarboxylic acid; ⊕, stimulation; ⊖, inhibition; Δψ, membrane potential.

(Fig. 19.11, circle 4). The increase in intracellular Ca^{2+} stimulates the fusion of insulin-containing exocytotic vesicles with the plasma membrane, resulting in insulin secretion (Fig. 19.11, circle 5). Thus, an increase in glucose levels within the β-cells initiates insulin release.

Other intracellular metabolites, particularly nicotinamide adenine dinucleotide phosphate (NADPH), have been proposed to play important roles in insulin release in response to glucose. This will be discussed further in later chapters.

C. Stimulation and Inhibition of Insulin Release

The release of insulin occurs within minutes after the pancreas is exposed to a high glucose concentration. The threshold for insulin release is approximately 80 mg of glucose/dL. Above 80 mg/dL, the rate of insulin release is not an all-or-nothing response but is proportional to the glucose concentration up to approximately 300 mg/dL. As insulin is secreted, the synthesis of new insulin molecules is stimulated, so that secretion is maintained until blood glucose levels fall. Insulin is rapidly removed from the circulation and degraded by the liver (and, to a lesser extent, by kidney and skeletal muscle), so blood insulin levels decrease rapidly once the rate of secretion slows.

Several factors other than the blood glucose concentration can modulate insulin release (Table 19.2). The pancreatic islets are innervated by the autonomic nervous system, including a branch of the vagus nerve. These neural signals help to coordinate insulin release with the secretory signals initiated by the ingestion of fuels. However, signals from the central nervous system are not required for insulin secretion.

Dianne A. has type 1 diabetes mellitus. This metabolic disorder is usually caused by antibody-mediated (autoimmune) destruction of the β-cells of the pancreas. Susceptibility to type 1 diabetes mellitus is, in part, conferred by a genetic defect in the human leukocyte antigen (HLA) region of β-cells that codes for the major histocompatibility complex II (MHC II). This protein presents an intracellular antigen to the cell surface for "self-recognition" by the cells involved in the immune response. Because of this defective protein, a cell-mediated immune response leads to varying degrees of β-cell destruction and eventually to dependence on exogenous insulin administration to control the levels of glucose in the blood.

Autonomous hypersecretion of insulin from a suspected pancreatic β-cell tumor (an insulinoma) can be demonstrated in several ways. The simplest test is to simultaneously draw blood for the measurement of both glucose and insulin at a time when the patient is spontaneously experiencing the characteristic adrenergic or neuroglycopenic symptoms of hypoglycemia. During such a test, **Connie C.'s** glucose levels fell to 45 mg/dL (normal = 80 to 100 mg/dL), and her ratio of insulin to glucose was far higher than normal. The elevated insulin levels markedly increased glucose uptake by the peripheral tissues, resulting in a dramatic lowering of blood glucose levels. In normal individuals, as blood glucose levels drop, insulin levels also drop. Insulin levels were determined by radioimmunoassay; see the "Biochemical Comments" in Chapter 41 for a description of this method.

TABLE 19.2 **Regulators of Insulin Release**	
REGULATOR	**EFFECT**
Major regulators	
Glucose	+
Minor regulators	
Amino acids	+
Neural input	+
Gut hormones[a]	+
Epinephrine (adrenergic)	−

+, stimulates; −, inhibits.
[a]Gut hormones that regulate fuel metabolism are discussed in Chapter 41.

A rare form of diabetes known as *maturity-onset diabetes of the young* (MODY) results from mutations in either pancreatic glucokinase or specific nuclear transcription factors. MODY type 2 is caused by a glucokinase mutation that results in an enzyme with reduced activity because of either an elevated K_m for glucose or a reduced V_{max} for the reaction. Because insulin release depends on normal glucose metabolism within the β-cell that yields a critical ATP/ADP ratio in the β-cell, individuals with this glucokinase mutation cannot significantly metabolize glucose unless glucose levels are higher than normal. Thus, although these patients can release insulin, they do so at higher than normal glucose levels and are, therefore, almost always in a hyperglycemic state. Interestingly, however, these patients are somewhat resistant to the long-term complications of chronic hyperglycemia. The mechanism for this seeming resistance is not well understood.

Neonatal diabetes is a very rare inherited disorder in which newborns develop diabetes within the first 3 months of life. The diabetes may be permanent, requiring lifelong insulin treatment, or transient. The most common mutation leading to permanent neonatal diabetes is in the *KCNJ11* gene, which encodes a subunit of the K^+_{ATP} channel in various tissues including the pancreas. This is an activating mutation, which keeps the K^+_{ATP} channel open, and less susceptible to ATP inhibition. If the K^+_{ATP} channel cannot be closed, activation of the Ca^{2+} channel will not occur and insulin secretion will be impaired.

Deborah S. is taking a sulfonylurea compound known as *glipizide* to treat her diabetes. The sulfonylureas act on the K^+_{ATP} channels on the surface of the pancreatic β-cells. The K^+_{ATP} channels contain pore-forming subunits (encoded by the *KCNJ11* gene) and regulatory subunits (the subunit to which sulfonylurea compounds bind, encoded by the *ABCC8* gene). The binding of the drug to the sulfonylurea receptor closes K^+ channels (as do elevated ATP levels), which, in turn, increases Ca^{2+} movement into the interior of the β-cell. This influx of calcium modulates the interaction of the insulin storage vesicles with the plasma membrane of the β-cell, resulting in the release of insulin into the circulation.

Patients have been described who have an activating mutation in the *ABCC8* gene (which would make it difficult to close the K^+_{ATP} channel), and, among other symptoms, the patients displayed neonatal diabetes. Activating mutations in the *KCNJ11* gene also have the same effect.

Certain amino acids also can stimulate insulin secretion, although the amount of insulin released during a high-protein meal is very much lower than that released by a high-carbohydrate meal. Gastric inhibitory polypeptide (GIP) and glucagonlike peptide 1 (GLP-1), gut hormones released after the ingestion of food, also aid in the onset of insulin release. Epinephrine, secreted in response to fasting, stress, trauma, and vigorous exercise, decreases the release of insulin. Epinephrine release signals energy use, which indicates that less insulin needs to be secreted, because insulin stimulates energy storage.

D. Synthesis and Secretion of Glucagon

Glucagon, a polypeptide hormone, is synthesized in the α-cells of the pancreas by cleavage of the much larger preproglucagon, a 160-amino acid peptide. Like insulin, preproglucagon is produced on the RER and is converted to proglucagon as it enters the lumen of the endoplasmic reticulum. Proteolytic cleavage at various sites produces the mature 29-amino acid glucagon (molecular weight = 3,500 Da) and larger glucagon-containing fragments (named GLP-1 and GLP-2). Glucagon is rapidly metabolized, primarily in the liver and kidneys. Its plasma half-life is only about 3 to 5 minutes.

Glucagon secretion is regulated principally by circulating levels of glucose and insulin. Increasing levels of each inhibit glucagon release. Glucose probably has both a direct suppressive effect on secretion of glucagon from the α-cell as well as an indirect effect, the latter being mediated by its ability to stimulate the release of insulin. The direction of blood flow in the islets of the pancreas carries insulin from the β-cells in the center of the islets to the peripheral α-cells, where it suppresses glucagon secretion.

Conversely, certain hormones stimulate glucagon secretion. Among these are the catecholamines (including epinephrine) and cortisol (Table 19.3).

Many amino acids also stimulate glucagon release (Fig. 19.12). Thus, the high levels of glucagon that would be expected in the fasting state do not decrease after a high-protein meal. In fact, glucagon levels may increase, stimulating gluconeogenesis in the absence of dietary glucose. The relative amounts of insulin and glucagon in the blood after a mixed meal depend on the composition of the meal because glucose stimulates insulin release, and amino acids stimulate glucagon release. However, amino acids also induce insulin secretion but not to the same extent that glucose does. Although this may seem paradoxical, it actually makes good sense. Insulin release stimulates amino acid uptake by tissues and enhances protein synthesis. However, because glucagon levels also increase in response to a protein meal, and the critical factor is the insulin-to-glucagon ratio, sufficient glucagon is released that gluconeogenesis is enhanced (at the expense of protein synthesis), and the amino acids that are taken up by the tissues serve as a substrate for gluconeogenesis. The synthesis of glycogen and triglycerides is also reduced when glucagon levels rise in the blood.

TABLE 19.3 **Regulators of Glucagon Release**	
REGULATOR	**EFFECT**
Major regulators	
Glucose	−
Insulin	−
Amino acids	+
Minor regulators	
Cortisol	+
Neural (stress)	+
Epinephrine	+

+, stimulates; −, inhibits.

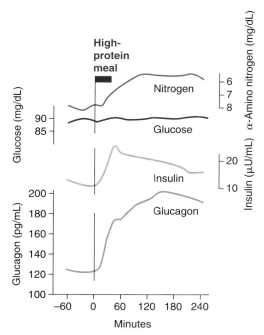

FIGURE 19.12   Release of insulin and glucagon in response to a high-protein meal. This figure shows the increase in the release of insulin and glucagon into the blood after an overnight fast followed by the ingestion of 100 g of protein (equivalent to a slice of roast beef). Insulin levels do not increase nearly as much as they do after a high-carbohydrate meal (see Fig. 19.8). The levels of glucagon, however, significantly increase above those present in the fasting state.

In fasting subjects, the average level of immunoreactive glucagon in the blood is 75 pg/mL and does not vary as much as insulin during the daily fasting–feeding cycle. However, only 30% to 40% of the measured immunoreactive glucagon is mature pancreatic glucagon. The rest is composed of larger immunoreactive fragments that are also produced in the pancreas or in the intestinal L-cells.

IV. Mechanisms of Hormone Action

For a hormone to affect the flux of substrates through a metabolic pathway, it must be able to change the rate at which that pathway proceeds by increasing or decreasing the rate of the slowest step(s). Either directly or indirectly, hormones affect the activity of specific enzymes or transport proteins that regulate the flux through a pathway. Thus, ultimately, the hormone must either cause the amount of the substrate for the enzyme to increase (if substrate supply is a rate-limiting factor), change the conformation at the active site by phosphorylating the enzyme, change the concentration of an allosteric effector of the enzyme, or change the amount of the protein by inducing or repressing its synthesis or by changing its turnover rate or location. Insulin, glucagon, and other hormones use all of these regulatory mechanisms to determine the rate of flux in metabolic pathways. The effects mediated by phosphorylation or changes in the kinetic properties of an enzyme occur rapidly, within minutes. In contrast, it may take hours for induction or repression of enzyme synthesis to change the amount of an enzyme in the cell.

The details of hormone action were described in Chapter 11 and are only summarized here.

A. Signal Transduction by Hormones that Bind to Plasma Membrane Receptors

Hormones initiate their actions on target cells by binding to specific receptors or binding proteins. In the case of polypeptide hormones (such as insulin and glucagon)

 Measurements of proinsulin and the connecting peptide between the α- and β-chains of insulin (C-peptide) in **Connie C.'s** blood during her hospital fast provided confirmation that she had an insulinoma. Insulin and C-peptide are secreted in approximately equal proportions from the β-cell, but C-peptide is not cleared from the blood as rapidly as insulin. Therefore, it provides a reasonably accurate estimate of the rate of insulin secretion. Plasma C-peptide measurements are also potentially useful in helping to figure out the type of diabetes mellitus or degree of insulin secretion in patients who are receiving exogenous insulin because exogenous insulin lacks the C-peptide.

 Patients with type 1 diabetes mellitus, such as **Dianne A.**, have almost undetectable levels of insulin in their blood. Patients with type 2 diabetes mellitus, such as **Deborah S.**, conversely, have normal or even elevated levels of insulin in their blood; however, the level of insulin in their blood is inappropriately low relative to their elevated blood glucose concentration. In type 2 diabetes mellitus, skeletal muscle, liver, and other tissues exhibit a resistance to the actions of insulin. As a result, insulin has a smaller than normal effect on glucose and fat metabolism in such patients. Levels of insulin in the blood must be higher than normal to maintain normal blood glucose levels. In the early stages of type 2 diabetes mellitus, these compensatory adjustments in insulin release may keep the blood glucose levels near the normal range. Over time, as the β-cells' capacity to secrete high levels of insulin declines, blood glucose levels increase and exogenous insulin becomes necessary.

 The physiologic importance of insulin's usual action of mediating the suppressive effect of glucose on glucagon secretion is apparent in patients with types 1 and 2 diabetes mellitus. Despite the presence of hyperglycemia, glucagon levels in such patients initially remain elevated (near fasting levels) either because of the absence of insulin's suppressive effect or because of the resistance of the α-cells to insulin's suppressive effect even in the face of adequate insulin levels in type 2 patients. Thus, these patients have inappropriately high glucagon levels, leading to the suggestion that diabetes mellitus is actually a "bi-hormonal" disorder.

During the "stress" of hypoglycemia, the autonomic nervous system stimulates the pancreas to secrete glucagon, which tends to restore the serum glucose level to normal. The increased activity of the adrenergic nervous system (through epinephrine) also alerts a patient, such as **Connie C.**, to the presence of increasingly severe hypoglycemia. Hopefully, this will induce the patient to ingest simple sugars or other carbohydrates, which, in turn, will also increase glucose levels in the blood. **Connie C.** gained 8 lb before resection of her pancreatic insulin-secreting adenoma through this mechanism.

and catecholamines (epinephrine and norepinephrine), the action of the hormone is mediated through binding to a specific receptor on the plasma membrane (see Chapter 11, Section III). The first message of the hormone is transmitted to intracellular enzymes by the activated receptor and an intracellular second messenger; the hormone does not need to enter the cell to exert its effects. (In contrast, steroid hormones such as cortisol and the thyroid hormone triiodothyronine [T_3] enter the cytosol and eventually move into the cell nucleus to exert their effects.)

The mechanism by which the message carried by the hormone ultimately affects the rate of the regulatory enzyme in the target cell is called *signal transduction*. The three basic types of signal transduction for hormones binding to receptors on the plasma membrane are (1) receptor coupling to adenylate cyclase, which produces cAMP; (2) receptor kinase activity; and (3) receptor coupling to hydrolysis of phosphatidylinositol bisphosphate (PIP_2). The hormones of metabolic homeostasis each use one of these mechanisms to carry out their physiologic effect. In addition, some hormones and neurotransmitters act through receptor coupling to gated ion channels (described in Chapter 11).

1. Signal Transduction by Insulin

Insulin initiates its action by binding to a receptor on the plasma membrane of insulin's many target cells (see Fig. 11.13). The insulin receptor has two types of subunits: the α-subunits to which insulin binds, and the β-subunits, which span the membrane and protrude into the cytosol. The cytosolic portion of the β-subunit has tyrosine kinase activity. On binding of insulin, the tyrosine kinase phosphorylates tyrosine residues on the β-subunit (autophosphorylation) as well as on several other enzymes within the cytosol. A principal substrate for phosphorylation by the receptor, insulin receptor substrate 1 (IRS-1), then recognizes and binds to various signal transduction proteins in regions referred to as *SH2 domains*. IRS-1 is involved in many of the physiologic responses to insulin through complex mechanisms that are the subject of intensive investigation. The basic tissue-specific cellular responses to insulin, however, can be grouped into five major categories: (1) insulin reverses glucagon-stimulated phosphorylation, (2) insulin works through a phosphorylation cascade that stimulates the phosphorylation of several enzymes, (3) insulin induces and represses the synthesis of specific enzymes, (4) insulin acts as a growth factor and has a general stimulatory effect on protein synthesis, and (5) insulin stimulates glucose and amino acid transport into cells (see Fig. IV.10 in the introduction to Section IV of this text).

Several mechanisms have been proposed for the action of insulin in reversing glucagon-stimulated phosphorylation of the enzymes of carbohydrate metabolism. From the student's point of view, the ability of insulin to reverse glucagon-stimulated phosphorylation occurs as if it were lowering cAMP and stimulating phosphatases that could remove those phosphates added by PKA. In reality, the mechanism is more complex and still is not fully understood.

2. Signal Transduction by Glucagon

The pathway for signal transduction by glucagon is one that is common to several hormones; the glucagon receptor is coupled to adenylate cyclase and cAMP production (see Fig. 11.10). Glucagon, through G-proteins, activates the membrane-bound adenylate cyclase, increasing the synthesis of the intracellular second messenger 3′,5′-cyclic AMP (cAMP) (see Fig. 11.18). cAMP activates PKA (cAMP-dependent protein kinase), which changes the activity of enzymes by phosphorylating them at specific serine residues. Phosphorylation activates some enzymes and inhibits others.

The G-proteins, which couple the glucagon receptor to adenylate cyclase, are proteins in the plasma membrane that bind guanosine triphosphate (GTP) and have dissociable subunits that interact with both the receptor and adenylate cyclase. In the absence of glucagon, the stimulatory G_s-protein complex binds guanosine diphosphate (GDP) but cannot bind to the unoccupied receptor or adenylate cyclase (see Fig. 11.17). Once glucagon binds to the receptor, the receptor also binds the G_s-complex, which then releases GDP and binds GTP. The α-subunit then dissociates from the β- and γ-subunits and binds to adenylate cyclase, thereby activating it. As the GTP on the α-subunit is hydrolyzed to GDP, the subunit dissociates and recomplexes with the β- and γ-subunits. Only continued occupancy of the glucagon receptor can keep adenylate cyclase active.

Although glucagon works by activating adenylate cyclase, a few hormones inhibit adenylate cyclase. In this case, the inhibitory G-protein complex is called a G_i-complex. cAMP is the intracellular second messenger for several hormones that regulate fuel metabolism. The specificity of the physiologic response to each hormone results from the presence of specific receptors for that hormone in target tissues. For example, glucagon activates glucose production from glycogen in liver but not in skeletal muscle because glucagon receptors are present in liver but are absent in skeletal muscle. However, skeletal muscle has adenylate cyclase, cAMP, and PKA, which can be activated by epinephrine binding to the $β_2$-receptors in the membranes of muscle cells. Liver cells also have epinephrine receptors.

cAMP is very rapidly degraded to AMP by a membrane-bound phosphodiesterase. The concentration of cAMP is thus very low in the cell, so changes in its concentration can occur rapidly in response to changes in the rate of synthesis. The amount of cAMP present at any time is a direct reflection of hormone binding and the activity of adenylate cyclase. It is not affected by ATP, ADP, or AMP levels in the cell.

cAMP transmits the hormone signal to the cell by activating PKA (cAMP-dependent protein kinase). As cAMP binds to the regulatory subunits of PKA, these subunits dissociate from the catalytic subunits, which are thereby activated (see Chapter 9, Fig. 9.12). Activated PKA phosphorylates serine residues of key regulatory enzymes in the pathways of carbohydrate and fat metabolism. Some enzymes are activated and others are inhibited by this change in phosphorylation state. The message of the hormone is terminated by the action of semispecific protein phosphatases that remove phosphate groups from the enzymes. The activity of the protein phosphatases is also controlled through hormonal regulation.

Changes in the phosphorylation state of proteins that bind to cAMP response elements (CREs) in the promoter region of genes contribute to the regulation of gene transcription by several cAMP-coupled hormones (see Chapter 16). For instance, cAMP response element–binding protein (CREB) is directly phosphorylated by PKA, a step essential for the initiation of transcription. Phosphorylation at other sites on CREB, by a variety of kinases, also may play a role in regulating transcription.

The mechanism for signal transduction by glucagon illustrates some of the important principles of hormonal signaling mechanisms. The first principle is that specificity of action in tissues is conferred by the receptor on a target cell for glucagon. In general, the major actions of glucagon occur in liver, adipose tissue, and certain cells of the kidney that contain glucagon receptors. The second principle is that signal transduction involves amplification of the first message. Glucagon and other hormones are present in the blood in very low concentrations. However, these minute concentrations of hormone are adequate to initiate a cellular response because the binding of one molecule of glucagon to one receptor ultimately activates many PKA molecules, each of which phosphorylates hundreds of downstream enzymes. The third principle involves integration of metabolic responses. For instance, the glucagon-stimulated phosphorylation of enzymes simultaneously activates glycogen degradation, inhibits glycogen synthesis, and inhibits glycolysis in the liver (see Fig. IV.10 in the introduction to Section IV of this text). The fourth principle involves augmentation and antagonism of signals. An example of augmentation involves the actions of glucagon and epinephrine (which is released during exercise). Although these hormones bind to different receptors, each can increase cAMP and stimulate glycogen degradation. A fifth principle is that of rapid signal termination. In the case of glucagon, both the termination of the G_s-protein activation and the rapid degradation of cAMP contribute to signal termination.

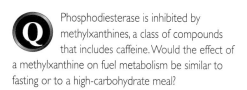

Phosphodiesterase is inhibited by methylxanthines, a class of compounds that includes caffeine. Would the effect of a methylxanthine on fuel metabolism be similar to fasting or to a high-carbohydrate meal?

Ann R., to stay thin, frequently fasts for prolonged periods, but she jogs every morning (see Chapter 2). The release of epinephrine and norepinephrine and the increase of glucagon and fall of insulin during her exercise provide coordinated and augmented signals that stimulate the release of fuels above the fasting levels. Fuel mobilization will occur, of course, only as long as she has fuel stored as triacylglycerols.

A Inhibition of phosphodiesterase by methylxanthine would increase cAMP and have the same effects on fuel metabolism as would an increase of glucagon and epinephrine, as in the fasted state. Increased fuel mobilization would occur through glycogenolysis (the release of glucose from glycogen) and through lipolysis (the release of fatty acids from triacylglycerols).

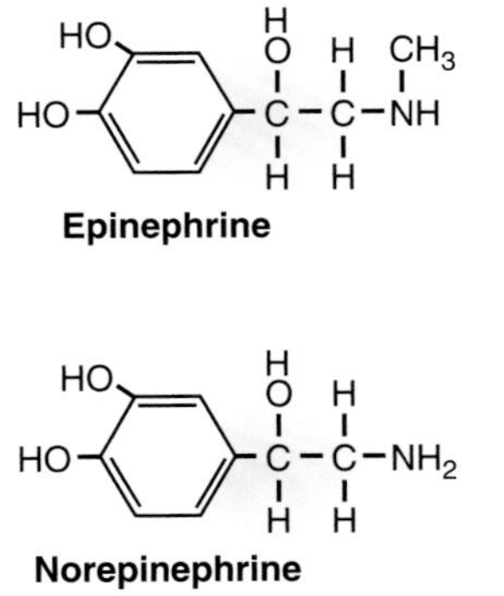

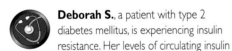

Epinephrine

Norepinephrine

FIGURE 19.13 Structure of epinephrine and norepinephrine. Epinephrine and norepinephrine are synthesized from tyrosine and act as both hormones and neurotransmitters. They are catecholamines, the term *catechol* referring to a ring structure containing two hydroxyl groups.

Deborah S., a patient with type 2 diabetes mellitus, is experiencing insulin resistance. Her levels of circulating insulin are normal to high, although inappropriately low for her elevated level of blood glucose. However, her insulin target cells, such as muscle and fat, do not respond as those of a nondiabetic subject would to this level of insulin. For most type 2 patients, the site of insulin resistance is subsequent to binding of insulin to its receptor; that is, the number of receptors and their affinity for insulin is near normal. However, the binding of insulin at these receptors does not elicit most of the normal intracellular effects of insulin discussed previously. Consequently, there is little stimulation of glucose metabolism and storage after a high-carbohydrate meal and little inhibition of hepatic gluconeogenesis.

B. Signal Transduction by Cortisol and Other Hormones that Interact with Intracellular Receptors

Signal transduction by the glucocorticoid cortisol and other steroids that have glucocorticoid activity, and by thyroid hormone, involves hormone binding to intracellular (cytosolic) receptors or binding proteins; thereafter, this hormone–binding protein complex, if not already in the nucleus, moves into the nucleus, where it interacts with chromatin. This interaction changes the rate of gene transcription in the target cells (see Chapter 16). The cellular responses to these hormones continue as long as the target cell is exposed to the specific hormones. Thus, disorders that cause a chronic excess in their secretion result in an equally persistent influence on fuel metabolism. For example, chronic stress such as that seen in prolonged sepsis may lead to varying degrees of glucose intolerance (hyperglycemia) if high levels of epinephrine and cortisol persist.

The effects of cortisol on gene transcription are usually synergistic to those of certain other hormones. For instance, the rates of gene transcription for some of the enzymes in the pathway for glucose synthesis from amino acids (gluconeogenesis) are induced by glucagon as well as by cortisol.

C. Signal Transduction by Epinephrine and Norepinephrine

Epinephrine and norepinephrine are catecholamines (Fig. 19.13). They can act as neurotransmitters or as hormones. A neurotransmitter allows a neural signal to be transmitted across the junction or synapse between the nerve terminal of a proximal nerve axon and the cell body of a distal neuron. A hormone, conversely, is released into the blood and travels in the circulation to interact with specific receptors on the plasma membrane or cytosol of cells of the target organ. The general effect of these catecholamines is to prepare us for fight or flight. Under these acutely stressful circumstances, these "stress" hormones increase fuel mobilization, cardiac output, blood flow, and so on, which enables us to meet these stresses. The catecholamines bind to adrenergic receptors (the term *adrenergic* refers to nerve cells or fibers that are part of the involuntary or autonomic nervous system, a system that uses norepinephrine as a neurotransmitter).

There are nine different types of adrenergic receptors: α_{1A}, α_{1B}, α_{1D}, α_{2A}, α_{2B}, α_{2C}, β_1, β_2, and β_3. Only the three β- and α_1-receptors are discussed here. The three β-receptors work through the adenylate cyclase–cAMP system, activating a G_s-protein, which activates adenylate cyclase, and eventually PKA. The β_1-receptor is the major adrenergic receptor in the human heart and is primarily stimulated by norepinephrine. On activation, the β_1-receptor increases the rate of muscle contraction, in part because of PKA-mediated phosphorylation of phospholamban (see Chapter 45). The β_2-receptor is present in liver, skeletal muscle, and other tissues and is involved in the mobilization of fuels (such as the release of glucose through glycogenolysis). It also mediates vascular, bronchial, and uterine smooth muscle contraction. Epinephrine is a much more potent agonist for this receptor than norepinephrine, whose major action is neurotransmission. The β_3-receptor is found predominantly in adipose tissue and to a lesser extent in skeletal muscle. Activation of this receptor stimulates fatty acid oxidation and thermogenesis, and agonists for this receptor may prove to be beneficial weight-loss agents. The α_1-receptors, which are postsynaptic receptors, mediate vascular and smooth muscle contraction. They work through the PIP_2 system (see Chapter 11, Section III.B.2) via activation of a G_q-protein, and phospholipase Cβ. This receptor also mediates glycogenolysis in liver.

CLINICAL COMMENTS

Deborah S. has type 2 diabetes mellitus, whereas **Dianne A.** has type 1 diabetes mellitus. Although the pathogenesis differs for these major forms of diabetes mellitus, both cause varying degrees of hyperglycemia. In type 1 diabetes mellitus, antibodies directed at a variety of proteins within the β-cells gradually destroy the pancreatic β-cells. As insulin-secretory capacity by the β-cells gradually diminishes below a critical level, the symptoms of chronic hyperglycemia develop rapidly.

In type 2 diabetes mellitus, these symptoms develop more subtly and gradually over the course of months or years. Eighty-five percent or more of type 2 patients are obese and, like **Ivan A.**, have a high waist–hip ratio with regard to adipose tissue disposition. This abnormal distribution of fat in the visceral (peri-intestinal) adipocytes is associated with reduced sensitivity of fat cells, muscle cells, and liver cells to the actions of insulin outlined previously. This insulin resistance can be diminished through weight loss, specifically in the visceral depots. The development of type 2 diabetes mellitus, coupled with obesity and high blood pressure, can lead to the metabolic syndrome, a common clinical entity that is discussed in more detail in Section IV of the text.

 Connie C. underwent an ultrasonographic (ultrasound) study of her upper abdomen, which showed a 2.6-cm mass in the midportion of her pancreas. With this finding, her physicians decided that further noninvasive studies would not be necessary before surgery and removal of the mass. At the time of surgery, a yellow-white 2.8-cm mass consisting primarily of insulin-rich β-cells was resected from her pancreas. No cytologic changes of malignancy were seen on microscopic examination of the surgical specimen, and no evidence of malignant behavior by the tumor (such as local metastases) was found. Connie had an uneventful postoperative recovery and no longer experienced the signs and symptoms of insulin-induced hypoglycemia.

BIOCHEMICAL COMMENTS

 Actions of Insulin. One of the important cellular responses to insulin is the reversal of glucagon-stimulated phosphorylation of enzymes. Mechanisms proposed for this action include the inhibition of adenylate cyclase, a reduction of cAMP levels, the stimulation of phosphodiesterase, the production of a specific protein (insulin factor), the release of a second messenger from a bound glycosylated phosphatidylinositol, and the phosphorylation of enzymes at a site that antagonizes PKA phosphorylation. Not all of these physiologic actions of insulin occur in each of the insulin-sensitive organs of the body.

Insulin also is able to antagonize the actions of glucagon at the level of specific induction or repression of key regulatory enzymes of carbohydrate metabolism. For instance, the rate of synthesis of messenger RNA (mRNA) for phosphoenolpyruvate carboxykinase, a key enzyme of the gluconeogenic pathway, is increased severalfold by glucagon (via cAMP) and decreased by insulin. Thus, all of the effects of glucagon, even the induction of certain enzymes, can be reversed by insulin. This antagonism is exerted through an insulin-sensitive hormone response element (IRE) in the promoter region of the genes. Insulin causes repression of the synthesis of enzymes that are induced by glucagon.

The general stimulation of protein synthesis by insulin (its mitogenic or growth-promoting effect) appears to occur through a general increase in rates of mRNA translation for a broad spectrum of structural proteins. These actions result from a phosphorylation cascade initiated by autophosphorylation of the insulin receptor and ending in the phosphorylation of subunits of proteins that bind to and inhibit eukaryotic protein synthesis initiation factors (eIFs). When phosphorylated, the inhibitory proteins are released from the eIFs, allowing translation of mRNA to be stimulated. In this respect, the actions of insulin are similar to those of other hormones that act as growth factors and that also have receptors with tyrosine kinase activity.

In addition to signal transduction, activation of the insulin receptor mediates the internalization of receptor-bound insulin molecules, increasing their subsequent degradation. Although unoccupied receptors can be internalized and eventually recycled to the plasma membrane, the receptor can be irreversibly degraded after prolonged occupation by insulin. The result of this process, referred to as *receptor downregulation*, is an attenuation of the insulin signal. The physiologic importance of receptor internalization on insulin sensitivity is poorly understood but could lead eventually to chronic hyperglycemia.

KEY CONCEPTS

- Glucose homeostasis is directed toward the maintenance of constant blood glucose levels.
- Insulin and glucagon are the two major hormones that regulate the balance between fuel mobilization and storage. They maintain blood glucose levels near 80 to 100 mg/dL, despite varying carbohydrate intake during the day.
- If dietary intake of all fuels is in excess of immediate need, it is stored as either glycogen or fat. Conversely, appropriately stored fuels are mobilized when demand requires.
- Insulin is released in response to carbohydrate ingestion and promotes glucose use as a fuel and glucose storage as fat and glycogen. Insulin secretion is regulated principally by blood glucose levels.
- Glucagon promotes glucose production via glycogenolysis (glycogen degradation) and gluconeogenesis (glucose synthesis from amino acids and other noncarbohydrate precursors).
- Glucagon release is regulated principally through suppression by rising levels of glucose and rising levels of insulin. Glucagon levels decrease in response to a carbohydrate meal and increase during fasting. Increased levels of glucagon relative to insulin stimulate the release of fatty acids from adipose tissue.
- Glucagon acts by binding to a receptor on the cell surface, which stimulates the synthesis of the intracellular second messenger, cAMP.
- cAMP activates PKA, which phosphorylates key regulatory enzymes, activating some and inhibiting others.
- Insulin acts via a receptor tyrosine kinase and leads to the dephosphorylation of the key enzymes phosphorylated in response to glucagon.
- Hormones that antagonize insulin action, known as *insulin counterregulatory hormones*, include glucagon, epinephrine, and cortisol.
- Diseases discussed in this chapter are summarized in Table 19.4.

TABLE 19.4 Diseases Discussed in Chapter 19

DISEASE OR DISORDER	ENVIRONMENTAL OR GENETIC	COMMENTS
Type 2 diabetes	Both	Emergence of insulin resistance, owing to a wide variety of causes; tissues do not respond to insulin as they normally would.
Insulinoma	Both	Periodic release of insulin from a tumor of the pancreatic β-cells, leading to hypoglycemic symptoms, which are accompanied by excessive appetite and weight gain.
Hyperglycemia	Both	Constantly elevated levels of glucose in the circulation owing to a wide variety of causes. Hyperglycemia leads to protein glycation and potential loss of protein function in a variety of tissues.
Type 1 diabetes	Both	No production of insulin by the pancreatic β-cells, owing to an autoimmune destruction of the β-cells. Hyperglycemia and ketoacidosis may result from the lack of insulin.
Maturity-onset diabetes of the young	Genetic	Forms of diabetes caused by specific mutations, such as a mutation in pancreatic glucokinase, which alters the set point for insulin release from the β-cells
Neonatal diabetes	Genetic	One cause of neonatal diabetes is a mutation in a subunit of the K^+ channel in various tissues. Such a mutation in the pancreas leads to permanent opening of the K^+ channel, keeping intracellular Ca^{2+} levels low, and difficulty in releasing insulin from the β-cells.

REVIEW QUESTIONS—CHAPTER 19

1. A patient with type 1 diabetes mellitus takes an insulin injection before eating dinner but then gets distracted and does not eat. Approximately 3 hours later, the patient becomes shaky, sweaty, and confused. These symptoms have occurred because of which one of the following?
   A. Increased glucagon release from the pancreas
   B. Decreased glucagon release from the pancreas
   C. High blood glucose levels
   D. Low blood glucose levels
   E. Elevated ketone-body levels

2. Concerning our patient in question 19.1, if the patient had fallen asleep before recognizing the symptoms, the patient could lose consciousness while sleeping. If that were to occur and paramedics were called to help the patient, the administration of which one of the following would help to reverse this effect?
   A. Insulin
   B. Normal saline
   C. Triglycerides
   D. Epinephrine
   E. Short-chain fatty acids

3. Caffeine is a potent inhibitor of the enzyme cAMP phosphodiesterase. Which one of the following consequences would you expect to occur in the liver after drinking two cups of strong espresso coffee?
   A. A prolonged response to insulin
   B. A prolonged response to glucagon
   C. An inhibition of PKA
   D. An enhancement of glycolytic activity
   E. A reduced rate of glucose export to the circulation

4. Assume that an increase in blood glucose concentration from 5 to 10 mM would result in insulin release by the pancreas. A mutation in pancreatic glucokinase can lead to MODY because of which one of the following within the pancreatic β-cell?
   A. A reduced ability to raise cAMP levels
   B. A reduced ability to raise ATP levels
   C. A reduced ability to stimulate gene transcription
   D. A reduced ability to activate glycogen degradation
   E. A reduced ability to raise intracellular lactate levels

5. Which one of the following organs has the highest demand for glucose as a fuel?
   A. Brain
   B. Muscle (skeletal)
   C. Heart
   D. Liver
   E. Pancreas

6. Glucagon release does not alter muscle metabolism because of which one of the following?
   A. Muscle cells lack adenylate cyclase.
   B. Muscle cells lack PKA.
   C. Muscle cells lack G-proteins.
   D. Muscle cells lack GTP.
   E. Muscle cells lack the glucagon receptor.

7. A male patient with fasting hypoglycemia experiences tremors, sweating, and a rapid heartbeat. These symptoms have been caused by the release of which one of the following hormones?
   A. Insulin
   B. Epinephrine
   C. Cortisol
   D. Glucagon
   E. Testosterone

8. A patient has tried many different "fad" diets to lose weight. Which one of the following meals would lead to the lowest level of circulating glucagon shortly after the meal?
   A. High-fat meal
   B. Low-protein meal
   C. Low-fat meal
   D. Low-carbohydrate meal
   E. High-carbohydrate meal

9. A 45-year-old patient was admitted to the hospital in a coma caused by severe hyperglycemia and was treated with insulin and fluids. He has been placed on long- and short-acting insulin injected daily to control his blood glucose levels. What test could be ordered at this point to determine if the patient has type 1 versus type 2 diabetes?
   A. C-peptide level
   B. Insulin level
   C. Insulin antibodies
   D. Proglucagon level
   E. Glucagon level

10. The patient in the previous question had very high blood glucose levels, and his urine also contained high blood glucose levels. The high blood glucose levels can lead to cerebral dysfunction owing to which one of the following?
    A. Dehydration
    B. Reduced lipid concentrations in the blood
    C. Increased lipid concentrations in the blood
    D. Hyperhydration
    E. High ammonia levels
    F. Low ammonia levels

ANSWERS

1. **The answer is D.** Once insulin is injected, glucose transport into the peripheral tissues will be enhanced. If the patient does not eat, the normal fasting level of glucose will drop even further resulting from the injection of insulin, which increases the movement of glucose into muscle and fat cells. The patient becomes hypoglycemic, as a result of which epinephrine is released from the adrenal medulla. This, in turn, leads to the signs and symptoms associated with high levels of epinephrine in the blood. Answers A and B are incorrect because as glucose levels drop, glucagon will be released from the pancreas to raise blood glucose levels, which would alleviate the symptoms. Answer E is incorrect because ketone body production does not produce hypoglycemic symptoms, nor would ketone bodies be significantly elevated only a few hours after the insulin shock the patient is experiencing.

2. **The answer is D.** When the patient took the insulin, the hormone stimulated glucose transport into the muscle and fat cells. This had the effect of lowering blood glucose levels, and, by not eating, the patient became severely hypoglycemic to the point that the blood glucose levels were below the K_m for the glucose transporters for the nervous system. The administration of epinephrine will stimulate the liver to release glucose, via glycogenolysis and gluconeogenesis, and will raise blood glucose levels sufficiently to overcome the insulin-induced hypoglycemia. The addition of insulin would only exacerbate the problem. Addition of triglycerides will not aid the nervous system because the fatty acids cannot cross the blood–brain barrier. Normal saline will not add nutrients for the nervous system. Short-chain fatty acids also cannot enter the nervous system.

3. **The answer is B.** When glucagon binds to its receptor, the enzyme adenylate cyclase is eventually activated (through the action of G-proteins), which raises cAMP levels in the cell. The cAMP phosphodiesterase opposes this rise in cAMP and hydrolyzes cAMP to 5'-AMP. If the phosphodiesterase is inhibited by caffeine, cAMP levels would stay elevated for an extended period of time, enhancing the glucagon response. The glucagon response in liver is to export glucose (thus, E is incorrect) and to inhibit glycolysis (thus, D is incorrect). cAMP activates PKA, making answer C incorrect as well. The effect of insulin is to reduce cAMP levels (thus, A is incorrect).

4. **The answer is B.** Insulin release is dependent on an increase in the ATP/ADP ratio within the pancreatic β-cell. In MODY, the mutation in glucokinase results in a less active glucokinase at glucose concentrations that normally stimulate insulin release. Thus, higher concentrations of glucose are required to stimulate glycolysis and the TCA cycle to effectively raise the ratio of ATP to ADP. Answer A is incorrect because cAMP levels

are not related to the mechanism of insulin release. Answer C is incorrect because initially transcription is not involved because insulin release is caused by exocytosis of preformed insulin in secretory vesicles. Answer D is incorrect because the pancreas will not degrade glycogen under conditions of high blood glucose, and answer E is incorrect because lactate does not play a role in stimulating insulin release.

5. **The answer is A.** The brain requires glucose because fatty acids cannot readily cross the blood–brain barrier to enter neuronal cells. Thus, glucose production is maintained at an adequate level to allow the brain to continue to burn glucose for its energy needs. The other organs listed as possible answers can switch to the use of alternative fuel sources (lactate, fatty acids, amino acids) and are not as dependent on glucose for their energy requirements as is the brain.

6. **The answer is E.** Muscle does not express glucagon receptors, so they are refractory to the actions of glucagon. Muscle does, however, contain GTP (made via the TCA cycle), G-proteins, PKA, and adenylate cyclase (epinephrine stimulation of muscle cells raises cAMP levels and activates PKA).

7. **The answer is B.** Insulin does lower blood glucose and cause hypoglycemia, but this would produce symptoms of fatigue, confusion, and blurred vision. When hypoglycemia is present, the body releases glucagon, cortisol, epinephrine, and norepinephrine to raise blood glucose levels. Epinephrine causes tremors, sweating, and elevated pulse rate (fight-or-flight response). Testosterone is not involved.

8. **The answer is E.** Carbohydrates are more rapidly absorbed and have the greatest and most rapid influence on elevating blood glucose levels, which stimulates insulin production and reduces glucagon secretion from the pancreas. In addition, both elevated blood glucose and elevated insulin levels suppress glucagon release. Many amino acids stimulate glucagon release, and a low-protein diet would still lead to glucagon secretion from the pancreas to a greater extent than a high-carbohydrate diet. High- or low-fat diets will not stimulate insulin release, and because gluconeogenesis is required to synthesize glucose under such diets, glucagon secretion would still be occurring.

9. **The answer is A.** Type 1 diabetes mellitus is caused by a lack of insulin (therefore, neither proinsulin nor C-peptide is produced as well), whereas type 2 diabetes mellitus is cellular resistance to secreted insulin (therefore, endogenous insulin and C-peptide are still produced in patients with type 2 diabetes). Measurement of an absolute insulin level would not be helpful because the patient is injecting insulin each day. However, if the patient is still producing insulin, he would also produce the C-peptide and would be classified as having

type 2 diabetes. If C-peptide levels are not detected, the patient is classified as having type 1 diabetes. Individuals with type 1 diabetes can have islet cell antibodies in their blood, but not insulin antibodies. The presence of antibodies against insulin in the blood would lead to a reduced response to insulin, or a form of type 2 diabetes. The measurement of glucagon or proglucagon levels would not differentiate type 1 from type 2 diabetes because both glucagon and proglucagon would still be produced in individuals with diabetes. The levels of glucagon secreted in both types of diabetes is similar.

10. **The answer is A.** The elevated glucose in the blood leads to an osmotic diuresis because water will leave cells to enter the blood and urine in order to reduce the glucose concentration in those fluids. As the water leaves the tissues and enters the urine, blood volume also decreases, leading to even higher blood glucose concentrations. The loss of water leads to severe dehydration and to reduced blood flow to the brain (because of reduced blood volume), which will lead to cerebral dysfunction. The brain cannot use lipids as an energy source, so altering lipid concentrations in the blood will not affect cerebral function. The cerebral dysfunction is actually occurring under higher than normal blood glucose concentrations; it is the reduced blood volume that leads to the dysfunction. Carbohydrates do not contain a nitrogen group, so they do not produce ammonia. High levels of ammonia can cause cerebral dysfunction, but it does not come about because of high blood glucose levels.

20

Cellular Bioenergetics: Adenosine Triphosphate and O_2

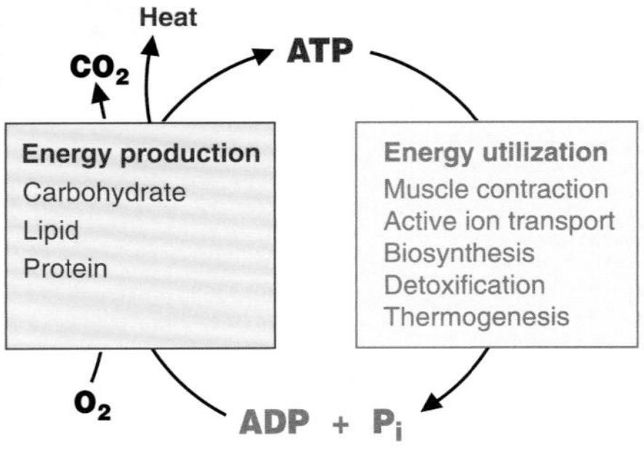

FIGURE 20.1 The ATP–ADP cycle. *ADP*, adenosine diphosphate; *ATP*, adenosine triphosphate; *P_i*, inorganic phosphate.

Bioenergetics refers to **cellular energy transformations**.

The ATP–ADP Cycle. In cells, the **chemical bond energy** of fuels is transformed into the physiologic responses that are necessary for life. The central role of the **high-energy phosphate bonds of adenosine triphosphate (ATP)** in these processes is summarized in the **ATP–ADP (adenosine diphosphate) cycle** (Fig. 20.1). To generate ATP through cellular respiration, fuels are degraded by oxidative reactions that transfer most of their **chemical bond energy** to **nicotinamide adenine dinucleotide** (NAD$^+$) and **flavin adenine dinucleotide** (FAD) to generate the reduced form of these coenzymes, **NADH** and **FAD(2H)**. When NADH and FAD(2H) are oxidized by oxygen (O_2) in the electron-transport chain (ETC), the energy is used to regenerate ATP in the process of **oxidative phosphorylation**. Energy available from cleavage of the high-energy phosphate bonds of ATP can be used directly for **mechanical work** (e.g., muscle contraction) or for **transport work** (e.g., a Na$^+$ gradient generated by **Na$^+$,K$^+$-ATPase**). It can also be used for **biochemical work** (energy-requiring chemical reactions), such as **anabolic pathways** (biosynthesis of large molecules such as proteins) or detoxification reactions. **Phosphoryl transfer** reactions, **protein conformational changes**, and the formation of **activated intermediates** containing **high-energy bonds** (e.g., uridine diphosphate [UDP]-sugars) facilitate these energy transformations. Energy released from foods that is not used for work against the environment is transformed into **heat**.

ATP Homeostasis. Fuel oxidation is regulated to maintain **ATP homeostasis** ("homeo," same; "stasis," state). Regardless of whether the level of cellular fuel use is high (with increased ATP consumption) or low (with decreased ATP consumption), the available ATP within the cell is maintained at a constant level by appropriate increases or decreases in the rate of fuel oxidation. Problems in ATP homeostasis and energy balance occur in obesity, hyperthyroidism, and myocardial infarction (MI).

Energy from Fuel Oxidation. Fuel oxidation is **exergonic**; it releases energy. The maximum quantity of energy released that is available for useful work (e.g., ATP synthesis) is called $\Delta G^{0'}$, the **change in Gibbs free energy** at pH 7.0 under standard conditions. Fuel oxidation has a **negative $\Delta G^{0'}$**; that is, the products have a lower chemical bond energy than the reactants, and their formation is energetically favored. ATP synthesis from ADP and inorganic phosphate (P_i) is **endergonic**: It requires energy and has a positive $\Delta G^{0'}$. To proceed in our cells, all pathways must have a negative $\Delta G^{0'}$. How is this accomplished for anabolic pathways such as glycogen synthesis? These metabolic pathways incorporate reactions that expend high-energy bonds to compensate for the energy-requiring steps. Because the $\Delta G^{0'}$ values for a sequence of reactions **are additive**, the overall pathway becomes energetically favorable.

Fuels are oxidized principally by donating electrons to NAD$^+$ and FAD, which then donate electrons to O_2 in the ETC. The **caloric value** of a fuel is related to its $\Delta G^{0'}$ for transfer of electrons to O_2, and its **reduction potential, E$^{0'}$** (a measure of its willingness to donate, or accept, electrons). Because fatty acids are more reduced than carbohydrates, they have a higher caloric value. The high affinity of O_2 for electrons (a high positive reduction potential) drives fuel oxidation forward, with release of energy that can be used for ATP synthesis in oxidative phosphorylation. However, smaller amounts of ATP can be generated without the use of O_2 in **anaerobic glycolysis**.

Fuel oxidation can also generate **NADPH**, which usually donates electrons to biosynthetic pathways and detoxification reactions. For example, in some reactions catalyzed by **oxygenases**, NADPH is the electron donor and O_2 is the electron acceptor.

THE WAITING ROOM

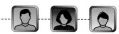

 Otto S. is a 26-year-old medical student who has completed his first year of medical school. He is 5 ft 10 in tall and began medical school weighing 154 lb, within his ideal weight range (see Chapter 1). By the time he finished his last examination in his first year, he weighed 187 lb. He had calculated his basal metabolic rate (BMR) at approximately 1,680 kilocalorie [kcal] and his energy expenditure for physical exercise equal to 30% of his BMR. He planned on returning to his pre–medical school weight in 6 weeks over the summer by eating 576 kcal less each day and playing 7 hours of tennis every day. However, he did a summer internship instead of playing tennis. When Otto started his second year of medical school, he weighed 210 lb.

 Stanley T. is a 26-year-old man who noted heat intolerance, with heavy sweating, heart palpitations, and tremulousness. Over the past 4 months, he has lost weight in spite of a good appetite. He is sleeping poorly and describes himself as feeling "jittery inside."

On physical examination, his heart rate is rapid (116 beats/minute) and he appears restless and fidgety. His skin feels warm, and he is perspiring profusely. A fine hand tremor is observed as he extends his arms in front of his chest. His thyroid gland appears to be diffusely enlarged and, on palpation, is approximately three times normal size. Thyroid function tests confirm that Mr. T.'s thyroid gland is secreting excessive amounts of the thyroid hormones tetraiodothyronine (T_4) and triiodothyronine (T_3), the major thyroid hormones present in the blood.

 Cora N. is a 64-year-old female who had a myocardial infarction (MI; often referred to as a "heart attack") 8 months ago. Although she has managed to lose 6 lb since the MI, she remains overweight and has not reduced the fat content of her diet adequately. The graded aerobic exercise program she started 5 weeks after her infarction is now followed irregularly, falling far short of the cardiac conditioning intensity prescribed by her cardiologist. She is readmitted to the hospital cardiac care unit after experiencing a severe "viselike pressure" in the midchest area while cleaning ice from the windshield of her car. The electrocardiogram shows evidence of a new anterior wall MI. Signs and symptoms of left ventricular failure are present.

I. Energy Available to Do Work

The basic principle of the ATP–ADP cycle is that fuel oxidation generates ATP, and hydrolysis of ATP to ADP provides the energy to perform most of the work required in the cell. ATP has, therefore, been called the *energy currency* of the cells. To keep up with the demand, we must constantly replenish our ATP supply through the use of oxygen (O_2) for fuel oxidation.

The amount of energy from ATP cleavage available to do useful work is related to the difference in energy levels between the products and substrates of the reaction and is called the change in *Gibbs free energy*, ΔG (Δ, difference; G, Gibbs free energy). In cells, the ΔG for energy production from fuel oxidation must be greater than the ΔG of energy-requiring processes, such as protein synthesis and muscle contraction, for life to continue.

 To assess for thyroid function, one must understand how the hormones T_3 and T_4 are released from the thyroid (see Chapter 41). The hypothalamus and the pituitary gland both monitor the level of free T_3 in the blood bathing them. When the concentration of free T_3 in the blood drops, the pituitary releases thyroid-stimulating hormone (TSH), which stimulates the thyroid to release T_3 and T_4. The pituitary is under the control of the hypothalamus, which releases TSH-releasing hormone (TSHRH) under the appropriate conditions. Thus, if one notices low serum T_3 or T_4 levels, it may represent a thyroid or pituitary problem. Understanding the physiology enables the appropriate tests to be run to determine where the defect lies.

T_3 and T_4 are measured using sensitive techniques that involve antibody recognition (radioimmunoassay; see Chapter 41). TSH levels can be determined in a similar fashion using a sandwich technique (which requires the use of two distinct antibodies that recognize TSH).

Through the appropriate interpretation of these tests, one can determine if thyroid or pituitary function is impaired and design treatment accordingly.

 Cora N. suffered a heart attack 8 months ago and had a significant loss of functional heart muscle. She occasionally gets pain while walking. The pain she is experiencing is called *angina pectoris* and is a crushing or constricting pain located in the center of the chest, often radiating to the neck or arms (see **Ann J.**, Chapters 6 and 7). The most common cause of angina is partial blockage of coronary arteries from atherosclerosis. The heart muscle cells beyond the block receive an inadequate blood flow and oxygen, and they die when ATP production falls too low.

 The heart is a specialist in the transformation of ATP chemical bond energy into mechanical work. Each single heartbeat uses approximately 2% of the ATP in the heart. If the heart were not able to regenerate ATP, all its ATP would be hydrolyzed in <1 minute. Because the amount of ATP required by the heart is so high, it must rely on the pathway of oxidative phosphorylation for generation of this ATP. In **Cora N.'s** heart, hypoxia (the lack of oxygen) is affecting her ability to generate ATP.

A. The High-Energy Phosphate Bonds of ATP

The amount of energy released or required by bond cleavage or formation is determined by the chemical properties of the substrates and products. The bonds between the phosphate groups in ATP are called *phosphoanhydride bonds* (Fig. 20.2). When these bonds are hydrolyzed, energy is released because the products of the reaction (ADP and phosphate) are more stable, with lower bond energies, than the reactants (ATP and water [H_2O]). The instability of the phosphoanhydride bonds arises from their negatively charged phosphate groups, which repel each other and strain the bonds between them. It takes energy to make the phosphate groups stay together. In contrast, there are fewer negative charges in ADP to repel each other. The phosphate group as a free anion is more stable than it is in ATP because of an increase in resonance structures (i.e., the electrons of the oxygen double bond are shared by all the oxygen atoms). As a consequence, ATP hydrolysis is energetically favorable and proceeds with release of energy as heat.

In the cell, ATP is not hydrolyzed directly. Energy released as heat from ATP hydrolysis cannot be transferred efficiently into energy-requiring processes such as biosynthetic reactions or maintenance of an ion gradient. Instead, cellular enzymes transfer the phosphate group to a metabolic intermediate or protein that is part of the energy-requiring process (a phosphoryl transfer reaction).

B. Change in Free Energy (ΔG) during a Reaction

How much energy can be obtained from ATP hydrolysis to do the work required in the cell? The maximum amount of useful energy that can be obtained from a reaction is called ΔG— the change in Gibbs free energy. The value of ΔG for a reaction can be influenced by the initial concentration of substrates and products, by temperature, pH, and by pressure. The ΔG^0 for a reaction refers to the energy change for a reaction starting at 1 M substrate and product concentrations and proceeding to equilibrium (equilibrium, by definition, occurs when there is no change in substrate and product concentrations with time). $\Delta G^{0'}$ is the value for ΔG^0 under standard conditions (pH = 7.0, [H_2O] = 55 M, and 25°C) as well as standard concentrations (Table 20.1).

$\Delta G^{0'}$ is equivalent to the chemical bond energy of the products minus that of the reactants, corrected for energy that has gone into entropy (an increase in amount of molecular disorder). This correction for change in entropy is very small for most

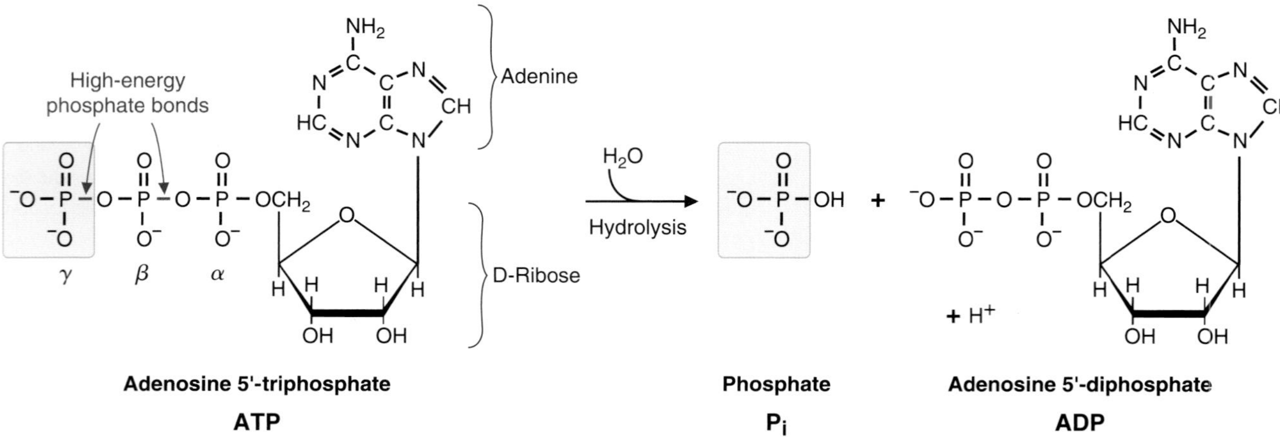

FIGURE 20.2 Hydrolysis of adenosine triphosphate (ATP) to adenosine diphosphate (ADP) and inorganic phosphate (P_i). Cleavage of the phosphoanhydride bonds between either the β- and γ-phosphates or between the α- and β-phosphates releases the same amount of energy, approximately 7.3 kcal/mol. However, hydrolysis of the phosphate–adenosine bond (a phosphoester bond) releases less energy (≈3.4 kcal/mol), and consequently, this bond is not considered a high-energy phosphate bond. During ATP hydrolysis, the change in disorder during the reaction is small, and so ΔG values at physiologic temperature (37°C) are similar to those at standard temperature (25°C). ΔG is affected by pH, which alters the ionization state of the phosphate groups of ATP and by the intracellular concentration of Mg^{2+} ions, which bind to the β- and γ-phosphate groups of ATP.

TABLE 20.1	Thermodynamic Expressions, Laws, and Constants
DEFINITIONS	
ΔG	Change in free energy, or Gibbs free energy
ΔG^0	Standard free-energy change, ΔG starting with 1 M concentrations of substrates and products
$\Delta G^{0'}$	Standard free-energy change at 25°C, pH 7.0
ΔH	Change in enthalpy, or heat content
ΔS	Change in entropy, or increase in disorder
K'_{eq}	Equilibrium constant at 25°C, pH 7.0, incorporating $[H_2O] = 55.5$ M and $[H^+] = 10^{-7}$ M in the constant
$\Delta E^{0'}$	Change in reduction potential
P	Biochemical symbol for a high-energy phosphate bond; that is, a bond that is hydrolyzed with the release of more than about 7 kcal/mol of heat

LAWS OF THERMODYNAMICS

First law of thermodynamics, the conservation of energy: In any physical or chemical change, the total energy of a system, including its surroundings, remains constant.
Second law of thermodynamics: The universe tends toward disorder. In all natural processes, the total entropy of a system always increases.

CONSTANTS

Units of ΔG and ΔH = cal/mol or joule (J)/mol: 1 cal = 4.18 J
T, absolute temperature: K, Kelvin = 273 + °C (25°C = 298°K)
R, universal gas constant: 1.98 cal/mol-K or 8.31 J/mol-K
F, Faraday constant: F = 23 kcal/mole-volt (V) or 96,500 J/V-mol
Units of $E^{0'}$, V

FORMULAS

$\Delta G = \Delta H - T\Delta S$
$\Delta G^{0'} = -RT \ln K_{eq}'$
$\Delta G^{0'} = -nF \Delta E^{0'}$
$\ln = 2.303 \log_{10}$

reactions that occur in cells, and thus, the $\Delta G^{0'}$ for hydrolysis of various chemical bonds reflects the amount of energy available from that bond.

The value -7.3 kcal/mol (-30.5 kilojoule [kJ]/mol) that is generally used for the $\Delta G^{0'}$ of ATP hydrolysis is thus the amount of energy available from hydrolysis of ATP, under standard conditions, that can be spent on energy-requiring processes; it defines the "monetary value" of our "ATP currency." Although the difference between cellular conditions (pH 7.3, 37°C) and standard conditions is very small, the difference between cellular concentrations of ATP, ADP, and P_i and the standard 1 M concentrations is huge and greatly affects the availability of energy in the cell.

C. Exothermic and Endothermic Reactions

The value of $\Delta G^{0'}$ tells you whether the reaction requires or releases energy, the amount of energy involved, and the ratio of products to substrates at equilibrium. The negative value for the $\Delta G^{0'}$ of ATP hydrolysis indicates that, if you begin with equimolar (1 M) concentrations of substrates and products, the reaction proceeds in the forward direction with the release of energy. From initial concentrations of 1 M, the ATP concentration will decrease, and ADP and P_i will increase until equilibrium is reached.

For a reaction in which a substrate S is converted to a product P, the ratio of the product concentration to the substrate concentration *at equilibrium* is given by

$$\Delta G^{0'} = -RT \ln[P]/[S] \qquad \textbf{Equation 20.1.}$$

Q The reaction catalyzed by phosphoglucomutase is reversible and functions in the synthesis of glycogen from glucose as well as the degradation of glycogen back to glucose. If the $\Delta G^{0'}$ for conversion of glucose 6-P to glucose 1-P is +1.65 kcal/mol, what is the $\Delta G^{0'}$ of the reverse reaction?

The $\Delta G^{0'}$ for the reverse reaction is −1.65 kcal. The change in free energy is the same for the forward and reverse directions but has opposite sign. Because negative $\Delta G^{0'}$ values indicate favorable reactions, this reaction under standard conditions favors the conversion of glucose 1-P to glucose 6-P.

TABLE 20.2	**A General Expression for ΔG**

To generalize the expression for ΔG, consider a reaction in which

$$aA + bB \leftrightarrows cC + dD$$

The lowercase letters denote that a moles of A will combine with b moles of B to produce c moles of C and d moles of D.

$$\Delta G^{0'} = -RT \ln K_{eq} = -RT \ln \frac{[C]^c_{eq}[D]^d_{eq}}{[A]^a_{eq}[B]^b_{eq}}$$

and, when not in equilibrium,

$$\Delta G = =\Delta G^{0'} + RT \ln \frac{[C]^c[D]^d}{[A]^a[B]^b}$$

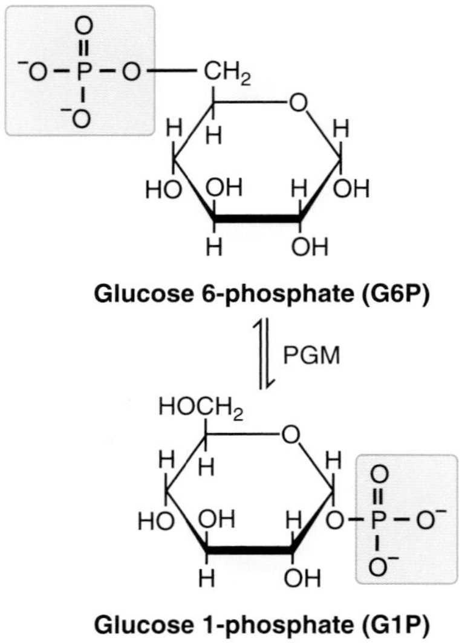

Table 20.2 indicates a more general form of this equation; R is the gas constant [1.98 cal/mol °K], and T is equal to the temperature in degrees Kelvin.

Thus, the difference in chemical bond energies of the substrate and product ($\Delta G^{0'}$) determines the concentration of each at equilibrium.

Reactions such as ATP hydrolysis are *exergonic* (releasing energy) or *exothermic* (releasing heat). Both exergonic and exothermic reactions have a negative $\Delta G^{0'}$ and release energy while proceeding in the forward direction to equilibrium. *Endergonic*, or *endothermic*, reactions have a positive $\Delta G^{0'}$ for the forward direction (the direction shown), and the backward direction is favored. For example, in the pathway of glycogen synthesis, phosphoglucomutase converts glucose 6-phosphate (glucose 6-P) to glucose 1-phosphate (glucose 1-P). Glucose 1-P has a higher phosphate bond energy than glucose 6-P because the phosphate is on the aldehyde carbon (Fig. 20.3). The $\Delta G^{0'}$ value for the forward direction (glucose 6-P → glucose 1-P) is therefore positive. Beginning at equimolar concentrations of both compounds, there is a net conversion of glucose 1-P back to glucose 6-P, and at equilibrium, the concentration of glucose 6-P is higher than glucose 1-P. The exact ratio is determined by the $\Delta G^{0'}$ for the reaction.

It is often said that a reaction with a negative $\Delta G^{0'}$ proceeds spontaneously in the forward direction, meaning that products accumulate at the expense of reactants. However, $\Delta G^{0'}$ is not an indicator of the velocity of the reaction or of the rate at which equilibrium can be reached. In the cell, the velocity of the reaction depends on the efficiency and amount of enzyme available to catalyze the reaction (see Chapter 9), so "spontaneously" in this context can be misleading.

The equations for calculating ΔG are based on the first law of thermodynamics (see Table 20.1). The change in chemical bond energy that occurs during a reaction is ΔH, the change in enthalpy of the reaction. At constant temperature and pressure, ΔH is equivalent to the chemical bond energy of the products minus that of the reactants. ΔG, the maximum amount of useful work available from a reaction, is equal to $\Delta H - T\Delta S$. $T\Delta S$ is a correction for the amount of energy that has gone into an increase in the entropy (disorder in arrangement of molecules) of the system. Thus, $\Delta G = \Delta H - T\Delta S$, where ΔH is the change in enthalpy, T is the temperature of the system in Kelvin, and ΔS is the change in entropy, or increased disorder of the system. ΔS is often negligible in reactions such as ATP hydrolysis, in which the numbers of substrates (H_2O, ATP) and products (ADP, P_i) are equal and no gas is formed. Under these conditions, the values for ΔG at physiologic temperature (37°C) are similar to those at standard temperature (25°C).

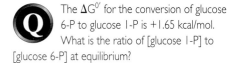

Glucose 6-phosphate (G6P)

PGM

Glucose 1-phosphate (G1P)

For G6P → G1P:
$\Delta G^{0'} = +1.6$ kcal/mol

$\Delta G^{0'} = -RT \ln \dfrac{[G1P]}{[G6P]}$

FIGURE 20.3 The phosphoglucomutase (PGM) reaction. The forward direction (formation of glucose 1-phosphate [G1P]) is involved in converting glucose to glycogen, and the reverse direction in converting glycogen to glucose 6-phosphate (G6P).

The $\Delta G^{0'}$ for the conversion of glucose 6-P to glucose 1-P is +1.65 kcal/mol. What is the ratio of [glucose 1-P] to [glucose 6-P] at equilibrium?

II. Energy Transformations to Do Mechanical and Transport Work

For work in the cell to be done, a mechanism must be available for converting the chemical bond energy of ATP into another form, such as a Na^+ gradient across a membrane. These energy transformations usually involve intermediate steps in which ATP is bound to a protein, and cleavage of the bound ATP results in a conformational change of the protein.

A. Mechanical Work

In *mechanical work*, the high-energy phosphate bond of ATP is converted into movement by changing the conformation of a protein (Fig. 20.4). For example, in contracting muscle fibers, the hydrolysis of ATP while it is bound to myosin ATPase changes the conformation of myosin so that it is in a "cocked" position, ready to associate with the sliding actin filament. Thus, exercising muscle fibers have almost a 100-fold higher rate of ATP use and caloric requirements than resting muscle fibers. Motor proteins, such as kinesins that transport chemicals along fibers, provide another example of mechanical work in a cell.

B. Transport Work

In *transport work*, called *active transport*, the high-energy phosphate bond of ATP is used to transport compounds against a concentration gradient (see Chapter 10, Fig. 10.10). In plasma membrane ATPases (P-ATPases) and vesicular ATPases (V-ATPases), the chemical bond energy of ATP is used to reversibly phosphorylate the transport protein and change its conformation. For example, as the Na^+,K^+-ATPase binds and cleaves ATP, it becomes phosphorylated and changes its conformation to release three Na^+ ions to the outside of the cell, thereby building up a higher extracellular than intracellular concentration of Na^+. Na^+ reenters the cell on cotransport proteins that drive the uptake of amino acids and many other compounds into the cell. Thus, Na^+ must be continuously transported back out. The expenditure of ATP for Na^+ transport occurs even while we sleep and is estimated to account for 10% to 30% of our BMR.

A large number of other active transporters also convert ATP chemical bond energy into an ion gradient (membrane potential). Vesicular ATPases pump protons into lysosomes. Ca^{2+}-ATPases in the plasma membrane move Ca^{2+} out of the cell against a concentration gradient. Similar Ca^{2+}-ATPases pump Ca^{2+} into the

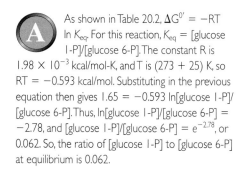

As shown in Table 20.2, $\Delta G^{0'} = -RT \ln K_{eq}$. For this reaction, $K_{eq} = $ [glucose 1-P]/[glucose 6-P]. The constant R is 1.98×10^{-3} kcal/mol-K, and T is (273 + 25) K, so RT = -0.593 kcal/mol. Substituting in the previous equation then gives $1.65 = -0.593 \ln$[glucose 1-P]/[glucose 6-P]. Thus, $\ln$[glucose 1-P]/[glucose 6-P] = -2.78, and [glucose 1-P]/[glucose 6-P] = $e^{-2.78}$, or 0.062. So, the ratio of [glucose 1-P] to [glucose 6-P] at equilibrium is 0.062.

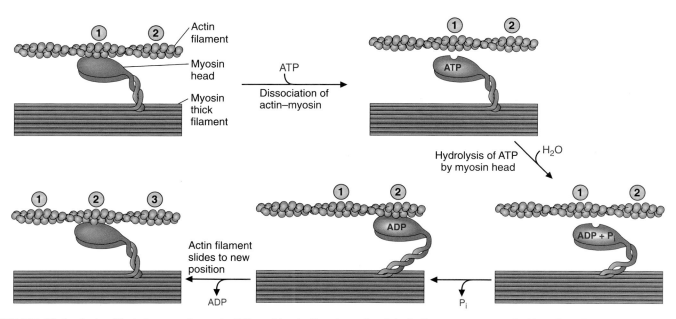

FIGURE 20.4 A simplified diagram of myosin ATPase. Muscle fiber is made of thick filaments composed of bundles of the protein myosin, and thin filaments composed of the protein actin (which is activated by Ca^{2+} binding). At many positions along the actin filament, a terminal domain of a myosin molecule, referred to as the "head," binds to a specific site on the actin. The myosin head has an ATP-binding site and is an ATPase; it can hydrolyze ATP to ADP and P_i. (*1*) As ATP binds to myosin, the conformation of myosin changes, and it dissociates from the actin. (*2*) Myosin hydrolyzes the ATP, again changing conformation. (*3*) When P_i dissociates, the myosin head reassociates with activated actin at a new position (position 2 in the figure). (*4*) As ADP dissociates, the myosin again changes conformation, or tightens. This change of conformation at multiple association points between actin and myosin slides the actin filament forward. *ADP*, adenosine diphosphate; *ATP*, adenosine triphosphate; P_i, inorganic phosphate.

Otto S. has not followed his proposed diet and exercise regimen and has been gaining weight. He has a positive caloric balance because his daily energy expenditure is less than his daily energy intake (see Chapter 2). Although the energy expenditure for physical exercise is only approximately 30% of the BMR in a sedentary individual, it can be 100% or more of the BMR in a person who exercises strenuously for several hours or more. The large increase in ATP use for muscle contraction during exercise accounts for its contribution to the daily energy expenditure.

In the thermodynamic perspective of energy expenditure, when energy intake to the body exceeds energy expended, the difference is effectively stored as fat.

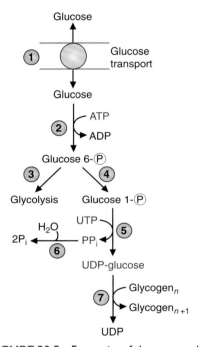

FIGURE 20.5 Energetics of glycogen synthesis. Compounds containing high-energy bonds are shown in *red*. (*1*) Glucose is transported into the cell. (*2*) Glucose phosphorylation uses the high-energy phosphate bond (~P) of adenosine triphosphate (ATP) in a phosphoryl transfer step. (*4*) Conversion of glucose 6-phosphate to glucose 1-phosphate by phosphoglucomutase. (*5*) Uridine diphosphate (UDP)-glucose pyrophosphorylase cleaves a ~P bond in uridine triphosphate (UTP), releasing pyrophosphate (PP$_i$) and forming UDP-glucose, an activated intermediate. (*6*) The pyrophosphate is hydrolyzed, releasing additional energy. (*7*) The phosphoester bond of UDP-glucose is cleaved during the addition of a glucosyl unit to the end of a glycogen polysaccharide chain. The UDP acts as the leaving group in this reaction. Glucose 6-phosphate also can be metabolized via glycolysis (*3*) when energy is required. *P$_i$*, inorganic phosphate.

lumen of the endoplasmic reticulum and the sarcoplasmic reticulum (in muscle). Thus, a considerable amount of energy is expended in maintaining a low cytoplasmic Ca^{2+} level.

III. Biochemical Work

The high-energy phosphate bonds of ATP are also used for *biochemical work*. Biochemical work occurs in *anabolic pathways*, which are pathways that synthesize large molecules (e.g., DNA, glycogen, triacylglycerols, proteins) from smaller compounds. Biochemical work also occurs when toxic compounds are converted to nontoxic compounds that can be excreted (e.g., the liver converts NH_4^+ ions to urea in the urea cycle). In general, formation of chemical bonds between two organic molecules (e.g., C–C bonds in fatty acid synthesis or C–N bonds in protein synthesis) requires energy and is therefore biochemical work. How do our cells get these necessary energy-requiring reactions to occur?

To answer this question, the next sections consider how energy is used to synthesize glycogen from glucose (Fig. 20.5). Glycogen is a storage polysaccharide consisting of glucosyl units linked together through glycosidic bonds. If an anabolic pathway, such as glycogen synthesis, were to have an overall positive $\Delta G^{0'}$, the cell would be full of glucose and intermediates of the pathway but very little glycogen would be formed. To avoid this, cells do biochemical work and spend enough of their ATP currency to give anabolic pathways an overall negative $\Delta G^{0'}$.

A. Adding ΔG^0 Values

Reactions in which chemical bonds are formed between two organic molecules are usually catalyzed by enzymes that transfer energy from cleavage of ATP in a phosphoryl transfer reaction or by enzymes that cleave a high-energy bond in an activated intermediate of the pathway. Because the $\Delta G^{0'}$ values in a reaction sequence are additive, the pathway acquires an overall negative $\Delta G^{0'}$, and the reactions in the pathway will occur to move toward an equilibrium state in which the concentration of final products is greater than that of the initial reactants.

1. Phosphoryl Transfer Reactions

One of the characteristics of Gibbs free energy is that ΔG^0 values for consecutive steps or reactions in a sequence can be added together to obtain a single value for the overall process. Thus, the high-energy phosphate bonds of ATP can be used to drive a reaction forward that would otherwise be highly unfavorable energetically. Consider, for example, synthesis of glucose 6-P from glucose, the first step in glycolysis and glycogen synthesis (see Fig. 20.5, circle 2). If the reaction were to proceed by addition of P$_i$ to glucose, glucose 6-P synthesis would have a positive $\Delta G^{0'}$ value of 3.3 kcal/mol (Table 20.3). However, when this reaction is coupled to cleavage of the high-energy ATP bond through a phosphoryl transfer reaction, the $\Delta G^{0'}$ for glucose 6-P synthesis acquires a net negative value of −4.0 kcal/mol, which can be calculated from the sum of the two reactions. Glucose 6-P cannot be transported back out of the cell, and, therefore, the net negative $\Delta G^{0'}$ for glucose 6-P synthesis helps the cell to trap glucose for its own metabolic needs.

TABLE 20.3 $\Delta G^{0'}$ for the Transfer of a Phosphate from ATP to Glucose	
Glucose + P$_i$ → G6P + H$_2$O	$\Delta G^{0'}$ = +3.3 kcal/mol
ATP + H$_2$O → ADP + P$_i$	$\Delta G^{0'}$ = −7.3 kcal/mol
Sum: glucose + ATP → G6P + ADP	$\Delta G^{0'}$ = −4.0 kcal/mol

ADP, adenosine diphosphate; ATP, adenosine triphosphate; G6P, glucose 6-phosphate; P$_i$, inorganic phosphate.

The net value for synthesis of glucose 6-P from glucose and ATP would be the same whether the two reactions are catalyzed by the same enzyme, are catalyzed by two separate enzymes, or are not catalyzed by an enzyme at all because the net value of glucose 6-P synthesis is dictated by the amount of energy in the chemical bonds being broken and formed.

2. Activated Intermediates in Glycogen Synthesis

To synthesize glycogen from glucose, energy is provided by the cleavage of three high-energy phosphate bonds in ATP, uridine triphosphate (UTP), and pyrophosphate (PP$_i$) (see Fig. 20.5, steps 2, 5, and 6). Energy transfer is facilitated by phosphoryl group transfer and by formation of an activated intermediate (UDP-glucose). Step 4, the conversion of glucose 6-P to glucose 1-P, has a positive $\Delta G^{0'}$. This step is pulled and pushed in the desired direction by the accumulation of substrate and removal of product in reactions that have a negative $\Delta G^{0'}$ from cleavage of high-energy bonds. In step 5, the UTP high-energy phosphate bond is cleaved to form the activated sugar, UDP-glucose (Fig. 20.6). This reaction is further facilitated by cleavage of the high-energy bond in the PP$_i$ (step 6) that is released in step 5 (approximately -7.7 kcal). In step 7, cleavage of the bond between UDP and glucose in the activated intermediate provides the energy for attaching the glucose moiety to the end of the glycogen molecule (approximately -3.3 kcal). In general, the amount of ATP phosphate bond energy used in an anabolic pathway, or detoxification pathway, must provide the pathway with an overall negative $\Delta G^{0'}$, so that the concentration of products is favored over that of reactants.

B. ΔG Depends on Substrate and Product Concentrations

$\Delta G^{0'}$ reflects the energy difference between reactants and products at specific concentrations (each at 1 M) and standard conditions (pH 7.0, 25°C). However, these are not the conditions prevailing in cells, in which variations from "standard conditions" are relevant to determining actual free-energy changes and hence the direction in which reactions are likely to occur. One aspect of free-energy changes contributing to the forward direction of anabolic pathways is the dependence of ΔG, the free-energy change of a reaction, on the initial substrate and product concentrations. Reactions in the cell with a positive $\Delta G^{0'}$ can proceed in the forward direction if the concentration of substrate is raised to high enough levels, or if the concentration of product is decreased to very low levels. Product concentrations can be very low if, for example, the product is rapidly used in a subsequent energetically favorable reaction, or if the product diffuses or is transported away.

I. The Difference between ΔG and ΔG$^{0'}$

The driving force toward equilibrium starting at any concentration of substrate and product is expressed by ΔG, and not by $\Delta G^{0'}$, which is the free-energy change to

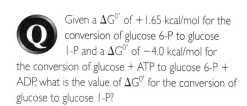

Given a $\Delta G^{0'}$ of $+1.65$ kcal/mol for the conversion of glucose 6-P to glucose 1-P and a $\Delta G^{0'}$ of -4.0 kcal/mol for the conversion of glucose + ATP to glucose 6-P + ADP, what is the value of $\Delta G^{0'}$ for the conversion of glucose to glucose 1-P?

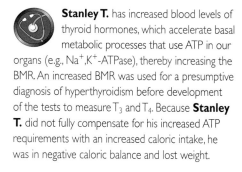

Stanley T. has increased blood levels of thyroid hormones, which accelerate basal metabolic processes that use ATP in our organs (e.g., Na$^+$,K$^+$-ATPase), thereby increasing the BMR. An increased BMR was used for a presumptive diagnosis of hyperthyroidism before development of the tests to measure T$_3$ and T$_4$. Because **Stanley T.** did not fully compensate for his increased ATP requirements with an increased caloric intake, he was in negative caloric balance and lost weight.

FIGURE 20.6 Uridine diphosphate (UDP)-glucose contains a high-energy pyrophosphate bond, shown in the *green box*.

Uridine diphosphate glucose (UDP-glucose)

$\Delta G^{0'}$ for the overall reaction is the sum of the individual reactions, or -2.35 kcal. The individual reactions are

Glucose + ATP $\rightarrow$ glucose 6-P + ADP

$\Delta G^{0'} = -4.0$ kcal/mol

glucose 6-P $\rightarrow$ glucose 1-P

$\Delta G^{0'} = +1.65$ kcal/mol

Therefore,

Glucose + ATP $\rightarrow$ glucose 1-P + ADP

$\Delta G^{0'} = -2.35$ kcal/mol

Thus, the cleavage of ATP has made the synthesis of glucose 1-P from glucose energetically favorable.

Approximately 70% of our resting daily energy requirement arises from work carried out by our largest organs: the heart, brain, kidneys, and liver. Using their rate of O_2 consumption and an assumption that for each mole of oxygen atom consumed, 2.5 mol of ATP are synthesized (see Chapter 24), it can be estimated that each of these organs is using and producing several times its own weight in ATP each day.

Estimated Daily Use of ATP (g ATP/g Tissue)	
Heart	16
Brain	6
Kidneys	24
Liver	6
Skeletal muscle (rest)	0.3
Skeletal muscle (running)	23.6

The heart, which rhythmically contracts, is using this ATP for mechanical work. In contrast, skeletal muscles in a resting individual use far less ATP per gram of tissue. The kidney has an ATP consumption per gram of tissue similar to that of the heart and uses this ATP largely for transport work to recover usable nutrients and to maintain pH and electrolyte balance. The brain, likewise, uses most of its ATP for transport work, maintaining the ion gradients necessary for conduction of nerve impulses. The liver, in contrast, has a high rate of ATP consumption and use to carry out metabolic work (biosynthesis and detoxification). **Otto S.** realizes that his resting daily energy requirement will remain constant, and for him to lose weight, he will have to eat less, exercise more, or both.

reach equilibrium starting with 1 M concentrations of substrate and product. For a reaction in which the substrate S is converted to the product P,

$$\Delta G = \Delta G^{0'} + RT \ln[P]/[S] \qquad \textbf{Equation 20.2.}$$

(See Table 20.2 for the general form of this equation.)

The expression for ΔG has two terms: $\Delta G^{0'}$, the energy change to reach equilibrium starting at equal and 1 M concentrations of substrates and products; and the second term, the energy change to reach equal concentrations of substrate and product starting from any initial concentration. (When [P] = [S] and [P]/[S] = 1, $\ln[P]/[S] = 0$, and $\Delta G = \Delta G^{0'}$.) The second term will be negative for all concentrations of substrate greater than product, and the greater the substrate concentration, the more negative this term will be. Thus, if the substrate concentration is suddenly raised high enough or the product concentration is decreased low enough, ΔG (the sum of the first and second terms) will also be negative, and conversion of substrate to product becomes thermodynamically favorable.

2. The Reversibility of the Phosphoglucomutase Reaction in the Cell

The effect of substrate and product concentration on ΔG and the direction of a reaction in the cell can be illustrated with conversion of glucose 6-P to glucose 1-P, the reaction catalyzed by phosphoglucomutase in the pathway of glycogen synthesis (see Fig. 20.3). The reaction has a small positive $\Delta G^{0'}$ for glucose 1-P synthesis ($+1.65$ kcal/mol) and, at equilibrium, the ratio of [glucose 1-P]/[glucose 6-P] is approximately 6/94 (which was determined using Equation 20.1). However, if another reaction uses glucose 1-P such that this ratio suddenly becomes 3/94, there is now a driving force for converting more glucose 6-P to glucose 1-P and restoring the equilibrium ratio. Substitution in Equation 20.2 gives ΔG, the driving force to equilibrium, as $+1.65 + RT \ln[\text{glucose 1-P}]/[\text{glucose 6-P}] = 1.65 + (-2.06) = -0.41$ kcal/mol, which is a negative value. Thus, a decrease in the ratio of product to substrate has converted the synthesis of glucose 1-P from a thermodynamically unfavorable to a thermodynamically favorable reaction that will proceed in the forward direction until equilibrium is reached.

C. Activated Intermediates with High-Energy Bonds

Many biochemical pathways form activated intermediates containing high-energy bonds to facilitate biochemical work. The term "high-energy bond" is a biologic term defined by the $\Delta G^{0'}$ for ATP hydrolysis; any bond that can be hydrolyzed with the release of approximately as much, or more, energy than ATP is called a *high-energy bond*. The high-energy bond in activated intermediates, such as UDP-glucose in glycogen synthesis, facilitate energy transfer.

Cells use guanosine triphosphate (GTP) and cytidine triphosphate (CTP), as well as UTP and ATP, to form activated intermediates. Different anabolic pathways generally use different nucleotides as their direct source of high-energy phosphate bonds: UTP is used for combining sugars, CTP in lipid synthesis, and GTP in protein synthesis.

The high-energy phosphate bonds of UTP, GTP, and CTP are energetically equivalent to ATP and are synthesized from ATP by nucleoside diphosphokinases and nucleoside monophosphokinases. For example, UTP is formed from UDP by a nucleoside diphosphokinase in the reaction

$$\text{ATP} + \text{UDP} \leftrightarrow \text{UTP} + \text{ADP}$$

ADP is converted back to ATP by the process of oxidative phosphorylation, using energy supplied by fuel oxidation.

Energy-requiring reactions often generate the nucleoside diphosphate ADP. Adenylate kinase, an important enzyme in cellular energy balance, is a nucleoside monophosphate kinase that transfers a phosphate from one ADP to another ADP to form ATP and adenosine monophosphate (AMP):

$$ADP + ADP \leftrightarrow AMP + ATP$$

This enzyme can thus regenerate ATP under conditions in which ATP use is required.

In addition to the nucleoside triphosphates, other compounds containing high-energy bonds are formed to facilitate energy transfer in anabolic and catabolic pathways (e.g., 1,3-bis-phosphoglycerate in glycolysis and acetyl coenzyme A [acetyl-CoA] in the tricarboxylic acid [TCA] cycle) (Fig. 20.7). Creatine phosphate contains a high-energy phosphate bond that allows it to serve as an energy reservoir for ATP synthesis and transport in muscle cells, neurons, and spermatozoa. A common feature of these molecules is that all of these high-energy bonds are "unstable," and their hydrolysis yields substantial free energy because the products are much more stable as a result of electron resonance within their structures.

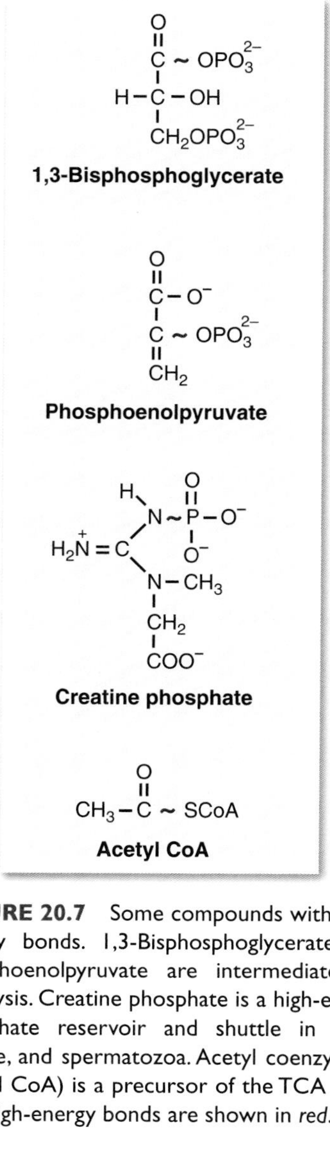

IV. Thermogenesis

According to the first law of thermodynamics, energy cannot be destroyed. Thus, energy from oxidation of a fuel (its caloric content) must be equal to the amount of heat released, the work performed against the environment, and the increase in order of molecules in our bodies. Some of the energy from fuel oxidation is converted into heat as the fuel is oxidized, and some heat is generated as ATP is used to do work. If we become less efficient in converting energy from fuel oxidation into ATP, or if we use an additional amount of ATP for muscular contraction, we will oxidize an additional amount of fuel to maintain ATP homeostasis (constant cellular ATP levels). With the oxidation of additional fuel, we release additional heat. Thus, heat production is a natural consequence of "burning fuel."

The term *thermogenesis* refers to energy expended for the purpose of generating heat in addition to that expended for ATP production. To maintain the body at 37°C despite changes in environmental temperature, it is necessary to regulate fuel oxidation and its efficiency (as well as heat dissipation). In shivering thermogenesis, we respond to sudden cold with asynchronous muscle contractions (shivers) that increase ATP use and therefore fuel oxidation and the release of energy as heat. In nonshivering thermogenesis (adaptive thermogenesis), the efficiency of converting energy from fuel oxidation into ATP is decreased. More fuel needs to be oxidized to maintain constant ATP levels, and thus, more heat is generated.

V. Energy from Fuel Oxidation

Fuel oxidation provides energy for bodily processes principally through generation of the reduced coenzymes nicotinamide adenine dinucleotide (NADH) and flavin adenine dinucleotide (FAD[2H]). They are used principally to generate ATP in oxidative phosphorylation. However, fuel oxidation also generates NADPH, which is most often used directly in energy-requiring processes. Carbohydrates also may be used to generate ATP through a nonoxidative pathway called *anaerobic glycolysis*.

A. Energy Transfer from Fuels through Oxidative Phosphorylation

Fuel oxidation is our major source of ATP and our major means of transferring energy from the chemical bonds of the fuels to cellular energy-requiring processes. The amount of energy available from a fuel is equivalent to the amount of heat that is generated when a fuel is burned. To conserve this energy for the generation of ATP, the process of cellular respiration transforms the energy from the chemical bonds of fuels into the reduction state of electron-accepting coenzymes, NAD^+ and FAD (Fig. 20.8, circle 1). As these compounds transfer electrons to O_2 in the ETC, most of this energy is transformed into an electrochemical gradient across the inner

FIGURE 20.7 Some compounds with high-energy bonds. 1,3-Bisphosphoglycerate and phosphoenolpyruvate are intermediates of glycolysis. Creatine phosphate is a high-energy phosphate reservoir and shuttle in brain, muscle, and spermatozoa. Acetyl coenzyme A (acetyl CoA) is a precursor of the TCA cycle. The high-energy bonds are shown in *red*.

1,3-Bisphosphoglycerate

Phosphoenolpyruvate

Creatine phosphate

Acetyl CoA

Stanley T. has increased thyroid hormone levels that increase his rate of ATP use and fuel oxidation. An excess of thyroid hormones also may affect the efficiency of ATP production, resulting in fewer ATP produced for a given level of O_2 consumption. The increased rate of ATP use and diminished efficiency stimulate oxidative metabolism, resulting in a much greater rate of heat production. The hyperthyroid patient, therefore, complains of constantly feeling hot (heat intolerance) and sweaty. (Perspiration allows dissipation of excess heat through evaporation from the skin surface.)

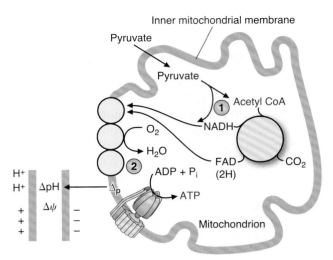

FIGURE 20.8 Overview of energy transformations in oxidative phosphorylation. The electrochemical potential gradient across the mitochondrial membrane (Δp) is represented by two components: the ΔpH, the proton gradient; and $\Delta \psi$, the membrane potential. The role of the electrochemical potential in oxidative phosphorylation is discussed in more depth in Chapter 24. *Acetyl CoA*, acetyl coenzyme A; *ADP*, adenosine diphosphate; *ATP*, adenosine triphosphate; *FAD(2H)*, reduced flavin adenine dinucleotide; *NADH*, reduced nicotinamide adenine dinucleotide; P_i, inorganic phosphate.

mitochondrial membrane (Fig. 20.8, circle 2). Much of the energy in the electrochemical gradient is used to regenerate ATP from ADP in oxidative phosphorylation (phosphorylation that requires O_2).

I. Oxidation–Reduction Reactions

Oxidation–reduction reactions always involve a pair of chemicals: an electron donor, which is oxidized in the reactions; and an electron acceptor, which is reduced in the reaction. In fuel metabolism, the fuel donates electrons and is oxidized, and NAD^+ and FAD accept electrons and are reduced.

To remember this, think of the acronym LEO GER: *L*oss of *E*lectrons = *O*xidation; *G*ain of *E*lectrons = *R*eduction. Compounds are oxidized in the body in essentially three ways: (1) the transfer of electrons from the compound as a hydrogen atom or a hydride ion, (2) the direct addition of oxygen from O_2, and (3) the direct donation of electrons (e.g., $Fe^{2+} \rightarrow Fe^{3+}$) (see Chapter 5). Fuel oxidation involves the transfer of electrons as a hydrogen atom or a hydride ion, and thus, reduced compounds have more hydrogen relative to oxygen than the oxidized compounds. Consequently, aldehydes are more reduced than acids, and alcohols are more reduced than aldehydes.

When is NAD^+, rather than FAD, used in a particular oxidation–reduction reaction? It depends on the chemical properties of the electron donor and the enzyme catalyzing the reaction. In oxidation reactions, NAD^+ accepts two electrons as a hydride ion to form NADH, and a proton (H^+) is released into the medium (Fig. 20.9). It is generally used for metabolic reactions involving oxidation of alcohols and aldehydes. In contrast, FAD accepts two electrons as hydrogen atoms, which are donated singly from separate atoms (e.g., formation of a double bond or a disulfide) (Fig. 20.10).

As the reduced coenzymes donate these electrons to O_2 through the ETC, they are reoxidized. The energy derived from reoxidation of NADH and FAD(2H) is available for the generation of ATP by oxidative phosphorylation. In our analogy of ATP as currency, the reduced coenzymes are our paychecks for oxidizing fuels. Because our cells spend ATP so fast, we must immediately convert our paychecks into ATP cash.

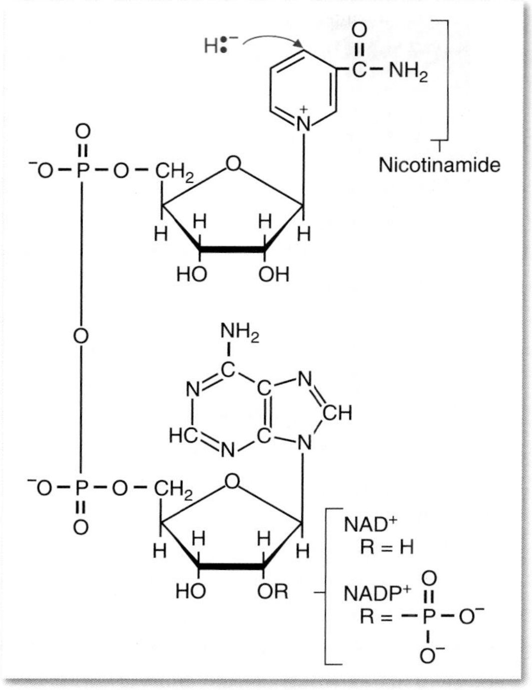

FIGURE 20.9 Reduction of nicotinamide adenine dinucleotide (NAD$^+$) and NADP$^+$. These structurally related coenzymes are reduced by accepting two electrons as H$^-$, the hydride ion.

2. Reduction Potential

Each oxidation–reduction reaction makes or takes a fixed amount of energy ($\Delta G^{0'}$), which is directly proportional to the $\Delta E^{0'}$ (the difference in reduction potentials of the oxidation–reduction pair). The *reduction potential* of a compound, $E^{0'}$, is a measure in volts of the energy change when that compound accepts electrons (becomes reduced); $-\Delta E^{0'}$ is the energy change when the compound donates electrons (becomes oxidized). $E^{0'}$ can be considered an expression of the willingness of the

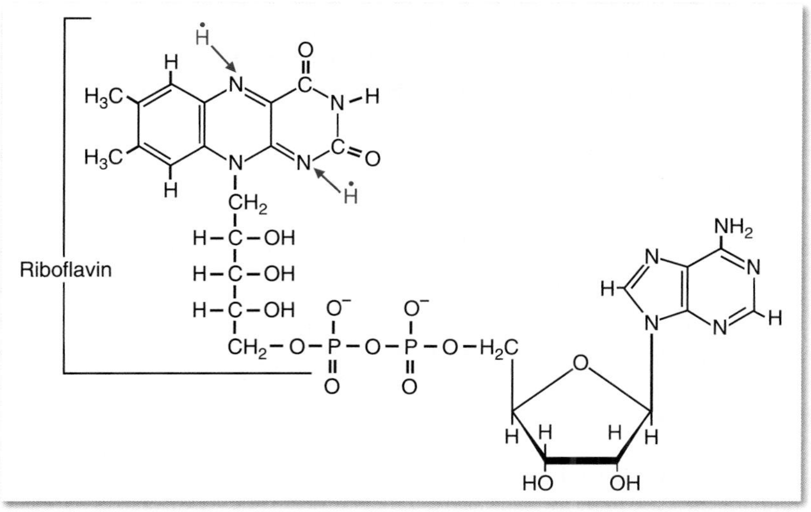

FIGURE 20.10 Reduction of flavin adenine dinucleotide (FAD). FAD accepts two electrons as two hydrogen atoms and is reduced. The reduced coenzyme is denoted in this text as *FAD(2H)* because it often accepts a total of two electrons one at a time, never going to the fully reduced form, FADH$_2$. Flavin mononucleotide consists of riboflavin with one phosphate group attached.

TABLE 20.4 Reduction Potentials of Some Oxidation–Reduction Half-Reactions	
REDUCTION HALF-REACTIONS	**$E^{0'}$ AT pH 7.0**
$\frac{1}{2}O_2 + 2H^+ + 2e^- \rightarrow H_2O$	0.816
Cytochrome a-Fe^{3+} + 1e^- → cytochrome a-Fe^{2+}	0.290
$CoQ + 2H^+ + 2e^- \rightarrow CoQ\text{-}H_2$	0.060
Fumarate + $2H^+$ + $2e^-$ → succinate	0.030
Oxaloacetate + $2H^+$ + $2e^-$ → malate	−0.102
Acetaldehyde + $2H^+$ + $2e^-$ → ethanol	−0.163
Pyruvate + $2H^+$ + $2e^-$ → lactate	−0.200
Riboflavin + $2H^+$ + $2e^-$ → riboflavin-H_2	−0.200
FAD + $2H^+$ + $2e^-$ → FAD(2H)	−0.220[a]
NAD^+ + $2H^+$ + $2e^-$ → NADH + H^+	−0.320
Acetate + $2H^+$ + $2e^-$ → acetaldehyde	−0.468

CoQ, coenzyme Q; FAD, flavin adenine dinucleotide; NAD, nicotinamide adenine dinucleotide.
[a]This is the value for free FAD; when FAD is bound to a protein, its value can be altered in either direction.

compound to accept electrons. Some examples of reduction potentials are shown in Table 20.4. Oxygen, which is the best electron acceptor, has the largest positive reduction potential (i.e., is the most willing to accept electrons and be reduced). As a consequence, the transfer of electrons from all compounds to O_2 is energetically favorable and occurs with energy release.

The more negative the reduction potential of a compound, the greater is the energy available for ATP generation when that compound passes its electrons to oxygen. The $\Delta G^{0'}$ for transfer of electrons from NADH to O_2 is greater than the transfer from FAD(2H) to O_2 (see the reduction potential values for NADH and FAD[2H] in Table 20.4). Thus, the energy available for ATP synthesis from NADH is approximately −53 kcal, and from the FAD-containing flavoproteins in the ETC is approximately −41 kcal.

To calculate the free-energy change of an oxidation–reduction reaction, the reduction potential of the electron donor (NADH) is added to that of the acceptor (O_2). The $\Delta E^{0'}$ for the net reaction is calculated from the sum of the half-reactions. For NADH donation of electrons, it is +0.320 V, opposite of that shown in Table 20.4 (remember, Table 20.4 shows the $E^{0'}$ for accepting electrons), and for O_2 acceptance, it is +0.816 V. The number of electrons being transferred is 2 (so, $n = 2$). The direct relationship between the energy changes in oxidation–reduction reactions and $\Delta G^{0'}$ is expressed by the Nernst equation

$$\Delta G^{0'} = -n\text{F}\,\Delta E^{0'} \qquad \text{Equation 20.3.}$$

where n is the number of electrons transferred and F is Faraday constant (23 kcal/mol-V). Thus, a value of approximately −53 kcal/mol is obtained for the energy available for ATP synthesis by transferring two electrons from NADH to O_2. The $\Delta E^{0'}$ for FAD(2H) to donate electrons to O_2 is 1.016 V, compared to a $\Delta E^{0'}$ of 1.136 V for electron transfer from NADH to O_2.

3. Caloric Values of Fuels

The caloric value of a food is related directly to its oxidation state, which is a measure of $\Delta G^{0'}$ for transfer of electrons from that fuel to O_2. The electrons donated by the fuel are from its C–H and C–C bonds. Fatty acids such as palmitate, $CH_3(CH_2)_{14}COOH$, have a caloric value of roughly 9 kcal/g. Glucose is already partially oxidized and has a caloric value of only about 4 kcal/g. The carbons, on average, contain fewer C–H bonds from which to donate electrons.

Otto S. decided to lose weight by decreasing his intake of fat and alcohol (ethanol) and increasing his intake of carbohydrates. Compare the structure of ethanol with that of glucose and fatty acids in the following figure. On the basis of their oxidation states, which compound provides the most energy (calories) per gram?

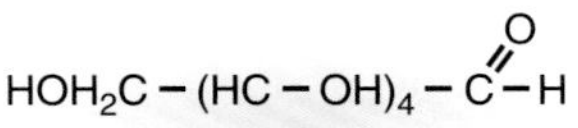

$HOH_2C - (HC - OH)_4 - \overset{\displaystyle O}{\underset{\displaystyle \|}{C}} - H$

Glucose

CH_3CH_2OH

Ethanol

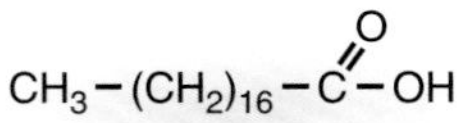

$CH_3 - (CH_2)_{16} - \overset{\displaystyle O}{\underset{\displaystyle \|}{C}} - OH$

A fatty acid

The caloric value of a food is applicable in humans only if our cells have enzymes that can oxidize that fuel by transferring electrons from the fuel to NAD^+, $NADP^+$, or FAD. When we burn wood in a fireplace, electrons are transferred from cellulose and other carbohydrates to O_2, releasing energy as heat. However, wood has no caloric content for humans; we cannot digest it and convert cellulose to a form that can be oxidized by our enzymes. Cholesterol, although it is a lipid, also has no caloric value for us because we cannot oxidize the carbons in its complex ring structure in reactions that generate NADH, FAD(2H), or NADPH.

B. NADPH in Oxidation–Reduction Reactions

$NADP^+$ is similar to NAD^+ and has the same reduction potential. However, $NADP^+$ has an extra phosphate group on the ribose, which affects its enzyme binding (see Fig. 20.9). Consequently, most enzymes use either NAD^+ or $NADP^+$ but seldom both. In certain reactions, fuels are oxidized by transfer of electrons to $NADP^+$ to form NADPH. For example, glucose 6-P dehydrogenase, in the pentose phosphate pathway, transfers electrons from glucose 6-P to $NADP^+$ instead of NAD^+. NADPH usually donates electrons to biosynthetic reactions such as fatty acid synthesis and to detoxification reactions that use oxygen directly. Consequently, the energy in its reduction potential is usually used in energy-requiring reactions without first being converted to ATP currency.

C. Anaerobic Glycolysis

Not all ATP is generated by fuel oxidation. In *anaerobic glycolysis*, glucose is degraded in reactions that form high-energy phosphorylated intermediates of the pathway (Fig. 20.11). These activated high-energy intermediates provide the energy for the generation of ATP from ADP without involving electron transfer to O_2. Therefore, this pathway is called *anaerobic glycolysis*, and ATP is generated from substrate-level phosphorylation rather than from oxidative phosphorylation (see Chapter 24). Anaerobic glycolysis is a critical source of ATP for cells that have a decreased O_2 supply either because they are physiologically designed that way (e.g., cells in the kidney medulla, rapidly working muscle, red blood cells) or because their supply of O_2 has been pathologically decreased (e.g., coronary artery disease).

VI. Oxygenases and Oxidases Not Involved in ATP Generation

Approximately 90% to 95% of the O_2 we consume is used by the terminal oxidase in the ETC for ATP generation via oxidative phosphorylation. The remainder of the O_2 is used directly by oxygenases and other oxidases, enzymes that oxidize a compound in the body by transferring electrons directly to O_2 (Fig. 20.12). The large positive reduction potential of O_2 makes all of these reactions extremely favorable thermodynamically, but the electronic structure of O_2 slows the speed of electron transfer. These enzymes, therefore, contain a metal ion that facilitates reduction of O_2.

A. Oxidases

Oxidases transfer electrons from the substrate to O_2, which is reduced to water (H_2O) or to hydrogen peroxide (H_2O_2). The terminal protein complex in the ETC, called *cytochrome oxidase*, is an oxidase because it accepts electrons donated to the chain by NADH and FAD(2H) and uses these to reduce O_2 to H_2O. Most of the other oxidases in the cell form H_2O_2 instead of H_2O and are called *peroxidases*. Peroxidases are generally confined to peroxisomes to protect DNA and other cellular components from toxic free radicals (compounds containing single electrons in an outer orbital) generated by H_2O_2.

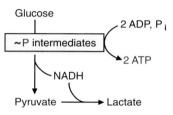

In palmitate and other fatty acids, most carbons are more reduced than those in glucose or ethanol (more of the carbons have electrons in C–H bonds). Therefore, fatty acids have the greatest caloric content per gram, 9 kcal. In glucose, the carbons have already formed bonds with oxygen, and fewer electrons in C–H bonds are available to generate energy. Thus, the complete oxidation of glucose provides roughly 4 kcal/g. In ethanol, one carbon is a methyl group with C–H bonds, and one has an –OH group. Therefore, the oxidation state is intermediate between those of glucose and fatty acids, and ethanol thus has a caloric value of 7 kcal/g.

Glucose → ~P intermediates → Pyruvate → Lactate
2 ADP, P_i → 2 ATP
NADH

Anaerobic glycolysis

FIGURE 20.11 Anaerobic glycolysis. Phosphate is transferred from high-energy intermediates of the pathway to adenosine diphosphate (ADP). Because nicotinamide adenine dinucleotide (NADH) from the pathway is reoxidized by reduction of pyruvate to lactate, no oxygen is required. *ATP*, adenosine triphosphate; P_i, inorganic phosphate.

Oxidases

$$O_2 + 4e^-, 4H^+ \longrightarrow 2H_2O$$
$$O_2 + SH_2 \longrightarrow S + H_2O_2$$

Mono-oxygenases

$$O_2 + S + \text{Electron donor–}XH_2 \longrightarrow$$
$$H_2O + \text{Electron donor–}X + S\text{–}OH$$

Dioxygenases

$$S + O_2 \longrightarrow SO_2$$

FIGURE 20.12 Oxidases and oxygenases. The fate of O_2 is shown in *red*. *S* represents an organic substrate.

B. Oxygenases

Oxygenases, in contrast to oxidases, incorporate one or both of the atoms of oxygen into the organic substrate (see Fig. 20.12). Monooxygenases, enzymes that incorporate one atom of oxygen into the substrate and the other into H_2O, are often named *hydroxylases* (e.g., phenylalanine hydroxylase, which adds a hydroxyl group to phenylalanine to form tyrosine) or mixed-function oxidases. Monooxygenases require an electron-donor substrate, such as NADPH; a coenzyme such as FAD, which can transfer single electrons; and a metal or similar compound that can form a reactive oxygen complex. They are usually found in the endoplasmic reticulum and occasionally in mitochondria. Dioxygenases, enzymes that incorporate both atoms of oxygen into the substrate, are used in the pathways for converting arachidonate into prostaglandins, thromboxanes, and leukotrienes.

VII. Energy Balance

Our total energy expenditure is equivalent to our O_2 consumption (Fig. 20.13). The *resting metabolic rate* (energy expenditure of a person at rest, at 25°C, after an overnight fast) accounts for approximately 60% to 70% of our total energy expenditure and O_2 consumption, and physical exercise accounts for the remainder. Of the resting metabolic rate, approximately 90% to 95% of O_2 consumption is used by the mitochondrial ETC, and only 5% to 10% is required for nonmitochondrial oxidases and oxygenases and is not related to ATP synthesis. Approximately 20% to 30% of the energy from this mitochondrial O_2 consumption is lost by proton leak back across the mitochondrial membrane, which dissipates the electrochemical gradient without ATP synthesis. The remainder of our O_2 consumption is used for ATPases that maintain ion gradients and for biosynthetic pathways.

ATP homeostasis refers to the ability of our cells to maintain constant levels of ATP despite fluctuations in the rate of use. Thus, increased use of ATP for exercise or biosynthetic reactions increases the rate of fuel oxidation. The major mechanism used is feedback regulation; all of the pathways of fuel oxidation that lead to generation of ATP are feedback-regulated by ATP levels or by compounds related to the concentration of ATP. In general, the less ATP is used, the less fuel will be oxidized to generate ATP.

According to the first law of thermodynamics, the energy (in calories) in our consumed fuel can never be lost. Consumed fuel is either oxidized to meet the energy

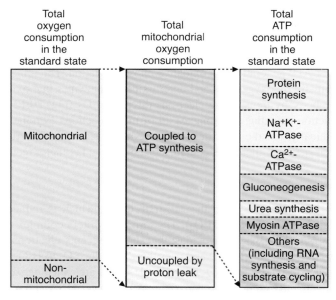

FIGURE 20.13 Estimated contribution of processes to energy use in standard state. (Reproduced, with permission, from Rolfe DF, Brown GC. Cellular energy utilization and molecular origin of standard metabolic rate in mammals. *Physiol Rev.* 1997;77:731–758.)

demands of the BMR plus exercise, or it is stored as fat. Thus, an intake of calories in excess of those expended results in weight gain. The simple statement, "If you eat too much and don't exercise, you will gain weight," is really a summary of the bioenergetics of the ATP–ADP cycle.

CLINICAL COMMENTS

Otto S. Otto S. visited his physician, who noted the increased weight. The physician recommended several diet modifications to Otto that would decrease the caloric content of his diet and pointed out the importance of exercise for weight reduction. He reminded Otto that the American Heart Association recommends at least 30 minutes of moderate-intensity aerobic activity at least 5 days per week or at least 25 minutes of vigorous aerobic activity at least 3 days per week. He also reminded Otto that he would want to be a role model for his patients. Otto decided to begin an exercise regimen that included at least 30 minutes of running and tennis at least 5 days a week.

Stanley T. Mr. T. exhibited the classical signs and symptoms of hyperthyroidism (increased secretion of the thyroid hormones T_3 and T_4; see Fig. 11.8 for the structure of T_3), including a goiter (enlarged thyroid gland). T_3 is the more active form of the hormone. T_4 is synthesized and secreted in approximately 10 times greater amounts than T_3. Liver and other cells contain an enzyme (a deiodinase) that removes one of the iodines from T_4, converting it to T_3. Thyroid function tests confirmed this diagnosis.

Thyroid hormones (principally T_3) modulate cellular energy production and use through their ability to increase gene transcription (see Fig. 16.13) of many proteins involved in intermediary metabolism, including enzymes in the TCA cycle and oxidative phosphorylation. They increase the rate of ATP use by the Na^+,K^+-ATPase and other enzymes. They also affect the efficiency of energy transformations, so that either more fuel must be oxidized to maintain a given level of ATP or more ATP must be expended to achieve the desired physiologic response. The loss of weight experienced by **Stanley T.**, in spite of a very good appetite, reflects his increased caloric requirements and less efficient use of fuels. The result is enhanced oxidation of adipose tissue stores as well as a catabolic effect on muscle and other protein-containing tissues. Through mechanisms that are not well understood, increased levels of thyroid hormone in the blood also increase the activity or "tone" of the sympathetic (adrenergic) nervous system. An activated sympathetic nervous system leads to a more rapid and forceful heartbeat (tachycardia and palpitations), increased nervousness (anxiety and insomnia), tremulousness (a sense of shakiness or jitteriness), and other symptoms.

Cora N. Cora N. was in left ventricular heart failure (LVF) when she presented to the hospital with her second heart attack in 8 months. The diagnosis of LVF was suspected, in part, by her rapid heart rate (104 beats/minute) and respiratory rate. On examining her lungs, her physician heard respiratory rales (or crackles) caused by inspired air bubbling in fluid that had filled her lung air spaces secondary to LVF. This condition is referred to as *congestive heart failure*.

Cora's rapid heart rate (tachycardia) resulted from a reduced capacity of her ischemic, failing left ventricular muscle to eject a normal amount of blood into the arteries leading away from the heart with each contraction. The resultant drop in intra-arterial pressure signaled a reflex response in the central nervous system that, in turn, caused an increase in heart rate in an attempt to bring the total amount of blood leaving the left ventricle each minute (the cardiac output) back toward a more appropriate level to maintain systemic blood pressure.

Initial treatment of Cora's congestive heart failure will include efforts to reduce the workload of the heart by decreasing blood volume (preload) with diuretics and decreasing her blood pressure, and the administration of oxygen by nasal cannula to increase the oxygen levels in her blood.

Congestive heart failure occurs when the weakened pumping action of the left ventricular heart muscle, often from ischemia, leads to a reduced blood flow from the heart to the rest of the body. This leads to an increase in blood volume in the vessels that bring oxygenated blood from the lungs to the left side of the heart. The pressure inside these pulmonary vessels eventually reaches a critical level, above which water from the blood moves down a "pressure gradient" from the capillary lumen into alveolar air spaces of the lung (transudation). The patient experiences shortness of breath as the fluid in the air spaces interferes with oxygen exchange from the inspired air into arterial blood, causing hypoxia. The hypoxia then stimulates the respiratory center in the central nervous system, leading to a more rapid respiratory rate in an effort to increase the oxygen content of the blood. As the patient inhales deeply, the physician hears gurgling/crackling sounds (known as *inspiratory rales*) with a stethoscope placed over the posterior lung bases. These sounds represent the bubbling of inspired air as it enters the fluid-filled pulmonary alveolar air spaces.

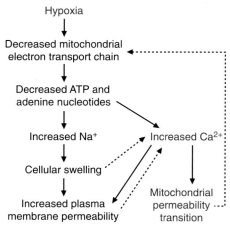

FIGURE 20.14 Hypoxia, Ca^{2+}, Na^+, and cell death. Without an adequate O_2 supply, decreased adenosine triphosphate (ATP) synthesis from oxidative phosphorylation results in an increase of cytoplasmic Na^+ and Ca^{2+} ions. Increased ion levels can trigger death cascades that involve increased permeability of the plasma membrane, loss of ion gradients, decreased cytosolic pH, mitochondrial Ca^{2+} overload, and a change in mitochondrial permeability called the *mitochondrial permeability transition*. The *solid lines* show the first sequence of events; the *dashed lines* show how these events feed back to accelerate the mitochondrial deterioration, making recovery of oxidative phosphorylation impossible.

BIOCHEMICAL COMMENTS

Active Transport and Cell Death. Most of us cannot remember when we first learned that we would die if we stopped breathing. But exactly how cells die from a lack of oxygen is an intriguing question. Hypoxia leads to both physical and transcriptional changes. Pathologists generally describe two histologically distinct types of cell death: necrosis and apoptosis (programmed cell death). Cell death from a lack of O_2, such as occurs during an MI, can be very rapid and is considered necrosis. The lack of ATP for the active transport of Na^+ and Ca^{2+} triggers some of the death cascades that lead to necrosis (Fig. 20.14).

The influx of Na^+ and loss of the Na^+ gradient across the plasma membrane is an early event accompanying ATP depletion during interruption of the O_2 supply. One consequence of the increased intracellular Na^+ concentration is that other transport processes driven by the Na^+ gradient are impaired. For example, the Na^+/H^+ exchanger, which normally pumps out H^+ generated from metabolism in exchange for extracellular Na^+, can no longer function, and intracellular pH may drop. The increased intracellular H^+ may impair ATP generation from anaerobic glycolysis. As a consequence of increased intracellular ion concentrations, H_2O enters the cells and hydropic swelling occurs. Swelling is accompanied by the release of creatine kinase MB subunits, troponin I, and troponin C into the blood. Some of these enzymes are measured in the blood to help diagnose an MI (see Chapters 6 and 7). Swelling is an early event and is considered a reversible stage of cell injury.

Normally, intracellular Ca^{2+} concentration is carefully regulated to fluctuate at low levels (intracellular Ca^{2+} concentration is $<10^{-7}$ M, compared to $\sim 10^{-3}$ M in extracellular fluid). Fluctuations of Ca^{2+} concentration at these low levels regulate myofibrillar contraction, energy metabolism, and other cellular processes. However, when Ca^{2+} concentration is increased above this normal range, it triggers cell death (necrosis). High Ca^{2+} concentrations activate a phospholipase that increases membrane permeability, resulting in further loss of ion gradients across the cell membrane. They also trigger opening of the mitochondrial permeability transition pore, which results in loss of mitochondrial function and further impairs oxidative phosphorylation.

Intracellular Ca^{2+} levels may increase as a result of cell swelling, the lack of ATP for ATP-dependent Ca^{2+} pumps, or the loss of the Na^+ gradient. Normally, Ca^{2+}-ATPases located in the plasma membrane pump Ca^{2+} out of the cell. Ca^{2+}-ATPases in the endoplasmic reticulum, and in the sarcoplasmic reticulum of heart and other muscles, sequester Ca^{2+} within the membranes, where it is bound by a low-affinity binding protein. Ca^{2+} is released from the sarcoplasmic reticulum in response to a nerve impulse, which signals contraction, and the increase of Ca^{2+} stimulates both muscle contraction and the oxidation of fuels. Within the heart, another Ca^{2+} transporter protein, the Na^+/Ca^{2+} exchange transporter, coordinates the efflux of Ca^{2+} in exchange for Na^+, so that Ca^{2+} is extruded with each contraction.

Hypoxia also induces the transcription of genes in an attempt to compensate for the hypoxic conditions. A family of transcription factors, known as *hypoxia-inducible factors* (HIFs), are activated under hypoxic conditions. These factors bind to hypoxia-responsive elements (promoter-proximal elements) in the regulatory region of target genes. More than 70 target genes are regulated by HIFs, including the gene for erythropoietin, which stimulates increased red blood cell production. Induction of these genes allows cells to adapt to and survive for some time under these hypoxic conditions.

KEY CONCEPTS

- *Bioenergetics* refers to cellular energy transformations.
- The high-energy phosphate bonds of ATP are a cell's primary source of energy.
- ATP is generated through cellular respiration, the oxidation of fuels to carbon dioxide and water.
- ATP can also be generated, at reduced levels, via anaerobic glycolysis (in the absence of O_2).
- The electrons captured from fuel oxidation generate NADH and FAD(2H), which are used to regenerate ATP via the process of oxidative phosphorylation.
- The energy available from ATP hydrolysis can be used for the following:
  - Mechanical work (muscle contraction)
  - Transport work (establishment of ion gradients across membranes)
  - Biochemical work (energy-requiring chemical reactions, including detoxification reactions)
- Energy released from fuel oxidation that is not used for work is transformed into and released as heat.
- The many pathways of fuel oxidation are coordinately regulated to maintain ATP homeostasis.
- $\Delta G^{0'}$ is the change in Gibbs free energy at pH 7.0 under standard conditions between the substrates and products of a reaction.
- Fuel oxidation has a negative $\Delta G^{0'}$; the products formed have less chemical energy than the reactants (an exergonic reaction pathway).
- ATP synthesis has a positive $\Delta G^{0'}$ and is endergonic; the reaction requires energy.
- Metabolic pathways have an overall negative $\Delta G^{0'}$, which is obtained by summing all of the $\Delta G^{0'}$ values for each reaction in the pathway.
- Oxidation–reduction reactions can be related to changes in free energy, the use of $E^{0'}$, the chemical's affinity for electrons. Compounds with higher $E^{0'}$ values have greater affinity for electrons than those with lower $E^{0'}$ values.
- Diseases discussed in this chapter are summarized in Table 20.5.

TABLE 20.5	Diseases Discussed in Chapter 20	
DISEASE OR DISORDER	**ENVIRONMENTAL OR GENETIC**	**COMMENTS**
Obesity	Both	Understanding daily caloric needs can enable one to gain or lose weight through alterations in exercise and eating habits.
Hyperthyroidism	Both	Thyroid hormone is important in regulating energy metabolism; excessive triiodothyronine (T_3) and tetraiodothyronine (T_4) release enhance metabolism, leading to weight loss and a greater rate of heat production.
Myocardial infarction (heart attack)	Both	The heart requires a constant level of energy, derived primarily from lactate, glucose, and fatty acids. This is necessary so that the rate of contraction can remain constant or increase during appropriate periods. Interference of oxygen flow to certain areas of the heart will reduce energy generation, leading to a myocardial infarction.

REVIEW QUESTIONS—CHAPTER 20

1. ATP is the cells' major chemical form of energy, and often it is converted to ADP during reactions, thereby releasing energy to allow the reaction to proceed in the forward direction. The highest energy phosphate bond in ATP is located between which of the following groups?
   A. Adenosine and phosphate
   B. Ribose and phosphate
   C. Ribose and adenine
   D. Two hydroxyl groups in the ribose ring
   E. Two phosphate groups

2. All cells require energy to survive, and the laws of thermodynamics need to be followed within biologic systems. Which one of the following bioenergetic terms or phrases is defined correctly?
   A. The first law of thermodynamics states that the universe tends toward a state of increased order.
   B. The second law of thermodynamics states that the total energy of a system remains constant.
   C. The change in enthalpy of a reaction is a measure of the total amount of heat that can be released from changes in the chemical bonds.
   D. $\Delta G^{0'}$ of a reaction is the standard free-energy change measured at 37°C and a pH of 7.4.
   E. A high-energy bond is a bond that releases >3 kcal/mol of heat when it is hydrolyzed.

3. In order for a cell to carry out its biologic functions, the intracellular reactions need to be directed to follow a certain pathway. Which one statement best describes the direction a chemical reaction will follow?
   A. A reaction with positive free energy will proceed in the forward direction if the substrate concentration is raised high enough.
   B. Under standard conditions, a reaction will proceed in the forward direction if the free energy $\Delta G^{0'}$ is positive.
   C. The direction of a reaction is independent of the initial substrate and product concentrations because the direction is determined by the change in free energy.
   D. The concentration of all of the substrates must be higher than that of all of the products for the reaction to proceed in the forward direction.
   E. The enzyme for the reaction must be working at >50% of its maximum efficiency for the reaction to proceed in the forward direction.

4. A patient, Mr. P., has just suffered a heart attack. As a consequence, his heart will display which one of the following changes?
   A. Increased intracellular O_2 concentration
   B. Increased intracellular ATP concentration
   C. Increased intracellular H^+ concentration
   D. Decreased intracellular Ca^{2+} concentration
   E. Decreased intracellular Na^+ concentration

5. Many biologic reactions are oxidation–reduction reactions that use a biologic electron carrier. Which one of the following statements correctly describes reduction of one of these electron carriers, NAD^+ or FAD?
   A. NAD^+ accepts two electrons as hydrogen atoms to form NAD(2H).
   B. NAD^+ accepts two electrons that are each donated from a separate atom of the substrate.
   C. NAD^+ accepts two electrons as a hydride ion to form NADH.
   D. FAD releases a proton as it accepts two electrons.
   E. FAD must accept two electrons at a time.

6. Active transport is necessary to move compounds into or out of the cell or mitochondria. Transport work can occur when ATP donates its phosphate group to a transport protein, thereby altering the conformation of that protein. Which one of the following mechanisms allows this conformational change to occur?
   A. A gain of ionic interactions, which alter tertiary and/or quaternary structure of the protein
   B. Loss of ionic interactions, thereby altering the proteins tertiary and/or quaternary structure
   C. Loss of hydrogen bonds in the primary structure of the protein
   D. Gain of hydrophobic interactions, leading to an alteration in the proteins tertiary and/or quaternary structure
   E. Loss of hydrophobic interactions, leading to an alteration in the proteins tertiary and/or quaternary structure

7. The $\Delta G^{0'}$ values are determined under standard biochemical conditions and reflect the energy either required, or released, as a particular reaction proceeds. Given the $\Delta G^{0'}$ values below, determine the overall $\Delta G^{0'}$ for the following reaction:

   creatine + ATP yields creatine phosphate + ADP

   The half reactions are

   ATP + H_2O yields ADP
   + inorganic phosphate $\Delta G^{0'} = -7.3$ kcal/mol
   Creatine phosphate + H_2O yields creatine
   + inorganic phosphate $\Delta G^{0'} = -10.3$ kcal/mol
   A. −3.0 kcal/mol
   B. −10.3 kcal/mol
   C. −17.6 kcal/mol
   D. +3.0 kcal/mol
   E. +10.3 kcal/mol
   F. +17.6 kcal/mol

8. When athletes expend vast amounts of energy, they are sometimes seen on the sidelines using supplemental oxygen. More than 90% of the O_2 we breathe is used for the generation of which one of the following?
   A. ATP
   B. ADP
   C. NAD^+
   D. FAD
   E. Acetyl-CoA

9. ATP is the cells' major energy-carrying molecule, and in order for a cell to survive, the cell must be able to regenerate ATP when ATP levels drop. Which one of the following statements accurately describes an aspect of ATP metabolism?
   A. ATP is more stable than ADP.
   B. ATP has more positively charged phosphate groups than ADP.

C. Phosphate groups repel each other, which in ATP leads to strained bond formation.
   D. Heat from ATP hydrolysis is used to drive energy requiring processes.
   E. ATP is hydrolyzed directly in the cell.

10. All physiologic processes in living cells require energy transformation. Which one of the following would be considered biochemical work using the high-energy phosphate bonds of ATP?
    A. Contracting muscle fibers
    B. Developing a Na^+ gradient across a membrane
    C. Transporting compounds against a concentration gradient
    D. Converting toxic compounds to nontoxic compounds in the liver
    E. Undergoing catabolic pathways

ANSWERS

1. **The answer is E.** Both of the high-energy phosphate bonds in ATP are located between phosphate groups (both the α- and β-phosphates, and the β- and γ-phosphates). The phosphate bond between the α-phosphate and ribose (or adenosine) is not a high-energy bond (thus, A and B are incorrect); and there is no phosphate between the ribose and adenine, or two hydroxyl groups in the ribose ring; therefore, answers C and D are incorrect.

2. **The answer is C.** The change in enthalpy, ΔH, is the total amount of heat that can be released in a reaction. The first law of thermodynamics states that the total energy of a system remains constant, and the second law of thermodynamics states the universe tends toward a state of disorder (thus, A and B are incorrect). Answer D is incorrect because $\Delta G^{0'}$ is the standard free-energy change measured at 25°C and a pH of 7. Answer E is incorrect because a high-energy bond releases more than about 7 kcal/mol of heat when it is hydrolyzed. The definition of a high-energy bond is based on the hydrolysis of one of the high-energy bonds of ATP.

3. **The answer is A.** The concentration of the substrates and products influence the direction of a reaction. Answer B is incorrect because reactions with a positive free energy, at 1 M concentrations of substrate and product, will proceed in the reverse direction. Answer C is incorrect because substrate and product concentrations do influence the free energy of a reaction. Answer D is incorrect because the free energy must be considered (in addition to the substrate and product concentrations) to determine the direction of a reaction. Answer E is false; an enzyme's efficiency does not influence the direction of a reaction.

4. **The answer is C.** A heart attack results in decreased pumping of blood, and thus a decreased O_2 supply to

the heart (thus, A is incorrect). The lack of O_2 leads to a lack of ATP (thus, B is incorrect) owing to an inability to perform oxidative phosphorylation. The lack of ATP impairs the working of Na^+,K^+-ATPase, which pumps sodium out of the cell in exchange for potassium. Therefore, intracellular levels of sodium will increase as Na^+ enters the cell through other transport mechanisms (thus, E is incorrect). The high intracellular sodium concentration then blocks the functioning of the Na^+/H^+ antiporter (which sends protons out of the cell in exchange for sodium). Because intracellular sodium is high, the driving force for this reaction is lost, which leads to increased intracellular H^+, or a lower intracellular pH (thus, C is correct). The intracellular pH also decreases because of glycolysis in the absence of O_2, which produces lactic acid. The loss of the sodium gradient, coupled with the lack of ATP, leads to increased calcium in the cell (thus, D is incorrect) owing to an inability to pump calcium out.

5. **The answer is C.** NAD^+ accepts two electrons as hydride ions to form NADH (thus, A and B are incorrect). Answers D and E are incorrect because FAD can accept two single electrons from separate atoms, together with protons, or FAD can accept a pair of electrons.

6. **The answer is A.** When a protein is phosphorylated, the most likely sites of phosphorylation are the hydroxyl groups of serine, threonine, or tyrosine. Prior to phosphorylation, those hydroxyl groups on the amino acid side chains can only participate in hydrogen bonds. When phosphorylated, the oxygen of the hydroxyl group is now covalently linked to the phosphate, which has two negative charges. This allows this group to form ionic bonds, which were not available prior to phosphorylation. The formation of ionic bonds then alters the tertiary and/or the quaternary structure of the protein. The addition of phosphate groups reduces the hydrophobicity

of this region of the protein, and the primary structure of the protein is the linear sequence of amino acids and does not involve hydrogen bond formation.

7. **The answer is D.** $\Delta G^{0'}$ values are additive for a series of reactions. In order to generate the overall reaction required, creatine + ATP yields ADP + creatine phosphate, the second reaction listed in the question needs to be reversed. Upon reversing a reaction, the sign of the standard free energy is reversed, in this case becoming +10.3 for the reaction creatine + inorganic phosphate yields creatine phosphate + H_2O. Upon summing the first reaction, and the reversed second reaction, the overall reaction is obtained and the $\Delta G^{0'} = 10.3 - 7.3$, or +3.0 kcal/mol.

8. **The answer is A.** More than 90% of the O_2 we breathe is used for cellular respiration, the overall process of transferring the electrons obtained from oxidizing fuels to oxygen in order to generate ATP. When ATP energy is needed, a high-energy phosphate bond of ATP is cleaved, forming ADP. NAD^+ and FAD are electron-accepting coenzymes that accept electrons from fuels as they are oxidized, and the electron carriers are reduced to NADH and FAD(2H). NADH and FAD(2H) donate their electrons to the electron transfer chain in order to generate ATP via oxidative phosphorylation. Generation of acetyl-CoA is only phase 1 of cellular respiration and does not by itself generate ATP. In phase 2, oxidation of acetyl-CoA in the TCA cycle collects energy as NADH and FAD(2H) in order to generate ATP.

9. **The answer is C.** The instability of the phosphoanhydride bonds arises from their negatively charged phosphate groups that repel each other and strain their bonds. ATP has more negatively charged phosphate groups (4) than ADP (3), reflective of ATP containing two high-energy bonds, and ADP containing one high-energy bond. In the cell, ATP is not hydrolyzed directly; rather, it is hydrolyzed in specific reactions that require energy to be pushed toward product formation. ATP is also used to form phosphate intermediates that are then substrates for other reactions in a metabolic pathway. The heat released from ATP hydrolysis is used for thermogenesis, but it cannot be used to drive other energy-requiring processes.

10. **The answer is D.** Biochemical work occurs in anabolic pathways (synthesizing large molecules) or when toxic compounds are converted to nontoxic compounds that can be excreted. Muscle fiber contraction is mechanical work and generating a sodium gradient, or transporting compounds against a concentration gradient, are considered transport work. Catabolic pathways lead to the generation of ATP.

Digestion, Absorption, and Transport of Carbohydrates

21

Carbohydrates are the largest source of dietary calories for most of the world's population. The major carbohydrates in the US diet are starch, lactose, and sucrose. The **starches amylose** and **amylopectin** are polysaccharides composed of hundreds to millions of glucosyl units linked together through α-1,4- and α-1,6-glycosidic bonds (Fig. 21.1). **Lactose** is a disaccharide composed of glucose and galactose, linked together through a β-1,4-glycosidic bond. **Sucrose** is a disaccharide composed of glucose and fructose, linked through an α-1,2-glycosidic bond. The digestive processes convert all of these dietary carbohydrates to their constituent monosaccharides by **hydrolyzing glycosidic bonds** between the sugars.

The digestion of starch begins in the mouth (Fig. 21.2). The **salivary** gland releases α-**amylase**, which converts starch to smaller polysaccharides called α-**dextrins**. Salivary α-amylase is inactivated by the acidity of the stomach (hydrochloric acid [HCl]). **Pancreatic α-amylase** and bicarbonate are secreted by the exocrine pancreas into the lumen of the small intestine, where bicarbonate neutralizes the gastric secretions. Pancreatic α-amylase continues the digestion of α-dextrins, converting them to disaccharides (**maltose**), trisaccharides (**maltotriose**), and oligosaccharides called **limit dextrins**. Limit dextrins usually contain four to nine glucosyl residues and an **isomaltose** branch (two glucosyl residues attached through an α-1,6-glycosidic bond).

The digestion of the disaccharides lactose and sucrose, as well as further digestion of maltose, maltotriose, and limit dextrins, occurs through **disaccharidases** attached to the membrane surface of the **brush border (microvilli)** of intestinal epithelial cells. **Glucoamylase** hydrolyzes the α-1,4-bonds of dextrins. The **sucrase–isomaltase complex** hydrolyzes sucrose, most of maltose, and almost all of the isomaltose formed by glucoamylase from limit dextrins. **Lactase-glycosylceramidase** (β-glycosidase) hydrolyzes the β-glycosidic bonds in **lactose** and **glycolipids**. A fourth disaccharidase complex, **trehalase**, hydrolyzes the bond (an α-1,1-glycosidic bond) between two glucosyl units in the sugar trehalose. The monosaccharides produced by these hydrolases (glucose, fructose, and galactose) are then transported into the intestinal epithelial cells.

Dietary fiber, composed principally of polysaccharides, cannot be digested by enzymes in the human intestinal tract. In the colon, dietary fiber and other nondigested carbohydrates may be converted to gases (H_2, CO_2, and methane) and short-chain fatty acids (principally acetic acid, propionic acid, and butyric acid) by bacteria in the colon.

Glucose, **galactose**, and **fructose** formed by the digestive enzymes are transported into the absorptive epithelial cells of the small intestine by protein-mediated **Na$^+$-dependent active transport** and **facilitative diffusion**. Monosaccharides are transported from these cells into the blood and circulate to the liver and peripheral tissues, where they are taken up by facilitative transporters. Facilitative transport of glucose across epithelial cells and other cell membranes is mediated by a family of **tissue-specific glucose transport proteins** (**GLUT 1 to GLUT 5**). The type of transporter found in each cell reflects the role of glucose metabolism in that cell.

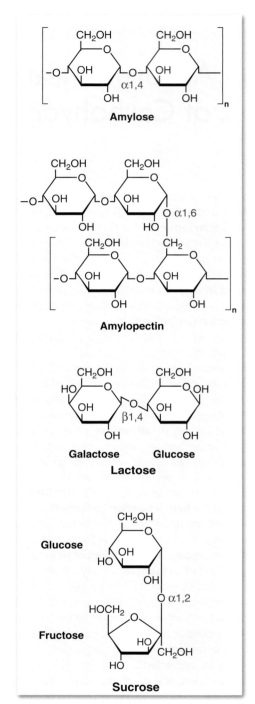

FIGURE 21.1 The structures of common dietary carbohydrates. For disaccharides and higher, the sugars are linked through glycosidic bonds between the anomeric carbon of one sugar and a hydroxyl group on another sugar. The glycosidic bond may be either α or β, depending on its position above or below the plane of the sugar containing the anomeric carbon. (See Chapter 5, Section II.A, to review terms used in the description of sugars.) The starch amylose is a polysaccharide of glucose residues linked with α-1,4-glycosidic bonds. Amylopectin is amylose with the addition of α-1,6-glycosidic branch points. Dietary sugars may be monosaccharides (single sugar residues), disaccharides (two sugar residues), oligosaccharides (several sugar residues), or polysaccharides (hundreds of sugar residues). For clarity, the hydrogen atoms are not shown in the figure.

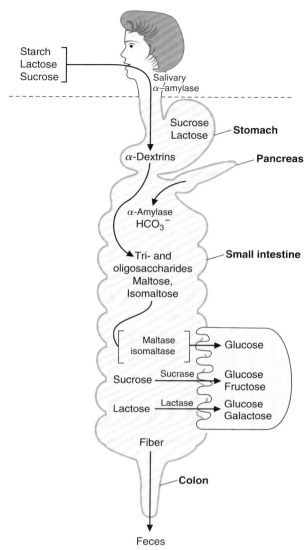

FIGURE 21.2   Overview of carbohydrate digestion. *Digestion* of the carbohydrates occurs first, followed by *absorption* of monosaccharides. Subsequent metabolic reactions occur after the sugars are absorbed.

THE WAITING ROOM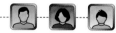

Denise V. is a 20-year-old exchange student from Nigeria who has noted gastrointestinal bloating, abdominal cramps, and intermittent diarrhea ever since arriving in the United States 6 months ago. A careful history shows that these symptoms occur most commonly about 45 minutes to 1 hour after eating breakfast but may occur after other meals as well. Dairy products, which were not a part of Denise's diet in Nigeria, were identified as the probable offending agent because her gastrointestinal symptoms disappeared when milk and milk products were eliminated from her diet.

Deborah S.'s fasting and postprandial blood glucose levels are frequently above the normal range in spite of good compliance with insulin therapy. Her physician has referred her to a dietician skilled in training diabetic patients in the successful application of an appropriate American Diabetes Association diet. As part of the program, Ms. S. is asked to incorporate foods containing fiber into her diet, such as whole grains (e.g., wheat, oats, corn), legumes (e.g., peas, beans, lentils), tubers (e.g., potatoes, peanuts), and fruits.

The dietary sugar in fruit juice and other sweets is sucrose, a disaccharide composed of glucose and fructose joined through their anomeric carbons. **Nina M.'s** symptoms of pain and abdominal distension are caused by an inability to digest sucrose or absorb fructose, which are converted to gas by colonic bacteria. The possibility of carbohydrate malabsorption was considered, and a hydrogen breath test was recommended.

Nina M. is a 13-month-old baby girl, the second child born to unrelated parents. Her mother had a healthy, full-term pregnancy, and Nina's birth weight was normal. She did not respond well to breastfeeding and was changed entirely to a formula based on cows' milk at 6 weeks. Between 9 and 18 weeks of age, she was admitted to the hospital twice with a history of screaming after feeding but was discharged after observation without a specific diagnosis. Elimination of cows' milk from her diet did not relieve her symptoms; Nina's mother reported that when Nina turned 1 year old and she introduced some fruit juice into her diet, the screaming bouts were worse, particularly after drinking juice. She also noticed that Nina frequently had gas and a distended abdomen. She was still thriving (weight >97th percentile), with no abnormal findings on physical examination. A stool sample was taken.

I. Dietary Carbohydrates

Carbohydrates are the largest source of calories in the average American diet and usually constitute 40% to 45% of our caloric intake. The plant starches *amylopectin* and *amylose*, which are present in grains, tubers, and vegetables, constitute approximately 50% to 60% of the carbohydrate calories consumed. These starches are polysaccharides, containing 10,000 to 1 million glucosyl units. In amylose, the glucosyl residues form a straight chain linked via α-1,4-glycosidic bonds; in amylopectin, the α-1,4-chains contain branches connected via α-1,6-glycosidic bonds (see Fig. 21.1). The other major sugar found in fruits and vegetables is *sucrose*, a disaccharide of glucose and fructose (see Fig. 21.1). Sucrose and small amounts of the monosaccharides *glucose* and *fructose* are the major natural sweeteners found in fruit, honey, and vegetables. *Dietary fiber*, the part of the diet that cannot be digested by human enzymes of the intestinal tract, is also composed principally of plant polysaccharides and a polymer called *lignin*.

Most foods derived from animals, such as meat or fish, contain very little carbohydrate except for small amounts of glycogen (which has a structure similar to amylopectin) and glycolipids. The major dietary carbohydrate of animal origin is lactose, a disaccharide composed of glucose and galactose that is found exclusively in milk and milk products (see Fig. 21.1). Sweeteners, in the form of sucrose and high-fructose corn syrup (starch, partially hydrolyzed and isomerized to fructose), also appear in the diet as additives to processed foods. On average, a person in the United States consumes 65 lb of added sucrose and 40 lb of high-fructose corn syrup solids per year.

Although all cells require glucose for metabolic functions, neither glucose nor other sugars are specifically required in the diet. Glucose can be synthesized from many amino acids found in dietary protein. Fructose, galactose, xylulose, and all the other sugars required for metabolic processes in the human can be synthesized from glucose.

II. Digestion of Dietary Carbohydrates

In the digestive tract, dietary polysaccharides and disaccharides are converted to monosaccharides by *glycosidases*, enzymes that hydrolyze the glycosidic bonds between the sugars. All of these enzymes exhibit some specificity for the sugar, the glycosidic bond (α or β), and the number of saccharide units in the chain. The monosaccharides formed by glycosidases are transported across the intestinal mucosal cells into the interstitial fluid and subsequently enter the bloodstream. Undigested carbohydrates enter the colon, where bacteria may ferment them.

A. Salivary and Pancreatic α-Amylase

The digestion of starch (amylopectin and amylose) begins in the mouth, where chewing mixes the food with saliva. The salivary glands secrete approximately 1 L of liquid per day into the mouth, containing *salivary α-amylase* and other components.

Starch blockers were marketed many years ago as a means of losing weight without having to exercise or reduce your daily caloric intake. Starch blockers were based on a protein found in beans, which blocked the action of amylase. Thus, as the advertisements proclaimed, one could eat a large amount of starch during a meal, and as long as you took the starch blocker, the starch would pass through the digestive tract without being metabolized. Unfortunately, this was too good to be true, and starch blockers were never shown to be effective in aiding weight loss. This was probably because of a combination of factors, such as inactivation of the inhibitor by the low pH in the stomach, and an excess of amylase activity as compared with the amount of starch blocker ingested. Recently, this issue has been revisited because a starch blocker from wheat has been developed that may work as advertised, although much more research is required to determine whether this amylase inhibitor will be safe and effective in humans. In addition, newer (and improved) preparations of the bean extract are also being readvertised.

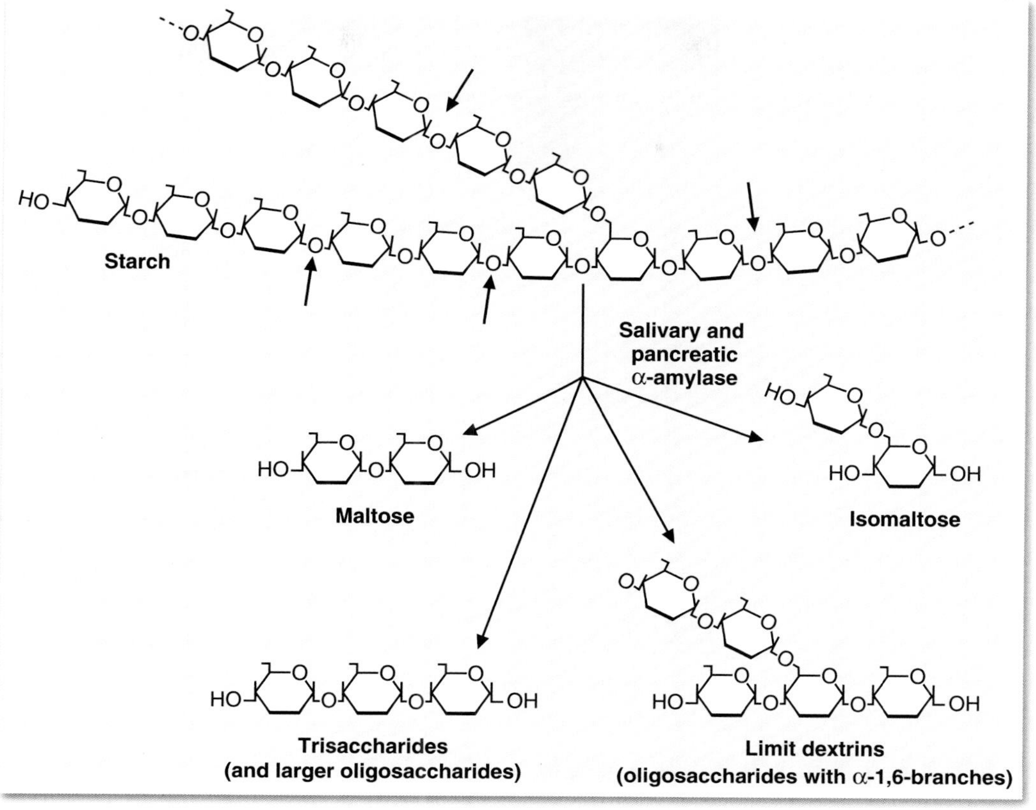

Starch

Salivary and pancreatic α-amylase

Maltose

Isomaltose

Trisaccharides (and larger oligosaccharides)

Limit dextrins (oligosaccharides with α-1,6-branches)

FIGURE 21.3 Action of salivary and pancreatic α-amylases.

α-Amylase is an *endoglycosidase*, which means that it hydrolyzes internal α-1,4-bonds between glucosyl residues at random intervals in the polysaccharide chains (Fig. 21.3). The shortened polysaccharide chains that are formed are called *α-dextrins*. Salivary α-amylase is largely inactivated by the acidity of the stomach contents, which contain HCl secreted by the parietal cells.

The acidic gastric juice enters the duodenum, the upper part of the small intestine, where digestion continues. Secretions from the exocrine pancreas (~1.5 L/day) flow down the pancreatic duct and also enter the duodenum. These secretions contain bicarbonate (HCO_3^-), which neutralizes the acidic pH of stomach contents, and digestive enzymes, including pancreatic α-amylase.

Pancreatic α-amylase continues to hydrolyze the starches and glycogen, forming the disaccharide maltose, the trisaccharide maltotriose, and oligosaccharides. These oligosaccharides, called *limit dextrins*, are usually four to nine glucosyl units long and contain one or more α-1,6-branches. The two glucosyl residues that contain the α-1,6-glycosidic bond eventually become the disaccharide isomaltose.

α-Amylase has no activity toward sugar-containing polymers other than glucose linked by α-1,4-bonds. α-Amylase displays no activity toward the α-1,6-bond at branch points and has little activity for the α-1,4-bond at the nonreducing end of a chain.

B. Disaccharidases of the Intestinal Brush-Border Membrane

The dietary disaccharides lactose and sucrose, as well as the products of starch digestion, are converted to monosaccharides by glycosidases attached to the membrane in the brush border of absorptive cells. The different glycosidase activities are found in four glycoproteins: glucoamylase, the sucrase–isomaltase complex, the smaller glycoprotein trehalase, and lactase-glucosylceramidase (Table 21.1). These glycosidases are collectively called the *small intestinal disaccharidases*, although glucoamylase is really an oligosaccharidase.

Amylase activity in the gut is abundant and is not normally rate-limiting for the process of digestion. Alcohol-induced pancreatitis or surgical removal of part of the pancreas can decrease pancreatic secretion. Pancreatic exocrine secretion into the intestine also can be decreased because of cystic fibrosis (as in **Susan F.**; see Chapter 17), in which mucus blocks the pancreatic duct, which eventually degenerates. However, pancreatic exocrine secretion can be decreased to 10% of normal and still not affect the rate of starch digestion because amylases are secreted in the saliva and pancreatic fluid in excessive amounts. In contrast, protein and fat digestion are more strongly affected in cystic fibrosis.

Acarbose is a U.S. Food and Drug Administration–approved drug that blocks the activities of pancreatic α-amylase and brush-border α-glucosidases (with a specificity for glucose). The drug is produced from a microorganism and is a unique tetrasaccharide. Acarbose can be used in patients with type 2 diabetes. It reduces the rate at which ingested carbohydrate reaches the bloodstream after a meal, but flatulence and diarrhea (caused by colonic bacterial metabolism of the nondigested sugars) are side effects of taking this drug, and thus, it is not used very often.

TABLE 21.1	The Different Forms of the Brush-Border Glycosidases	
COMPLEX	**CATALYTIC SITES**	**PRINCIPAL ACTIVITIES**
β-Glucoamylase	α-Glucosidase	Split α-1,4-glycosidic bonds between glucosyl units, beginning sequentially with the residue at the tail end (nonreducing end) of the chain. This is an exoglycosidase. Substrates include amylose, amylopectin, glycogen, and maltose.
	β-Glucosidase	Same as above but with slightly different specificities and affinities for the substrates
Sucrase	Sucrase–maltase	Splits sucrose, maltose, and maltotriose
Isomaltase	Isomaltase–maltase	Splits α-1,-6-bonds in several limit dextrins as well as the α-1,4-bonds in maltose and maltotriose
β-Glycosidase	Glucosyl–ceramidase	Splits β-glycosidic bonds between glucose or galactose and hydrophobic residues, such as the glycolipids glucosylceramide and galactosylceramide; also known as *phlorizin hydrolase* for its activity on an artificial substrate
	Lactase	Splits the β-1,4-bond between glucose and galactose; to a lesser extent also splits the β-1,4-bond between some cellulose disaccharides
Trehalase	Trehalase	Splits bond in trehalose, which is two glucosyl units linked α-1,1 through their anomeric carbons

Q Can the glycosidic bonds of the structure shown here be hydrolyzed by α-amylose?

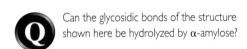

I. Glucoamylase

Glucoamylase and the sucrase–isomaltase complex have similar structures and exhibit a great deal of sequence homogeneity. A membrane-spanning domain near the N terminus attaches the protein to the luminal membrane. The long polypeptide chain forms two globular domains, each with a catalytic site. In glucoamylase, the two catalytic sites have similar activities, with only small differences in substrate specificity. The protein is heavily glycosylated, with oligosaccharides that protect it from digestive proteases.

Glucoamylase is an *exoglycosidase* that is specific for the α-1,4-bonds between glucosyl residues (Fig. 21.4A). It begins at the nonreducing end of a polysaccharide or limit dextrin, and it sequentially hydrolyzes the bonds to release glucose monosaccharides. It will digest a limit dextrin down to isomaltose, the glucosyl disaccharide with an α-1,6-branch, that is subsequently hydrolyzed principally by the isomaltase activity in the sucrase–isomaltase complex.

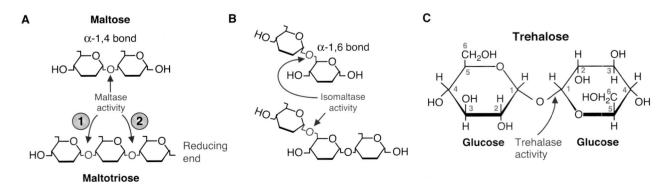

FIGURE 21.4 **A.** Glucoamylase activity. Glucoamylase is an α-1,4-exoglycosidase that initiates cleavage at the nonreducing end of the sugar. Thus, for maltotriose, the bond labeled *1* is hydrolyzed first, which then allows the bond at position 2 to be the next one hydrolyzed. **B.** Isomaltase activity. *Arrows* indicate the α-1,6-bonds that are cleaved. **C.** Trehalose. This disaccharide contains two glucose moieties linked by an unusual bond that joins their anomeric carbons. It is cleaved by trehalase.

2. Sucrase–Isomaltase Complex

The structure of the sucrase–isomaltase complex is similar to that of glucoamylase, and these two proteins have a high degree of sequence homology. However, after the single polypeptide chain of sucrase–isomaltase is inserted through the membrane and the protein protrudes into the intestinal lumen, an intestinal protease clips it into two separate subunits that remain attached to each other through noncovalent interactions. Each subunit has a catalytic site that differs in substrate specificity from the other through noncovalent interactions. The sucrase–maltase site accounts for approximately 100% of the intestine's ability to hydrolyze sucrose in addition to maltase activity; the isomaltase–maltase site accounts for almost all of the intestine's ability to hydrolyze α-1,6-bonds (see Fig. 21.4B), in addition to maltase activity. Together, these sites account for approximately 80% of the maltase activity of the small intestine. The remainder of the maltase activity is found in the glucoamylase complex.

3. Trehalase

Trehalase is only half as long as the other disaccharidases and has only one catalytic site. It hydrolyzes the glycosidic bond in trehalose, a disaccharide composed of two glucosyl units linked by an α-bond between their anomeric carbons (see Fig. 21.4C). Trehalose, which is found in insects, algae, mushrooms, and other fungi, is not currently a major dietary component in the United States. However, unwitting consumption of trehalose can cause nausea, vomiting, and other symptoms of severe gastrointestinal distress if consumed by an individual deficient in the enzyme. Trehalase deficiency was discovered when a woman became very sick after eating mushrooms and was initially thought to have α-amanitin poisoning.

4. β-Glycosidase Complex (Lactase-Glucosylceramidase)

The β-glycosidase complex is another large glycoprotein found in the brush border that has two catalytic sites extending in the lumen of the intestine. However, its primary structure is very different from that of the other enzymes, and it is attached to the membrane through its carboxyl end by a phosphatidylglycan anchor (see Fig. 10.6). The lactase catalytic site hydrolyzes the β-bond connecting glucose and galactose in lactose (a β-galactosidase activity; Fig. 21.5). The major activity of the other catalytic site in humans is the β-bond between glucose or galactose and ceramide in glycolipids (this catalytic site is sometimes called *phlorizin hydrolase*, named for its ability to hydrolyze an artificial substrate).

5. Location Within the Intestine

The production of maltose, maltotriose, and limit dextrins by pancreatic α-amylase occurs in the duodenum, the most proximal portion of the small intestine. Sucrase–isomaltase activity is highest in the jejunum, where the enzymes can hydrolyze sucrose and the products of starch digestion. β-Glycosidase activity is also highest in the jejunum. Glucoamylase activity increases progressively along the length of the small intestine, and its activity is highest in the ileum. Thus, it presents a final opportunity for digestion of starch oligomers that have escaped amylase and disaccharidase activities at the more proximal regions of the intestine.

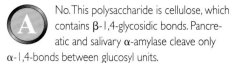

No. This polysaccharide is cellulose, which contains β-1,4-glycosidic bonds. Pancreatic and salivary α-amylase cleave only α-1,4-bonds between glucosyl units.

Individuals with genetic deficiencies of the sucrase–isomaltase complex show symptoms of sucrose intolerance but are able to digest normal amounts of starch in a meal without problems. The maltase activity in the glucoamylase complex, and residual activity in the sucrase–isomaltase complex (which is normally present in excess of need), is apparently sufficient to digest normal amounts of dietary starch.

Q Which of the bonds in the structure shown here are hydrolyzed by the sucrase–isomaltase complex? Which by glucoamylase?

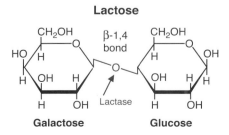

Lactose

CH₂OH β-1,4 bond   CH₂OH

Galactose   Glucose

FIGURE 21.5 Lactase activity. Lactase is a β-galactosidase. It cleaves the β-galactoside lactose, the major sugar in milk, forming galactose and glucose.

A Bonds (*1*) and (*3*) would first be hydrolyzed by glucoamylase. Bond (*2*) requires isomaltase. Bonds (*4*) and (*5*) can then be hydrolyzed by the sucrase–isomaltase complex or by the glucoamylase complex, all of which can convert maltotriose and maltose to glucose.

C. Metabolism of Sugars by Colonic Bacteria

Not all of the starch ingested as part of foods is normally digested in the small intestine (Fig. 21.6). Starches that are high in amylose, or are less well-hydrated (e.g., starch in dried beans), are resistant to digestion and enter the colon. Dietary fiber and undigested sugars also enter the colon. Here, colonic bacteria rapidly metabolize the saccharides, forming gases, short-chain fatty acids, and lactate. The major short-chain fatty acids formed are acetic acid (two carbons), propionic acid (three carbons), and butyric acid (four carbons). The short-chain fatty acids are absorbed by the colonic mucosal cells and can provide a substantial source of energy for these cells. The major gases formed are hydrogen gas (H_2), carbon dioxide (CO_2), and methane (CH_4). These gases are released through the colon, resulting in flatulence, or through the breath. Incomplete products of digestion in the intestines increase the retention of water in the colon, resulting in diarrhea.

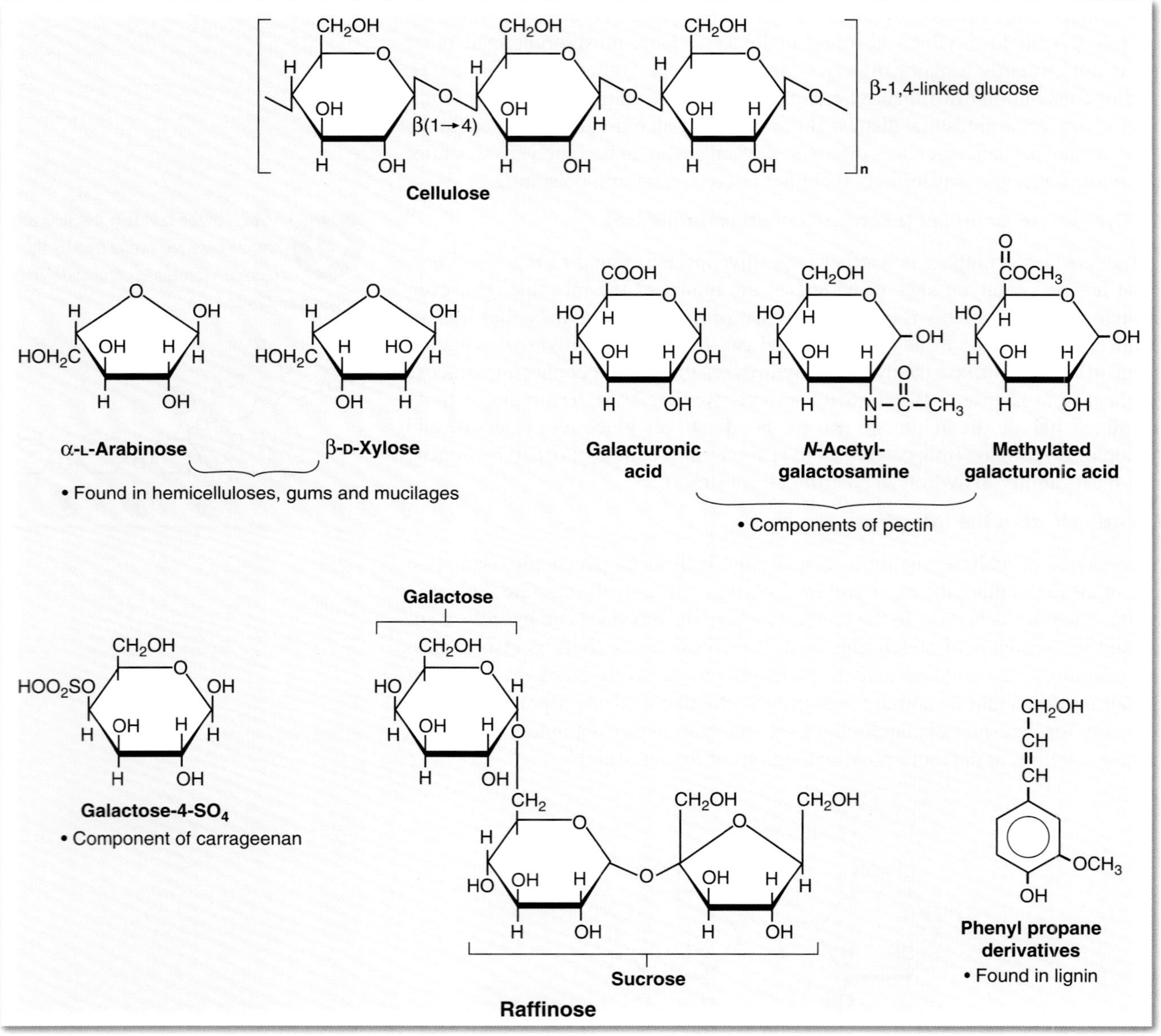

FIGURE 21.6 Some indigestible carbohydrates. These compounds are components of dietary fiber.

D. Lactose Intolerance

Lactose intolerance refers to a condition of pain, nausea, and flatulence after the ingestion of foods containing lactose, most notably dairy products. Although lactose intolerance is often caused by low levels of lactase, it also can be caused by intestinal injury (defined in the following text).

1. Nonpersistent and Persistent Lactase

Lactase activity increases in the human from about 6 to 8 weeks of gestation, and it rises during the late gestational period (21 to 32 weeks) through full term. It remains high for about 1 month after birth and then begins to decline. For most of the world's population, lactase activity decreases to adult levels at approximately 5 to 7 years of age. Adult levels are <10% of those present in infants. These populations have *adult hypolactasia* (formerly called *adult lactase deficiency*) and exhibit the lactase nonpersistence phenotype. In people who are derived mainly from Western Northern Europeans, and milk-dependent Nomadic tribes of Saharan Africa, the levels of lactase remain at, or only slightly below, infant levels throughout adulthood (lactase persistence phenotype). Thus, adult hypolactasia is the normal condition for most of the world's population (Table 21.2).

In contrast, *congenital lactase deficiency* is a severe autosomal-recessive inherited disease in which lactase activity is significantly reduced or totally absent. The disorder presents as soon as the newborn is fed breast milk or lactose-containing formula, resulting in watery diarrhea, weight loss, and dehydration. Treatment consists of removal of lactose from the diet, which allows for normal growth and development to occur.

2. Intestinal Injury

Intestinal diseases that injure the absorptive cells of the intestinal villi diminish lactase activity along the intestine, producing a condition known as *secondary lactase deficiency*. Kwashiorkor (protein malnutrition), colitis, gastroenteritis, tropical and nontropical sprue, and excessive alcohol consumption fall into this category. These diseases also affect other disaccharidases, but sucrase, maltase, isomaltase, and glucoamylase activities are usually present at such excessive levels that there are no pathologic effects. Lactase is usually the first activity lost and the last to recover.

Nina M. was given a hydrogen breath test, a test measuring the amount of hydrogen gas released after consuming a test dose of sugar. In this test, the patient breathes into a portable meter or a collecting bag attached to a nonportable device. The larger, nonportable devices measure the hydrogen in the breath via gas chromatography. The portable devices measure the hydrogen gas produced using hydrogen-specific electrodes and measuring a current that is created when hydrogen comes into contact with the electrode. The association of Nina's symptoms with her ingestion of fruit juices suggests that she might have a problem resulting from low sucrase activity or an inability to absorb fructose. Her ability to thrive and her adequate weight gain suggest that any deficiencies of the sucrase–isomaltase complex must be partial and do not result in a functionally important reduction in maltase activity (maltase activity is also present in the glucoamylase complex). Her urine tested negative for sugar, suggesting that the problem is in digestion or absorption because only sugars that are absorbed and enter the blood can be found in urine. The basis of the hydrogen breath test is that if a sugar is not absorbed, it is metabolized in the intestinal lumen by bacteria that produce various gases including hydrogen. The test can be accompanied by measurements of the amount of sugar that appear in the blood or feces, and acidity of the feces.

TABLE 21.2 Prevalence of Late-Onset Lactase Deficiency	
GROUP	**PREVALENCE (%)**
US Population	
Asians	100
American Indians (Oklahoma)	95
Black Americans	81
Mexican Americans	56
White Americans	24
Other Populations	
Ibo, Yoruba (Nigeria)	89
Italians	71
Aborigines (Australia)	67
Greeks	53
Danes	3
Dutch	0

Reproduced with permission from Büller HA, Grand RJ. Lactose intolerance. *Annu Rev Med.* 1990;41:141–148. Copyright © 1990 by Annual Reviews, Inc.

Lactose intolerance can either be the result of a primary deficiency of lactase production in the small bowel (as is the case for **Denise V.**), or it can be secondary to an injury to the intestinal mucosa, where lactase is normally produced. The lactose that is not absorbed is converted by colonic bacteria to lactic acid, methane gas (CH_4), and H_2 gas (see the following figure). The osmotic effect of the lactose and lactic acid in the bowel lumen is responsible for the diarrhea that is often seen as part of this syndrome. Similar symptoms can result from sensitivity to milk proteins (milk intolerance) or from the malabsorption of other dietary sugars.

In adults suspected of having a lactase deficiency, the diagnosis is usually made inferentially when avoidance of all dairy products results in relief of symptoms and a rechallenge with these foods reproduces the characteristic syndrome. If the results of these measures are equivocal, however, the malabsorption of lactose can be determined more specifically by measuring the H_2 content of the patient's breath after a test dose of lactose has been consumed.

Denise V.'s symptoms did not appear if she took available over-the-counter tablets containing lactase when she ate dairy products.

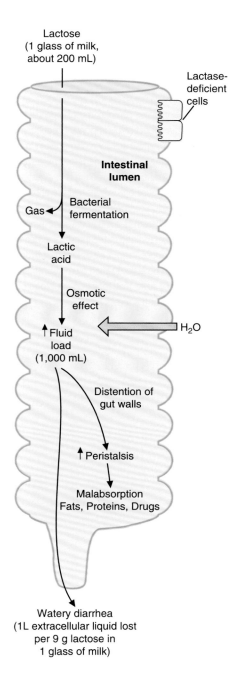

Lactose
(1 glass of milk,
about 200 mL)

Lactase-
deficient
cells

Intestinal
lumen

Gas — Bacterial
fermentation

Lactic
acid

Osmotic
effect

↑Fluid
load
(1,000 mL)

H_2O

Distention of
gut walls

↑ Peristalsis

Malabsorption
Fats, Proteins, Drugs

Watery diarrhea
(1L extracellular liquid lost
per 9 g lactose in
1 glass of milk)

III. Dietary Fiber

Dietary fiber is the portion of the diet resistant to digestion by human digestive enzymes. It consists principally of plant materials that are polysaccharide derivatives and lignan (see Fig. 21.6). The components of fiber are often divided into the categories of soluble and insoluble fiber, according to their ability to dissolve in water. Insoluble fiber consists of three major categories: cellulose, hemicellulose, and lignins. Soluble fiber categories include pectins, mucilages, and gums (Table 21.3). Although human enzymes cannot digest fiber, the bacterial flora in the normal human gut may metabolize the more soluble dietary fibers to gases and short-chain fatty acids, much as they do undigested starch and sugars. Some of these fatty acids may be absorbed and used by the colonic epithelial cells of the gut, and some may travel to the liver through the hepatic portal vein. We may obtain as much as 10% of our total calories from compounds produced by bacterial digestion of substances in our digestive tract.

The 2015 Dietary Guideline Advisory Committee issued guidelines for fiber ingestion—anywhere from 22 to 34 g/day in adults, depending on the age and sex of the individual. No distinction was made between soluble and insoluble fibers. Adult males between the ages of 19 and 30 years require 34 g of fiber per day. Males between 31 and 50 years of age require 30.8 g of fiber per day. Males older than 51 years of age are recommended to consume 28 g of fiber per day. Adult women between 19 and 30 years of age require 28 g/day. Women between the ages of 31 and 50 years of age are recommended to consume 25.2 g of fiber per day. Women older than 51 years of age are recommended to consume 22 g of fiber per day. These numbers are increased during pregnancy and lactation. One beneficial effect of fiber is seen in diverticular disease in which sacs or pouches may develop in the colon

TABLE 21.3 Types of Fiber in the Diet		
CLASSICAL NOMENCLATURE	**CLASSES OF COMPOUNDS**	**DIETARY SOURCES**
Insoluble Fiber		
Cellulose	Polysaccharide composed of glucosyl residues linked β-1,4	Whole-wheat flour, unprocessed bran, vegetables
Hemicelluloses	Polymers of arabinoxylans or galactomannans	Bran cereals, whole grains,
Lignin	Noncarbohydrate, polymeric derivatives of phenylpropane	Fruits and edible seeds, mature vegetables
Water-Soluble Fiber (or Dispersible)		
Pectic substances	Galacturonans, arabinogalactans, β-glucans, arabinoxylans	Apples, strawberries, carrots, citrus
Gums	Galactomannans, arabinogalactans	Oats, legumes, guar, barley
Mucilages	Wide range of branched and substituted galactans	Flax seed, psyllium, mustard seed

because of a weakening of the muscle and submucosal structures. Fiber is thought to "soften" the stool, thereby reducing pressure on the colonic wall and enhancing expulsion of feces.

Certain types of soluble fiber have been associated with disease prevention. For example, pectins may lower blood cholesterol levels by binding bile acids. β-Glucan (obtained from oats) has also been shown, in some studies, to reduce cholesterol levels through a reduction in bile acid resorption in the intestine (see Chapter 32). Pectins also may have a beneficial effect in the diet of individuals with diabetes mellitus by slowing the rate of absorption of simple sugars and preventing high blood glucose levels after meals. However, each of the beneficial effects that have been related to "fiber" is relatively specific for the type of fiber and the physical form of the food that contains the fiber. This factor, along with many others, has made it difficult to obtain conclusive results from studies of the effects of fiber on human health.

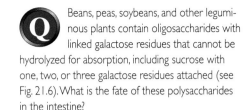

Beans, peas, soybeans, and other leguminous plants contain oligosaccharides with linked galactose residues that cannot be hydrolyzed for absorption, including sucrose with one, two, or three galactose residues attached (see Fig. 21.6). What is the fate of these polysaccharides in the intestine?

IV. Absorption of Sugars

Once the carbohydrates have been split into monosaccharides, the sugars are transported across the intestinal epithelial cells and into the blood for distribution to all tissues. Not all complex carbohydrates are digested at the same rate within the intestine, and some carbohydrate sources lead to a near-immediate rise in blood glucose levels after ingestion, whereas others slowly raise blood glucose levels over an extended period after ingestion. The *glycemic index* of a food is an indication of how rapidly blood glucose levels rise after consumption. Glucose and maltose have the highest glycemic indices (defined as 100). Table 21.4 indicates the glycemic index for a variety of food types. Although there is no need to memorize this table, note that cornflakes and potatoes have high glycemic indices, whereas yogurt and skim milk have particularly low glycemic indices.

The glycemic response to ingested foods depends not only on the glycemic index of the foods but also on the fiber and fat content of the food as well as its method of preparation. Highly glycemic carbohydrates can be consumed before and

TABLE 21.4 Glycemic Indices of Selected Foods, with Values Adjusted to Glucose of 100			
Breads		**Legumes**	
Whole wheat	74	Soya beans	16
Specialty grain bread	53	Lentils	32
Pasta		Chick peas	28
Spaghetti, white, boiled	49	Kidney beans (dried)	24
Cereal Grains		Peanuts	15
Barley	28	**Fruit**	
White rice (boiled)	73	Banana	51
Brown rice (boiled)	68	Apple	36
Sweet corn	52	Apple juice	41
Breakfast Cereals		Orange	43
Wheat flake biscuits	69	Watermelon	76
Cornflakes	81	**Sugars**	
Muesli	57	Maltose	105
Snacks		Fructose	15
Popcorn	65	Glucose	100
Chocolate	40	Honey	61
Root Vegetables		Sucrose	65
Potatoes (instant, mash)	87	**Dairy Products**	
Potato (new, white, boiled)	78	Ice cream	51
Potato, French fries	63	Whole milk	39
Sweet potato, boiled	63	Skim milk	37
		Yogurt, fruit	41

Data from Atkinson FS, Foster-Powell K, Brand-Miller JC. International tables of glycemic index and glycemic load values. *Diabetes Care.* 2008;31(12):2281–2283.

These sugars are not digested well by the human intestine but form good sources of energy for the bacteria of the gut. These bacteria convert the sugars to H_2, lactic acid, and short-chain fatty acids. The amount of gas released after a meal containing beans is especially notorious.

The dietitian explained to **Deborah S.** the rationale for a person with diabetes to follow a carbohydrate-controlled diet using meal-planning tools such as carbohydrate counting (www.diabetes.org, click on *Food and Fitness*). It is important for Deborah to add a variety of fibers, particularly soluble fiber, to her diet. The gel-forming, water-retaining pectins and gums found in foods such as oatmeal, nuts, beans, lentils, and apples delay gastric emptying and retard the rate of absorption of disaccharides and monosaccharides, thus reducing the rate at which blood glucose levels rise. Although research has shown that the total amount of carbohydrate is most influential on blood glucose levels, the quality of carbohydrate—the glycemic index of foods—may also need to be considered for optimal maintenance of blood glucose levels in people with diabetes. Consumption of a low-glycemic-index diet results in a lower rise in blood glucose levels after eating, which can be more easily controlled by exogenous insulin. For example, **Ms. S.** is advised to eat pasta and barley (glycemic indices of 49 and 28, respectively) instead of potatoes (glycemic index of 63 to 87, depending on the method of preparation) and to incorporate breakfast cereals composed of wheat bran, barley, and oats into her morning routine. Because the total amount and the type of carbohydrate influence blood glucose levels, Deborah is advised to consume lower glycemic index foods in appropriate portions.

after exercise because their metabolism results in a rapid entry of glucose into the blood, where it is then immediately available for use by muscle cells. Low-glycemic carbohydrates enter the circulation slowly and can be used to best advantage if consumed before exercise, such that as exercise progresses, glucose is slowly being absorbed from the intestine into the circulation, where it can be used to maintain blood glucose levels during the exercise period.

A. Absorption by the Intestinal Epithelium

Glucose is transported through the absorptive cells of the intestine by facilitated diffusion and by Na^+-dependent facilitated transport. (See Chapter 10 for a description of transport mechanisms.) The glucose molecule is extremely polar and cannot diffuse through the hydrophobic phospholipid bilayer of the cell membrane. Each hydroxyl group of the glucose molecule forms at least two hydrogen bonds with water molecules, and random movement would require energy to dislodge the polar hydroxyl groups from their hydrogen bonds and to disrupt the van der Waals forces between the hydrocarbon tails of the fatty acids in the membrane phospholipid. Glucose, therefore, enters the absorptive cells by binding to transport proteins, membrane-spanning proteins that bind the glucose molecule on one side of the membrane and release it on the opposite side. Two types of glucose transport proteins are present in the intestinal absorptive cells: the Na^+-dependent glucose transporters and the facilitative glucose transporters (Fig. 21.7).

1. Na^+-Dependent Transporters

Na^+-dependent glucose transporters, which are located on the luminal side of the absorptive cells, enable these cells to concentrate glucose from the intestinal lumen. A low intracellular Na^+ concentration is maintained by a Na^+,K^+-ATPase on the serosal (blood) side of the cell that uses the energy from adenosine triphosphate (ATP) cleavage to pump Na^+ out of the cell into the blood. Thus, the transport of glucose from a low concentration in the lumen to a high concentration in the cell is promoted by the cotransport of Na^+ from a high concentration in the lumen to a low concentration in the cell (secondary active transport). Similar transporters are found in the epithelial cells of the kidney, which are thus able to transport glucose against its concentration gradient.

2. Facilitative Glucose Transporters

Facilitative glucose transporters, which do not bind Na^+, are located on the serosal side of the cells. Glucose moves via the facilitative transporters from the high concentration inside the cell to the lower concentration in the blood without the expenditure of energy. In addition to the Na^+-dependent glucose transporters, facilitative transporters for glucose also exist on the luminal side of the absorptive cells. The best characterized facilitative glucose transporters found in the plasma membranes of cells (referred to as *GLUT 1* to *GLUT 5*) are described in Table 21.5. One common structural theme to these proteins is that they all contain 12 membrane-spanning domains. Note that the sodium-linked transporter on the luminal side of the intestinal epithelial cell is not a member of the GLUT family.

The epithelial cells of the kidney, which reabsorb glucose from the lumen of the renal tubule back into the blood, have Na^+-dependent glucose transporters similar to those of intestinal epithelial cells. They are thus also able to transport glucose against its concentration gradient. Other types of cells use mainly facilitative glucose transporters that carry glucose down its concentration gradient.

3. Galactose and Fructose Absorption through Glucose Transporters

Galactose is absorbed through the same mechanisms as glucose. It enters the absorptive cells on the luminal side via the Na^+-dependent glucose transporters and facilitative glucose transporters and is transported through the serosal side on the facilitative glucose transporters.

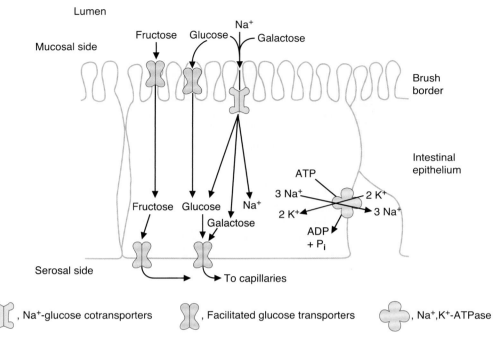

FIGURE 21.7 Na$^+$-dependent and facilitative transporters in the intestinal epithelial cells. Both glucose and fructose are transported by the facilitated glucose transporters on the luminal and serosal sides of the absorptive cells. Glucose and galactose are transported by the Na$^+$-glucose cotransporters on the luminal (mucosal) side of the absorptive cells. *ADP*, adenosine diphosphate; *ATP*, adenosine triphosphate; *P$_i$*, inorganic phosphate.

Fructose both enters and leaves absorptive epithelial cells by facilitated diffusion, apparently via transport proteins that are part of the GLUT family. The transporter on the luminal side has been identified as GLUT 5. Although this transporter can transport glucose, it has a much higher activity with fructose (see Fig. 21.7). Other fructose transport proteins also may be present. For reasons as yet unknown, fructose is absorbed at a much more rapid rate when it is ingested as sucrose than when it is ingested as a monosaccharide.

TABLE 21.5 Properties of the GLUT 1 to GLUT 5 Isoforms of the Glucose Transport Proteins		
TRANSPORTER	**TISSUE DISTRIBUTION**	**COMMENTS**
GLUT 1	Human erythrocyte Blood–brain barrier Blood–retinal barrier Blood–placental barrier Blood–testis barrier	Expressed in cell types with barrier functions; a high-affinity glucose transport system
GLUT 2	Liver Kidney Pancreatic β-cell Serosal surface of intestinal mucosa cells	A high-capacity, low-affinity transporter May be used as the glucose sensor in the pancreas
GLUT 3	Brain (neurons)	Major transporter in the central nervous system; a high-affinity system
GLUT 4	Adipose tissue Skeletal muscle Heart muscle	Insulin-sensitive transporter; in the presence of insulin, the number of GLUT 4 transporters increases on the cell surface; a high-affinity system
GLUT 5	Intestinal epithelium Spermatozoa	This is actually a fructose transporter.

Genetic techniques have identified additional GLUT transporters (GLUT 6 to GLUT 12), but the roles of these transporters have not yet been fully described.

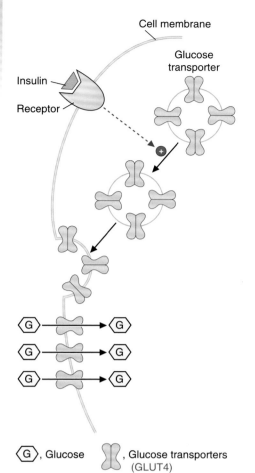

FIGURE 21.8 Stimulation by insulin of glucose transport into muscle and adipose cells. Binding of insulin to its cell membrane receptor causes vesicles containing glucose transport proteins to move from inside the cell to the cell membrane.

B. Transport of Monosaccharides into Tissues

The properties of the GLUT transport proteins differ among tissues, reflecting the function of glucose metabolism in each tissue. In most cell types, the rate of glucose transport across the cell membrane is not rate-limiting for glucose metabolism. This is because the isoform of transporter present in these cell types has a relatively low K_m for glucose (i.e., a low concentration of glucose will result in half the maximal rate of glucose transport) or is present in relatively high concentration in the cell membrane so that the intracellular glucose concentration reflects that in the blood. Because the enzyme that initially metabolizes glucose in these (named *hexokinase*; see Chapter 22) cells has an even lower K_m for glucose (0.05 to 0.10 mM), variations in blood glucose levels do not affect the intracellular rate of glucose metabolism. However, in several tissues, the rate of transport becomes rate limiting when the serum level of glucose is low or when low levels of insulin signal the absence of dietary glucose.

The erythrocyte (red blood cell) is an example of a tissue in which glucose transport is not rate-limiting. Although the glucose transporter (GLUT 1) has a K_m of 1 to 7 mM, it is present in extremely high concentrations, constituting approximately 5% of all membrane proteins. Consequently, as the blood glucose levels fall from a postprandial level of 140 mg/dL (7.5 mM) to the normal fasting level of 80 mg/dL (4.5 mM), or even the hypoglycemic level of 40 mg/dL (2.2 mM), the supply of glucose is still adequate for the rates at which glucose-dependent metabolic pathways operate.

In the liver, the K_m for the glucose transporter (GLUT 2) is relatively high compared with that of other tissues, probably ≥ 15 mM. This is in keeping with the liver's role as the organ that maintains blood glucose levels. Thus, the liver will convert glucose into other energy storage molecules only when blood glucose levels are high, such as the time immediately after ingesting a meal. In muscle and adipose tissue, the transport of glucose is greatly stimulated by insulin. The mechanism involves the recruitment of glucose transporters (specifically, GLUT 4) from intracellular vesicles into the plasma membrane (Fig. 21.8). In adipose tissue, the stimulation of glucose transport across the plasma membrane by insulin increases its availability for the synthesis of fatty acids and glycerol from the glycolytic pathway. In skeletal muscle, the stimulation of glucose transport by insulin increases its availability for energy generation (glycolysis) and glycogen synthesis.

V. Glucose Transport through the Blood–Brain Barrier and into Neurons

A hypoglycemic response is elicited by a decrease of blood glucose concentration to some point between 18 and 54 mg/dL (1 and 3 mM). The hypoglycemic response is a result of a decreased supply of glucose to the brain and starts with light-headedness and dizziness and may progress to coma. The slow rate of transport of glucose through the blood–brain barrier (from the blood into the cerebrospinal fluid) at low levels of glucose is thought to be responsible for this neuroglycopenic response. Glucose transport from the cerebrospinal fluid across the plasma membranes of neurons is rapid and is not rate-limiting for ATP generation from glycolysis.

In the brain, the endothelial cells of the capillaries have extremely tight junctions, and glucose must pass from the blood into the extracellular cerebrospinal fluid by GLUT 1 transporters in the endothelial cell membranes (Fig. 21.9) and then through the basement membrane. Measurements of the overall process of glucose transport from the blood into the brain (mediated by GLUT 3 on neural cells) show a $K_{m,app}$ of 7 to 11 mM and a maximal velocity not much greater than the rate of glucose use by the brain. Thus, decreases of blood glucose below the fasting level of 80 to 90 mg/dL (~5 mM) are likely to significantly affect the rate of glucose metabolism in the brain because of reduced glucose transport into the brain.

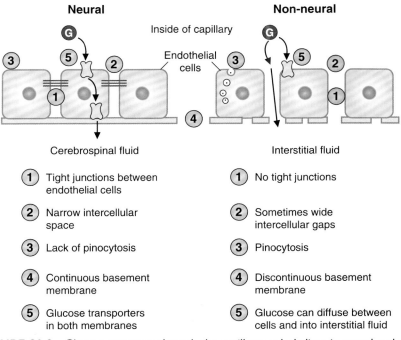

Neural	Non-neural

Inside of capillary

Endothelial cells

Cerebrospinal fluid

Interstitial fluid

Neural	Non-neural
1 Tight junctions between endothelial cells	**1** No tight junctions
2 Narrow intercellular space	**2** Sometimes wide intercellular gaps
3 Lack of pinocytosis	**3** Pinocytosis
4 Continuous basement membrane	**4** Discontinuous basement membrane
5 Glucose transporters in both membranes	**5** Glucose can diffuse between cells and into interstitial fluid

FIGURE 21.9 Glucose transport through the capillary endothelium in neural and non-neural tissues. Characteristics of transport in each type of tissue are listed by numbers that refer to the *numbers* in the drawing. *G*, glucose.

CLINICAL COMMENTS

Denise V. One out of five Americans experiences some form of gastrointestinal discomfort from 30 minutes to 12 hours after ingesting lactose-rich foods. Most become symptomatic when they consume more than 25 g of lactose at one time (e.g., 8 oz of milk or its equivalent). **Denise V.'s** symptoms were caused by her "new" diet in this country, which included a glass of milk in addition to the milk she used on her cereal with breakfast each morning.

Management of lactose intolerance includes a reduction or avoidance of lactose-containing foods, depending on the severity of the deficiency of intestinal lactase. Hard cheeses (cheddar, Swiss, Jarlsberg) are low in lactose and may be tolerated by patients with only moderate lactase deficiency. Yogurt with "live and active cultures" printed on the package contains bacteria that release free lactases when the bacteria are lysed by gastric acid and proteolytic enzymes. The free lactases then digest the lactose. Commercially available milk products that have been hydrolyzed with a lactase enzyme provide a 70% reduction in total lactose content, which may be adequate to prevent digestive symptoms in mildly affected patients. Tablets and capsules containing lactase are also available and should be taken 30 minutes before meals.

Many adults who have a lactase deficiency develop the ability to ingest small amounts of lactose in dairy products without experiencing symptoms. This adaptation probably involves an increase in the population of colonic bacteria that can cleave lactose and not a recovery or induction of human lactase synthesis. For many individuals, dairy products are the major dietary source of calcium, and their complete elimination from the diet can lead to osteoporosis. Therefore, other dietary sources such as beans, almonds, tofu, turnip greens, kale, and calcium-fortified juices/beverages or calcium supplements should be recommended. Lactose, however, is used as a "filler" or carrying agent in >1,000 prescription and over-the-counter drugs in this country. People with lactose intolerance often unwittingly ingest lactose with their medications.

Deborah S. Patients with poorly controlled diabetes, such as **Deborah S.**, frequently have elevations in serum glucose levels (hyperglycemia). This is often attributable to a lack of circulating, active insulin, which normally stimulates glucose uptake (through the recruitment of GLUT 4 transporters from the endoplasmic reticulum to the plasma membrane) by the peripheral tissues (heart, muscle, and adipose tissue). Without uptake by these tissues, glucose tends to accumulate within the bloodstream, leading to hyperglycemia.

Nina M. The large amount of H_2 produced on fructose ingestion suggested that **Nina M.'s** problem was one of a deficiency in fructose transport into the absorptive cells of the intestinal villi. If fructose were being absorbed properly, the fructose would not have traveled to the colonic bacteria, which metabolized the fructose to generate the hydrogen gas. If there was a concern for deficiencies of the sucrase–isomaltase complex, a jejunal biopsy could be done; it would allow the measurement of lactase, sucrase, maltase, and trehalase activities. Genetic testing for the presence of a mutation in one of these proteins is also becoming available. Although Nina had no sugar in her urine, malabsorption of disaccharides can result in their appearance in the urine if damage to the intestinal mucosal cells allows their passage into the interstitial fluid. When Nina was placed on a diet free of fruit juices and other foods containing fructose, she did well and could tolerate small amounts of pure sucrose.

More than 50% of the adult population is estimated to be unable to absorb fructose in high doses (50 g), and >10% cannot completely absorb 25 g of fructose. These individuals, like those with other disorders of fructose metabolism, must avoid fruits and other foods that contain high concentrations of fructose.

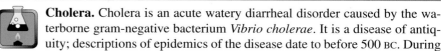

BIOCHEMICAL COMMENTS

Cholera. Cholera is an acute watery diarrheal disorder caused by the waterborne gram-negative bacterium *Vibrio cholerae*. It is a disease of antiquity; descriptions of epidemics of the disease date to before 500 BC. During epidemics, the infection is spread by large numbers of *Vibrio* that enter water sources from the voluminous liquid stools and contaminate the environment, particularly in areas of extreme poverty where plumbing and modern waste-disposal systems are primitive or nonexistent. **Dennis V.** experienced cholera after eating contaminated shellfish (see Chapter 10).

After being ingested, the *V. cholerae* organisms attach to the brush border of the intestinal epithelium and secrete an exotoxin that binds irreversibly to a specific chemical receptor (G_{M1} ganglioside) on the cell surface. This exotoxin catalyzes an adenosine diphosphate (ADP)-ribosylation reaction that increases adenylate cyclase activity and thus cyclic adenosine monophosphate (cAMP) levels in the enterocyte. As a result, the normal absorption of sodium, anions, and water from the gut lumen into the intestinal cell is markedly diminished. The exotoxin also stimulates the crypt cells to secrete chloride, accompanied by cations and water, from the bloodstream into the lumen of the gut. The resulting loss of solute-rich diarrheal fluid may, in severe cases, exceed 1 L/hour, leading to rapid dehydration and even death.

The therapeutic approach to cholera takes advantage of the fact that the Na^+-dependent transporters for glucose and amino acids are not affected by the cholera exotoxin. As a result, coadministration of glucose and Na^+ by mouth results in the uptake of glucose and Na^+, accompanied by chloride and water, thereby partially correcting the ion deficits and fluid loss. Amino acids and small peptides are also absorbed by Na^+-dependent cotransport involving transport proteins distinct from the Na^+-dependent glucose transporters. Therefore, addition of protein to the glucose–sodium replacement solution enhances its effectiveness and markedly decreases the severity of the diarrhea. Adjunctive antibiotic therapy also shortens the diarrheal phase of cholera but does not decrease the need for the oral replacement therapy outlined earlier.

KEY CONCEPTS

- The major carbohydrates in the American diet are starch, lactose, and sucrose.
- Starch is a polysaccharide composed of many glucose units linked together through α-1,4- and α-1,6-glycosidic bonds.
- Lactose is a disaccharide composed of glucose and galactose.
- Sucrose is a disaccharide composed of glucose and fructose.
- Digestion converts all dietary carbohydrates to their respective monosaccharides.
- Amylase digests starch; it is found in the saliva and pancreas, which releases it into the lumen of the small intestine.
- Intestinal epithelial cells contain disaccharidases, which cleave lactose, sucrose, and digestion products of starch into monosaccharides.
- Dietary fiber is composed of polysaccharides that cannot be digested by human enzymes.
- Monosaccharides are transported into the absorptive intestinal epithelial cells via active transport systems.
- Monosaccharides released into the blood via the intestinal epithelial cells are recovered by tissues that use facilitative transporters.
- Diseases discussed in this chapter are summarized in Table 21.6.

TABLE 21.6 Diseases Discussed in Chapter 21		
DISEASE OR DISORDER	**ENVIRONMENTAL OR GENETIC**	**COMMENTS**
Lactose intolerance	Both	Reduced levels of lactase on the intestinal epithelial cell surface lead to reduced lactose digestion in the intestinal lumen, providing substrate for flora in the large intestine. Metabolism of the lactose by these bacteria leads to the generation of organic acids and gases.
Type 2 diabetes	Both	Healthy diets with controlled intake of carbohydrates will be beneficial in managing blood glucose levels.
Fructose malabsorption	Genetic	Inability to absorb fructose in the small intestine, leading to colonic bacteria metabolism of fructose and the generation of organic acids and gases
Cholera	Environmental	Increased cAMP levels in the intestinal epithelial cells lead to inhibition of ion transport and significant water extrusion from the affected cells, leading to severe diarrhea.

REVIEW QUESTIONS—CHAPTER 21

1. The facilitative transporter that is most responsible for transporting fructose from the blood into cells is which one of the following?
   A. GLUT 1
   B. GLUT 2
   C. GLUT 3
   D. GLUT 4
   E. GLUT 5

2. A patient with alcoholism developed pancreatitis that affected his exocrine pancreatic function. He exhibited discomfort after eating a high-carbohydrate meal. The patient most likely had a reduced ability to digest which one of the following?
   A. Starch
   B. Lactose
   C. Fiber
   D. Sucrose
   E. Maltose

3. A man with type 1 diabetes neglects to take his insulin injections while on a weekend vacation. Cells found within which tissue will be most greatly affected by this mistake?
   A. Brain
   B. Liver
   C. Muscle
   D. Red blood cells
   E. Pancreas

4. After digestion of a piece of cake that contains flour, milk, and sucrose as its primary ingredients, the major carbohydrate products that enter the blood are which of the following?
   A. Glucose
   B. Fructose and galactose
   C. Galactose and glucose
   D. Fructose and glucose
   E. Glucose, galactose, and fructose

5. A patient has a genetic defect that causes intestinal epithelial cells to produce disaccharidases of much lower activity than normal. Compared with a normal person, after eating a bowl of oatmeal and milk sweetened with table sugar, this patient will exhibit higher levels of which of the following?
   A. Maltose, sucrose, and lactose in the stool
   B. Starch in the stool
   C. Galactose and fructose in the blood
   D. Glycogen in the muscles
   E. Insulin in the blood

6. The majority of calories in the US diet are derived from carbohydrates, which can contain a variety of glycosidic bonds. Which one of the following carbohydrates contains glucosyl units linked through α-1,6 glycosidic bonds?
   A. Amylose
   B. Amylopectin
   C. Lactose
   D. Sucrose
   E. Maltose

7. A patient has increased her dietary fiber intake in an effort to decrease constipation. She has recently noticed abdominal cramping and bloating as well as increased flatulence. Which one of the following best explains why this is happening?
   A. Human enzymes in the small intestine break down the fiber and produce H_2, CO_2, and methane as byproducts.
   B. Bacteria in the small intestine can convert fiber to H_2, CO_2, and methane.

C. Viruses in the unwashed vegetables convert fiber to H_2, CO_2, and methane.
   D. Bacteria in the colon can convert fiber to H_2, CO_2, and methane.
   E. Human enzymes in the colon can convert fiber to H_2, CO_2, and methane.

8. A newly diagnosed patient with diabetes avoided table sugar because he knew he had "sugar diabetes," but he continued to consume fruits, fruit drinks, milk, honey, and vegetables, with the result being poor diabetic control. The diet the patient was following contained carbohydrate primarily in which form? Choose the one best answer.
   A. Sucrose
   B. Glucose
   C. Fructose
   D. Lactose
   E. Xylulose

9. A 10-year-old patient had 3 days of severe diarrhea after developing a viral gastroenteritis. Now, whenever she drinks milk, she experiences nausea, abdominal pain, and flatulence. She never had this happen before after drinking milk. Which one of the following would be the best advice for this patient?
   A. She should never consume milk products again.
   B. Her children will have lactose deficiency at birth.
   C. Her ability to drink milk should return in a few days.
   D. She has developed viral gastroenteritis again and should receive antibiotics.
   E. The cause of the symptoms is a defect in the colon.

10. A runner wanted to "carb load" just before a race, and she wanted to pick something to eat that has a high glycemic index. Which one of the following foods should the runner pick?
   A. Ice cream
   B. Malted milk balls
   C. Oatmeal cookies
   D. Spaghetti
   E. Potato chips

ANSWERS

1. **The answer is E.** The GLUT 5 transporter has a much higher affinity for fructose than glucose and is the facilitator of choice for fructose uptake by cells. The other GLUT transporters do not transport fructose to any significant extent.

2. **The answer is A.** The pancreas produces α-amylase, which digests starch in the intestinal lumen. If pancreatic

α-amylase cannot enter the lumen because of pancreatitis, the starch will not be digested to a significant extent. (The salivary α-amylase begins the process, but only for the time during which the food is in the mouth, because the acidic conditions of the stomach destroy the salivary activity.) The discomfort arises from the bacteria in the intestine digesting the starch and producing acids and gases. Lactose, sucrose, and maltose are all disaccharides that would be cleaved by the intestinal disaccharidases located on the brush border of the intestinal epithelial cells (thus, B, D, and E are incorrect). These activities might be slightly reduced because the pancreas would also have difficulty excreting bicarbonate to the intestine, and the low pH of the stomach contents might reduce the activity of these enzymes. However, these enzymes are present in excess and will eventually digest the disaccharides. Fiber cannot be digested by human enzymes, so answer C is incorrect.

3. **The answer is C.** Insulin is required to stimulate glucose transport into muscle and fat cells but not into brain, liver, pancreas, or red blood cells. Thus, muscle would be feeling the effects of glucose deprivation and would be unable to replenish its own glycogen supplies as a result of its inability to extract blood glucose, even though blood glucose levels would be high.

4. **The answer is E.** Flour contains starch, which leads to glucose production in the intestine. Milk contains lactose, a disaccharide of glucose and galactose, which is split by lactase in the small intestine. Sucrose is a disaccharide of glucose and fructose, which is split by sucrase in the small intestine. Thus, glucose, galactose, and fructose are all available in the lumen of the small intestine for transport through the intestinal epithelial cells and into the circulation.

5. **The answer is A.** Salivary and pancreatic α-amylase will partially digest starch to glucose, but maltose and disaccharides will pass through the intestine and exit with the stool as a result of the limited activity of the brush-border enzymes. Because the amylase enzymes are working, there will only be normal levels of starch in the stool (thus, B is incorrect). Not all available glucose is entering the blood, so less insulin will be released by the pancreas (thus, E is incorrect), which will lead to less glucose uptake by the muscles and less glycogen production (thus, D is incorrect). Because neither lactose nor sucrose can be digested to a large extent in the intestinal lumen under these conditions, it would be difficult to have elevated levels of galactose or fructose in the blood (thus, C is incorrect).

6. **The answer is B.** The starch amylopectin is a branched polysaccharide of glucosyl units linked through α-1,4 glycosidic bonds with α-1,6 glycosidic bonds as branchpoints. The straight-chained starch amylose and the disaccharide maltose are both linked through α-1,4 glycosidic bonds. The disaccharide sucrose contains a 1,2-glycosidic bond between glucose and fructose, whereas lactose contains a β-1,4-glycosidic bond between galactose and glucose.

7. **The answer is D.** Human enzymes cannot digest dietary fiber. However, bacteria in the colon can convert fiber to short-chain fatty acids, H_2, CO_2, and methane. These gases give the symptoms of bloating, cramping, and excess gas (flatulence). Viruses do not metabolize fiber.

8. **The answer is A.** Sucrose and small amounts of glucose and fructose are the major natural sweeteners in fruit, honey, and vegetables. Lactose is the sugar found in milk and milk-derived products. Xylulose is a component of the pentose phosphate pathway, and its levels in fruits and vegetables are low.

9. **The answer is C.** With viral gastroenteritis, the cells lining the brush borders of the small intestine can be sloughed off into the lumen of the intestine, resulting in temporary lactose intolerance owing to the lack of lactase activity. Once these cells regenerate, the symptoms should disappear. She does not have congenital lactase deficiency, so her children will not inherit a defect in lactose metabolism. Antibiotics have no effect on viral illnesses and should not be given for viral gastroenteritis.

10. **The answer is B.** Maltose (glucose α-1,4-glucose) has the highest glycemic index and would most rapidly raise blood sugar levels after ingestion. Malted grains and malted milk are high in maltose. All the other foods listed exhibit a glycemic index that is only about half the glycemic index of maltose, and the glucose derived from that food would require more time to reach the blood than the glucose derived from maltose.

Generation of Adenosine Triphosphate from Glucose, Fructose, and Galactose: Glycolysis

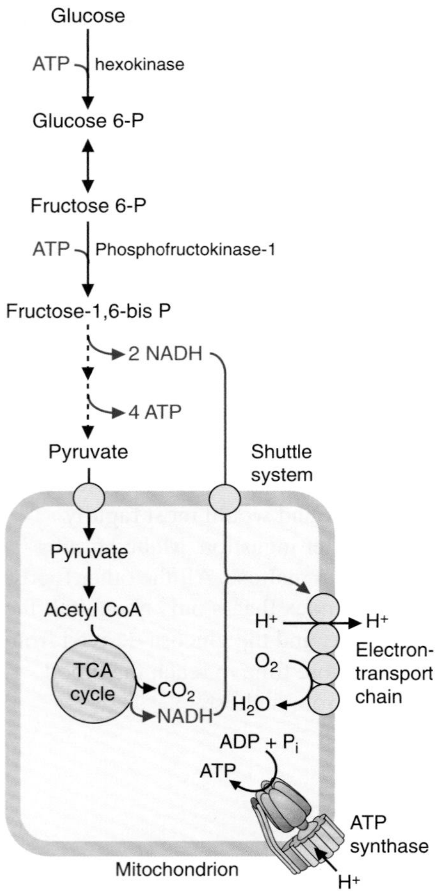

FIGURE 22.1 Overview of glycolysis and the tricarboxylic acid (TCA) cycle. *Acetyl CoA*, acetyl coenzyme A; *ADP*, adenosine diphosphate; *ATP*, adenosine triphosphate; *Fructose 6-P*, fructose 6-phosphate; *Fructose-1,6-bis P*, fructose 1,6-bisphosphate; *Glucose 6-P*, glucose 6-phosphate; *NADH*, reduced nicotinamide adenine dinucleotide; P_i, inorganic phosphate.

Glucose is the universal fuel for human cells. Every cell type in humans is able to generate adenosine triphosphate (ATP) from glycolysis, the pathway in which glucose is oxidized and cleaved to form pyruvate. The importance of glycolysis in our fuel economy is related to the availability of glucose in the blood as well as the ability of glycolysis to generate ATP in both the presence and absence of O_2. Glucose is the major sugar in our diet and the sugar that circulates in the blood to ensure that all cells have a continuous fuel supply. The brain uses glucose almost exclusively as a fuel.

Glycolysis begins with the phosphorylation of glucose to glucose 6-phosphate (**glucose 6-P**) by **hexokinase** (**HK**). In subsequent steps of the pathway, one glucose 6-P molecule is oxidized to two **pyruvate** molecules with generation of two molecules of **nicotinamide adenine dinucleotide** (**NADH**) (Fig. 22.1). A net generation of two molecules of ATP occurs through direct transfer of **high-energy phosphate** from intermediates of the pathway to adenosine diphosphate (ADP) (**substrate-level phosphorylation**).

Glycolysis occurs in the **cytosol** and generates cytosolic NADH. Because NADH cannot cross the inner mitochondrial membrane, its reducing equivalents are transferred to the electron-transport chain (ETC) by either the **malate–aspartate shuttle** or the **glycerol 3-phosphate shuttle** (see Fig. 22.1). Pyruvate is then oxidized completely to CO_2 by pyruvate dehydrogenase (PDH) and the tricarboxylic acid (TCA) cycle (see Chapter 23). Complete **aerobic oxidation** of glucose to CO_2 can generate approximately **30 to 32 mol of ATP per mole of glucose**.

When cells have a limited supply of oxygen (e.g., the kidney medulla), or few or no mitochondria (e.g., the red cell), or greatly increased demands for ATP (e.g., skeletal muscle during high-intensity exercise), they rely on **anaerobic glycolysis** for generation of ATP. In anaerobic glycolysis, **lactate dehydrogenase** (**LDH**) oxidizes the NADH generated from glycolysis by reducing pyruvate to **lactate** (Fig. 22.2). Because O_2 is not required to reoxidize the NADH, the pathway is referred to as anaerobic. The energy yield from anaerobic glycolysis (2 mol of ATP per mole of glucose) is much lower than the yield from aerobic oxidation. The lactate (lactic acid) is released into the blood. Under pathologic conditions that cause **hypoxia**, tissues may generate enough lactic acid to cause **lactic acidemia**.

In each cell, glycolysis is regulated to ensure that **ATP homeostasis** is maintained, without using more glucose than necessary. In most cell types, **hexokinase**, the first enzyme of glycolysis, is inhibited by glucose 6-P (see Fig. 22.1). Thus, glucose is not taken up and phosphorylated by a cell unless glucose 6-P enters a metabolic pathway, such as glycolysis or glycogen synthesis. The control of glucose 6-P entry into glycolysis occurs at phosphofructokinase-1 (**PFK-1**), the rate-limiting enzyme of the pathway. PFK-1 is **allosterically inhibited** by **ATP** and **allosterically activated** by adenosine monophosphate (**AMP**). AMP increases in the cytosol as ATP is hydrolyzed by energy-requiring reactions.

Glycolysis has functions in addition to ATP production. For example, in liver and adipose tissue, this pathway generates pyruvate as a precursor for **fatty acid biosynthesis**. Glycolysis also provides precursors for the synthesis of compounds such as amino acids and five-carbon sugar phosphates.

Although glucose is at the center of carbohydrate metabolism and is the major dietary sugar, other sugars in the diet are converted to intermediates of glucose metabolism, and their fates parallel that of glucose.

Fructose, the second most common sugar in the adult diet, is ingested principally as the monosaccharide or as part of **sucrose** (Fig. 22.3). It is metabolized principally in the liver (and to a lesser extent in the small intestine and kidney) by phosphorylation at the 1-position to form **fructose 1-phosphate** (fructose 1-P), followed by conversion to intermediates of the glycolytic pathway. The major products of its metabolism in liver are, therefore, the same as for glucose (including lactate, blood glucose, and glycogen). **Essential fructosuria (fructokinase deficiency)** and **hereditary fructose intolerance** (a deficiency of the fructose 1-P cleavage by **aldolase B**) are inherited disorders of fructose metabolism.

Fructose synthesis from glucose in the **polyol pathway** occurs in seminal vesicles and other tissues. **Aldose reductase** converts glucose to the sugar alcohol sorbitol (a polyol), which is then oxidized to fructose. In the lens of the eye, elevated levels of **sorbitol** in diabetes mellitus may contribute to formation of **cataracts**.

Galactose is ingested principally as **lactose**, which is converted to galactose and glucose in the intestine. **Galactose** is converted to glucose principally in the liver. It is phosphorylated to galactose 1-phosphate (galactose 1-P) by **galactokinase** and activated to a UDP-sugar by **galactosyl uridylyltransferase**. The metabolic pathway subsequently generates glucose 1-P. **Classical galactosemia**, a deficiency of galactosyl uridylyltransferase, results in the accumulation of galactose 1-P in the liver and the inhibition of hepatic glycogen metabolism and other pathways that require UDP sugars. Cataracts can occur from accumulation of galactose in the blood, which is converted to **galactitol** (the sugar alcohol of galactose) in the lens of the eye.

THE WAITING ROOM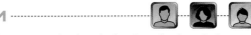

 Linda F. is a 68-year-old woman who is admitted to the hospital emergency department with very low blood pressure (80/40 mm Hg) caused by an acute hemorrhage from a previously diagnosed ulcer of the stomach. Linda's bleeding stomach ulcer has reduced her effective blood volume severely enough to compromise her ability to perfuse (deliver blood to) her tissues. She is also known to have chronic obstructive pulmonary disease (COPD) as a result of 42 years of smoking two packs of cigarettes per day. Her respiratory rate is rapid and labored, her skin is cold and clammy, and her lips are slightly blue (cyanotic). She appears anxious and moderately confused.

As appropriate emergency measures are taken to stabilize her and elevate her blood pressure, blood is sent for immediate blood typing and cross-matching, so that blood transfusions can be started. A battery of laboratory tests is ordered, including venous hemoglobin, hematocrit, and an arterial blood gas, which includes an arterial pH, partial pressures of oxygen (P_{O_2}) and carbon dioxide (P_{CO_2}), bicarbonate, and oxygen saturation. Results show that the hemorrhaging and COPD have resulted in hypoxemia, with decreased oxygen delivery to her tissues and both a respiratory and a metabolic acidosis.

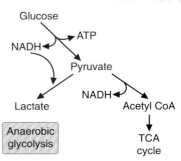

FIGURE 22.2 Anaerobic glycolysis (shown in *red*). The conversion of glucose to lactate generates 2 adenosine triphosphate (ATP) from substrate-level phosphorylation. Because there is no net generation of reduced nicotinamide adenine dinucleotide (NADH), there is no need for O_2, and thus, the pathway is anaerobic. *Acetyl CoA*, acetyl coenzyme A; *TCA*, tricarboxylic acid.

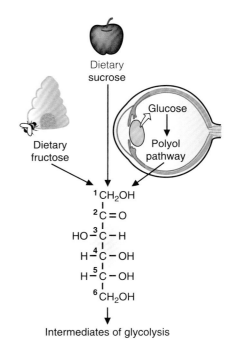

FIGURE 22.3 Fructose. The sugar fructose is found in the diet as the free sugar in foods such as honey or as a component of the disaccharide sucrose in fruits and sweets. It also can be synthesized from glucose via the polyol pathway. In the lens of the eye, the polyol pathway contributes to the formation of cataracts. Fructose is metabolized by conversion to intermediates of glycolysis.

The hematocrit (the percentage of the volume of blood occupied by packed red blood cells) and hemoglobin content (grams of hemoglobin in 100 mL of blood) are measured to determine whether the oxygen-carrying capacity of the blood is adequate. Both values can be decreased by conditions that interfere with erythropoiesis (the synthesis of red blood cells in bone marrow), such as iron deficiency. They also can be decreased during chronic bleeding as interstitial fluid replaces the lost blood volume and dilutes out the red blood cells but not during immediate acute hemorrhage. The P_{CO_2} and P_{O_2} are the partial pressures of CO_2 and O_2 in the blood. The P_{O_2} and oxygen saturation determine whether adequate oxygen is available for tissues. Measurement of the P_{CO_2} and bicarbonate can distinguish between a metabolic and a respiratory acidosis (see Chapter 4).

Otto S., a 26-year-old medical student, had gained weight during his first sedentary year in medical school. During his second year, he began watching his diet, jogging for an hour four times each week, and playing tennis twice a week. He has decided to compete in a 5-km race. To prepare for the race, he begins training with wind sprints—bouts of alternately running and walking.

Ivan A. is a 56-year-old morbidly obese accountant (see Chapters 1 through 3). He decided to see his dentist because he felt excruciating pain in his teeth when he ate ice cream. He really likes sweets and keeps hard candy in his pocket. The dentist noted from Mr. A.'s history that he had numerous cavities as a child in his baby teeth. At this visit, the dentist found cavities in two of Mr. A.'s teeth.

Candice S. is an 18-year-old girl who presented to her physician for a precollege physical examination. While taking her medical history, the doctor learned that she carefully avoided eating all fruits and any foods that contained table sugar. She related that from a very early age, she had learned that these foods caused severe weakness and symptoms suggestive of low blood sugar such as tremulousness and sweating. Her medical history also indicated that her mother had told her that once she started drinking and eating more than breast milk, she became an irritable baby who often cried incessantly, especially after meals, and vomited frequently. At these times, Candice's abdomen had become distended, and she became drowsy and apathetic. Her mother had intuitively eliminated certain foods from Candice's diet, after which the severity and frequency of these symptoms diminished.

Erin G. is the third child in her family, with a normal pregnancy and vaginal delivery at home like her older siblings. Her mother was unable to get to the initial pediatrician visit because she was busy with all her young children, but she noticed that Erin began vomiting 3 days after birth, usually within 30 minutes after breastfeeding. She finally brought Erin to the pediatrician at 3 weeks, when she noticed her child's eyes were yellow. She also reported that her abdomen became distended at these times and she became irritable and cried frequently. The doctor agreed that Erin was slightly jaundiced. He also noted an enlargement of her liver and questioned the possibility of early cataract formation in the lenses of Erin's eyes. He ordered liver and kidney function tests and did two separate dipstick urine tests in his office, one designed to measure only glucose in the urine and the other capable of detecting any of the reducing sugars.

I. Glycolysis

Glycolysis is one of the principal pathways for generating ATP in cells and is present in all cell types. The central role of glycolysis in fuel metabolism is related to its ability to generate ATP with, and without, oxygen. The oxidation of glucose to pyruvate generates ATP from *substrate-level phosphorylation* (the transfer of phosphate from high-energy intermediates of the pathway to ADP) and NADH. Subsequently, the pyruvate may be oxidized to CO_2 in the TCA cycle and ATP generated from electron transfer to oxygen in *oxidative phosphorylation* (see Chapter 23). However, if the pyruvate and NADH from glycolysis are converted to lactate (*anaerobic glycolysis*), ATP can be generated in the absence of oxygen, via substrate-level phosphorylation.

Glucose is readily available from our diet, internal glycogen stores, and the blood. Carbohydrate provides 50% or more of the calories in most diets, and glucose is the major carbohydrate. Other dietary sugars, such as fructose and galactose, are oxidized by conversion to intermediates of glycolysis. Glucose is stored in cells as glycogen, which can provide an internal source of fuel for glycolysis in emergency situations (e.g., decreased supply of fuels and oxygen during ischemia, caused by a reduced blood flow). Insulin and other hormones maintain blood glucose at a constant level (glucose homeostasis), thereby ensuring that glucose is always available to cells that depend on glycolysis for generation of ATP.

After a high-carbohydrate meal, glucose is the major fuel for almost all tissues. Exceptions include intestinal mucosal cells, which transport glucose from the gut into the blood, and cells in the proximal convoluted tubule of the kidney, which return glucose from the renal filtrate to the blood. During fasting, the brain continues to oxidize glucose because it has a limited capacity for the oxidation of fatty acids or other fuels. Cells also continue to use glucose for the portion of their ATP generation that must be met by anaerobic glycolysis because of either a limited oxygen supply or a limited capacity for oxidative phosphorylation (e.g., the red blood cell).

In addition to serving as an anaerobic and aerobic source of ATP, glycolysis is an anabolic pathway that provides biosynthetic precursors. For example, in liver and adipose tissue, this pathway generates pyruvate as a precursor for fatty acid biosynthesis. Glycolysis also provides precursors for the synthesis of compounds such as amino acids and of nucleotides. The integration of glycolysis with other anabolic pathways is discussed in Chapter 34.

A. The Reactions of Glycolysis

The glycolytic pathway, which cleaves 1 mol of glucose to 2 mol of the three-carbon compound pyruvate, consists of a preparative phase and an ATP-generating phase. In the initial *preparative phase* of glycolysis, glucose is phosphorylated twice by ATP to form fructose 1,6-bisphosphate (fructose 1,6-bisP) (Fig. 22.4). The ATP expenditure in the beginning of the preparative phase is sometimes called *priming the pump* because this initial use of 2 mol of ATP per mole of glucose results in the production of 4 mol of ATP per mole of glucose in the ATP-generating phase.

In the *ATP-generating phase*, fructose 1,6-bisP is split into two triose phosphates. Glyceraldehyde 3-phosphate (glyceraldehyde 3-P; a triose phosphate) is oxidized by NAD$^+$ and phosphorylated using inorganic phosphate (P$_i$). The high-energy phosphate bond generated in this step is transferred to ADP to form ATP. The remaining phosphate is also rearranged to form another high-energy phosphate bond that is transferred to ADP. Because 2 mol of triose phosphate were formed, the yield from the ATP-generating phase is 4 ATP and 2 NADH. The result is a net yield of 2 mol of ATP, 2 mol of NADH, and 2 mol of pyruvate per mole of glucose.

1. Conversion of Glucose to Glucose 6-Phosphate

Glucose metabolism begins with transfer of a phosphate from ATP to glucose to form glucose 6-P (Fig. 22.5). Phosphorylation of glucose commits it to metabolism within the cell because glucose 6-P cannot be transported back across the plasma membrane. The phosphorylation reaction is irreversible under physiologic conditions because the reaction has a high negative ΔG$^{0'}$. Phosphorylation does not, however, commit glucose to glycolysis.

Glucose 6-P is a branch point in carbohydrate metabolism. It is a precursor for almost every pathway that uses glucose, including glycolysis, the pentose phosphate pathway (see Chapter 27), and glycogen synthesis (see Chapter 26). From the opposite point of view, it also can be generated from other pathways of carbohydrate metabolism, such as glycogenolysis (breakdown of glycogen), the pentose phosphate pathway, and gluconeogenesis (the synthesis of glucose from noncarbohydrate sources).

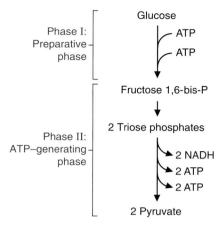

FIGURE 22.4 Phases of the glycolytic pathway. *ATP*, adenosine triphosphate; *Fructose-1,6-bis P*, fructose 1,6-bisphosphate; *NADH*, reduced nicotinamide adenine dinucleotide.

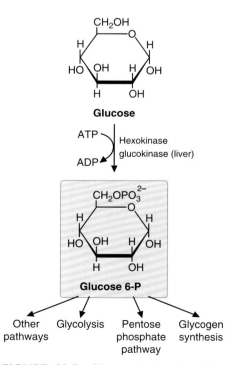

FIGURE 22.5 Glucose 6-phosphate (glucose 6-P) metabolism. *ADP*, adenosine diphosphate; *ATP*, adenosine triphosphate.

Hexokinases, the enzymes that catalyze the phosphorylation of glucose, are a family of tissue-specific isoenzymes that differ in their kinetic properties. The isoenzyme found in liver and β-cells of the pancreas has a much higher K_m than other hexokinases and is called *glucokinase*. In many cells, some of the hexokinase is bound to porins in the outer mitochondrial membrane (voltage-dependent anion channels; see Chapter 24), which gives these enzymes first access to newly synthesized ATP as it exits the mitochondria.

2. Conversion of Glucose 6-Phosphate to the Triose Phosphates

In the remainder of the preparative phase of glycolysis, glucose 6-P is isomerized to fructose 6-phosphate (fructose 6-P), again phosphorylated, and subsequently cleaved into two three-carbon fragments (Fig. 22.6). The isomerization, which positions a keto group next to carbon 3, is essential for the subsequent cleavage of the bond between carbons 3 and 4.

The next step of glycolysis, phosphorylation of fructose 6-P to fructose 1,6-bisP by PFK-1, is generally considered the first committed step of the pathway. This phosphorylation requires ATP and is thermodynamically and kinetically irreversible. Therefore, PFK-1 irrevocably commits glucose to the glycolytic pathway. PFK-1 is a regulated enzyme in cells, and its regulation controls the entry of glucose into glycolysis. Like hexokinase, it exists as tissue-specific isoenzymes whose regulatory properties match variations in the role of glycolysis in different tissues.

Fructose 1,6-bisP is cleaved into two phosphorylated three-carbon compounds (triose phosphates) by aldolase (see Fig. 22.6). Dihydroxyacetone phosphate (DHAP) and glyceraldehyde 3-P are the products. DHAP is isomerized to glyceraldehyde 3-P by triose phosphate isomerase. *Aldolase* is named for the mechanism of the forward reaction, which is an aldol cleavage, and the mechanism of the reverse reaction, which is an aldol condensation. The enzyme exists as tissue-specific isoenzymes, which all catalyze the cleavage of fructose 1,6-bisP but differ in their specificities for fructose 1-P. The enzyme uses a lysine residue at the active site to form a covalent bond with the substrate during the course of the reaction. Inability to form this covalent linkage inactivates the enzyme.

Thus, at this point in glycolysis, for every mole of glucose that enters the pathway, 2 mol of glyceraldehyde 3-P are produced and continue through the pathway.

3. Oxidation and Substrate-Level Phosphorylation

In the next part of the glycolytic pathway, glyceraldehyde 3-P is oxidized and phosphorylated so that subsequent intermediates of glycolysis can donate phosphate to ADP to generate ATP. The first reaction in this sequence, catalyzed by glyceraldehyde-3-P dehydrogenase, is really the key to the pathway (see Fig. 22.6). This enzyme oxidizes the aldehyde group of glyceraldehyde 3-P to an enzyme-bound carboxyl group and transfers the electrons to NAD^+ to form NADH. The oxidation step is dependent on a cysteine residue at the active site of the enzyme, which forms a high-energy thioester bond during the course of the reaction. The high-energy intermediate immediately accepts a P_i to form the high-energy acyl phosphate bond in 1,3-bisphosphoglycerate (1,3-BPG), releasing the product from the cysteine residue on the enzyme. This high-energy phosphate bond is the start of *substrate-level phosphorylation* (the formation of a high-energy phosphate bond where none previously existed, without the use of oxygen).

In the next reaction, the phosphate in this bond is transferred to ADP to form ATP by 3-phosphoglycerate kinase. The energy of the acyl phosphate bond is high enough (~10 kcal/mol) so that transfer to ADP is an energetically favorable process. 3-Phosphoglycerate is also a product of this reaction.

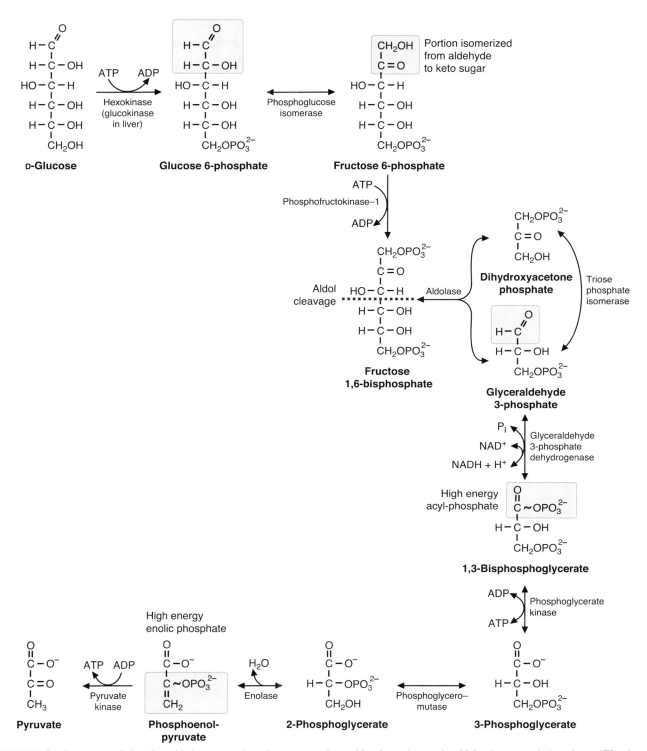

FIGURE 22.6 Reactions of glycolysis. High-energy phosphates are indicated by the *red squiggles*. *ADP*, adenosine diphosphate; *ATP*, adenosine triphosphate; *NAD*⁺, nicotinamide adenine dinucleotide; *P*ᵢ, inorganic phosphate.

To transfer the remaining low-energy phosphoester on 3-phosphoglycerate to ADP, it must be converted into a high-energy bond. This conversion is accomplished by moving the phosphate to the second carbon (forming 2-phosphoglycerate) and then removing water to form phosphoenolpyruvate (PEP). The enolphosphate bond is a high-energy bond (its hydrolysis releases ~14 kcal/mol of energy), so the transfer of phosphate to ADP by pyruvate kinase is energetically favorable (see Fig. 22.6) and not reversible. This final reaction converts PEP to pyruvate.

4. Summary of the Glycolytic Pathway

The overall net reaction in the glycolytic pathway is

$$\text{Glucose} + 2\,NAD^+ + 2\,P_i + 2\,ADP \rightarrow 2\,\text{pyruvate} + 2\,NADH + 4\,H^+ + 2\,ATP + 2\,H_2O$$

The pathway occurs with an overall negative $\Delta G^{0'}$ of approximately -22 kcal/mol. Therefore, it cannot be reversed without the expenditure of energy.

B. Fructose

Fructose is found in the diet as a component of sucrose in fruit, as a free sugar in honey, and in high-fructose corn syrup (see Fig. 22.3). Fructose enters epithelial cells and other types of cells by facilitated diffusion on the GLUT 5 transporter. It is metabolized to intermediates of glycolysis. Problems with fructose absorption and metabolism are relatively more common than with other sugars.

1. Fructose Metabolism

Fructose is metabolized by conversion to glyceraldehyde 3-P and DHAP, which are intermediates of glycolysis (Fig. 22.7). The steps parallel those of glycolysis. The first step in the metabolism of fructose, as with glucose, is phosphorylation. Fructokinase, the major kinase involved, phosphorylates fructose at the 1-position. Fructokinase has a high V_{max} and rapidly phosphorylates fructose as it enters the cell. The fructose 1-P formed is not an intermediate of glycolysis but rather is cleaved by aldolase B to DHAP (an intermediate of glycolysis)

 When individuals with defects of aldolase B ingest fructose, the extremely high levels of fructose 1-P that accumulate in the liver and kidney cause several adverse effects. Hypoglycemia results from inhibition of glycogenolysis and gluconeogenesis. Glycogen phosphorylase (and possibly phosphoglucomutase and other enzymes of glycogen metabolism) are inhibited by the accumulated fructose 1-P. Aldolase B is required for glucose synthesis from glyceraldehyde 3-P and DHAP, and its low activity in aldolase B–deficient individuals is further decreased by the accumulated fructose 1-P. The inhibition of gluconeogenesis results in lactic acidosis.

The accumulation of fructose 1-P also substantially depletes the intracellular phosphate pools. The fructokinase reaction uses ATP at a rapid rate such that the mitochondria regenerate ATP rapidly, which leads to a drop in free phosphate levels. The low levels of phosphate release inhibition of AMP deaminase, which converts AMP to inosine monophosphate (IMP). The nitrogenous base of IMP (hypoxanthine) is degraded to uric acid. The lack of phosphate and depletion of adenine nucleotides lead to a loss of ATP, further contributing to the inhibition of biosynthetic pathways, including gluconeogenesis.

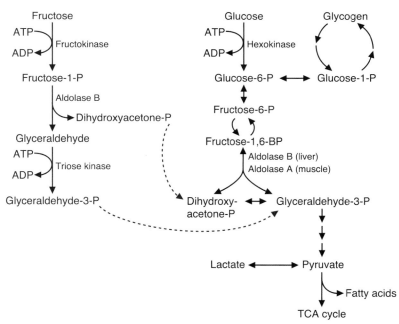

FIGURE 22.7 Fructose metabolism. The pathway for the conversion of fructose to dihydroxyacetone phosphate (dihydroxyacetone-P) and glyceraldehyde 3-phosphate (glyceraldehyde-3-P) is shown in *red*. These two compounds are intermediates of glycolysis and are converted in the liver principally to glucose, glycogen, or fatty acids. In the liver, aldolase B cleaves both fructose 1-phosphate (fructose-1-P) in the pathway for fructose metabolism, and fructose 1,6-bisphosphate (fructose-1,6-BP) in the pathway for glycolysis. *ADP*, adenosine diphosphate; *ATP*, adenosine triphosphate; *Fructose-6-P*, fructose 6-phosphate; *Glucose-1-P*, glucose 1-phosphate; *Glucose-6-P*, glucose 6-phosphate; *TCA*, tricarboxylic acid.

and glyceraldehyde. Glyceraldehyde is then phosphorylated to glyceraldehyde 3-P by triose kinase. DHAP and glyceraldehyde 3-P are intermediates of the glycolytic pathway and can proceed through it to pyruvate, the TCA cycle, and fatty acid synthesis. Alternatively, these intermediates can also be converted to glucose by gluconeogenesis. In other words, the fate of fructose parallels that of glucose.

The metabolism of fructose occurs principally in the liver, and to a lesser extent in the small intestinal mucosa and proximal epithelium of the renal tubule, because these tissues have both fructokinase and aldolase B. Aldolase exists as several isoforms: aldolases A, B, and C and fetal aldolase. Although all of these aldolase isoforms can cleave fructose 1,6-bisP, the intermediate of glycolysis, only aldolase B can also cleave fructose 1-P. Aldolase A, present in muscle and most other tissues, and aldolase C, present in brain, have almost no ability to cleave fructose 1-P. Fetal aldolase, present in the liver before birth, is similar to aldolase C.

Aldolase B is the rate-limiting enzyme of fructose metabolism, although it is not a rate-limiting enzyme of glycolysis. It has a much lower affinity for fructose 1-P than fructose 1,6-bisP and is very slow at physiologic levels of fructose 1-P. As a consequence, after ingesting a high dose of fructose, normal individuals accumulate fructose 1-P in the liver while it is slowly converted to glycolytic intermediates. Individuals with hereditary fructose intolerance (a deficiency of aldolase B) accumulate much higher amounts of fructose 1-P in their livers.

Other tissues also have the capacity to metabolize fructose but do so much more slowly. The hexokinase isoforms present in muscle, adipose tissue, and other tissues can convert fructose to fructose 6-P but react much more efficiently with glucose. As a result, fructose phosphorylation is very slow in the presence of physiologic levels of intracellular glucose and glucose 6-P.

2. Synthesis of Fructose in the Polyol Pathway

Fructose can be synthesized from glucose in the *polyol pathway*. The polyol pathway is named for the first step of the pathway, in which sugars are reduced to the sugar alcohol by the enzyme aldose reductase (Fig. 22.8). Glucose is reduced to the sugar alcohol sorbitol, and sorbitol is then oxidized to fructose. This pathway is present in seminal vesicles, which synthesize fructose for the seminal fluid. Spermatozoa use fructose as a major fuel source while in the seminal fluid and then switch to glucose once in the female reproductive tract. Use of fructose is thought to prevent acrosomal breakdown of the plasma membrane (and consequent activation) while the spermatozoa are still in the seminal fluid.

The polyol pathway is present in many tissues, but its function in all tissues is not understood. Aldose reductase is relatively nonspecific, and its major function may be the metabolism of an aldehyde sugar other than glucose. The activity of this enzyme can lead to major problems in the lens of the eye where it is responsible for the production of sorbitol from glucose and galactitol from galactose. When the concentration of glucose or galactose is elevated in the blood, their respective sugar alcohols are synthesized in the lens more rapidly than they are removed, resulting in increased osmotic pressure within the lens.

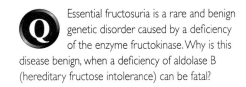

Essential fructosuria is a rare and benign genetic disorder caused by a deficiency of the enzyme fructokinase. Why is this disease benign, when a deficiency of aldolase B (hereditary fructose intolerance) can be fatal?

The accumulation of sorbitol in muscle and nerve tissues may contribute to the peripheral neuropathy characteristic of patients with poorly controlled diabetes mellitus. This is one of the many reasons it is so important for **Dianne A.** (who has type 1 diabetes mellitus) and **Deborah S.** (who has type 2 diabetes mellitus) to achieve good glycemic control.

The accumulation of sugars and sugar alcohols in the lens of patients with hyperglycemia (e.g., diabetes mellitus) results in the formation of cataracts. Glucose levels are elevated and increase the synthesis of sorbitol and fructose. As a consequence, a high osmotic pressure is created in the lens. The high glucose and fructose levels also result in nonenzymatic glycosylation of lens proteins. The result of the increased osmotic pressure and the glycosylation of the lens protein is an opaque cloudiness of the lens known as a *cataract*. **Erin G.** seemed to have an early cataract, probably caused by the accumulation of galactose and its sugar alcohol galactitol.

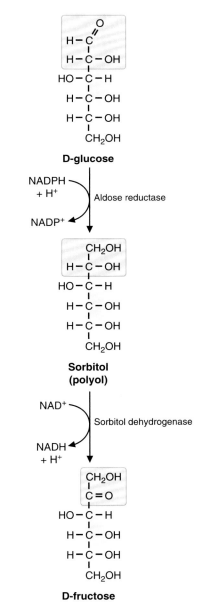

FIGURE 22.8 The polyol pathway converts glucose to fructose. NAD^+, nicotinamide adenine dinucleotide.

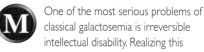

In essential fructosuria, fructose cannot be converted to fructose 1-P. This condition is benign because no toxic metabolites of fructose accumulate in the liver, and the patient remains nearly asymptomatic. Some of the ingested fructose is slowly phosphorylated by hexokinase in nonhepatic tissues and metabolized by glycolysis, and some appears in the urine. There is no renal threshold for fructose; the appearance of fructose in the urine (fructosuria) does not require a high fructose concentration in the blood.

Hereditary fructose intolerance, conversely, results in the accumulation of fructose 1-P and fructose. By inhibiting glycogenolysis and gluconeogenesis, the high levels of fructose 1-P caused the hypoglycemia that **Candice S.** experienced as an infant when she became apathetic and drowsy, and as an adult when she experienced sweating and tremulousness.

C. Galactose Metabolism: Conversion to Glucose 1-Phosphate

Dietary galactose is metabolized principally by phosphorylation to galactose 1-P and then conversion to UDP-galactose and glucose 1-P (Fig. 22.9). The phosphorylation of galactose, again an important first step in the pathway, is carried out by a specific kinase, galactokinase. The formation of UDP-galactose is accomplished by attack of the phosphate oxygen on galactose 1-P on the α-phosphate of UDP-glucose, releasing glucose 1-P while forming UDP-galactose. The enzyme that catalyzes this reaction is galactose 1-P uridylyltransferase. The UDP-galactose is then converted to UDP-glucose by the reversible UDP-glucose epimerase (the configuration of the hydroxyl group on carbon 4 is reversed in this reaction). The net result of this sequence of reactions is that galactose is converted to glucose 1-P, at the expense of one high-energy bond of ATP. The sum of these reactions is indicated in the following equations:

$$(1)\ \text{Galactose} + \text{ATP} \xrightarrow{\text{Galactokinase}} \text{galactose 1-P} + \text{ADP}$$

$$(2)\ \text{Galactose 1-P} + \text{UDP-glucose} \xrightarrow[\text{Uridylyltransferase}]{\text{Galactose1-P}} \text{UDP-galactose} + \text{glucose 1-P}$$

$$(3)\ \text{UDP-galactose} \xrightarrow{\text{UDP-glucose epimerase}} \text{UDP-glucose}$$

$$\text{Net equation: Galactose} + \text{ATP} \rightarrow \text{Glucose 1-P} + \text{ADP}$$

The enzymes for galactose conversion to glucose 1-P are present in many tissues, including the adult erythrocyte, fibroblasts, and fetal tissues. The liver has high activity of these enzymes and can convert dietary galactose to blood glucose and glycogen. The fate of dietary galactose, like that of fructose, therefore, parallels that of glucose. The ability to metabolize galactose is even greater in infants than in adults. Newborn infants ingest up to 1 g of galactose per kilogram per feeding (as lactose). Yet, the rate of metabolism is so high that the blood level in the systemic circulation is <3 mg/dL, and none of the galactose is lost in the urine.

One of the most serious problems of classical galactosemia is irreversible intellectual disability. Realizing this problem, **Erin G.'s** physician wanted to begin immediate dietary therapy. A test that measures galactose-1-P uridylyltransferase in erythrocytes was ordered. This test is an enzymatic assay that mixes the unknown sample (in this case, a lysate from red blood cells, which contain the enzyme) with galactose 1-P, UDP-glucose, and NADP$^+$ in the presence of excess phosphoglucomutase and glucose-6-P dehydrogenase. As the uridylyltransferase converts galactose 1-P to UDP-galactose and glucose 1-phosphate (glucose 1-P), the glucose 1-P is rapidly converted to glucose 6-P by phosphoglucomutase. The glucose 6-P is then converted to 6-phosphogluconate and NADPH by glucose-6-P dehydrogenase. The resulting increase in absorbance at 340 nm allows a determination of the initial uridylyltransferase activity. The enzyme activity in **Erin G.'s** red blood cells was virtually absent, confirming the diagnosis of classical galactosemia.

Erin G.'s urine was negative for glucose when measured with the glucose oxidase strip but was positive for the presence of a reducing sugar. The reducing sugar was identified as galactose. Her liver function tests showed an increase in serum bilirubin and in several liver enzymes. Albumin was present in her urine. These findings and the clinical history increased her physician's suspicion that Erin had classical galactosemia.

Classical galactosemia is caused by a deficiency of galactose-1-P uridylyltransferase. In this disease, galactose 1-P accumulates in tissues, and galactose is elevated in the blood and urine. This condition differs from the rarer deficiency of galactokinase (nonclassical galactosemia), in which galactosemia and galactosuria occur but galactose 1-P is not formed. Both enzyme defects result in cataracts from galactitol formation by aldose reductase in the polyol pathway. Aldose reductase has a relatively high K_m for galactose, approximately 12 to 20 mM, so galactitol is formed only in galactosemic patients who have eaten galactose. Galactitol is not further metabolized and diffuses out of the lens very slowly. Thus, hypergalactosemia is even more likely to cause cataracts than hyperglycemia. **Erin G.**, although she is only 3 weeks old, appeared to have early cataracts forming in the lenses of her eyes.

One of the most serious problems of classical galactosemia is an irreversible intellectual disability. Realizing the problem, Erin G.'s physician wanted to begin immediate dietary therapy. A test that measures galactose 1-P uridylyltransferase activity in erythrocytes was ordered. The enzyme activity was virtually absent, confirming the diagnosis of classical galactosemia.

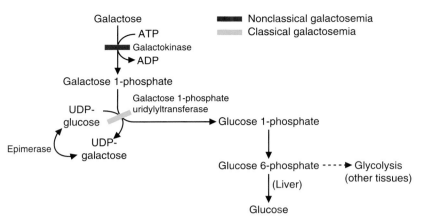

FIGURE 22.9 Metabolism of galactose. Galactose is phosphorylated to galactose 1-phosphate (galactose 1-P) by galactokinase. Galactose 1-P reacts with uridine diphosphate (UDP)-glucose to release glucose 1-phosphate (glucose 1-P). Galactose thus can be converted to blood glucose, enter glycolysis, or enter any of the metabolic routes of glucose. In classical galactosemia, a deficiency of galactose-1-P uridylyltransferase (shown in *green*) results in the accumulation of galactose 1-P in tissues and the appearance of galactose in the blood and urine. In nonclassical galactosemia, a deficiency of galactokinase (shown in *red*) results in the accumulation of galactose. *ADP*, adenosine diphosphate; *ATP*, adenosine triphosphate.

D. Oxidative Fates of Pyruvate and NADH

The NADH produced from glycolysis must be continuously reoxidized back to NAD^+ to provide an electron acceptor for the glyceraldehyde-3-P dehydrogenase reaction and prevent product inhibition. Without oxidation of this NADH, glycolysis cannot continue. There are two alternate routes for oxidation of cytosolic NADH (Fig. 22.10). One route is aerobic, involving shuttles that transfer reducing equivalents across the mitochondrial membrane (see Chapter 23 for details of the shuttle systems) and ultimately to the ETC and oxygen (see Fig. 22.10A). The other route is anaerobic (without the use of oxygen). In anaerobic glycolysis, NADH is reoxidized in the cytosol by LDH, which reduces pyruvate to lactate (see Fig. 22.10B).

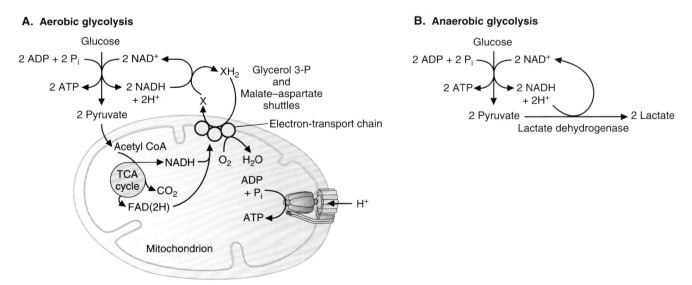

FIGURE 22.10 Alternate fates of pyruvate. **A.** The pyruvate produced by glycolysis enters mitochondria and is oxidized to CO_2 and H_2O. The reducing equivalents in nicotinamide adenine dinucleotide (NADH) enter mitochondria via a shuttle system. **B.** Pyruvate is reduced to lactate in the cytosol, thereby using the reducing equivalents in NADH. *Acetyl CoA*, acetyl coenzyme A; *ADP*, adenosine diphosphate; *ATP*, adenosine triphosphate; *FAD(2H)*, reduced flavin adenine dinucleotide; *Glycerol 3-P*, glycerol 3-phosphate; *P_i*, inorganic phosphate; *TCA*, tricarboxylic acid.

The confusion experienced by **Linda F.** in the emergency department is caused by an inadequate delivery of oxygen to the brain. Neurons have very high ATP requirements, and most of this ATP is provided by aerobic oxidation of glucose to pyruvate in glycolysis and by pyruvate oxidation to CO_2 in the TCA cycle. The brain has little or no capacity to oxidize fatty acids, so its glucose consumption is high (~125 to 150 g/day in the adult). Its oxygen demands are also high. If cerebral oxygen supply were completely interrupted, the brain would last only 10 seconds. The only reason that consciousness lasts longer during anoxia or asphyxia is that there is still some oxygen in the lungs and in circulating blood. A decrease of blood flow to approximately one-half of the normal rate results in a loss of consciousness.

Glycolysis

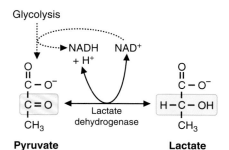

FIGURE 22.11 Lactate dehydrogenase reaction. Pyruvate, which may be produced by glycolysis, is reduced to lactate. The reaction, which occurs in the cytosol, requires reduced nicotinamide adenine dinucleotide (NADH) and is catalyzed by lactate dehydrogenase. This reaction is readily reversible.

The dental caries in **Ivan A.'s** mouth were caused principally by the low pH generated from lactic acid production by oral bacteria. Below a pH of 5.5, decalcification of tooth enamel and dentine occurs. Lactobacilli and *Streptococcus mutans* are major contributors to this process because almost all of their energy is derived from the conversion of glucose or fructose to lactic acid, and they are able to grow well at the low pH generated by this process. Mr. A.'s dentist explained that bacteria in his dental plaque could convert all the sugar in his candy into acid in <20 minutes. The acid is buffered by bicarbonate and other buffers in saliva, but saliva production decreases in the evening. Thus, the acid could dissolve the hydroxyapatite in his tooth enamel during the night.

The fate of pyruvate depends on the route used for NADH oxidation. If NADH is reoxidized in a shuttle system, pyruvate can be used for other pathways, one of which is oxidation to acetyl coenzyme A and entry into the TCA cycle for complete oxidation. Alternatively, in anaerobic glycolysis, pyruvate is reduced to lactate and diverted away from other potential pathways. Thus, the use of the shuttle systems allows for more ATP to be generated than by anaerobic glycolysis, by both oxidizing the cytoplasmically derived NADH in the ETC and by allowing pyruvate to be oxidized completely to CO_2.

The reason that shuttles are required for the oxidation of cytosolic NADH by the ETC is that the inner mitochondrial membrane is impermeable to NADH, and no transport protein exists that can translocate NADH across this membrane directly.

E. Anaerobic Glycolysis

When the oxidative capacity of a cell is limited (e.g., such as in the red blood cell, which has no mitochondria), the pyruvate and NADH produced from glycolysis cannot be oxidized aerobically. The NADH is, therefore, oxidized to NAD^+ in the cytosol by reduction of pyruvate to lactate. This reaction is catalyzed by LDH (Fig. 22.11). The net reaction for anaerobic glycolysis is

$$\text{Glucose} + 2\,\text{ADP} + 2\,\text{P}_i \rightarrow 2\,\text{lactate} + 2\,\text{ATP} + 2\,\text{H}_2\text{O} + 2\,\text{H}^+$$

1. Acid Production in Anaerobic Glycolysis

Anaerobic glycolysis results in acid production in the form of H^+. Glycolysis forms pyruvic acid, which is reduced to *lactic acid*. At an intracellular pH of 7.35, lactic acid dissociates to form the carboxylate anion *lactate* and H^+ (the pK_a for lactic acid is 3.85). Lactate and the H^+ are both transported out of the cell into interstitial fluid by a transporter on the plasma membrane and eventually diffuse into the blood. If the amount of lactate generated exceeds the buffering capacity of the blood, the pH drops below the normal range, resulting in lactic acidosis (see Chapter 4).

2. Tissues Dependent on Anaerobic Glycolysis

Many tissues, including red and white blood cells, the kidney medulla, the tissues of the eye, and skeletal muscles, rely on anaerobic glycolysis for at least a portion of their ATP requirements (Table 22.1). Tissues (or cells) that are heavily dependent on anaerobic glycolysis usually have a low ATP demand, high levels of glycolytic enzymes, and few capillaries, such that oxygen must diffuse over a greater distance to reach target cells. The lack of mitochondria, or the increased rate of glycolysis, is often related to some aspect of cell function. For example, the mature red blood cell has no mitochondria because oxidative metabolism might interfere with its function

TABLE 22.1 Major Tissue Sites of Lactate Production in a Resting Man (an Average 70-kg Man Consumes about 300 g of Carbohydrate per Day)	
DAILY LACTATE PRODUCTION (g/day)	
Total lactate production	115
Red blood cells	29
Skin	20
Brain	17
Skeletal muscle	16
Renal medulla	15
Intestinal mucosa	8
Other tissues	10

in transporting oxygen bound to hemoglobin. Some of the lactic acid generated by anaerobic glycolysis in skin is secreted in sweat, where it acts as an antibacterial agent. Many large tumors use anaerobic glycolysis for ATP production and lack capillaries in their core.

In tissues with some mitochondria, both aerobic and anaerobic glycolysis occur simultaneously. The relative proportion of the two pathways depends on the mitochondrial oxidative capacity of the tissue and its oxygen supply and may vary among cell types within the same tissue because of cell distance from the capillaries. When a cell's energy demand exceeds the capacity of the rate of the ETC and oxidative phosphorylation to produce ATP, glycolysis is activated, and the increased NADH/NAD$^+$ ratio will direct excess pyruvate into lactate. Because under these conditions PDH, the TCA cycle, and the ETC are operating as fast as they can, anaerobic glycolysis is meeting the need for additional ATP.

3. Fate of Lactate

Lactate released from cells undergoing anaerobic glycolysis is taken up by other tissues (primarily the liver, heart, and skeletal muscle) and oxidized back to pyruvate. In the liver, the pyruvate is used to synthesize glucose (gluconeogenesis), which is returned to the blood. The cycling of lactate and glucose between peripheral tissues and liver is called the *Cori cycle* (Fig. 22.12).

In many other tissues, lactate is oxidized to pyruvate, which is then oxidized to CO$_2$ in the TCA cycle. Although the equilibrium of the LDH reaction favors lactate production, flux occurs in the opposite direction if NADH is being rapidly oxidized in the ETC (or is being used for gluconeogenesis):

$$\text{Lactate} + \text{NAD}^+ \rightarrow \text{pyruvate} + \text{NADH} + \text{H}^+$$

The heart, with its huge mitochondrial content and oxidative capacity, is able to use lactate released from other tissues as a fuel. During exercise such as bicycle riding, lactate released into the blood from skeletal muscles in the leg might be used by resting skeletal muscles in the arm. In the brain, glial cells and astrocytes produce lactate, which is used by neurons or released into the blood.

LDH is a tetramer composed of A subunits (also called *M subunits*, for skeletal muscle form) and B subunits (also called *H subunits*, for heart). Different tissues produce different amounts of the two subunits, which then combine randomly to form five different tetramers (M4, M3H1, M2H2, M1H3, and H4). These isoenzymes differ only slightly in their properties, but the kinetic properties of the M4 form facilitate conversion of pyruvate to lactate in skeletal muscle, whereas the H4 form facilitates conversion of lactate to pyruvate in the heart for energy generation.

 In response to the hypoxemia caused by **Linda F.'s** COPD, she has increased levels of hypoxia-inducible factor-1 (HIF-1) in her tissues. HIF-1 is a gene transcription factor found in tissues throughout the body (including brain, heart, kidney, lung, liver, pancreas, skeletal muscle, and white blood cells) which plays a homeostatic role in coordinating tissue responses to hypoxia. Each tissue will respond with a subset of the following changes. HIF-1 increases transcription of the genes for many of the glycolytic enzymes, including PFK-1, enolase, phosphoglycerate kinase, and LDH. HIF-1 also increases synthesis of several proteins that enhance oxygen delivery to tissues, including erythropoietin, which increases the generation of red blood cells in bone marrow; vascular endothelial growth factor, which regulates angiogenesis (formation of blood vessels); and inducible nitric oxide synthase, which synthesizes nitric oxide, a vasodilator. As a consequence, Ms. F. was able to maintain hematocrit and hemoglobin levels that were on the high side of the normal range, and her tissues had an increased capacity for anaerobic glycolysis.

 The tissues of the eye are also partially dependent on anaerobic glycolysis.

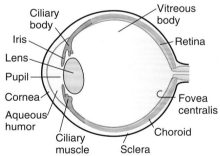

The eye contains cells that transmit or focus light, and these cells, therefore, cannot be filled with opaque structures such as mitochondria or densely packed capillary beds. The corneal epithelium generates most of its ATP aerobically from its few mitochondria but still metabolizes some glucose anaerobically. Oxygen is supplied by diffusion from the air. The lens of the eye is composed of fibers that must remain birefringent to transmit and focus light, so mitochondria are nearly absent. The small amount of ATP required (principally for ion balance) can readily be generated from anaerobic glycolysis even though the energy yield is low. The lens is able to pick up glucose and release lactate into the vitreous body and aqueous humor. It does not need oxygen and has no use for capillaries.

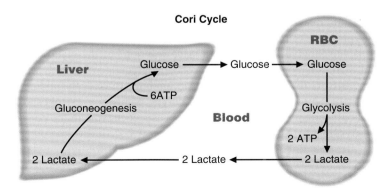

FIGURE 22.12 The Cori cycle. Glucose, produced in the liver by gluconeogenesis, is converted by glycolysis in muscle, red blood cells (RBC), and many other cells, to lactate. Lactate returns to the liver and is reconverted to glucose by gluconeogenesis. *ATP*, adenosine triphosphate.

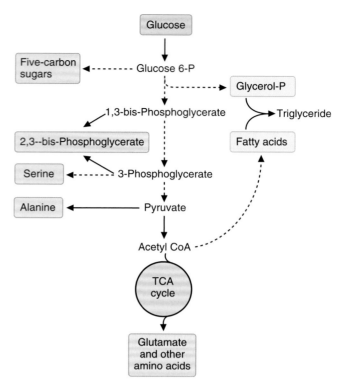

FIGURE 22.13 Biosynthetic functions of glycolysis. Compounds formed from intermediates of glycolysis are shown in the *boxes*. These pathways are discussed in later chapters. *Dotted lines* indicate that more than one step is required for the conversion shown in the figure. *Acetyl CoA*, acetyl coenzyme A; *Glucose 6-P*, glucose 6-phosphate; *Glycerol-P*, glycerol phosphate; *TCA*, tricarboxylic acid.

II. Other Functions of Glycolysis

Glycolysis, in addition to providing ATP, generates precursors for biosynthetic pathways (Fig. 22.13). Intermediates of the pathway can be converted to ribose 5-phosphate, the sugar incorporated into nucleotides such as ATP. Other sugars, such as UDP-glucose, mannose, and sialic acid, are also formed from intermediates of glycolysis. Serine is synthesized from 3-phosphoglycerate, and alanine from pyruvate. The backbone of triacylglycerols, glycerol 3-P, is derived from DHAP in the glycolytic pathway.

The liver is the major site of biosynthetic reactions in the body. In addition to those pathways mentioned previously, the liver synthesizes fatty acids from the pyruvate generated by glycolysis. It also synthesizes glucose from lactate, glycerol 3-P, and amino acids in the gluconeogenic pathway, which is basically a reversal of glycolysis. Consequently, in liver, many of the glycolytic enzymes exist as isoenzymes with properties suited for these functions.

The bisphosphoglycerate shunt is a "side reaction" of the glycolytic pathway in which 1,3-BPG is converted to 2,3-bisphosphoglycerate (2,3-BPG). Red blood cells form 2,3-BPG to serve as an allosteric inhibitor of oxygen binding to heme (see Chapter 42). 2,3-BPG reenters the glycolytic pathway via dephosphorylation to 3-phosphoglycerate. 2,3-BPG also functions as a coenzyme in the conversion of 3-phosphoglycerate to 2-phosphoglycerate by the glycolytic enzyme phosphoglyceromutase. Because 2,3-BPG is not depleted by its role in this catalytic process, most cells need only very small amounts.

III. Regulation of Glycolysis by the Need for Adenosine Triphosphate

The principles of pathway regulation are summarized in Table 22.2. In pathways that are subject to feedback regulation, the first step of the pathway must be

TABLE 22.2   **Generalizations on the Regulation of Metabolic Pathways**
1. Regulation matches function. The type of regulation use depends on the function of the pathway. Tissue-specific isozymes may allow the features of regulatory enzymes to match somewhat different functions of the pathway in different tissues.
2. Regulation of metabolic pathways occurs at rate-limiting steps—the slowest steps—in the pathway. These are reactions in which a small change of rate will affect the flux through the whole pathway.
3. Regulation usually occurs at the first committed step of a pathway or at metabolic branch points. In human cells, most pathways are interconnected with other pathways and have regulatory enzymes for every branch point.
4. Regulatory enzymes often catalyze physiologically irreversible reactions. These are also the steps that differ in biosynthetic and degradative pathways.
5. Many pathways have feedback regulation; that is, the end product of the pathway controls the rate of its own synthesis. Feedback regulation may involve inhibition of an early step in the pathway (feedback inhibition) or regulation of gene transcription.
6. Human cells use compartmentation to control access of substrate and activators or inhibitors to different enzymes.
7. Hormonal regulation integrates responses in pathways requiring more than one tissue. Hormones generally regulate fuel metabolism by a. Changing the phosphorylation state of enzymes b. Changing the amount of enzyme present by changing its rate of synthesis (often induction or repression of mRNA synthesis) or degradation c. Changing the concentration of an activator or inhibitor

regulated so that precursors flow into alternative pathways if product is not needed. Another generalization concerning regulation of metabolic pathways is that it occurs at the enzyme that catalyzes the rate-limiting (slowest) step in a pathway (see Table 22.2).

One of the major functions of glycolysis is the generation of ATP, so the pathway is regulated to maintain ATP homeostasis in all cells. PFK-1 and PDH (see Chapter 23), which links glycolysis and the TCA cycle, are both major regulatory sites that respond to feedback indicators of the rate of ATP use (Fig. 22.14). The supply of glucose 6-P for glycolysis is tissue-dependent and can be regulated at the steps of glucose transport into cells, glycogenolysis (the degradation of glycogen to form glucose), or the rate of glucose phosphorylation by hexokinase isoenzymes. Other regulatory mechanisms integrate the ATP-generating role of glycolysis with its anabolic roles.

All of the regulatory enzymes of glycolysis exist as tissue-specific isoenzymes, which alter the regulation of the pathway to match variations in conditions and needs in different tissues. For example, in the liver, an isoenzyme of pyruvate kinase introduces an additional regulatory site in glycolysis that contributes to the inhibition of glycolysis when the reverse pathway, gluconeogenesis, is activated.

A. Relationships among ATP, ADP, and AMP Concentrations

The AMP levels within the cytosol provide a better indicator of the rate of ATP use than the ATP concentration itself (Fig. 22.15). The concentration of AMP in the cytosol is determined by the equilibrium position of the adenylate kinase reaction, which catalyzes the following reaction:

$$2\,ADP \leftrightarrow AMP + ATP$$

The equilibrium is such that hydrolysis of ATP to ADP in energy-requiring reactions increases both the ADP and AMP contents of the cytosol. However, ATP is present in much higher quantities than AMP or ADP, so a small decrease of ATP concentration in the cytosol causes a much larger percentage increase in the small AMP pool. In skeletal muscles, for instance, ATP levels are approximately 5 mM and decrease by no more than 20% during strenuous exercise (see Fig. 22.15). At the same time, ADP levels may increase by 50%, and AMP levels, which are in the micromolar range, may increase by 300%. AMP activates several metabolic pathways, including glycolysis, glycogenolysis, and fatty acid oxidation (particularly in muscle tissues) to ensure that ATP homeostasis is maintained.

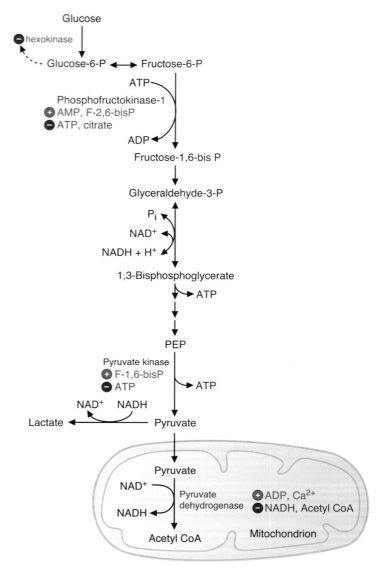

FIGURE 22.14 Major sites of regulation in the glycolytic pathway. Hexokinase and phosphofructokinase-1 are the major regulatory enzymes in skeletal muscle. The activity of pyruvate dehydrogenase in the mitochondrion determines whether pyruvate is converted to lactate or to acetyl coenzyme A (acetyl CoA). The regulation shown for pyruvate kinase occurs only for the liver (L) isoenzyme. *ADP*, adenosine diphosphate; *AMP*, adenosine monophosphate; *ATP*, adenosine triphosphate; *Fructose-6-P*, fructose 6-phosphate; *Fructose-1,6-bis P and F-1,6-bisP*, fructose 1,6-bisphosphate; *F-2,6-bisP*, fructose 2,6-bisphosphate; *Glucose-6-P*, glucose 6-phosphate; *Glyceraldehyde-3-P*, glyceraldehyde 3-phosphate; *NADH*, reduced nicotinamide adenine dinucleotide; *PEP*, phosphoenolpyruvate; *TCA*, tricarboxylic acid.

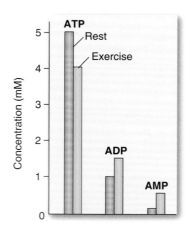

FIGURE 22.15 Changes in adenosine triphosphate (ATP), adenosine diphosphate (ADP), and adenosine monophosphate (AMP) concentrations in skeletal muscle during exercise. The concentration of ATP decreases by only ~20% during exercise, and the concentration of ADP rises. The concentration of AMP, produced by the adenylate kinase reaction, increases manyfold and serves as a sensitive indicator of decreasing ATP levels.

B. Regulation of Hexokinases

Hexokinases exist as tissue-specific isoenzymes whose regulatory properties reflect the role of glycolysis in different tissues. In most tissues, hexokinase is a low-K_m enzyme with a high affinity for glucose (see Chapter 9). It is inhibited by physiologic concentrations of its product, glucose 6-P (see Fig. 22.14). If glucose 6-P does not enter glycolysis or another pathway, it accumulates and decreases the activity of hexokinase. In the liver, the isoenzyme glucokinase is a high-K_m enzyme that is not readily inhibited by glucose 6-P. Thus, glycolysis can continue in the liver even when energy levels are high, so that anabolic pathways, such as the synthesis of the major energy-storage compounds, glycogen and fatty acids, can occur. Hepatic glucokinase, however, does bind to the glucokinase regulatory protein (GKRP) when glucose levels in the hepatocyte are low. When GKRP binds to glucokinase, the complex translocates to the nucleus, removing glucokinase (and its enzymatic activity) from the cytoplasm. As glucose levels eventually rise in the hepatocyte, the complex reenters the cytoplasm, and the glucokinase is released from the GKRP such that glucokinase can phosphorylate glucose and initiate the glycolytic pathway.

C. Regulation of Phosphofructokinase-1

PFK-1 is the rate-limiting enzyme of glycolysis and controls the rate of glucose 6-P entry into glycolysis in most tissues. PFK-1 is an allosteric enzyme that has a total of six binding sites: Two are for substrates (Mg-ATP and fructose 6-P) and four are allosteric regulatory sites (see Fig. 22.14). The allosteric regulatory sites occupy a physically different domain on the enzyme than the catalytic site. When an allosteric effector binds, it changes the conformation at the active site and may activate or inhibit the enzyme (see also Chapter 9). The allosteric sites for PFK-1 include an inhibitory site for MgATP, an inhibitory site for citrate and other anions, an allosteric activation site for AMP, and an allosteric activation site for fructose 2,6-bisphosphate (fructose 2,6-bisP) and other bisphosphates. Several different tissue-specific isoforms of PFK-1 are affected in different ways by the concentration of these substrates and allosteric effectors, but all contain these four allosteric sites.

Three different types of PFK-1 isoenzyme subunits exist: M (muscle), L (liver), and C (common). The three subunits show variable expression in different tissues, with some tissues having more than one type. For example, mature human muscle expresses only the M subunit, the liver expresses principally the L subunit, and erythrocytes express both the M and the L subunits. The C subunit is present in highest levels in platelets, placenta, kidney, and fibroblasts but is relatively common to most tissues. Both the M and L subunits are sensitive to AMP and ATP regulation, but the C subunits are much less so. Active PFK-1 is a tetramer, composed of four subunits. Within muscle, the M4 form predominates; but within tissues that express multiple isoenzymes of PFK-1, heterotetramers can form that have full activity.

1. Allosteric Regulation of PFK-1 by AMP and ATP

ATP binds to two different sites on the enzyme, the substrate-binding site and an allosteric-inhibitory site. Under physiologic conditions in the cell, the ATP concentration is usually high enough to saturate the substrate-binding site and inhibit the enzyme by binding to the ATP allosteric site. This effect of ATP is opposed by AMP, which binds to a separate allosteric-activator site (Fig. 22.16). For most of the PFK-1 isoenzymes, the binding of AMP increases the affinity of the enzyme for fructose 6-P (e.g., it shifts the kinetic curve to the left). Thus, increases in AMP concentration can greatly increase the rate of the enzyme (see Fig. 22.16), particularly when fructose 6-P concentrations are low.

2. Regulation of PFK-1 by Fructose 2,6-Bisphosphate

Fructose 2,6-bisP is also an allosteric activator of PFK-1 that opposes ATP inhibition. Its effect on the rate of activity of PFK-1 is qualitatively similar to that of AMP, but it has a separate binding site. Fructose 2,6-bisP is *not* an intermediate of glycolysis but is synthesized by an enzyme that phosphorylates fructose 6-P at the 2-position. The enzyme is, therefore, named phosphofructokinase-2 (PFK-2); it is a bifunctional enzyme with two separate domains, a kinase domain and a phosphatase domain. At the kinase domain, fructose 6-P is phosphorylated to fructose 2,6-bisP; and at the phosphatase domain, fructose 2,6-bisP is hydrolyzed back to fructose 6-P. PFK-2 is regulated through changes in the ratio of activity of the two domains. For example, in skeletal muscles, high concentrations of fructose 6-P activate the kinase and inhibit the phosphatase, thereby increasing the concentration of fructose 2,6-bisP and activating glycolysis.

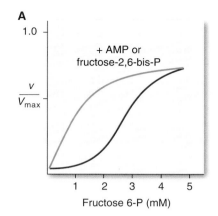

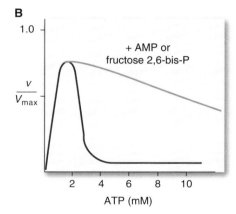

FIGURE 22.16 Regulation of phosphofructokinase-1 (PFK-1) by adenosine monophosphate (AMP), adenosine triphosphate (ATP), and fructose 2,6-bisphosphate (fructose 2,6-bisP). **A.** AMP and fructose 2,6-bisP activate PFK-1. **B.** ATP, as a substrate, increases the rate of the reaction at low concentrations but allosterically inhibits the enzyme at high concentrations. *fructose 6-P,* fructose 6-phosphate.

 Otto S. has started high-intensity exercise that will increase the production of lactate in his exercising skeletal muscles. In skeletal muscles, the amount of aerobic versus anaerobic glycolysis that occurs varies with intensity of the exercise, with duration of the exercise, with the type of skeletal muscle fiber involved, and with the level of training. Human skeletal muscles are usually combinations of type I fibers (called *fast glycolytic fibers,* or *white muscle fibers*) and type IIb fibers (called *slow oxidative fibers,* or *red muscle fibers*). The designation *fast* or *slow* refers to their rate of shortening, which is determined by the isoenzyme of myosin ATPase present. Compared with glycolytic fibers, oxidative fibers have a higher content of mitochondria and myoglobin, which gives them a red color. The gastrocnemius, a muscle in the leg used for running, has a high content of type IIb fibers. However, these fibers will still produce lactate during sprints when the ATP demand exceeds their oxidative capacity.

Under ischemic conditions, AMP levels within the heart increase rapidly because of the lack of ATP production via oxidative phosphorylation. The increase in AMP levels activates the AMP-activated protein kinase, which phosphorylates the heart isoenzyme of PFK-2 to activate its kinase activity. This results in increased levels of fructose 2,6-bisP, which activates PFK-1 along with AMP so that the rate of glycolysis can increase to compensate for the lack of ATP production via aerobic means.

Several methods can be used to determine lactate levels in blood. Two of the most common use enzymatic methods are given. The first is the conversion of lactate to pyruvate (which also converts NAD$^+$ to NADH) in the presence of LDH. Because NADH has considerable light absorption at 340 nm (and NAD$^+$ does not), one can follow the increase in absorbance at this wavelength as the reaction proceeds and determine the levels of lactate that were initially present in the sample. To ensure that all of the lactate is measured, hydrazine is added to the reaction; the hydrazine reacts with the pyruvate to remove the product of the LDH reaction, which forces the reaction to go to completion. The second enzymatic procedure that is commonly used employs lactate oxidase, which converts lactate, in the presence of oxygen, to pyruvate and hydrogen peroxide. In this case, a second enzymatic reaction measures the amount of hydrogen peroxide produced (which removes the product of the lactate oxidase reaction, ensuring completion of the reaction). This second reaction uses peroxidase and a chromogen, which is converted to a colored product as the hydrogen peroxide is removed. The amount of colored product produced allows lactate levels to be determined accurately. Both procedures have been automated for use in the clinical laboratory.

During **Cora N.'s** myocardial infarction (see Chapter 20), the ischemic area in her heart had a limited supply of oxygen and bloodborne fuels. The absence of oxygen for oxidative phosphorylation would decrease the levels of ATP and increase those of AMP, an activator of PFK-1 and the AMP-dependent protein kinase, resulting in a compensatory increase of anaerobic glycolysis and lactate production. However, obstruction of a vessel leading to her heart would decrease lactate removal, resulting in a decrease of intracellular pH. Under these conditions, at very low pH levels, glycolysis is inhibited and unable to compensate for the lack of oxidative phosphorylation.

PFK-2 also can be regulated through phosphorylation by serine–threonine protein kinases. The liver isoenzyme contains a phosphorylation site near the amino terminus that decreases the activity of the kinase and increases the phosphatase activity. This site is phosphorylated by the cAMP-dependent protein kinase (protein kinase A) and is responsible for decreased levels of liver fructose 2,6-bisP during fasting conditions (as modulated by circulating glucagon levels, which is discussed in detail in Chapters 19 and 28). The cardiac isoenzyme contains a phosphorylation site near the carboxyl terminus that can be phosphorylated in response to adrenergic activators of contraction (such as norepinephrine) and by increased AMP levels. Phosphorylation at this site increases the kinase activity and increases fructose 2,6-bisP levels, thereby contributing to the activation of glycolysis.

3. Allosteric Inhibition of PFK-1 at the Citrate Site

The function of the citrate-anion allosteric site is to integrate glycolysis with other pathways. For example, the inhibition of PFK-1 by citrate (an intermediate of the Krebs TCA cycle; see Chapter 23) may play a role in decreasing glycolytic flux in the heart during the oxidation of fatty acids.

D. Regulation of Pyruvate Kinase

Pyruvate kinase exists as tissue-specific isoenzymes, designated as R (red blood cells), L (liver), and M1/M2 (muscle and other tissues). The M1 form present in brain, heart, and muscle contains no allosteric sites, and pyruvate kinase does not contribute to the regulation of glycolysis in these tissues (these tissues also do not undergo significant gluconeogenesis). However, the liver isoenzyme can be inhibited through phosphorylation by the cAMP-dependent protein kinase and by several allosteric effectors that contribute to the inhibition of glycolysis during fasting conditions. These allosteric effectors include activation by fructose 1,6-bisP, which ties the rate of pyruvate kinase to that of PFK-1, and inhibition by ATP, which signifies high energy levels.

IV. Lactic Acidemia

Lactate production is a normal part of metabolism. In the absence of disease, elevated lactate levels in the blood are associated with anaerobic glycolysis during exercise. In lactic acidosis, lactic acid accumulates in blood to levels that significantly affect the pH (lactate levels >5 mM and a decrease of blood pH <7.2). A further discussion of lactic acidemia occurs in Chapter 24, after learning about oxidative phosphorylation.

CLINICAL COMMENTS

Linda F. was admitted to the hospital with severe hypotension caused by an acute hemorrhage. Her plasma lactic acid level was elevated and her arterial pH was low. The underlying mechanism for Ms. F.'s derangement in acid–base balance is a severe reduction in the amount of oxygen delivered to her tissues for cellular respiration (hypoxemia). Several concurrent processes contributed to this lack of oxygen. The first was her severely reduced blood pressure caused by a brisk hemorrhage from a bleeding gastric ulcer. The blood loss led to hypoperfusion and, therefore, reduced delivery of oxygen to her tissues. This led to increased lactate production from anaerobic glycolysis and an elevation of serum lactate to almost 10 times the normal levels. The marked reduction in the number of red blood cells in her circulation caused by blood loss further compromised oxygen delivery. Her preexisting COPD added to her hypoxemia by decreasing her ventilation and, therefore, the transfer of oxygen to her blood (low P_{O_2}). In addition, her COPD led to retention of carbon dioxide (high P_{CO_2}), which caused a respiratory acidosis because the retained CO_2 interacted with water to form carbonic acid (H_2CO_3), which dissociates to H^+ and bicarbonate. The reduction in her arterial pH to 7.18

(reference range = 7.35 to 7.45), therefore, resulted from both a mild respiratory acidosis (elevated P_{CO_2}) and a more profound metabolic acidosis (elevated serum lactate levels).

Otto S. In skeletal muscles, lactate production occurs when the need for ATP exceeds the capacity of the mitochondria for oxidative phosphorylation. Thus, increased lactate production accompanies an increased rate of the TCA cycle. The extent to which skeletal muscles use aerobic versus anaerobic glycolysis to supply ATP varies with the intensity of exercise. During low-intensity exercise, the rate of ATP use is lower, and fibers can generate this ATP from oxidative phosphorylation, with the complete oxidation of glucose to CO_2. However, when **Otto S.** sprints, a high-intensity exercise, the ATP demand exceeds the rate at which the ETC and the TCA cycle can generate ATP from oxidative phosphorylation. The increased AMP level signals the need for additional ATP and stimulates PFK-1. The $NADH/NAD^+$ ratio directs the increase in pyruvate production toward lactate. The fall in pH causes muscle fatigue and pain. As Otto trains, the amounts of mitochondria and myoglobin in his skeletal muscle fibers increase, and these fibers rely less on anaerobic glycolysis.

Ivan A. Ivan A. had two sites of dental caries: one on a smooth surface and one in a fissure. The decreased pH resulting from lactic acid production by lactobacilli, which grow anaerobically within the fissure, is a major cause of fissure caries. *Streptococcus mutans* plays a major role in smooth-surface caries because it secretes dextran, an insoluble polysaccharide, which forms the base for plaque. *S. mutans* contains dextran-sucrase, a glucosyltransferase that transfers glucosyl units from dietary sucrose (the glucose–fructose disaccharide in sugar and sweets) to form the $\alpha(1{\rightarrow}6)$ and $\alpha(1{\rightarrow}3)$ linkages between the glucosyl units in dextran. Dextran-sucrase is specific for sucrose and does not catalyze the polymerization of free glucose, or glucose from other disaccharides or polysaccharides. Thus, sucrose is responsible for the cariogenic potential of candy. The sticky water-insoluble dextran mediates the attachment of *S. mutans* and other bacteria to the tooth surface. This also keeps the acids produced from these bacteria close to the enamel surface. Fructose from sucrose is converted to intermediates of glycolysis and is rapidly metabolized to lactic acid. Other bacteria present in the plaque produce different acids from anaerobic metabolism, such as acetic acid and formic acid. The decrease in pH that results initiates demineralization of the hydroxyapatite of the tooth enamel. **Ivan A.'s** caries in his baby teeth could have been caused by sucking on bottles containing fruit juice. The sugar in fruit juice is also sucrose, and babies who fall asleep with a bottle of fruit juice or milk (milk can also decrease the pH) in their mouth may develop caries. Rapid decay of these baby teeth can harm the development of their permanent teeth.

Candice S. Hereditary fructose intolerance (HFI) is caused by a low level of fructose 1-P aldolase activity in aldolase B. Aldolase B is an isozyme of fructose 1,6-bisP aldolase that is also capable of cleaving fructose 1-P. In people of European descent, the most common defect is a single missense mutation in exon 5 (G → C), resulting in an amino acid substitution (Ala → Pro). As a result of this substitution, a catalytically impaired aldolase B is synthesized in abundance. The exact prevalence of HFI in the United States is not established but is approximately 1 per 15,000 to 25,000 population. The disease is transmitted by an autosomal-recessive inheritance pattern.

When affected patients such as Candice ingest fructose, fructose is converted to fructose 1-P. Because of the deficiency of aldolase B, fructose 1-P cannot be further metabolized to dihydroxyacetone phosphate and glyceraldehyde and accumulates in those tissues that have fructokinase (liver, kidney, and small intestine). Fructose is detected in the urine with the reducing sugar test (see the "Methods" comment in Chapter 5). A DNA screening test (based on the generation of a new restriction site by the mutation) now provides a safe method to confirm a diagnosis of HFI.

In infants and small children, the major symptoms include poor feeding, vomiting, intestinal discomfort, and failure to thrive. The greater the ingestion of dietary fructose, the more severe is the clinical reaction. The result of prolonged ingestion of fructose is ultrastructural changes in the liver and kidney that result in hepatic and renal failure. Hereditary fructose intolerance is usually a disease of infancy because adults with fructose intolerance who have survived avoid the ingestion of fruits, table sugar, and other sweets.

Before the metabolic toxicity of fructose was appreciated, substitution of fructose for glucose in intravenous solutions, and of fructose for sucrose in enteral tube feeding or diabetic diets, was frequently recommended. (*Enteral* tube feeding refers to tubes placed into the gut; *parenteral* tube feeding refers to tubes placed into a vein, feeding intravenously.) Administration of intravenous fructose to patients with diabetes mellitus or other forms of insulin resistance avoided the hyperglycemia found with intravenous glucose, possibly because fructose metabolism in the liver bypasses the insulin-regulated step at phosphofructokinase-1. However, because of the unregulated flow of fructose through glycolysis, intravenous fructose feeding frequently resulted in lactic acidosis (see Fig. 22.7). In addition, the fructokinase reaction is very rapid, and tissues became depleted of ATP and phosphate when large quantities of fructose were metabolized over a short period. This led to cell death. Fructose is less toxic in the diet or in enteral feeding because of the relatively slow rate of fructose absorption.

 Erin G. has galactosemia, which is caused by a deficiency of galactose-1-P uridylyltransferase; it is one of the most common genetic diseases. Galactosemia is an autosomal-recessive disorder of galactose metabolism that occurs in about 1 in 60,000 newborns. All of the states in the United States screen newborns for this disease because failure to begin immediate treatment results in intellectual disability. Failure to thrive is the most common initial clinical symptom. Vomiting or diarrhea occurs in most patients, usually starting within a few days of beginning milk ingestion. Signs of deranged liver function, jaundice or hepatomegaly, are present almost as frequently after the first week of life. The jaundice of intrinsic liver disease may be accentuated by the severe hemolysis in some patients. Cataracts have been observed within a few days of birth.

Management of patients requires eliminating galactose from the diet. Failure to eliminate this sugar results in progressive liver failure and death. In infants, artificial milk made from casein or soybean hydrolysate is used.

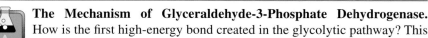

BIOCHEMICAL COMMENTS

The Mechanism of Glyceraldehyde-3-Phosphate Dehydrogenase. How is the first high-energy bond created in the glycolytic pathway? This is the work of the glyceraldehyde-3-P dehydrogenase reaction, which converts glyceraldehyde 3-P to 1,3-BPG. This reaction can be considered to be two separate half-reactions: the first being the oxidation of glyceraldehyde 3-P to 3-phosphoglycerate, and the second being the addition of inorganic phosphate (P_i) to 3-phosphoglycerate to produce 1,3-BPG. The $\Delta G^{0'}$ for the first reaction is approximately -12 kcal/mol; for the second reaction, it is approximately $+12$ kcal/mol. Thus, although the first half-reaction is extremely favorable, the second half-reaction is unfavorable and does not proceed under cellular conditions. So how does the enzyme help this reaction to proceed? This is accomplished through the enzyme forming a covalent bond with the substrate, using an essential cysteine residue at the active site to form a high-energy thioester linkage during the course of the reaction (Fig. 22.17). Thus, the energy that would be released as heat in the oxidation of glyceraldehyde 3-P to 3-phosphoglycerate is conserved in the thioester linkage that is formed (such that the $\Delta G^{0'}$ of the formation of the thioester intermediate from glyceraldehyde 3-P is close to zero). Then, replacement of the sulfur

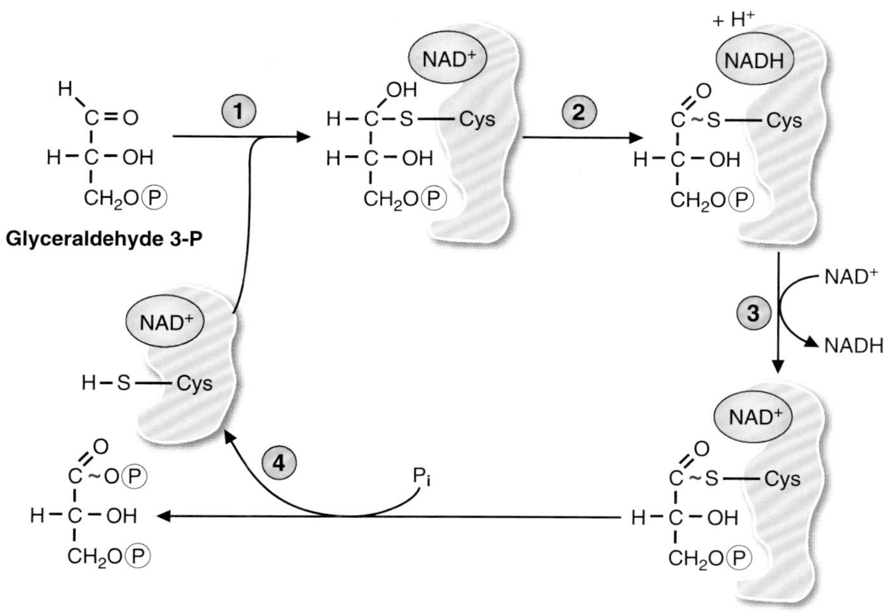

FIGURE 22.17 Mechanism of the glyceraldehyde 3-phosphate (glyceraldehyde-3-P) dehydrogenase reaction. (*1*) The enzyme forms a covalent linkage with the substrate, using a cysteine (Cys) group at the active site. The enzyme also contains bound nicotinamide adenine dinucleotide (NAD$^+$) close to the active site. (*2*) The substrate is oxidized, forming a high-energy thioester linkage (in *red*) and NADH. (*3*) NADH has a low affinity for the enzyme and is replaced by a new molecule of NAD$^+$. (*4*) Inorganic phosphate (P$_i$) attacks the thioester linkage, releasing the product 1,3-bisphosphoglycerate and regenerating the active enzyme in a form ready to initiate another reaction.

with P$_i$ to form the final product, 1,3-BPG, is relatively straightforward, as the $\Delta G^{0'}$ for that conversion is also close to zero, and the acylphosphate bond retains the energy from the oxidation of the aldehyde. This is one example of how covalent catalysis by an enzyme can result in the conservation of energy between different bond types.

KEY CONCEPTS

- Glycolysis is the pathway in which glucose is oxidized and cleaved to form pyruvate.
- The enzymes of glycolysis are in the cytosol.
- Glucose is the major sugar in our diet; all cells can use glucose for energy.
- Glycolysis generates two molecules of ATP through substrate-level phosphorylation, and two molecules of NADH.
- The cytosolic NADH generated via glycolysis transfers its reducing equivalents to mitochondrial NAD$^+$ via shuttle systems across the inner mitochondrial membrane.
- The pyruvate generated during glycolysis can enter the mitochondria and be oxidized completely to CO$_2$ by pyruvate dehydrogenase and the TCA cycle.
- Anaerobic glycolysis generates energy in cells with a limited supply of oxygen or few mitochondria.
- Under anaerobic conditions, pyruvate is reduced to lactate by NADH, thereby regenerating the NAD$^+$ required for glycolysis to continue.
- Glycolysis is regulated to ensure that ATP homeostasis is maintained.
- The key regulated enzymes of glycolysis are hexokinase, phosphofructokinase-1, and pyruvate kinase.
- Fructose is ingested principally as the monosaccharide or as part of sucrose. Fructose metabolism generates fructose 1-phosphate, which is then converted to intermediates of the glycolytic pathway.

- Galactose is ingested principally as lactose, which is converted to glucose and galactose in the intestine. Galactose metabolism generates, first, galactose 1-phosphate, which is converted to UDP-galactose. The end product is glucose 1-phosphate, which is isomerized to glucose 6-phosphate, which then enters glycolysis.
- The energy yield through glycolysis for both fructose and galactose is the same as for glucose metabolism.
- Diseases discussed in this chapter are summarized in Table 22.3.

TABLE 22.3 Diseases Discussed in Chapter 22		
DISEASE OR DISORDER	**ENVIRONMENTAL OR GENETIC**	**COMMENTS**
Chronic obstructive pulmonary disease	Both	Can lead to inefficient energy production in the nervous system owing to reduced oxygen delivery to the tissue
Obesity	Both	Lactate production via anaerobic glycolysis in the muscle occurs during vigorous exercise
Dental caries	Environmental	Effects of carbohydrate metabolism on oral flora and acid production
Lactic acidemia	Both	Elevated lactic acid owing to mutations in a variety of enzymes involved in carbohydrate and energy metabolism
Hereditary fructose intolerance	Genetic	Lack of aldolase B, leading to an accumulation of fructose 1-P after fructose ingestion. The increased levels of fructose 1-P interfere with glycogen metabolism and can lead to hypoglycemia.
Galactosemia	Genetic	Mutations in either galactokinase or galactose 1-P uridylyltransferase, leading to elevated galactose and/or galactose 1-P levels. This can lead to cataract formation (high galactose) and intellectual disability (elevated galactose 1-P levels) if not treated early in life.

Fructose 1-P, fructose 1-phosphate; galactose 1-P, galactose 1-phosphate.

REVIEW QUESTIONS—CHAPTER 22

1. Glucose is the body's universal fuel, which can be used by virtually all tissues. A major role of glycolysis is which one of the following?
   A. To synthesize glucose
   B. To generate energy
   C. To produce FAD(2H)
   D. To synthesize glycogen
   E. To use ATP to generate heat

2. Glycolysis generates energy such that cells have a source of energy to survive. Starting with glyceraldehyde 3-P and synthesizing one molecule of pyruvate, the net yield of ATP and NADH would be which one of the following?
   A. 1 ATP, 1 NADH
   B. 1 ATP, 2 NADH
   C. 1 ATP, 4 NADH
   D. 2 ATP, 1 NADH
   E. 2 ATP, 2 NADH
   F. 2 ATP, 4 NADH

   G. 3 ATP, 1 NADH
   H. 3 ATP, 2 NADH
   I. 3 ATP, 4 NADH

3. Glycogen is the body's storage form of glucose. When glycogen is degraded, glucose 1-P is formed. Glucose 1-P can then be isomerized to glucose 6-P. Starting with glucose 1-P and ending with two molecules of pyruvate, what is the net yield of glycolysis in terms of ATP and NADH formed?
   A. 1 ATP, 1 NADH
   B. 1 ATP, 2 NADH
   C. 1 ATP, 3 NADH
   D. 2 ATP, 1 NADH
   E. 2 ATP, 2 NADH
   F. 2 ATP, 3 NADH
   G. 3 ATP, 1 NADH
   H. 3 ATP, 2 NADH
   I. 3 ATP, 3 NADH

4. Every human cell has the capacity to use glycolysis for energy production. Which one of the following statements correctly describes an aspect of glycolysis?
   A. ATP is formed by oxidative phosphorylation.
   B. Two molecules of ATP are used in the beginning of the pathway.
   C. Pyruvate kinase is the rate-limiting enzyme.
   D. One molecule of pyruvate and three molecules of CO_2 are formed from the oxidation of one glucose molecule.
   E. The reactions take place in the matrix of the mitochondria.

5. Fructose is the second most common sugar in the human adult diet and its metabolism parallels glycolysis. Which one of the following substances is found in both the fructose metabolic pathway and the glycolytic pathway?
   A. Glucose 1-P
   B. Fructose 1-P
   C. Fructose 6-P
   D. Fructose 1,6-bisP
   E. Glyceraldehyde 3-P

6. A 4-week-old baby is being seen by the pediatrician because of frequent vomiting after meals and tenderness in the abdomen. Upon examination, the physician noted an enlarged liver and a hint of cataract formation in both of the child's eyes. A urine dipstick test for a reducing sugar gave a positive result. Blood glucose levels were slightly below normal. The compound that reacted with the urine dipstick test was most likely which one of the following?
   A. Glucose
   B. Fructose
   C. Lactose
   D. Maltose
   E. Galactose

7. Considering the child discussed in the previous question, measurement of which single intracellular metabolite would allow a determination of the enzyme deficiency?
   A. Glucose 6-P
   B. Fructose 6-P
   C. Galactose 1-P
   D. Fructose 1-P
   E. UDP-glucose

8. Metformin is a medication used in treating diabetes mellitus type 2. One of its actions is to decrease hepatic gluconeogenesis. A theoretical concern with this medication was lactic acidosis, which in practice does not occur in patients taking metformin. Which one of the following explains why lactic acidosis does not occur with the use of this medication?
   A. The Cori cycle overcomes the lactate buildup in the liver.
   B. Red blood cells use lactate as fuel.
   C. Renal medullary cells use lactate as fuel.
   D. The heart uses lactate as fuel.
   E. The eye uses lactate as fuel.

9. Because glucose has several metabolic routes it might take once it arrives in the cytoplasm, which one of the following reactions would commit the glucose to following the glycolytic pathway?
   A. Glucose to glucose 1-P
   B. Glucose to glucose 6-P
   C. Fructose 6-P to fructose 1,6-bisP
   D. Fructose 1,6-bisP to dihydroxyacetone phosphate and glyceraldehyde 3-P
   E. Glucose 1-P to glucose 6-P

10. The red blood cells require ATP in order to maintain ion gradients across their membrane. In the absence of these ion gradients, the red blood cells will swell and burst, bringing about a hemolytic anemia. Red cells generate their energy via which one of the following?
    A. Substrate-level phosphorylation
    B. TCA cycle
    C. Oxidative phosphorylation
    D. Electron transfer to oxygen
    E. Oxidation of glucose to CO_2 and H_2O

ANSWERS

1. **The answer is B.** The major roles of glycolysis are to generate energy and to produce precursors for other biosynthetic pathways. Gluconeogenesis is the pathway that generates glucose (thus, A is incorrect); FAD(2H) is produced in the mitochondria by a variety of reactions but not glycolysis (thus, C is incorrect); glycogen synthesis occurs under conditions in which glycolysis is inhibited (thus, D is incorrect); and glycolysis does not hydrolyze ATP to generate heat (that is caused by nonshivering thermogenesis; thus, E is incorrect).

2. **The answer is D.** By starting with glyceraldehyde 3-P, the energy-requiring steps of glycolysis are bypassed. Thus, as glyceraldehyde 3-P is converted to pyruvate, two molecules of ATP will be produced (at the phosphoglycerate kinase and pyruvate kinase steps) and one molecule of NADH will be produced (at the glyceraldehyde-3-P dehydrogenase step).

3. **The answer is H.** Glucose 1-P is isomerized to glucose 6-P, which then enters glycolysis. This skips the hexokinase step, which uses 1 ATP. Thus, starting from glucose 1-P, one would get the normal 2 ATP and 2 NADH; but with one less ATP used in the priming steps, the total yield would be 3 ATP and 2 NADH.

4. **The answer is B.** The pathway consumes 2 ATP at the beginning of the pathway and produces 4 ATP at the end of the pathway for each molecule of glucose. Therefore,

the net energy production is 2 ATP for each molecule of glucose. Glycolysis synthesizes ATP via substrate-level phosphorylation, not oxidative phosphorylation (thus, A is incorrect) and synthesizes two molecules of pyruvate in the process (thus, D is incorrect). The pathway is cytosolic (thus, D is incorrect), and the rate-limiting step is the one catalyzed by phosphofructokinase-1 (thus, C is incorrect).

5. **The answer is E.** Fructose 1-P is found only in fructose metabolism. Glucose 1-P is derived from glycogen degradation. Fructose 6-P and fructose 1,6-bisP are found in glycolysis but not in fructose metabolism. Both fructose and glucose are converted to glyceraldehyde 3-P, and this is where the two pathways intersect. Their continued metabolism is identical from this point on.

6. **The answer is E.** The child has a form of galactosemia in which galactose cannot be metabolized, such that free galactose enters the blood and is excreted via the urine. The below-normal blood glucose levels indicate that glucose is not being excreted in the urine. The high levels of galactose lead to galactose entering the lens of the eye, where it is converted to galactitol via aldose reductase, trapping the galactitol in the lens. This leads to an osmotic imbalance across the lens, resulting in swelling and cataract formation. High levels of fructose do not lead to cataract formation. Lactose is a disaccharide that is cleaved to glucose and galactose in the small intestine, such that lactose does not enter the blood. Maltose is another disaccharide (glucose-glucose) that does not enter the blood.

7. **The answer is C.** The child either has classical galactosemia (caused by a deficiency of galactose 1-P uridylyltransferase) or nonclassical galactosemia (caused by a deficiency of galactokinase). Measurement of galactose 1-P levels would enable one to determine if galactokinase were deficient (if it were, galactose 1-P levels

would be low) or if galactose 1-P uridylyltransferase were defective (in which case galactose 1-P levels would be elevated). Measurement of the other compounds listed would not allow for a determination as to whether galactokinase or galactose 1-P uridylyltransferase were defective.

8. **The answer is D.** Metformin interrupts the Cori cycle (gluconeogenesis in the liver using lactate, derived from the muscle, as a source of carbons). The heart, with its huge mitochondrial content and oxidative capacity, uses lactate as fuel and easily metabolizes the excess lactate (which is why heart failure is a contraindication to the use of metformin; otherwise, lactic acidosis would occur). The red blood cells, renal medullary cells, and tissues of the eye all use anaerobic glycolysis to generate energy, producing lactate, but cannot use lactate as a fuel.

9. **The answer is C.** The committed step for glycolysis is the one catalyzed by phosphofructokinase-1, which converts fructose 6-P to fructose 1,6-bisP. Glucose is not directly converted to glucose 1-P (glucose 1-P); glucose must first be phosphorylated to glucose 6-P and then isomerized to glucose 1-P. Glucose 6-P has other potential fates (glycogen synthesis, hexose monophosphate shunt), so the generation of glucose 6-P from glucose does not commit the sugar to the glycolytic pathway. Aldolase cleaves fructose 1,6-bisP into 2 triose phosphates, but this is not considered the committed step of glycolysis.

10. **The answer is A.** Red blood cells do not contain mitochondria and can only generate energy via anaerobic mechanisms. Without mitochondria, aerobic glycolysis cannot occur through the TCA cycle or oxidative phosphorylation of glucose to CO_2 and H_2O. Only anaerobic glycolysis can occur with production of lactate and production of ATP by substrate-level phosphorylation. The ETC occurs within the mitochondria.

Tricarboxylic Acid Cycle

The **tricarboxylic acid cycle** (TCA cycle) accounts for more than two-thirds of the adenosine triphosphate (ATP) generated from fuel oxidation. The pathways for oxidation of fatty acids, glucose, amino acids, acetate, and ketone bodies all generate **acetyl coenzyme A** (acetyl-CoA), which is the substrate for the TCA cycle. As the activated two-carbon acetyl group is oxidized to two molecules of CO_2, energy is conserved as reduced **nicotinamide adenine dinucleotide (NADH)** and **flavin adenine dinucleotide (FAD[2H])**, and guanosine triphosphate (**GTP**) (Fig. 23.1). NADH and FAD(2H) subsequently donate electrons to O_2 via the electron-transport chain (ETC), with the generation of ATP from oxidative phosphorylation. Thus, the TCA cycle is central to energy generation from **cellular respiration**.

Within the TCA cycle, the oxidative decarboxylation of α-ketoglutarate is catalyzed by the multisubunit **α-ketoglutarate dehydrogenase complex**, which contains the coenzymes **thiamin pyrophosphate (TPP)**, **lipoate**, and **FAD**. A similar complex, the **pyruvate dehydrogenase complex (PDC)**, catalyzes the oxidation of pyruvate to acetyl-CoA, thereby providing a link between the pathways of glycolysis and the TCA cycle (see Fig. 23.1)

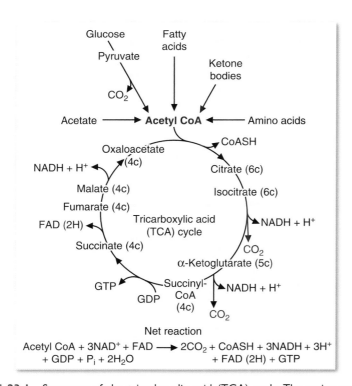

FIGURE 23.1 Summary of the tricarboxylic acid (TCA) cycle. The major pathways of fuel oxidation generate acetyl coenzyme A (acetyl-CoA), which is the substrate for the TCA cycle. The number of carbons in each intermediate of the cycle is indicated in *parentheses* by the name of the compound. *CoASH*, coenzyme A; *GDP*, guanosine diphosphate; *GTP*, guanosine triphosphate; *FAD*, flavin adenine dinucleotide; *NAD*, nicotinamide adenine dinucleotide; *P_i*, inorganic phosphate.

The two-carbon acetyl group is the ultimate source of the electrons that are transferred to NAD^+ and FAD and also the carbon in the two CO_2 molecules that are produced. Oxaloacetate is used and regenerated in each turn of the cycle (see Fig. 23.1). However, when cells use intermediates of the TCA cycle for biosynthetic reactions, the carbons of oxaloacetate must be replaced by **anaplerotic** (filling up) reactions, such as the **pyruvate carboxylase reaction**.

The TCA cycle occurs in the mitochondrion, where its flux is tightly coordinated with the rate of the ETC and oxidative phosphorylation through **feedback regulation that reflects the demand for ATP**. The rate of the TCA cycle is increased when ATP use in the cell is increased through the response of several enzymes to adenosine diphosphate (**ADP**) **levels**, the **NADH/NAD$^+$ ratio**, the rate of FAD(2H) oxidation, or the **Ca2$^+$ concentration**. For example, **isocitrate dehydrogenase is allosterically activated by ADP**.

There are two general consequences to impaired functioning of the TCA cycle: (1) an inability to generate ATP from fuel oxidation and (2) an accumulation of TCA cycle precursors. For example, inhibition of pyruvate oxidation in the TCA cycle results in its reduction to lactate, which can cause **lactic acidosis**. The most common situation leading to an impaired function of the TCA cycle is a relative lack of oxygen to accept electrons in the ETC.

THE WAITING ROOM

 Otto S., a 26-year-old medical student, has faithfully followed his diet and aerobic exercise program of daily tennis and jogging (see Chapter 20). He has lost a total of 33 lb and is just 23 lb from his college weight of 154 lb. His exercise capacity has markedly improved; he can run for a longer time at a faster pace before noting shortness of breath or palpitations of his heart. Even his test scores in his medical school classes have improved.

 Ann R. suffers from anorexia nervosa (see Chapters 1, 3, and 9). In addition to a low body weight and decreased muscle mass, glycogen, and fat stores, she has iron-deficiency anemia (see Chapter 16). She has started to gain weight and is trying a daily exercise program. However, she constantly feels weak and tired. When she walks, she feels pain in her calf muscles. On this visit to her nutritionist, they discuss the vitamin content of her diet and its role in energy metabolism.

 Al M. has been hospitalized for congestive heart failure (see Chapter 8) and for head injuries sustained while driving under the influence of alcohol (Chapters 9 and 10). He completed an alcohol detoxification program, enrolled in a local Alcoholics Anonymous (AA) group, and began seeing a psychologist. During this time, his alcohol-related neurologic and cardiac manifestations of alcohol toxicity and thiamin deficiency partially cleared. However, in spite of the support he was receiving, he began drinking excessive amounts of alcohol again while eating poorly. Three weeks later, he was readmitted with symptoms of "high-output" heart failure, sometimes referred to as *wet beriberi* or as the *beriberi heart* when related to thiamin deficiency.

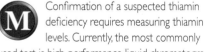 Confirmation of a suspected thiamin deficiency requires measuring thiamin levels. Currently, the most commonly used test is high-performance liquid chromatography (HPLC) analysis to quantify the levels of both free thiamin and the active form, TPP, in blood. In the past, a standard assay was used that determined whether thiamin levels were sufficient for metabolic processes by using the enzyme transketolase, which requires TPP for activity (see Chapter 27). Transketolase can be obtained from red blood cells, making sample collection relatively straightforward. The measurement of transketolase activity is done in the absence and presence of exogenous TPP. If the difference in activity levels is >25%, then a thiamin deficiency was confirmed.

I. Overview of the Tricarboxylic Acid Cycle

The TCA cycle is frequently called the *Krebs cycle* because Sir Hans Krebs first formulated its reactions into a cycle. It is also called the *citric acid cycle* because citrate was one of the first compounds known to participate. The most common name for this pathway, the *tricarboxylic acid* or *TCA cycle*, denotes the involvement of the tricarboxylates citrate and isocitrate.

In order for the body to generate large amounts of ATP, the major pathways of fuel oxidation generate acetyl-CoA, which is the substrate for the TCA cycle. In the first step of the TCA cycle, the acetyl portion of acetyl-CoA combines with the four-carbon intermediate oxaloacetate to form citrate (six carbons), which is rearranged to form isocitrate. In the next two oxidative decarboxylation reactions, electrons are transferred to NAD^+ to form NADH, and two molecules of electron-depleted CO_2 are released. Subsequently, a high-energy phosphate bond in GTP is generated from substrate-level phosphorylation. In the remaining portion of the TCA cycle, succinate is oxidized to oxaloacetate with the generation of one FAD(2H) and one NADH. The *net* reaction of the TCA cycle, which is the sum of the equations for individual steps, shows that the two carbons of the acetyl group have been oxidized to two molecules of CO_2, with conservation of energy as three molecules of NADH, one of FAD(2H), and one of GTP.

The TCA cycle requires a large number of vitamins and minerals to function. These include niacin (NAD^+), riboflavin (FAD and flavin mononucleotide [FMN]), pantothenic acid (coenzyme A), thiamin, Mg^{2+}, Ca^{2+}, Fe^{2+}, and phosphate.

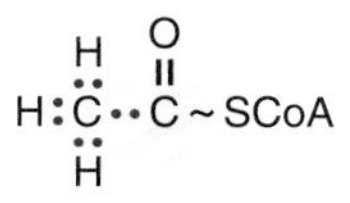

II. Reactions of the Tricarboxylic Acid Cycle

In the TCA cycle, the two-carbon acetyl group of acetyl-CoA is oxidized to two CO_2 molecules (see Fig. 23.1). The function of the cycle is to conserve the energy from this oxidation, which it accomplishes principally by transferring electrons from intermediates of the cycle to NAD^+ and FAD. The eight electrons donated by the acetyl group (four from each carbon) eventually end up in three molecules of NADH and one of FAD(2H) (Fig. 23.2). As a consequence, ATP can be generated from oxidative phosphorylation when NADH and FAD(2H) donate these electrons to O_2 via the ETC.

Initially, the acetyl group is incorporated into *citrate*, an intermediate of the TCA cycle (Fig. 23.3). As citrate progresses through the cycle to *oxaloacetate*, it is oxidized by four dehydrogenases (isocitrate dehydrogenase, α-ketoglutarate dehydrogenase, succinate dehydrogenase, and malate dehydrogenase), which remove electron-containing hydrogen or hydride atoms from a substrate and transfer them to electron-accepting coenzymes such as NAD^+ or FAD. The isomerase aconitase rearranges electrons in citrate, thereby forming isocitrate, to facilitate an electron transfer to NAD^+. An iron cofactor in aconitase facilitates the isomerization.

Although no oxygen is introduced into the TCA cycle, the two molecules of CO_2 produced have more oxygen than the acetyl group. These oxygen atoms are ultimately derived from the carbonyl group of acetyl-CoA, two molecules of water added by fumarase and citrate synthase, and the PO_4^{2-} added to GDP.

The overall yield of energy-containing compounds from the TCA cycle is three NADH, one FAD(2H), and one GTP. The high-energy phosphate bond of GTP is generated from substrate-level phosphorylation catalyzed by succinate thiokinase (succinyl coenzyme A [succinyl-CoA] synthetase). As the NADH and FAD(2H) are reoxidized in the ETC, approximately 2.5 ATP are generated for each NADH, and 1.5 ATP for the FAD(2H) (see Chapter 24). Consequently, the net energy yield from the TCA cycle and oxidative phosphorylation is about 10 high-energy phosphate bonds for each acetyl group oxidized.

A. Formation and Oxidation of Isocitrate

The TCA cycle begins with condensation of the activated acetyl group and oxaloacetate to form the six-carbon intermediate citrate, a reaction that is catalyzed by the enzyme citrate synthase (see Fig. 23.3). Synthases, in general, catalyze the condensation of two organic molecules to form a carbon–carbon bond in the absence of high-energy phosphate bond energy. A synthetase catalyzes the same type of reaction but requires high-energy phosphate bonds to complete the reaction. Because oxaloacetate is regenerated with each turn of the cycle, it is not really considered a substrate of the cycle or a source of electrons or carbon.

FIGURE 23.2 The acetyl group of acetyl coenzyme A (acetyl-CoA). Acetyl-CoA donates eight electrons to the tricarboxylic acid cycle, which are shown in *red*, and two carbons. The high-energy bond is shown by a ~. The acetyl group is the ultimate source of the carbons in the two molecules of CO_2 that are produced, and the source of electrons in the one molecule of reduced flavin adenine dinucleotide (FAD[2H]) and three molecules of reduced nicotinamide adenine dinucleotide (NADH), which have each accepted two electrons. However, the same carbon atoms and electrons that enter from one molecule of acetyl-CoA do not leave as CO_2, NADH, or FAD(2H) within the same turn of the cycle. SCoA, coenzyme A.

Otto S.'s exercise program increases his rate of ATP use and his rate of fuel oxidation in the TCA cycle. The TCA cycle generates NADH and FAD(2H), and the electron-transport chain transfers electrons from NADH and FAD(2H) to O_2, thereby creating the electrochemical potential that drives ATP synthesis from ADP. As ATP is used in the cell, the rate of the electron-transport chain increases. The TCA cycle and other fuel oxidative pathways respond by increasing their rates of NADH and FAD(2H) production.

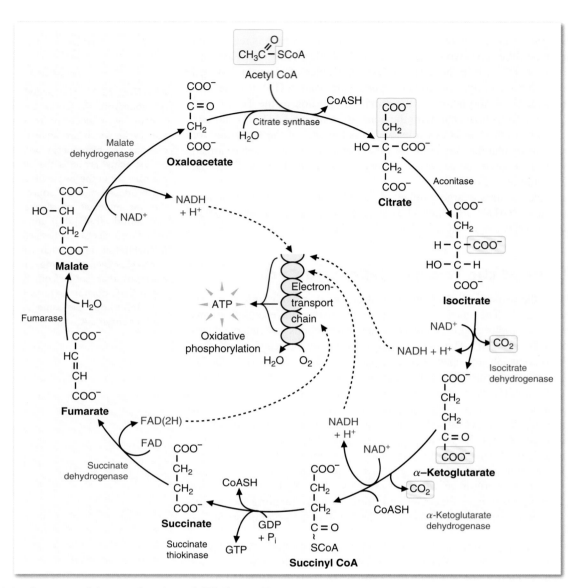

FIGURE 23.3 Reactions of the tricarboxylic acid (TCA) cycle. The oxidation–reduction enzymes and coenzymes are shown in *red*. Entry of the two carbons of acetyl coenzyme A (acetyl-CoA) into the TCA cycle are indicated with the *green box*. The carbons released as CO_2 are shown with *yellow boxes*. *ATP*, adenosine triphosphate; *CoASH*, coenzyme A; *FAD*, flavin adenine dinucleotide; *GDP*, guanosine diphosphate; *GTP*, guanosine triphosphate; *NAD*, nicotinamide adenine dinucleotide; *Pi*, inorganic phosphate; *SCoA*, coenzyme A.

In the next step of the TCA cycle, the hydroxyl (alcohol) group of citrate is moved to an adjacent carbon so that it can be oxidized to form a keto group. The isomerization of citrate to isocitrate is catalyzed by the enzyme aconitase, which is named for an intermediate of the reaction. The enzyme isocitrate dehydrogenase catalyzes the oxidation of the alcohol group and the subsequent cleavage of the carboxyl group to release CO_2 (an oxidation followed by a decarboxylation), forming α-ketoglutarate.

B. α-Ketoglutarate to Succinyl Coenzyme A

The next step of the TCA cycle is the oxidative decarboxylation of α-ketoglutarate to succinyl-CoA, catalyzed by the α-ketoglutarate dehydrogenase complex (see Fig. 23.3). The dehydrogenase complex contains the coenzymes TPP, lipoic acid, and FAD.

In this reaction, one of the carboxyl groups of α-ketoglutarate is released as CO_2, and the adjacent keto group is oxidized to the level of an acid, which then combines with the sulfhydryl group of coenzyme A (CoASH) to form succinyl-CoA (see Fig. 23.3). Energy from the reaction is conserved principally in the reduction state of NADH, with a smaller amount present in the high-energy thioester bond of succinyl-CoA.

C. Generation of Guanosine Triphosphate

Energy from the succinyl-CoA thioester bond is used to generate GTP from guanosine diphosphate (GDP) and inorganic phosphate (P_i) in the reaction catalyzed by succinate thiokinase (also known as *succinyl-CoA synthetase*, for the reverse reaction) (see Fig. 23.3). This reaction is an example of substrate-level phosphorylation. By definition, *substrate-level phosphorylation* is the formation of a high-energy phosphate bond where none previously existed without the use of molecular O_2 (in other words, *not* oxidative phosphorylation). The high-energy phosphate bond of GTP is energetically equivalent to that of ATP and can be used directly for energy-requiring reactions like protein synthesis.

D. Oxidation of Succinate to Oxaloacetate

Up to this stage of the TCA cycle, two carbons have been stripped of their available electrons and released as CO_2. Two pairs of these electrons have been transferred to two NAD^+, and one GTP has been generated. However, two additional pairs of electrons arising from acetyl-CoA still remain in the TCA cycle as part of succinate. The remaining steps of the TCA cycle transfer these two pairs of electrons to FAD and NAD^+ and add H_2O, thereby regenerating oxaloacetate.

The sequence of reactions converting succinate to oxaloacetate begins with the oxidation of succinate to fumarate (see Fig. 23.3). Single electrons are transferred from the two adjacent $-CH_2-$ methylene groups of succinate to an FAD bound to succinate dehydrogenase, thereby forming the double bond of fumarate. From the reduced enzyme-bound FAD, the electrons are passed into the ETC. A hydroxyl group and a proton from water add to the double bond of fumarate, converting it to malate. In the last reaction of the TCA cycle, the alcohol group of malate is oxidized to a keto group through the donation of electrons to NAD^+.

With regeneration of oxaloacetate, the TCA cycle is complete; the chemical bond energy, carbon, and electrons donated by the acetyl group have been converted to CO_2, NADH, FAD(2H), GTP, and heat.

The succinate-to-oxaloacetate sequence of reactions—oxidation through formation of a double bond, addition of water to the double bond, and oxidation of the resultant alcohol to a ketone—is found in many oxidative pathways in the cell, such as the pathways for the oxidation of fatty acids and oxidation of the branched-chain amino acids.

III. Coenzymes of the Tricarboxylic Acid Cycle

The enzymes of the TCA cycle rely heavily on coenzymes for their catalytic function. Isocitrate dehydrogenase and malate dehydrogenase use NAD^+ as a coenzyme, and succinate dehydrogenase uses FAD. Citrate synthase catalyzes a reaction that uses a CoA derivative, acetyl-CoA. The α-ketoglutarate dehydrogenase complex uses TPP, lipoate, and FAD as bound coenzymes, and NAD^+ and CoASH are used as substrates. Each of these coenzymes has unique structural features that enable it to fulfill its role in the TCA cycle.

A. Flavin Adenine Dinucleotide and Nicotinamide Adenine Dinucleotide

Both FAD and NAD^+ are electron-accepting coenzymes. Why is FAD used in some reactions and NAD^+ in others? Their unique structural features enable FAD and

Q From Figure 23.3, which enzymes in the TCA cycle release CO_2? How many moles of oxaloacetate are consumed in the TCA cycle for each mole of CO_2 produced?

 Ann R. has been malnourished for some time and has developed subclinical deficiencies of many vitamins, including riboflavin. The coenzymes FAD and FMN are synthesized from the vitamin riboflavin. Riboflavin is actively transported into cells, where the enzyme flavokinase adds a phosphate to form FMN. FAD synthetase then adds AMP to form FAD. FAD is the major coenzyme in tissues and is generally found tightly bound to proteins, with about 10% being covalently bound. Its turnover in the body is very slow, and people can live for long periods on low intakes without displaying any signs of a riboflavin deficiency.

A Isocitrate dehydrogenase releases the first CO_2, and α-ketoglutarate dehydrogenase releases the second CO_2. There is no net consumption of oxaloacetate in the TCA cycle—the first step uses an oxaloacetate, and the last step produces one. The use and regeneration of oxaloacetate is the "cycle" part of the TCA cycle.

Q One of **Otto S.'s** tennis partners told him that he had heard about a health food designed for athletes that contained succinate. The advertisement made the claim that succinate would provide an excellent source of energy during exercise because it could be metabolized directly without oxygen. Do you see anything wrong with this statement?

NAD^+ to act as electron acceptors in different types of reactions and to play different physiologic roles in the cell. FAD is able to accept single electrons (H•) and forms a half-reduced single-electron intermediate (Fig. 23.4). It thus participates in reactions in which single electrons are transferred independently from two different atoms, which occurs in double-bond formation (e.g., succinate to fumarate) and disulfide bond formation (e.g., lipoate to lipoate disulfide in the α-ketoglutarate dehydrogenase reaction). In contrast, NAD^+ accepts a pair of electrons as the hydride ion (H^-), which is attracted to the carbon opposite the positively charged pyridine ring (Fig. 23.5). This occurs, for example, in the oxidation of alcohols to ketones by malate dehydrogenase and isocitrate dehydrogenase. The nicotinamide ring accepts a hydride ion from the C−H bond, and the alcoholic hydrogen is released into the medium as a positively charged proton, H^+.

The free-radical, single-electron forms of FAD are very reactive, and FADH can lose its electron through exposure to water or the initiation of chain reactions. As a consequence, FAD must remain very tightly, sometimes covalently, attached to its enzyme while it accepts and transfers electrons to another group bound on the enzyme. Because FAD interacts with many functional groups on amino acid side chains in the active site, the $E^{0'}$ for enzyme-bound FAD varies greatly and can be greater or much less than that of NAD^+. In contrast, NAD^+ and NADH are more like substrate and product than coenzymes.

NADH plays a regulatory role in balancing energy metabolism that FAD(2H) cannot because FAD(2H) remains attached to its enzyme. Free NAD^+ binds to a dehydrogenase and is reduced to NADH, which is then released into the medium, where it can bind and inhibit a different dehydrogenase. Consequently, oxidative enzymes are controlled by the NADH/NAD^+ ratio and do not generate NADH faster than it can be reoxidized in the ETC. The regulation of the TCA cycle and other

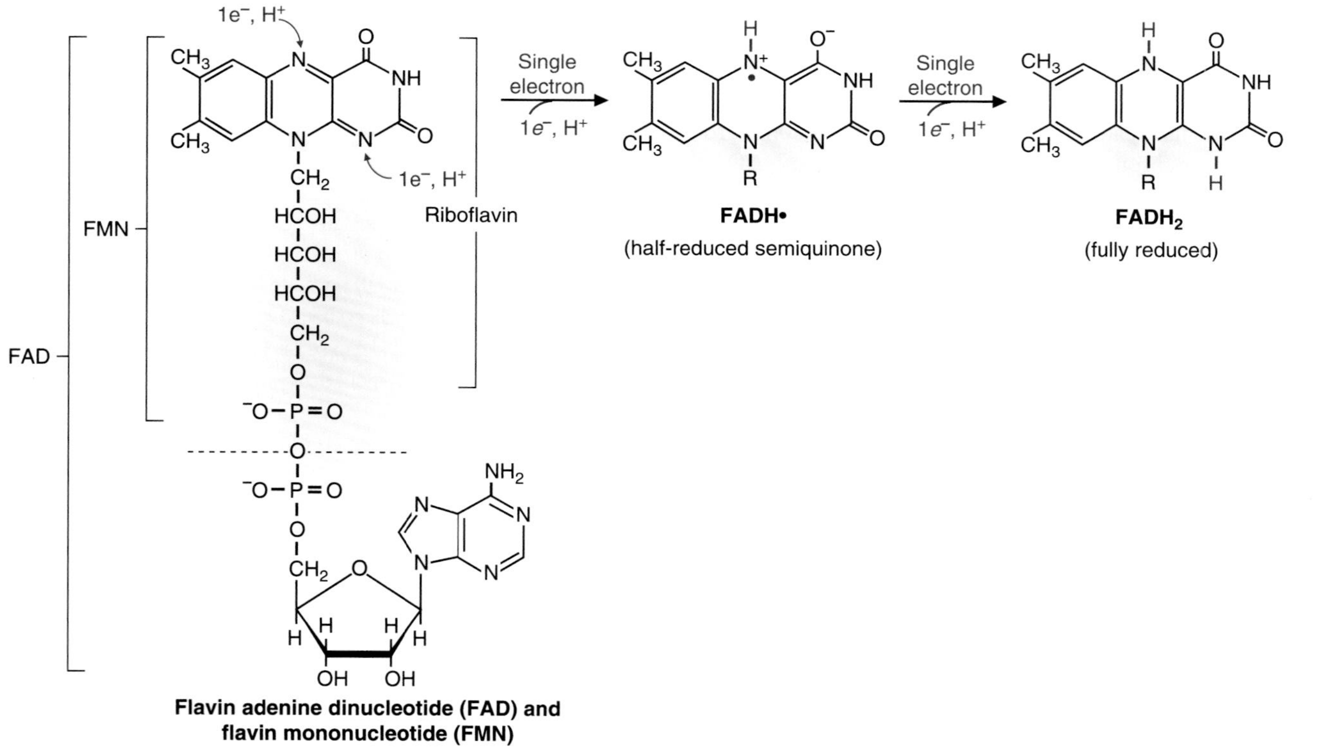

FIGURE 23.4 One-electron steps in the reduction of flavin adenine dinucleotide (FAD). When FAD and flavin mononucleotide (FMN) accept single electrons (e), they are converted to the half-reduced *semiquinone*, a semistable free-radical form. They can also accept two electrons to form the fully reduced form, FADH$_2$. However, in most dehydrogenases, FADH$_2$ is never formed. Instead, the first electron is shared with a group on the protein as the next electron is transferred. Therefore, in this text, overall acceptance of two electrons by FAD has been denoted by the more general abbreviation *FAD(2H)*.

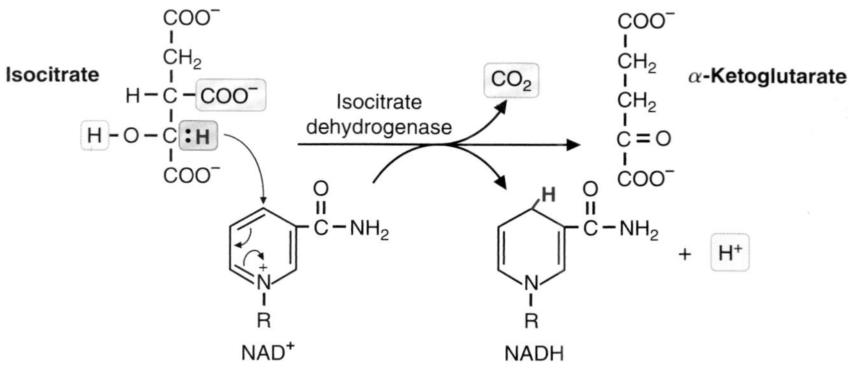

Isocitrate $\qquad$ **α-Ketoglutarate**

Isocitrate dehydrogenase

CO_2

$+$ H^+

NAD^+ $\qquad$ $NADH$

FIGURE 23.5 Oxidation and decarboxylation of isocitrate. The alcohol group (C—OH) is oxidized to a ketone, with the C—H electrons donated to nicotinamide adenine dinucleotide (NAD$^+$) as the hydride ion. Subsequent electron shifts in the pyridine ring remove the positive charge. The H of the —OH group dissociates into water as a proton, H$^+$. NAD$^+$, the electron acceptor, is reduced.

pathways of fuel oxidation by the NADH/NAD$^+$ ratio is part of the mechanism for coordinating the rate of fuel oxidation to the rate of ATP use.

B. Role of Coenzyme A in the Tricarboxylic Acid Cycle

CoASH, the acylation coenzyme, participates in reactions through the formation of a thioester bond between the sulfur (S) of CoASH and an acyl group (e.g., acetyl-CoA, succinyl-CoA) (Fig. 23.6). The complete structure of CoASH and its vitamin precursor, pantothenate, is shown in Figure 8.9A. A thioester bond differs from a typical oxygen ester bond because sulfur, unlike oxygen, does not share its electrons and participate in resonance formations. One of the consequences of this feature of sulfur chemistry is that the carbonyl carbon, the α-carbon, and the β-carbon of the acyl group in a CoA thioester can be activated for participation in different types of reactions (e.g., in the citrate synthase reaction, the α-carbon methyl group is activated for condensation with oxaloacetate; see Figs. 23.3 and 23.6A). Another consequence is that the thioester bond is a high-energy bond that has a large negative $\Delta G^{0\prime}$ of hydrolysis (approximately -13 kcal/mol).

A

$CH_3 - C{\sim}SCoA$
Acetyl CoA

OAA $\qquad$ HS-CoA

Citrate synthase

$HO - C - CH_2 - C - O^-$

Citrate

B

$^-O - C - CH_2 - CH_2 - C{\sim}SCoA$
Succinyl CoA

GDP $\qquad$ GTP

P$_i$ $\qquad$ CoASH

$^-O - C - CH_2 - CH_2 - C - O^-$
Succinate

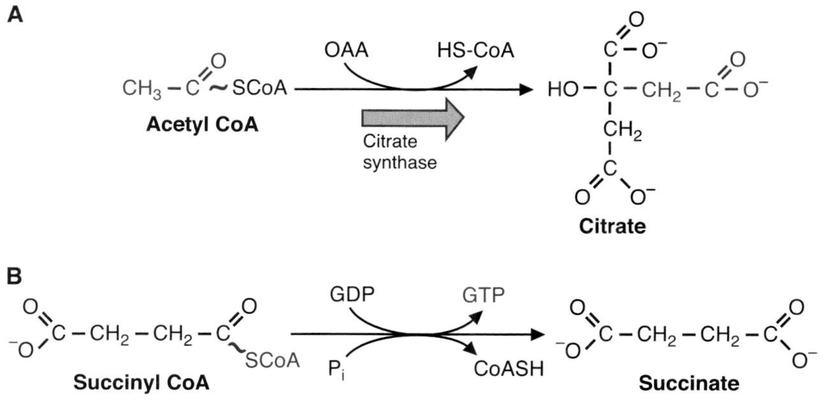

FIGURE 23.6 Use of the high-energy thioester bond of acyl coenzyme As. Energy transformations are shown in *red*. **A.** The energy released by hydrolysis of the thioester bond of acetyl coenzyme A in the citrate synthase reaction contributes a large negative $\Delta G^{0\prime}$ to the forward direction of the tricarboxylic acid cycle. **B.** The energy of the succinyl coenzyme A thioester bond is used for the synthesis of the high-energy phosphate bond of guanosine triphosphate (GTP). *CoASH*, coenzyme A; *GDP*, guanosine diphosphate; *OAA*, oxaloacetate; *P$_i$*, inorganic phosphate; *SCoA*, coenzyme A.

 The claim that succinate oxidation can produce energy without oxygen is wrong. It is probably based on the fact that succinate is oxidized to fumarate by the donation of electrons to FAD. However, ATP can be generated from this process only when these electrons are donated to oxygen in the ETC. The energy generated by the electron-transport chain is used for ATP synthesis in the process of oxidative phosphorylation. After the covalently bound FAD(2H) is oxidized back to FAD by the electron-transport chain, succinate dehydrogenase can oxidize another succinate molecule. If oxygen was not present, the FAD(2H) would remain reduced, and the enzyme could no longer convert succinate to fumarate.

Coenzyme A (CoASH) is synthesized from the vitamin pantothenate in a sequence of reactions that phosphorylate pantothenate, add the sulfhydryl portion of coenzyme A from cysteine, and then add AMP and an additional phosphate group from ATP (see Fig. 8.9A). Pantothenate is widely distributed in foods (*pantos* means "everywhere"), so it is unlikely that **Ann R.** has developed a pantothenate deficiency. Although coenzyme A is required in approximately 100 different reactions in mammalian cells, no Recommended Daily Allowance has been established for pantothenate, in part because indicators have not yet been found that specifically and sensitively reflect a deficiency of this vitamin in humans. The reported symptoms of pantothenate deficiency (fatigue, nausea, and loss of appetite) are characteristic of vitamin deficiencies in general.

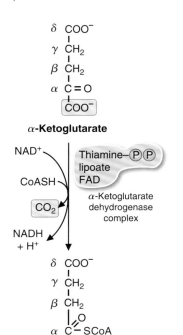

α-Ketoglutarate

Succinyl CoA

FIGURE 23.7 Oxidative decarboxylation of α-ketoglutarate. The α-ketoglutarate dehydrogenase complex oxidizes α-ketoglutarate to succinyl coenzyme A (succinyl CoA). The carboxyl group is released as CO_2. The keto group on the α-carbon is oxidized and then forms the acyl coenzyme A thioester, succinyl-CoA. The α, β, γ, and δ on succinyl-CoA refer to the sequence of atoms in α-ketoglutarate. *CoASH*, coenzyme A; *FAD*, flavin adenine dinucleotide; *NAD*, nicotinamide adenine dinucleotide; *SCoA*, coenzyme A.

Q The $E^{0'}$ for FAD-accepting electrons is −0.219 (see Table 19.4). The $E^{0'}$ for NAD^+ accepting electrons is −0.32. Thus, transfer of electrons from FAD(2H) to NAD^+ is energetically unfavorable. How do the α-keto acid dehydrogenase complexes allow this electron transfer to occur?

The energy from cleavage of the high-energy thioester bonds of succinyl-CoA and acetyl-CoA is used in two different ways in the TCA cycle. When the succinyl-CoA thioester bond is cleaved by succinate thiokinase, the energy is used directly for activating an enzyme-bound phosphate that is transferred to GDP (see Fig. 23.6B). In contrast, when the thioester bond of acetyl-CoA is cleaved in the citrate synthase reaction, the energy is released, giving the reaction a large negative $\Delta G^{0'}$ of −7.7 kcal/mol. The large negative $\Delta G^{0'}$ for citrate formation helps to keep the TCA cycle going in the forward direction.

C. The α-Ketoacid Dehydrogenase Complexes

The *α-ketoglutarate dehydrogenase complex* is one of a three-member family of similar α-keto acid dehydrogenase complexes. The other members of this family are the *PDC* and the *branched-chain amino acid α-keto acid dehydrogenase complex*. Each of these complexes is specific for a different α-keto acid structure. In the sequence of reactions catalyzed by the complexes, the α-keto acid is decarboxylated (i.e., releases the carboxyl group as CO_2) (Fig. 23.7). The keto group is oxidized to the level of a carboxylic acid and then combined with CoASH to form an acyl-CoA thioester (e.g., succinyl-CoA).

All of the α-keto acid dehydrogenase complexes are huge enzyme complexes composed of multiple subunits of three different enzymes, designated as E_1, E_2, and E_3 (Fig. 23.8). E_1 is an α-keto acid decarboxylase that contains TPP; it cleaves off the carboxyl group of the α-keto acid. E_2 is a transacylase-containing lipoate; it transfers the acyl portion of the α-keto acid from thiamin to CoASH. E_3 is dihydrolipoyl dehydrogenase, which contains FAD; it transfers electrons from reduced lipoate to NAD^+. The collection of three enzyme activities into one huge complex enables the product of one enzyme to be transferred to the next enzyme without loss of energy. Complex formation also increases the rate of catalysis because the substrates for E_2 and E_3 remain bound to the enzyme complex.

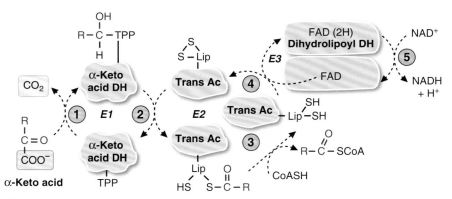

FIGURE 23.8 Mechanism of α-keto acid dehydrogenase complexes (including α-ketoglutarate dehydrogenase, pyruvate dehydrogenase, and the branched-chain α-keto acid dehydrogenase complex). R represents the portion of the α-keto acid that begins with the β-carbon. In α-ketoglutarate, R is CH_2–CH_2–COOH. In pyruvate, R is −CH_3. The individual steps in the oxidative decarboxylation of α-keto acids are catalyzed by three different subunits: E_1, α-keto acid decarboxylase (α-ketoglutarate decarboxylase); E_2, transacylase (*trans*-succinylase); and E_3, dihydrolipoyl dehydrogenase. (*1*) Thiamin pyrophosphate (TPP) on E_1 decarboxylates the α-keto acid and forms a covalent intermediate with the remaining portion. (*2*) The acyl portion of the α-keto acid is transferred by TPP on E_1 to lipoate on E_2, which is a transacylase. (*3*) E_2 transfers the acyl group from lipoate to CoASH. Note how lipoate is reduced during this conversion. The lipoyl disulfide bond has been reduced to sulfhydryl groups (dihydrolipoate). (*4*) E_3, dihydrolipoyl dehydrogenase transfers the electrons from reduced lipoate to its tightly bound FAD molecule, thereby oxidizing lipoate back to its original disulfide form. (*5*) The electrons are then transferred from FAD(2H) to NAD^+ to form NADH. *DH*, dehydrogenase; *FAD*, flavin adenine dinucleotide; *Lip*, lipoate; *NAD*, nicotinamide adenine dinucleotide; *Trans Ac*, transacylase.

1. Thiamin Pyrophosphate in the α-Ketoglutarate Dehydrogenase Complex

TPP is synthesized from the vitamin thiamin by the addition of pyrophosphate (see Fig. 8.8). The pyrophosphate group binds magnesium, which binds to amino acid side chains on the enzyme. This binding is relatively weak for a coenzyme, so thiamin turns over rapidly in the body, and a deficiency can develop rapidly in individuals who are on thiamin-free or low-thiamin diets.

The general function of TPP is the cleavage of a carbon–carbon bond next to a keto group. In the α-ketoglutarate, pyruvate, and branched-chain α-keto acid dehydrogenase complexes, the functional carbon on the thiazole ring forms a covalent bond with the α-keto carbon, thereby cleaving the bond between the α-keto carbon and the adjacent carboxylic acid group (see Fig. 8.8 for the mechanism of this reaction). TPP is also a coenzyme for transketolase in the pentose phosphate pathway, where it similarly cleaves the carbon–carbon bond next to a keto group. In thiamin deficiency, α-ketoglutarate, pyruvate, and other α-keto acids accumulate in the blood.

2. Lipoate

Lipoate is a coenzyme found only in α-keto acid dehydrogenase complexes. It is synthesized in humans from carbohydrate and amino acids, and it does not require a vitamin precursor. Lipoate is attached to the transacylase enzyme through its carboxyl group, which is covalently bound to the terminal $-NH_2$ of a lysine in the protein (Fig. 23.9). At its functional end, lipoate contains a disulfide group that accepts electrons when it binds the acyl fragment of α-ketoglutarate. It can thus act like a long, flexible $-CH_2-$ arm of the enzyme that reaches over to the decarboxylase to pick up the acyl fragment from thiamin and transfer it to the active site containing bound CoASH. It then swings over to dihydrolipoyl dehydrogenase to transfer electrons from the lipoyl sulfhydryl groups to FAD.

3. Flavin Adenine Dinucleotide and Dihydrolipoyl Dehydrogenase

FAD on dihydrolipoyl dehydrogenase accepts electrons from the lipoyl sulfhydryl groups and transfers them to bound NAD^+. FAD thus accepts and transfers electrons

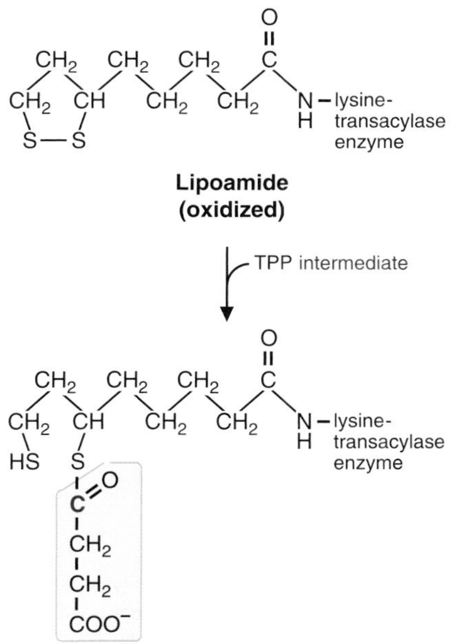

The $E^{0'}$ values were calculated in a test tube under standard conditions. When FAD is bound to an enzyme, as it is in the α-keto acid dehydrogenase complexes, amino acid side chains can alter its $E^{0'}$ value. Thus, the transfer of electrons from the bound FAD(2H) to NAD^+ in dihydrolipoyl dehydrogenase is actually energetically favorable.

In **Al M.'s** heart failure, which is caused by a dietary deficiency of the vitamin thiamin, pyruvate dehydrogenase, α-ketoglutarate dehydrogenase, and the branched-chain α-keto acid dehydrogenase complexes are less functional than normal. Because heart muscle, skeletal muscle, and nervous tissue have high rates of ATP production from the NADH produced by the oxidation of pyruvate to acetyl-CoA and of acetyl-CoA to CO_2 in the TCA cycle, these tissues present with the most obvious signs of thiamin deficiency.

In Western societies, gross thiamin deficiency is most often associated with alcoholism. The mechanism for active absorption of thiamin is strongly and directly inhibited by alcohol. Subclinical deficiency of thiamin from malnutrition or anorexia may be common in the general population and is usually associated with multiple vitamin deficiencies.

Arsenic poisoning is caused by the presence of a large number of different arsenious compounds that are effective metabolic inhibitors. Acute accidental or intentional arsenic poisoning requires high doses and involves arsenate (AsO_4^{2-}) and arsenite (AsO_3^{2-}). Arsenite, which is 10 times more toxic than arsenate, binds to neighboring sulfhydryl groups, such as those in dihydrolipoate and in nearby cysteine pairs (vicinal) found in α-keto acid dehydrogenase complexes and in succinic dehydrogenase. Arsenate weakly inhibits enzymatic reactions involving phosphate, including the enzyme glyceraldehyde 3-phosphate dehydrogenase in glycolysis (see Chapter 22). Thus, both aerobic and anaerobic ATP production can be inhibited. The low doses of arsenic compounds found in water supplies are a major public health concern but are associated with increased risk of cancer rather than direct toxicity.

FIGURE 23.9 Function of lipoate. Lipoate is attached to the ε-amino group of a lysine side chain of the transacylase enzyme (E_2). The oxidized lipoate disulfide form is reduced as it accepts the acyl group from thiamin pyrophosphate (TPP) attached to E_1. The example shown is for the α-ketoglutarate dehydrogenase complex.

without leaving its binding site on the enzyme. The direction of the reaction is favored by interactions of FAD with groups on the enzyme, which change its reduction potential, and by the overall release of energy from cleavage and oxidation of α-ketoglutarate.

IV. Energetics of the Tricarboxylic Acid Cycle

Like all metabolic pathways, the TCA cycle operates with an overall net negative $\Delta G^{0'}$ (Fig. 23.10). The conversion of substrates to products is, therefore, energetically favorable. However, some of the reactions, such as the malate dehydrogenase reaction, have a positive value.

The net standard free-energy change for the TCA cycle, $\Delta G^{0'}$, can be calculated from the sum of the $\Delta G^{0'}$ values for the individual reactions. The $\Delta G^{0'}$, −13 kcal, is the amount of energy lost as heat. It can be considered the amount of energy spent to ensure that oxidation of the acetyl group to CO_2 goes to completion. This value is surprisingly small. However, oxidation of NADH and FAD(2H) in the ETC helps to make acetyl oxidation more energetically favorable and pulls the TCA cycle forward.

A. Overall Efficiency of the Tricarboxylic Acid Cycle

The reactions of the TCA cycle are extremely efficient in converting energy in the chemical bonds of the acetyl group to other forms. The total amount of energy available from the acetyl group is about 228 kcal/mol (the amount of energy that could be released from complete combustion of 1 mol of acetyl groups to CO_2 in an experimental chamber). The products of the TCA cycle (NADH, FAD[2H], and GTP) contain about 207 kcal (Table 23.1). Thus, the TCA cycle reactions are able to conserve about 90% of the energy available from the oxidation of acetyl-CoA.

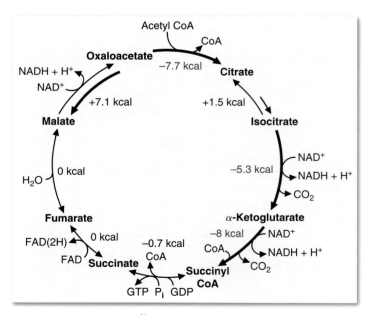

FIGURE 23.10 Approximate $\Delta G^{0'}$ values for the reactions in the tricarboxylic acid cycle, given for the forward direction. The reactions with *large* negative $\Delta G^{0'}$ values are shown in *red*. The standard free-energy change ($\Delta G^{0'}$) refers to the free-energy change for conversion of 1 mol of substrate to 1 mol of product at pH 7.0 under standard conditions. *Acetyl CoA,* acetyl coenzyme A; *FAD,* flavin adenine dinucleotide; *GDP,* guanosine diphosphate; *GTP,* guanosine triphosphate; *NAD,* nicotinamide adenine dinucleotide; *P_i,* inorganic phosphate; *Succinyl CoA,* succinyl coenzyme A.

TABLE 23.1 Energy Yield of the Tricarboxylic Acid Cycle	
kcal/mol	
3 NADH: 3 × 53 =	159
1 FAD(2H) =	41
1 GTP =	7
Sum =	207

FAD, flavin adenine dinucleotide; GTP, guanosine triphosphate; NAD, nicotinamide adenine dinucleotide. The values given for energy yield from NADH and FAD(2H) are based on the equation $\Delta G = -nF\,\Delta E^{0'}$, explained in Chapter 19.

B. Thermodynamically and Kinetically Reversible and Irreversible Reactions

Three reactions in the TCA cycle have large negative values for $\Delta G^{0'}$ that strongly favor the forward direction: the reactions catalyzed by citrate synthase, isocitrate dehydrogenase, and α-ketoglutarate dehydrogenase (see Fig. 23.10). Within the TCA cycle, these reactions are physiologically irreversible for two reasons: The products do not rise to high enough concentrations under physiologic conditions to overcome the large negative $\Delta G^{0'}$ values, and the enzymes involved catalyze the reverse reaction very slowly. These reactions make the major contribution to the overall negative $\Delta G^{0'}$ for the TCA cycle and keep it going in the forward direction.

In contrast to these irreversible reactions, the reactions catalyzed by aconitase and malate dehydrogenase have a positive $\Delta G^{0'}$ for the forward direction and are thermodynamically and kinetically reversible. Because aconitase is rapid in both directions, equilibrium values for the concentration ratio of products to substrates is maintained, and the concentration of citrate is about 23 times that of isocitrate. The accumulation of citrate instead of isocitrate facilitates transport of excess citrate to the cytosol, where it can provide a source of acetyl-CoA for pathways like fatty acid and cholesterol synthesis. It also allows citrate to serve as an inhibitor of citrate synthase when flux through isocitrate dehydrogenase is decreased. Likewise, the equilibrium constant of the malate dehydrogenase reaction favors the accumulation of malate over oxaloacetate, resulting in a low oxaloacetate concentration that is influenced by the NADH/NAD$^+$ ratio. Thus, there is a net flux of oxaloacetate toward malate in the liver during fasting (as a result of fatty acid oxidation, which raises the NADH/NAD$^+$ ratio), and malate can then be transported out of the mitochondria to provide a substrate for gluconeogenesis.

Otto S. had difficulty losing weight because human fuel use is too efficient. His adipose tissue fatty acids are being converted to acetyl-CoA, which is being oxidized in the TCA cycle, thereby generating NADH and FAD(2H). The energy in these compounds is used for ATP synthesis from oxidative phosphorylation. If his fuel use were less efficient and his ATP yield were lower, he would have to oxidize much greater amounts of fat to get the ATP he needs for exercise.

V. Regulation of the Tricarboxylic Acid Cycle

The oxidation of acetyl-CoA in the TCA cycle and the conservation of this energy as NADH and FAD(2H) is essential for generation of ATP in almost all tissues in the body. Despite changes in the supply of fuels, type of fuels in the blood, or rate of ATP use, cells maintain ATP homeostasis (a constant level of ATP). The rate of the TCA cycle, like that of all fuel oxidation pathways, is principally regulated to correspond to the rate of the ETC, which is regulated by the ATP/ADP ratio and the rate of ATP use (see Chapter 24). The major sites of regulation are shown in Figure 23.11.

Two major messengers feed information on the rate of ATP use back to the TCA cycle: (1) the phosphorylation state of ATP, as reflected in ATP and ADP levels; and (2) the reduction state of NAD$^+$, as reflected in the ratio of NADH/NAD$^+$. Within the cell, even within the mitochondrion, the total adenine nucleotide pool (adenosine monophosphate [AMP], ADP, plus ATP) and the total NAD pool (NAD$^+$ plus NADH) are relatively constant. Thus, an increased rate of ATP use results in a small decrease of ATP concentration and an increase of ADP. Likewise, increased NADH oxidation to NAD$^+$ by the ETC increases the rate of pathways that produce NADH. Under normal physiologic conditions, the TCA cycle and other oxidative pathways respond so rapidly to increased ATP demand that the ATP concentration does not significantly change.

As **Otto S.** exercises, his myosin ATPase hydrolyzes ATP to provide the energy for movement of myofibrils. The decrease of ATP and increase of ADP stimulates the electron-transport chain to oxidize more NADH and FAD(2H). The TCA cycle is stimulated to provide more NADH and FAD(2H) to the electron-transport chain. The activation of the TCA cycle occurs through a decrease of the NADH/NAD$^+$ ratio, an increase of ADP concentration, and an increase of Ca^{2+}. Although regulation of the transcription of genes for TCA cycle enzymes is too slow to respond to changes of ATP demands during exercise, the number and size of mitochondria increase during training. Thus, Otto S. is increasing his capacity for fuel oxidation as he trains.

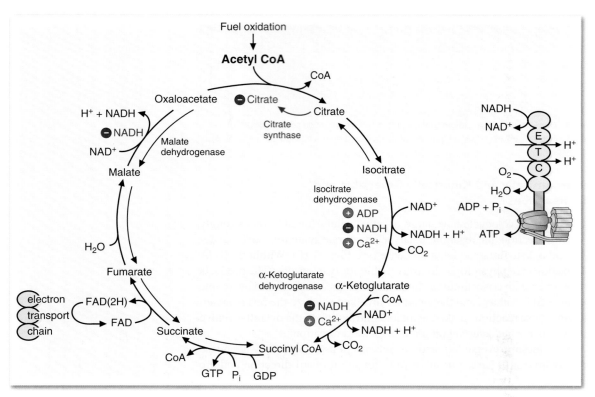

FIGURE 23.11 Major regulatory interactions in the tricarboxylic acid (TCA) cycle. The rate of adenosine triphosphate (ATP) hydrolysis controls the rate of ATP synthesis, which controls the rate of reduced nicotinamide adenine dinucleotide (NADH) oxidation in the electron-transport chain (ETC). All NADH and reduced flavin adenine dinucleotide (FAD[2H]) produced by the cycle donate electrons to this chain (shown on the *right*). Thus, oxidation of acetyl coenzyme A in the TCA cycle can go only as fast as electrons from NADH enter the electron-transport chain, which is controlled by the ATP and adenosine diphosphate (ADP) content of the cells. The ADP and NADH concentrations feed information on the rate of oxidative phosphorylation back to the TCA cycle. Isocitrate dehydrogenase (DH), α-ketoglutarate DH, and malate DH are inhibited by increased NADH concentration. The NADH/NAD$^+$ ratio changes the concentration of oxaloacetate. Citrate is a product inhibitor of citrate synthase. ADP is an allosteric activator of isocitrate DH. During muscular contraction, increased Ca^{2+} concentrations activate isocitrate DH and α-ketoglutarate DH (as well as pyruvate DH). *Acetyl CoA*, acetyl coenzyme A; *GDP*, guanosine diphosphate; *GTP*, guanosine triphosphate; *P$_i$*, inorganic phosphate; *Succinyl CoA*, succinyl coenzyme A.

A. Regulation of Citrate Synthase

Citrate synthase, which is the first enzyme of the TCA cycle, is a simple enzyme that has no allosteric regulators. Its rate is controlled principally by the concentration of oxaloacetate, its substrate, and the concentration of citrate, a product inhibitor, that is competitive with oxaloacetate (see Fig. 23.11). The malate–oxaloacetate equilibrium favors malate, so the oxaloacetate concentration is very low inside the mitochondrion, and is below the apparent K_m (see Chapter 9, Section II.A.1) of citrate synthase. When the NADH/NAD$^+$ ratio decreases, the ratio of oxaloacetate to malate increases. When isocitrate dehydrogenase is activated, the concentration of citrate decreases, thus relieving the product inhibition of citrate synthase. Hence, both increased oxaloacetate and decreased citrate levels regulate the response of citrate synthase to conditions established by the ETC and oxidative phosphorylation. In the liver, the NADH/NAD$^+$ ratio helps determine whether acetyl-CoA enters the TCA cycle or goes into the alternative pathway for ketone body synthesis.

B. Allosteric Regulation of Isocitrate Dehydrogenase

Isocitrate dehydrogenase, which consists of eight subunits, is considered one of the rate-limiting steps of the TCA cycle, and it is allosterically activated by ADP and inhibited by NADH (Fig. 23.12). In the absence of ADP, the enzyme exhibits positive cooperativity; as isocitrate binds to one subunit, other subunits are converted to an active conformation (see Chapter 9, Section III.A, on allosteric enzymes). In the presence of ADP, all of the subunits are in their active conformation, and isocitrate binds more readily. Consequently, the apparent $K_{m,app}$ (the $S_{0.5}$) shifts to a much lower value. Thus, at the concentration of isocitrate found in the mitochondrial matrix, a small change in the concentration of ADP can produce a large change in the rate of the isocitrate dehydrogenase reaction. Small changes in the concentration of the product, NADH, and of the cosubstrate, NAD^+, also affect the rate of the enzyme more than they would a nonallosteric enzyme.

C. Regulation of α-Ketoglutarate Dehydrogenase

The α-ketoglutarate dehydrogenase complex, although not an allosteric enzyme, is product-inhibited by NADH and succinyl-CoA and may also be inhibited by GTP (see Fig. 23.11). Thus, both α-ketoglutarate dehydrogenase and isocitrate dehydrogenase respond directly to changes in the relative levels of ADP and hence the rate at which NADH is oxidized by electron transport. Both of these enzymes are also activated by Ca^{+2}. In contracting heart muscle, and possibly other muscle tissues, the release of Ca^{+2} from the sarcoplasmic reticulum during muscle contraction may provide an additional activation of these enzymes when ATP is being rapidly hydrolyzed.

D. Regulation of Tricarboxylic Acid Cycle Intermediates

Regulation of the TCA cycle serves two functions: It ensures that NADH is generated fast enough to maintain ATP homeostasis, and it regulates the concentration of TCA cycle intermediates. For example, in the liver, a decreased rate of isocitrate dehydrogenase increases citrate concentration, which stimulates citrate efflux to the cytosol. In the cytosol, citrate can act as an inhibitor of PFK-1 as well as activating fatty acid synthesis and providing a substrate for fatty acid synthesis (see Chapter 31). Citrate efflux from the mitochondria sends the message that energy levels are high within the mitochondria. Several regulatory interactions occur in the TCA cycle, in addition to those mentioned previously, that control the levels of TCA intermediates and their flux into pathways that adjoin the TCA cycle.

VI. Precursors of Acetyl Coenzyme A

Compounds enter the TCA cycle as acetyl-CoA or as an intermediate that can be converted to malate or oxaloacetate. Compounds that enter as acetyl-CoA are oxidized to CO_2. Compounds that enter as TCA cycle intermediates replenish intermediates that have been used in biosynthetic pathways, such as gluconeogenesis or heme synthesis, but cannot be fully oxidized to CO_2.

A. Sources of Acetyl Coenzyme A

Acetyl-CoA serves as a common point of convergence for the major pathways of fuel oxidation. It is generated directly from the β-oxidation of fatty acids and degradation of the ketone bodies β-hydroxybutyrate and acetoacetate (Fig. 23.13). It is also formed from acetate, which can arise from the diet or from ethanol oxidation. Glucose and other carbohydrates enter glycolysis, a pathway common to all cells, and are oxidized to pyruvate. The amino acids alanine and serine are also converted to pyruvate. Pyruvate is oxidized to acetyl-CoA by the PDC complex. Several amino acids, such as leucine and isoleucine, are also oxidized to acetyl-CoA. Thus, the final oxidation of acetyl-CoA to CO_2 in the TCA cycle is the last step in all the major pathways of fuel oxidation.

B. Pyruvate Dehydrogenase Complex

The PDC oxidizes pyruvate to acetyl-CoA, thus linking glycolysis and the TCA cycle. In the brain, which is dependent on the oxidation of glucose to CO_2 to fulfill its ATP needs, regulation of the PDC is a life-and-death matter.

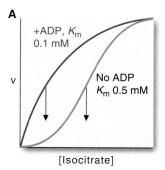

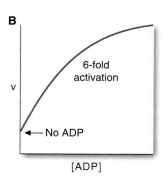

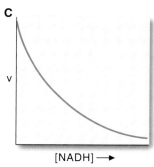

FIGURE 23.12 Allosteric regulation of isocitrate dehydrogenase. Isocitrate, nicotinamide adenine dinucleotide (NAD^+), and NADH bind in the active site; adenosine diphosphate (ADP) and Ca^{2+} are activators and bind to separate allosteric sites. **A.** A graph of velocity versus isocitrate concentration shows positive cooperativity (sigmoid curve) in the absence of ADP. The allosteric activator ADP changes the curve into one closer to a rectangular hyperbola, and decreases the K_m ($S_{0.5}$) for isocitrate. **B.** The allosteric activation by ADP is not an all-or-nothing response. The extent of activation by ADP depends on its concentration. **C.** Increases in the concentration of product, NADH, decrease the velocity of the enzyme through effects on the allosteric activation.

Deficiencies of the PDC, although rare, are among the most common inherited diseases leading to lactic acidemia and, similar to pyruvate carboxylase deficiency, are grouped into the category of Leigh disease (subacute necrotizing encephalopathy). When PDC is defective, pyruvate will accumulate and ATP production will drop. The low ATP will stimulate glycolysis (see Chapter 22) to proceed anaerobically, and to do so, pyruvate is reduced to lactate. In its severe form, PDC deficiency presents with overwhelming lactic acidosis at birth, with death in the neonatal period. In a second form of presentation, the lactic acidemia is moderate, but there is profound psychomotor disability with increasing age. In many cases, concomitant damage to the brainstem and basal ganglia lead to death in infancy. The neurologic symptoms arise because the brain has a very limited ability to use fatty acids as a fuel and is, therefore, dependent on glucose metabolism for its energy supply.

The most common PDC genetic defects are in the gene for the α-subunit of E_1. The E_1 α-gene is X-linked. Because of its importance in central nervous system metabolism, pyruvate dehydrogenase deficiency is a problem in both males and females, even if the female is a carrier. For this reason, it is classified as an X-linked dominant disorder.

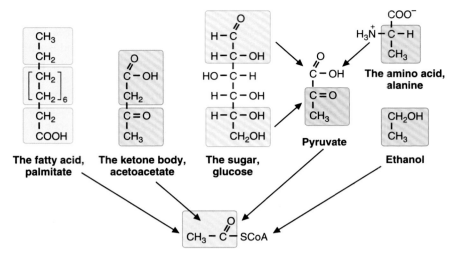

FIGURE 23.13 Origin of the acetyl group from various fuels. Acetyl coenzyme A (acetyl-CoA) is derived from the oxidation of fuels. The portions of fatty acids, ketone bodies, glucose, pyruvate, the amino acid alanine, and ethanol that are converted to the acetyl group of acetyl-CoA are shown in *boxes*. SCoA, coenzyme A.

I. Structure of the Pyruvate Dehydrogenase Complex

The PDC belongs to the α-ketoacid dehydrogenase complex family and thus shares structural and catalytic features with the α-ketoglutarate dehydrogenase complex and the branched-chain α-ketoacid dehydrogenase complex (Fig. 23.14). It contains the same three basic types of catalytic subunits: (1) pyruvate decarboxylase subunits that bind TPP (E_1), (2) transacetylase subunits that bind lipoate (E_2), and (3) dihydrolipoyl dehydrogenase subunits that bind FAD (E_3) (see Fig. 23.8). Although the E_1 and E_2 enzymes in PDC are relatively specific for pyruvate, the same dihydrolipoyl dehydrogenase participates in all of the α-ketoacid dehydrogenase complexes. In addition to these three types of subunits, the PDC complex contains one additional subunit, an E_3-binding protein (E_3BP). Each functional component of the PDC complex is present in multiple copies (e.g., bovine heart PDC has 30 subunits of E_1, 60 subunits of E_2, and 6 subunits each of E_3 and E_3BP). The E_1 enzyme is itself a tetramer of two different types of subunits, α and β.

2. Regulation of the Pyruvate Dehydrogenase Complex

PDC activity is controlled principally through phosphorylation by pyruvate dehydrogenase kinase, which inhibits the enzyme, and dephosphorylation by pyruvate dehydrogenase phosphatase, which activates it (Fig. 23.15). Pyruvate dehydrogenase kinase and pyruvate dehydrogenase phosphatase are regulatory subunits within the PDC complex and act only on the complex. PDC kinase transfers a phosphate from ATP to specific serine hydroxyl (Ser-OH) groups on pyruvate decarboxylase (E_1). PDC phosphatase removes these phosphate groups by hydrolysis. Phosphorylation of just one serine on the PDC E_1 α-subunit can decrease its activity by >99%. PDC kinase is present in complexes as tissue-specific isozymes that vary in their regulatory properties.

PDC kinase is itself inhibited by ADP and pyruvate. Thus, when rapid ATP use results in an increase of ADP, or when activation of glycolysis increases pyruvate levels, PDC kinase is inhibited and PDC remains in an active, nonphosphorylated form. PDC phosphatase requires Ca^{2+} for full activity. In the heart, increased intramitochondrial Ca^{2+} during rapid contraction activates the phosphatase, thereby increasing the amount of active, nonphosphorylated PDC.

PDC is also regulated through inhibition by its products, acetyl-CoA and NADH. This inhibition is stronger than regular product inhibition because their

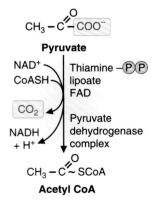

FIGURE 23.14 The pyruvate dehydrogenase complex catalyzes the oxidation of the α-keto acid pyruvate to acetyl coenzyme A. *Acetyl CoA*, acetyl coenzyme A; *CoASH*, coenzyme A; *FAD*, flavin adenine dinucleotide; *NAD*, nicotinamide adenine dinucleotide; *SCoA*, coenzyme A.

binding to PDC stimulates its phosphorylation to the inactive form. The substrates of the enzyme, CoASH and NAD$^+$, antagonize this product inhibition. Thus, when an ample supply of acetyl-CoA for the TCA cycle is already available from fatty acid oxidation, acetyl-CoA and NADH build up and dramatically decrease their own further synthesis by PDC.

PDC can also be activated rapidly through a mechanism involving insulin, which plays a prominent role in adipocytes. In many tissues, insulin may, over time, slowly increase the amount of PDC present.

The rate of other fuel oxidation pathways that feed into the TCA cycle is also increased when ATP use increases. Insulin, other hormones, and diet control the availability of fuels for these oxidative pathways.

3. Pyruvate Dehydrogenase Complex Regulation and Glycolysis

PDC is also regulated principally by the rate of ATP use through rapid phosphorylation to an inactive form (see Fig. 23.15). Thus, in a normally respiring cell, with an adequate supply of oxygen, glycolysis and the TCA cycle are activated together, and glucose can be completely oxidized to carbon dioxide. However, when tissues do not have an adequate supply of oxygen to meet their ATP demands, the increased NADH/NAD$^+$ ratio inhibits pyruvate dehydrogenase, but AMP activates glycolysis. A proportion of the pyruvate is then reduced to lactate to allow glycolysis to continue.

VII. Tricarboxylic Acid Cycle Intermediates and Anaplerotic Reactions

A. Tricarboxylic Acid Cycle Intermediates are Precursors for Biosynthetic Pathways

The intermediates of the TCA cycle serve as precursors for a variety of different pathways present in different cell types (Fig. 23.16). This is particularly important in the central metabolic role of the liver. The TCA cycle in the liver is often called an *open cycle* because there is such a high efflux of intermediates. After a high-carbohydrate meal, citrate efflux and cleavage to acetyl-CoA provides acetyl units for cytosolic fatty acid synthesis. During fasting, gluconeogenic precursors are converted to malate, which leaves the mitochondria for cytosolic gluconeogenesis. The liver also uses TCA cycle intermediates to synthesize carbon skeletons of amino

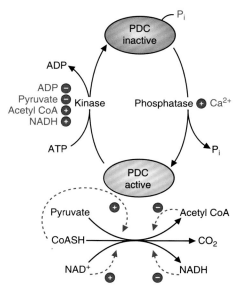

FIGURE 23.15 Regulation of pyruvate dehydrogenase complex (PDC). PDC kinase, a subunit of the enzyme, phosphorylates PDC at a specific serine residue, thereby converting PDC to an inactive form. The kinase is inhibited by adenine diphosphate (ADP) and pyruvate. PDC phosphatase, another subunit of the enzyme, removes the phosphate, thereby activating PDC. The phosphatase is activated by Ca^{2+}. When the substrates pyruvate and coenzyme A (CoASH) are bound to PDC, the kinase activity is inhibited and PDC is active. When the products acetyl coenzyme A and NADH bind to PDC, the kinase activity is stimulated, and the enzyme is phosphorylated to the inactive form. E$_1$ and the kinase exist as tissue-specific isozymes with overlapping tissue specificity and somewhat different regulatory properties. *Acetyl CoA*, acetyl coenzyme A; *ATP*, adenosine triphosphate; *CoASH*, coenzyme A; *NAD*, nicotinamide adenine dinucleotide; *P$_i$*, inorganic phosphate.

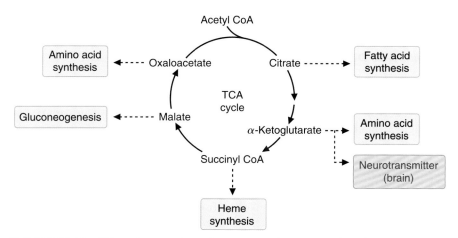

FIGURE 23.16 Efflux of intermediates from the tricarboxylic acid (TCA) cycle. In the liver, TCA cycle intermediates are continuously withdrawn into the pathways of fatty acid synthesis, amino acid synthesis, gluconeogenesis, and heme synthesis. In the brain, α-ketoglutarate is converted to glutamate and γ-aminobutyric acid (GABA), both of which are neurotransmitters. *Acetyl CoA*, acetyl coenzyme A; *Succinyl CoA*, succinyl coenzyme A.

Pyruvate carboxylase deficiency is one of the genetic diseases grouped together under the clinical manifestations of Leigh's disease. In the mild form, the patient presents early in life with delayed development and a mild-to-moderate lactic acidemia (similar to PDC defects, pyruvate will accumulate when pyruvate decarboxylase is defective). Patients who survive have severe intellectual disabilities, and there is a loss of cerebral neurons. In the brain, pyruvate carboxylase is present in the astrocytes, which use TCA cycle intermediates to synthesize glutamine. This pathway is essential for neuronal survival. The major cause of the lactic acidemia is that cells dependent on pyruvate carboxylase for an anaplerotic supply of oxaloacetate cannot oxidize pyruvate in the TCA cycle (because of low oxaloacetate levels), and the liver cannot convert pyruvate to glucose (because the pyruvate carboxylase reaction is required for this pathway to occur), so the excess pyruvate is converted to lactate.

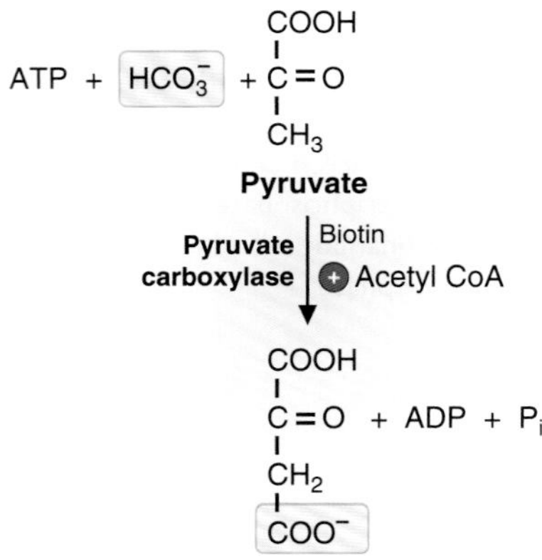

FIGURE 23.17 Pyruvate carboxylase reaction. Pyruvate carboxylase adds a carboxyl group from bicarbonate (which is in equilibrium with CO_2) to pyruvate to form oxaloacetate. Biotin is used to activate and transfer the CO_2. The energy to form the covalent biotin$-CO_2$ complex is provided by the high-energy phosphate bond of adenosine triphosphate (ATP), which is cleaved in the reaction. The enzyme is activated by acetyl coenzyme A. *Acetyl CoA,* acetyl coenzyme A; *ADP,* adenosine diphosphate; P_i, inorganic phosphate.

acids. Succinyl-CoA may be removed from the TCA cycle to form heme in cells of the liver and bone marrow. In the brain, α-ketoglutarate is converted to glutamate and then to γ-aminobutyric acid (GABA), a neurotransmitter. In skeletal muscle, α-ketoglutarate is converted to glutamine, which is transported through the blood to other tissues.

Pyruvate, citrate, α-ketoglutarate and malate, ADP, ATP, and phosphate (as well as many other compounds) have specific transporters in the inner mitochondrial membrane that transport compounds between the mitochondrial matrix and cytosol in exchange for a compound of similar charge. In contrast, CoASH, acetyl-CoA, other CoA derivatives, NAD^+ and NADH, and oxaloacetate are not transported at a metabolically significant rate. To obtain cytosolic acetyl-CoA, many cells transport citrate to the cytosol, where it is cleaved to acetyl-CoA and oxaloacetate by citrate lyase.

B. Anaplerotic Reactions

Removal of any of the intermediates from the TCA cycle removes the four carbons that are used to regenerate oxaloacetate during each turn of the cycle. With depletion of oxaloacetate, it is impossible to continue oxidizing acetyl-CoA. To enable the TCA cycle to keep running, cells have to supply enough four-carbon intermediates from degradation of carbohydrate or certain amino acids to compensate for the rate of removal. Pathways or reactions that replenish the intermediates of the TCA cycle are referred to as *anaplerotic* ("filling up").

1. Pyruvate Carboxylase

Pyruvate carboxylase is one of the major anaplerotic enzymes in the cell. It catalyzes the addition of CO_2 to pyruvate to form oxaloacetate (Fig. 23.17). Like most carboxylases, pyruvate carboxylase contains biotin (a vitamin), which forms a covalent intermediate with CO_2 in a reaction that requires ATP and Mg^{2+} (see Fig. 8.9). The activated CO_2 is then transferred to pyruvate to form the carboxyl group of oxaloacetate.

Pyruvate carboxylase is found in many tissues, such as liver, brain, adipocytes, and fibroblasts, where its function is anaplerotic. Its concentration is high in liver and kidney cortex, where there is a continuous removal of oxaloacetate and malate from the TCA cycle to enter the gluconeogenic pathway.

Pyruvate carboxylase is activated by acetyl-CoA and inhibited by high concentrations of many acyl-CoA derivatives. As the concentration of oxaloacetate is depleted through the efflux of TCA cycle intermediates, the rate of the citrate synthase reaction decreases and acetyl-CoA concentration rises. The acetyl-CoA then activates pyruvate carboxylase to synthesize more oxaloacetate.

2. Amino Acid Degradation

The pathways for oxidation of many amino acids convert their carbon skeletons into five- and four-carbon intermediates of the TCA cycle that can regenerate oxaloacetate (Fig. 23.18). Alanine and serine carbons can enter through pyruvate carboxylase (see Fig. 23.18, circle 1). In all tissues with mitochondria (except for, surprisingly, the liver), oxidation of the two branched-chain amino acids isoleucine and valine to succinyl-CoA forms a major anaplerotic route (see Fig. 23.18, circle 3). In the liver, other compounds forming propionyl-CoA (e.g., methionine, threonine, and odd-chain-length or branched fatty acids) also enter the TCA cycle as succinyl-CoA. In most tissues, glutamine is taken up from the blood, converted to glutamate, and then oxidized to α-ketoglutarate, forming another major anaplerotic route (see Fig. 23.18, circle 2). However, the TCA cycle cannot be resupplied with intermediates of fatty acid oxidation of even-chain-length, or ketone body oxidation, both of which only produce acetyl-CoA. In the TCA cycle, two carbons are lost from citrate before succinyl-CoA is formed, so there is no net conversion of acetyl carbon to oxaloacetate.

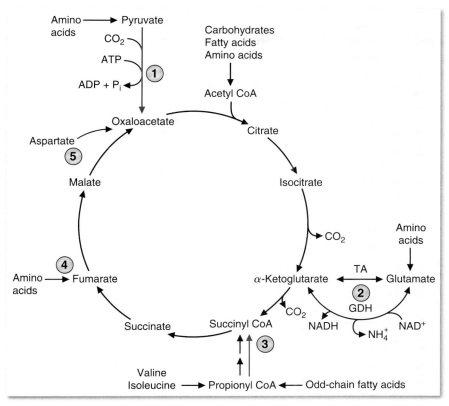

FIGURE 23.18 Major anaplerotic pathways of the tricarboxylic acid (TCA) cycle. (*1*) and (*3*) (*red arrows*) are the two major anaplerotic pathways. (*1*) Pyruvate carboxylase. (*2*) Glutamate is reversibly converted to α-ketoglutarate by transaminases (TA) and glutamate dehydrogenase (GDH) in many tissues. (*3*) The carbon skeletons of valine and isoleucine, a three-carbon unit from odd-chain fatty acid oxidation, and several other compounds enter the TCA cycle at the level of succinyl coenzyme A. Other amino acids are also degraded to fumarate (*4*) and oxaloacetate (*5*), principally in the liver. *Acetyl CoA*, acetyl coenzyme A; *ADP*, adenosine diphosphate; *ATP*, adenosine triphosphate; *NAD*, nicotinamide adenine dinucleotide; P_i, inorganic phosphate. *Propionyl CoA*, propionyl coenzyme A; *Succinyl CoA*, succinyl coenzyme A.

CLINICAL COMMENTS

Otto S. is experiencing the benefits of physical conditioning. A variety of functional adaptations in the heart, lungs, vascular system, and skeletal muscle occur in response to regular graded exercise. The pumping efficiency of the heart increases, allowing greater cardiac output with fewer beats per minute and at a lower rate of oxygen use. The lungs extract a greater percentage of oxygen from the inspired air, allowing fewer respirations per unit of activity. The vasodilatory capacity of the arterial beds in skeletal muscle increases, promoting greater delivery of oxygen and fuels to exercising muscle. Concurrently, the venous drainage capacity in muscle is enhanced, ensuring that lactic acid will not accumulate in contracting tissues. These adaptive changes in physiologic responses are accompanied by increases in the number, size, and activity of skeletal muscle mitochondria, along with the content of TCA cycle enzymes and components of the electron-transport chain. These changes markedly enhance the oxidative capacity of exercising muscle.

In skeletal muscle and other tissues, ATP is generated by anaerobic glycolysis when the rate of aerobic respiration is inadequate to meet the rate of ATP use. Under these circumstances, the rate of pyruvate production exceeds the cell's capacity to oxidize NADH in the electron-transport chain and hence to oxidize pyruvate in the TCA cycle. The excess pyruvate is reduced to lactate. Because lactate is an acid, its accumulation affects the muscle and causes pain and swelling.

Ann R. is experiencing fatigue for several reasons. She has iron-deficiency anemia, which affects iron-containing hemoglobin in her red blood cells, iron in aconitase and succinate dehydrogenase, as well as iron in the heme proteins of the electron-transport chain. She may also be experiencing the consequences of multiple vitamin deficiencies, including thiamin, riboflavin, and niacin (the vitamin precursor of NAD^+). It is less likely, but possible, that she also has subclinical deficiencies of pantothenate (the precursor of coenzyme A) or biotin. As a result, Ann's muscles must use glycolysis as their primary source of energy, which results in sore muscles.

Riboflavin deficiency generally occurs in conjunction with other deficiencies of water-soluble vitamins. The classic deficiency symptoms are *cheilosis* (inflammation of the corners of the mouth), *glossitis* (magenta tongue), and *seborrheic* ("greasy") dermatitis. It is also characterized by sore throat, edema of the pharyngeal and oral mucous membranes, and normochromic, normocytic anemia. However, it is not known whether the glossitis and dermatitis are actually caused by multiple vitamin deficiencies.

Riboflavin has a wide distribution in foods, and small amounts are present as coenzymes in most plant and animal tissues. Eggs, lean meats, milk, broccoli, and enriched breads and cereals are especially good sources. A portion of our niacin requirement can be met by synthesis from tryptophan. Meat (especially red meat), liver, legumes, milk, eggs, alfalfa, cereal grains, yeast, and fish are good sources of niacin and tryptophan.

Beriberi, now known to be caused by thiamin deficiency, was attributed to lack of a nitrogenous component in food by Takaki, a Japanese surgeon, in 1884. In 1890, Eijkman, a Dutch physician working in Java, noted that the polyneuritis associated with beriberi could be prevented by rice bran that had been removed during polishing. Thiamin is present in the bran portion of grains, and it is abundant in pork and legumes. In contrast to most vitamins, milk and milk products, seafood, fruits, and vegetables are *not* good sources of thiamin.

Al M. presents a second time with an alcohol-related high-output form of heart failure from thiamin deficiency that is sometimes referred to as *wet beriberi* or as the *beriberi heart* (see Chapter 9). The word *wet* refers to the fluid retention, which may eventually occur when left ventricular contractility is so compromised that cardiac output, although initially relatively "high," cannot meet the "demands" of the peripheral vascular beds, which have dilated in response to the thiamin deficiency.

The cardiomyopathy is the result of the persistent high output required because of the dilated peripheral vasculature and is also likely related to a reduction in the normal biochemical function of the vitamin thiamin in heart muscle. Inhibition of the α-keto acid dehydrogenase complexes causes accumulation of α-keto acids in heart muscle (and in blood), which may result in a chemically induced cardiomyopathy. Impairment of two other functions of thiamin may also contribute to the cardiomyopathy. TTP serves as the coenzyme for transketolase in the pentose phosphate pathway, and pentose phosphates accumulate in thiamin deficiency. In addition, thiamin triphosphate (a different coenzyme form) may function in Na^+ conductance channels.

Immediate treatment with large doses (50 to 100 mg) of intravenous thiamin may produce a measurable decrease in cardiac output and increase in peripheral vascular resistance as early as 30 minutes after the initial injection. Dietary supplementation of thiamin is not as effective because ethanol consumption interferes with thiamin absorption. Because ethanol also affects the absorption of most water-soluble vitamins, or their conversion to the coenzyme form, **Al M.** was also given a bolus containing a multivitamin supplement.

BIOCHEMICAL COMMENTS

Compartmentation of Mitochondrial Enzymes. The mitochondrion forms a structural, functional, and regulatory compartment within the cell. The inner mitochondrial membrane is impermeable to anions and cations, and compounds can cross the membrane only on specific transport proteins. The enzymes of the TCA cycle, therefore, have more direct access to products of the previous reaction in the pathway than they would if these products were able to diffuse throughout the cell. Complex formation between enzymes also restricts access to pathway intermediates. Malate dehydrogenase and citrate synthase may form a loosely associated complex. The multienzyme pyruvate dehydrogenase and α-ketoglutarate dehydrogenase complexes are examples of substrate channeling by tightly bound enzymes; only the transacylase enzyme has access to the thiamin-bound intermediate of the reaction, and only lipoamide dehydrogenase has access to reduced lipoic acid.

Compartmentation plays an important role in regulation. The close association between the rate of the electron-transport chain and the rate of the TCA cycle is maintained by their mutual access to the same pool of NADH and NAD^+ in the mitochondrial matrix. NAD^+, NADH, CoASH, and acyl-CoA derivatives have no transport proteins and cannot cross the mitochondrial membrane. Thus, all of the dehydrogenases compete for the same NAD^+ molecules and are inhibited when NADH rises. Likewise, accumulation of acyl-CoA derivatives (e.g., acetyl-CoA) within the mitochondrial matrix affects other CoA-using reactions, either by competing at the active site or by limiting CoASH availability.

 Import of Nuclear-Encoded Proteins. All mitochondrial matrix proteins, such as the TCA cycle enzymes, are encoded by the nuclear genome. They are imported into the mitochondrial matrix as unfolded proteins that are pushed and pulled through channels in the outer and inner mitochondrial membranes (Fig. 23.19). Proteins destined for the mitochondrial matrix have either a targeting N-terminal presequence of about 23 amino acids that includes several positively charged amino acid residues, or an internal mitochondrial localizing signal. The mitochondrial matrix proteins are synthesized on free ribosomes in the cytosol and maintain an unfolded conformation by binding to heat-shock protein 70 (hsp 70) chaperonins. This basic presequence binds to a receptor in a *translocase* of the *outer* *membrane* (TOM) complex (see Fig. 23.19, Circle 1). The TOM complexes consist of channel proteins, assembly proteins, and receptor proteins with different specificities (e.g., TOM23 binds the matrix protein presequence). Negatively charged acidic residues on the receptors and in the channel pore assist in translocation of the matrix protein through the channel, presequence first.

The matrix preprotein is translocated across the inner membrane through a *translocases* of the *inner* *membrane* (TIM) complex (see Fig. 23.19, Circle 2). Insertion of the preprotein into the TIM channel is driven by the potential difference across the membrane, $\Delta\Psi$. Mitochondrial hsp 70 (mthsp 70), which is bound to the matrix side of the TIM complex, binds the incoming preprotein and may "ratchet" it through the membrane. ATP is required for binding of mthsp 70 to the TIM complex and again for the subsequent dissociation of the mthsp 70 and the matrix preprotein. In the matrix, the preprotein may require another heat-shock protein, hsp 60, for proper folding. The final step in the import process is cleavage of the signal sequence by a matrix-processing protease (see Fig. 23.19, Circle 3).

Proteins of the inner mitochondrial membrane are imported through a similar process, using TOM and TIM complexes containing different protein components.

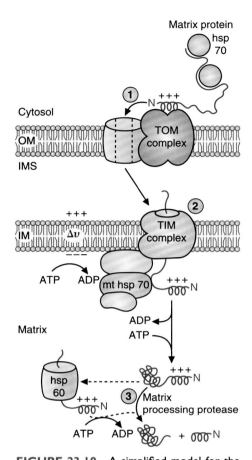

FIGURE 23.19 A simplified model for the import of nuclear-encoded proteins into the mitochondrial matrix. The matrix preprotein with its positively charged N-terminal presequence is shown in *red*. *ADP*, adenosine diphosphate; *ATP*, adenosine triphosphate; *hsp*, heat-shock protein; *OM*, outer mitochondrial membrane; *IMS*, intermembrane space; *IM*, inner mitochondrial membrane; *TOM*, translocases of the outer mitochondrial membrane; *TIM*, translocases of the inner mitochondrial membrane; *mthsp 70*, mitochondrial heat-shock protein 70.

KEY CONCEPTS

- The tricarboxylic acid (TCA) cycle accounts for more than two-thirds of the adenosine triphosphate (ATP) generated from fuel oxidation.
- All of the enzymes required for the TCA cycle are in the mitochondria.
- Acetyl coenzyme A (acetyl-CoA), generated from fuel oxidation, is the substrate for the TCA cycle.
- Acetyl-CoA, when oxidized via the cycle, generates CO_2, reduced electron carriers, and guanosine triphosphate.
- The reduced electron carriers (NADH, FAD[2H]) donate electrons to O_2 via the electron-transport chain, which leads to ATP generation from oxidative phosphorylation.

- The cycle requires several cofactors to function properly, some of which are derived from vitamins. These include thiamin pyrophosphate (derived from vitamin B_1), flavin adenine dinucleotide (derived from vitamin B_2, riboflavin), and coenzyme A (derived from pantothenic acid).
- Intermediates of the TCA cycle are used for many biosynthetic reactions and are replaced by anaplerotic (refilling) reactions within the cell.
- The cycle is carefully regulated within the mitochondria by energy and the levels of reduced electron carriers. As energy levels decrease, the rate of the cycle increases.
- Impaired functioning of the TCA cycle leads to an inability to generate ATP from fuel oxidation and an accumulation of TCA cycle precursors.
- Diseases discussed in this chapter are summarized in Table 23.2.

TABLE 23.2 **Diseases Discussed in Chapter 23**		
DISEASE OR DISORDER	**ENVIRONMENTAL OR GENETIC**	**COMMENTS**
Obesity	Both	Increased physical activity, without increasing caloric intake, will lead to weight loss and increased exercise capacity. One effect of increased aerobic exercise is increasing the number and size of mitochondria in the muscle cells.
Anorexia nervosa	Both	Patients who have been malnourished for some time may exhibit subclinical deficiencies in many vitamins, including riboflavin and niacin, factors required for energy generation.
Congestive heart failure linked to alcoholism	Both	Thiamin deficiency, brought about by chronic alcohol ingestion, leads to dilation of the blood vessels, inefficient energy production by the heart, and failure to adequately pump blood throughout the body. The vitamin B_1 deficiency reduces the activity of pyruvate dehydrogenase and the tricarboxylic acid cycle, severely restricting adenosine triphosphate generation.
Arsenic poisoning	Environmental	Arsenite inhibits enzymes and cofactors with free adjacent sulfhydryl groups (lipoic acid is a target of arsenite), whereas arsenate acts as a phosphate analog and inhibits substrate-level phosphorylation reactions.
Leigh disease (subacute necrotizing encephalopathy)	Genetic	Deficiencies of the pyruvate dehydrogenase complex (PDC), as well as of pyruvate carboxylase, are inherited disorders leading to lactic acidemia. In its most severe form, PDC deficiency presents with overwhelming lactic acidosis at birth, with death in the neonatal period. Even in less severe forms, neurologic symptoms arise because of the brain's dependence on glucose metabolism for energy. The most common PDC deficiency is X-linked, in the α-subunit of the pyruvate decarboxylase (E_1) subunit. Pyruvate carboxylase deficiency also leads to intellectual disability.

REVIEW QUESTIONS—CHAPTER 23

1. An individual displays lactic acidemia as well as a reduced activity of α-ketoglutarate dehydrogenase activity. The most likely single enzymatic mutation that leads to these changes would be in which one of the following proteins?
   A. The E_3 subunit of pyruvate dehydrogenase
   B. The E_1 subunit of pyruvate dehydrogenase
   C. The E_2 subunit of pyruvate dehydrogenase
   D. Lactate dehydrogenase
   E. Pyruvate carboxylase

2. A patient diagnosed with thiamin deficiency exhibited fatigue and muscle cramps. The muscle cramps have been related to an accumulation of metabolic acids. Which one of the following metabolic acids is most likely to accumulate in a thiamin deficiency?
   A. Isocitric acid
   B. Pyruvic acid
   C. Succinic acid
   D. Malic acid
   E. Oxaloacetic acid

3. Succinate dehydrogenase differs from all other enzymes in the TCA cycle in that it is the only enzyme that displays which one of the following characteristics?
   A. It is embedded in the inner mitochondrial membrane.
   B. It is inhibited by NADH.
   C. It contains bound FAD.
   D. It contains Fe–S centers.
   E. It is regulated by a kinase.

4. During exercise, stimulation of the TCA cycle results principally from which one of the following?
   A. Allosteric activation of isocitrate dehydrogenase by increased NADH
   B. Allosteric activation of fumarase by increased ADP
   C. A rapid decrease in the concentration of four-carbon intermediates
   D. Product inhibition of citrate synthase
   E. Stimulation of the flux through several enzymes by a decreased NADH/NAD$^+$ ratio

5. A deficiency of which one of the following compounds would lead to an inability to produce coenzyme A?
   A. Niacin
   B. Riboflavin
   C. Vitamin A
   D. Pantothenate
   E. Vitamin C

6. One of the major roles of the TCA cycle is to generate reduced cofactors for ATP production from oxidative phosphorylation. The compound donating the net eight electrons to the cofactors is which one of the following?
   A. Pyruvate
   B. Acetyl-CoA
   C. Lactate
   D. Oxaloacetate
   E. Phosphoenolpyruvate

7. Atherosclerosis can narrow the coronary arteries, leading to decreased blood flow and hypoxia of cardiac cells (cardiomyocytes). This causes the patient to experience angina. Which one of the following is likely to occur in the cardiomyocytes during the hypoxic event?
   A. The TCA cycle in the cytosol is greatly impaired.
   B. Pyruvate oxidation is increased.
   C. Lactate cannot be used as a fuel.
   D. Citrate accumulates.
   E. Succinyl-CoA accumulates.

8. A distance runner is training for her half marathon and as part of the training is allowing her muscles to use fatty acids as a fuel source. Fatty acids are converted to acetyl-CoA in the mitochondria, at which point the acetyl-CoA can be oxidized in the TCA cycle to generate reduced cofactors. Which one of the following correctly describes how the acetyl-CoA is metabolized in the mitochondria?
   A. One molecule of acetyl-CoA produces two molecules of CO_2, three molecules of NADH, one molecule of FAD(2H) and one molecule of ATP.
   B. All of the energy for high-energy phosphate bonds is derived from oxidative phosphorylation.
   C. NAD$^+$ is the only electron acceptor in the cycle.
   D. Substrate-level phosphorylation generates one high-energy phosphate bond during the cycle.
   E. The TCA cycle requires large amounts of vitamins C and D as coenzymes.

9. At birth, a full-term male neonate was found to be severely acidotic. His condition was found to result from an X-linked dominant mutation of the α-subunit of E_1 in the PDC. Compared with a healthy neonate in the same dietary state, what would be the consequences of this mutation?
   A. An increase in plasma concentrations of lactate and pyruvate
   B. A higher ATP/ADP ratio in cells of the brain
   C. A decrease in the rate of glycolysis in brain cells
   D. An increase in the activity of the electron-transfer chain in brain cells
   E. An increase in plasma acetyl-CoA levels

10. A pyruvate carboxylase deficiency will lead to lactic acidemia because of which one of the following?
    A. An accumulation of acetyl-CoA in the mitochondria
    B. Allosteric activation of lactate dehydrogenase
    C. An accumulation of NADH in the mitochondrial matrix
    D. Allosteric activation of the PDC
    E. An accumulation of ATP in the matrix

1. **The answer is A.** The E_3 subunit of pyruvate dehydrogenase, the dihydrolipoyl dehydrogenase activity (with bound FAD), is shared among all the α-keto acid dehydrogenases. Thus, with this mutation, both pyruvate dehydrogenase activity and α-ketoglutarate dehydrogenase activity would be defective. This defect would then lead to an accumulation of pyruvate (because pyruvate dehydrogenase activity is reduced), and the accumulated pyruvate is converted to lactate (to regenerate NAD^+ to allow glycolysis to continue), leading to an elevation of lactate in the bloodstream and a lowering of blood pH (lactic acidemia). A defect in pyruvate carboxylase will also result in an elevation of pyruvate levels, and lactic acidemia, but there would be no defect in α-ketoglutarate dehydrogenase activity with a pyruvate carboxylase deficiency. The E_1 and E_2 subunits of pyruvate dehydrogenase are unique to pyruvate dehydrogenase, and are not shared with any other enzymes, so defects in these subunits will lead to lactic acidemia but would not affect α-ketoglutarate dehydrogenase. A defect in lactate dehydrogenase would result in an inability to produce lactate, and lactic acidemia would not result from a defect in that enzyme.

2. **The answer is B.** TTP is a required coenzyme for the α-ketoglutarate dehydrogenase and pyruvate dehydrogenase complexes. With these complexes inactive, pyruvic acid and α-ketoglutaric acid accumulate and dissociate to generate the anion and H^+. Because α-ketoglutarate is not listed as an answer, the only possible answer is pyruvate.

3. **The answer is A.** Succinate dehydrogenase is the only TCA cycle enzyme located in the inner mitochondrial membrane. The other enzymes are in the mitochondrial matrix. Answer B is incorrect because succinate dehydrogenase is not regulated by NADH. Answer C is incorrect because α-ketoglutarate dehydrogenase also contains a bound FAD (the difference is that the FAD[2H] in α-ketoglutarate dehydrogenase donates its electrons to NAD^+, whereas the FAD[2H] in succinate dehydrogenase donates its electrons directly to the electron-transfer chain). Answer D is incorrect because both succinate dehydrogenase and aconitase have Fe–S centers. Answer E is incorrect because succinate dehydrogenase is not regulated by a kinase. Kinases regulate enzymes by phosphorylation (e.g., the regulation of pyruvate dehydrogenase occurs through reversible phosphorylation).

4. **The answer is E.** NADH decreases during exercise in order to generate energy for the exercise (if it were increased, it would inhibit the cycle and slow it down); thus, the $NADH/NAD^+$ ratio is decreased, and the lack of NADH activates flux through isocitrate dehydrogenase, α-ketoglutarate dehydrogenase, and malate dehydrogenase. Isocitrate dehydrogenase is inhibited by NADH, so answer A is not correct. Fumarase is not regulated; thus,

answer B is incorrect. The four-carbon intermediates of the cycle are regenerated during each turn of the cycle, so their concentrations do not decrease (thus, C is incorrect). Product inhibition of citrate synthase would slow the cycle and not generate more energy (hence, D is incorrect).

5. **The answer is D.** Pantothenate is the vitamin precursor of coenzyme A. Niacin is the vitamin precursor of NAD, and riboflavin is the vitamin precursor of FAD and FMN. Vitamins A and C are used with only minor modifications, if any, and are not involved in any TCA cycle reactions.

6. **The answer is B.** The net equation of the TCA cycle, in terms of carbon atoms, is that acetyl-CoA is converted to two molecules of CO_2. The eight electrons associated with the two carbon atoms of acetyl-CoA are removed and placed in three molecules of NADH and one molecule of FAD(2H). The TCA cycle does not generate reduced cofactors from pyruvate, lactate, oxaloacetate, or phosphoenolpyruvate. Those compounds would need to be converted to acetyl-CoA in order for the cycle to generate the reduced cofactors.

7. **The answer is C.** With hypoxia, the TCA cycle would slow down because of the accumulation of NADH (which cannot donate electrons to oxygen) caused by the lack of oxygen. The high NADH inhibits pyruvate dehydrogenase, so pyruvate will accumulate, and the high levels of pyruvate will block lactate from being converted to pyruvate (the lactate dehydrogenase reaction), leading to lactate accumulation. Because the operation of the TCA cycle is greatly reduced, citrate and succinyl-CoA will not be produced, so they will not accumulate. The enzymes of the TCA cycle are located in the mitochondria, not in the cytoplasm.

8. **The answer is D.** GTP is generated from substrate-level phosphorylation during the TCA cycle (not ATP). Mitochondrial ATP is generated by oxidative phosphorylation, using the electrons from the electron carriers NADH and FAD(2H). The TCA cycle requires some B vitamins but not vitamins C or D. One molecule of acetyl-CoA (two carbons) produces 2 CO_2, 3 NADH, 1 FAD(2H), and 1 GTP (not ATP).

9. **The answer is A.** A deficiency of the E_1 subunit of pyruvate dehydrogenase would decrease conversion of pyruvate to acetyl-CoA, leading to an accumulation of pyruvate. Pyruvate is converted to lactate to allow glycolysis to continue to generate ATP from substrate-level phosphorylation. The pyruvate to lactate conversion regenerates the NAD^+, which is required for glycolysis to proceed. Cells of the brain have a high ATP requirement and are highly dependent on glycolysis and pyruvate oxidation in the TCA cycle to meet this demand for ATP. Without pyruvate oxidation in the TCA cycle, glycolysis will try to produce ATP as fast as possible (because

of an increase of AMP levels, which activates PFK-1); however, the amount of ATP produced by glycolysis alone is not sufficient to meet the brain's needs. Thus, the ATP/ADP ratio actually decreases. Even though the brain cells are low in ATP levels, the decreased production of acetyl-CoA from pyruvate will not provide sufficient substrate to substantially increase the activity of the electron-transfer chain in brain cells. Fatty acids do not cross the blood–brain barrier, so ketone body oxidation would be required to increase acetyl-CoA levels within the mitochondria to allow rapid functioning of the TCA cycle. Acetyl-CoA is not produced from glucose when pyruvate dehydrogenase is defective, and acetyl-CoA cannot be exported to the circulation.

10. **The answer is A.** When pyruvate carboxylase is deficient, pyruvate cannot be converted to oxaloacetate, thereby reducing the ability to replenish TCA cycle intermediates as they are being used for other pathways. As oxaloacetate levels decrease, acetyl-CoA cannot be converted to citrate, and acetyl-CoA will accumulate within the mitochondria. The elevated acetyl-CoA inhibits pyruvate dehydrogenase, which, coupled with the reduced activity of pyruvate carboxylase, leads to pyruvate accumulation in the cytoplasm. The increased pyruvate is then converted to lactic acid, leading to lactic acidemia. Pyruvate is not an allosteric activator of lactate dehydrogenase. Because the TCA cycle is slowed owing to lack of oxaloacetate, NADH is not accumulating in the mitochondrial matrix, nor is ATP. Pyruvate is not an activator of the pyruvate dehydrogenase complex (NAD^+ and free coenzyme A are the primary activators, along with ADP).

Oxidative Phosphorylation and Mitochondrial Function

Energy from fuel oxidation is converted to the high-energy phosphate bonds of adenosine triphosphate (ATP) by the process of **oxidative phosphorylation**. Most of the energy from oxidation of fuels in the tricarboxylic acid (TCA) cycle and other pathways is conserved in the form of the reduced electron-accepting coenzymes, nicotinamide adenine dinucleotide (NADH) and flavin adenine dinucleotide (FAD[2H]). The **electron-transport chain** (ETC) oxidizes **NADH** and **FAD(2H)** and donates the electrons to O_2, which is reduced to H_2O (Fig. 24.1). Energy from reduction of O_2 is used for phosphorylation of adenosine diphosphate (ADP) to ATP by **ATP synthase** (**F_0F_1-ATPase**). The net yield of oxidative phosphorylation is approximately 2.5 mol of ATP per mole of NADH oxidized, or 1.5 mol of ATP per mole of FAD(2H) oxidized.

Chemiosmotic Model of Adenosine Triphosphate Synthesis. The **chemiosmotic model** explains how energy from transport of electrons to O_2 is transformed into the high-energy phosphate bond of ATP (see Fig. 24.1). Basically, the ETC contains three large **protein complexes** (**I**, **III**, and **IV**) that span the inner mitochondrial membrane. As electrons pass through these complexes in a series of oxidation–reduction reactions, protons are transferred from the mitochondrial matrix to the cytosolic side of the inner mitochondrial membrane. The pumping of protons generates an **electrochemical gradient** (Δp) across the membrane composed of the membrane potential and the proton gradient. ATP synthase contains a proton pore that spans the inner mitochondrial membrane and a catalytic headpiece that protrudes into the matrix. As protons are driven into the matrix through the pore, they change the conformation of the headpiece, which releases ATP from one site and catalyzes formation of ATP from ADP and inorganic phosphate (P_i) at another site.

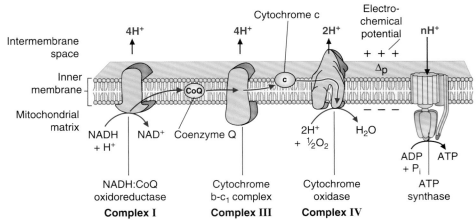

FIGURE 24.1 Oxidative phosphorylation. *Red arrows* show the path of electron transport from nicotinamide adenine dinucleotide (NADH) to O_2. As electrons pass through the chain, protons are pumped from the mitochondrial matrix to the intermembrane space, thereby establishing an electrochemical potential gradient, Δp, across the inner mitochondrial membrane. The positive and negative charges on the membrane denote the membrane potential ($\Delta\psi$). Δp drives protons into the matrix through a pore in ATP synthase, which uses the energy to form adenosine triphosphate (ATP) from adenosine diphosphate (ADP) and inorganic phosphate (P_i). *CoQ*, coenzyme Q.

Deficiencies of Electron Transport. In cells, complete transfer of electrons from NADH and FAD(2H) through the chain to O_2 is necessary for ATP generation. Impaired transfer through any complex can have pathologic consequences. Fatigue can result from iron-deficiency **anemia**, which decreases **Fe** for **Fe–S centers** and **cytochromes**. **Cytochrome c_1 oxidase**, which contains the **O_2-binding site**, is inhibited by **cyanide**. **Mitochondrial DNA** (**mtDNA**), which is maternally inherited, encodes some of the subunits of the ETC complexes and ATP synthase. **OXPHOS diseases** are caused by **mutations** in **nuclear DNA** or **mtDNA** that decrease mitochondrial capacity for oxidative phosphorylation.

Regulation of Oxidative Phosphorylation. The rate of the ETC is **coupled** to the rate of ATP synthesis by the transmembrane electrochemical gradient. As ATP is used for energy-requiring processes and ADP levels increase, proton influx through the ATP synthase pore generates more ATP, and the ETC responds to restore Δp. In **uncoupling**, protons return to the matrix by a mechanism that bypasses the ATP synthase pore, and the energy is released as heat. **Proton leakage**, **chemical uncouplers**, and regulated **uncoupling proteins** increase our metabolic rate and heat generation.

Mitochondria and Cell Death. Although oxidative phosphorylation is a mitochondrial process, most ATP use occurs outside of the mitochondrion. ATP synthesized from oxidative phosphorylation is actively transported from the matrix to the intermembrane space by **adenine nucleotide translocase** (**ANT**). **Porins form voltage-dependent anion channels** (**VDACs**) through the outer mitochondrial membrane for the diffusion of H_2O, ATP metabolites, and other ions. Under certain types of stress, ANT, VDACs, and other proteins form a nonspecific open channel known as the **mitochondrial permeability transition pore**. This pore is associated with events that lead rapidly to **necrotic cell death**.

THE WAITING ROOM

 Cora N. was recovering uneventfully from her heart attack 1 month earlier (see Chapter 20), when she won the Georgia state lottery. When she heard her number announced over the television, she experienced crushing chest pain and grew short of breath. Her family called 911 and she was rushed to the hospital emergency department.

On initial examination, her blood pressure was extremely high and her heart rhythm irregular. Cora is experiencing yet another myocardial infarction. An electrocardiogram showed unequivocal evidence of severe lack of oxygen (ischemia) in the muscles of the anterior and lateral walls of her heart. Life-support measures including nasal oxygen were initiated. An intravenous drip of nitroglycerin, a vasodilating agent, was started in an effort to reduce her hypertension (it will also help to decrease her "preload" by vasodilating the vessels going to the heart). She was also given a β-blocker, which will also help decrease her blood pressure as well as decrease the work of her heart by slowing her heart rate. She also required a small amount of intravenous nitroprusside to help lower her blood pressure. After her blood pressure was well controlled, and because the hospital did not have a cardiac catheterization laboratory and a transfer to a hospital with a cath lab was not possible, a decision was made to administer intravenous tissue plasminogen activator (TPA) in an attempt to break up any intracoronary artery blood clots in vessels supplying the ischemic myocardium (thrombolytic therapy).

Stanley T. A ^{123}I thyroid uptake and scan performed on **Stanley T.** confirmed that his hyperthyroidism was the result of Graves disease (see Chapter 20). *Graves disease*, also known as *diffuse toxic goiter*, is an autoimmune genetic disorder caused by the generation of human thyroid-stimulating immunoglobulins. These immunoglobulins stimulate growth of the thyroid gland (goiter) and excess secretion of the thyroid hormones triiodothyronine (T_3) and tetraiodothyronine (T_4). Because heat production is increased under these circumstances, Mr. T.'s heat intolerance and sweating were growing worse with time.

 Cora N. is experiencing a second myocardial infarction. Ischemia (low blood flow) has caused hypoxia (low levels of oxygen) in the threatened area of her heart muscle, resulting in inadequate generation of ATP for the maintenance of low intracellular Na^+ and Ca^{2+} levels (see Chapter 20). As a consequence, the myocardial cells in that specific location have become swollen and the cytosolic proteins creatine kinase (MB isoform) and troponin (heart isoform) have leaked into the blood. (See **Ann J.**, Chapters 6 and 7).

An electromyogram measures the electrical potential of muscle cells both at rest and while contracting. Electrodes are inserted through the skin and into the muscle, and baseline recordings (no contraction) are obtained, followed by measurements of electrical activity when the muscle contracts. The electrode is retracted a small amount, and the measurements are repeated. This occurs for up to 10 to 20 measurements, thereby sampling, many distinct areas of the muscle. Under normal conditions, muscles at rest will have minimal electrical activity, which increases significantly as the muscle contracts. Electromyograms that deviate from the norm suggest an underlying pathology interfering with membrane polarization–depolarization as the nerve cells instruct the muscle cells to contract.

Charles F., who has a follicular-type non-Hodgkin lymphoma, was being treated with the anthracycline drug doxorubicin (see Chapter 16). During the course of his treatment, he developed biventricular heart failure. Although doxorubicin is a highly effective anticancer agent against a wide variety of human tumors, its clinical use is limited by a specific, cumulative, dose-dependent cardiotoxicity. Impairment of mitochondrial function may play a major role in this toxicity. Doxorubicin binds to cardiolipin, a lipid component of the inner membrane of mitochondria, where it might directly affect components of oxidative phosphorylation. Doxorubicin inhibits succinate oxidation, inactivates cytochrome oxidase, interacts with CoQ, adversely affects ion pumps, and inhibits ATP synthase, resulting in decreased ATP levels and mildly swollen mitochondria. It decreases the ability of the mitochondria to sequester Ca^{2+} and increases free radicals (highly reactive single-electron forms), leading to damage of the mitochondrial membrane (see Chapter 25). It also might affect heart function indirectly through other mechanisms.

Isabel S., an intravenous drug user, appeared to be responding well to her multidrug regimens to treat pulmonary tuberculosis and HIV (see Chapters 12, 13, 14, and 17). In the past 6 weeks, however, she has developed increasing weakness in her extremities to the point that she has difficulty carrying light objects or walking. Physical examination indicates a diffuse proximal and distal muscle weakness associated with muscle atrophy. The muscles are not painful on motion but are mildly tender to palpation. The blood level of the muscle enzymes creatine phosphokinase and aldolase are elevated. An electromyogram revealed a generalized reduction in the muscle action potentials, suggestive of a primary myopathic process. Proton spectroscopy of her brain and upper spinal cord showed no anatomic or biochemical abnormalities. The diffuse and progressive skeletal muscle weakness was out of proportion to that expected from her HIV or tuberculosis. This information led her physicians to consider other etiologies.

I. Oxidative Phosphorylation

Generation of ATP from *oxidative phosphorylation* requires an electron donor (NADH or FAD[2H]), an electron acceptor (O_2), and an intact inner mitochondrial membrane that is impermeable to protons, all the components of the ETC and ATP synthase. It is regulated by the rate of ATP use.

Most cells are dependent on oxidative phosphorylation for ATP homeostasis. During oxygen deprivation from ischemia (low blood flow), an inability to generate energy from the ETC results in increased permeability of this membrane and mitochondrial swelling. Mitochondrial swelling is a key element in the pathogenesis of irreversible cell injury, leading to cell lysis and death (necrosis).

A. Overview of Oxidative Phosphorylation

Our understanding of oxidative phosphorylation is based on the *chemiosmotic hypothesis*, which proposes that the energy for ATP synthesis is provided by an electrochemical gradient across the inner mitochondrial membrane. This electrochemical gradient is generated by the components of the ETC, which pump protons across the inner mitochondrial membrane as they sequentially accept and donate electrons (see Fig. 24.1). The final acceptor is O_2, which is reduced to H_2O.

1. Electron Transfer from NADH to O_2

In the *ETC*, electrons donated by NADH or FAD(2H) are passed sequentially through a series of electron carriers embedded in the inner mitochondrial membrane. Each of the components of the ETC is reduced as it accepts an electron and then oxidized as it passes the electrons to the next member of the chain. From NADH, electrons are transferred sequentially through *NADH:CoQ oxidoreductase* (complex I, also known as *NADH dehydrogenase*), *coenzyme Q* (CoQ), the *cytochrome b–c_1 complex* (complex III), *cytochrome c*, and finally, *cytochrome c oxidase* (complex IV). NADH:CoQ oxidoreductase, the cytochrome b–c_1 complex, and cytochrome c oxidase are multisubunit protein complexes that span the inner mitochondrial membrane. CoQ is a lipid-soluble quinone that is not protein-bound and is free to diffuse in the lipid membrane. It transports electrons from complex I to complex III and is an intrinsic part of the proton pump for each of these complexes. Cytochrome c is a small protein in the intermembrane space that transfers electrons from the b–c_1 complex to cytochrome oxidase. The terminal complex, cytochrome c oxidase, contains the binding site for O_2. As O_2 accepts electrons from the chain, it is reduced to H_2O.

2. The Electrochemical Potential Gradient

At each of the three large membrane-spanning complexes in the chain, electron transfer is accompanied by proton pumping across the membrane. There is an energy drop of approximately 16 kilocalories (kcal) in reduction potential as electrons pass through each of these complexes, which provides the energy required to move protons against a concentration gradient. The membrane is impermeable to protons, so they cannot diffuse through the lipid bilayer back into the matrix. Thus, in actively respiring mitochondria, the intermembrane space and cytosol may be approximately 0.75 pH unit lower than the matrix.

The transmembrane movement of protons generates an electrochemical gradient with two components: the membrane potential (the external face of the membrane is charged positive relative to the matrix side) and the proton gradient (the intermembrane space has a higher proton concentration and is, therefore, more acidic than the matrix) (Fig. 24.2). The electrochemical gradient is sometimes called the *proton motive force* because it is the energy that pushes the protons to reenter the matrix to equilibrate on both sides of the membrane. The protons are attracted to the more negatively charged matrix side of the membrane, where the pH is more alkaline.

3. Adenosine Triphosphate Synthase

ATP synthase (F_0F_1-ATPase), the enzyme that generates ATP, is a multisubunit enzyme that contains an inner membrane portion (F_0) and a stalk and headpiece (F_1) that project into the matrix (Fig. 24.3). The 12 c-subunits in the membrane form a rotor that is attached to a central asymmetric shaft composed of the ε- and γ-subunits. The headpiece is composed of three $\alpha\beta$-subunit pairs. Each β-subunit contains a catalytic site for ATP synthesis. The headpiece is held stationary by a δ-subunit attached to a long b-subunit connected to subunit a in the membrane.

The influx of protons through the proton channel turns the rotor. The proton channel is formed by the c-subunits on one side and the a-subunit on the other side. Although the channel is continuous, it has two offset portions, one portion open directly to the intermembrane space and one portion open directly to the matrix. In the current model, each c-subunit contains a glutamyl carboxyl group that extends into the proton channel. Because this carboxyl group accepts a proton from the

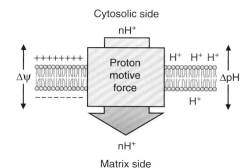

FIGURE 24.2 Proton motive force (electrochemical gradient) across the inner mitochondrial membrane. The proton motive force consists of a membrane potential, $\Delta\psi$, and a proton gradient, denoted by ΔpH for the difference in pH across the membrane. The electrochemical potential is called the *proton motive force* because it represents the potential energy driving protons to return to the more negatively charged alkaline matrix.

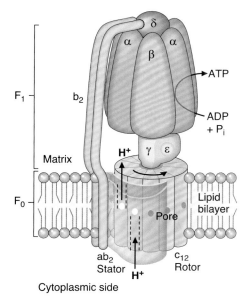

FIGURE 24.3 Adenosine triphosphate (ATP) synthase (F_0F_1-ATPase). Note that the matrix side of the mitochondrial inner membrane is at the *top* of the figure.

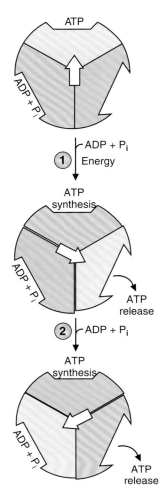

FIGURE 24.4 Binding-change mechanism for adenosine triphosphate (ATP) synthesis. The three αβ-subunit pairs of the ATP synthase headpiece have binding sites that can exist in three different conformations, depending on the position of the γ-stalk subunit. (*1*) When adenosine diphosphate (ADP) + inorganic phosphate (Pᵢ) bind to an open site and the proton influx rotates the γ-spindle (*white arrow*), the conformation of the subunits change and ATP is released from one site. (ATP dissociation is thus the energy-requiring step.) Bound ADP and Pᵢ combine to form ATP at another site. (2) As the ADP + Pᵢ bind to the new open site, and the γ-shaft rotates, the conformations of the sites change again and ATP is released. ADP and Pᵢ combine to form another ATP.

 Although iron-deficiency anemia is characterized by decreased levels of hemoglobin and other iron-containing proteins in the blood, the iron-containing cytochromes and Fe–S centers of the ETC in tissues such as skeletal muscle are affected as rapidly. Fatigue in iron-deficiency anemia, in patients such as **Ann R.** (see Chapter 16), results in part from the lack of electron transport for ATP production.

intermembrane space, the c-subunit rotates into the hydrophobic lipid membrane. The rotation exposes a different proton-containing c-subunit to the portion of the channel that is open directly to the matrix side. Because the matrix has a lower proton concentration, the glutamyl carboxylic acid group releases a proton into the matrix portion of the channel. Rotation is completed by an attraction between the negatively charged glutamyl residue and a positively charged arginyl group on the a-subunit.

According to the binding-change mechanism, as the asymmetric shaft rotates to a new position, it forms different binding associations with the αβ-subunits (Fig. 24.4). The new position of the shaft alters the conformation of one β-subunit so that it releases a molecule of ATP and another subunit spontaneously catalyzes synthesis of ATP from Pᵢ, one proton, and ADP. Thus, energy from the electrochemical gradient is used to change the conformation of the ATP synthase subunits so that the newly synthesized ATP is released.

B. Oxidation–Reduction Components of the Electron-Transport Chain

Electron transport to O_2 occurs via a series of oxidation–reduction steps in which each successive component of the chain is reduced as it accepts electrons and oxidized as it passes electrons to the next component of the chain. The oxidation–reduction components of the chain include flavin mononucleotide (FMN), Fe–S centers, CoQ, and Fe in cytochromes b, c_1, c, a, and a_3. Copper (Cu) is also a component of cytochromes a and a_3 (Fig. 24.5). With the exception of CoQ, all of these electron acceptors are tightly bound to the protein subunits of the carriers. FMN, like FAD, is synthesized from the vitamin riboflavin (see Fig. 20.10).

The reduction potential of each complex of the chain is at a lower energy level than the previous complex, so energy is released as electrons pass through each complex. This energy is used to move protons against their concentration gradient, so they become concentrated on the cytosolic side of the inner membrane.

1. NADH:CoQ Oxidoreductase

NADH:CoQ oxidoreductase (also named *NADH dehydrogenase*) is an enormous 42-subunit complex that contains a binding site for NADH, several FMN and iron–sulfur (Fe–S) center binding proteins, and binding sites for CoQ (see Fig. 24.5). An FMN accepts two electrons from NADH and is able to pass single electrons to the Fe–S centers. Fe–S centers, which are able to delocalize single electrons into large orbitals, transfer electrons to and from CoQ. Fe–S centers are also present in other enzyme systems—such as proteins within the cytochrome b–c_1 complex, which transfer electrons to CoQ—and in aconitase in the TCA cycle.

2. Succinate Dehydrogenase and Other Flavoproteins

In addition to NADH:CoQ oxidoreductase, *succinate dehydrogenase* and other flavoproteins in the inner mitochondrial membrane also pass electrons to CoQ (see Fig. 24.5). Succinate dehydrogenase is part of the TCA cycle and also a component of complex II of the ETC. *Electron-transferring flavoprotein* (ETF):CoQ oxidoreductase accepts electrons from ETF, which acquires them from fatty acid oxidation and other pathways. Both of these flavoproteins have Fe–S centers. Glycerol 3-phosphate dehydrogenase is a flavoprotein that is part of a shuttle for reoxidizing cytosolic NADH (see Section I.E).

The free-energy drop in electron transfer between NADH and CoQ of approximately −13 to −14 kcal is able to support movement of four protons. However, the FAD in succinate dehydrogenase (as well as ETF:CoQ oxidoreductase and glycerol 3-phosphate dehydrogenase) is at roughly the same redox potential as CoQ, and no energy is released as they transfer electrons to CoQ. These proteins do not span the membrane and consequently do not have a proton pumping mechanism.

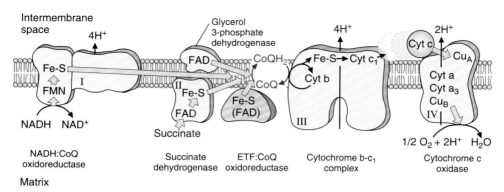

FIGURE 24.5   Components of the electron-transport chain. Nicotinamide adenine dinucleotide:coenzyme Q (NADH:CoQ) oxidoreductase (complex I) spans the membrane and has a proton-pumping mechanism involving CoQ. The electrons go from CoQ to the cytochrome b–c₁ complex (complex III); electron transfer does *not* involve complex II. Succinate dehydrogenase (complex II), glycerol 3-phosphate dehydrogenase, and electron-transferring flavoprotein (ETF):CoQ oxidoreductase all transfer electrons to CoQ, but they do not span the membrane and do not have proton pumping mechanisms. As CoQ accepts electrons and protons from the matrix side, it is converted to CoQH₂. Electrons are transferred from complex III to complex IV (cytochrome c oxidase) by cytochrome c, a small cytochrome in the intermembrane space that has reversible binding sites on the b–c₁ complex and cytochrome c oxidase. *FMN,* flavin mononucleotide.

3. Coenzyme Q

CoQ is the only component of the ETC that is not protein-bound. The large hydrophobic side chain of 10 isoprenoid units (50 carbons) confers lipid solubility, and CoQ is able to diffuse freely through the lipids of the inner mitochondrial membrane (Fig. 24.6). When the oxidized quinone form accepts a single electron (to form the semiquinone), it forms a free radical (a compound with a single electron in an orbital). The transfer of single electrons makes it the major site for generation of toxic oxygen free radicals in the body (see Chapter 25).

The semiquinone can accept a second electron and two protons from the matrix side of the membrane to form the fully reduced quinone. The mobility of CoQ in the membrane, its ability to accept one or two electrons, and its ability to accept and donate protons enable it to participate in the proton pumps for both complexes I and III as it shuttles electrons between them (see Section I.C). CoQ is also called *ubiquinone* (the ubiquitous quinone), because quinones with similar structures are found in all plants and animals.

4. Cytochromes

The remaining components in the ETC are cytochromes (see Fig. 24.5). Each cytochrome is a protein that contains a bound heme (i.e., an Fe atom bound to a porphyrin nucleus similar in structure to the heme in hemoglobin) (Fig. 24.7).

Because of differences in the protein component of the cytochromes and small differences in the heme structure, each heme has a different reduction potential. The cytochromes of the b–c₁ complex have a higher energy level than those of cytochrome oxidase (a and a₃). Thus, energy is released by electron transfer between

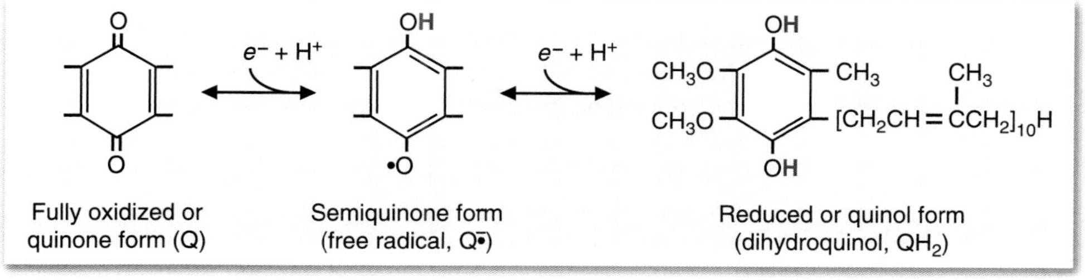

FIGURE 24.6   Structure of coenzyme Q (CoQ). CoQ contains a quinone with a long lipophilic side chain comprising 10 isoprenoid units (thus, it is sometimes called CoQ₁₀). CoQ can accept one electron (e⁻) to become the half-reduced form, or two e⁻ to become fully reduced.

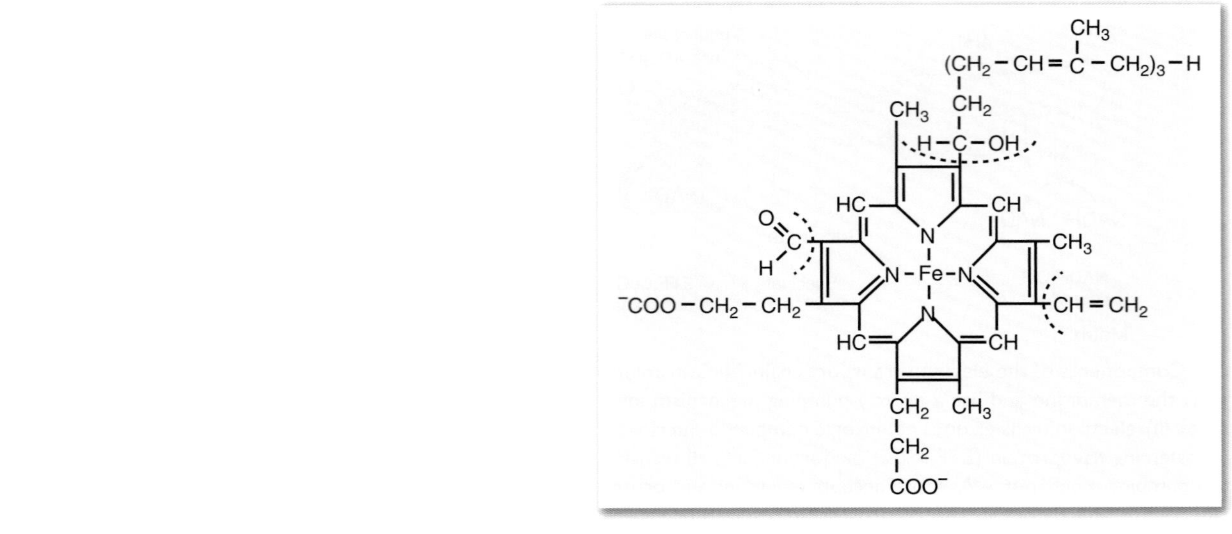

FIGURE 24.7 Heme A. Heme A is found in cytochromes a and a_3. Cytochromes are proteins that contain a heme chelated with an iron atom. Hemes are derivatives of protoporphyrin IX. Each cytochrome has a heme with different modifications of the side chains (indicated with *dashed lines*), resulting in a slightly different reduction potential and, consequently, a different position in the sequence of electron transfer.

Q The iron in the heme in hemoglobin, unlike the iron in the heme of cytochromes, never changes its oxidation state (it is Fe^{2+} in hemoglobin). If the iron in hemoglobin were to become oxidized (Fe^{3+}), the oxygen-binding capacity of the molecule would be lost. What accounts for this difference in iron oxidation states between hemoglobin and cytochromes?

complexes III and IV. The iron atoms in the cytochromes are in the Fe^{3+} state. As they accept an electron, they are reduced to Fe^{2+}. As they are reoxidized to Fe^{3+}, the electrons pass to the next component of the ETC.

5. Copper and the Reduction of Oxygen

The last cytochrome complex is cytochrome oxidase, which passes electrons from cytochrome c to O^2 (see Fig. 24.5). It contains cytochromes a and a_3 and the oxygen-binding site. A whole oxygen molecule, O_2, must accept four electrons to be reduced to two H_2O molecules. Bound copper (Cu^+) ions in the cytochrome oxidase complex facilitate the collection of the four electrons and the reduction of O_2.

Cytochrome oxidase has a much lower K_m for O_2 than myoglobin (the heme-containing intracellular oxygen carrier) or hemoglobin (the heme-containing oxygen transporter in the blood). Thus, O_2 is "pulled" from the erythrocyte to myoglobin, and from myoglobin to cytochrome oxidase, where it is reduced to H_2O.

C. Pumping of Protons

One of the tenets of the chemiosmotic theory is that energy from the oxidation–reduction reactions of the ETC is used to transport protons from the matrix to the intermembrane space. This proton pumping is generally facilitated by the vectorial arrangement of the membrane-spanning complexes. Their structure allows them to pick up electrons and protons on one side of the membrane and release protons on the other side of the membrane as they transfer an electron to the next component of the chain. The direct physical link between proton movement and electron transfer can be illustrated by an examination of the Q cycle for the b–c_1 complex (Fig. 24.8). The Q cycle involves a double cycle of CoQ reduction and oxidation. CoQ accepts two protons at the matrix side together with two electrons; it then releases protons into the intermembrane space while donating one electron back to another component of the cytochrome b–c_1 complex and one to cytochrome c.

The mechanism for pumping protons at the NADH:CoQ oxidoreductase complex is not well understood, but it involves a Q cycle in which the Fe–S centers and

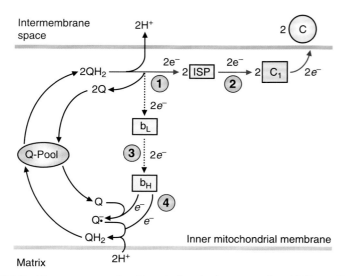

Normally, the protein structures binding the heme either protect the iron from oxidation (such as the globin proteins) or allow oxidation to occur (such as happens in the cytochromes). However, in hemoglobin M, a rare hemoglobin variant found in the human population, a tyrosine is substituted for the histidine at position F8 in the normal hemoglobin A. This tyrosine stabilizes the Fe^{3+} form of heme, and these subunits cannot bind oxygen. This is a lethal condition if it is homozygous.

FIGURE 24.8 The proton motive Q cycle for the b–c$_I$ complex. (*1*) From $2QH_2$, electrons go down two different paths: One path is through an Fe–S center protein (ISP) toward cytochrome c (*red arrows*). Another path is "backward" to one of the b cytochromes (*dashed arrows*). (*2*) Electrons are transferred from ISP through cytochrome c$_I$. Cytochrome c, which is in the intermembrane space, binds to the b–c$_I$ complex to accept an electron. (*3*) Returning electrons go through another b cytochrome and are directed toward the matrix. (*4*) At the matrix side, electrons and $2H^+$ are accepted by Q. Q, coenzyme Q; $Q^{\cdot-}$, coenzyme Q semiquinone; QH_2, coenzyme Q hydroquinone.

FMN might participate. However, transmembrane proton movement at cytochrome c oxidase probably involves direct transport of the proton through a series of bound water molecules or amino acid side chains in the protein complex, a mechanism that has been described as a *proton wire*.

The significance of the direct link between the electron transfer and proton movement is that one cannot occur without the other (the processes are said to be "coupled"). Thus, when protons are not being used for ATP synthesis, the proton gradient and the membrane potential build up. This "proton backpressure" controls the rate of proton pumping, which controls electron transport and O_2 consumption.

D. Energy Yield from the Electron-Transport Chain

The overall free-energy release from oxidation of NADH by O_2 is approximately −53 kcal, and from FAD(2H), it is approximately −41 kcal. This ΔG^0 is so negative that the chain is never reversible; we never synthesize oxygen from H_2O. The negative ΔG^0 also drives NADH and FAD(2H) formation from the pathways of fuel oxidation, such as the TCA cycle and glycolysis, to completion.

Overall, each NADH donates two electrons, equivalent to the reduction of one-half of an O_2 molecule. A generally (but not universally) accepted estimate of the stoichiometry of ATP synthesis is that four protons are pumped at complex I, four protons at complex III, and two at complex IV. With three protons translocated for each ATP synthesized, and one proton for each phosphate transported into the matrix (see Section IV.A of this chapter), an estimated 2.5 ATPs are formed for each NADH oxidized, and 1.5 ATPs are formed for each of the other FAD(2H)-containing flavoproteins that donate electrons to CoQ. (This calculation neglects the basal proton leak.) Thus, only approximately 30% of the energy available from NADH and FAD(2H) oxidation by O_2 is used for ATP synthesis. Some of the remaining energy in the electrochemical potential is used for the transport of anions and Ca^{2+} into the mitochondrion. The remainder of the energy is released as heat. Consequently, the ETC is also our major source of heat.

Cora N. has a lack of oxygen in the anterior and lateral walls of her heart caused by severe ischemia (lack of blood flow) resulting from blockage of the coronary arteries supplying blood to this area of her heart. The arteries are blocked by a clot at the site of ruptured atherosclerotic plaques. The limited availability of O_2 to act as an electron acceptor will decrease proton pumping and generation of an electrochemical potential gradient across the inner mitochondrial membrane of ischemic cells. As a consequence, the rate of ATP generation in these specific areas of her heart will decrease, thereby triggering events that lead to irreversible cell injury.

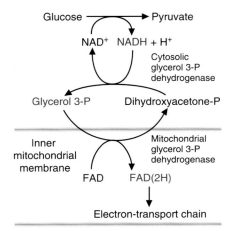

FIGURE 24.9 Glycerol 3-phosphate (glycerol 3-P) shuttle. Because nicotinamide adenine dinucleotide (NAD$^+$) and NADH cannot cross the mitochondrial membrane, shuttles transfer the reducing equivalents into mitochondria. Dihydroxyacetone phosphate (DHAP) is reduced to glycerol 3-P by cytosolic glycerol 3-P dehydrogenase, using cytosolic NADH produced in glycolysis. Glycerol 3-P then reacts in the inner mitochondrial membrane with mitochondrial glycerol 3-P dehydrogenase, which transfers the electrons to flavin adenine dinucleotide (FAD) and regenerates DHAP, which returns to the cytosol. The electron-transport chain transfers the electrons to O$_2$, which generates approximately 1.5 adenosine triphosphates (ATPs) for each FAD(2H) that is oxidized.

E. Cytoplasmic NADH

There is no transport system for cytoplasmic NADH to cross the inner mitochondrial membrane, or for mitochondrial NADH to enter the cytoplasm. However, there are two shuttle systems to transport the electrons from NADH (cytoplasmic) to NAD$^+$ (mitochondrial). NADH can be reoxidized to NAD$^+$ in the cytosol by a reaction that transfers the electrons to dihydroxyacetone phosphate (DHAP) in the glycerol 3-phosphate (glycerol 3-P) shuttle or to oxaloacetate in the malate–aspartate shuttle. The NAD$^+$ that is formed in the cytosol returns to glycolysis, whereas glycerol 3-P or malate carry the reducing equivalents that are ultimately transferred across the inner mitochondrial membrane. Thus, these shuttles transfer electrons and not NADH per se.

1. Glycerol 3-Phosphate Shuttle

The glycerol 3-P shuttle is the major shuttle in most tissues. In this shuttle, cytosolic NAD$^+$ is regenerated by cytoplasmic glycerol 3-P dehydrogenase, which transfers electrons from NADH to DHAP to form glycerol 3-P (Fig. 24.9). Glycerol 3-P then diffuses through the outer mitochondrial membrane to the inner mitochondrial membrane, where the electrons are donated to a membrane-bound FAD-containing glycerophosphate dehydrogenase. This enzyme, like succinate dehydrogenase, ultimately donates electrons to CoQ, resulting in an energy yield of approximately 1.5 ATPs from oxidative phosphorylation. DHAP returns to the cytosol to continue the shuttle. The sum of the reactions in this shuttle system is simply

$$\text{NADH}_{\text{cytosol}} + \text{H}^+ + \text{FAD}_{\text{mitochondria}} \rightarrow \text{NAD}^+{}_{\text{cytosol}} + \text{FAD(2H)}_{\text{mitochondria}}$$

2. Malate–Aspartate Shuttle

Many tissues contain both the glycerol 3-P shuttle and the malate–aspartate shuttle. In the malate–aspartate shuttle (Fig. 24.10), cytosolic NAD$^+$ is regenerated by cytosolic malate dehydrogenase, which transfers electrons from NADH to cytosolic oxaloacetate to form malate. Malate is transported across the inner mitochondrial membrane by a specific translocase, which exchanges malate for α-ketoglutarate. In the matrix, malate is oxidized back to oxaloacetate by mitochondrial malate dehydrogenase, and NADH is generated. This NADH can donate electrons to the ETC

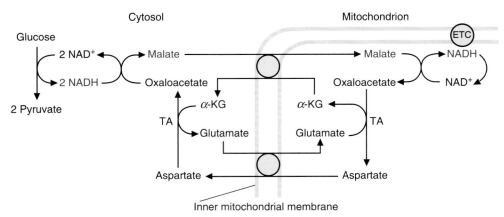

FIGURE 24.10 Malate–aspartate shuttle. Reduced nicotinamide adenine dinucleotide (NADH) produced by glycolysis reduces oxaloacetate (OAA) to malate, which crosses the mitochondrial membrane and is reoxidized to OAA. The mitochondrial NADH donates electrons to the electron-transport chain, with 2.5 adenosine triphosphates (ATPs) generated for each NADH. To complete the shuttle, OAA must return to the cytosol, although it cannot be transported directly on a translocase. Instead, it is transaminated to aspartate, which is then transported out to the cytosol, where it is transaminated back to OAA. The translocators exchange compounds in such a way that the shuttle is completely balanced. *TA,* transamination reaction. α-*KG,* α-ketoglutarate; *ETC,* electron-transport chain.

with generation of approximately 2.5 mol of ATP per mole of NADH. The newly formed oxaloacetate cannot pass back through the inner mitochondrial membrane under physiologic conditions, so aspartate is used to return the oxaloacetate carbon skeleton to the cytosol. In the matrix, transamination reactions transfer an amino group to oxaloacetate to form aspartate, which is transported out to the cytosol (using an aspartate–glutamate exchange translocase) and converted back to oxaloacetate through another transamination reaction. The sum of all the reactions of this shuttle system is simply

$$NADH_{cytosol} + NAD^+_{matrix} \rightarrow NAD^+_{cytosol} + NADH_{matrix}$$

3. Energy Yield of Aerobic versus Anaerobic Glycolysis

In both aerobic and anaerobic glycolysis, each mole of glucose generates 2 mol of ATP, 2 mol of NADH, and 2 mol of pyruvate. The energy yield from anaerobic glycolysis (1 mol of glucose to 2 mol of lactate) is only 2 mol of ATP per mole of glucose, as the NADH is recycled to NAD^+ by reducing pyruvate to lactate. Neither the NADH nor the pyruvate produced is thus used for further energy generation. However, when oxygen is available and cytosolic NADH can be oxidized via a shuttle system, pyruvate can also enter the mitochondria and be completely oxidized to CO_2 via pyruvate dehydrogenase (PDH) and the TCA cycle. The oxidation of pyruvate via this route generates roughly 12.5 mol of ATP per mole of pyruvate. If the cytosolic NADH is oxidized by the glycerol 3-P shuttle, approximately 1.5 mol of ATP are produced per NADH. If, instead, the NADH is oxidized by the malate–aspartate shuttle, approximately 2.5 mol are produced. Thus, the two moles of NADH produced during glycolysis can lead to 3 to 5 mol of ATP being produced, depending on which shuttle system is used to transfer the reducing equivalents. Because each mole of pyruvate produced can give rise to 12.5 mol of ATP, altogether 30 to 32 mol of ATP can be produced from 1 mol of glucose oxidized to carbon dioxide.

To produce the same amount of ATP per unit time from anaerobic glycolysis as from the complete aerobic oxidation of glucose to CO_2, anaerobic glycolysis must occur approximately 15 times faster and use approximately 15 times more glucose. Cells achieve this high rate of glycolysis by expressing high levels of glycolytic enzymes. In certain skeletal muscles and in most cells during hypoxic crises, high rates of glycolysis are associated with rapid degradation of internal glycogen stores to supply the required glucose 6-phosphate.

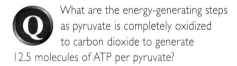 What are the energy-generating steps as pyruvate is completely oxidized to carbon dioxide to generate 12.5 molecules of ATP per pyruvate?

F. Respiratory Chain Inhibition and Sequential Transfer

In the cell, electron flow in the ETC must be sequential from NADH or a flavoprotein all the way to O_2 to generate ATP (see Fig. 24.5). In the absence of O_2 (anoxia), there is no ATP generated from oxidative phosphorylation because electrons back up in the chain. Even complex I cannot pump protons to generate the electrochemical gradient because every molecule of CoQ already has electrons that it cannot pass down the chain without an O_2 to accept them at the end. The action of the respiratory chain inhibitor *cyanide*, which binds to cytochrome oxidase, is similar to that of anoxia: It prevents proton pumping by all three complexes. Complete inhibition of the b–c_1 complex prevents pumping at cytochrome oxidase because there is no donor of electrons; it prevents pumping at complex I because there is no electron acceptor. Although complete inhibition of any one complex inhibits proton pumping at all of the complexes, partial inhibition of proton pumping can occur when only a fraction of the molecules of a complex contains bound inhibitor. The partial inhibition results in a partial decrease of the maximal rate of ATP synthesis. Table 24.1 lists chemical inhibitors of oxidative phosphorylation and indicates the steps within either electron transport or ATP synthesis at which they act.

 Intravenous nitroprusside rapidly lowers elevated blood pressure through its direct vasodilating action. Fortunately, it was required in **Cora N.'s** case only for a short time. During prolonged infusions of 24 to 48 hours or more, nitroprusside slowly breaks down to produce cyanide, an inhibitor of the cytochrome c oxidase complex. Because small amounts of cyanide are detoxified in the liver by conversion to thiocyanate, which is excreted in the urine, the conversion of nitroprusside to cyanide can be monitored by following blood thiocyanate levels.

(A) In the complete oxidation of pyruvate to carbon dioxide, four steps generate NADH (PDH, isocitrate dehydrogenase, α-ketoglutarate dehydrogenase, and malate dehydrogenase). One step generates FAD(2H) (succinate dehydrogenase) and one substrate-level phosphorylation (succinate thiokinase). Thus, because each NADH generates 2.5 ATPs, the overall contribution by NADH is 10 ATP molecules. The FAD(2H) generates an additional 1.5 ATPs, and the substrate-level phosphorylation provides one more. Therefore, $10 + 1.5 + 1 = 12.5$ molecules of ATP.

TABLE 24.1	Inhibitors of Oxidative Phosphorylation	
INHIBITOR	**SITE OF INHIBITION**	
Rotenone, Amytal	Transfer of electrons from complex I to coenzyme Q	
Antimycin C	Transfer of electrons from complex III to cytochrome c	
Carbon monoxide (CO)	Transfer of electrons from complex IV to oxygen	
Cyanide (CN)	Transfer of electrons through complex IV to oxygen	
Atractyloside	Inhibits the adenine nucleotide translocase (ANT)	
Oligomycin	Inhibits proton flow through the F_0 component of the adenosine triphosphate (ATP) synthase	
Dinitrophenol	An uncoupler; facilitates proton transfer across the inner mitochondrial membrane	
Valinomycin	A potassium ionophore; facilitates potassium ion transfer across the inner mitochondrial membrane	

II. OXPHOS Diseases

Clinical diseases involving components of oxidative phosphorylation (referred to as *OXPHOS diseases*) are among the most commonly encountered degenerative diseases. The clinical pathology may be caused by gene mutations in either mtDNA or nuclear DNA (nDNA) that encode proteins required for normal oxidative phosphorylation.

A. Mitochondrial DNA and OXPHOS Diseases

The mtDNA is a small double-stranded circular DNA consisting of 16,569 nucleotide pairs. It encodes 13 subunits of the complexes involved in oxidative phosphorylation: 7 of the 42 subunits of complex I (NADH:CoQ oxidoreductase complex), 1 of the 11 subunits of complex III (cytochrome b–c_1 complex), 3 of 13 of the subunits of complex IV (cytochrome oxidase), and 2 subunits of the F_0 portion ATP–synthase complex. In addition, mtDNA encodes the necessary components for translation of its messenger RNA (mRNA): a large and small ribosomal (rRNA) and 22 transfer RNAs (tRNAs). Mutations in mtDNA have been identified as deletions, duplications, or point mutations. Disorders associated with these mutations are outlined in Table 24.2.

Cyanide binds to the Fe^{3+} in the heme of the cytochrome aa_3 component of cytochrome c oxidase and prevents electron transport to O_2. Mitochondrial respiration and energy production cease, and cell death occurs rapidly. The central nervous system is the primary target for cyanide toxicity. Acute inhalation of high concentrations of cyanide (e.g., smoke inhalation during a fire) provokes a brief central nervous system stimulation followed rapidly by convulsion, coma, and death. Acute exposure to lower amounts can cause light-headedness, breathlessness, dizziness, numbness, and headaches.

Cyanide is present in the air as hydrogen cyanide (HCN), in soil and water as cyanide salts (e.g., NaCN), and in foods as cyanoglycosides. Most of the cyanide in the air usually comes from automobile exhaust. Examples of populations with potentially high exposures include active and passive smokers, people who are exposed to house or other building fires, residents who live near cyanide- or thiocyanate-containing hazardous waste sites, and workers involved in several manufacturing processes (e.g., photography, pesticide application).

Cyanoglycosides such as amygdalin are present in edible plants such as almonds, pits from stone fruits (e.g., apricots, peaches, plums, cherries), sorghum, cassava, soybeans, spinach, lima beans, sweet potatoes, maize, millet, sugar cane, and bamboo shoots.

HCN is released from cyanoglycosides by β-glucosidases present in the plant or in intestinal bacteria. Small amounts are inactivated in the liver principally by rhodanase, which converts it to thiocyanate.

In the United States, toxic amounts of cyanoglycosides have been ingested as ground apricot pits, either as a result of their promotion as a health food or as a treatment for cancer. The drug Laetrile (amygdalin) was used as a cancer therapeutic agent, although it was banned in the United States because it was ineffective and potentially toxic. Commercial fruit juices made from unpitted fruit could provide toxic amounts of cyanide, particularly in infants or children. In countries in which cassava is a dietary staple, improper processing results in retention of its high cyanide content at potentially toxic levels.

Amygdalin, a cyanoglycoside

TABLE 24.2   Examples of OXPHOS Diseases Arising from Mitochondrial DNA Mutations

SYNDROME	CHARACTERISTIC SYMPTOMS	mtDNA MUTATION
I. mtDNA Rearrangements in which Genes are Deleted or Duplicated		
Kearns-Sayre syndrome	Onset before 20 years of age, characterized by ophthalmoplegia, atypical retinitis pigmentosa, mitochondrial myopathy, and one of the following: cardiac conduction defect, cerebellar syndrome, or elevated CSF proteins	Deletion of contiguous segments of tRNA and OXPHOS polypeptides, or duplication mutations consisting of tandemly arranged normal mtDNA and an mtDNA with a deletion mutation
Pearson syndrome	Systemic disorder of oxidative phosphorylation that predominantly affects bone marrow	Deletion of contiguous segments of tRNA and OXPHOS polypeptides, or duplication mutations consisting of tandemly arranged normal mtDNA and a mtDNA with a deletion mutation
II. mtDNA Point Mutations in tRNA or Ribosomal RNA Genes		
Myoclonic epilepsy and ragged red fiber disease (MERRF)	Progressive myoclonic epilepsy, a mitochondrial myopathy with ragged red fibers, and a slowly progressive dementia; onset of symptoms: late childhood to adult	$tRNA^{Lys}$
Mitochondrial myopathy, encephalomyopathy, lactic acidosis, and strokelike episodes (MELAS)	Progressive neurodegenerative disease characterized by strokelike episodes first occurring between 5 and 15 years of age and a mitochondrial myopathy	80%–90% mutations in $tRNA^{Leu}$
III. mtDNA Missense Mutations in OXPHOS Polypeptides		
Leigh disease (subacute necrotizing encephalopathy)	Mean age of onset, 1.5–5 years; clinical manifestations include optic atrophy, ophthalmoplegia, nystagmus, respiratory abnormalities, ataxia, hypotonia, spasticity, and developmental delay or regression	7%–20% of cases have mutations in F_0 subunits of the F_0F_1-ATPase.
Leber hereditary optic neuropathy (LHON)	Late onset, acute optic atrophy	90% of European and Asian cases result from mutation in NADH dehydrogenase.

mtDNA, mitochondrial DNA; CSF, cerebrospinal fluid; NADH, reduced nicotinamide adenine dinucleotide; tRNA, transfer RNA; OXPHOS, oxidative phosphorylation.

The genetics of mutations in mtDNA are defined by maternal inheritance, replicative segregation, threshold expression, a high mtDNA mutation rate, and the accumulation of somatic mutations with age. The maternal inheritance pattern reflects the exclusive transmission of mtDNA from the mother to her children. The egg contains approximately 300,000 molecules of mtDNA packaged into mitochondria. These are retained during fertilization, whereas those of the sperm do not enter the egg or are lost. Usually, some mitochondria are present that have the mutant mtDNA and some have normal (wild-type) DNA. As cells divide during mitosis and meiosis, mitochondria replicate by fission, but various amounts of mitochondria with mutant and wild-type DNA are distributed to each daughter cell (replicative segregation). Thus, any cell can have a mixture of mitochondria, each with mutant or wild-type mtDNAs (termed *heteroplasmy*). The mitotic and meiotic segregation of the heteroplasmic mtDNA mutation results in variable oxidative phosphorylation deficiencies between patients with the same mutation, and even among a patient's own tissues.

 Oxidative phosphorylation (OXPHOS) is responsible for producing most of the ATP that our cells require. The genes responsible for the polypeptides that comprise the OXPHOS complexes within the mitochondria are located within either the nDNA or the mtDNA. A broad spectrum of human disorders (the OXPHOS diseases) may result from genetic mutations or nongenetic alterations (spontaneous mutations) in either the nDNA or the mtDNA. Increasingly, such changes appear to be responsible for at least some aspects of common disorders, such as Parkinson disease, dilated and hypertrophic cardiomyopathies, diabetes mellitus, Alzheimer disease, depressive disorders, and a host of less well-known clinical entities.

Q Decreased activity of the electron-transport chain can result from inhibitors as well as from mutations in mtDNA and nuclear DNA. Why does an impairment of the ETC result in lactic acidosis?

A patient experienced spontaneous muscle jerking (myoclonus) in her mid-teens, and her condition progressed over 10 years to include debilitating myoclonus, neurosensory hearing loss, dementia, hypoventilation, and mild cardiomyopathy. Energy metabolism was affected in the central nervous system, heart, and skeletal muscle, resulting in lactic acidosis. A history indicated that the patient's mother, her grandmother, and two maternal aunts had symptoms involving either nervous or muscular tissue (clearly a case of maternal inheritance). However, no other relative had identical symptoms. The symptoms and history of the patient are those of myoclonic epileptic ragged red fiber disease (MERRF). The affected tissues (central nervous system and muscle) are two of the tissues with the highest ATP requirements. Most cases of MERRF are caused by a point mutation in mitochondrial tRNA^{Lys} (mtRNA^{Lys}). The mitochondria, obtained by muscle biopsy, are enlarged and show abnormal patterns of cristae. The muscle tissue also shows ragged red fibers.

The disease pathology usually becomes worse with age because a small amount of normal mitochondria might confer normal function and exercise capacity while the patient is young. As the patient ages, somatic (spontaneous) mutations in mtDNA accumulate from the generation of free radicals within the mitochondria (see Chapter 25). These mutations frequently become permanent partly because mtDNA does not have access to the same repair mechanisms available for nDNA (high mutation rate). Even in normal individuals, somatic mutations result in a decline of oxidative phosphorylation capacity with age (accumulation of somatic mutations with age). At some stage, the ATP-generating capacity of a tissue falls below the tissue-specific threshold for normal function (threshold expression). In general, symptoms of these defects appear in one or more of the tissues with the highest ATP demands: nervous tissue, heart, skeletal muscle, and kidney.

B. Other Genetic Disorders of Oxidative Phosphorylation

Genetic mutations also have been reported for mitochondrial proteins that are encoded by nuclear DNA. Most of the estimated 1,000 proteins required for oxidative phosphorylation are encoded by nuclear DNA, whereas mtDNA encodes only 13 subunits of the oxidative phosphorylation complexes (including ATP synthase). Nuclear DNA encodes the additional 70 or more subunits of the oxidative phosphorylation complexes as well as the ANT and other anion translocators. Coordinate regulation of expression of nuclear and mtDNA, import of proteins into the mitochondria, assembly of the complexes, and regulation of mitochondrial fission are nuclear-encoded. The nuclear respiratory factors (NRF-1 and NRF-2) are nuclear transcription factors that bind to and activate promotor regions of the nuclear genes that encode subunits of the respiratory chain complexes, including cytochrome c. They also activate the transcription of the nuclear gene for the mitochondrial transcription factor (mTF)-A. The protein product of this gene translocates into the mitochondrial matrix, where it stimulates transcription and replication of the mitochondrial genome.

Nuclear DNA mutations differ from mtDNA mutations in several important respects. These mutations do not show a pattern of maternal inheritance but are usually autosomal recessive. The mutations are uniformly distributed to daughter cells and, therefore, are expressed in all tissues containing the allele for a particular tissue-specific isoform. However, phenotypic expression will still be most apparent in tissues with high ATP requirements.

C. Lactic Acidosis

Lactic acidosis generally results from a greatly increased NADH/NAD$^+$ ratio in tissues (Fig. 24.11). The increased NADH concentration prevents pyruvate oxidation in the TCA cycle and directs pyruvate to lactate. To compensate for the decreased ATP production from oxidative metabolism, phosphofructokinase-1, and, therefore, the entire glycolytic pathway, is activated. For example, consumption of large amounts of alcohol, which is rapidly oxidized in the liver and increases NADH levels, can result in lactic acidosis. Hypoxia in any tissue increases lactate production as cells attempt to compensate for a lack of O_2 for oxidative phosphorylation.

Several other problems that interfere with either the ETC or pyruvate oxidation in the TCA cycle result in lactic acidemia (see Fig. 24.11). For example, OXPHOS diseases (inherited deficiencies in subunits of complexes in the ETC, such as myoclonic epilepsy with ragged-red fibers [MERRF]) increase the NADH/NAD$^+$ ratio and inhibit PDH (see Chapter 23). Pyruvate accumulates and is converted to lactate to allow glycolytic ATP production to proceed. Similarly, impaired PDH activity from an inherited deficiency of E_1 (the decarboxylase subunit of the complex), or

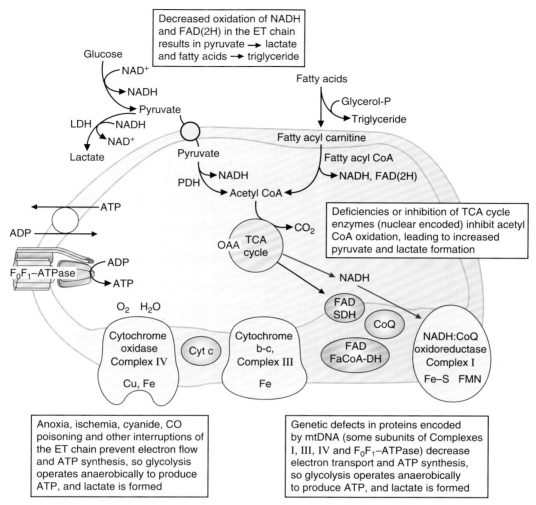

FIGURE 24.11 Pathways leading to lactic acidemia. *Acetyl CoA*, acetyl coenzyme A; *ADP*, adenosine diphosphate; *ATP*, adenosine triphosphate; *CoQ*, coenzyme Q; *Cyt c*, cytochrome c; *DH*, dehydrogenase; *ET*, electron transport; *FAD*, flavin adenine dinucleotide; *FMN*, flavin mononucleotide; *Glycerol-P*, glycerol 3-phosphate; *LDH*, lactate dehydrogenase; *mtDNA*, mitochondrial DNA; *NAD*, nicotinamide adenine dinucleotide; *OAA*, oxalo-acetate; *PDH*, pyruvate dehydrogenase; *SDH*, succinate dehydrogenase; *TCA*, tricarboxylic acid.

from severe thiamin deficiency, increases blood lactate levels (see Chapter 23). Pyruvate carboxylase deficiency also can result in lactic acidosis (see Chapter 23) also because of an accumulation of pyruvate.

Lactic acidosis can also result from inhibition of lactate use in gluconeogenesis (e.g., hereditary fructose intolerance, which is caused by a defective aldolase gene). If other pathways that use glucose 6-phosphate are blocked, glucose 6-phosphate can be shunted into glycolysis and lactate production (e.g., glucose 6-phosphate deficiency).

III. Coupling of Electron Transport and Adenosine Triphosphate Synthesis

The electrochemical gradient couples the rate of the ETC to the rate of ATP synthesis. Because electron flow requires proton pumping, electron flow cannot occur faster than protons are used for ATP synthesis (coupled oxidative phosphorylation) or returned to the matrix by a mechanism that short-circuits the ATP synthase pore (uncoupling).

 The effect of inhibition of electron transport is an impaired oxidation of pyruvate, fatty acids, and other fuels. In many cases, the inhibition of mitochondrial electron transport results in higher-than-normal levels of lactate and pyruvate in the blood and an increased lactate:pyruvate ratio. NADH oxidation requires the complete transfer of electrons from NADH to O_2, and a defect anywhere along the chain will result in the accumulation of NADH and a decrease in NAD^+. The increase in NADH/NAD^+ inhibits PDH and causes the accumulation of pyruvate. It also increases the conversion of pyruvate to lactate (anaerobic glycolysis), and elevated levels of lactate appear in the blood. A large number of genetic defects of the proteins in respiratory chain complexes have, therefore, been classified together as *congenital lactic acidosis*.

How does shivering generate heat?

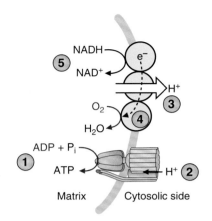

Matrix   Cytosolic side

FIGURE 24.12 The concentration of adenosine diphosphate (ADP) (or the phosphate potential, [ATP]/[ADP][P_i]) controls the rate of oxygen consumption. (*1*) ADP is phosphorylated to adenosine triphosphate (ATP) by ATP synthase. (*2*) The release of the ATP requires proton flow through ATP synthase into the matrix. (*3*) The use of protons from the intermembrane space for ATP synthesis decreases the proton gradient. (*4*) As a result, the electron-transport chain pumps more protons, and oxygen is reduced to H_2O. (*5*) As reduced nicotinamide adenine dinucleotide (NADH) donates electrons to the electron-transport chain, NAD^+ is regenerated and returns to the tricarboxylic acid cycle or other NADH-producing pathways. P_i, inorganic phosphate.

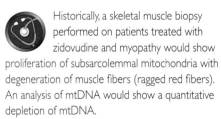

Historically, a skeletal muscle biopsy performed on patients treated with zidovudine and myopathy would show proliferation of subsarcolemmal mitochondria with degeneration of muscle fibers (ragged red fibers). An analysis of mtDNA would show a quantitative depletion of mtDNA.

Isabel S. was being treated for HIV with a multidrug regimen including a nucleoside analog reverse transcriptase inhibitor. One of the first drugs of this class was zidovudine (azidothymidine, AZT), which also can act as an inhibitor of the mtDNA polymerase (polymerase γ). A review of the drug's potential adverse effects showed that rarely it may cause varying degrees of mtDNA depletion in different tissues, including skeletal muscle. The depletion may cause a severe mitochondrial myopathy, including ragged red fiber accumulation within the skeletal muscle cells associated with ultrastructural abnormalities in their mitochondria. This can occur with all drugs in this class, but it is much less common with the newer ones.

A. Regulation through Coupling

As ATP chemical bond energy is used by energy-requiring reactions, ADP and P_i concentrations increase. The more ADP present to bind to the ATP synthase, the greater will be proton flow through the ATP synthase pore from the intermembrane space to the matrix. Thus, as ADP levels rise, proton influx increases, and the electrochemical gradient decreases (Fig. 24.12). The proton pumps of the ETC respond with increased proton pumping and electron flow to maintain the electrochemical gradient. The result is increased O_2 consumption. The increased oxidation of NADH in the ETC and the increased concentration of ADP stimulate the pathways of fuel oxidation, such as the TCA cycle, to supply more NADH and FAD(2H) to the ETC. For example, during exercise, we use more ATP for muscle contraction, consume more oxygen, oxidize more fuel (which means burn more calories), and generate more heat from the ETC. If we rest, the rate of ATP use decreases, proton influx decreases, the electrochemical gradient increases, and proton backpressure decreases the rate of the ETC. NADH and FAD(2H) cannot be oxidized as rapidly in the ETC, and consequently, their buildup inhibits the enzymes that generate them.

The system is poised to maintain very high levels of ATP at all times. In most tissues, the rate of ATP use is nearly constant over time. However, in skeletal muscles, the rates of ATP hydrolysis change dramatically as the muscle goes from rest to rapid contraction. Even under these circumstances, ATP concentration decreases by only approximately 20% because it is so rapidly regenerated. In the heart, Ca^{2+} activation of TCA cycle enzymes provides an extra push to NADH generation so that neither ATP nor NADH levels fall as ATP demand is increased. The ETC has a very high capacity and can respond very rapidly to any increase in ATP use.

B. Uncoupling Adenosine Triphosphate Synthesis from Electron Transport

When protons leak back into the matrix without going through the ATP synthase pore, they dissipate the electrochemical gradient across the membrane without generating ATP. This phenomenon is called *uncoupling* oxidative phosphorylation. It occurs with chemical compounds, known as *uncouplers*, and it occurs physiologically with uncoupling proteins (UCPs) that form proton conductance channels through the membrane. Uncoupling of oxidative phosphorylation results in increased oxygen consumption and heat production as electron flow and proton pumping attempt to maintain the electrochemical gradient.

1. Chemical Uncouplers of Oxidative Phosphorylation

Chemical uncouplers, also known as *proton ionophores*, are lipid-soluble compounds that rapidly transport protons from the cytosolic to the matrix side of the inner mitochondrial membrane (Fig. 24.13). Because the proton concentration is higher in the intermembrane space than in the matrix, uncouplers pick up protons from the intermembrane space. Their lipid solubility enables them to diffuse through the inner mitochondrial membrane while carrying protons and release these protons on the matrix side. The rapid influx of protons dissipates the electrochemical potential gradient; therefore, the mitochondria are unable to synthesize ATP. Eventually, mitochondrial integrity and function are lost.

2. Uncoupling Proteins and Thermogenesis

UCPs form channels through the inner mitochondrial membrane that are able to conduct protons from the intermembrane space to the matrix, thereby short-circuiting ATP synthase.

UCP1 (thermogenin) is associated with heat production in brown adipose tissue. The major function of brown adipose tissue is nonshivering thermogenesis, whereas the major function of white adipose tissue is the storage of triacylglycerols

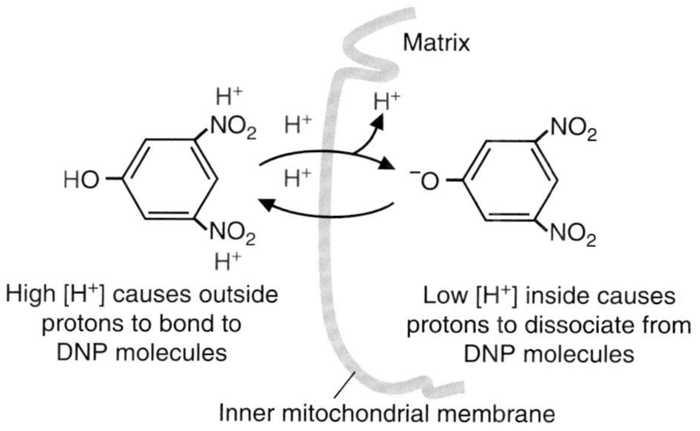

Matrix

High [H⁺] causes outside
protons to bond to
DNP molecules

Low [H⁺] inside causes
protons to dissociate from
DNP molecules

Inner mitochondrial membrane

FIGURE 24.13 Action of uncouplers. Dinitrophenol (DNP) is lipid-soluble and can therefore diffuse across the membrane. It has a dissociable proton with a pK_a near 7.2. Thus, in the intermembrane space where [H⁺] is high (pH low), DNP picks up a proton, which it carries across the membrane. At the lower proton concentration of the matrix, the H⁺ dissociates. As a consequence, cells cannot maintain their electrochemical gradient or synthesize adenosine triphosphate (ATP). DNP was once recommended in the United States as a weight-loss drug, based on the principle that decreased [ATP] and increased electron transport stimulate fuel oxidation. However, several deaths resulted from its use.

A Shivering results from muscle contraction, which increases the rate of ATP hydrolysis. As a consequence of proton entry for ATP synthesis, the ETC is stimulated. Oxygen consumption increases, as does the amount of energy lost as heat by the electron-transport chain.

in lipid droplets. The brown color arises from the large number of mitochondria that participate. Human infants, who have little voluntary control over their environment and may kick their blankets off at night, have brown fat deposits along the neck, the breastplate, between the scapulae, and around the kidneys to protect them from cold. However, there is very little brown fat in most adults.

In response to cold, sympathetic nerve endings release norepinephrine, which activates a lipase in brown adipose tissue that releases fatty acids from triacylglycerols (Fig. 24.14). Fatty acids serve as a fuel for the tissue (i.e., are oxidized to generate the electrochemical potential gradient and ATP) and participate directly in the proton conductance channel by activating UCP1 along with reduced CoQ. When UCP1 is activated by fatty acids, it transports protons from the cytosolic side of the inner mitochondrial membrane back into the mitochondrial matrix without

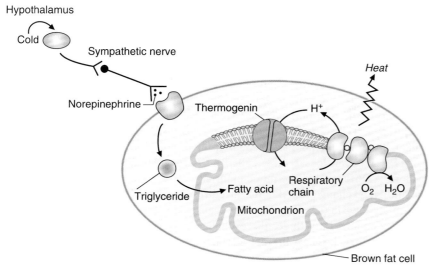

FIGURE 24.14 Brown fat is a tissue specialized for nonshivering thermogenesis. Cold or excessive food intake stimulates the release of norepinephrine from the sympathetic nerve endings. As a result, a lipase is activated that releases fatty acids for oxidation. The proton conductance protein thermogenin is activated, and protons are brought into the matrix. This stimulates the electron-transport chain, which increases its rate of NADH and FAD(2H) oxidation and produces more heat.

Salicylate, which is a degradation product of aspirin in humans, is lipid-soluble and has a dissociable proton. In high concentrations, as in salicylate poisoning, salicylate is able to partially uncouple mitochondria. The decline of ATP concentration in the cell and consequent increase of AMP in the cytosol stimulates glycolysis. The overstimulation of the glycolytic pathway (see Chapter 22) results in increased levels of lactic acid in the blood and a metabolic acidosis. Fortunately, **Dennis V.** did not develop this consequence of aspirin poisoning (see Chapter 4).

ATP generation. Thus, it partially uncouples oxidative phosphorylation and generates additional heat.

The UCPs exist as a family of proteins: *UCP1* (thermogenin) is expressed in brown adipose tissue; *UCP2* is found in most cells; *UCP3* is found principally in skeletal muscle; and *UCP4* and *UCP5* are found in the nervous system. These are highly regulated proteins that, when activated, increase the amount of energy from fuel oxidation that is being released as heat. However, recent data indicate that this may not be the primary role of UCP2 and UCP3. It has been hypothesized that UCP3 acts as a transport protein to remove fatty acid anions and lipid peroxides from the mitochondria, thereby reducing the risk of forming oxygen free radicals (see Chapter 25) and thus decreasing the occurrence of mitochondrial and cell injury.

3. Proton Leak and Resting Metabolic Rate

A low level of proton leak across the inner mitochondrial membrane occurs in our mitochondria all the time, and our mitochondria thus are normally partially uncoupled. It has been estimated that >20% of our resting metabolic rate is the energy expended to maintain the electrochemical gradient dissipated by our basal proton leak (also referred to as *global proton leak*). Some of the proton leak results from permeability of the membrane associated with proteins embedded in the lipid bilayer. An unknown amount may result from UCPs.

IV. Transport through Inner and Outer Mitochondrial Membranes

Most of the newly synthesized ATP that is released into the mitochondrial matrix must be transported out of the mitochondria, where it is used for energy-requiring processes such as active ion transport, muscle contraction, or biosynthetic reactions. Likewise, ADP, phosphate, pyruvate, and other metabolites must be transported into the matrix. This requires transport of compounds through both the inner and outer mitochondrial membranes.

A. Transport through the Inner Mitochondrial Membrane

The inner mitochondrial membrane forms a tight permeability barrier to all polar molecules, including ATP, ADP, P_i, anions such as pyruvate, and cations such as Ca^{2+}, H^+, and K^+. Yet the process of oxidative phosphorylation depends on rapid and continuous transport of many of these molecules across the inner mitochondrial membrane (Fig. 24.15). Ions and other polar molecules are transported across the inner mitochondrial membrane by specific protein translocases that nearly balance charge during the transport process. Most of the exchange transport is a form of active transport that generally uses energy from the electrochemical potential gradient, either the membrane potential or the proton gradient.

ATP–ADP translocase (also called *ANT*, for *a*denine *n*ucleotide *t*ranslocase) transports ATP formed in the mitochondrial matrix to the intermembrane space in a specific 1:1 exchange for ADP produced from energy-requiring reactions outside of the mitochondria (see Fig. 24.15). Because ATP contains four negative charges and ADP contains only three, the exchange is promoted by the electrochemical potential gradient because the net effect is the transport of one negative charge from the matrix to the cytosol. Similar antiports exist for most metabolic anions. In contrast, P_i and pyruvate are transported into the mitochondrial matrix on specific transporters called *symports* together with a proton. A specific transport protein for Ca^{2+} uptake, called the Ca^{2+} *uniporter*, is driven by the electrochemical potential gradient, which is negatively charged on the matrix side of the membrane relative to the cytosolic side. Other transporters include the dicarboxylate transporter (phosphate–malate exchange), the tricarboxylate transporter (citrate–malate exchange),

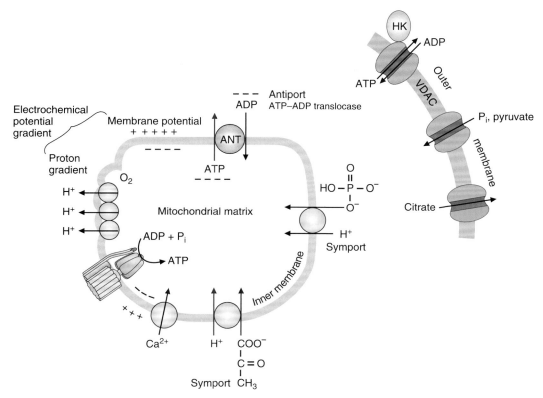

FIGURE 24.15 Transport of compounds across the inner and outer mitochondrial membranes. The electrochemical potential gradient drives the transport of ions across the inner mitochondrial membrane on specific translocases. Each translocase is composed of specific membrane-spanning helices that bind only specific compounds (adenine nucleotide translocase [ANT]). In contrast, the outer membrane contains relatively large unspecific pores called voltage-dependent anion channels (VDACs) through which a wide range of ions diffuse. These bind cytosolic proteins such as hexokinase (HK), which enables HK to have access to newly exported adenosine triphosphate (ATP). *ADP*, adenosine diphosphate; *P$_i$*, inorganic phosphate.

the aspartate–glutamate transporter, and the malate–α-ketoglutarate transporter (the last two as seen previously in the malate-aspartate shuttle for transferring reducing equivalents across the inner mitochondrial membrane).

B. Transport through the Outer Mitochondrial Membrane

Whereas the inner mitochondrial membrane is highly impermeable, the outer mitochondrial membrane is permeable to compounds with a molecular weight up to approximately 6,000 Da because it contains large nonspecific pores called *VDACs* that are formed by mitochondrial porins (see Fig. 24.15). Unlike most transport proteins, which are membrane-spanning helices with specific binding sites, VDACs are composed of porin homodimers that form a β-barrel with a relatively large nonspecific water-filled pore through the center. These channels are "open" at low transmembrane potential, with a preference for anions such as phosphate, chloride, pyruvate, citrate, and adenine nucleotides. VDACs thus facilitate translocation of these anions between the intermembrane space and the cytosol. Several cytosolic kinases, such as the hexokinase that initiates glycolysis, bind to the cytosolic side of the channel, where they have ready access to newly synthesized ATP.

C. The Mitochondrial Permeability Transition Pore

The mitochondrial permeability transition involves the opening of a large nonspecific pore (called the *mitochondrial permeability transition pore* [MPTP]) through the inner mitochondrial membrane and outer membranes at sites where they form a

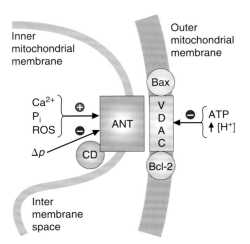

FIGURE 24.16 The mitochondrial permeability transition pore (MPTP). In the MPTP, adenine nucleotide translocase (ANT) is thought to complex with the voltage-dependent anion channel (VDAC). The conformation of ANT is regulated by cyclophilin D (CD), and Ca^{2+}. The change to an open pore is activated by Ca^{2+}, depletion of adenine nucleotides, and reactive oxygen species (ROS) that alter SH groups. It is inhibited by the electrochemical potential gradient (Δp), by cytosolic ATP, and by a low cytosolic pH. VDACs bind several proteins, including BCl-2 and Bax, which regulate apoptosis. Binding of proapoptotic members of the BCl-2 family to VDAC may change the permeability of the outer membrane so as to either favor, or block, events leading to apoptosis (such as cytochrome c release; see "Biochemical Comments" and Chapter 18).

junction (Fig. 24.16). In one model of the MPTP the basic components of the pore are ANT, the VDAC, and cyclophilin D (CD; which is a *cis–trans* isomerase for the proline peptide bond). Normally, ANT is a closed pore that functions specifically in a 1:1 exchange of matrix ATP for ADP in the intermembrane space. However, increased mitochondrial matrix Ca^{2+}, excess phosphate, or reactive oxygen species (ROS), which form oxygen or oxygen–nitrogen radicals, can activate opening of the pore. Conversely, ATP on the cytosolic side of the pore (and possibly a pH <7.0) and a membrane potential across the inner membrane protect against pore opening. Opening of the MPTP can be triggered by ischemia (hypoxia), which results in a temporary lack of O_2 for maintaining the proton gradient and ATP synthesis. When the proton gradient is not being generated by the ETC, ATP synthase runs backward and hydrolyzes ATP in an attempt to restore the gradient, thus rapidly depleting cellular levels of ATP. As ATP is hydrolyzed to ADP, the ADP is converted to adenine, and the nucleotide pool is no longer able to protect against pore opening. This can lead to a downward spiral of cellular events. A lack of ATP for maintaining the low mitochondrial Ca^{2+} can contribute to pore opening. When the MPTP opens, protons flood in, and maintaining a proton gradient becomes impossible. Anions and cations enter the matrix, mitochondrial swelling ensues, and the mitochondria become irreversibly damaged. The result is cell lysis and death (necrosis).

CLINICAL COMMENTS

Cora N. Thrombolysis stimulated by intravenous recombinant TPA restored O_2 to **Cora N.'s** heart muscle and successfully decreased the extent of ischemic damage. The rationale for the use of TPA within 4 to 6 hours after the onset of a myocardial infarction relates to the function of the normal intrinsic fibrinolytic system (see Chapter 43). This system is designed to dissolve unwanted intravascular clots through the action of the enzyme plasmin, a protease that digests the fibrin matrix within the clot. TPA stimulates the conversion of plasminogen to its active form, plasmin. The result is a lysis of the thrombus and improved blood flow through the previously obstructed vessel, allowing fuels and oxygen to reach the heart cells. The human TPA protein administered to Mrs. N. is produced by recombinant DNA technology (see Chapter 17). This treatment rapidly restored oxygen supply to her heart.

Stanley T. Mr. T. could be treated with antithyroid drugs, by subtotal resection of the thyroid gland, or with radioactive iodine. Successful treatment normalizes thyroid hormone secretion, and all of the signs, symptoms, and metabolic alterations of hyperthyroidism quickly subside.

Isabel S. In the case of **Isabel S.**, there was a concern for a myopathic process superimposed on her HIV and her pulmonary tuberculosis, either of which could have caused progressive weakness. In addition, she could have been suffering from a congenital mtDNA myopathy, symptomatic only as she ages. If she was being treated with zidovudine (AZT), an older drug not used very commonly anymore, her myopathy could have been caused by a disorder of oxidative phosphorylation induced by AZT. The lamivudine she was taking has rarely caused this myopathy. A systematic diagnostic process finally led her physician to conclude that she had HIV-associated myopathy.

BIOCHEMICAL COMMENTS

Mitochondria and Apoptosis. The loss of mitochondrial integrity is a major route initiating apoptosis (see Chapter 18, Section V). The intermembrane space contains procaspases 2, 3, and 9, which are proteolytic enzymes that are in the zymogen form (i.e., they must be proteolytically cleaved to be active). It also contains apoptosis-initiating factor (AIF) and caspase-activated DNase (CAD). AIF has a nuclear targeting sequence and is transported into the nucleus under appropriate conditions. Once AIF is inside the nucleus, it initiates chromatin condensation and degradation. Cytochrome c, which is loosely bound to the inner mitochondrial membrane, may also enter the intermembrane space when the electrochemical potential gradient is lost. The release of cytochrome c and the other proteins into the cytosol initiates apoptosis (see Chapter 18).

What is the trigger for the release of cytochrome c and the other proteins from the mitochondria? The VDAC pore is not large enough to allow the passage of proteins. Several theories have been proposed, each supported and contradicted by experimental evidence. One is that Bax (a member of the Bcl-2 family of proteins that forms an ion channel in the outer mitochondrial membrane) allows the entry of ions into the intermembrane space, causing swelling of this space and rupture of the outer mitochondrial membrane. Another theory is that Bax and VDAC (which is known to bind Bax and other Bcl-2 family members) combine to form an extremely large pore, much larger than is formed by either alone. Finally, it is possible that the MPTP or ANT participate in rupture of the outer membrane but that they close in a way that still provides the energy for apoptosis.

KEY CONCEPTS

- The reduced cofactors generated during fuel oxidation donate their electrons to the mitochondrial electron-transport chain.
- The electron-transport chain transfers the electrons to O_2, which is reduced to water.
- As electrons travel through the electron-transport chain, protons are transferred from the mitochondrial matrix to the cytosolic side of the inner mitochondrial membrane.
- The asymmetric distribution of protons across the inner mitochondrial membrane generates an electrochemical gradient across the membrane.
- The electrochemical gradient consists of a change in pH (ΔpH) across the membrane and a difference in charge ($\Delta\Psi$) across the membrane.

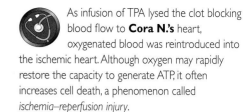

As infusion of TPA lysed the clot blocking blood flow to **Cora N.'s** heart, oxygenated blood was reintroduced into the ischemic heart. Although oxygen may rapidly restore the capacity to generate ATP, it often increases cell death, a phenomenon called *ischemia–reperfusion injury.*

During ischemia, several factors may protect heart cells against irreversible injury and cell death until oxygen is reintroduced. The stimulation of anaerobic glycolysis in the cytosol generates ATP without oxygen as glucose is converted to lactic acid. Lactic acid decreases cytosolic pH. Both cytosolic ATP and a lowering of the pH protect against opening of the MPTP. In addition, Ca^{2+} uptake by mitochondria requires a membrane potential, and it is matrix Ca^{2+} that activates opening of the MPTP. Thus, depending on the severity of the ischemic insult, the MPTP may not open, or may open and reseal, until oxygen is reintroduced. Then, depending on the sequence of events, reestablishment of the proton gradient, mitochondrial uptake of Ca^{2+}, or an increase of pH >7.0 may activate the MPTP before the cell has recovered. In addition, the reintroduction of O_2 generates oxygen free radicals, particularly through free-radical forms of CoQ in the ETC. These also may open the MPTP. The role of free radicals in ischemia–reperfusion injury is discussed in more detail in Chapter 25.

In addition to increased transcription of genes that encode TCA cycle enzymes and certain other enzymes of fuel oxidation, thyroid hormones increase the level of the uncoupling proteins UCP2 and UCP3. In hyperthyroidism, the efficiency with which energy is derived from the oxidation of these fuels is significantly less than normal. As a consequence of the increased rate of the ETC, hyperthyroidism results in increased heat production. Patients with hyperthyroidism, such as **Stanley T.**, complain of constantly feeling hot and sweaty.

- Proton entry into the mitochondrial matrix is energetically favorable and drives the synthesis of ATP via the ATP synthase.
- Respiration (oxygen consumption) is normally coupled to ATP synthesis; if one process is inhibited, the other is also inhibited.
- Uncouplers allow respiration to continue in the absence of ATP synthesis, as the energy inherent in the proton gradient is released as heat.
- OXPHOS diseases are caused by mutations in either nuclear or mitochondrial DNA that lead to a decrease in mitochondrial capacity for synthesizing ATP via oxidative phosphorylation.
- As the inner mitochondrial membrane is impermeable to virtually all biochemical compounds, transport systems exist to allow entry and exit of appropriate metabolites.
- The transfer of cytoplasmic reducing equivalents into the mitochondria occurs via shuttle systems; either the glycerol 3-phosphate shuttle or the malate-aspartate shuttle.
- Under appropriate stress, mitochondria will generate a nonspecific channel across both the inner and outer membranes that is known as the *mitochondrial permeability transition pore*. The opening of the pore is associated with events that lead to necrotic cell death.
- Diseases discussed in this chapter are summarized in Table 24.3.

TABLE 24.3	Diseases Discussed in Chapter 24	
DISEASE OR DISORDER	**ENVIRONMENTAL OR GENETIC**	**COMMENTS**
Myocardial infarction	Both	The lack of oxygen in the anterior and lateral walls of the heart is caused by severe ischemia owing to clots formed within certain coronary arteries at the site of ruptured atherosclerotic plaques. The limited availability of oxygen to act as an electron acceptor decreases the proton motive force across the inner mitochondrial membrane of ischemic cells. This leads to reduced adenosine triphosphate (ATP) generation, triggering events that lead to irreversible cell injury.
Hyperthyroidism	Both	Graves disease is an autoimmune genetic disorder caused by the generation of human thyroid-stimulating immunoglobulins. These immunoglobulins stimulate growth of the thyroid gland and excess secretion of the thyroid hormones triiodothyronine (T_3) and tetraiodothyronine (T_4).
HIV treatment complication	Environmental	One of the first drugs used to treat HIV was zidovudine (ZDV), formerly called azidothymidine (AZT) a nucleoside analog reverse transcriptase inhibitor. This class of drugs can act as an inhibitor of mitochondrial DNA polymerase. Under rare conditions, it can lead to a depletion of mitochondrial DNA in cells, leading to a severe mitochondrial myopathy.
Iron-deficiency anemia	Environmental	Lack of iron for heme synthesis, leading to reduced oxygen delivery to cells, and reduced iron in the electron-transfer chain, leading to muscle weakness.
Cyanide poisoning	Environmental	Cyanide binds to the Fe^{3+} in the heme of cytochrome aa_3, a component of cytochrome oxidase. Mitochondrial respiration and energy production cease, and cell death occurs rapidly.
Mitochondrial disorders	Genetic	Many types of mutations, leading to altered mitochondrial function and reduced energy production, caused by mutations in the mitochondrial DNA. See Table 24.2 for a full listing of these disorders.

1. Consider the following experiment. Carefully isolated liver mitochondria are incubated in the presence of a limiting amount of malate. Three minutes after adding the substrate, cyanide is added, and the reaction is allowed to proceed for another 7 minutes. At this point, which of the following components of the electron-transfer chain will be in an oxidized state?
   A. Complex I
   B. Complex II
   C. Complex III
   D. CoQ
   E. Cytochrome c

2. Consider the following experiment. Carefully isolated liver mitochondria are placed in a weakly buffered solution. Malate is added as an energy source, and an increase in oxygen consumption confirms that the ETC is functioning properly within these organelles. Valinomycin and potassium are then added to the mitochondrial suspension. Valinomycin is a drug that allows potassium ions to freely cross the inner mitochondrial membrane. What is the effect of valinomycin on the proton motive force that had been generated by the oxidation of malate?
   A. The proton motive force will be reduced to a value of zero.
   B. There will be no change in the proton motive force.
   C. The proton motive force will be increased.
   D. The proton motive force will be decreased but to a value greater than zero.
   E. The proton motive force will be decreased to a value less than zero.

3. Dinitrophenol, which was once tested as a weight-loss agent, acts as an uncoupler of oxidative phosphorylation by which one of the following mechanisms?
   A. Activating the H^+-ATPase
   B. Activating CoQ
   C. Blocking proton transport across the inner mitochondrial membrane
   D. Allowing for proton exchange across the inner mitochondrial membrane
   E. Enhancing oxygen transport across the inner mitochondrial membrane

4. A 25-year-old woman presents with chronic fatigue. A series of blood tests is ordered, and the results suggest that her red blood cell count is low because of iron-deficiency anemia. Such a deficiency would lead to fatigue because of which one of the following?
   A. Her decrease in Fe–S centers is impairing the transfer of electrons in the ETC.
   B. She is not producing enough H_2O in the electron-transport chain, leading to dehydration, which has resulted in fatigue.
   C. Iron forms a chelate with NADH and FAD(2H) that is necessary for them to donate their electrons to the ETC.

   D. Iron acts as a cofactor for α-ketoglutarate dehydrogenase in the TCA cycle, a reaction required for the flow of electrons through the ETC.
   E. Iron accompanies the protons that are pumped from the mitochondrial matrix to the cytosolic side of the inner mitochondrial membrane. Without iron, the proton gradient cannot be maintained to produce adequate ATP.

5. Which one of the following would be expected for a patient with an OXPHOS disease?
   A. A high ATP:ADP ratio in the mitochondria
   B. A high $NADH:NAD^+$ ratio in the mitochondria
   C. A deletion on the X chromosome
   D. A high activity of complex II of the ETC
   E. A defect in the integrity of the inner mitochondrial membrane

6. A 5-year-old boy was eating paint chips from the windowsill in his 125-year-old home, and he developed an anemia. Bloodwork indicated high levels of lead, which interfere with heme synthesis. Reduced heme synthesis would have little effect on the function of which one of the following proteins or complexes?
   A. Myoglobin
   B. Hemoglobin
   C. Complex I
   D. Complex III
   E. Complex IV

7. Rotenone, an inhibitor of NADH dehydrogenase, was originally used for fishing. When it was sprinkled on a lake, fish would absorb it through their gills and die. Until recently, it was used in the United States as an organic pesticide and was recommended for tomato plants. It was considered nontoxic to mammals and birds, neither of which can readily absorb it. What effect would rotenone have on ATP production by heart mitochondria, if it could be absorbed?
   A. There would be no reduction in ATP production.
   B. There would be a 95% reduction in ATP production.
   C. There would be a 10% reduction in ATP production.
   D. There would be a 50% reduction in ATP production.
   E. There would be a 50% increase in ATP production.

8. In order for cells to function properly, energy is required; for most cells, the energy is primarily derived from the high-energy phosphate bonds of ATP, which is produced through oxidative phosphorylation. Which one of the following is a key component of oxidative phosphorylation?
   A. Using NADH and FAD(H2) to accept electrons as substrates are oxidized.
   B. Creating a permeable inner mitochondrial membrane to allow mitochondrial ATP to enter the cytoplasm as it is made.
   C. An ATP synthase to synthesize ATP
   D. An ATP synthetase to synthesize ATP
   E. A source of electrons, which is usually oxygen in most tissues

9. Carefully isolated intact mitochondria were incubated with a high-salt solution, which is capable of disrupting noncovalent interactions between molecules at the membrane surface. After washing the mitochondria, pyruvate and oxygen were added to initiate electron flow. Oxygen consumption was minimal under these conditions because of the loss of which one of the following components from the electron-transfer chain?
   A. Complex I
   B. CoQ
   C. Complex III
   D. Cytochrome C
   E. Complex IV

10. UCPs allow oxidation to be uncoupled from phosphorylation. Assume that a drug company has developed a reagent that can activate several UCPs with the goal being the development of a weight-loss drug. A potential side effect of this drug could be which one of the following?
   A. Decreased oxidation of acetyl coenzyme A
   B. Decreased glycolytic rate
   C. Increase in body temperature
   D. Increased ATP production by the ATP synthase
   E. Inhibition of the ETC

ANSWERS

1. **The answer is B.** For a component to be in the oxidized state, it must have donated, or never received, electrons. Complex II will metabolize succinate to produce fumarate (generating FAD[2H]), but no succinate is available in this experiment. Thus, complex II never sees any electrons and is always in an oxidized state. The substrate malate is oxidized to oxaloacetate, generating NADH, which donates electrons to complex I of the ETC. These electrons are transferred to CoQ, which donates electrons to complex III, to cytochrome c, and then to complex IV. Cyanide will block the transfer of electrons from complex IV to oxygen, so all previous complexes containing electrons will be backed up and the electrons will be "stuck" in the complexes, making these components reduced. Thus, answers A and C through E must be incorrect.

2. **The answer is D.** The proton motive force consists of two components, a ΔpH, and a $\Delta\psi$ (electrical component). The addition of valinomycin and potassium will destroy the electrical component but not the pH component. Thus, the proton motive force will decrease but will still be greater than zero. Thus, the other answers are all incorrect.

3. **The answer is D.** Dinitrophenol equilibrates the proton concentration across the inner mitochondrial membrane, thereby destroying the proton motive force. Thus, none of the other answers is correct.

4. **The answer is A.** A deficiency of Fe–S centers in the ETC would impair the transfer of electrons down the chain and reduce ATP production by oxidative phosphorylation. Answer B is incorrect because the decreased production of water from the ETC is not of sufficient magnitude to cause her to become dehydrated. Answer C is incorrect because iron does not form a chelate with NADH and FAD(2H). Answer D is incorrect because iron is not a cofactor for α-ketoglutarate dehydrogenase. Answer E is incorrect because iron does not accompany the protons that make up the proton gradient.

5. **The answer is B.** NADH would not be reoxidized as efficiently by the ETC, and the NADH/NAD$^+$ ratio would increase. Answer A is incorrect because ATP would not be produced at a high rate. Therefore, ADP would build up and the ATP:ADP ratio would be low. Answer C is incorrect because OXPHOS diseases can be caused by mutations in nuclear or mtDNA, and not all OXPHOS proteins are encoded by the X chromosome. Answer D is incorrect because, depending on the nature of the mutation, the activity of complex II of the ETC might be normal or decreased, but there is no reason to expect increased activity. Answer E is incorrect because the integrity of the inner mitochondrial membrane would not necessarily be affected. It could be, but it would not be expected for all patients with OXPHOS disorders.

6. **The answer is C.** Heme is required for the synthesis of cytochromes. Complex I, although containing iron, does so in iron–sulfur centers and contains no cytochromes. Complexes III and IV contain cytochromes, whereas myoglobin and hemoglobin contain heme as the oxygen binding component of those proteins. Defects in heme synthesis, then, would have a negative impact on the function of complexes III and IV, as well as hemoglobin and myoglobin, without greatly affecting the functioning of complex I.

7. **The answer is B.** Because rotenone inhibits the oxidation of NADH, it would completely block the generation of the electrochemical potential gradient in vivo and, therefore, it would block ATP generation. In the presence of rotenone, NADH would accumulate and NAD$^+$ concentrations would decrease. Although the mitochondria might still be able to oxidize compounds like succinate, which transfer electrons to FAD, no succinate would be produced in vivo if the NAD$^+$-dependent dehydrogenases of the TCA cycle were inhibited. Thus, very shortly after rotenone administration, there would not be any substrates available for the electron transfer chain, and NADH dehydrogenase would be blocked, so

oxidative phosphorylation would be completely inhibited. If glucose supplies were high, anaerobic glycolysis could provide some ATP, but not nearly enough to keep the heart pumping. Anaerobic glycolysis produces 2 ATP per glucose molecule, compared with 32 ATP molecules generated by oxidative phosphorylation, which is a reduction of approximately 95%.

8. **The answer is C.** NAD$^+$ and FAD are electron acceptors and NADH and FAD(2H) are electron donors. Oxygen is the terminal electron acceptor and is not an electron donor. The inner mitochondrial membrane must be impermeable to most compounds, including protons; otherwise, the proton gradient that drives ATP synthesis could not be created or maintained. The enzyme ATP synthase contains a proton pore that spans the inner mitochondrial membrane and a catalytic headpiece that protrudes into the matrix. Protons are driven through the pore and change the conformation of the subunits in the headpiece, thereby producing ATP. If protons enter the mitochondria other ways then through the pore, no ATP is generated by the ATP synthase (partial uncoupling). A synthetase is an enzyme that uses high-energy phosphate bonds (usually from ATP) to catalyze its reaction, and the ATP synthase creates high-energy phosphate bonds and does not use them.

9. **The answer is D.** Complexes I, III, and IV are protein complexes that span the inner mitochondrial membrane, and their location within the membrane would not be disrupted by a high-salt solution. Cytochrome c is a small protein in the intermembrane space that binds to the inner mitochondrial membrane through noncovalent interactions. High salt can dislodge cytochrome c from the inner membrane, and the mitochondria would become cytochrome c–deficient. Electron flow would stop in the absence of cytochrome c owing to an inability to transfer electrons from complexes III to complex IV. CoQ is a lipid-soluble quinone that diffuses in the lipid membrane, and it would not be removed from the membrane by a high-salt solution.

10. **The answer is C.** Uncouplers uncouple oxidation from phosphorylation such that oxygen consumption is increased, there is an increased flow of electrons through the electron-transfer chain, but ATP synthesis via oxidative phosphorylation is diminished. ATP production is reduced owing to the reduction in the size of the proton gradient across the inner mitochondrial membrane because the UCPs allow protons to enter the matrix of the mitochondria without going through the ATP synthase. Because the energy of electron transfer is no longer being used to generate a proton gradient, it is released as heat, and an individual taking such a drug would be expected to exhibit an increased body temperature. Owing to the uncoupling, the oxidation of acetyl coenzyme A (acetyl-CoA) would increase, as would the glycolytic rate, in attempts to generate ATP for the cell. The ATP synthase would be producing less ATP, and glycolysis would be producing more ATP. The weight loss would come about because of the inefficiency in ATP generation via acetyl-CoA oxidation, as more fatty acids would have to be metabolized in order to generate a certain amount of ATP from the acetyl-CoA derived from the fatty acids.

Oxygen Toxicity and Free-Radical Injury

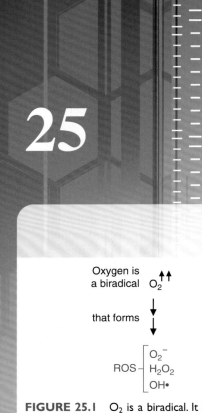

Oxygen is a biradical O_2

that forms

$ROS \begin{cases} O_2^- \\ H_2O_2 \\ OH\bullet \end{cases}$

FIGURE 25.1 O_2 is a biradical. It has two antibonding electrons with parallel spins, (*parallel arrows*). It has a tendency to form toxic reactive oxygen species (ROS), such as superoxide (O_2^-), the nonradical hydrogen peroxide (H_2O_2), and the hydroxyl radical (OH•).

O_2 is both essential to human life and **toxic**. We are dependent on O_2 for oxidation reactions in the pathways of adenosine triphosphate (ATP) generation, detoxification, and biosynthesis. However, when O_2 accepts single electrons, it is transformed into highly reactive **oxygen radicals** that damage cellular lipids, proteins, and DNA. Damage by reactive oxygen radicals contributes to cellular death and degeneration in a wide range of diseases (Table 25.1).

Radicals are compounds that contain a single electron, usually in an outside orbital. Oxygen is a **biradical**, a molecule that has two unpaired electrons in separate orbitals (Fig. 25.1). Through several enzymatic and nonenzymatic processes that routinely occur in cells, O_2 accepts **single electrons** to form **reactive oxygen species** (**ROS**). ROS are highly reactive oxygen radicals or compounds that are readily converted in cells to these reactive radicals. The ROS formed by reduction of O_2 are the radical **superoxide** (O_2^-), the nonradical **hydrogen peroxide** (H_2O_2), and the **hydroxyl radical** (**OH•**).

ROS may be generated nonenzymatically or enzymatically as accidental by-products or major products of reactions. Superoxide may be generated nonenzymatically from coenzyme Q (CoQ) or from metal-containing enzymes (e.g., **cytochrome P450**, **xanthine oxidase**, and reduced nicotinamide adenine dinucleotide phosphate [**NADPH**] **oxidase**). The highly toxic hydroxyl radical is formed nonenzymatically from superoxide in the presence of Fe^{2+} or Cu^+ by the **Fenton reaction** and from hydrogen peroxide in the **Haber–Weiss reaction**.

Oxygen radicals and their derivatives can be deadly to cells. The hydroxyl radical causes oxidative damage to proteins and DNA. It also forms **lipid peroxides** and **malondialdehyde** from membrane lipids containing **polyunsaturated fatty acids**. In some cases, free-radical damage is the direct cause of a disease state (e.g., tissue damage initiated by exposure to ionizing radiation). In **neurodegenerative diseases**, such as Parkinson disease, or in ischemia–reperfusion injury, ROS may perpetuate the cellular damage caused by another process.

TABLE 25.1 Some Disease States Associated with Free-Radical Injury	
Atherogenesis	Cerebrovascular disorders
Emphysema/bronchitis	Ischemia–reperfusion injury
Duchenne-type muscular dystrophy	Neurodegenerative disorders
Pregnancy/preeclampsia	Amyotrophic lateral sclerosis (Lou Gehrig disease)
Retrolental fibroplasia	
Cervical cancer	Alzheimer disease
Alcohol-induced liver disease	Down syndrome
Hemodialysis	Ischemia–reperfusion injury following stroke
Diabetes	OXPHOS diseases (mitochondrial DNA disorders)
Acute renal failure	Multiple sclerosis
Aging	Parkinson disease

OXPHOS, oxidative phosphorylation.

Oxygen radicals are joined in their destructive damage by the free-radical nitric oxide (NO) and the ROS **hypochlorous acid** (**HOCl**). NO combines with O_2 or superoxide to form **reactive nitrogen–oxygen species** (**RNOS**), such as the non-radical peroxynitrite or the radical **nitrogen dioxide**. RNOS are present in the environment (e.g., cigarette smoke) and are generated in cells. During phagocytosis of invading microorganisms, cells of the immune system produce O_2^-, HOCl, and NO through the actions of **NADPH oxidase**, **myeloperoxidase**, and **inducible nitric oxide synthase**, respectively. In addition to killing phagocytosed invading microorganisms, these toxic metabolites may damage surrounding tissue components.

Cells **protect** themselves against damage by ROS and other radicals through **repair processes**, **compartmentalization** of free-radical production, **defense enzymes**, and **endogenous and exogenous antioxidants** (**free-radical scavengers**). The defense enzyme **superoxide dismutase** (**SOD**) removes the superoxide free radical. Catalase and glutathione peroxidase remove hydrogen peroxide and lipid peroxides. **Vitamin E**, **vitamin C**, and **plant flavonoids** act as **antioxidants**. **Oxidative stress** occurs when the rate of ROS generation exceeds the capacity of the cell for their removal (Fig. 25.2).

THE WAITING ROOM

 Two years ago, **Les G.**, a 62-year-old man, noted an increasing tremor of his right hand when sitting quietly (resting tremor). The tremor disappeared if he actively used this hand to do purposeful movement. As this symptom progressed, he also complained of stiffness in his muscles that slowed his movements (bradykinesia). His wife noticed a change in his gait; he had begun taking short, shuffling steps and leaned forward as he walked (postural imbalance). He often appeared to be staring ahead with a rather immobile facial expression. She noted a tremor of his eyelids when he was asleep and, recently, a tremor of his legs when he was at rest. Because of these progressive symptoms and some subtle personality changes (anxiety and emotional lability), she convinced Les to see their family doctor.

The doctor suspected that her patient probably had primary or idiopathic parkinsonism (Parkinson disease) and referred Mr. G. to a neurologist. In Parkinson disease, neurons of the substantia nigra pars compacta, containing the pigment melanin and the neurotransmitter dopamine, degenerate.

 Cora N. had done well since the successful lysis of blood clots in her coronary arteries with the use of intravenous recombinant tissue plasminogen activator (TPA) (see Chapters 20 and 24). This therapy quickly relieved the crushing chest pain (angina) she had experienced when she won the lottery. At her first office visit after her discharge from the hospital, Cora's cardiologist told her she had developed multiple premature contractions of the ventricular muscle of her heart as the clots were being lysed. This process could have led to a life-threatening arrhythmia known as *ventricular tachycardia* or *ventricular fibrillation*. However, Cora's arrhythmia responded quickly to pharmacologic suppression and did not recur during the remainder of her hospitalization.

I. O_2 and the Generation of Reactive Oxygen Species

The generation of *ROS* from O_2 in our cells is a natural, everyday occurrence. The electrons that contribute to their formation are usually derived from reduced electron carriers of the electron-transport chain (ETC). ROS are formed as accidental products of nonenzymatic and enzymatic reactions. Occasionally, they are deliberately synthesized in enzyme-catalyzed reactions. Ultraviolet radiation and pollutants in the air can increase formation of toxic oxygen-containing compounds.

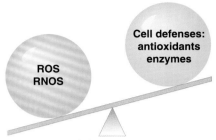

FIGURE 25.2 Oxidative stress. Oxidative stress occurs when the rate of reactive oxygen species (ROS) and reactive nitrogen–oxygen species (RNOS) production overbalances the rate of their removal by cellular defense mechanisms. These defense mechanisms include several enzymes and antioxidants. Antioxidants usually react nonenzymatically with ROS.

 The basal ganglia are part of a neuronal feedback loop that modulates and integrates the flow of information from the cerebral cortex to the motor neurons of the spinal cord. The neostriatum is the major input structure from the cerebral cortex. The substantia nigra pars compacta consists of neurons that provide integrative input to the neostriatum through pigmented neurons that use dopamine as a neurotransmitter (the nigrostriatal pathway). Integrated information feeds back to the basal ganglia and to the cerebral cortex to control voluntary movement. In Parkinson disease, a decrease in the amount of dopamine reaching the basal ganglia results in the movement disorder.

 In ventricular tachycardia, rapid premature beats from an irritative focus in ventricular muscle occur in runs of varying duration. Persistent ventricular tachycardia compromises cardiac output, leading to death. This arrhythmia can result from severe ischemia (lack of blood flow) in the ventricular muscle of the heart caused by clots forming at the site of a ruptured atherosclerotic plaque. However, **Cora N.'s** rapid beats began during the infusion of tissue TPA as the clot was lysed. Thus, they probably resulted from reperfusing a previously ischemic area of her heart with oxygenated blood. This phenomenon is known as *ischemia–reperfusion injury*, and it is caused by cytotoxic ROS derived from oxygen in the blood that reperfuses previously hypoxic cells. Ischemia–reperfusion injury also may occur when tissue oxygenation is interrupted during surgery or transplantation.

Catecholamine (epinephrine, norepinephrine, dopamine) measurements, which were ordered for **Mr. G.**, use either serum or a 25-hour urine collection as samples for assay. After appropriate removal of cells and/or particulate matter, the sample is placed over an ion-exchange high-pressure liquid chromatography (HPLC) column and the eluate from the column is analyzed by sensitive electrochemical detection. Through comparison with retention times of standard catecholamines on the column, the various catecholamine species can be clearly resolved from each other. The electrochemical detection uses electrodes that are oxidized by the samples, and the amplitude current that is generated via the redox reaction allows one to determine the concentration of catecholamines in the specimen.

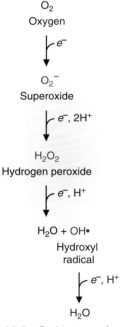

FIGURE 25.3 Reduction of oxygen by four one-electron steps. The four one-electron reduction steps for O_2 progressively generate superoxide, hydrogen peroxide, and the hydroxyl radical plus water. Superoxide is sometimes written O_2^- to better illustrate its single unpaired electron. H_2O_2, the half-reduced form of O_2, has accepted two electrons and is, therefore, not an oxygen radical. e^-, electron.

A. The Radical Nature of O_2

A *radical*, by definition, is a molecule that has a single unpaired electron in an orbital. A *free radical* is a radical that is capable of independent existence. (Radicals formed in an enzyme active site during a reaction, for example, are not considered free radicals unless they can dissociate from the protein to interact with other molecules.) Radicals are highly reactive and initiate chain reactions by extracting an electron from a neighboring molecule to complete their own orbitals. Although the transition metals (e.g., Fe, Cu, Mo) have single electrons in orbitals, they are not usually considered free radicals because they are relatively stable, do not initiate chain reactions, and are bound to proteins in the cell.

The oxygen molecule is a *biradical*, which means it has two single electrons in different orbitals. These electrons cannot both travel in the same orbital because they have parallel spins (they spin in the same direction). Although oxygen is very reactive from a thermodynamic standpoint, its single electrons cannot react rapidly with the paired electrons found in the covalent bonds of organic molecules. As a consequence, O_2 reacts slowly through the acceptance of single electrons in reactions that require a catalyst (such as a metal-containing enzyme).

Because the two unpaired electrons in oxygen have the same (parallel) spin, they are called *antibonding electrons*. In contrast, carbon–carbon and carbon–hydrogen bonds each contain two electrons, which have antiparallel spins and form a thermodynamically stable pair. As a consequence, O_2 cannot readily oxidize a covalent bond because one of its electrons would have to flip its spin around to make new pairs. The difficulty in changing spins is called *spin restriction*. Without spin restriction, organic life forms could not have developed in the oxygen atmosphere on earth because they would be spontaneously oxidized by O_2.

O_2 is capable of accepting a total of four electrons, which reduces it to water (Fig. 25.3). When O_2 accepts one electron, *superoxide* is formed. Superoxide is still a radical because it has one unpaired electron remaining. This reaction is not thermodynamically favorable and requires a moderately strong reducing agent that can donate single electrons (e.g., the radical form of coenzyme Q [CoQH•] in the ETC). When superoxide accepts an electron, it is reduced to *hydrogen peroxide* (H_2O_2), which is not a radical. The *hydroxyl radical* is formed in the next one-electron reduction step in the reduction sequence. Finally, acceptance of the last electron reduces the hydroxyl radical to H_2O.

B. Characteristics of Reactive Oxygen Species

ROS are oxygen-containing compounds that are highly reactive free radicals or compounds that are readily converted to these oxygen free radicals in the cell. The major oxygen metabolites produced by one-electron reduction of oxygen (superoxide, hydrogen peroxide, and the hydroxyl radical) are classified as ROS (Table 25.2).

Reactive free radicals extract electrons (usually as hydrogen atoms) from other compounds to complete their own orbitals, thereby initiating free-radical chain reactions. The hydroxyl radical is probably the most potent of the ROS. It initiates chain reactions that form lipid peroxides and organic radicals and adds directly to compounds. The superoxide anion is also highly reactive, but it has limited lipid solubility and cannot diffuse far. However, it can generate the more reactive hydroxyl and hydroperoxy radicals by reacting nonenzymatically with hydrogen peroxide in the Haber–Weiss reaction (Fig. 25.4).

Hydrogen peroxide, although not actually a radical, is a weak oxidizing agent that is classified as an ROS because it can generate the hydroxyl radical (OH•). Transition metals, such as Fe^{2+} or Cu^+, catalyze formation of the hydroxyl radical from hydrogen peroxide in the nonenzymatic Fenton reaction (see Fig. 25.4). Because hydrogen peroxide is lipid-soluble, it can diffuse through membranes and generate OH• at localized Fe^{2+}- or Cu^+-containing sites, such as the ETC within the mitochondria. Hydrogen peroxide is also the precursor of hypochlorous acid (HOCl), a powerful oxidizing agent that is produced endogenously and enzymatically by phagocytic cells. To decrease occurrence of the Fenton reaction, accessibility to transition metals, such as Fe^{2+} and Cu^+, are highly restricted in cells or in

TABLE 25.2	**Reactive Oxygen Species and Reactive Nitrogen–Oxygen Species**
REACTIVE SPECIES	**PROPERTIES**
Superoxide anion (O_2^-)	Produced by the electron-transport chain and at other sites. Cannot diffuse far from the site of origin. Generates other **reactive oxygen species**.
Hydrogen peroxide (H_2O_2)	Not a free radical but can generate free radicals by reaction with a transition metal (e.g., Fe^{2+}). Can diffuse into and through cell membranes.
Hydroxyl radical (OH•)	The most reactive species in attacking biologic molecules. Produced from H_2O_2 in the Fenton reaction in the presence of Fe^{2+} or Cu^+.
Organic radicals (RO•, R•, R–S)	Organic free radicals (R denotes the remainder of the compound). Produced from ROH, RH (e.g., at the carbon of a double bond in a fatty acid), or RSH OH• attack.
Peroxy radical (RCOO•)	An organic peroxy radical, such as occurs during lipid degradation (also denoted LOO•).
Hypochlorous acid (HOCl)	Produced in neutrophils during the respiratory burst to destroy invading organisms. Toxicity is through halogenation and oxidation reactions. Attacking species is OCl^-.
Singlet oxygen ($O_2^{\downarrow\uparrow}$)	Oxygen with antiparallel spins. Produced at high oxygen tensions from absorption of ultraviolet light. Decays so fast that it is probably not a significant in vivo source of toxicity.
Nitric oxide (NO)	**Reactive nitrogen–oxygen species** (RNOS). A free radical produced endogenously by nitric oxide synthase. Binds to metal ions. Combines with O_2 or other oxygen-containing radicals to produce additional RNOS.
Peroxynitrite ($ONOO^-$)	RNOS. A strong oxidizing agent that is not a free radical. It can generate nitrogen dioxide (NO_2), which is a radical.

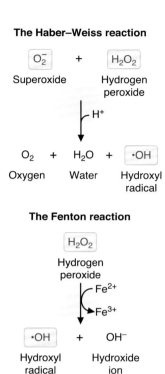

The Haber–Weiss reaction

O_2^- Superoxide + H_2O_2 Hydrogen peroxide

H^+

O_2 Oxygen + H_2O Water + •OH Hydroxyl radical

The Fenton reaction

H_2O_2 Hydrogen peroxide

Fe^{2+}
Fe^{3+}

•OH Hydroxyl radical + OH^- Hydroxide ion

FIGURE 25.4 Generation of the hydroxyl radical by the nonenzymatic Haber–Weiss and Fenton reactions. In the simplified versions of these reactions shown here, the transfer of single electrons generates the hydroxyl radical. Reactive oxygen species are shown in the *boxes*. In addition to Fe^{2+}, Cu^+ and many other metals can also serve as single-electron donors in the Fenton reaction.

the body as a whole. Events that release iron from cellular storage sites, such as a crushing injury, are associated with increased free-radical injury.

Organic radicals are generated when superoxide or the hydroxyl radical indiscriminately extract electrons from other molecules. Organic peroxy radicals are intermediates of chain reactions, such as lipid peroxidation. Other organic radicals, such as the ethoxy radical, are intermediates of enzymatic reactions that escape into solution (see Table 25.2).

An additional group of oxygen-containing radicals, termed RNOS, contains nitrogen as well as oxygen. These radicals are derived principally from the free radical nitric oxide (NO), which is produced endogenously by the enzyme nitric oxide synthase. NO combines with O_2 or superoxide to produce additional RNOS.

C. Major Sources of Primary Reactive Oxygen Species in the Cell

ROS are constantly being formed in the cell; approximately 3% to 5% of the oxygen we consume is converted to oxygen free radicals. Some are produced as accidental by-products of normal enzymatic reactions that escape from the active site of metal-containing enzymes during oxidation reactions. Others, such as hydrogen peroxide, are physiologic products of oxidases in peroxisomes. Deliberate production of toxic free radicals occurs during the inflammatory response. Drugs, natural radiation, air pollutants, and other chemicals also can increase formation of free radicals in cells.

1. Generation of Superoxide

One of the major sites of superoxide generation is CoQ in the mitochondrial ETC (Fig. 25.5). The one-electron reduced form of CoQ (CoQH•) is free within the membrane and can accidentally transfer an electron to dissolved O_2, thereby forming superoxide. In contrast, when O_2 binds to cytochrome oxidase and accepts electrons, none of the O_2 radical intermediates is released from the enzyme, and no ROS are generated.

 With insufficient oxygen, **Cora N.'s** ischemic heart muscle mitochondria were unable to maintain cellular ATP levels, resulting in high intracellular Na^+ and Ca^{2+} levels. The reduced state of the electron carriers in the absence of oxygen, and loss of mitochondrial ion gradients or membrane integrity, leads to increased superoxide production once oxygen becomes available during reperfusion. The damage can be self-perpetuating, especially if iron bound to components of the ETC becomes available for the Fenton reaction, or the mitochondrial permeability transition is activated.

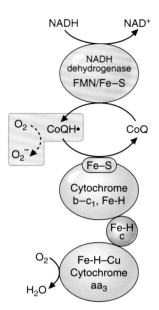

FIGURE 25.5 Generation of superoxide by coenzyme Q (CoQ) in the electron-transport chain. In the process of transporting electrons to O_2, some of the electrons escape when CoQH• accidentally interacts with O_2 to form superoxide. *Fe-H* represents the Fe-heme center of the cytochromes. *FMN*, flavin mononucleotide; *NAD*, nicotinamide adenine dinucleotide.

2. Oxidases, Oxygenases, and Peroxidases

Most of the oxidases, peroxidases, and oxygenases in the cell bind O_2 and transfer single electrons to it via a metal. Free-radical intermediates of these reactions may be accidentally released before the reduction is complete.

Cytochrome P450 enzymes are a major source of free radicals "leaked" from reactions. Because these enzymes catalyze reactions in which single electrons are transferred to O_2 and an organic substrate, the possibility of accidentally generating and releasing free-radical intermediates is high (see Chapters 20 and 24). Induction of P450 enzymes by alcohol, drugs, or chemical toxicants leads to increased cellular injury. As an example, carbon tetrachloride (CCl_4), which is used as a solvent in the dry-cleaning industry, is converted by cytochrome P450 to a highly reactive free radical that has caused hepatocellular necrosis in workers in that industry. When the enzyme-bound CCl_4 accepts an electron, it dissociates into CCl_3• and Cl. The CCl_3• radical, which cannot continue through the P450 reaction sequence, "leaks" from the enzyme active site and initiates chain reactions in the surrounding polyunsaturated lipids of the endoplasmic reticulum. These reactions spread into the plasma membrane and to proteins, eventually resulting in cell swelling, accumulation of lipids, and cell death. When substrates for cytochrome P450 enzymes are not present, its potential for destructive damage is diminished by repression of gene transcription.

Hydrogen peroxide and lipid peroxides are generated enzymatically as major reaction products by several oxidases present in peroxisomes, mitochondria, and the endoplasmic reticulum. For example, monoamine oxidase, which oxidatively degrades the neurotransmitter dopamine, generates H_2O_2 at the mitochondrial membrane of certain neurons. Peroxisomal fatty acid oxidase generates H_2O_2 rather than FAD(2H) during the oxidation of very-long-chain fatty acids (see Chapter 30). Xanthine oxidase, an enzyme of purine degradation that can reduce O_2 to O_2^- or H_2O_2 in the cytosol, is thought to be a major contributor to ischemia–reperfusion injury, especially in intestinal mucosal and endothelial cells. Lipid peroxides are also formed enzymatically as intermediates in the pathways for synthesis of many eicosanoids, including leukotrienes and prostaglandins.

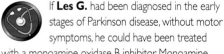

If **Les G.** had been diagnosed in the early stages of Parkinson disease, without motor symptoms, he could have been treated with a monoamine oxidase B inhibitor. Monoamine oxidase is a copper-containing enzyme that inactivates dopamine in neurons, producing H_2O_2. The drug was originally administered to inhibit dopamine degradation. However, current theory suggests that the effectiveness of the drug is also related to a decrease of free-radical formation within the cells of the basal ganglia. The dopaminergic neurons involved are particularly susceptible to the cytotoxic effects of ROS and RNOS that may arise from H_2O_2.

3. Ionizing Radiation

Cosmic rays that continuously bombard the earth, radioactive chemicals, and X-rays are forms of *ionizing radiation*. Ionizing radiation has a high enough energy level that it can split water into hydroxyl and hydrogen radicals, thus leading to radiation damage to the skin, mutations, cancer, and cell death. It also may generate organic radicals through direct collision with organic cellular components.

II. Oxygen Radical Reactions with Cellular Components

Oxygen radicals produce cellular dysfunction by reacting with lipids, proteins, carbohydrates, and DNA to extract electrons (summarized in Fig. 25.6). Evidence of free-radical damage has been described in >100 disease states. In some of these diseases, free-radical damage is the primary cause of the disease; in others, it enhances complications of the disease.

A. Membrane Attack: Formation of Lipid and Lipid Peroxy Radicals

Chain reactions that form lipid free radicals and lipid peroxides in membranes make a major contribution to ROS-induced injury (Fig. 25.7). An initiator (such as a hydroxyl radical produced locally in the Fenton reaction) begins the chain reaction. It extracts a hydrogen atom, preferably from the double bond of a polyunsaturated fatty acid in a membrane lipid. The chain reaction is propagated when O_2 adds to form lipid peroxy radicals and lipid peroxides. Eventually, lipid degradation occurs, forming such products as malondialdehyde (from fatty acids with three or more double bonds) and ethane and pentane (from the ω-terminal carbons of three- and six-carbon fatty acids, respectively). Malondialdehyde appears in the blood and urine and is used as an indicator of free-radical damage.

 Production of ROS by xanthine oxidase in endothelial cells may be enhanced during ischemia–reperfusion in **Cora N.'s** heart. In undamaged tissues, xanthine oxidase exists as a dehydrogenase that uses NAD^+ rather than O_2 as an electron acceptor in the pathway for degradation of purines (hypoxanthine $\rightarrow$ xanthine $\rightarrow$ uric acid; see Chapter 39). When O_2 levels decrease, phosphorylation of ADP to ATP decreases, and degradation of ADP and adenine through xanthine oxidase increases. In the process, xanthine dehydrogenase is converted to an oxidase. As long as O_2 levels are below the high K_m of the enzyme for O_2, little damage is done. However, during reperfusion, when O_2 levels return to normal, xanthine oxidase generates H_2O_2 and O_2^- at the site of injury.

 The appearance of lipofuscin granules in many tissues increases during aging. The pigment lipofuscin (from the Greek *lipos*, for lipids, and the Latin *fuscus*, for dark) consists of a heterogeneous mixture of cross-linked polymerized lipids and protein formed by reactions between amino acid residues and lipid peroxidation products, such as malondialdehyde. These cross-linked products are probably derived from peroxidatively damaged cell organelles that were autophagocytized by lysosomes but could not be digested. When these dark pigments appear on the skin of the hands in aged individuals, they are referred to as "liver spots," a traditional hallmark of aging. In **Les G.** and other patients with Parkinson disease, lipofuscin appears as Lewy bodies in degenerating neurons.

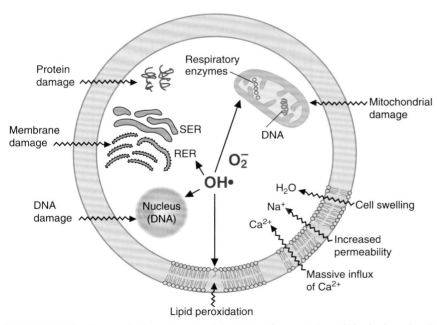

FIGURE 25.6 Free radical–mediated cellular injury. Superoxide and the hydroxyl radical initiate lipid peroxidation in the cellular, mitochondrial, nuclear, and endoplasmic reticulum membranes. The increase in cellular permeability results in an influx of Ca^{2+}, which causes further mitochondrial damage. The cysteine sulfhydryl groups and other amino acid residues on proteins are oxidized and degraded. Nuclear and mitochondrial DNA can be oxidized, resulting in strand breaks and other types of damage. Reactive nitrogen–oxygen species (nitric oxide [NO], NO_2, and peroxynitrites) have similar effects. *RER*, rough endoplasmic reticulum; *SER*, smooth endoplasmic reticulum.

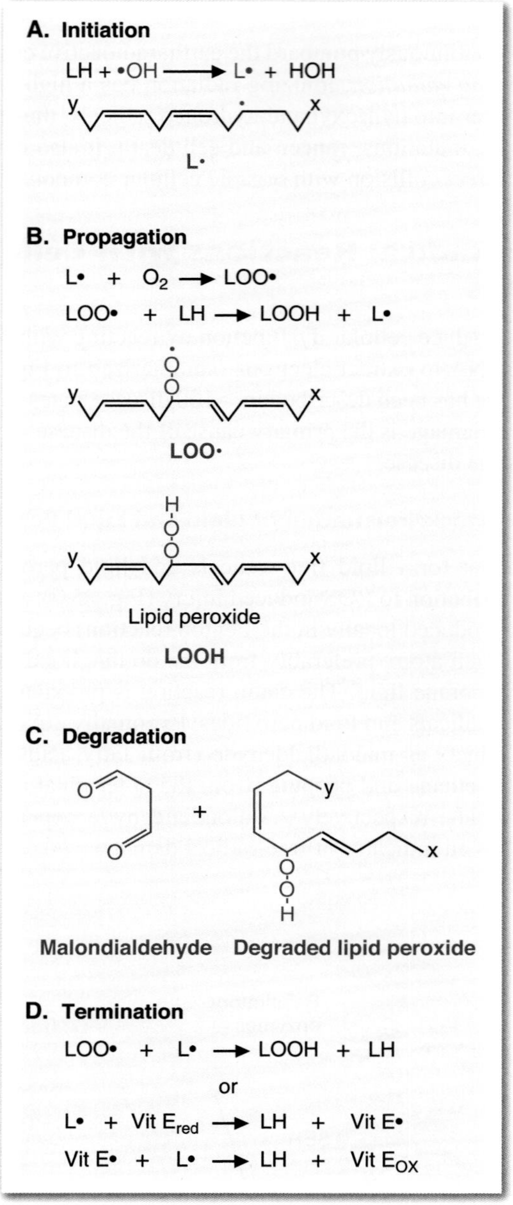

FIGURE 25.7 Lipid peroxidation: a free-radical chain reaction. **A.** Lipid peroxidation is initiated by a hydroxyl or other radical that extracts a hydrogen atom from a polyunsaturated lipid (LH), thereby forming a lipid radical (L•). **B.** The free-radical chain reaction is propagated by reaction with O_2, forming the lipid peroxy radical (LOO•) and lipid peroxide (LOOH). **C.** Rearrangements of the single electron result in degradation of the lipid. Malondialdehyde, one of the compounds formed, is soluble and appears in blood. **D.** The chain reaction can be terminated by reduced vitamin E (Vit E_{red}) and other lipid-soluble antioxidants that donate single electrons. Two subsequent reduction steps form a stable, oxidized antioxidant.

Peroxidation of lipid molecules invariably changes or damages lipid molecular structure. In addition to the self-destructive nature of membrane lipid peroxidation, the aldehydes that are formed can cross-link proteins. When the damaged lipids are the constituents of biologic membranes, the cohesive lipid bilayer arrangement and stable structural organization is disrupted (see Fig. 25.6). Disruption of mitochondrial membrane integrity may result in further free-radical production.

B. Proteins and Peptides

In proteins, the amino acids proline, histidine, arginine, cysteine, and methionine are particularity susceptible to hydroxyl radical attack and oxidative damage. As a consequence of oxidative damage, the protein may fragment or residues cross-link with other residues. Free-radical attack on protein cysteine residues can result in cross-linking and formation of aggregates that prevents their degradation. However, oxidative damage increases the susceptibility of other proteins to proteolytic digestion.

Free-radical attack and oxidation of the cysteine sulfhydryl residues of the tripeptide glutathione (γ-glutamylcysteinylglycine; see Section V.A.3) increases oxidative damage throughout the cell. Glutathione is a major component of cellular defense against free-radical injury, and its oxidation reduces its protective effects.

 Evidence of protein damage shows up in many diseases, particularly those associated with aging. In patients with cataracts, proteins in the lens of the eye exhibit free-radical damage and contain methionine sulfoxide residues and tryptophan degradation products.

C. DNA

Oxygen-derived free radicals are also a major source of DNA damage. Approximately 20 types of oxidatively altered DNA molecules have been identified. The nonspecific binding of Fe^{2+} to DNA facilitates localized production of the hydroxyl radical, which can cause base alterations in the DNA (one example is generating 8-hydroxyguanine from guanine, in the presence of the hydroxyl radical). It also can attack the deoxyribose backbone and cause strand breaks. This DNA damage can be repaired to some extent by the cell (see Chapter 12) or minimized by apoptosis of the cell.

III. Nitric Oxide and Reactive Nitrogen–Oxygen Species

NO is an oxygen-containing free radical that, like O_2, is both essential to life and toxic. NO has a single electron and therefore binds to other compounds that contain single electrons, such as Fe^{3+}. As a gas, NO diffuses through the cytosol and lipid membranes and into cells. At low concentrations, it functions physiologically as a neurotransmitter and as a hormone that causes vasodilation. At high concentrations, however, it combines with O_2 or with superoxide to form additional reactive and toxic species that contain both nitrogen and oxygen (RNOS). RNOS are involved in neurodegenerative diseases such as Parkinson disease and in chronic inflammatory diseases such as rheumatoid arthritis.

 Nitroglycerin, in tablet form, is often given to patients with coronary artery disease who experience ischemia-induced chest pain (angina). The nitroglycerin decomposes in the blood, forming nitric oxide, a potent vasodilator. This decreases the preload (blood return to the heart) by dilating the veins and therefore eases the work of the heart and also increases blood flow to the heart by dilating arteries, which relieves the angina.

A. Nitric Oxide Synthase

At low concentrations, NO serves as a neurotransmitter or as a hormone. It is synthesized from arginine by NO synthases (Fig. 25.8). As a gas, it is able to diffuse through water and lipid membranes and into target cells. In the target cell, it exerts its physiologic effects by high-affinity binding to Fe-heme in the enzyme guanylyl cyclase, thereby activating a signal transduction cascade. However, NO is rapidly inactivated by nonspecific binding to many molecules, and therefore, cells that produce NO need to be close to the target cells.

The body has three different tissue-specific isoforms of NO synthase, each encoded by a different gene: neuronal nitric oxide synthase (nNOS, isoform I), inducible nitric oxide synthase (iNOS, isoform II), and endothelial nitric oxide synthase (eNOS, isoform III). nNOS and eNOS are tightly regulated by the concentration of Ca^{2+} to produce the small amounts of NO required for its role as a neurotransmitter and hormone. In contrast, iNOS is present in many cells of the immune system and cell types with a similar lineage, such as macrophages and brain astroglia. This isoenzyme of NO synthase is regulated principally by induction of gene transcription and not by changes in Ca^{2+} concentration. It produces high and toxic levels of NO to assist in killing invading microorganisms. It is these very high levels of NO that are associated with generation of RNOS and NO toxicity.

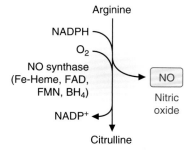

FIGURE 25.8 Nitric oxide synthase (NOS) synthesizes the free radical nitric oxide (NO). Like cytochrome P450 enzymes, NOS uses Fe-heme, flavin adenine dinucleotide (FAD), and flavin mononucleotide (FMN) to transfer single electrons from reduced nicotinamide adenine dinucleotide phosphate (NADPH) to O_2. NOS also requires the cofactor tetrahydrobiopterin (BH_4).

B. Nitric Oxide Toxicity

The toxic actions of NO can be divided into two categories: direct toxic effects resulting from binding to Fe-containing proteins, and indirect effects mediated by compounds formed when NO combines with O_2 or with superoxide to form RNOS.

1. Direct Toxic Effects of Nitric Oxide

NO, as a radical, exerts direct toxic effects by combining with Fe-containing compounds that also have single electrons. Major destructive sites of attack include Fe–S centers (e.g., ETC complexes I through III, aconitase) and Fe-heme proteins (e.g., hemoglobin and ETC cytochromes). However, there is usually little damage because NO is present in low concentrations and Fe-heme compounds are present in excess capacity. NO can cause serious damage, however, through direct inhibition of respiration in cells that are already compromised through oxidative phosphorylation diseases or ischemia.

2. Reactive Nitrogen–Oxygen Species Toxicity

When NO is present in very high concentrations (e.g., during inflammation), it combines nonenzymatically with superoxide to form peroxynitrite ($ONOO^-$), or with O_2 to form dinitrogen trioxide (N_2O_3) (Fig. 25.9). Peroxynitrite, although it is not a free radical, is a strong oxidizing agent that is stable and directly toxic. It can diffuse through the cell and lipid membranes to interact with a wide range of targets, including the methionine side chain in proteins and –SH groups (e.g., Fe–S centers in the ETC). It also breaks down to form additional RNOS, including the free-radical nitrogen dioxide (NO_2), which is an effective initiator of lipid peroxidation. Peroxynitrite products also react (nitration) with aromatic rings, forming compounds

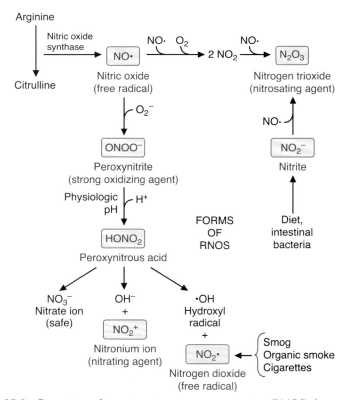

FIGURE 25.9 Formation of reactive nitrogen–oxygen species (RNOS) from nitric oxide (NO). RNOS are shown in *red*. The type of damage caused by each RNOS is shown in *parentheses*. Of all the nitrogen–oxygen–containing compounds shown, only nitrate is relatively nontoxic. Nitrogen dioxide (NO_2) is one of the toxic agents present in smog, automobile exhaust, gas ranges, pilot lights, cigarette smoke, and smoke from forest fires or burning buildings.

such as nitrotyrosine or nitroguanosine. N_2O_3, which can be derived from either NO_2 or nitrite, is the agent of nitrosative stress, and it nitrosylates sulfhydryl and similarly reactive groups in the cell. Nitrosylation usually interferes with the proper functioning of the protein or lipid that has been modified. Thus, RNOS can do as much oxidative and free-radical damage as non–nitrogen-containing ROS, as well as nitrating and nitrosylating compounds. The result is widespread and includes inhibition of a large number of enzymes, mitochondrial lipid peroxidation, inhibition of the ETC and energy depletion, single-stranded or double-stranded breaks in DNA, and modification of bases in DNA.

IV. Formation of Free Radicals during Phagocytosis and Inflammation

In response to infectious agents and other stimuli, phagocytic cells of the immune system (neutrophils, eosinophils, and monocytes/macrophages) exhibit a rapid consumption of O_2 called the *respiratory burst*. The respiratory burst is a major source of superoxide, hydrogen peroxide, the hydroxyl radical, HOCl, and RNOS. The generation of free radicals is part of the human antimicrobial defense system and is intended to destroy invading microorganisms, tumor cells, and other cells targeted for removal.

A. Reduced Nicotinamide Adenine Dinucleotide Phosphate Oxidase

The respiratory burst results from the activity of NADPH oxidase, which catalyzes the transfer of an electron from NADPH to O_2 to form superoxide (Fig. 25.10). NADPH oxidase is assembled from cytosolic as well as membranous proteins recruited into the phagolysosome membrane as it surrounds an invading microorganism.

 In patients with chronic granulomatous disease, phagocytes have genetic defects in NADPH oxidase. NADPH oxidase, of which there are several isozymes, generally has six different subunits (two in the cell membrane, α and β, which together form flavoprotein b_{558}, and four recruited from the cytosol, which include the small GTPase Rac, as well as a complex of $p47^{phox}$, $p67^{phox}$, and $p40^{phox}$); the genetic defect may be in any of four of the genes that encode these subunits. The membrane catalytic β-subunit of NADPH oxidase is a 91-kDa flavocytochrome glycoprotein. It transfers electrons from bound NADPH to FAD, which transfers them to the Fe-heme components. The membranous α-subunit (p22) is required for stabilization. The cytosolic proteins are required for assembly of the complex. The 91-kDa β-subunit is affected most often in X-linked chronic granulomatous disease, whereas the α-subunit is affected in a rare autosomal-recessive form. The cytosolic subunits p47 and p67 are affected most often in patients with the autosomal-recessive form of granulomatous disease. In addition to their enhanced susceptibility to bacterial and fungal infections, these patients suffer from an apparent dysregulation of normal inflammatory responses.

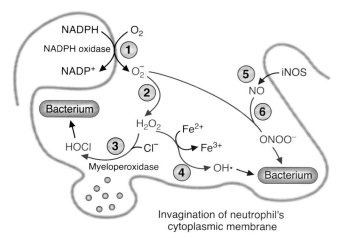

FIGURE 25.10 Production of reactive oxygen species (ROS) during the phagocytic respiratory burst by activated neutrophils. (*1*) Activation of reduced nicotinamide adenine dinucleotide phosphate (NADPH) oxidase on the outer side of the plasma membrane initiates the respiratory burst with the generation of superoxide. During phagocytosis, the plasma membrane invaginates, and superoxide is released into the vacuole space. (*2*) Superoxide (either spontaneously or enzymatically via superoxide dismutase [SOD]) generates H_2O_2. (*3*) Granules containing myeloperoxidase are secreted into the phagosome, where myeloperoxidase generates hypochlorous acid (HOCl) and other halides. (*4*) H_2O_2 can also generate the hydroxyl radical from the Fenton reaction. (*5*) Inducible nitric oxide synthase (iNOS) may be activated and generate nitric oxide (NO). (*6*) NO combines with superoxide to form peroxynitrite, which may generate additional reactive nitrogen–oxygen species. The result is an attack on the membranes and other components of phagocytosed cells, and eventual lysis. The whole process is referred to as the *respiratory burst* because it lasts only 30 to 60 minutes and consumes O_2.

Superoxide is released into the intramembranous space of the phagolysosome, where it is generally converted to hydrogen peroxide and other ROS that are effective against bacteria and fungal pathogens. Hydrogen peroxide is formed by SOD, which may come from the phagocytic cell or from the invading microorganism.

B. Myeloperoxidase and Hypochlorous Acid

The formation of HOCl from H_2O_2 is catalyzed by myeloperoxidase, a heme-containing enzyme that is present only in phagocytic cells of the immune system (predominantly neutrophils). The HOCl rapidly dissociates and loses a proton.

$$H_2O_2 + Cl^- + H^+ \xrightarrow{\text{Myeloperoxidase}} HOCl + H_2O \xrightarrow{\text{Dissociation}} {}^-OCl + H^+ + H_2O$$

Myeloperoxidase contains two Fe-hemelike centers, which give it the green color seen in pus. HOCl is a powerful toxin that destroys bacteria within seconds through halogenation and oxidation reactions. It oxidizes many Fe- and S-containing groups (e.g., sulfhydryl groups, Fe–S centers, ferredoxin, heme-proteins, methionine), oxidatively decarboxylates and deaminates proteins, and cleaves peptide bonds. Aerobic bacteria under attack rapidly lose membrane transport, possibly because of damage to ATP synthase or electron transport chain components (which reside in the plasma membrane of bacteria).

C. Reactive Nitrogen–Oxygen Species and Inflammation

When human neutrophils of the immune system are activated to produce NO, NADPH oxidase is also activated. NO reacts rapidly with superoxide to generate peroxynitrite, which forms additional RNOS. NO also may be released into the surrounding medium to combine with superoxide in target cells.

In several disease states, free-radical release by neutrophils or macrophages during inflammation contributes to injury in the surrounding tissues. During stroke or myocardial infarction, phagocytic cells that move into the ischemic area to remove dead cells may increase the area and extent of damage. The self-perpetuating mechanism of radical release by neutrophils during inflammation and immune-complex formation may explain some of the features of chronic inflammation in patients with rheumatoid arthritis. As a result of free-radical release, the immunoglobulin G (IgG) proteins present in the synovial fluid are partially oxidized, which improves their binding with the rheumatoid antibody. This binding, in turn, stimulates the neutrophils to release more free radicals.

V. Cellular Defenses against Oxygen Toxicity

Our defenses against oxygen toxicity fall into the categories of antioxidant defense enzymes, dietary and endogenous antioxidants (free-radical scavengers), cellular compartmentalization, metal sequestration, and repair of damaged cellular components. The antioxidant defense enzymes react with ROS and cellular products of free-radical chain reactions to convert them to nontoxic products.

Dietary antioxidants, such as vitamin E and flavonoids, and endogenous antioxidants, such as urate, can terminate free-radical chain reactions. *Defense through compartmentalization* refers to separation of species and sites involved in ROS generation from the rest of the cell (Fig. 25.11). For example, many of the enzymes that produce hydrogen peroxide are sequestered in peroxisomes with a high content of antioxidant enzymes. Metals are bound to a wide range of proteins within the blood and in cells, preventing their participation in the Fenton reaction. Iron, for example, is tightly bound to its storage protein, ferritin, and cannot react with hydrogen peroxide. Repair mechanisms for DNA and for removal of oxidized fatty acids from membrane lipids are available to the cell. Oxidized amino acids on proteins are continuously repaired through protein degradation and resynthesis of new proteins.

During **Cora N.'s** myocardial ischemia (decreased blood flow), the ability of her heart to generate ATP from oxidative phosphorylation was compromised. The damage appeared to accelerate when oxygen was first reintroduced (reperfused) into the tissue. During ischemia, Co Q and the other single-electron components of the ETC become saturated with electrons. When oxygen is reintroduced (reperfusion), electron donation to O_2 to form superoxide is increased. The increase of superoxide results in enhanced formation of hydrogen peroxide and the hydroxyl radical. Macrophages in the area clean up cell debris from ischemic injury and produce nitric oxide, which may further damage mitochondria by generating RNOS that attack Fe–S centers and cytochromes in the ETC. These radicals, which increase in concentration when oxygen is introduced into the system, may actually amplify the damage done by the original ischemic event and increase the infarct size.

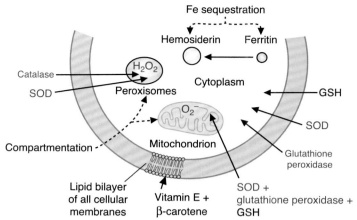

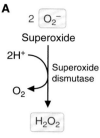

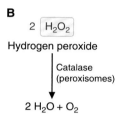

FIGURE 25.11 Compartmentalization of free-radical defenses. Various defenses against reactive oxygen species (ROS) are found in the various subcellular compartments of the cell. The location of free-radical defense enzymes (shown in *red*) matches the type and amount of ROS generated in each subcellular compartment. The highest activities of these enzymes are found in the liver, adrenal gland, and kidney, where mitochondrial and peroxisomal contents are high, and cytochrome P450 enzymes are found in abundance in the smooth endoplasmic reticulum. The enzymes superoxide dismutase (SOD) and gluta-thione (GSH) peroxidase are present as isozymes in the various compartments. Another form of compartmentalization involves the sequestration of Fe, which is stored as mobiliz-able Fe in ferritin. Excess Fe is stored in nonmobilizable hemosiderin deposits. GSH is a nonenzymatic antioxidant.

A. Antioxidant Scavenging Enzymes

The enzymatic defense against ROS includes SOD, catalase, and glutathione peroxidase.

1. Superoxide Dismutase

Conversion of superoxide anion to hydrogen peroxide and O_2 (dismutation) by SOD is often called the *primary defense* against oxidative stress because superoxide is such a strong initiator of chain reactions (Fig. 25.12A). SOD exists as three isoen-zyme forms, a $Cu^+–Zn^{2+}$ form present in the cytosol, a Mn^{2+} form present in mi-tochondria, and a $Cu^+–Zn^{2+}$ form found extracellularly. The activity of $Cu^+–Zn^{2+}$ SOD is increased by chemicals or conditions (such as hyperbaric oxygen) that in-crease the production of superoxide.

2. Catalase

Hydrogen peroxide, once formed, must be reduced to water to prevent it from forming the hydroxyl radical in the Fenton reaction or the Haber–Weiss reaction (see Fig. 25.4) One of the enzymes that is capable of reducing hydrogen peroxide is catalase (see Fig. 25.12B). Catalase is found principally in peroxisomes and to a lesser extent in the cytosol and microsomal fraction of the cell. The highest activities are found in tissues with a high peroxisomal content (kidney and liver). In cells of the immune system, catalase serves to protect the cell against its own respiratory burst.

3. Glutathione Peroxidase and Glutathione Reductase

Glutathione (γ-glutamylcysteinylglycine) is one of the body's principal means of protecting against oxidative damage (see also Chapter 27). Glutathione is a tripep-tide composed of glutamate, cysteine, and glycine, with the amino group of cys-teine joined in peptide linkage to the γ-carboxyl group of glutamate (Fig. 25.13). In reactions that are catalyzed by glutathione peroxidases, the reactive sulfhydryl groups reduce hydrogen peroxide to water and lipid peroxides to nontoxic alco-hols. In these reactions, two glutathione molecules are oxidized to form a single

FIGURE 25.12 **A.** Superoxide dismutase converts superoxide to hydrogen peroxide, which is nontoxic unless it is converted to other reac-tive oxygen species (ROS). **B.** Catalase converts two molecules of hydrogen peroxide to two molecules of water and one molecule of oxygen. (ROS is shown in a *yellow box*.)

The intracellular form of the $Cu^+–Zn^{2+}$ SOD is encoded by the *SOD1* gene. To date, 58 mutations in this gene have been discovered in individuals affected by familial amyotrophic lateral sclerosis (ALS, or Lou Gehrig disease). How a mutation in this gene leads to the symptoms of this disease has yet to be understood. It is important to note that only 5% to 10% of the total cases of diagnosed ALS are caused by the familial form. Recent work has indicated that mutations in enzymes involved in RNA processing also lead to familial and sporadic ALS.

Why does the cell need a high content of SOD in mitochondria?

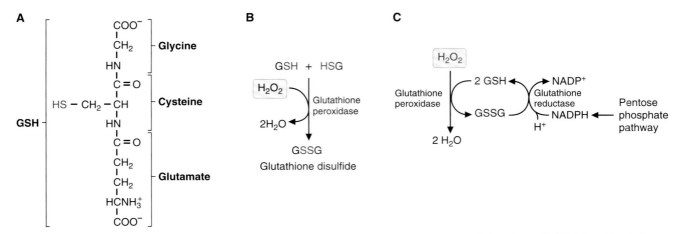

FIGURE 25.13 Glutathione peroxidase reduces hydrogen peroxide to water. **A.** The structure of glutathione (GSH). The sulfhydryl group of GSH, which is oxidized to a disulfide, is shown in *red*. **B.** Glutathione peroxidase transfers electrons from GSH to hydrogen peroxide. **C.** GSH redox cycle. Glutathione reductase regenerates reduced GSH. (Reactive oxygen species is shown in the *yellow box*.)

molecule, glutathione disulfide. The sulfhydryl groups are also oxidized in nonenzymatic chain-terminating reactions with organic radicals.

Glutathione peroxidases exist as a family of selenium enzymes with somewhat different properties and tissue locations. Within cells, they are found principally in the cytosol and mitochondria and are the major means for removing H_2O_2 produced outside of peroxisomes. They contribute to our dietary requirement for selenium and account for the protective effect of selenium in the prevention of free-radical injury.

Once oxidized glutathione (GSSG) is formed, it must be reduced back to the sulfhydryl form by glutathione reductase in a redox cycle (see Fig. 25.13C). Glutathione reductase contains a flavin adenine dinucleotide (FAD) and catalyzes transfer of electrons from NADPH to the disulfide bond of GSSG. NADPH is thus essential for protection against free-radical injury. The major source of NADPH for this reaction is the pentose phosphate pathway (see Chapter 27).

B. Nonenzymatic Antioxidants (Free-Radical Scavengers)

Free-radical scavengers convert free radicals to a nonradical, nontoxic form in nonenzymatic reactions. Most free-radical scavengers are antioxidants, compounds that neutralize free radicals by donating a hydrogen atom (with its one electron) to the radical. Antioxidants, therefore, reduce free radicals and are themselves oxidized in the reaction. Dietary free-radical scavengers (e.g., vitamin E, ascorbic acid, carotenoids, flavonoids), as well as endogenously produced free-radical scavengers (e.g., urate, melatonin), have a common structural feature, which is a conjugated double-bond system that may be an aromatic ring.

 Mitochondria are major sites for generation of superoxide from the interaction of Co Q and O_2. The Mn^{2+} SOD present in mitochondria is not regulated through induction/repression of gene transcription, presumably because the rate of superoxide generation is always high. Mitochondria also have a high content of glutathione and glutathione peroxidase and can thus convert H_2O_2 to H_2O and prevent lipid peroxidation.

 Premature infants with low levels of lung surfactant (see Chapter 31) require oxygen therapy. The level of oxygen must be closely monitored to prevent ROS-induced retinopathy and subsequent blindness (the retinopathy of prematurity) and to prevent bronchial pulmonary dysplasia. The tendency for these complications to develop is enhanced by the possibility of low levels of SOD and vitamin E in the premature infant.

 Selenium (Se) is present in human proteins principally as selenocysteine (cysteine with the sulfur group replaced by Se, abbreviated sec). This amino acid functions in catalysis and has been found in 11 or more human enzymes, including the 4 enzymes of the glutathione peroxidase family. Se is supplied in the diet as selenomethionine from plants (methionine with the Se replacing the sulfur), selenocysteine from animal foods, and inorganic Se. Se from all of these sources can be converted to selenophosphate. Selenophosphate reacts with a unique tRNA-containing bound serine to form a selenocysteine-tRNA, which incorporates selenocysteine into the appropriate protein as it is being synthesized. Se homeostasis in the body is controlled principally through regulation of its secretion as methylated Se. The current dietary requirement is approximately 70 μg/day for adult males and 55 μg/day for females. Deficiency symptoms reflect diminished antioxidant defenses and include symptoms of vitamin E deficiency.

I. Vitamin E

Vitamin E (α-tocopherol), the most widely distributed antioxidant in nature, is a lipid-soluble antioxidant vitamin that functions principally to protect against lipid peroxidation in membranes (see Fig. 25.11). Vitamin E comprises several tocopherols that differ in their methylation pattern. Among these, α-tocopherol is the most potent antioxidant and is present in the largest amounts in our diet (Fig. 25.14).

Vitamin E is an efficient antioxidant and nonenzymatic terminator of free-radical chain reactions, and it has little pro-oxidant activity. When vitamin E donates an electron to a lipid peroxy radical, it is converted to a free-radical form that is stabilized by resonance. If this free-radical form were to act as a pro-oxidant and abstract an electron from a polyunsaturated lipid, it would be oxidizing that lipid and actually propagate the free-radical chain reaction. The chemistry of vitamin E is such that it has a much greater tendency to donate a second electron and go to the fully oxidized form.

Vitamin E is found in the diet in the lipid fractions of some vegetable oils and in liver, egg yolks, and cereals. It is absorbed together with lipids, and fat malabsorption results in symptomatic deficiencies. Vitamin E circulates in the blood in lipoprotein particles. Its deficiency causes neurologic symptoms, probably because the polyunsaturated lipids in myelin and other membranes of the nervous system are particularly sensitive to free-radical injury. Epidemiologic evidence suggests that individuals with a higher intake of foods containing vitamin E, β-carotene, and vitamin C have a somewhat lower risk of cancer and certain other ROS-related diseases than do individuals on diets that are deficient in these vitamins. However, studies in which well-nourished populations were given supplements of these antioxidant vitamins found either no effects or harmful effects compared with the beneficial effects from eating foods containing a wide variety of antioxidant compounds. Of the pure chemical supplements tested, there is evidence only for the efficacy of vitamin E. In two clinical trials, β-carotene (or β-carotene + vitamin A) was associated with a higher incidence of lung cancer among smokers and higher mortality rates. In one study, vitamin E intake was associated with a higher incidence of hemorrhagic stroke (possibly because of vitamin K mimicry).

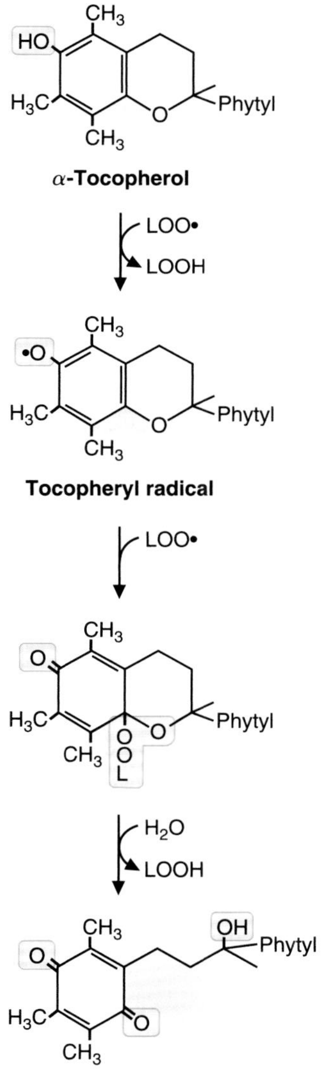

FIGURE 25.14 Vitamin E (α-tocopherol) terminates free-radical lipid peroxidation by donating single electrons to lipid peroxy radicals (LOO•) to form the more stable lipid peroxide, LOOH. In so doing, the α-tocopherol is converted to the fully oxidized tocopheryl quinone.

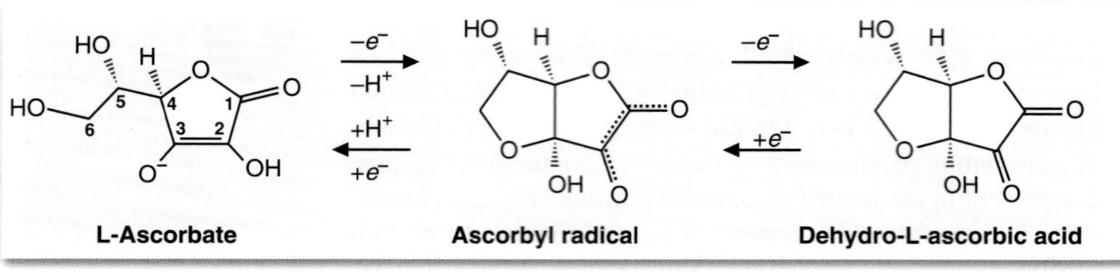

FIGURE 25.15   L-Ascorbate (the reduced form) donates single electrons (e^-) to free radicals or disulfides in two steps as it is oxidized to dehydro-L-ascorbic acid. Its principal role in free-radical defense is probably regeneration of vitamin E. However, it also may react with superoxide, hydrogen peroxide, hypochlorite, the hydroxyl and peroxy radicals, and nitrogen dioxide.

Age-related macular degeneration (AMD) is the leading cause of blindness in the United States among people older than 50 years of age, and it affects as many as 15 million people in the United States. In AMD, visual loss is related to oxidative damage to the retinal pigment epithelium (RPE) and the choriocapillaris epithelium. The photoreceptor/retinal pigment complex is exposed to sunlight, it is bathed in near-arterial levels of oxygen, and the membranes contain high concentrations of polyunsaturated fatty acids, all of which are conducive to oxidative damage. Lipofuscin granules, which accumulate in the RPE throughout life, may serve as photosensitizers, initiating damage by absorbing blue light and generating singlet oxygen (an energetically excited form of oxygen) that forms other radicals. Dark sunglasses are protective. Epidemiologic studies showed that the intake of lutein and zeaxanthin in dark-green leafy vegetables (e.g., spinach, collard greens) also may be protective. Lutein and zeaxanthin accumulate in the macula and protect against free-radical damage by absorbing blue light and quenching singlet oxygen.

2. Ascorbic Acid

Although ascorbate (vitamin C) is an oxidation–reduction coenzyme that functions in collagen synthesis and other reactions, it also plays a role in free-radical defense. Reduced ascorbate can regenerate the reduced form of vitamin E by donating electrons in a redox cycle (Fig. 25.15). It is water-soluble and circulates unbound in blood and extracellular fluid, where it has access to the lipid-soluble vitamin E present in membranes and lipoprotein particles.

3. Carotenoids

Carotenoids is a term applied to β-carotene (the precursor of vitamin A) and similar compounds with functional oxygen-containing substituents on the rings, such as zeaxanthin and lutein. These compounds can exert antioxidant effects as well as quench singlet O_2 (singlet oxygen is a highly ROS in which there are no unpaired electrons in the outer orbitals, but there is one orbital that is completely empty). Epidemiologic studies have shown a correlation between diets that are high in fruits and vegetables and health benefits, leading to the hypothesis that carotenoids might slow the progression of cancer, atherosclerosis, and other degenerative diseases by acting as chain-breaking antioxidants. However, in clinical trials, β-carotene supplements had either no effect or an undesirable effect. Its ineffectiveness may be the result of the pro-oxidant activity of the free-radical form.

In contrast, epidemiologic studies relating the intake of lutein and zeaxanthin with decreased incidence of AMD have received progressive support. These two carotenoids are concentrated in the macula (the central portion of the retina) and are called the *macular carotenoids*.

4. Other Dietary Antioxidants

Flavonoids are a group of structurally similar compounds that contain two spatially separate aromatic rings and are found in red wine, green tea, chocolate, and other plant-derived foods. Flavonoids have been hypothesized to contribute to our free-radical defenses in several ways. Some flavonoids inhibit enzymes responsible for superoxide anion production, such as xanthine oxidase. Others efficiently chelate Fe and Cu, making it impossible for these metals to participate in the Fenton reaction. They also may act as free-radical scavengers by donating electrons to superoxide or lipid peroxy radicals, or they may stabilize free radicals by complexing with them.

It is difficult to tell how much dietary flavonoids contribute to our free-radical defense system; they have a high pro-oxidant activity and are poorly absorbed. Nonetheless, we generally consume large amounts of flavonoids ($\sim$800 mg/day), and there is evidence that they can contribute to the maintenance of vitamin E as an antioxidant.

5. Endogenous Antioxidants

Several compounds that are synthesized endogenously for other functions, or as urinary excretion products, also function nonenzymatically as free-radical antioxidants. Uric acid is formed from the degradation of purines and is released into extracellular fluids, including blood, saliva, and lung lining fluid. Together with protein thiols, it accounts for the major free-radical trapping capacity of plasma. It is particularly important in the upper airways, where there are few other antioxidants. It can directly scavenge hydroxyl radicals, oxyheme oxidants formed between the reaction of hemoglobin and peroxy radicals, and peroxy radicals themselves. Having acted as a scavenger, uric acid produces a range of oxidation products that are subsequently excreted.

Melatonin, which is a secretory product of the pineal gland, is a neurohormone that functions in regulation of our circadian rhythm, light–dark signal transduction, and sleep induction. In addition to these receptor-mediated functions, it functions as a nonenzymatic free-radical scavenger that donates an electron (as hydrogen) to "neutralize" free radicals. It also can react with ROS and RNOS to form addition products, thereby undergoing suicidal transformations. Its effectiveness is related to both its lack of pro-oxidant activity and its joint hydrophilic/hydrophobic nature, which allows it to pass through membranes and the blood–brain barrier.

CLINICAL COMMENTS

Les G. has "primary" parkinsonism. The pathogenesis of this disease is not well established and may be multifactorial (Fig. 25.16). Recent work has identified several genes, which, when mutated and inactive, lead to rare familial Parkinson disease and others that affect the risk for Parkinson disease. The major clinical disturbances in Parkinson disease are a result of dopamine depletion in the neostriatum, resulting from degeneration of dopaminergic neurons whose cell bodies reside in the substantia nigra pars compacta. The decrease in dopamine production is the result of severe degeneration of these nigrostriatal neurons. Although the agent that initiates the disease is unknown, a variety of studies support a role for free radicals in Parkinson disease (mitochondrial dysfunction), along with alterations in the ubiquitin–proteasome pathway of protein degradation. Within these neurons, dopamine turnover is increased, dopamine levels are lower, glutathione is decreased, and lipofuscin (Lewy bodies) is increased. Iron levels are higher, and ferritin, the storage form of iron, is lower. Furthermore, the disease is mimicked by the compound 1-methyl-4-phenylpyridinium (MPP^+), an inhibitor of NADH:CoQ oxidoreductase that increases superoxide production in these neurons and decreases ATP production. Analysis of mitochondria from patients with Parkinson disease indicate a 30% to 40% reduction in complex I activity. The reduced ATP levels may affect the ubiquitin–proteasome pathway negatively, reducing protein degradation and linking these two pathways, which can lead to Parkinson disease. Even so, it is not known whether oxidative stress makes a primary or secondary contribution to the disease process.

Drug therapy is based on the severity of the disease. Several options are available. In the early phases of the disease if symptoms are mild, a monoamine oxidase B inhibitor can be used that inhibits dopamine degradation and decreases hydrogen peroxide formation. In later stages of the disease or more symptomatic stages, patients are treated with levodopa (L-DOPA), a precursor of dopamine, sometimes in combination with the monoamine oxidase B inhibitor.

Cora N. experienced angina caused by severe ischemia in the ventricular muscle of her heart. The ischemia was caused by clots that formed at the site of atherosclerotic plaques within the lumen of the coronary arteries. When TPA was infused to dissolve the clots, the ischemic area of her heart was reperfused with oxygenated blood, resulting in ischemia–reperfusion injury. In her case, the reperfusion injury resulted in some short runs of ventricular tachycardia.

During ischemia, several events occur simultaneously in cardiomyocytes. A decreased O_2 supply results in decreased ATP generation from mitochondrial oxidative phosphorylation and inhibition of cardiac muscle contraction. As a consequence, cytosolic AMP levels increase, activating anaerobic glycolysis and lactic acid production. If ATP levels are inadequate to maintain Na^+,K^+-ATPase activity, intracellular Na^+ increases, resulting in cellular swelling, a further increase in H^+ concentration, and increases of cytosolic and subsequently mitochondrial Ca^{2+} levels.

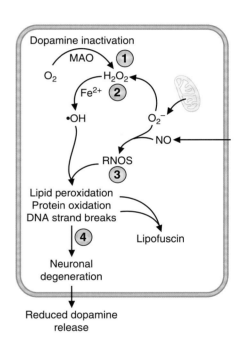

FIGURE 25.16 A model for the role of reactive oxygen species and reactive nitrogen–oxygen species (RNOS) in neuronal degradation in Parkinson disease. (*1*) Dopamine levels are reduced by monoamine oxidase (MAO), which generates H_2O_2. (*2*) Superoxide also can be produced by mitochondria, which superoxide dismutase (SOD) will convert to H_2O_2. Iron levels increase, which allows the Fenton reaction to proceed, generating hydroxyl radicals. (*3*) Nitric oxide (NO), produced by inducible nitric oxide synthase, reacts with superoxide to form RNOS. (*4*) The RNOS and hydroxyl radical lead to radical chain reactions that result in lipid peroxidation, protein oxidation, the formation of lipofuscin, and neuronal degeneration. The end result is a reduced production and release of dopamine, which leads to the clinical symptoms observed.

The decrease in ATP and increase in Ca^{2+} may open the mitochondrial permeability transition pore, resulting in permanent inhibition of oxidative phosphorylation. Damage to lipid membranes is further enhanced by Ca^{2+} activation of phospholipases.

Reperfusion with O_2 allows recovery of oxidative phosphorylation, provided that the mitochondrial membrane has maintained some integrity and the mitochondrial transition pore can close. However, it also increases generation of free radicals. The transfer of electrons from $CoQ\bullet$ to O_2 to generate superoxide is increased. Endothelial production of superoxide by xanthine oxidase also may increase. These radicals may go on to form the hydroxyl radical, which can enhance the damage to components of the ETC and mitochondrial lipids as well as activate the mitochondrial permeability transition. As macrophages move into the area to clean up cellular debris, they may generate nitric oxide and superoxide, thus introducing peroxynitrite and other free radicals into the area. Depending on the route and timing involved, the acute results may be cell death through necrosis, with slower cell death through apoptosis in the surrounding tissue.

Currently, an intense study of ischemic insults to a variety of animal organs is underway, in an effort to discover ways of preventing reperfusion injury. These include methods designed to increase endogenous antioxidant activity, to reduce the generation of free radicals, and, finally, to develop exogenous antioxidants that, when administered before reperfusion, would prevent its injurious effects. Preconditioning tissues to hypoxia is also a viable option to reducing reperfusion injury. Each of these approaches has met with some success, but their clinical application awaits further refinement. With the growing number of invasive procedures aimed at restoring arterial blood flow through partially obstructed coronary vessels, such as clot lysis, balloon or laser angioplasty, and coronary artery bypass grafting, development of methods to prevent ischemia–reperfusion injury will become increasingly urgent.

In **Cora N.'s** case, oxygen was restored before permanent impairment of oxidative phosphorylation had occurred and the stage of irreversible injury was reached.

BIOCHEMICAL COMMENTS

Oxidases, the Tricarboxylic Acid Cycle, and Cancer. The advent of whole genome sequencing (see Chapter 17) has allowed a large number of tumor cells to be analyzed for mutations in the genome. Surprisingly, certain types of tumors contained mutations in enzymes related to the tricarboxylic acid (TCA) cycle (see Chapter 23). Enzymes identified include succinate dehydrogenase, which was found in familial paraganglioma cells (this mutation is a loss of activity, in which succinate will accumulate); fumarase deficiency was found in multiple cutaneous and uterine leiomyomas and exhibited autosomal dominant behavior (in this mutation, fumarate will accumulate); and certain isozymes of isocitrate dehydrogenase, in which a gain of function mutation enables the enzyme to produce 2-hydroxyglutarate instead of α-ketoglutarate, is found in gliomas and acute myeloid leukemia (AML). The accumulation of succinate, fumarate, or 2-hydroxyglutarate, in a manner described in the following paragraphs, leads to an alteration in gene expression and oxygen sensing, which, in part, leads to tumor formation.

α-Ketoglutarate, in addition to being a key intermediate in the TCA cycle, is also required for vitamin C–dependent hydroxylation reactions (see Chapter 5). Enzymes catalyzing such reactions include N-methyllysine hydroxylase (the first step in demethylating histones) and methylcytosine demethylase (the first step in demethylating 5-methylcytosine, found in the promoter of genes which are usually inactivated). The reaction catalyzed by these enzymes is oxygen + α-ketoglutarate + substrate to be hydroxylated yields succinate + CO_2 + hydroxylated product.

Isocitrate dehydrogenase exists as three different isozymes: IDH1, IDH2, and IDH3. IDH3 is the mitochondrial version, requires NAD^+, and is part of the TCA cycle. Mutations in IDH3 do not lead to tumor formation. IDH1 and IDH2 are $NADP^+$-dependent isozymes, with IDH1 being located in the cytoplasm, and IDH2 in the mitochondria. If IDH1 or IDH2 contains a mutation that alters a key arginine residue at the active site, the enzyme will use α-ketoglutarate as a substrate (instead of isocitrate) and generate 2-hydroxyglutarate as the product.

As described in Chapter 16, histone methylation occurs on the *N*-terminal tails of histones and is a component of the epigenetic regulation of gene expression. These methylation events can either activate or inhibit expression of a gene, depending on the gene. The enzyme *N*-methyllysine hydroxylase is the first step in the demethylation of the tails. The methyl group becomes hydroxylated, and the carbon is then lost in the form of formaldehyde, which is picked up by the one carbon carrier tetrahydrofolate. If 2-hydroxyglutarate has accumulated, it will bind to the active site of *N*-methyllysine hydroxylase, inhibiting the enzyme, and not allowing histone demethylation to occur. Similarly, if succinate has accumulated owing to a mutation in succinate dehydrogenase or fumarase, succinate will inhibit the hydroxylation reaction because of product inhibition (recall that succinate is a product of the hydroxylase).

In a similar fashion, the removal of methyl groups from cytosine in promoter regions of genes requires an initial hydroxylation reaction (the enzyme is methylcytosine dioxygenase) which is similarly inhibited by 2-hydroxyglutarate, succinate, or fumarate. This leads to a constant state of hypermethylation of the genome, and altered gene expression. In cases of AML the methylation pattern of the genome resembles that of stem cells and not that of differentiated blood cells.

The mutations in the TCA cycle enzymes and isozymes also affect the degradation of the transcription factor hypoxia inducible factor (HIF). Under conditions of low oxygen concentration, HIF binds to DNA regulatory elements to induce genes in response to low-oxygen conditions, such as an increase in expression of glycolytic enzymes. HIF activity is regulated, in part, by proline hydroxylation (which requires α-ketoglutarate). An inability to hydroxylate the proline residue (because of 2-hydroxyglutarate, succinate, or fumarate accumulation) leads to HIF being active for extended period of times, altering gene transcription and leading to cell proliferation.

Laboratory experiments using inhibitors of the altered IDH molecules are in progress, and drugs have been developed that are candidates for clinical trials. Some of the drugs developed led to reversal of both DNA and histone hypermethylation, and induced cellular differentiation, in cultured cells containing tumor-inducing IDH-2 mutations.

KEY CONCEPTS

- Oxygen radical generation contributes to cellular death and degeneration in a variety of diseases.
- Radical damage occurs via electron extraction from a biologic molecule, creating a chain reaction of radical propagation.
- Reactive oxygen species (ROS) include superoxide, hydrogen peroxide, and the hydroxyl radical.
- ROS can be produced either enzymatically or nonenzymatically.
- ROS cause damage by oxidatively damaging DNA, proteins, and lipids, leading to mutations and cell death.
- Other radical species include nitric oxide (NO) and hypochlorous acid (HOCl).
- NO reacts with oxygen or superoxide to form a family of reactive nitrogen species (RNOS).
- The immune response normally produces radical species (superoxide, HOCl, NO) to destroy invading microorganisms. Escape of radicals from the immune cells during this protective event can damage surrounding tissues.
- Cellular defense mechanisms against radical damage include defense enzymes, antioxidants, and compartmentalization of free radicals.
- Cellular defense enzymes include superoxide dismutase, catalase, and glutathione peroxidase.
- Antioxidants include vitamins E and C and plant flavonoids.
- Diseases discussed in this chapter are summarized in Table 25.3.

TABLE 25.3   Diseases Discussed in Chapter 25

DISEASE OR DISORDER	ENVIRONMENTAL OR GENETIC	COMMENTS
Free-radical disease	Both	Damage caused to proteins and lipids owing to free-radical generation may lead to cellular dysfunction.
Parkinson disease	Both	Inability to convert tyrosine to DOPA; DOPA treatment can temporarily reverse tremors and other symptoms.
Myocardial infarction	Both	The lack of oxygen in the walls of the heart is caused by severe ischemia owing to clots forming within certain coronary arteries at the site of ruptured atherosclerotic plaques. The limited availability of oxygen to act as an electron acceptor decreases the proton motive force across the inner mitochondrial membrane of ischemic cells. This leads to reduced adenosine triphosphate generation, triggering events that lead to irreversible cell injury. Further damage to the heart muscle can occur because of free-radical generation after oxygen is reintroduced to the cells that were temporarily ischemic, a process known as *ischemia–reperfusion injury*.
Chronic granulomatous disease	Genetic	This disorder occurs owing to a reduced activity of nicotinamide adenine dinucleotide phosphate oxidase, leading to a reduction in the oxidative burst by neutrophils, coupled with a dysregulated immune response to bacteria and fungi.
Respiratory distress syndrome of a newborn	Both	Either mutations in surfactant or lack of surfactant production in newborns; lungs have difficulty inflating and compressing.
Amyotrophic lateral sclerosis (ALS)	Both	The familial form of ALS is caused by mutations in superoxide dismutase, leading to difficulty in disposing of superoxide radicals, which leads to cell damage owing to excessive **reactive oxygen species**.
Age-related macular degeneration	Both	Oxidative damage occurs in the retinal pigment epithelium, leading first to reduced vision and then to blindness.

REVIEW QUESTIONS—CHAPTER 25

1. Which one of the following vitamins or enzymes is unable to protect against free-radical damage?
   A. β-Carotene
   B. Glutathione peroxidase
   C. SOD
   D. Vitamin B_6
   E. Vitamin C
   F. Vitamin E

2. SOD is one of the body's primary defense mechanisms against oxidative stress. The enzyme catalyzes which one of the following reactions?
   A. $O_2^- + e^- + 2H+ \rightarrow H_2O_2$
   B. $2O_2^- + 2H^+ \rightarrow H_2O_2 + O_2$
   C. $O_2^- + HO\bullet + H+ \rightarrow CO_2 + H_2O$
   D. $H_2O_2 + O_2 \rightarrow 4H_2O$
   E. $O_2^- + H_2O_2 + H+ \rightarrow 2H_2O + O_2$

3. The mechanism of vitamin E as an antioxidant is best described by which one of the following?
   A. Vitamin E binds to free radicals and sequesters them from the contents of the cell.
   B. Vitamin E participates in the oxidation of the radicals.
   C. Vitamin E participates in the reduction of the radicals.
   D. Vitamin E forms a covalent bond with the radicals, thereby stabilizing the radical state.
   E. Vitamin E inhibits enzymes that produce free radicals.

4. An accumulation of hydrogen peroxide in a cellular compartment can be converted to dangerous radical forms in the presence of which metal?
   A. Selenium
   B. Iron
   C. Manganese
   D. Magnesium
   E. Molybdenum

5. The level of oxidative damage to mitochondrial DNA is 10 times greater than that to nuclear DNA. This could be, in part, because of which one of the following?
   A. SOD is present in the mitochondria.
   B. The nucleus lacks glutathione.
   C. The nuclear membrane presents a barrier to ROS.
   D. The mitochondrial membrane is permeable to ROS.
   E. Mitochondrial DNA lacks histones.

6. A patient with chronic granulomatous disease, who is complaining of fever, dermatitis, and diarrhea, is seen in your clinic. The genetic form of this disease results in the inability to generate, primarily, which one of the following?
   A. Superoxide
   B. Hydrogen peroxide
   C. Reduced glutathione
   D. Hypochlorous acid
   E. Nitric oxide

7. You diagnose a patient with ALS, and you discover that his father also had the disease. The patient most likely had a mutation that leads to the inability to detoxify which one of the following?
   A. Oxidized glutathione
   B. Hydrogen peroxide
   C. Nitric oxide
   D. Hydroxyl radical
   E. Superoxide

8. Nitroglycerin and other medications used for treating erectile dysfunction work by forming NO, a potent vasodilator (in low concentrations). In high concentrations, NO can produce RNOS that are involved in which one of the following diseases?
   A. Ischemic heart disease
   B. Infertility
   C. Viral infections
   D. Fungal infections
   E. Rheumatoid arthritis

9. An individual taking xenobiotics, such as alcohol, medications, and other foreign chemicals, can increase their risk for free-radical injury through which one of the following mechanisms?
   A. Reaction of O_2 with CoQ
   B. Induction of oxidases in peroxisomes
   C. Induction of enzymes containing cytochrome P450
   D. Production of ionizing radiation
   E. Production of hydrogen peroxide in the manufacturing process, such that hydrogen peroxide is present in the ingested materials

10. A balanced diet contains antioxidant molecules that help to protect cells from free-radical injury. Which one of the following foods would contain high levels of an antioxidant?
    A. Citrus fruits
    B. Enriched bread
    C. Dairy products
    D. Energy drinks
    E. Green leafy vegetables

ANSWERS

1. **The answer is D.** Pyridoxal phosphate is a water-soluble vitamin that is important for amino acid and glycogen metabolism but has no role in protecting against free-radical damage. Ascorbate (vitamin C), vitamin E, and β-carotene can all react with free radicals to terminate chain propagation, whereas SOD uses the superoxide radical as a substrate and converts it to hydrogen peroxide, and glutathione peroxidase removes hydrogen peroxide from the cell, converting it to water.

2. **The answer is B.** SOD combines two superoxide radicals to produce hydrogen peroxide and molecular oxygen. None of the other reactions is correct.

3. **The answer is C.** Vitamin E donates an electron and proton to the radical, thereby converting the radical to a stable form (LOO• → LOOH). The vitamin thus prevents the free radical from oxidizing another compound by extracting an H from that compound and propagating a free-radical chain reaction. The radical form of vitamin E generated is relatively stable and actually donates another electron and proton to a second free radical, forming oxidized vitamin E.

4. **The answer is B.** The Fenton reaction is the nonenzymatic donation of an electron from Fe^{2+} to H_2O_2 to produce Fe^{3+}, the hydroxyl radical, and hydroxide ion. Only Fe^{2+} or Cu^{1+} can be used in this reaction; thus, the other answers are incorrect.

5. **The answer is E.** Histones coat nuclear DNA and protect it from damage by radicals. Mitochondrial DNA lacks histones, so when radicals are formed, the DNA can be easily oxidized. Answers A and B are nonsensical; SOD reduces radical concentrations, so the fact that it is present in the mitochondria should help to protect the DNA from damage, not enhance it. Glutathione also protects against radical damage, and if the nucleus lacks it, then one would expect higher levels of nuclear DNA damage, not reduced levels. ROS can diffuse across membranes, so answers C and D are incorrect. Other factors that increase mitochondrial DNA damage relative to nuclear DNA are the proximity of mitochondrial DNA to the membrane, and the fact that most radical species are formed from CoQ, which is found within the mitochondria.

6. **The answer is A.** The familial form of chronic granulomatous disease is caused by reduced activity of NADPH

oxidase, which generates superoxide from oxygen during the respiratory burst in neutrophils, designed to destroy engulfed bacteria. Once superoxide is generated, other oxygen radicals can be generated (such as hydrogen peroxide), but the generation of superoxide is the primary event. Hypochlorous acid is also generated during the respiratory burst, but the enzyme required is myeloperoxidase, which is not defective in chronic granulomatous disease. Nitric oxide is generated by nitric oxide synthase and is not mutated in chronic granulomatous disease. Reduced glutathione is the protective form of glutathione and can be generated using glutathione peroxidase or glutathione reductase, neither of which is defective in chronic granulomatous disease.

7. **The answer is E.** The familial form of ALS (Lou Gehrig disease) is caused by an inherited mutation in SOD. In the absence of SOD, increased oxidative damage is possible to the neurons because of the accumulation of superoxide, the substrate for SOD. Catalase will reduce hydrogen peroxide levels, whereas glutathione peroxidase will convert reduced glutathione to oxidized glutathione, using hydrogen peroxide as an electron donor. Nitric oxide does not accumulate in Lou Gehrig disease. The hydroxyl radical may accumulate because of the accumulation of superoxide, but the hydroxyl radical is not the direct cause of the disease.

8. **The answer is E.** RNOS are involved in neurodegenerative diseases such as Parkinson and in chronic inflammatory diseases such as rheumatoid arthritis. Although RNOS has a minor role in neutrophils (bacterial infections), ROS are strongly involved in fungal and viral infections as well as ischemic heart disease and infertility.

9. **The answer is C.** Most xenobiotics (e.g., alcohol, medications, other chemicals) induce the cytochrome P450 family of enzymes to metabolize the xenobiotic. During the reactions catalyzed by this family of enzymes, free radicals are sometimes generated and released from the enzyme complex, which can lead to intracellular protein and lipid damage. The ingestion of alcohol, medications, and other chemicals do not increase the frequency of oxygen reacting with CoQ, nor do they induce oxidases in peroxisomes or produce ionizing radiation. Hydrogen peroxide is not produced in the manufacturing of alcohol, most medications, or most chemicals.

10. **The answer is A.** Vitamins C and E and perhaps A act as antioxidants. Citrus fruits are high in vitamin C. Enriched bread is high in niacin and folate. Fortified dairy products are high in vitamin D (although raw milk is not), and green leafy vegetables are high in vitamin K and folate. Energy drinks usually have sugar, caffeine, and B vitamins.

Formation and Degradation of Glycogen

Glycogen is the storage form of glucose found in most types of cells. It is composed of glucosyl units linked by **α-1,4-glycosidic bonds**, with **α-1,6-branches** occurring roughly every 8 to 10 glucosyl units (Fig. 26.1). The liver and skeletal muscle contain the largest glycogen stores.

The formation of glycogen from glucose is an energy-requiring pathway that begins, like most of glucose metabolism, with the phosphorylation of glucose to **glucose 6-phosphate**. Glycogen synthesis from glucose 6-phosphate involves the formation of uridine diphosphate glucose (**UDP-glucose**) and the transfer of glucosyl units from UDP-glucose to the ends of the glycogen chains by the enzyme **glycogen synthase**. Once the chains reach approximately 11 glucosyl units, a **branching enzyme** moves 6 to 8 units to form an α-(1,6)-branch.

Glycogenolysis, the pathway for glycogen degradation, is not the reverse of the biosynthetic pathway. The degradative enzyme **glycogen phosphorylase** removes glucosyl units one at a time from the ends of the glycogen chains, converting them to **glucose 1-phosphate** without resynthesizing UDP-glucose or uridine triphosphate (UTP). A **debranching enzyme** removes the glucosyl residues near each branch point.

Liver glycogen serves as a source of **blood glucose**. To generate glucose, the glucose 1-phosphate produced from glycogen degradation is converted to glucose 6-phosphate. **Glucose 6-phosphatase**, an enzyme found only in liver and kidney, converts glucose 6-phosphate to free glucose, which then enters the blood.

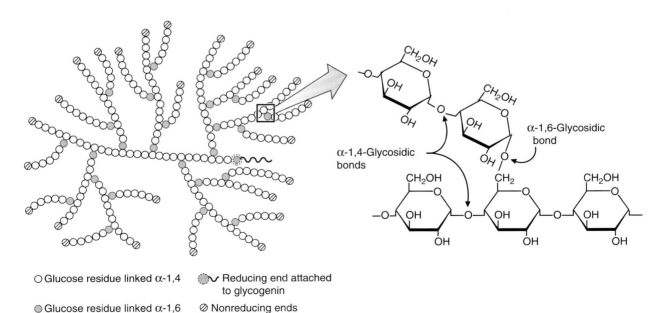

○ Glucose residue linked α-1,4

● Glucose residue linked α-1,6

🔵〰 Reducing end attached to glycogenin

⊘ Nonreducing ends

FIGURE 26.1 Glycogen structure. Glycogen is composed of glucosyl units linked by α-1,4-glycosidic bonds and α-1,6-glycosidic bonds. The branches occur more frequently in the center of the molecule and less frequently in the periphery. The anomeric carbon that is not attached to another glucosyl residue (the reducing end) is attached to the protein glycogenin by a glycosidic bond. The hydrogen atoms have been omitted from this figure for clarity.

525

Glycogen synthesis and degradation are regulated in liver by **hormonal changes** that signal the need for blood glucose (see Chapter 19). The body maintains fasting blood glucose levels at approximately 80 mg/dL to ensure that the brain and other tissues that are dependent on glucose for the generation of adenosine triphosphate (ATP) have a continuous supply. The lack of dietary glucose, signaled by a decrease of the **insulin/glucagon ratio**, activates liver glycogenolysis and inhibits glycogen synthesis. **Epinephrine**, which signals an increased use of blood glucose and other fuels for exercise or emergency situations, also activates liver glycogenolysis. The hormones that regulate liver glycogen metabolism work principally through changes in the **phosphorylation** state of glycogen synthase in the biosynthetic pathway and glycogen phosphorylase in the degradative pathway.

In skeletal muscle, glycogen supplies glucose 6-phosphate for ATP synthesis in the glycolytic pathway. Muscle glycogen phosphorylase is stimulated during exercise by the increase of **adenosine monophosphate** (**AMP**), an **allosteric activator** of the enzyme, and also by phosphorylation. The phosphorylation is stimulated by **calcium** released during contraction and by epinephrine, the fight-or-flight hormone. Glycogen synthesis is activated in resting muscles by the elevation of insulin after carbohydrate ingestion.

The neonate must rapidly adapt to an intermittent fuel supply after birth. Once the umbilical cord is clamped, the supply of glucose from the maternal circulation is interrupted. The combined effect of epinephrine and glucagon on the liver glycogen stores of the neonate rapidly restores glucose levels to normal.

THE WAITING ROOM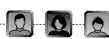

 A newborn baby girl, **Gretchen C.**, was born after a 38-week gestation. Her 36-year-old mother developed a significant viral infection that resulted in a prolonged severe loss of appetite with nausea in the month preceding delivery, leading to minimal food intake. Fetal bradycardia (slower than normal fetal heart rate) was detected at the end of each uterine contraction of labor, a sign of possible fetal distress, and the baby was delivered emergently.

At birth, Gretchen was cyanotic (a bluish discoloration caused by a lack of adequate oxygenation of tissues) and limp. She responded to several minutes of assisted ventilation. Her Apgar score of 3 was low at 1 minute after birth, but it improved to a score of 7 at 5 minutes. The Apgar score is an objective estimate of the overall condition of the newborn, determined at both 1 and 5 minutes after birth. A score of 7, 8, or 9 is normal. The highest score of 10 is less common.

Physical examination in the nursery at 10 minutes showed a thin, malnourished female newborn. Her body temperature was slightly low, her heart rate was rapid, and her respiratory rate of 55 breaths/minute was elevated. Gretchen's birth weight was only 2,100 g, compared with a normal value of >2,500 g. Her length was 47 cm, and her head circumference was 33 cm (low normal). The laboratory reported that Gretchen's serum glucose level when she was unresponsive was 14 mg/dL. A glucose value <40 mg/dL (2.5 mM) is considered to be abnormal in newborn infants.

At 5 hours of age, she was apneic (not breathing) and unresponsive. Ventilatory resuscitation was initiated and a cannula placed in the umbilical vein. Blood for a glucose level was drawn through this cannula, and 5 mL of a 20% glucose solution was injected. Gretchen slowly responded to this therapy.

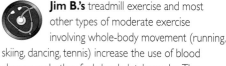 **Jim B.'s** treadmill exercise and most other types of moderate exercise involving whole-body movement (running, skiing, dancing, tennis) increase the use of blood glucose and other fuels by skeletal muscles. The blood glucose is normally supplied by the stimulation of liver glycogenolysis and gluconeogenesis.

Jim B., a 19-year-old body builder, was rushed to the hospital emergency department in a coma. One-half hour earlier, his mother had heard a loud crashing sound in the basement where Jim had been lifting weights and completing his daily workout on the treadmill. She found her son on the floor having severe jerking movements of all muscles (a grand mal seizure).

In the emergency department, the doctors learned that despite the objections of his family and friends, Jim regularly used androgens, other anabolic steroids, and insulin in an effort to bulk up his muscle mass.

On initial physical examination, he was comatose, with occasional involuntary jerking movements of his extremities. Foamy saliva dripped from his mouth. He had bitten his tongue and had lost bowel and bladder control at the height of the seizure.

The laboratory reported a serum glucose level of 18 mg/dL (extremely low). The intravenous infusion of 5% glucose (5 g of glucose per 100 mL of solution), which had been started earlier, was increased to 10%. In addition, 50 g of glucose was given over 30 seconds through the intravenous tubing.

I. Structure of Glycogen

Glycogen, the storage form of glucose, is a branched glucose polysaccharide composed of chains of glucosyl units linked by α-1,4-bonds with α-1,6-branches every 8 to 10 residues (see Fig. 26.1). In a molecule of this highly branched structure, only one glucosyl residue has an anomeric carbon that is not linked to another glucose residue. This anomeric carbon at the beginning of the chain is attached to the protein glycogenin. The other ends of the chains are called *nonreducing ends* (see Chapter 5). The branched structure permits rapid degradation and rapid synthesis of glycogen because enzymes can work on several chains simultaneously from the multiple nonreducing ends.

Glycogen is present in tissues as polymers of very high molecular weight (10^7 to 10^8 Da) collected together in glycogen particles. The enzymes involved in glycogen synthesis and degradation and some of the regulatory enzymes are bound to the surface of the glycogen particles.

II. Function of Glycogen in Skeletal Muscle and Liver

Glycogen is found in most cell types, where it serves as a reservoir of glucosyl units for ATP generation from glycolysis.

Glycogen is degraded mainly to *glucose 1-phosphate* (glucose 1-P), which is converted to *glucose 6-phosphate* (glucose 6-P). In skeletal muscle and other cell types, glucose 6-P enters the glycolytic pathway (Fig. 26.2). Glycogen is an extremely important fuel source for skeletal muscle when ATP demands are high and when glucose 6-P is used rapidly in anaerobic glycolysis. In many other cell types, the small glycogen reservoir serves a similar purpose; it is an emergency fuel source that supplies glucose for the generation of ATP in the absence of oxygen or during restricted blood flow. In general, glycogenolysis and glycolysis are activated together in these cells.

Glycogen serves a very different purpose in liver than in skeletal muscle and other tissues (see Fig. 26.2). Liver glycogen is the first and immediate source of glucose for the maintenance of blood glucose levels. In the liver, the glucose 6-P that is generated from glycogen degradation is hydrolyzed to glucose by *glucose 6-phosphatase*, an enzyme that is present only in the liver and kidneys. Glycogen degradation thus provides a readily mobilized source of blood glucose as dietary glucose decreases or as exercise increases the use of blood glucose by muscles.

The pathways of glycogenolysis and gluconeogenesis in the liver both supply blood glucose, and, consequently, these two pathways are activated together by glucagon. Gluconeogenesis, the synthesis of glucose from amino acids and other gluconeogenic precursors (discussed in detail in Chapter 28), also forms glucose 6-P, so that glucose 6-phosphatase serves as a "gateway" to the blood for both pathways (see Fig. 26.2).

Regulation of glycogen synthesis serves to prevent futile cycling and waste of ATP. *Futile cycling* (or substrate cycling) refers to a situation in which a substrate is converted to a product through one pathway, and the product is converted back to the substrate through another pathway. Because the biosynthetic pathway is

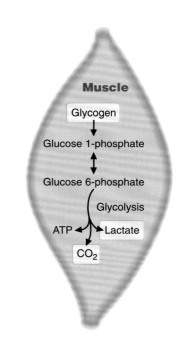

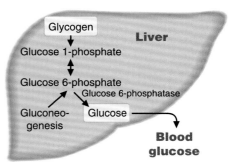

FIGURE 26.2 Glycogenolysis in skeletal muscle and liver. Glycogen stores serve different functions in muscle cells and liver. In the muscle and most other cell types, glycogen stores serve as a fuel source for the generation of adenosine triphosphate (ATP). In the liver, glycogen stores serve as a source of blood glucose.

energy-requiring, futile cycling results in a waste of high-energy phosphate bonds. Thus, glycogen synthesis is activated when glycogen degradation is inhibited, and vice versa.

III. Synthesis and Degradation of Glycogen

Glycogen synthesis, like almost all the pathways of glucose metabolism, begins with the phosphorylation of glucose to glucose 6-P by hexokinase or, in the liver, glucokinase (Fig. 26.3). Glucose 6-P is the precursor of glycolysis, the pentose phosphate pathway, and pathways for the synthesis of other sugars. In the pathway for glycogen synthesis, glucose 6-P is converted to glucose 1-P by phosphoglucomutase, a reversible reaction.

Glycogen is both formed from and degraded to glucose 1-P, but the biosynthetic and degradative pathways are separate and involve different enzymes (see Fig. 26.3). The biosynthetic pathway is an energy-requiring pathway; high-energy phosphate from UTP is used to activate the glucosyl residues to UDP-glucose (Fig. 26.4). In the degradative pathway, the glycosidic bonds between the glucosyl residues in glycogen are simply cleaved by the addition of phosphate to produce glucose 1-P (or water to produce free glucose), and UDP-glucose is not resynthesized. The existence of separate pathways for the formation and degradation of important compounds is a common theme in metabolism. Because the synthesis and degradation pathways use different enzymes, one can be activated while the other is inhibited.

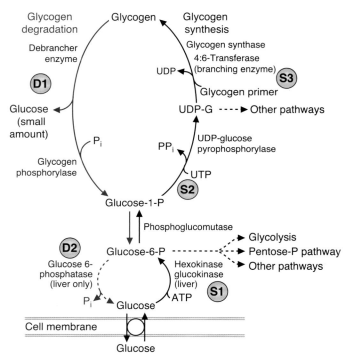

FIGURE 26.3 Scheme of glycogen synthesis and degradation. (*S1*) Glucose 6-phosphate (glucose 6-P) is formed from glucose by hexokinase in most cells, and glucokinase in the liver. It is a metabolic branch point for the pathways of glycolysis, the pentose phosphate pathway, and glycogen synthesis. (*S2*) Uridine diphosphate (UDP)-glucose (UDP-G) is synthesized from glucose 1-phosphate (glucose 1-P). UDP-glucose is the branch point for glycogen synthesis and other pathways that require the addition of carbohydrate units. (*S3*) Glycogen synthesis is catalyzed by glycogen synthase and the branching enzyme. (*D1*) Glycogen degradation is catalyzed by glycogen phosphorylase and a debrancher enzyme. (*D2*) Glucose 6-phosphatase in the liver (and, to a small extent, the kidney) generates free glucose from glucose 6-P. *ATP*, adenosine triphosphate; *P_i*, inorganic phosphate; *PP_i*, pyrophosphate; *UTP*, uridine triphosphate.

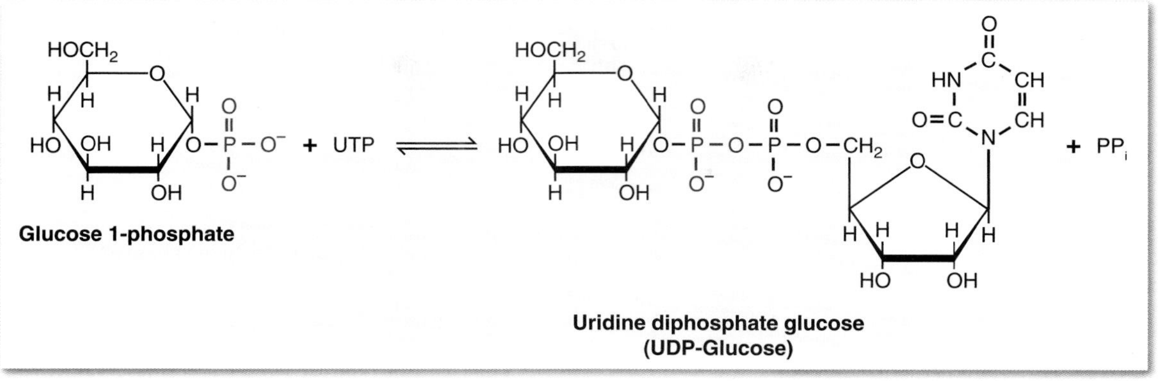

FIGURE 26.4 Formation of uridine diphosphate (UDP)-glucose. The high-energy phosphate bond of uridine triphosphate (UTP) provides the energy for the formation of a high-energy bond in UDP-glucose. Pyrophosphate (PP_i), released by the reaction, is cleaved to two inorganic phosphate (P_i).

A. Glycogen Synthesis

Glycogen synthesis requires the formation of α-1,4-glycosidic bonds to link glucosyl residues in long chains and the formation of an α-1,6-branch every 8 to 10 residues (Fig. 26.5). Most of glycogen synthesis occurs through the lengthening of the polysaccharide chains of a preexisting glycogen molecule (a glycogen primer) in which the reducing end of the glycogen is attached to the protein glycogenin. To lengthen the glycogen chains, glucosyl residues are added from UDP-glucose to the nonreducing ends of the chain by glycogen synthase. The anomeric carbon of each glucosyl residue is attached in an α-1,4-bond to the hydroxyl on carbon 4 of the terminal glucosyl residue. When the chain reaches approximately 11 residues in length, a 6- to 8-residue piece is cleaved by amylo-4,6-transferase (also known as *branching enzyme*) and reattached to a glucosyl unit by an α-1,6-bond. Both chains continue to lengthen until they are long enough to produce two new branches. This process continues, producing highly branched molecules. *Glycogen synthase*, the enzyme that attaches the glucosyl residues in α-1,4-bonds, is the regulated step in the pathway. Branching of glycogen serves two major roles: increased sites for synthesis and degradation, and enhancing the solubility of the molecule.

The synthesis of new glycogen primer molecules also occurs. Glycogenin, the protein to which glycogen is attached, glycosylates itself (autoglycosylation) by attaching the glucosyl residue of UDP-glucose to the hydroxyl side chain of a serine residue in the protein. The protein then extends the carbohydrate chain (using UDP-glucose as the substrate) until the glucosyl chain is long enough to serve as a substrate for glycogen synthase.

B. Glycogen Degradation

Glycogen is degraded by two enzymes, *glycogen phosphorylase* and the *debrancher enzyme* (Fig. 26.6). Glycogen degradation is a phosphorolysis reaction (breaking of a bond using a phosphate ion as a nucleophile). Enzymes that catalyze phosphorolysis reactions are named phosphorylase. Because more than one type of phosphorylase exists, the substrate usually is included in the name of the enzyme, such as glycogen phosphorylase or purine nucleoside phosphorylase.

The enzyme glycogen phosphorylase starts at the nonreducing end of a chain and successively cleaves glucosyl residues by adding phosphate to the anomeric carbon of the terminal glycosidic bond, thereby releasing glucose 1-P and producing a free 4′-hydroxyl group on the glucose residue now at the end of the glycogen chain. However, glycogen phosphorylase cannot act on the glycosidic bonds of the four glucosyl residues closest to a branch point because the branching chain sterically hinders a proper fit into the catalytic site of the enzyme. The debrancher enzyme,

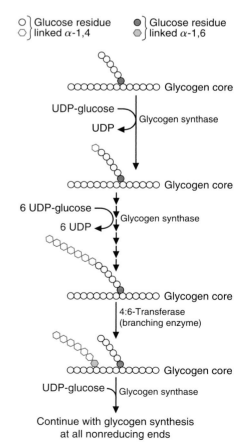

FIGURE 26.5 Glycogen synthesis. See text for details. *UDP*, uridine diphosphate.

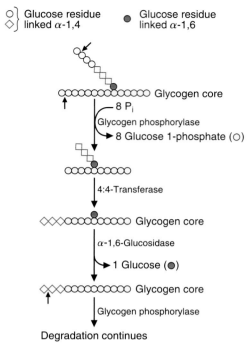

FIGURE 26.6 Glycogen degradation. See text for details. P_i, inorganic phosphate.

which catalyzes the removal of the four residues closest to the branch point, has two catalytic activities: It acts as a transferase and as an α-1,6-glucosidase. As a transferase, the debrancher first removes a unit containing three glucose residues and adds it to the end of a longer chain by an α-1,4-glycosidic bond. The one glucosyl residue remaining at the α-1,6-branch is hydrolyzed by the amylo-1,6-glucosidase activity of the debrancher, resulting in the release of free glucose. Thus, one glucose and approximately seven to nine glucose 1-P residues are released for every branchpoint.

Some degradation of glycogen also occurs within lysosomes when glycogen particles become surrounded by membranes that then fuse with the lysosomal membranes. A lysosomal α-glucosidase hydrolyzes this glycogen to glucose.

A genetic defect of lysosomal glucosidase, called *type II glycogen storage disease*, or Pompe disease, leads to the accumulation of glycogen particles in large, membrane-enclosed residual bodies, which disrupt the function of liver and muscle cells. The disorder can be treated with enzyme replacement therapy (Lumizyme [alglucosidase alfa], Sanofi Genzyme, Cambridge, MA), which requires periodic enzyme infusions for the life of the patient. In the absence of treatment, the disorder is fatal.

 In order to confirm a diagnosis of phosphorylase deficiency (in either muscle or liver), a biopsy must be obtained, followed by a sensitive assay for phosphorylase activity within the biopsied tissue. There are several procedures to do this. The first is to incubate glycogen, inorganic phosphate, and a sample of the extracted biopsy tissue. If phosphorylase activity is present, glucose 1-P will be produced. One can determine the amount of glucose 1-P produced by converting it to glucose 6-P, using the enzyme phosphoglucomutase. The glucose 6-P levels are then measured by the conversion of glucose 6-P to 6-phosphogluconate using the enzyme glucose 6-P dehydrogenase. Glucose 6-P dehydrogenase requires nicotinamide adenine dinucleotide ($NADP^+$), generating NADPH during the course of the reaction. The formation of NADPH can be followed spectrophotometrically as the absorbance at 340 nm will increase as NADPH is produced, and the increase in NADPH levels will be directly proportional to the amount of glucose 1-P produced by phosphorylase. A second assay to measure phosphorylase activity uses radioactive glycogen as a substrate. The labeled glycogen is incubated with inorganic phosphate and sample extract, generating labeled glucose 1-P. The radioactive glucose 1-P is then separated from the glycogen and measured. A variation of this method is to use ^{32}P-labeled inorganic phosphate and measure the radioactive glucose 1-P produced. A third assay for phosphorylase activity is to measure the reverse reaction (glycogen synthesis). Under appropriate conditions, the phosphorylase reaction can go backward, in which the glucose residue from glucose 1-P is added to an existing glycogen chain, releasing inorganic phosphate. The phosphate produced using this method is then measured in a sensitive spectrophotometric assay.

TABLE 26.1 Glycogen Storage Diseases

TYPE	ENZYME AFFECTED	PRIMARY ORGAN INVOLVED	MANIFESTATIONS[a]
O	Glycogen synthase	Liver	Hypoglycemia, hyperketonemia, failure to thrive, early death
I[b]	Glucose 6-phosphatase (von Gierke disease)	Liver	Enlarged liver and kidney, growth failure, severe fasting hypoglycemia, acidosis, lipemia, thrombocyte dysfunction
II	Lysosomal α-glucosidase (Pompe disease): may see clinical symptoms in childhood, juvenile, or adult life stages, depending on the nature of the mutation	All organs with lysosomes	Infantile form: early-onset progressive muscle hypotonia, cardiac failure, death before age 2 years. Juvenile form: later-onset myopathy with variable cardiac involvement. Adult form: limb-girdle muscular dystrophy–like features. Glycogen deposits accumulate in lysosomes.
III	Amylo-1,6-glucosidase (debrancher): form IIIa is the liver and muscle enzymes, form IIIb is a liver-specific form, and IIIc a muscle-specific form	Liver, skeletal muscle, heart	Fasting hypoglycemia; hepatomegaly in infancy and some myopathic features. Glycogen deposits have short outer branches.
IV	Amylo-4,6-glucosidase (branching enzyme) (Andersen disease)	Liver	Hepatosplenomegaly; symptoms may arise from a hepatic reaction to the presence of a foreign body (glycogen with long outer branches); usually fatal
V	Muscle glycogen phosphorylase (McArdle disease) (expressed as either adult or infantile form)	Skeletal muscle	Exercise-induced muscular pain, cramps, and progressive weakness, sometimes with myoglobinuria
VI[c]	Liver glycogen phosphorylase (Hers disease) and its activating system (includes mutations in liver phosphorylase kinase and liver protein kinase A)	Liver	Hepatomegaly, mild hypoglycemia; good prognosis
VII	Phosphofructokinase-1 (Tarui syndrome)	Muscle, red blood cells	As in type V; in addition, enzymopathic hemolysis
XI	GLUT 2 (glucose/galactose transporter); Fanconi-Bickel syndrome	Intestine, pancreas, kidney, liver	Glycogen accumulation in liver and kidney; rickets, growth retardation, glucosuria

[a]All of these diseases except type O are characterized by increased glycogen deposits.

[b]Glucose 6-phosphatase is composed of several subunits that also transport glucose, glucose 6-phosphate, phosphate, and pyrophosphate across the endoplasmic reticulum membranes. Therefore, there are several subtypes of this disease, corresponding to defects in the different subunits. Type Ia is a lack of glucose 6-phosphatase activity, type Ib is a lack of glucose 6-phosphate translocase activity, type Ic is a lack of phosphotranslocase activity, and type Id is a lack of glucose translocase activity.

[c]Glycogen storage diseases IX (hepatic phosphorylase kinase) and X (hepatic protein kinase A) have been reclassified to VI, which now refers to the hepatic glycogen phosphorylase activating system.

Sources: Parker PH, Ballew M, Greene HL. Nutritional management of glycogen storage disease. Annu Rev Nutr. 1993;13:83–109. Copyright © 1993 by Annual Reviews, Inc.; Shin YS. Glycogen storage disease: clinical, biochemical and molecular heterogeneity. Semin Pediatr Neurol. 2006;13:115–120; Ozen H. Glycogen storage diseases: new perspectives. World J Gastroenterol. 2007;13:2541–2553.

IV. Disorders of Glycogen Metabolism

A series of inborn errors of metabolism, the glycogen storage diseases, result from deficiencies in the enzymes of glycogenolysis (Table 26.1). The diseases are labeled I through XI, and O. Several disorders have different subtypes, as indicated in the legend to Table 26.1. Glycogen phosphorylase, the key regulatory enzyme of glycogen degradation, is encoded by different genes in the muscle and liver (tissue-specific isozymes), and thus, a person may have a defect in one and not the other.

Q Why do you think that a genetic deficiency in muscle glycogen phosphorylase (McArdle disease) is a mere inconvenience, whereas a deficiency of liver glycogen phosphorylase (Hers disease) can be lethal?

V. Regulation of Glycogen Synthesis and Degradation

The regulation of glycogen synthesis in different tissues matches the function of glycogen in each tissue. Liver glycogen serves principally for the support of blood glucose during fasting or during extreme need (e.g., exercise), and the degradative and biosynthetic pathways are regulated principally by changes in the insulin/glucagon ratio and by blood glucose levels, which reflect the availability of dietary

Muscle glycogen is used within the muscle to support exercise. Thus, an individual with McArdle disease (type V glycogen storage disease) experiences no symptoms except unusual fatigue and muscle cramps during exercise. These symptoms may be accompanied by myoglobinuria and release of muscle creatine kinase into the blood.

Liver glycogen is the first reservoir for the support of blood glucose levels, and a deficiency in glycogen phosphorylase or any of the other enzymes of liver glycogen degradation can result in fasting hypoglycemia. The hypoglycemia is usually mild because patients can still synthesize glucose from gluconeogenesis (see Table 26.1).

Maternal blood glucose readily crosses the placenta to enter the fetal circulation. During the last 9 or 10 weeks of gestation, glycogen formed from maternal glucose is deposited in the fetal liver under the influence of the insulin-dominated hormonal milieu of that period. At birth, maternal glucose supplies cease, causing a temporary physiologic drop in glucose levels in the newborn's blood, even in normal healthy infants. This drop serves as one of the signals for glucagon release from the newborn's pancreas, which, in turn, stimulates glycogenolysis. As a result, the glucose levels in the newborn return to normal.

Healthy full-term babies have adequate stores of liver glycogen to survive short periods (12 hours) of caloric deprivation provided that other aspects of fuel metabolism are normal. Because **Gretchen C.'s** mother was markedly anorexic during the critical period when the fetal liver is normally synthesizing glycogen from glucose supplied in the maternal blood, Gretchen's liver glycogen stores were below normal. Thus, because fetal glycogen is the major source of fuel for the newborn in the early hours of life, Gretchen became profoundly hypoglycemic within 5 hours of birth because of her low levels of stored carbohydrate.

TABLE 26.2	Regulation of Liver and Muscle Glycogen Stores	
STATE	**REGULATORS**	**RESPONSE OF TISSUE**
Liver		
Fasting	Blood: glucagon ↑ Insulin ↓ Tissue: cAMP ↑	Glycogen degradation ↑ Glycogen synthesis ↓
Carbohydrate meal	Blood: glucagon ↓ Insulin ↑ Glucose ↑ Tissue: cAMP ↓ Glucose ↑	Glycogen degradation ↓ Glycogen synthesis ↑
Exercise and stress	Blood: epinephrine ↑ Tissue: cAMP ↑ Ca^{2+}–calmodulin ↑	Glycogen degradation ↑ Glycogen synthesis ↓
Muscle		
Fasting (rest)	Blood: insulin ↓	Glycogen synthesis ↓ Glucose transport ↓
Carbohydrate meal (rest)	Blood: insulin ↑	Glycogen synthesis ↑ Glucose transport ↑
Exercise	Blood: epinephrine ↑ Tissue: AMP ↑ Ca^{2+}–calmodulin ↑ cAMP ↑	Glycogen synthesis ↓ Glycogen degradation ↑ Glycolysis ↑

↑, increased compared with other physiologic states; ↓, decreased compared with other physiologic states; AMP, adenosine monophosphate; cAMP, cyclic AMP.

glucose (Table 26.2). Degradation of liver glycogen is also activated by epinephrine, which is released in response to exercise, hypoglycemia, or other stress situations in which there is an immediate demand for blood glucose. In contrast, in skeletal muscles, glycogen is a reservoir of glucosyl units for the generation of ATP from glycolysis and glucose oxidation. As a consequence, muscle glycogenolysis is regulated principally by AMP, which signals a lack of ATP, and by Ca^{2+} released during contraction. Epinephrine, which is released in response to exercise and other stress situations, also activates skeletal muscle glycogenolysis. The glycogen stores of resting muscle decrease very little during fasting.

A. Regulation of Glycogen Metabolism in Liver

Liver glycogen is synthesized after a carbohydrate meal when blood glucose levels are elevated, and it is degraded as blood glucose levels decrease. When an individual eats a carbohydrate-containing meal, blood glucose levels immediately increase, insulin levels increase, and glucagon levels decrease (see Fig. 19.8). The increase of blood glucose levels and the rise of the insulin/glucagon ratio inhibit glycogen degradation and stimulate glycogen synthesis. The immediate increased transport of glucose into peripheral tissues, and storage of blood glucose as glycogen helps to bring circulating blood glucose levels back to the normal range, 80 to 100 mg/dL, of the fasted state. As the length of time after a carbohydrate-containing meal increases, insulin levels decrease and glucagon levels increase. The fall of the insulin/glucagon ratio results in inhibition of the biosynthetic pathway and activation of the degradative pathway. As a result, liver glycogen is rapidly degraded to glucose, which is released into the blood.

Although glycogenolysis and gluconeogenesis are activated together by the same regulatory mechanisms, glycogenolysis responds more rapidly, with a greater outpouring of glucose. A substantial proportion of liver glycogen is degraded within the first few hours after eating (30% after 4 hours) (Table 26.3). The rate

| | GLYCOGEN CONTENT | RATE OF GLYCOGENOLYSIS |
LENGTH OF FAST (h)	(μmol/g liver)	(μmol/kg-min)
0	300	—
2	260	4.3
4	216	4.3
24	42	1.7
64	16	0.3

TABLE 26.3   Effect of Fasting on Liver Glycogen Content in Humans

of glycogenolysis decreases significantly in a prolonged fast as the liver glycogen supplies dwindle. Liver glycogen stores are therefore a rapidly rebuilt and degraded store of glucose, ever responsive to small and rapid changes of blood glucose levels.

1. Nomenclature of Enzymes Metabolizing Glycogen

Both glycogen phosphorylase and glycogen synthase will be covalently modified to regulate their activity. When activated by covalent modification, glycogen phosphorylase is referred to as *glycogen phosphorylase a* (remember *a* for *active*); when the covalent modification is removed and the enzyme is inactive, it is referred to as *glycogen phosphorylase b*. Glycogen synthase, when it is not covalently modified, is active and can be designated *glycogen synthase a* or *glycogen synthase I* (the *I* stands for *independent* of modifiers for activity). When glycogen synthase is covalently modified, it is inactive, in the form of *glycogen synthase b* or *glycogen synthase D* (for *dependent* on a modifier for activity).

2. Regulation of Liver Glycogen Metabolism by Insulin and Glucagon

Insulin and glucagon regulate liver glycogen metabolism by changing the phosphorylation state of glycogen phosphorylase in the degradative pathway and glycogen synthase in the biosynthetic pathway. An increase of glucagon and decrease of insulin during the fasting state initiates a cyclic adenosine monophosphate (cAMP)-directed phosphorylation cascade, which results in the phosphorylation of glycogen phosphorylase to an active enzyme and the phosphorylation of glycogen synthase to an inactive enzyme (Fig. 26.7). As a consequence, glycogen degradation is stimulated and glycogen synthesis is inhibited.

3. Activation of a Phosphorylation Cascade by Glucagon

Glucagon regulates glycogen metabolism through its intracellular second messenger cAMP and protein kinase A (PKA) (see Chapter 19). Glucagon, by binding to its cell membrane receptor, transmits a signal through G-proteins that activates adenylate cyclase, causing cAMP levels to increase (see Fig. 26.7). cAMP binds to the regulatory subunits of PKA, which dissociate from the catalytic subunits. The catalytic subunits of PKA are activated by the dissociation and phosphorylate the enzyme phosphorylase kinase, activating it. Phosphorylase kinase is the protein kinase that converts the inactive liver glycogen phosphorylase b to the active glycogen phosphorylase a by transferring a phosphate from ATP to a specific serine residue on the phosphorylase subunits. The addition of the phosphate triggers a conformational change in the enzyme, thereby activating it. As a result of the activation of glycogen phosphorylase, glycogenolysis is stimulated.

4. Inhibition of Glycogen Synthase by Glucagon-Directed Phosphorylation

When glycogen degradation is activated by the cAMP-stimulated phosphorylation cascade, glycogen synthesis is simultaneously inhibited. The enzyme glycogen synthase is also phosphorylated by PKA, but this phosphorylation results in a less active form, glycogen synthase b.

Q A patient was diagnosed as an infant with type III glycogen storage disease, a deficiency of debrancher enzyme (see Table 26.1). The patient had hepatomegaly (an enlarged liver) and experienced bouts of mild hypoglycemia. To diagnose the disease, glycogen was obtained from the patient's liver by biopsy after the patient had fasted overnight and was compared with normal glycogen. The glycogen samples were treated with a preparation of commercial glycogen phosphorylase and commercial debrancher enzyme. The amounts of glucose 1-P and glucose produced in the assay were then measured. The ratio of glucose 1-P to glucose for the normal glycogen sample was 9:1, and the ratio for the patient was 3:1. Can you explain these results?

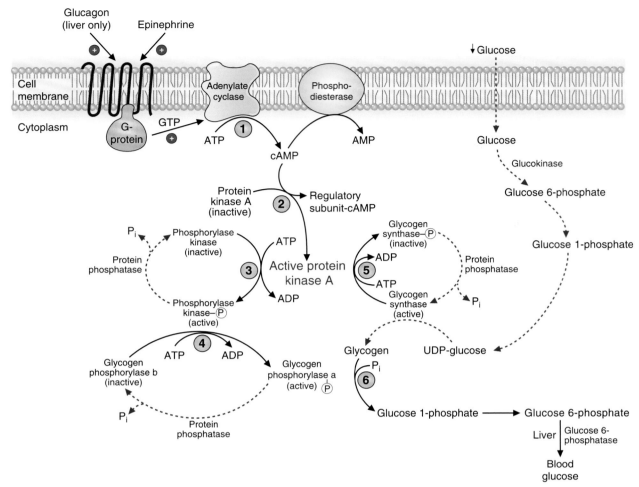

FIGURE 26.7 Regulation of glycogen synthesis and degradation in the liver. (*1*) Glucagon binding to the serpentine glucagon receptor or epinephrine binding to a serpentine β-receptor in the liver activates adenylate cyclase, via G-proteins, which synthesizes cyclic adenosine monophosphate (cAMP) from adenosine triphosphate (ATP). (2) cAMP binds to protein kinase A (PKA; cAMP-dependent protein kinase), thereby activating the catalytic subunits. (3) PKA activates phosphorylase kinase by phosphorylation. (4) Phosphorylase kinase adds a phosphate to specific serine residues on glycogen phosphorylase b, thereby converting it to the active glycogen phosphorylase a. (5) PKA also phosphorylates glycogen synthase, thereby decreasing its activity. (6) As a result of the inhibition of glycogen synthase and the activation of glycogen phosphorylase, glycogen is degraded to glucose 1-phosphate. The *red dashed lines* denote reactions that are decreased in the livers of fasting individuals. *ADP*, adenosine diphosphate; *GTP*, guanosine triphosphate; *P_i*, inorganic phosphate; *UDP*, uridine diphosphate.

A With a deficiency of debrancher enzyme but normal levels of glycogen phosphorylase, the glycogen chains of the patient could be degraded in vivo only to within four residues of the branch point. When the glycogen samples were treated with the commercial preparation containing normal enzymes, one glucose residue was released for each α-1,6-branch. However, in the patient's glycogen sample, with the short outer branches, three glucose 1-Ps and one glucose residue were obtained for each α-1,6-branch. Normal glycogen has 8 to 10 glucosyl residues per branch and thus gives a ratio of approximately 9 mol of glucose 1-P to 1 mol of glucose.

The phosphorylation of glycogen synthase is far more complex than glycogen phosphorylase. Glycogen synthase has multiple phosphorylation sites and is acted on by up to 10 different protein kinases. Phosphorylation by PKA does not, by itself, inactivate glycogen synthase. Instead, phosphorylation by PKA facilitates the subsequent addition of phosphate groups by other kinases, and these inactivate the enzyme. A term that has been applied to changes of activity resulting from multiple phosphorylations is *hierarchical* or *synergistic* phosphorylation; the phosphorylation of one site makes another site more reactive and easier to phosphorylate by a different protein kinase.

Most of the enzymes that are regulated by phosphorylation have multiple phosphorylation sites. Glycogen phosphorylase, which has only one serine per subunit and can be phosphorylated only by phosphorylase kinase, is the exception. For some enzymes, the phosphorylation sites are antagonistic, and phosphorylation initiated by one hormone counteracts the effects of other hormones. For other enzymes, the phosphorylation sites are synergistic, and phosphorylation at one site stimulated by one hormone can act synergistically with phosphorylation at another site.

5. Regulation by Protein Phosphatases

At the same time that PKA and phosphorylase kinase are adding phosphate groups to enzymes, the protein phosphatases that remove this phosphate are inhibited. Protein phosphatases remove the phosphate groups, bound to serine or other residues of enzymes, by hydrolysis. Hepatic protein phosphatase 1 (hepatic PP-1), one of the major protein phosphatases involved in glycogen metabolism, removes phosphate groups from phosphorylase kinase, glycogen phosphorylase, and glycogen synthase. During fasting, hepatic PP-1 is inactivated by several mechanisms. One is dissociation from the glycogen particle, such that the substrates are no longer available to the phosphatase. A second is the binding of inhibitor proteins, such as the protein called *inhibitor-1*, which, when phosphorylated by a glucagon (or epinephrine)-directed mechanism, binds to and inhibits phosphatase action. Insulin indirectly activates hepatic PP-1 through its own signal transduction cascade initiated at the insulin receptor tyrosine kinase.

PP-1 will bind to proteins that target the phosphatase to glycogen particles. There are four such targeting proteins: G_M, G_L, R6, and R5/PTG (*protein targeting to glycogen*). G_M is found in the heart and skeletal muscle, G_L is found primarily in the liver, whereas R5/PTG and R6 are found in most tissues. The targeting subunits all bind to the same hydrophobic site on PP-1, leading to just one targeting subunit bound per PP-1 molecule. The targeting subunits allow for compartmentalized activation of PP-1 under the appropriate conditions, whereas other tissues, or cellular compartments, may still express an inhibited PP-1. Regulation of the phosphatase involves complex interactions between the target enzymes, the targeting subunits, the phosphatase, and protein inhibitor 1 and will not be considered further.

6. Insulin in Liver Glycogen Metabolism

Insulin is antagonistic to glucagon in the degradation and synthesis of glycogen. The glucose level in the blood is the signal that controls the secretion of insulin and glucagon. Glucose stimulates insulin release and suppresses glucagon release; after a high-carbohydrate meal, one increases while the other decreases. However, insulin levels in the blood change to a greater degree with the fasting–feeding cycle than do the glucagon levels, and thus, insulin is considered the principal regulator of glycogen synthesis and degradation. The role of insulin in glycogen metabolism is often overlooked because the mechanisms by which insulin reverses all of the effects of glucagon on individual metabolic enzymes is still under investigation. In addition to the activation of hepatic PP-1 through the insulin-receptor tyrosine kinase phosphorylation cascade, insulin may activate the phosphodiesterase that converts cAMP to AMP, thereby decreasing cAMP levels and inactivating PKA. Regardless of the mechanisms involved, insulin is able to reverse all of the effects of glucagon and is the most important hormonal regulator of blood glucose levels.

7. Blood Glucose Levels and Glycogen Synthesis and Degradation

When an individual eats a high-carbohydrate meal, glycogen degradation immediately stops. Although the changes in insulin and glucagon levels are relatively rapid (10 to 15 minutes), the direct inhibitory effect of rising glucose levels on glycogen degradation is even more rapid. Glucose, as an allosteric effector, inhibits liver glycogen phosphorylase a by stimulating dephosphorylation of this enzyme. As insulin levels rise and glucagon levels fall, cAMP levels decrease and PKA reassociates with its inhibitory subunits and becomes inactive. The protein phosphatases are activated, and phosphorylase a and glycogen synthase D are dephosphorylated. The collective result of these effects is rapid inhibition of glycogen degradation and rapid activation of glycogen synthesis.

8. Epinephrine and Calcium in the Regulation of Liver Glycogen

Epinephrine, the fight-or-flight hormone, is released from the adrenal medulla in response to neural signals reflecting an increased demand for glucose. To flee from a dangerous

Most of the enzymes that are regulated by phosphorylation also can be converted to the active conformation by allosteric effectors. Glycogen synthase b, the less active form of glycogen synthase, can be activated by the accumulation of glucose 6-P above physiologic levels. The activation of glycogen synthase by glucose 6-P may be important in individuals with glucose 6-phosphatase deficiency, a disorder known as *type I* or *von Gierke glycogen storage disease* (see Table 26.1). When glucose 6-P produced from gluconeogenesis accumulates in the liver, it activates glycogen synthesis even though the individual may be hypoglycemic and have low insulin levels. Glucose 1-P is also elevated, resulting in the inhibition of glycogen phosphorylase. As a consequence, large glycogen deposits accumulate in certain tissues, including the liver, and hepatomegaly occurs.

An inability of liver and muscle to store glucose as glycogen contributes to the hyperglycemia in patients, such as **Dianne A.**, with type 1 diabetes mellitus and in patients, such as **Deborah S.**, with type 2 diabetes mellitus. The absence of insulin in patients with type 1 diabetes mellitus and the high levels of glucagon result in decreased activity of glycogen synthase. Glycogen synthesis in skeletal muscles of type 1 patients is also limited by the lack of insulin-stimulated glucose transport. Insulin resistance in type 2 patients has the same effect.

An injection of insulin suppresses glucagon release and alters the insulin/glucagon ratio. The result is rapid uptake of glucose into skeletal muscle and rapid conversion of glucose to glycogen in skeletal muscle and liver.

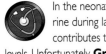

In the neonate, the release of epinephrine during labor and birth normally contributes to restoring blood glucose levels. Unfortunately, **Gretchen C.** did not have adequate liver glycogen stores to support a rise in her blood glucose levels.

situation, skeletal muscles use increased amounts of blood glucose to generate ATP. As a result, liver glycogenolysis must be stimulated. In the liver, epinephrine stimulates glycogenolysis through two different types of receptors, the α- and β-agonist receptors.

a. Epinephrine Acting at β-Receptors

Epinephrine, acting at the β-receptors, transmits a signal through G-proteins to adenylate cyclase, which increases cAMP and activates PKA. Hence, regulation of glycogen degradation and synthesis in liver by epinephrine and glucagon are similar (see Fig. 26.7).

b. Epinephrine Acting at α-Receptors

Epinephrine also binds to α-receptors in the hepatocyte. This binding activates glycogenolysis and inhibits glycogen synthesis principally by increasing the Ca^{2+} levels in the liver. The effects of epinephrine at the α-agonist receptor are mediated by the phosphatidylinositol bisphosphate (PIP_2)-Ca^{2+} signal transduction system, one of the principal intracellular second-messenger systems used by many hormones (Fig. 26.8) (see Chapter 11).

In the PIP_2-Ca^{2+} signal transduction system, the signal is transferred from the epinephrine receptor to membrane-bound phospholipase C by G-proteins. Phospholipase C hydrolyzes PIP_2 to form diacylglycerol (DAG) and inositol trisphosphate (IP_3). IP_3 stimulates the release of Ca^{2+} from the endoplasmic reticulum. Ca^{2+} and DAG activate protein kinase C. The amount of calcium bound to one of the calcium-binding proteins, calmodulin, is also increased.

Ca^{2+}–calmodulin associates as a subunit with several enzymes and modifies their activities. It binds to inactive phosphorylase kinase, thereby partially activating this enzyme. (The fully activated enzyme is both bound to the Ca^{2+}–calmodulin subunit and phosphorylated.) Phosphorylase kinase then phosphorylates glycogen phosphorylase b, thereby activating glycogen degradation. Ca^{2+}–calmodulin is also a modifier protein that activates one of the glycogen synthase kinases (Ca^{2+}–calmodulin synthase kinase). Protein kinase C, Ca^{2+}–calmodulin synthase kinase, and phosphorylase kinase all phosphorylate glycogen synthase at different serine residues on the enzyme, thereby inhibiting glycogen synthase and thus glycogen synthesis.

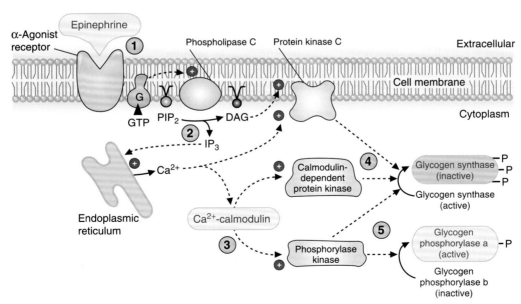

FIGURE 26.8 Regulation of glycogen synthesis and degradation by epinephrine and Ca^{2+}. (*1*) The effect of epinephrine binding to α-agonist receptors in liver transmits a signal via G-proteins to phospholipase C, which hydrolyzes phosphatidylinositol bisphosphate (PIP_2) to diacylglycerol (DAG) and inositol trisphosphate (IP_3). (*2*) IP_3 stimulates the release of Ca^{2+} from the endoplasmic reticulum. (*3*) Ca^{2+} binds to the modifier protein calmodulin, which activates calmodulin-dependent protein kinase and phosphorylase kinase. Both Ca^{2+} and DAG activate protein kinase C. (*4*) These three kinases phosphorylate glycogen synthase at different sites and decrease its activity. (*5*) Phosphorylase kinase phosphorylates glycogen phosphorylase b to the active form. It therefore activates glycogenolysis as well as inhibiting glycogen synthesis. *GTP*, guanosine triphosphate.

The effect of epinephrine in the liver, therefore, enhances or is synergistic with the effects of glucagon. Epinephrine release during bouts of hypoglycemia or during exercise can stimulate hepatic glycogenolysis and inhibit glycogen synthesis very rapidly.

B. Regulation of Glycogen Synthesis and Degradation in Skeletal Muscle

The regulation of glycogenolysis in skeletal muscle is related to the availability of ATP for muscular contraction. Skeletal muscle glycogen produces glucose 1-P and a small amount of free glucose. Glucose 1-P is converted to glucose 6-P, which is committed to the glycolytic pathway; the absence of glucose 6-phosphatase in skeletal muscle prevents conversion of the glucosyl units from glycogen to blood glucose. Skeletal muscle glycogen is therefore degraded only when the demand for ATP generation from glycolysis is high. The highest demands occur during anaerobic glycolysis, which requires more moles of glucose for each ATP produced than oxidation of glucose to CO_2 (see Chapter 24). Anaerobic glycolysis occurs in tissues that have fewer mitochondria, a higher content of glycolytic enzymes, and higher levels of glycogen or in those that have fast-twitch glycolytic fibers. It occurs most frequently at the onset of exercise—before vasodilation occurs to bring in bloodborne fuels. The regulation of skeletal muscle glycogen degradation, therefore, must respond very rapidly to the need for ATP, indicated by the increase in AMP.

The regulation of skeletal muscle glycogen synthesis and degradation differs from that in liver in several important respects:

1. Glucagon has no effect on muscle, and thus, glycogen levels in muscle do not vary with the fasting/feeding state.
2. AMP is an allosteric activator of the muscle isozyme of glycogen phosphorylase but not liver glycogen phosphorylase (Fig. 26.9).

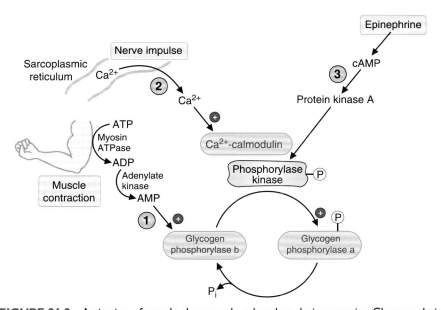

FIGURE 26.9 Activation of muscle glycogen phosphorylase during exercise. Glycogenolysis in skeletal muscle is initiated by muscle contraction, neural impulses, and epinephrine. (*1*) Adenosine monophosphate (AMP) produced from the degradation of adenosine triphosphate (ATP) during muscular contraction allosterically activates glycogen phosphorylase b. (*2*) The neural impulses that initiate contraction release Ca^{2+} from the sarcoplasmic reticulum. The Ca^{2+} binds to calmodulin, which is a modifier protein that activates phosphorylase kinase. (*3*) Phosphorylase kinase is also activated through phosphorylation by protein kinase A. The formation of cyclic AMP (cAMP) and the resultant activation of protein kinase A are initiated by the binding of epinephrine to plasma membrane receptors. *ADP*, adenosine diphosphate; *P_i*, inorganic phosphate.

Jim B. gradually regained consciousness with continued infusions of high-concentration glucose titrated to keep his serum glucose level between 120 and 160 mg/dL. Although he remained somnolent and moderately confused over the next 12 hours, he was eventually able to tell his physicians that he had self-injected approximately 25 units of regular (short-acting) insulin every 6 hours while eating a high-carbohydrate diet for the last 2 days preceding his seizure. Normal subjects under basal conditions secrete an average of 40 U of insulin daily. He had last injected insulin just before exercising. An article in a body-building magazine that he had read recently cited the anabolic effects of insulin on increasing muscle mass. He had purchased the insulin and necessary syringes from the same underground drug source from whom he regularly bought his anabolic steroids.

Normally, muscle glycogenolysis supplies the glucose required for the kinds of high-intensity exercise that require anaerobic glycolysis, such as weightlifting. Jim's treadmill exercise also uses blood glucose, which is supplied by liver glycogenolysis. The high serum insulin levels, resulting from the injection he gave himself just before his workout, activated both glucose transport into skeletal muscle and glycogen synthesis, while inhibiting glycogen degradation. His exercise, which would continue to use blood glucose, could normally be supported by breakdown of liver glycogen. However, glycogen synthesis in his liver was activated, and glycogen degradation was inhibited by the insulin injection.

3. The effects of Ca^{2+} in muscle result principally from the release of Ca^{2+} from the sarcoplasmic reticulum after neural stimulation and not from epinephrine-stimulated uptake.
4. Glucose is not a physiologic inhibitor of glycogen phosphorylase a in muscle.
5. Glycogen is a stronger feedback inhibitor of muscle glycogen synthase than of liver glycogen synthase, resulting in a smaller amount of stored glycogen per gram weight of muscle tissue.

However, the effects of epinephrine-stimulated phosphorylation by PKA on skeletal muscle glycogen degradation and glycogen synthesis are similar to those occurring in liver (see Fig. 26.7).

Muscle glycogen phosphorylase is a genetically distinct isoenzyme of liver glycogen phosphorylase and contains an amino acid sequence that has a purine nucleotide-binding site. When AMP binds to this site, it changes the conformation at the catalytic site to a structure very similar to that in the phosphorylated enzyme. Thus, hydrolysis of ATP to adenosine diphosphate (ADP) and the consequent increase of AMP generated by adenylate kinase during muscular contraction can directly stimulate glycogenolysis to provide fuel for the glycolytic pathway. AMP also stimulates glycolysis by activating phosphofructokinase-1, so this one effector activates both glycogenolysis and glycolysis. The activation of the Ca^{2+}–calmodulin subunit of phosphorylase kinase by the Ca^{2+} released from the sarcoplasmic reticulum during muscle contraction also provides a direct and rapid means of stimulating glycogen degradation.

CLINICAL COMMENTS

Gretchen C. Gretchen C.'s hypoglycemia illustrates the importance of glycogen stores in the neonate. At birth, the fetus must make two major adjustments in the way fuels are used: It must adapt to using a greater variety of fuels than were available in utero, and it must adjust to intermittent feeding. In utero, the fetus receives a relatively constant supply of glucose from the maternal circulation through the placenta, producing a level of glucose in the fetus that approximates 75% of maternal blood levels. With regard to the hormonal regulation of fuel use in utero, fetal tissues function in an environment dominated by insulin, which promotes growth. During the last 10 weeks of gestation, this hormonal milieu leads to glycogen formation and storage. At birth, the infant's diet changes to one containing greater amounts of fat and lactose (galactose and glucose in equal ratio), presented at intervals rather than in a constant fashion. At the same time, the neonate's need for glucose is relatively larger than that of the adult because the newborn's ratio of brain to liver weight is greater. Thus, the infant has even greater difficulty maintaining glucose homeostasis than the adult.

At the moment that the umbilical cord is clamped, the normal neonate is faced with a metabolic problem: The high insulin levels of late fetal existence must be quickly reversed to prevent hypoglycemia. This reversal is accomplished through the secretion of the counterregulatory hormones epinephrine and glucagon. Glucagon release is triggered by the normal decline of blood glucose after birth. The neural response that stimulates the release of both glucagon and epinephrine is activated by the anoxia, cord clamping, and tactile stimulation that are part of a normal delivery. These responses have been referred to as the "normal sensor function" of the neonate.

Within 3 to 4 hours of birth, these counterregulatory hormones reestablish normal serum glucose levels in the newborn's blood through their glycogenolytic and gluconeogenic actions. The failure of Gretchen's normal "sensor function" was partly the result of maternal malnutrition, which resulted in an inadequate deposition of glycogen in Gretchen's liver before birth. The consequence was a serious degree of postnatal hypoglycemia.

The ability to maintain glucose homeostasis during the first few days of life also depends on the activation of gluconeogenesis and the mobilization of fatty acids.

Fatty acid oxidation in the liver not only promotes gluconeogenesis (see Chapter 28), it also generates ketone bodies. The neonatal brain has an enhanced capacity to use ketone bodies relative to that of infants (4-fold) and adults (40-fold). This ability is consistent with the relatively high fat content of breast milk.

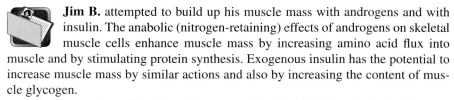 **Jim B.** attempted to build up his muscle mass with androgens and with insulin. The anabolic (nitrogen-retaining) effects of androgens on skeletal muscle cells enhance muscle mass by increasing amino acid flux into muscle and by stimulating protein synthesis. Exogenous insulin has the potential to increase muscle mass by similar actions and also by increasing the content of muscle glycogen.

The most serious side effect of exogenous insulin administration is the development of severe hypoglycemia, such as occurred in Jim's case. The immediate adverse effect relates to an inadequate flow of fuel (glucose) to the metabolizing brain. When hypoglycemia is extreme, the patient may suffer a seizure and, if the hypoglycemia worsens, irreversible brain damage may occur. If prolonged, the patient will lapse into a coma and die.

BIOCHEMICAL COMMENTS

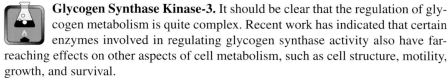 **Glycogen Synthase Kinase-3.** It should be clear that the regulation of glycogen metabolism is quite complex. Recent work has indicated that certain enzymes involved in regulating glycogen synthase activity also have far-reaching effects on other aspects of cell metabolism, such as cell structure, motility, growth, and survival.

The best example of this is glycogen synthase kinase-3 (GSK-3). The enzyme was first identified as being an inhibitor of glycogen synthase. *GSK-3* refers to two isozymes: GSK3α and GSK3β. GSK-3 has been identified as a kinase that can phosphorylate >60 different proteins, including a large number of transcription factors. GSK-3 activity is also itself regulated by phosphorylation.

GSK-3 activity is reduced by phosphorylation of a serine residue near its amino terminus. PKA, Akt, and protein kinase C can all catalyze this inhibitory phosphorylation event. GSK-3 is most active on protein substrates that have already been phosphorylated by other kinases (the substrates are said to be primed for further phosphorylation events). For example, GSK-3 will add phosphates to glycogen synthase but only after glycogen synthase had been phosphorylated by PKA.

GSK-3 binds to several proteins that sequester GSK-3 in certain pathways. This includes the Wnt signaling pathway, disruption of which is a significant component of colon cancer, the Patched–Smoothened signal transduction pathway (see Chapter 18), and the phosphorylation of microtubule-associated proteins, which leads to altered cell motility. Activation of GSK-3 has also been linked to apoptosis, although GSK-3 activity is also required for cell survival.

One of the effects of insulin is to phosphorylate GSK-3, via activation of Akt, rendering the GSK-3 inactive. Loss of activity of GSK-3 will lead to activation of glycogen synthase activity and the pathways of energy storage. In animal models of type 2 diabetes, there is a loss of inhibitory control of GSK-3, leading to greater-than-normal GSK-3 activity, which antagonizes insulin action (promoting insulin resistance, a hallmark of type 2 diabetes). Studies in rats have shown that inhibitors of GSK-3 lowered blood glucose levels and stimulated glucose transport into muscles of insulin-resistant animals. Inappropriate stimulation of GSK-3 has also been implicated in Alzheimer disease.

Current research concerning GSK-3 is geared toward understanding all of the roles of GSK-3 in cell growth and survival and to decipher its actions in the multitude of multiprotein complexes with which it is associated. Inhibitors of GSK-3 are being examined as possible agents to treat diabetes, but interpretation of results is difficult because of the multitude of roles GSK-3 plays within cells. It is possible that in the future, such drugs will be available to treat type 2 diabetes.

KEY CONCEPTS

- Glycogen is the storage form of glucose, composed of glucosyl units linked by α-1,4-glycosidic bonds with α-1,6-branches occurring about every 8 to 10 glucosyl units.
- Glycogen synthesis requires energy.
- Glycogen synthase transfers a glucosyl residue from the activated intermediate UDP-glucose to the nonreducing ends of existing glycogen chains during glycogen synthesis. The branching enzyme creates α-1,6-linkages in the glycogen chain.
- Glycogenolysis is the degradation of glycogen. Glycogen phosphorylase catalyzes a phosphorolysis reaction, using exogenous inorganic phosphate to break α-1,4-linkages at the ends of glycogen chains, releasing glucose 1-phosphate. The debranching enzyme hydrolyzes the α-1,6-linkages in glycogen, releasing free glucose.
- Liver glycogen supplies blood glucose.
- Glycogen synthesis and degradation are regulated in the liver by hormonal changes that signify either a deficiency of or an excess of blood glucose.
- Lack of dietary glucose, signaled by a decrease of the insulin/glucagon ratio, activates liver glycogenolysis and inhibits glycogen synthesis. Epinephrine also activates liver glycogenolysis.
- Glucagon and epinephrine release lead to phosphorylation of glycogen synthase (inactivating it) and glycogen phosphorylase (activating it).
- Glycogenolysis in muscle supplies glucose 6-phosphate for ATP synthesis in the glycolytic pathway.
- Muscle glycogen phosphorylase is allosterically activated by AMP as well as by phosphorylation.
- Increases in sarcoplasmic Ca^{2+} stimulates phosphorylation of muscle glycogen phosphorylase.
- Diseases discussed in this chapter are summarized in Table 26.4.

TABLE 26.4   **Diseases Discussed in Chapter 26**

DISEASE OR DISORDER	ENVIRONMENTAL OR GENETIC	COMMENTS
Newborn hypoglycemia	Environmental	Poor maternal nutrition may lead to inadequate glycogen levels in the newborn, resulting in hypoglycemia during the early fasting period after birth.
Insulin overdose	Environmental	Insulin taken without carbohydrate ingestion will lead to severe hypoglycemia, owing to stimulation of glucose uptake by peripheral tissues, leading to insufficient glucose in the circulation for proper functioning of the nervous system.
Glycogen storage diseases	Genetic	These have been summarized in Table 26.1. They affect storage and use of glycogen, with different levels of severity, from mild to fatal.

REVIEW QUESTIONS—CHAPTER 26

1. Under conditions of glucagon release, the degradation of liver glycogen normally produces which one of the following?
   A. More glucose than glucose 1-P
   B. More glucose 1-P than glucose
   C. Equal amounts of glucose and glucose 1-P
   D. Neither glucose nor glucose 1-P
   E. Only glucose 1-P

2. A patient has large deposits of liver glycogen, which, after an overnight fast, had shorter-than-normal branches. This abnormality could be caused by a defective form of which one of the following proteins or activities?
   A. Glycogen phosphorylase
   B. Glucagon receptor
   C. Glycogenin
   D. Amylo-1,6-glucosidase
   E. Amylo-4,6-transferase

3. An adolescent patient with a deficiency of muscle phosphorylase was examined while exercising her forearm by squeezing a rubber ball. Compared with a normal person performing the same exercise, this patient would exhibit which one of the following?
   A. Exercise for a longer time without fatigue
   B. Have increased glucose levels in blood drawn from her forearm
   C. Have decreased lactate levels in blood drawn from her forearm
   D. Have lower levels of glycogen in biopsy specimens from her forearm muscle
   E. Hyperglycemia

4. In a glucose tolerance test, an individual in the basal metabolic state ingests a large amount of glucose. If the individual is normal, this ingestion should result in which one of the following?
   A. An enhanced glycogen synthase activity in the liver
   B. An increased ratio of glycogen phosphorylase a to glycogen phosphorylase b in the liver
   C. An increased rate of lactate formation by red blood cells
   D. An inhibition of PP-1 activity in the liver
   E. An increase of cAMP levels in the liver

5. Consider a person with type 1 diabetes who has neglected to take insulin for the past 72 hours and also has not eaten much. Which one of the following best describes the activity level of hepatic enzymes involved in glycogen metabolism under these conditions?

	Glycogen Synthase	Phosphorylase Kinase	Glycogen Phosphorylase
A	Active	Active	Active
B	Active	Active	Inactive
C	Active	Inactive	Inactive
D	Inactive	Inactive	Inactive
E	Inactive	Active	Inactive
F	Inactive	Active	Active

6. Assume that an individual carries a mutation in muscle PKA such that the protein is refractory to high levels of cAMP. Glycogen degradation in the muscle would occur, then, under which one of the following conditions?
   A. High levels of intracellular calcium
   B. High levels of intracellular glucose
   C. High levels of intracellular glucose 6-P
   D. High levels of intracellular glucose 1-P
   E. High levels of intracellular magnesium

7. Without a steady supply of glucose to the bloodstream, a patient would become hypoglycemic and, if blood glucose levels get low enough, experience seizures or even a coma. Which one of the following is necessary for the maintenance of normal blood glucose?
   A. Muscle glucose 6-P
   B. Liver glucose 6-P
   C. Glycogen in the heart
   D. Glycogen in the brain
   E. Glycogen in the muscle

8. Glycogen is the storage form of glucose, and its synthesis and degradation is carefully regulated. Which one statement below correctly describes glycogen synthesis and/or degradation?
   A. UDP-glucose is produced in both the synthesis and degradation of glycogen.
   B. Synthesis requires the formation of α-1,4 branches every 8 to 10 residues.
   C. Energy, in the form of ATP, is used to produce UDP-glucose.
   D. Glycogen is both formed from and degrades to glucose 1-P.
   E. The synthesis and degradation of glycogen use the same enzymes, so they are reversible processes.

9. Mutations in various enzymes can lead to the glycogen storage diseases. Which one statement is true of the glycogen storage diseases?
   A. All except type O are fatal in infancy or childhood.
   B. All except type O involve the liver.
   C. All except type O produce hepatomegaly.
   D. All except type O produce hypoglycemia.
   E. All except type O produce increased glycogen deposits.

10. A baby weighing 7.5 lb was delivered at 40 weeks of gestation by normal spontaneous vaginal delivery. At 1 hour, the baby's blood glucose level was determined to be 50 mg/dL and at 2 hours post-birth was 80 mg/dL. These glucose numbers indicate which process?
    A. Maternal malnutrition
    B. Glycogen storage disease
    C. Normal physiologic change
    D. Insulin was given to the baby.
    E. IV dextrose 50 was given to the baby.

ANSWERS

1. **The answer is B.** Glycogen phosphorylase produces glucose 1-P; the debranching enzyme hydrolyzes branch points and thus releases free glucose. Ninety percent of the glycogen contains α-(1,4)-bonds, and only 10% are α-(1,6)-bonds, so more glucose 1-P will be produced than glucose.

2. **The answer is D.** If, after fasting, the branches were shorter than normal, glycogen phosphorylase must be functional and capable of being activated by glucagon (thus, A and B are incorrect). The branching enzyme (amylo-4,6-transferase) is also normal because branch points are present within the glycogen (thus, E is incorrect). Because glycogen is also present, glycogenin is present in order to build the carbohydrate chains, indicating that C is incorrect. If the debranching activity is abnormal (the amylo-1,6-glucosidase), glycogen phosphorylase would break the glycogen down up to four residues from branch points and would then stop. With no debranching activity, the resultant glycogen would contain the normal number of branches, but the branched chains would be shorter than normal.

3. **The answer is C.** The patient has McArdle disease, a glycogen storage disease caused by a deficiency of muscle glycogen phosphorylase. Because she cannot degrade glycogen to produce energy for muscle contraction, she becomes fatigued more readily than a normal person (thus, A is incorrect), the glycogen levels in her muscle will be higher than normal as a result of the inability to degrade them (thus, D is incorrect), and her blood lactate levels will be lower because of the lack of glucose for entry into glycolysis. She will, however, draw on the glucose in her circulation for energy, so her forearm blood glucose levels will be decreased (thus B is incorrect), and because the liver is not affected, blood glucose levels can be maintained by liver glycogenolysis (thus, E is incorrect).

4. **The answer is A.** After ingestion of glucose, insulin levels rise, cAMP levels within the cell drop (thus, E is incorrect), and PP-1 is activated (thus, D is incorrect). Glycogen phosphorylase a is converted to glycogen phosphorylase b by the phosphatase (thus, B is incorrect), and glycogen synthase is activated by the phosphatase. Red blood cells continue to use glucose at their normal rate; hence, lactate formation will remain the same (thus, C is incorrect).

5. **The answer is F.** In the absence of insulin, glucagon-stimulated activities predominate. This leads to the activation of PKA, the phosphorylation and inactivation of glycogen synthase, the phosphorylation and activation of phosphorylase kinase, and the phosphorylation and activation of glycogen phosphorylase.

6. **The answer is A.** Calcium activates a calmodulin subunit in phosphorylase kinase which will allow phosphorylase kinase to phosphorylate, and activate, glycogen phosphorylase. Glucose is an allosteric inhibitor of glycogen phosphorylase a in liver but has no effect in muscle. Glucose 1-P has no effect on muscle phosphorylase, whereas glucose 6-P is an allosteric inhibitor of muscle glycogen phosphorylase a. The levels of magnesium have no effect on muscle glycogen phosphorylase activity. Normally, glucagon or epinephrine would activate the cAMP-dependent PKA, but this is not occurring under these conditions.

7. **The answer is B.** Glycogen in the liver provides glucose for the circulation. Glycogen in the heart, brain, or muscle cannot provide glucose for the circulation. In the liver, glucose 6-phosphatase hydrolyzes glucose 6-P to glucose, which is released into the bloodstream. The liver generates glucose 6-P from either glycogen degradation or gluconeogenesis. Muscle does not contain glucose 6-phosphatase.

8. **The answer is D.** Glycogen is both formed from and degrades to glucose 1-P. A high-energy phosphate bond from UTP is required to produce UDP-glucose in glycogen synthesis, but UDP-glucose is not resynthesized when glycogen is degraded. The pathways of glycogen synthesis and degradation use different enzymes and are not reversible reactions. In this way, the pathways can be regulated independently.

9. **The answer is E.** Type O glycogen storage disease is caused by a reduced level of liver glycogen synthase activity, so in this disease, very little liver glycogen is formed so glycogen deposits would not be found in the liver. All of the other glycogen storage diseases are characterized by glycogen deposits. Not all are fatal, some are mild, and some have an adult-onset form. Some glycogen storage disorders involve the liver, whereas others involve the muscle. Only those involving the liver will produce hepatomegaly and hypoglycemia.

10. **The answer is C.** At birth, maternal glucose supply to the baby ceases, causing a temporary physiologic drop in glucose even in normal healthy infants. This drop signals glycogenolysis in the newborn liver, returning the blood glucose to normal levels. Exogenous insulin would precipitously drop the blood glucose into hypoglycemic levels, and an exogenous bolus of dextrose would raise blood glucose levels above normal levels. This physiologic drop does not necessarily mean maternal malnutrition or evidence of a glycogen storage disease.

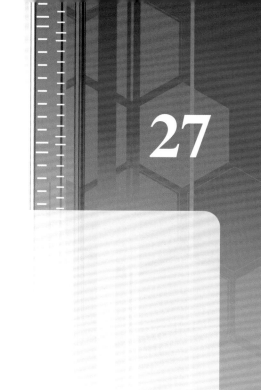

Pentose Phosphate Pathway and the Synthesis of Glycosides, Lactose, Glycoproteins, and Glycolipids

27

Glucose is used in several pathways other than glycolysis and glycogen synthesis. The **pentose phosphate pathway** (also known as the hexose monophosphate shunt, or HMP shunt) consists of both **oxidative** and **nonoxidative** components (Fig. 27.1). In the oxidative pathway, glucose 6-phosphate (glucose 6-P) is oxidized to **ribulose 5-phosphate** (ribulose 5-P), carbon dioxide (CO_2), and reduced nicotinamide adenine dinucleotide phosphate (**NADPH**). Ribulose 5-P, a pentose, can be converted to **ribose 5-phosphate** (ribose 5-P) for nucleotide biosynthesis. The NADPH is used for reductive pathways, such as **fatty acid biosynthesis**, **detoxification** of drugs by monooxygenases, and the **glutathione defense system** against injury by reactive oxygen species (ROS).

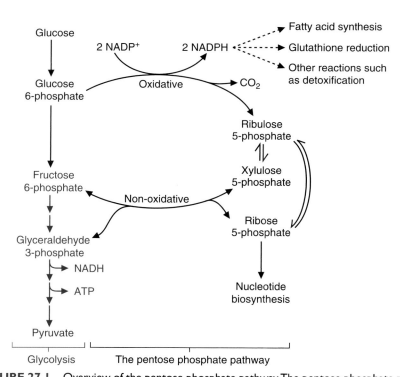

FIGURE 27.1 Overview of the pentose phosphate pathway. The pentose phosphate pathway generates reduced nicotinamide adenine dinucleotide phosphate (NADPH) for reactions that require reducing equivalents (electrons) or ribose 5-phosphate for nucleotide biosynthesis. Glucose 6-phosphate is a substrate for both the pentose phosphate pathway and glycolysis. The five-carbon sugar intermediates of the pentose phosphate pathway are reversibly interconverted to intermediates of glycolysis. The portion of glycolysis that is not part of the pentose phosphate pathway is shown in *red*. *ATP*, adenosine triphosphate.

In the nonoxidative phase of the pathway, ribulose 5-P is converted to ribose 5-P and to intermediates of the glycolytic pathway. This portion of the pathway is reversible; therefore, ribose 5-P can also be formed from intermediates of glycolysis. One of the enzymes involved in these sugar interconversions, **transketolase**, uses **thiamin pyrophosphate** as a coenzyme.

The sugars produced by the pentose phosphate pathway enter glycolysis as fructose 6-phosphate (fructose 6-P) and glyceraldehyde 3-phosphate (glyceraldehyde 3-P), and their further metabolism in the glycolytic pathway generates NADH, adenosine triphosphate (ATP), and pyruvate. The overall equation for the conversion of glucose 6-P to fructose 6-P and glyceraldehyde 3-P through both the oxidative and nonoxidative reactions of the pentose phosphate pathway is

$$3 \text{ Glucose 6-P} + 6 \text{ NADP}^+ \rightarrow 3 \text{ CO}_2 + 6 \text{ NADPH} + 6 \text{ H}^+ \\ + 2 \text{ fructose 6-P} + \text{glyceraldehyde 3-P}$$

As had been seen previously in glycogen synthesis, several pathways for interconversion of sugars or the formation of sugar derivatives use activated sugars attached to nucleotides. Both uridine diphosphate **(UDP)-glucose** and **UDP-galactose** are used for **glycosyltransferase** reactions in many systems. Lactose, for example, is synthesized from UDP-galactose and glucose in the mammary gland. UDP-glucose also can be oxidized to form UDP-glucuronate, which is used to form **glucuronide derivatives** of bilirubin and xenobiotic compounds. Glucuronide derivatives are generally more readily excreted in urine or bile than the parent compound.

In addition to serving as fuel, carbohydrates are often found in **glycoproteins** (carbohydrate chains attached to proteins) and **glycolipids** (carbohydrate chains attached to lipids). **Nucleotide sugars** are used to donate sugar residues for the formation of the glycosidic bonds in both glycoproteins and glycolipids. These carbohydrate groups have many different types of functions.

Glycoproteins contain short chains of carbohydrates (oligosaccharides) that are usually branched. These oligosaccharides are generally composed of glucose, galactose, and their amino derivatives. In addition, mannose, L-fucose, and *N*-acetylneuraminic acid (NANA) are frequently present. The carbohydrate chains grow by the sequential addition of sugars to a **serine** or **threonine** residue of the protein. Nucleotide sugars are the precursors. Branched carbohydrate chains also may be attached to the amide nitrogen of **asparagine** in the protein. In this case, the chains are synthesized on **dolichol phosphate** and subsequently transferred to the protein. Glycoproteins are found in mucus, in the blood, in compartments within the cell (such as lysosomes), in the extracellular matrix, and embedded in the cell membrane with the carbohydrate portion extending into the extracellular space.

Glycolipids belong to the class of sphingolipids. They are synthesized from nucleotide sugars that add monosaccharides sequentially to the hydroxymethyl group of the lipid ceramide (related to sphingosine). They often contain branches of NANA produced from cytidine monophosphate (CMP)-NANA. They are found in the cell membrane with the carbohydrate portion extruding from the cell surface. These carbohydrates, as well as some of the carbohydrates of glycoproteins, serve as **cell recognition factors**.

 Blood typing in a clinical lab uses antibodies that recognize either the A antigen, the B antigen, or the Rh(D) antigen. Each antigen is distinctive, in part, because of the different carbohydrate chains attached to the protein. The blood sample is mixed with each antibody individually. If cell clumping (agglutination) occurs, the red blood cells are expressing the carbohydrate that is recognized by the antibody (recall from Chapter 7 that antibodies are bivalent; the agglutination occurs because one arm of the antibody binds to antigen on one cell, whereas the other arm binds to antigen on a second cell, thereby bringing the cells together). If neither the A nor B antibodies cause agglutination, the blood type is O, indicating a lack of either antigen.

THE WAITING ROOM

After **Al M.** had been released from the hospital, where he had been treated for thiamin deficiency, he quickly fell off the wagon and injured his arm after falling down in the street while intoxicated. Two days after hurting his arm, Al's friends took him to the hospital when he developed a fever of 101.5°F. One of the physicians noticed that one of the lacerations on Mr. M.'s arm was red and swollen, with some pus drainage. The pus was cultured and gram-positive cocci were found and identified as *Staphylococcus aureus*. Because his friends stated that he had an allergy to penicillin, and because of the concern over methicillin-resistant

S. aureus, Al was started on a course of the antibiotic combination of trimethoprim and sulfamethoxazole (TMP/sulfa). To his friends' knowledge, he had never been treated with a sulfa drug previously.

On the third day of therapy with TMP/sulfa for his infection, Mr. M. was slightly jaundiced. His hemoglobin level had fallen by 3.5 g/dL from its value at admission, and his urine was red-brown because of the presence of free hemoglobin. Mr. M. had apparently suffered acute hemolysis (lysis or destruction of some of his red blood cells) induced by his infection and exposure to the sulfa drug.

 To help support herself through medical school, **Edna R.** works evenings in a hospital blood bank. She is responsible for ensuring that compatible donor blood is available to patients who need blood transfusions. As part of her training, Edna has learned that the external surfaces of all blood cells contain large numbers of antigenic determinants. These determinants are often glycoproteins or glycolipids that differ from one individual to another. As a result, all blood transfusions expose the recipient to many foreign immunogens. Most of these, fortunately, do not induce antibodies, or they induce antibodies that elicit little or no immunologic response. For routine blood transfusions, therefore, tests are performed only for the presence of antigens that determine whether the patient's blood type is A, B, AB, or O and Rh(D)-positive or -negative.

 Jay S.'s psychomotor development has become progressively more abnormal (see Chapter 15). At 2 years of age, he is obviously severely developmentally delayed and nearly blind. His muscle weakness has progressed to the point that he cannot sit up or even crawl. As the result of a weak cough reflex, he is unable to clear his normal respiratory secretions and has had recurrent respiratory infections.

I. The Pentose Phosphate Pathway

The *pentose phosphate pathway* is essentially a scenic bypass route around the first stage of glycolysis that generates NADPH and ribose 5-P (as well as other pentose sugars). Glucose 6-P is the common precursor for both pathways. The oxidative first stage of the pentose phosphate pathway generates 2 mol of NADPH per mole of glucose 6-P oxidized. The second stage of the pentose phosphate pathway generates ribose 5-P and converts unused intermediates to fructose 6-P and glyceraldehyde 3-P in the glycolytic pathway (see Fig. 27.1). All cells require NADPH for reductive detoxification, and most cells require ribose 5-P for nucleotide synthesis. Consequently, the pathway is present in all cells. The enzymes reside in the cytosol, as do the enzymes of glycolysis.

A. Oxidative Phase of the Pentose Phosphate Pathway

In the oxidative first phase of the pentose phosphate pathway, glucose 6-P undergoes an oxidation and decarboxylation to a pentose sugar, ribulose 5-P (Fig. 27.2). The first enzyme of this pathway, glucose 6-P dehydrogenase, oxidizes the aldehyde at carbon 1 and reduces NADP$^+$ to NADPH. The gluconolactone that is formed is rapidly hydrolyzed to 6-phosphogluconate, a sugar acid with a carboxylic acid group at carbon 1. The next oxidation step releases this carboxyl group as CO_2, with the electrons being transferred to NADP$^+$. This reaction is mechanistically very similar to the one catalyzed by isocitrate dehydrogenase in the tricarboxylic acid (TCA) cycle. Thus, 2 mol of NADPH per mole of glucose 6-P are formed from this portion of the pathway.

NADPH, rather than NADH, is generally used in the cell in pathways that require the input of electrons for reductive reactions, because the ratio of NADPH/NADP$^+$ is much greater than the NADH/NAD$^+$ ratio. The NADH generated from fuel oxidation

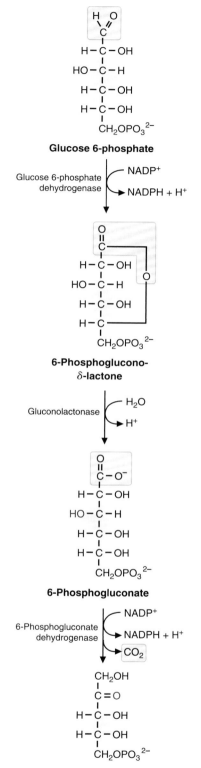

FIGURE 27.2 Oxidative portion of the pentose phosphate pathway. Carbon 1 of glucose 6-phosphate is oxidized to an acid and then released as CO_2 in an oxidation followed by a decarboxylation reaction. Each of the oxidation steps generate a reduced nicotinamide adenine dinucleotide phosphate (NADPH).

M The transketolase activity of red blood cells can be used to measure thiamin nutritional status and diagnose the presence of thiamin deficiency. The activity of transketolase is measured in the presence and absence of added thiamin pyrophosphate. If the thiamin intake of a patient is adequate, the addition of thiamin pyrophosphate does not increase the activity of transketolase because it already contains bound thiamin pyrophosphate. If the patient is thiamin-deficient, transketolase activity will be low, and adding thiamin pyrophosphate will greatly stimulate the reaction. In Chapter 24, **Al M.** was diagnosed as having beriberi heart disease, resulting from thiamin deficiency, by direct measurement of thiamin, which is the more commonly used test currently.

Q How does the net energy yield from the metabolism of 3 mol of glucose 6-P through the pentose phosphate pathway to pyruvate compare with the yield of 3 mol of glucose 6-P through glycolysis?

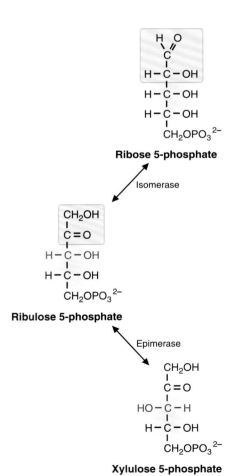

FIGURE 27.3 Ribulose 5-phosphate can be epimerized (to xylulose 5-phosphate, shown in *red*) or isomerized (to ribose 5-phosphate, shown in the *yellow box*).

is rapidly oxidized back to NAD$^+$ by NADH dehydrogenase in the electron-transport chain, so the level of NADH in the cell is very low.

NADPH can be generated from several reactions in the liver and other tissues but not red blood cells. For example, in tissues with mitochondria, an energy-requiring transhydrogenase located near the complexes of the electron-transport chain can transfer reducing equivalents from NADH to NADP$^+$ to generate NADPH.

NADPH, however, cannot be oxidized directly by the electron-transport chain, and the ratio of NADPH to NADP$^+$ in cells is >1. The reduction potential of NADPH, therefore, can contribute to the energy needed for biosynthetic processes and provide a constant source of reducing power for detoxification reactions.

The ribulose 5-P formed from the action of the two oxidative steps is isomerized to produce ribose 5-P (a ketose-to-aldose conversion, similar to fructose 6-P being isomerized to glucose 6-P). The ribose 5-P can then enter the pathway for nucleotide synthesis, if needed, or it can be converted to glycolytic intermediates, as described in the following section for the nonoxidative phase of the pentose phosphate pathway. The pathway through which the ribose 5-P travels is determined by the needs of the cell at the time of its synthesis.

B. Nonoxidative Phase of the Pentose Phosphate Pathway

The nonoxidative reactions of this pathway are *reversible reactions* that allow intermediates of glycolysis (specifically, glyceraldehyde 3-P and fructose 6-P) to be converted to five-carbon sugars (such as ribose 5-P), and vice versa. The needs of the cell determine in which direction this pathway proceeds. If the cell has produced ribose 5-P but does not need to synthesize nucleotides, then the ribose 5-P is converted to glycolytic intermediates. If the cell still requires NADPH, the ribose 5-P is converted back into glucose 6-P using nonoxidative reactions (see the next section). And finally, if the cell already has a high level of NADPH but needs to produce nucleotides, the oxidative reactions of the pentose phosphate pathway are inhibited, and the glycolytic intermediates fructose 6-P and glyceraldehyde 3-P are used to produce the five-carbon sugars using exclusively the nonoxidative phase of the pentose phosphate pathway.

1. Conversion of Ribulose 5-Phosphate to Glycolytic Intermediates

The nonoxidative portion of the pentose phosphate pathway consists of a series of rearrangement and transfer reactions that first convert ribulose 5-P to ribose 5-P and xylulose 5-phosphate (xylulose 5-P), and then the ribose 5-P and xylulose 5-P are converted to intermediates of the glycolytic pathway. The enzymes involved are an epimerase, an isomerase, transketolase, and transaldolase.

The epimerase and isomerase convert ribulose 5-P to two other five-carbon sugars (Fig. 27.3). The isomerase converts ribulose 5-P to ribose 5-P. The epimerase changes the stereochemical position of one hydroxyl group (at carbon 3), converting ribulose 5-P to xylulose 5-P.

Transketolase transfers two-carbon fragments of keto sugars (sugars with a keto group at carbon 2) to other sugars. Transketolase picks up a two-carbon fragment from xylulose 5-P by cleaving the carbon–carbon bond between the keto group and the adjacent carbon, thereby releasing glyceraldehyde 3-P (Fig. 27.4). The two-carbon fragment is covalently bound to thiamin pyrophosphate, which transfers it to the aldehyde carbon of another sugar, forming a new ketose. The role of thiamin pyrophosphate here is thus very similar to its role in the oxidative decarboxylation of pyruvate and α-ketoglutarate (see Chapter 24, Section III.C). Two reactions in the pentose phosphate pathway use transketolase: In the first, the two-carbon keto fragment from xylulose 5-P is transferred to ribose 5-P to form sedoheptulose 7-phosphate (sedoheptulose 7-P); and in the other, a two-carbon keto fragment (usually derived from xylulose 5-P) is transferred to erythrose 4-phosphate (erythrose 4-P) to form fructose 6-P.

Transaldolase transfers a three-carbon keto fragment from sedoheptulose 7-P to glyceraldehyde 3-P to form erythrose 4-P and fructose 6-P (Fig. 27.5). The aldol cleavage occurs between the two hydroxyl carbons adjacent to the keto group (on carbons 3 and 4 of the sugar). This reaction is similar to the aldolase reaction in glycolysis, and the enzyme uses an active amino group, from the side chain of lysine, to catalyze the reaction.

The net result of the metabolism of 3 mol of ribulose 5-P in the pentose phosphate pathway is the formation of 2 mol of fructose 6-P and 1 mol of glyceraldehyde 3-P, which then continue through the glycolytic pathway with the production of NADH, ATP, and pyruvate. Because the pentose phosphate pathway begins with glucose 6-P and feeds back into the glycolytic pathway, it is sometimes called the *HMP shunt* (a shunt or a pathway for glucose 6-P). The reaction sequence starting from glucose 6-P and involving both the oxidative and nonoxidative phases of the pathway is shown in Figure 27.6.

(A) The net energy yield from 3 mol of glucose 6-P metabolized through the pentose phosphate pathway and then the last portion of the glycolytic pathway is 6 mol of NADPH, 3 mol of CO_2, 5 mol of NADH, 8 mol of ATP, and 5 mol of pyruvate. In contrast, the metabolism of 3 mol of glucose 6-P through glycolysis is 6 mol of NADH, 9 mol of ATP, and 6 mol of pyruvate.

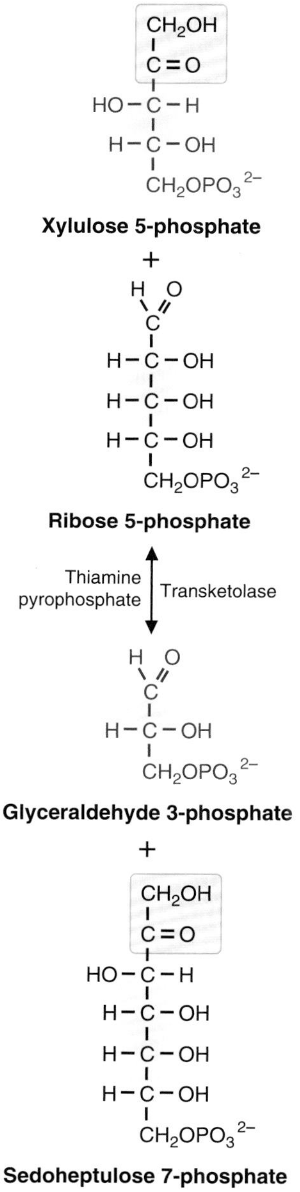

FIGURE 27.4 Two-carbon unit transferred by transketolase. Transketolase cleaves the bond next to the keto group and transfers the two-carbon keto fragment to an aldehyde. Thiamin pyrophosphate carries the two-carbon fragment, forming a covalent bond with the carbon of the keto group.

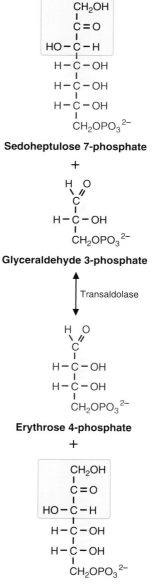

FIGURE 27.5 Transaldolase transfers a three-carbon fragment that contains an alcohol group next to a keto group.

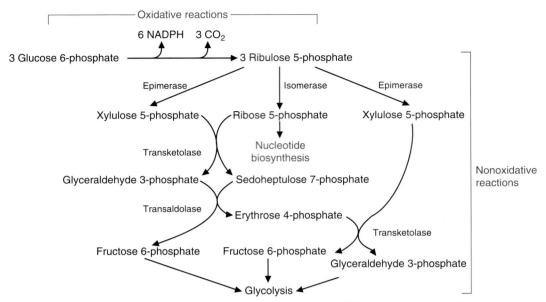

FIGURE 27.6 A balanced sequence of reactions in the pentose phosphate pathway. The interconversion of sugars in the pentose phosphate pathway results in conversion of three glucose 6-phosphate to six reduced nicotinamide adenine dinucleotide phosphate (NADPH), three CO_2, two fructose 6-phosphate, and one glyceraldehyde 3-phosphate.

2. Generation of Ribose 5-Phosphate from Intermediates of Glycolysis

The reactions catalyzed by the epimerase, isomerase, transketolase, and transaldolase are all reversible reactions under physiologic conditions. Thus, ribose 5-P required for purine and pyrimidine nucleotide synthesis can be generated from intermediates of the glycolytic pathway, as well as from the oxidative phase of the pentose phosphate pathway. The sequence of reactions that generate ribose 5-P from intermediates of glycolysis is as follows:

(1) Fructose 6-P + glyceraldehyde 3-P $\xleftrightarrow{\text{Transketolase}}$ Erythrose 4-P + xylulose 5-P

(2) Erythrose 4-P + fructose 6-P $\xleftrightarrow{\text{Transaldolase}}$ Sedoheptulose 7-P + glyceraldehyde 3-P

(3) Sedoheptulose 7-P + glyceraldehyde 3-P $\xleftrightarrow{\text{Transketolase}}$ Ribose 5-P + xylulose 5-P

(4) 2 Xylulose 5-P $\xleftrightarrow{\text{Epimerase}}$ 2 Ribulose 5-P

(5) 2 Ribulose 5-P $\xleftrightarrow{\text{Isomerase}}$ 2 Ribose 5-P

Net equation: 2 Fructose 6-P + glyceraldehyde 3-P $\leftrightarrow$ 3 Ribose 5-P

C. Role of the Pentose Phosphate Pathway in Generation of NADPH

In general, the oxidative phase of the pentose phosphate pathway is the major source of NADPH in cells. NADPH provides the reducing equivalents for biosynthetic reactions and for oxidation–reduction reactions involved in protection against the toxicity of ROS (see Chapter 25). The glutathione-mediated defense against oxidative stress is common to all cell types (including red blood cells), and the requirement for NADPH to maintain levels of reduced glutathione probably accounts for the universal distribution of the pentose phosphate pathway among different types of cells. Figure 27.7 illustrates the importance of this pathway in maintaining the membrane integrity of the red blood cells. NADPH is also used for anabolic pathways, such as fatty acid synthesis, cholesterol synthesis, and fatty acid chain elongation (Table 27.1). It is the source of reducing equivalents for cytochrome P450 hydroxylation

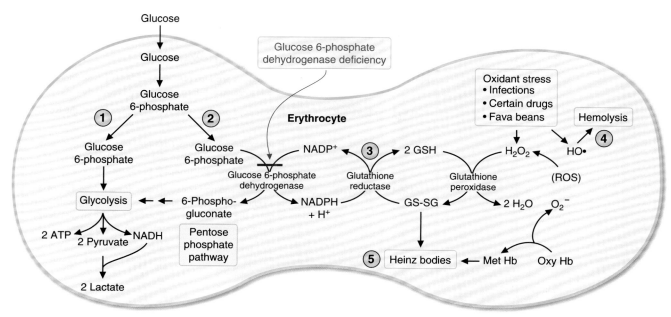

FIGURE 27.7 Hemolysis caused by reactive oxygen species (ROS). (*1*) Maintenance of the integrity of the erythrocyte membrane depends on its ability to generate adenosine triphosphate (ATP) and reduced nicotinamide adenine dinucleotide (NADH) from glycolysis. (2) NADPH is generated by the pentose phosphate pathway. (3) NADPH is used for the reduction of oxidized glutathione (GSSG) to reduced glutathione (GSH). Glutathione is necessary for the removal of hydrogen peroxide (H_2O_2) and lipid peroxides generated by ROS. (4) In the erythrocytes of healthy individuals, the continuous generation of superoxide ion from the nonenzymatic oxidation of hemoglobin provides a source of ROS. The glutathione defense system is compromised by glucose 6-phosphate dehydrogenase deficiency, infections, certain drugs, and the purine glycosides of fava beans. (5) As a consequence, Heinz bodies, aggregates of cross-linked hemoglobin, form on the cell membranes and subject the cell to mechanical stress as it tries to go through small capillaries. The action of the ROS on the cell membrane as well as mechanical stress from the lack of deformability result in hemolysis. *Met Hb*, methemoglobin; *Oxy Hb*, oxyhemoglobin.

of aromatic compounds, steroids, alcohols, and drugs. The highest concentrations of glucose 6-P dehydrogenase are found in phagocytic cells, where NADPH oxidase uses NADPH to form superoxide from molecular oxygen. The superoxide then generates hydrogen peroxide, which kills the microorganisms taken up by the phagocytic cells (see Chapter 25).

The entry of glucose 6-P into the pentose phosphate pathway is controlled by the cellular concentration of NADPH. NADPH is a strong product inhibitor of glucose 6-P dehydrogenase, the first enzyme of the pathway. As NADPH is oxidized in other pathways, the product inhibition of glucose 6-P dehydrogenase is relieved, and the rate of the enzyme is accelerated to produce more NADPH.

In the liver, the synthesis of fatty acids from glucose is a major route of NADPH reoxidation. The synthesis of liver glucose 6-P dehydrogenase, like the key enzymes of glycolysis and fatty acid synthesis, is induced by the increased

TABLE 27.1	**Pathways that Require Reduced Nicotinamide Adenine Dinucleotide Phosphate**

Detoxification
- Reduction of oxidized glutathione
- Cytochrome P450 monooxygenases

Reductive synthesis
- Fatty acid synthesis
- Fatty acid chain elongation
- Cholesterol synthesis
- Neurotransmitter synthesis
- Deoxynucleotide synthesis
- Superoxide synthesis

 Doctors suspected that the underlying factor in the destruction of **Al M.'s** red blood cells was an X-linked defect in the gene that codes for glucose 6-P dehydrogenase. The red blood cell is dependent on this enzyme for a source of NADPH to maintain reduced levels of glutathione, one of its major defenses against oxidative stress (see Chapter 25). Glucose 6-P dehydrogenase deficiency is the most common known enzymopathy, affecting approximately 7% of the world's population and about 2% of the US population. Most glucose 6-P dehydrogenase–deficient individuals are asymptomatic but can undergo an episode of hemolytic anemia if they are exposed to certain drugs or to certain types of infections, or if they ingest fava beans. When questioned, **Al M.** replied that he did not know what a fava bean was and had no idea whether he was sensitive to them.

TABLE 27.2 Cellular Needs Dictate the Direction of the Pentose Phosphate Pathway Reactions	
CELLULAR NEED	**DIRECTION OF PATHWAY**
NADPH only	Oxidative reactions produce NADPH; nonoxidative reactions convert ribulose 5-P to glucose 6-P to produce more NADPH.
NADPH + ribose 5-P	Oxidative reactions produce NADPH and ribose 5-P; the isomerase converts ribulose 5-P to ribose 5-P.
Ribose 5-P only	Only the nonoxidative reactions. High NADPH inhibits glucose 6-P dehydrogenase, so transketolase and transaldolase are used to convert fructose 6-P and glyceraldehyde 3-P to ribose 5-P.
NADPH and pyruvate	Both the oxidative and nonoxidative reactions are used. The oxidative reactions generate NADPH and ribulose 5-P. The nonoxidative reactions convert the ribulose 5-P to fructose 6-P and glyceraldehyde 3-P, and glycolysis converts these intermediates to pyruvate.

fructose 6-P, fructose 6- phosphate; glucose 6-P, glucose 6-phosphate; glyceraldehyde 3-P, glyceraldehyde 3-phosphate; NADPH, reduced nicotinamide adenine dinucleotide phosphate; ribose 5-P, ribose 5-phosphate; ribulose 5-P, ribulose 5-phosphate;

insulin:glucagon ratio after a high-carbohydrate meal. A summary of the possible routes that glucose 6-P may follow using the pentose phosphate pathway is presented in Table 27.2.

II. Interconversions Involving Nucleotide Sugars

Activated sugars attached to nucleotides are converted to other sugars; oxidized to sugar acids; and joined to proteins, lipids, or other sugars through *glycosidic bonds*.

A. Reactions of Uridine Diphosphate-Glucose

UDP-glucose is an activated sugar nucleotide that is a precursor of glycogen and lactose; UDP-glucuronate and glucuronides; and the carbohydrate chains in proteoglycans, glycoproteins, and glycolipids (Fig. 27.8). Both proteoglycans and glycosaminoglycans are discussed further in Chapter 47. In the synthesis of many of the carbohydrate portions of these compounds, a sugar is transferred from the

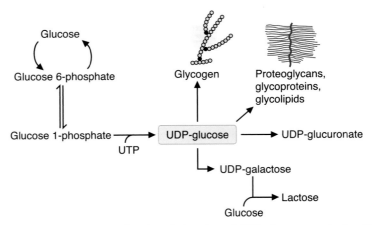

FIGURE 27.8 An overview of uridine diphosphate (UDP)-glucose metabolism. The activated glucose moiety of UDP-glucose can be attached by a glycosidic bond to other sugars, as in glycogen or the sugar oligosaccharide and polysaccharide side chains of proteoglycans, glycoproteins, and glycolipids. UDP-glucose also can be oxidized to UDP-glucuronate, or epimerized to UDP-galactose, a precursor of lactose. *UTP*, uridine triphosphate.

UDP-glucose

— Protein—OH

Glycosyltransferase

→ UDP

Glycosylated protein

FIGURE 27.9 Glycosyltransferases. These enzymes transfer sugars from nucleotide sugars to nucleophilic amino acid residues on proteins, such as the hydroxyl group of serine or the amide group of asparagine. Other transferases transfer specific sugars from a nucleotide sugar to a hydroxyl group of other sugars. The bond formed between the anomeric carbon of the sugar and the nucleophilic group of another compound is a glycosidic bond. *UDP*, uridine diphosphate.

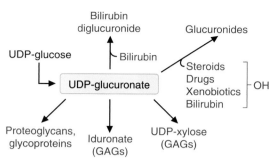

FIGURE 27.10 Metabolic routes of uridine diphosphate (UDP)-glucuronate. UDP-glucuronate is formed from UDP-glucose (shown in *black*). Glucuronate from UDP-glucuronate is incorporated into glycosaminoglycans (GAGs), where certain of the glucuronate residues are converted to iduronate (see Chapter 47). UDP-glucuronate is a precursor of UDP-xylose, another sugar residue incorporated into GAGs. Glucuronate is also transferred to the carboxyl groups of bilirubin or the alcohol groups of steroids, drugs, and xenobiotics to form glucuronides. The "-ide" in the name glucuronide denotes that these compounds are glycosides. Xenobiotics are pharmacologically, endocrinologically, or toxicologically active substances not produced endogenously and, therefore, are foreign to an organism. Drugs are an example of xenobiotics.

nucleotide sugar to an alcohol or other nucleophilic group to form a glycosidic bond (Fig. 27.9). The use of UDP as a leaving group in this reaction provides the energy for formation of the new bond. The enzymes that form glycosidic bonds are sugar transferases (e.g., glycogen synthase is a glucosyltransferase). Transferases are also involved in the formation of the glycosidic bonds in bilirubin glucuronides, proteoglycans, and lactose.

B. Uridine Diphosphate-Glucuronate: A Source of Negative Charges

One of the major routes of UDP-glucose metabolism is the formation of *UDP-glucuronate*, which serves as a precursor of other sugars and of glucuronides (Fig. 27.10). Glucuronate is formed by the oxidation of the alcohol on carbon 6 of glucose to an acid (through two oxidation states) by an NAD^+-dependent dehydrogenase (Fig. 27.11). Glucuronate is also present in the diet and can be formed from the degradation of inositol (the sugar alcohol that forms inositol trisphosphate [IP_3]), an intracellular second messenger for many hormones.

C. Glucuronides: A Source of Negative Charges

The function of glucuronate in the excretion of bilirubin, drugs, xenobiotics, and other compounds containing a hydroxyl group is to add negative charges and increase their solubility. Bilirubin is a degradation product of heme that is formed in the reticuloendothelial system and is only slightly soluble in plasma. It is transported, bound to albumin, to the liver. In the liver, glucuronate residues are transferred from UDP-glucuronate to two carboxyl groups on bilirubin, sequentially forming bilirubin monoglucuronide and bilirubin diglucuronide, the "conjugated" forms of bilirubin (Fig. 27.12). The more soluble bilirubin diglucuronide (as compared with unconjugated bilirubin) is then actively transported into the bile for excretion.

Many xenobiotics, drugs, steroids, and other compounds with hydroxyl groups and low solubility in water are converted to glucuronides in a similar fashion by glucuronyltransferases present in the endoplasmic reticulum and cytoplasm of the liver and kidney (Table 27.3). This is one of the major conjugation pathways for excretion of these compounds.

 What is the difference in structure between 6-phosphogluconate and glucuronic acid?

 A failure of the liver to transport, store, or conjugate bilirubin results in the accumulation of unconjugated bilirubin in the blood. Jaundice (or icterus), the yellowish tinge to the skin and the whites of the eyes (sclerae) experienced by **Erin G.** (see Chapter 22), occurs when plasma becomes supersaturated with bilirubin (>2 to 2.5 mg/dL), and the excess diffuses into tissues. When bilirubin levels are measured in the blood (see Chapter 6), one can either measure indirect bilirubin (this is the nonconjugated form of bilirubin, which is bound to albumin), direct bilirubin (the conjugated, water-soluble form), or total bilirubin (the sum of the direct and indirect levels). If total bilirubin levels are high, then a determination of direct and indirect bilirubin is needed to appropriately determine a cause for the elevation of total bilirubin.

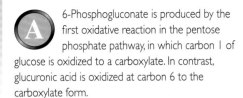

6-Phosphogluconate is produced by the first oxidative reaction in the pentose phosphate pathway, in which carbon 1 of glucose is oxidized to a carboxylate. In contrast, glucuronic acid is oxidized at carbon 6 to the carboxylate form.

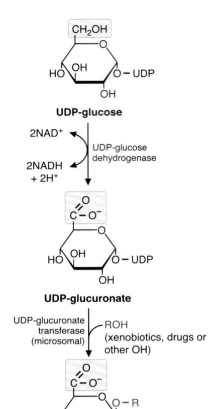

UDP-glucose

2NAD⁺

UDP-glucose dehydrogenase

2NADH + 2H⁺

UDP-glucuronate

UDP-glucuronate transferase (microsomal)

ROH (xenobiotics, drugs or other OH)

+ UDP

Glucuronide

Bile or urine

FIGURE 27.11 Formation of glucuronate and glucuronides. A glycosidic bond is formed between the anomeric hydroxyl of glucuronate (at carbon 1) and the hydroxyl group of a nonpolar compound. The negatively charged carboxyl group of the glucuronate increases the water solubility and allows otherwise nonpolar compounds to be excreted in the urine or bile. The hydrogen atoms have been omitted from the figure for clarity. *NAD*, nicotinamide adenine dinucleotide; *UDP*, uridine diphosphate.

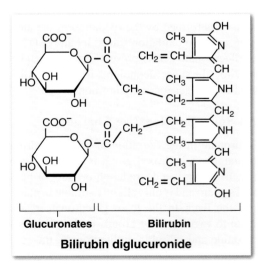

Glucuronates   Bilirubin

Bilirubin diglucuronide

FIGURE 27.12   Formation of bilirubin diglucuronide. A glycosidic bond is formed between the anomeric hydroxyl of glucuronate and the carboxylate groups of bilirubin. The addition of the hydrophilic carbohydrate group and the negatively charged carboxyl group of the glucuronate increases the water solubility of the conjugated bilirubin and allows the otherwise insoluble bilirubin to be excreted in the urine or bile. The hydrogen atoms on the sugars have been omitted from the figure for clarity.

TABLE 27.3 Examples of Compounds Degraded and Excreted as Urinary Glucuronides

Estrogen (female sex hormone)
Progesterone (steroid hormone)
Triiodothyronine (thyroid hormone)
Acetylaminofluorene (xenobiotic carcinogen)
Meprobamate (drug for sleep)
Morphine (painkiller)

Glucuronate, once formed, can reenter the pathways of glucose metabolism through reactions that eventually convert it to D-xylulose 5-P, an intermediate of the pentose phosphate pathway. In most mammals other than humans, an intermediate of this pathway is the precursor of ascorbic acid (vitamin C). Humans, however, are deficient in this pathway and cannot synthesize vitamin C.

D. Synthesis of Uridine Diphosphate-Galactose and Lactose from Glucose

Lactose is synthesized from UDP-galactose and glucose (Fig. 27.13). However, galactose is not required in the diet for lactose synthesis because galactose can be synthesized from glucose.

1. Conversion of Glucose to Galactose

Galactose and glucose are *epimers*; they differ only in the stereochemical position of one hydroxyl group, at carbon 4. Thus, the formation of UDP-galactose from UDP-glucose is an *epimerization* (Fig. 27.14). The epimerase does not actually transfer the hydroxyl group; it oxidizes the hydroxyl to a ketone by transferring electrons to NAD$^+$ and then donates electrons back to re-form the alcohol group on the other side of the carbon.

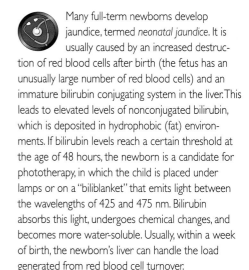

Many full-term newborns develop jaundice, termed *neonatal jaundice*. It is usually caused by an increased destruction of red blood cells after birth (the fetus has an unusually large number of red blood cells) and an immature bilirubin conjugating system in the liver. This leads to elevated levels of nonconjugated bilirubin, which is deposited in hydrophobic (fat) environments. If bilirubin levels reach a certain threshold at the age of 48 hours, the newborn is a candidate for phototherapy, in which the child is placed under lamps or on a "biliblanket" that emits light between the wavelengths of 425 and 475 nm. Bilirubin absorbs this light, undergoes chemical changes, and becomes more water-soluble. Usually, within a week of birth, the newborn's liver can handle the load generated from red blood cell turnover.

High concentrations of galactose 1-phosphate (galactose 1-P) inhibit phosphoglucomutase, the enzyme that converts glucose 6-P to glucose 1-P. How can this inhibition account for the hypoglycemia and jaundice that accompany galactose 1-P uridylyltransferase deficiency?

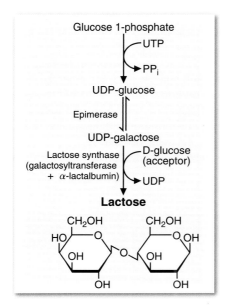

FIGURE 27.13 Lactose synthesis. Lactose is a disaccharide composed of galactose and glucose. Uridine diphosphate (UDP)-galactose for the synthesis of lactose in the mammary gland is usually formed from the epimerization of UDP-glucose. Lactose synthase catalyzes the attack of the C4 alcohol group of glucose on the anomeric carbon of the galactose, releasing UDP and forming a glycosidic bond. Lactose synthase is composed of a galactosyltransferase and α-lactalbumin, which is a regulatory subunit. *PP$_i$*, pyrophosphate; *UTP*, uridine triphosphate.

FIGURE 27.14 Epimerization of uridine diphosphate (UDP)-glucose to UDP-galactose. The epimerization of glucose to galactose occurs on UDP-sugars. The epimerase uses nicotinamide adenine dinucleotide (NAD$^+$) to oxidize the alcohol to a ketone, and then it reduces the ketone back to an alcohol. The reaction is reversible; glucose being converted to galactose forms galactose for lactose synthesis, and galactose being converted to glucose is part of the pathway for the metabolism of dietary galactose. The hydrogen atoms have been omitted for clarity.

A The inhibition of phosphoglucomutase by galactose 1-P results in hypoglycemia by interfering with both the formation of UDP-glucose (the glycogen precursor) and the degradation of glycogen back to glucose 6-P. Ninety percent of glycogen degradation leads to glucose 1-P, which can only be converted to glucose 6-P by phosphoglucomutase. When phosphoglucomutase activity is inhibited, less glucose 6-P production occurs, and hence, less glucose is available for export. Thus, the stored glycogen is only approximately 10% efficient in raising blood glucose levels, and hypoglycemia results. UDP-glucose levels are reduced because glucose 1-P is required to synthesize UDP-glucose, and in the absence of phosphoglucomutase activity, glucose 6-P (derived from either the glucokinase reaction or gluconeogenesis) cannot be converted to glucose 1-P. This prevents the formation of UDP-glucuronate, which is necessary to convert bilirubin to the diglucuronide form for transport into the bile. Bilirubin accumulates in tissues, giving them a yellow color (jaundice).

Q A pregnant woman who was extremely lactose intolerant asked her physician if she would still be able to breastfeed her infant even though she could not drink milk or dairy products. What advice should she be given?

2. Lactose Synthesis

Lactose is unique in that it is synthesized only in the mammary gland of the adult female for short periods during lactation. Lactose synthase, an enzyme present in the endoplasmic reticulum of the lactating mammary gland, catalyzes the last step in lactose biosynthesis, the transfer of galactose from UDP-galactose to glucose (see Fig. 27.13). Lactose synthase has two protein subunits, a galactosyltransferase and α-lactalbumin. α-Lactalbumin is a modifier protein synthesized after parturition (childbirth) in response to the hormone prolactin. This enzyme subunit lowers the K_m of the galactosyltransferase for glucose from 1,200 to 1 mM, thereby increasing the rate of lactose synthesis. In the absence of α-lactalbumin, galactosyltransferase transfers galactosyl units to glycoproteins.

E. Formation of Sugars for Glycolipid and Glycoprotein Synthesis

The transferases that produce the oligosaccharide and polysaccharide side chains of glycolipids and attach sugar residues to proteins are specific for the sugar moiety and for the donating nucleotide (e.g., UDP, CMP, or guanosine diphosphate [GDP]). Some of the sugar nucleotides used for *glycoprotein*, *proteoglycan* (see Chapter 47), and *glycolipid* formation are listed in Table 27.4. They include the derivatives of glucose and galactose that we have already discussed, as well as acetylated amino sugars and derivatives of mannose. The reason for the large variety of sugars attached to proteins and lipids is that they have relatively specific and different functions, such as targeting a protein toward a membrane; providing recognition sites on the cell surface for other cells, hormones, or viruses; or acting as lubricants or molecular sieves (see Chapter 47).

The pathways for use and formation of many of these sugars are summarized in Figure 27.15. Note that many of the steps are reversible so that glucose and other dietary sugars enter a common pool from which the diverse sugars can be formed.

The amino sugars are all derived from glucosamine 6-phosphate (glucosamine 6-P). To synthesize glucosamine 6-P an amino group is transferred from the amide of glutamine to fructose 6-P (Fig. 27.16). Amino sugars, such as glucosamine, can then be *N*-acetylated by an acetyltransferase. *N*-Acetyltransferases are present in the endoplasmic reticulum and cytosol and provide another means of chemically modifying sugars, metabolites, drugs, and xenobiotic compounds. Individuals may vary greatly in their capacity for acetylation reactions.

Mannose is found in the diet in small amounts. Like galactose, it is an epimer of glucose, and mannose and glucose are interconverted by epimerization reactions at carbon 2. The interconversion can take place either at the level of fructose 6-P to mannose 6-phosphate (mannose 6-P) or at the level of the derivatized sugars (see Fig. 27.15). *N*-Acetylmannosamine is the precursor of NANA (a sialic acid) and GDP-mannose is the precursor of GDP-fucose (see Fig. 27.15). The negative charge on NANA is obtained by the addition of a three-carbon carboxyl moiety from phosphoenolpyruvate.

TABLE 27.4 Examples of Sugar Nucleotides that are Precursors for Transferase Reactions	
UDP-glucose	
UDP-galactose	
UDP-glucuronic acid	
UDP-xylose	
UDP-*N*-acetylglucosamine	
UDP-*N*-acetylgalactosamine	
CMP-*N*-acetylneuraminic acid	
GDP-fucose	
GDP-mannose	

CMP, cytidine monophosphate; GDP, guanosine diphosphate; UDP, uridine diphosphate.

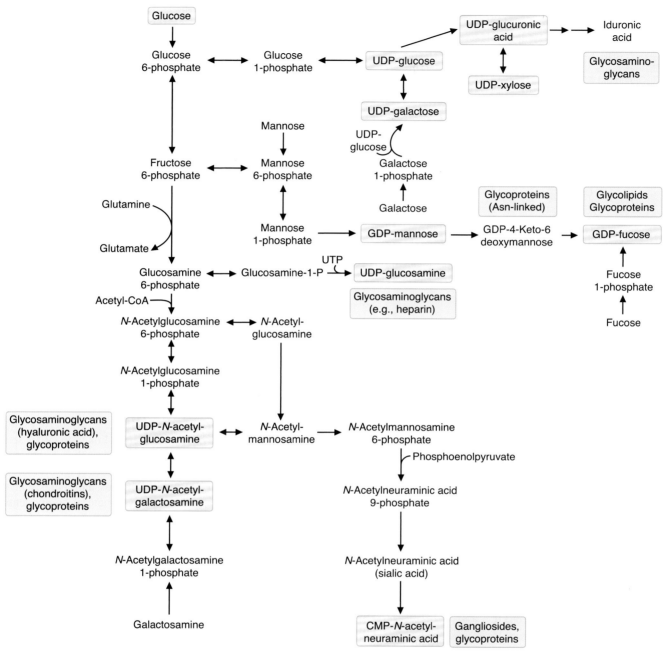

FIGURE 27.15 Pathways for the interconversion of sugars. All of the different sugars found in glycosaminoglycans, gangliosides, and other compounds in the body can be synthesized from glucose. Dietary glucose, fructose, galactose, mannose, and other sugars enter a common pool from which other sugars are derived. The activated sugar is transferred from the nucleotide sugar, shown in *yellow boxes*, to form a glycosidic bond with another sugar or amino acid residue. The *green box* next to each nucleotide sugar lists some of the compounds that contain the sugar. Iduronic acid, in the *upper right* corner of the diagram, is formed only after glucuronic acid is incorporated into a glycosaminoglycan (which is discussed in more detail in Chapter 47). *Acetyl-CoA*, acetyl coenzyme A; *CMP*, cytidine monophosphate; *GDP*, guanosine diphosphate; *UDP*, uridine diphosphate; *UTP*, uridine triphosphate.

Although the lactose in dairy products is a major source of galactose, the ingestion of lactose is not required for lactation. UDP-galactose in the mammary gland is derived principally from the epimerization of glucose. Dairy products are, however, a major dietary source of Ca^{2+}, so breastfeeding mothers need increased Ca^{2+} from another source.

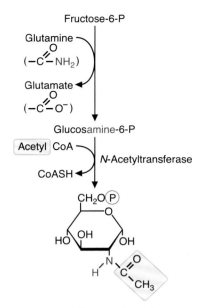

N-Acetylglucosamine-6-P

FIGURE 27.16 The formation of *N*-acetylglucosamine 6-phosphate (*N*-acetylglucosamine 6-P). The amino sugar is formed by a transfer of the amino group from the amide of glutamine to a carbon of the sugar. The amino group is acetylated by the transfer of an acetyl group from acetyl coenzyme A (acetyl CoA). The hydrogen atoms from the sugar have been omitted for clarity. *CoASH*, coenzyme A; *Fructose 6-P*, fructose 6-phosphate; *Glucosamine 6-P*, glucosamine 6-phosphate.

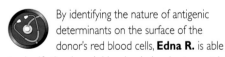 By identifying the nature of antigenic determinants on the surface of the donor's red blood cells, **Edna R.** is able to classify the donor's blood as belonging to certain specific blood groups. These antigenic determinants are located in the oligosaccharides of the glycoproteins and glycolipids of the cell membranes. The most important blood group in humans is the ABO group, which comprises two antigens, A and B. Individuals with the A antigen on their cells belong to blood group A. Those with B belong to group B, and those with both A and B belong to group AB. The absence of both the A and B antigens results in blood type O (see Fig. 27.23).

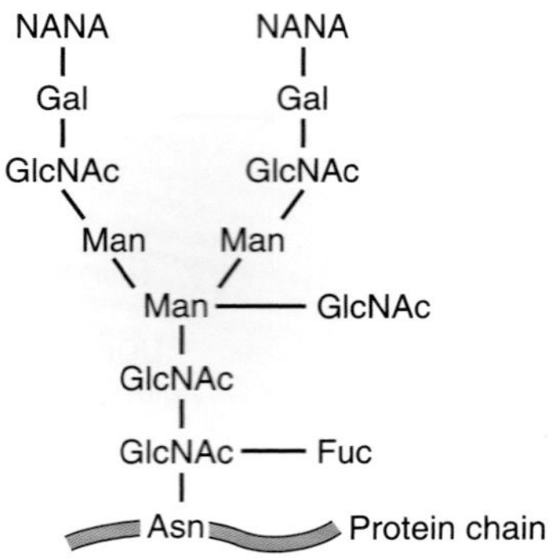

FIGURE 27.17 An example of a branched glycoprotein. *Fuc*, fucose; *Gal*, galactose; *GlcNAc*, N-acetylglucosamine; *Man*, mannose; *NANA*, N-acetylneuraminic acid.

Salivary mucin

-O- = Sialic acid
-O- = N-Acetylglucosamine

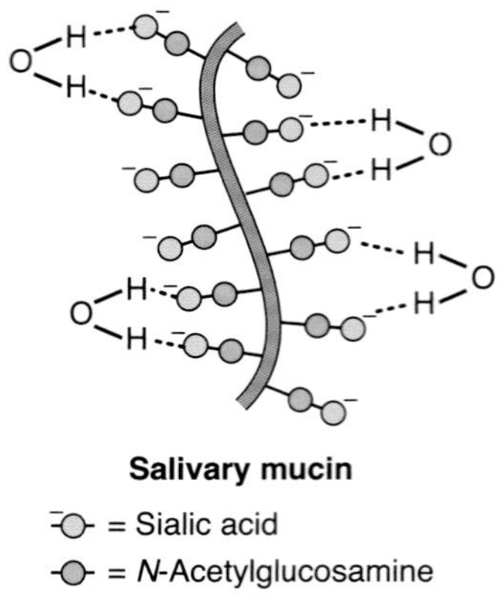

FIGURE 27.18 Structure of salivary mucin. The sugars form hydrogen bonds with water. Sialic acid provides a negatively charged carboxylate group. The protein is extremely large, and the negatively charged sialic acids extend the carbohydrate chains (by charge repulsion) so the molecules occupy a large space. All of the salivary glycoproteins contain O-linked sugars. N-Acetylneuraminic acid is a sialic acid.

III. Glycoproteins

A. Structure and Function

Glycoproteins contain short carbohydrate chains covalently linked to either serine/threonine or asparagine residues in the protein. These oligosaccharide chains are often branched and they do not contain repeating disaccharides (Fig. 27.17). Most proteins in the blood are glycoproteins. They serve as hormones, antibodies, enzymes (including those of the blood clotting cascade), and as structural components of the extracellular matrix. Collagen contains galactosyl units and disaccharides composed of galactosyl-glucose attached to hydroxylysine residues (see Chapter 47). The secretions of mucus-producing cells, such as salivary mucin, are glycoproteins (Fig. 27.18).

Although most glycoproteins are secreted from cells, some are segregated in lysosomes, where they serve as the lysosomal enzymes that degrade various types of cellular and extracellular material. Other glycoproteins are produced like secretory proteins, but hydrophobic regions of the protein remain attached to the cell membrane, and the carbohydrate portion extends into the extracellular space (also see Chapter 15, Section VIII). These glycoproteins serve as receptors for compounds such as hormones, as transport proteins, and as cell attachment and cell–cell recognition sites. Bacteria and viruses also bind to these sites.

B. Synthesis

The protein portion of glycoproteins is synthesized on ribosomes attached to the endoplasmic reticulum (ER). The carbohydrate chains are attached to the protein in the lumen of the ER and the Golgi complex. In some cases, the initial sugar is added to a serine or a threonine residue in the protein, and the carbohydrate chain is extended by the sequential addition of sugar residues to the nonreducing end. As seen in Table 27.4, UDP-sugars are the precursors for the addition of four of the seven sugars that are usually found in glycoproteins—glucose, galactose, *N*-acetylglucosamine, and *N*-acetylgalactosamine. GDP-sugars are the precursors for the addition of mannose and L-fucose, and CMP-NANA is the precursor for NANA. Dolichol phosphate (Fig. 27.19) (which is synthesized from isoprene

FIGURE 27.19 Structure of dolichol phosphate. In humans, the isoprene unit (in *brackets*) is repeated approximately 17 times ($n = \sim 17$).

$$O^- - \overset{\overset{O}{\|}}{P} - O - \overset{\overset{O}{\|}}{P} - O - CH_2 - CH_2 - \overset{\overset{H}{|}}{\underset{CH_3}{C}} - CH_2 - \left[CH_2 - CH = \overset{\overset{CH_3}{|}}{C} - CH_2 \right]_n - CH_2 - CH = \overset{\overset{CH_3}{|}}{C} - CH_3$$

units, as discussed in Chapter 32) is involved in transferring branched sugar chains to the amide nitrogen of asparagine residues. Sugars are removed and added as the glycoprotein moves from the ER through the Golgi complex (Fig. 27.20). As discussed in Chapter 10, the carbohydrate chain is used as a targeting marker for lysosomal enzymes.

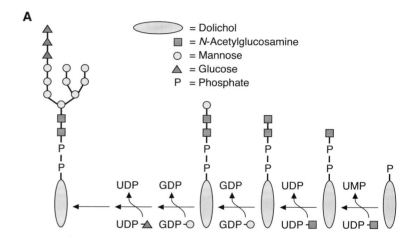

A

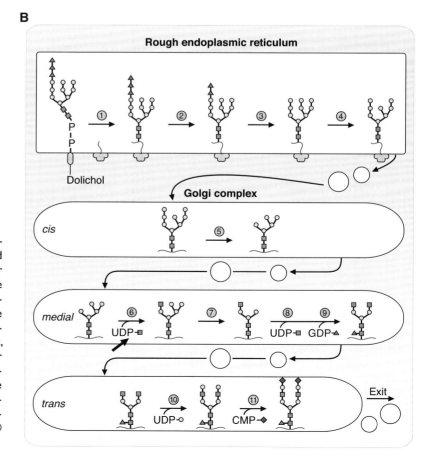

B

FIGURE 27.20 Action of dolichol phosphate in synthesizing the high-mannose form of oligosaccharides (**A**) and the processing of these carbohydrate groups (**B**). Transfer of the branched oligosaccharide from dolichol phosphate to a protein in the lumen of the rough endoplasmic reticulum (RER) *(step 1)* and processing of the oligosaccharide *(steps 2–11)*. Steps 1 through 4 occur in the RER. The glycoprotein is transferred in vesicles to the Golgi complex, where further modifications of the oligosaccharides occur *(steps 5–11)*. CMP, cytidine monophosphate; GDP, guanosine diphosphate; UDP, uridine diphosphate; UMP, uridine monophosphate. (**B** modified with permission from Kornfeld R, Kornfeld S. Assembly of asparagine-linked oligosaccharides. *Annu Rev Biochem.* 1985;54:631–664. Copyright © 1985 by Annual Reviews, Inc.)

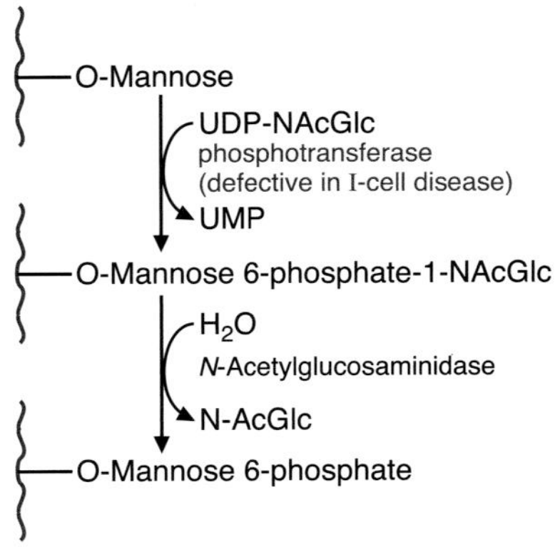

```
{———O-Mannose
{        ┌—UDP-NAcGlc
{        │   phosphotransferase
{        │   (defective in I-cell disease)
{        └↘UMP
{———O-Mannose 6-phosphate-1-NAcGlc
{        ┌—H₂O
{        │   N-Acetylglucosaminidase
{        └↘N-AcGlc
{———O-Mannose 6-phosphate
{
```

FIGURE 27.21 Synthesis of mannose 6-phosphate on the oligosaccharide of lysosomal proteins. The pathway for phosphorylating a mannose residue within the protein-attached oligosaccharide requires two steps. The first is a transfer of *N*-acetylglucosamine phosphate to the mannose residue, and the second is the release of *N*-acetylglucosamine from the intermediate product, leaving the phosphate behind on the mannose residue. *NAcGlc*, N-acetylglucosamine; *UDP*, uridine diphosphate; *UMP*, uridine monophosphate.

I-cell (inclusion cell) disease is a rare condition in which lysosomal enzymes lack the mannose phosphate marker that targets them to lysosomes. The enzyme that is deficient in I-cell disease is a phosphotransferase located in the Golgi apparatus (Fig. 27.21). The phosphotransferase has the unique ability to recognize lysosomal proteins because of their three-dimensional structure, such that they can all be appropriately tagged for transport to the lysosomes. Consequently, as a result of the lack of mannose phosphate, lysosomal enzymes are secreted from the cells. Because lysosomes lack their normal complement of enzymes, undegraded molecules accumulate within the nonfunctional lysosomes inside these cells, forming inclusion bodies.

IV. Glycolipids

A. Function and Structure

Glycolipids are derivatives of the lipid sphingosine. These *sphingolipids* include the *cerebrosides* and the *gangliosides* (Fig. 27.22; see also Chapter 5, Fig. 5.20). They contain ceramide, with carbohydrate moieties attached to its hydroxymethyl group.

Glycolipids are involved in intercellular communication. Oligosaccharides of identical composition are present in both the glycolipids and glycoproteins associated with the cell membrane, where they serve as cell recognition factors. For example, carbohydrate residues in these oligosaccharides are the antigens of the ABO blood group substances (Fig. 27.23).

B. Synthesis

Cerebrosides are synthesized from ceramide and UDP-glucose or UDP-galactose. They contain a single sugar (a monosaccharide). Gangliosides contain oligosaccharides produced from UDP-sugars and CMP-NANA, which is the precursor for

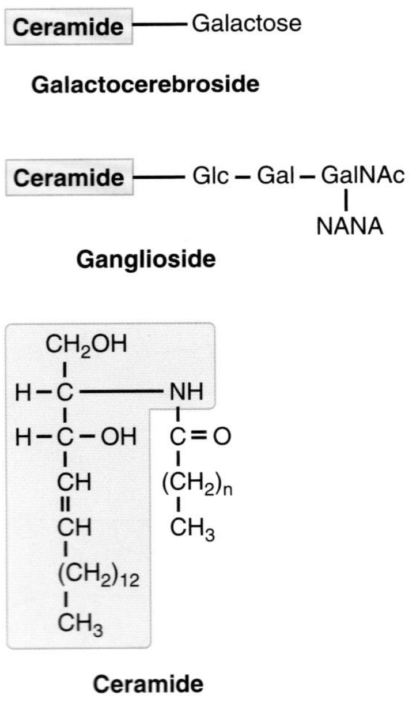

```
Ceramide ——— Galactose

        Galactocerebroside

Ceramide ——— Glc – Gal – GalNAc
                        |
                       NANA

        Ganglioside

┌─────────────────┐
│   CH₂OH         │
│    |            │
│ H–C———————NH    │
│    |       |    │
│ H–C–OH    C=O   │
│    |       |    │
│   CH      (CH₂)ₙ│
│   ‖        |    │
│   CH      CH₃   │
│    |            │
│  (CH₂)₁₂        │
│    |            │
│   CH₃           │
└─────────────────┘

        Ceramide
```

FIGURE 27.22 Structures of cerebrosides and gangliosides. In these glycolipids, sugars are attached to ceramide (shown *below* the glycolipids). The *boxed portion* of ceramide is sphingosine, from which the name "sphingolipids" is derived. *GalNAc*, N-acetylgalactosamine; *NANA*, N-acetylneuraminic acid.

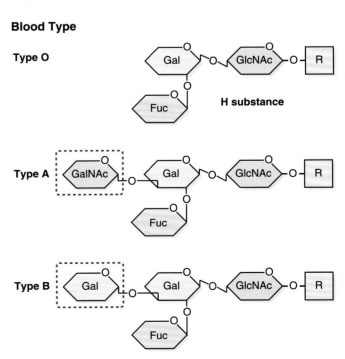

FIGURE 27.23 Structures of the blood group substances. Note that these structures are the same except that type A has *N*-acetylgalactosamine (GalNAc) at the nonreducing end, type B has galactose (Gal), and type O has neither. *R* is either a protein or the lipid ceramide. Each antigenic determinant is boxed. *Fuc*, fucose; *Gal*, galactose; *GlcNAc*, N-acetylglucosamine.

TABLE 27.5	Defective Enzymes in the Gangliosidoses	
DISEASE	**ENZYME DEFICIENCY**	**ACCUMULATED LIPID**[a]
Fucosidosis	α-Fucosidase	Cer-Glc-Gal-GalNAc-Gal:Fuc H-isoantigen
Generalized gangliosidosis	GM₁-β-galactosidase	Cer-Glc-Gal(NeuAc)-GalNAc:Gal GM₁ ganglioside
Tay-Sachs disease	Hexosaminidase A	Cer-Glc-Gal(NeuAc):GalNAc GM₂ ganglioside
Tay-Sachs variant or Sandhoff disease	Hexosaminidase A and B	Cer-Glc-Gal-Gal:GalNAc globoside plus GM₂ ganglioside
Fabry disease	α-Galactosidase	Cer-Glc-Gal:Gal globotriaosylceramide
Ceramide lactoside lipidosis	Ceramide lactosidase (β-galactosidase)	Cer-Glc:Gal ceramide lactoside
Metachromatic leukodystrophy	Arylsulfatase A	Cer-Gal:OSO₃³⁻ sulfogalactosylceramide
Krabbe disease	β-Galactosidase	Cer:Gal galactosylceramide
Gaucher disease	β-Glucosidase	Cer:Glc glucosylceramide
Niemann-Pick disease	Sphingomyelinase	Cer:P-choline sphingomyelin
Farber disease	Ceramidase	Acyl:sphingosine ceramide

Cer, ceramide; Fuc, fucose; Gal, galactose; Glc, glucose; NeuAc, N-acetylneuraminic acid; P-choline, phosphocholine.

[a]The colon indicates the bond that cannot be broken because of the enzyme deficiency associated with the disease.

the NANA residues that branch from the linear chain. The synthesis of the sphingolipids is described in more detail in Chapter 31. Defects in the degradation of sphingolipids lead to the sphingolipidoses (also known as the *gangliosidoses*), as outlined in Table 27.5.

Sphingolipids are produced in the Golgi complex. Their lipid component becomes part of the membrane of the secretory vesicle that buds from the *trans* face of the Golgi. After the vesicle membrane fuses with the cell membrane, the lipid component of the glycolipid remains in the outer layer of the cell membrane, and the carbohydrate component extends into the extracellular space. Sometimes, the carbohydrate component is used as a recognition signal for foreign proteins; for example, cholera toxin (which affected **Dennis V.**; see Chapter 10) binds to the carbohydrate portion of the GM₁-ganglioside to allow its catalytic subunit to enter the cell.

 The blood group substances are oligosaccharide components of glycolipids and glycoproteins found in most cell membranes. Those located on red blood cells have been studied extensively. A single genetic locus with two alleles determines an individual's blood type. These genes encode glycosyltransferases involved in the synthesis of the oligosaccharides of the blood group substances.

Most individuals can synthesize the H substance, an oligosaccharide that contains a fucose linked to a galactose at the nonreducing end of the blood group substance (see Fig. 27.23). Type A individuals produce an N-acetylgalactosamine transferase (encoded by the A gene) that attaches N-acetylgalactosamine to the galactose residue of the H substance. Type B individuals produce a galactosyltransferase (encoded by the B gene) that links galactose to the galactose residue of the H substance. Type AB individuals have both alleles and produce both transferases. Thus, some of the oligosaccharides of their blood group substances contain N-acetylgalactosamine and some contain galactose. Type O individuals produce a defective transferase, and, therefore, they do not attach either N-acetylgalactosamine or galactose to the H substance. Thus, individuals of blood type O have only the H substance.

CLINICAL COMMENTS

 Al M. Al M.'s pus culture, sent on the second day of his admission for fever from a cut on his arm, grew out *S. aureus*. This organism can be resistant to a variety of antibiotics, so TMP/sulfa treatment was initiated. Unfortunately, it appeared that Mr. M. had suffered an acute hemolysis (lysis or destruction of some of his red blood cells), probably induced by exposure to the sulfa drug and his infection with *S. aureus*. The hemoglobin that escaped from the lysed red blood cells was filtered by his kidneys and appeared in his urine.

By mechanisms that are not fully delineated, certain drugs (such as sulfa drugs and antimalarials), a variety of infectious agents, and exposure to fava beans can cause red blood cell destruction in individuals with a genetic deficiency of glucose 6-P dehydrogenase. Presumably, these patients cannot generate enough reduced NADPH to defend against the ROS. Although erythrocytes lack most of the other enzymatic sources of NADPH for the glutathione antioxidant system, they do have the defense mechanisms provided by the antioxidant vitamins E and C and catalase. Thus, individuals who are not totally deficient in glucose 6-P dehydrogenase remain asymptomatic unless an additional oxidative stress, such as an infection, generates additional oxygen radicals.

Some drugs, such as the antimalarial primaquine and the sulfonamide that Mr. M. is taking, affect the ability of red blood cells to defend against oxidative stress. Fava beans, which look like fat string beans and are sometimes called *broad beans*, contain the purine glycosides vicine and isouramil. These compounds react with glutathione. It has been suggested that cellular levels of reduced glutathione (GSH) decrease to such an extent that critical sulfhydryl groups in some key proteins cannot be maintained in reduced form.

The highest prevalence rates for glucose 6-P dehydrogenase deficiency are found in tropical Africa and Asia, in some areas of the Middle East and the Mediterranean, and in Papua New Guinea. The geographic distribution of this deficiency is similar to that of sickle cell trait and is probably also related to the relative resistance it confers against the malaria parasite.

Because individuals with this deficiency are asymptomatic unless they are exposed to an "oxidant challenge," the clinical course of the hemolytic anemia is usually self-limited if the causative agent is removed. However, genetic polymorphism accounts for a substantial variability in the severity of the disease. Severely affected patients may have a chronic hemolytic anemia and other sequelae even without known exposure to drugs, infection, and other causative factors. In such patients, neonatal jaundice is also common and can be severe enough to cause death.

Al M.'s antibiotic was changed and his infection, and symptoms caused by the lack of glucose 6-P dehydrogenase deficiency, abated.

 Edna R. During her stint in the hospital blood bank, **Edna R.** learned that the importance of the ABO blood group system in transfusion therapy is based on two principles (Table 27.6): (1) Antibodies to A and to B antigens occur naturally in the blood serum of people whose red blood cell surfaces lack the corresponding antigen (i.e., individuals with A antigens on their red blood cells have B antibodies in their serum, and vice versa). These antibodies may arise as a result of previous exposure to cross-reacting antigens in bacteria and foods or to blood transfusions. (2) Antibodies to A and B are usually present in high titers and are capable of activating the entire complement system. As a result, these antibodies may cause intravascular destruction of a large number of incompatible red blood cells given inadvertently during a blood transfusion. Individuals with type AB blood have both A and B antigens and do not produce antibodies to either. Hence, they are "universal" recipients. They can safely receive red blood cells from individuals of A, B, AB, or O blood type. (However, they cannot safely receive serum from these individuals, because it contains antibodies to A or B antigens.) Those with type O blood do not have either antigen. They are "universal" donors; that is, their red cells can safely be infused into type A, B, O, or AB individuals. (However, their serum contains antibodies to both A and B antigens and cannot be given safely to recipients with those antigens.)

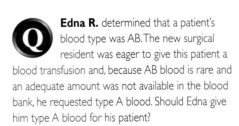 **Edna R.** determined that a patient's blood type was AB. The new surgical resident was eager to give this patient a blood transfusion and, because AB blood is rare and an adequate amount was not available in the blood bank, he requested type A blood. Should Edna give him type A blood for his patient?

TABLE 27.6	Characteristics of the ABO Blood Groups			
RED CELL TYPE	**O**	**A**	**B**	**AB**
Possible genotypes	OO	AA or AO	BB or BO	AB
Antibodies in serum	Anti-A and B	Anti-B	Anti-A	None
Frequency (in whites)	45%	40%	10%	5%
Can accept blood types	O	A, O	B, O	A, B, AB, O

The second important red blood cell group is the Rh group. It is important because one of its antigenic determinants, the D antigen, is a very potent immunogen, stimulating the production of a large number of antibodies. The unique carbohydrate composition of the glycoproteins that constitute the antigenic determinants on red blood cells in part contributes to the relative immunogenicity of the A, B, and Rh(D) red blood cell groups in human blood.

 Jay S. Tay-Sachs disease, the problem afflicting **Jay S.**, is an autosomal-recessive disorder that is rare in the general population (1 in 300,000 births), but its prevalence in Jews of Eastern European (Ashkenazi) extraction (who make up 90% of the Jewish population in the United States) is much higher (1 in 3,600 births). One in 28 Ashkenazi Jews carries this defective gene. Its presence can be discovered by measuring the serum hexosaminidase A enzymatic activity or by recombinant DNA techniques.

Carriers of the affected gene have a reduced but functional level of this enzyme that normally hydrolyzes a specific bond between an N-acetyl-D-galactosamine and a D-galactose residue in the polar head of the ganglioside.

No effective therapy is available. Enzyme replacement has met with little success because of the difficulties in getting the enzyme across the blood–brain barrier.

Tay-Sachs disease, which is one of the gangliosidoses, is a multifaceted disorder. The sphingolipidoses, which include Fabry and Gaucher diseases, affect mainly the brain, the skin, and the reticuloendothelial system (e.g., liver and spleen). In these diseases, complex lipids accumulate. Each of these lipids contains a ceramide as part of its structure (see Table 27.5). The rate at which the lipid is synthesized is normal. However, the lysosomal enzyme required to degrade it is not very active, either because it is made in deficient quantities as a result of a mutation in a gene that specifically codes for the enzyme or because a critical protein required to activate the enzyme is deficient. Because the lipid cannot be degraded, it accumulates and causes degeneration of the affected tissues, with progressive malfunction, such as the psychomotor deficits that occur as a result of the central nervous system involvement seen in most of these storage diseases.

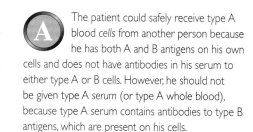 The patient could safely receive type A blood *cells* from another person because he has both A and B antigens on his own cells and does not have antibodies in his serum to either type A or B cells. However, he should not be given type A *serum* (or type A whole blood), because type A serum contains antibodies to type B antigens, which are present on his cells.

BIOCHEMICAL COMMENTS

Biochemistry of Tay-Sachs Disease. Hexosaminidase A, the defective enzyme in Tay-Sachs disease, is actually composed of two subunits, an α- and a β-chain. The stoichiometry is currently considered to be αβ (a dimer). The α-subunit is coded for by the *HexA* gene, whereas the β-subunit is coded for by the *HexB* gene. In Tay-Sachs disease, the α-subunit is defective, and hexosaminidase A activity is lost. However, the β-subunit can form active dimers in the absence of the α-subunit, and this activity, named hexosaminidase B, which cleaves the glycolipid globoside, retains activity in children with Tay-Sachs disease. Thus, children with Tay-Sachs disease accumulate the ganglioside GM$_2$ but not globoside (Fig. 27.24).

Mutation of the *HexB* gene, and production of a defective β-subunit, leads to inactivation of both hexosaminidase A and B activity. Such a mutation leads to Sandhoff disease. Both activities are lost because both activities require a functional β-subunit. The clinical course of this disease is similar to Tay-Sachs but with an accelerated timetable because of the initial accumulation of both GM$_2$ and globoside in the lysosomes.

A third type of mutation also can lead to disease symptoms similar to those of Tay-Sachs disease. Children were identified with Tay-Sachs symptoms, but when both hexosaminidase A and B activities were measured in a test tube, they were normal. This disease, ultimately named Sandhoff activator disease, is caused by a mutation in a protein that is needed to activate hexosaminidase A activity. In the absence of the activator, hexosaminidase A activity is minimal, and GM$_2$ initially accumulates in lysosomes. This mutation has no effect on hexosaminidase B activity.

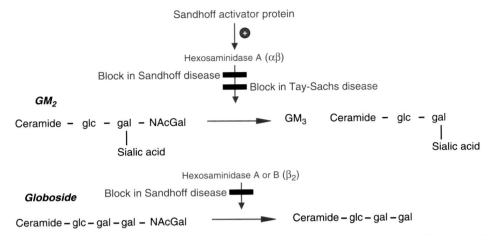

FIGURE 27.24 Substrate specificities of hexosaminidase A, B, and the function of the activator protein. Defects in the β-subunit inactivate both HexA and HexB activities, leading to GM$_2$ and globoside accumulation. A defect in Sandhoff activator protein also leads to GM$_2$ accumulation, as HexA activity is reduced. Defects in the α-subunit inactivate only HexA activity, such that HexB activity toward globoside is unaffected. *Gal*, galactose; *Glc*, glucose; *NAcGal*, N-acetylgalactosamine.

When a glycolipid cannot be degraded because of an enzymatic mutation, it accumulates in residual bodies (vacuoles that contain material that lysosomal enzymes cannot digest). Normal cells contain a small number of residual bodies, but in diseases of lysosomal enzymes, large numbers of residual bodies accumulate within the cell, eventually interfering with normal cell function.

In 70% of the cases of Tay-Sachs disease in people of Ashkenazi Jewish background, exon 11 of the gene for the α-chain of hexosaminidase A contains a mutation. The normal gene sequence encodes a protein with the amino acids Arg-Ile-Ser-Tyr-Gly-Pro-Asp in this region, as shown here:

$$5' - \text{CGTATATCCTATGGCCCTGAC}$$
Arg – Ile – Ser – Tyr – Gly – Pro – Asp

The mutant DNA sequence for this area is

$$5' - \text{CGTATATC}\underline{\text{TATC}}\text{CTATGGCCCTGAC}$$
Arg – Ile – Ser – Ile – Leu – Trp – Pro – Stop

A four-base insertion (*underlined*) occurs in the mutated gene, which alters the reading frame of the protein and also introduces a premature stop codon farther down the protein, so no functional α-subunit can be produced.

KEY CONCEPTS

- The pentose phosphate pathway consists of both oxidative and nonoxidative reactions.
- The oxidative steps of the pentose phosphate pathway generate reduced nicotinamide adenine dinucleotide phosphate (NADPH) and ribulose 5-phosphate from glucose 6-phosphate.
  - Ribulose 5-phosphate is converted to ribose 5-phosphate for nucleotide biosynthesis.
  - NADPH is used as reducing power for biosynthetic pathways.
- The nonoxidative steps of the pentose phosphate pathway reversibly convert five-carbon sugars to fructose 6-phosphate and glyceraldehyde 3-phosphate.

- The needs of the cell dictate whether the cell will use the oxidative reactions of the pentose phosphate pathway, the non-oxidative reactions, or both sets of reactions.
- Reactions between sugars or the formation of sugar derivatives use sugars activated by attachment to nucleotides (a nucleotide sugar).
- Uridine diphosphate (UDP)-glucose and UDP-galactose are substrates for many glycosyltransferase reactions.
- Lactose is formed from UDP-galactose and glucose.
- UDP-glucose is oxidized to UDP-glucuronate, which forms glucuronide derivatives of various hydrophobic compounds, making them more readily excreted in urine or bile than the parent compound.
- Glycoproteins and glycolipids contain various types of carbohydrate residues.
- The carbohydrates in glycoproteins can be either *O*-linked or *N*-linked and are synthesized in the endoplasmic reticulum and the Golgi apparatus.
- For *O*-linked carbohydrates, the carbohydrates are added sequentially (via nucleotide sugar precursors), beginning with a sugar linked to the hydroxyl group of the amino acid side chains of serine or threonine.
- For *N*-linked carbohydrates, the branched carbohydrate chain is first synthesized on dolichol phosphate and then transferred to the amide nitrogen of an asparagine residue of the protein.
- Glycolipids belong to the class of sphingolipids that add carbohydrate groups to the base ceramide one at a time from nucleotide sugars.
- Defects in the degradation of glycosphingolipids leads to a class of lysosomal diseases known as the *sphingolipidoses*.
- Table 27.7 summarizes the diseases discussed in this chapter.

TABLE 27.7   Diseases Discussed in Chapter 27

DISEASE OR DISORDER	ENVIRONMENTAL OR GENETIC	COMMENTS
Blood transfusions	Environmental/genetic	Blood typing is dependent on antigens on the cell surface, particularly the carbohydrate content of the antigen.
Tay-Sachs disease	Genetic	Lack of hexosaminidase A activity, leading to an accumulation of GM_2 ganglioside in the lysosomes
Jaundice	Both	Lack of ability to conjugate bilirubin with glucuronic acid in the liver
Sphingolipidoses	Genetic	Defects in ganglioside and sphingolipid degradation, as summarized in Table 27.5
Glucose 6-phosphate dehydrogenase deficiency	Genetic, X-linked	Lack of glucose 6-phosphate dehydrogenase activity leads to hemolytic anemia in the presence of strong oxidizing agents.

REVIEW QUESTIONS—CHAPTER 27

1. Which one of the following best describes a mother with galactosemia caused by a deficiency of galactose 1-P uridylyltransferase?
   A. She can convert galactose to UDP-galactose for lactose synthesis during lactation.
   B. She can form galactose 1-P from galactose.
   C. She can use galactose as a precursor to glucose production.
   D. She can use galactose to produce glycogen.
   E. She will have lower-than-normal levels of serum galactose after drinking milk.

2. The immediate carbohydrate precursors for glycolipid and glycoprotein synthesis are which of the following?
   A. Sugar phosphates
   B. Sugar acids
   C. Sugar alcohols

D. Nucleotide sugars

E. Acyl-sugars

3. A newborn is diagnosed with neonatal jaundice. In this patient, the bilirubin produced lacks which one of the following carbohydrates?

A. Glucose

B. Gluconate

C. Glucuronate

D. Galactose

E. Galactitol

4. The nitrogen donor for the formation of amino sugars is which one of the following?

A. Ammonia

B. Asparagine

C. Glutamine

D. Adenine

E. Dolichol

5. Which one of the following glycolipids would accumulate in a patient with Sandhoff disease?

A. GM_1

B. Lactosyl-ceramide

C. Globoside

D. Glucocerebroside

E. GM_3

6. A defect in which one of the following enzymes would severely affect an individual's ability to specifically metabolize galactose?

A. UDP-glucose pyrophosphorylase

B. Hexokinase

C. Glucose 6-P dehydrogenase

D. Triose kinase

E. Pyruvate carboxylase

7. A woman, shortly after giving birth to her first child, was discovered to be unable to synthesize lactose. Analysis of various glycoproteins in her serum indicated that there was no defect in the carbohydrate chains, nor was the carbohydrate content of her cell-surface glycolipids altered. This woman may have a mutation in which one of the following enzymes or class of enzymes?

A. A glucosyltransferase

B. A galactosyltransferase

C. Lactase

D. α-Lactalbumin

E. A lactosyltransferase

8. A 27-year-old man of Mediterranean descent developed hemolytic anemia after being prescribed a drug that is a potent oxidizing agent. The anemia results from which one of the following?

A. A lowered concentration of oxidized glutathione

B. A lowered concentration of reduced glutathione

C. Increased production of NADPH

D. A reduction of hydrogen peroxide levels

E. An increase in the production of glucose 6-P

9. A patient's blood is being typed by exposing it to either type A or type B antibodies. Which result would be expected if the patient had type AB blood?

A. No reaction to A antibodies

B. No reaction to B antibodies

C. No reaction to either A or B antibodies

D. Reaction to both A and B antibodies

E. A reaction to A antibodies but not to B antibodies

10. Inherited defects in the pentose phosphate shunt pathway could lead to which one of the following?

A. Ineffective oxidative phosphorylation caused by dysfunctional mitochondria

B. An inability to carry out reductive detoxification

C. An inability to produce fructose 6-P and glyceraldehyde 3-P for five-carbon sugar biosynthesis

D. An inability to generate NADH for biosynthetic reactions

E. An inability to generate NADH to protect cells from ROS

ANSWERS

1. **The answer is B.** Galactose metabolism requires the phosphorylation of galactose to galactose 1-P, which is then converted to UDP-galactose (which is the step that is defective in the patient), and then epimerized to UDP-glucose. Although the mother cannot convert galactose to lactose because of the enzyme deficiency, she can make UDP-glucose from glucose 6-P, and once she has made UDP-glucose, she can epimerize it to form UDP-galactose and can synthesize lactose (thus, A is incorrect). However, because of her enzyme deficiency, the mother cannot convert galactose 1-P to UDP-galactose or UDP-glucose, so the dietary galactose cannot be used for glycogen synthesis or glucose production (thus, C and D are incorrect). After ingesting milk, the galactose levels will be elevated in the serum because of the metabolic block in the cells (thus, E is incorrect).

2. **The answer is D.** Nucleotide sugars, such as UDP-glucose, UDP-galactose, and CMP-sialic acid, donate sugars to the growing carbohydrate chain. The other activated sugars listed do not contribute to glycolipid or glycoprotein synthesis.

3. **The answer is C.** Bilirubin is conjugated with glucuronic acid residues to enhance its solubility. Glucuronic acid is glucose oxidized at position 6; gluconic acid is glucose oxidized at position 1 and is generated by the HMP shunt pathway. The activated form of glucuronic acid is UDP-glucuronate.

4. **The answer is C.** Glutamine donates the amide nitrogen to fructose 6-P to form glucosamine 6-P. None of

the other nitrogen-containing compounds (A, B, and D) donate their nitrogen to carbohydrates. Dolichol contains no nitrogens and is the carrier for carbohydrate chain synthesis of *N*-linked glycoproteins.

5. **The answer is C.** Sandhoff disease is a deficiency of both hexosaminidase A and B activity, resulting from loss of activity of the β-subunit in both of these enzymes. The degradative step at which amino sugars need to be removed from the glycolipids would be defective, such that globoside and GM_2 accumulate in this disease. The other answers are incorrect; GM_1 does contain an amino sugar, but it is converted to GM_2 before the block in Sandhoff disease is apparent.

6. **The answer is A.** Galactose is phosphorylated by galactokinase and the galactose 1-P formed reacts with UDP-glucose to form glucose 1-P and UDP-galactose. The enzyme that catalyzes this reaction is galactose 1-P uridylyltransferase. UDP-glucose is absolutely required for further galactose metabolism. UDP-glucose is formed from UTP and glucose 1-P by the enzyme UDP-glucose pyrophosphorylase, so a deficiency in this enzyme would lead to reduced galactose metabolism, caused by a lack of UDP-glucose. Galactose is phosphorylated by galactokinase, not by hexokinase. Glucose 6-P dehydrogenase is not required for galactose metabolism; it converts glucose 6-P to 6-phosphogluconate in the first step of the HMP shunt pathway. Triose kinase is also not required for galactose metabolism because this enzyme converts glyceraldehyde to glyceraldehyde 3-P. Pyruvate carboxylase is also not required for galactose metabolism, because it converts pyruvate to oxaloacetate.

7. **The answer is D.** Lactose synthase is composed of two subunits, a galactosyltransferase and α-lactalbumin. In the absence of α-lactalbumin, the galactosyltransferase is active in glycoprotein and glycolipid synthesis but is relatively inactive for lactose synthesis. At birth, α-lactalbumin is induced and alters the specificity of the galactosyltransferase such that lactose can now be synthesized. Because glycoprotein and glycolipid synthesis was normal, the mutation could not be in the galactosyltransferase subunit. Lactase is the enzyme that digests lactose in the intestine, and a lactosyltransferase enzyme, if such an enzyme did exist, would not answer the question, because it would require lactose as a sub-

strate. A glucosyltransferase is not required for lactose synthesis (lactose synthase is).

8. **The answer is B.** The patient has glucose 6-P dehydrogenase deficiency and cannot generate NADPH from glucose 6-P. In the red blood cells, which lack mitochondria, this is the only pathway through which NADPH can be generated. In the absence of NADPH, the molecule which protects against oxidative damage (glutathione) is oxidized preferentially to protect membrane lipids and proteins. There is only limited glutathione in the membrane, so once it is oxidized, it needs to be converted back to reduced glutathione (the protective form). The enzyme that does this, glutathione reductase, requires NADPH to supply the electrons to reduce the oxidized glutathione. In the absence of NADPH, the glutathione cannot be reduced, and the protection offered by reduced glutathione is eliminated, leading to membrane damage and cell lysis. Because the life of a red cell is so short (120 days in circulation), there is usually sufficient glutathione to protect the cell in the absence of an exogenous oxidizing agent. However, once such an agent is present (such as a drug), the red cells are easily lysed, leading to the anemia. The hemolytic anemia is not caused by a lowering of hydrogen peroxide levels nor by an increase in the production of glucose 6-P.

9. **The answer is D.** A person with type AB blood would carry both the A and B antigens, so the blood cells would bind to antibodies directed against either the type A antigen or the type B antigen. Type O blood, which does not express either the type A or type B antigens, would not react with either antibody. Type A blood would react to antibodies to antigen A but not to antigen B. Type B blood would react to antibodies to antigen B but not to antibodies directed against antigen A.

10. **The answer is B.** The pentose phosphate pathway is operative in the cytosol of all cells because all cells require NADPH for reductive detoxification. NADPH is also used for fatty-acid synthesis and detoxification of medications. NADPH does not donate electrons to complex I of the electron-transfer chain, so oxidative phosphorylation would not be impaired. Fructose 6-P and glyceraldehyde 3-P can be generated via glycolysis; the pentose phosphate pathway is not required for their synthesis. NADPH is used for both biosynthetic reactions and to protect cells from ROS, not NADH (which is generated via glycolysis).

28 Gluconeogenesis and Maintenance of Blood Glucose Levels

During fasting, many of the reactions of glycolysis are reversed as the liver produces glucose to maintain blood glucose levels. This process of **glucose production** is called **gluconeogenesis**.

Gluconeogenesis, which occurs primarily in the liver, is the pathway for the synthesis of glucose from compounds other than carbohydrates. In humans, the major precursors of glucose are **lactate**, **glycerol**, and **amino acids**, particularly **alanine**. Except for three key sequences, the reactions of gluconeogenesis are reversals of the steps of glycolysis (Fig. 28.1). The sequences of gluconeogenesis that do not use enzymes of glycolysis involve the irreversible, regulated steps of glycolysis. These three sequences are the conversion of (1) pyruvate to phosphoenolpyruvate (PEP), (2) fructose 1,6-bisphosphate to fructose 6-phosphate, and (3) glucose 6-phosphate to glucose.

Some tissues of the body, such as the brain and red blood cells, cannot synthesize glucose on their own but depend on glucose for energy. On a long-term basis, most tissues also require glucose for other functions, such as synthesis of the ribose moiety of nucleotides or the carbohydrate portion of glycoproteins and glycolipids. Therefore, to survive, humans must have mechanisms for maintaining blood glucose levels.

After a meal containing carbohydrates, blood glucose levels rise (Fig. 28.2). Some of the glucose from the diet is stored in the liver as **glycogen**. After 2 or 3 hours of fasting, this glycogen begins to be degraded by the process of **glycogenolysis**, and glucose is released into the blood. As glycogen stores decrease, **adipose triacylglycerols** are also degraded, providing **fatty acids** as an alternative fuel and glycerol for the synthesis of glucose by gluconeogenesis. Amino acids are also released from the muscle to serve as gluconeogenic precursors.

During an overnight fast, blood glucose levels are maintained by both glycogenolysis and gluconeogenesis. However, after approximately 30 hours of fasting, liver glycogen stores are mostly depleted. Subsequently, gluconeogenesis is the only source of blood glucose.

Changes in the metabolism of glucose that occur during the switch from the fed to the fasting state are regulated by the hormones **insulin** and **glucagon**. Insulin is elevated in the fed state, and glucagon is elevated during fasting. Insulin stimulates the **transport** of glucose into certain cells such as those in muscle and adipose tissue. Insulin also alters the activity of key enzymes that regulate metabolism, stimulating the storage of fuels. Glucagon counters the effects of insulin, stimulating the release of stored fuels and the conversion of lactate, amino acids, and glycerol to glucose.

Blood glucose levels are maintained not only during fasting but also during exercise, when muscle cells take up glucose from the blood and oxidize it for energy. During exercise, the liver supplies glucose to the blood by the processes of glycogenolysis and gluconeogenesis.

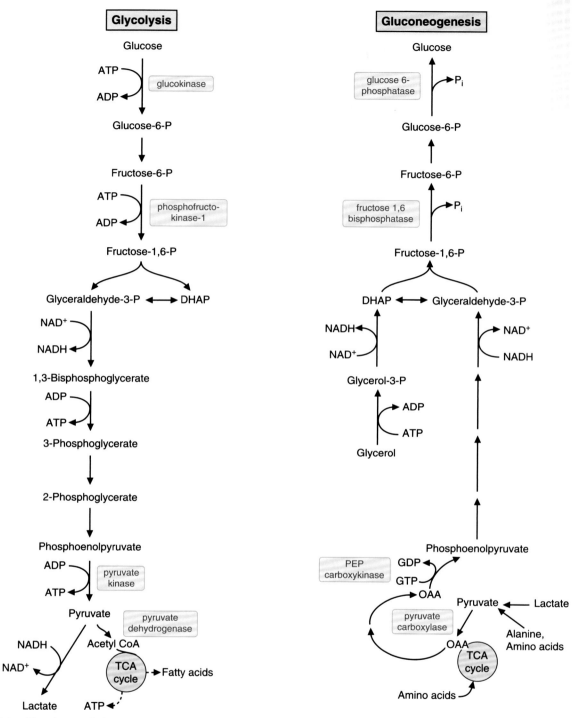

FIGURE 28.1   Glycolysis and gluconeogenesis in the liver. The gluconeogenic pathway is almost the reverse of the glycolytic pathway, except for three reaction sequences. At these three steps, the reactions are catalyzed by different enzymes. The energy requirements of these reactions differ, and one pathway can be activated while the other is inhibited. The steps for which enzyme names are indicated are the irreversible steps of those pathways. All other steps are reversible, although for clarity this is not indicated in the figure. *Acetyl CoA*, acetyl coenzyme A; *ADP*, adenosine diphosphate; *ATP*, adenosine triphosphate; *DHAP*, dihydroxyacetone phosphate; *Fructose-1,6-P*, fructose 1,6-bisphosphate; *Fructose-6-P*, fructose 6-phosphate; *GDP*, guanosine diphosphate; *Glucose-6-P*, glucose 6-phosphate; *Glyceraldehyde-3-P*, glyceraldehyde 3-phosphate; *Glycerol-3-P*, glycerol 3-phosphate; *GTP*, guanosine triphosphate; *NAD*, nicotinamide adenine dinucleotide; *OAA*, oxaloacetate; *PEP*, phosphoenolpyruvate; *P$_i$*, inorganic phosphate; *TCA*, tricarboxylic acid.

Fed

Dietary carbohydrate

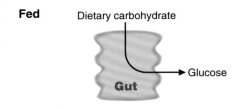

Glucose

Gut

Fasting

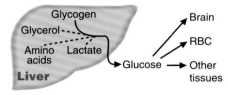

Glycogen → Brain

Glycerol

Amino acids — Lactate → RBC

Liver → Glucose → Other tissues

Starved

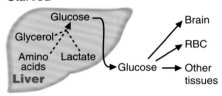

Glucose → Brain

Glycerol

Amino acids — Lactate → RBC

Liver → Glucose → Other tissues

FIGURE 28.2 Sources of blood glucose in the fed, fasting, and starved states. *RBC*, red blood cells.

 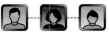
 Al M., a known alcoholic, was brought to the emergency department by his landlady, who stated that he had been drinking heavily for the past week. During this time, his appetite had gradually diminished, and he had not eaten any food for the past 3 days. He was confused, combative, tremulous, and sweating profusely. His speech was slurred. His heart rate was rapid (110 beats/minute). As his blood pressure was being determined, he had a grand mal seizure. His blood glucose, drawn just before the onset of the seizure, was 28 mg/dL or 1.6 mM (reference range for overnight fasting blood glucose, 80 to 100 mg/dL or 4.4 to 5.6 mM). His blood ethanol level drawn at the same time was 295 mg/dL (intoxication level, i.e., "confused" stage, 150 to 300 mg/dL).

 Emma W. presented to the emergency department 3 days after being discharged from the hospital following a 7-day admission for a severe asthma exacerbation. She was intubated and required high-dose intravenous *methylprednisolone* (a synthetic anti-inflammatory glucocorticoid) for the first 4 days of her stay. After 3 additional days on oral prednisone, she was discharged on substantial pharmacologic doses of this steroid and instructed to return to her physician's office in 5 days. She presented now with marked *polyuria* (increased urination), *polydipsia* (increased thirst), and muscle weakness. Her blood glucose was 275 mg/dL or 15 mM (reference range, 80 to 100 mg/dL or 4.4 to 5.6 mM).

 Dianne A. took her morning insulin but then didn't feel well, so she did not eat and took a nap. When her friend came over later, she was unresponsive. The friend called an ambulance, and Dianne was rushed to the hospital emergency department in a coma. Her pulse and blood pressure at admission were normal. Her skin was flushed and slightly moist. Her respirations were slightly slow.

 Ann R. continues to resist efforts on the part of her psychiatrist and family physician to convince her to increase her caloric intake. Her body weight varies between 97 and 99 lb, far below the desirable weight for a woman who is 5 ft 7 in tall. In spite of her severe diet, her fasting blood glucose levels range from 55 to 70 mg/dL. She denies having any hypoglycemic symptoms.

 Otto S. has complied with his calorie-restricted diet and aerobic exercise program. He has lost another 7 lb and is closing in on his goal of weighing 154 lb. He notes increasing energy during the day, and he remains alert during lectures and assimilates the lecture material noticeably better than he did before starting his weight-loss and exercise program. He jogs for 45 minutes each morning before breakfast.

I. Glucose Metabolism in the Liver

Glucose serves as a fuel for most tissues of the body. It is the major fuel for certain tissues such as the brain and red blood cells. After a meal, food is the source of blood glucose. The liver oxidizes glucose and stores the excess as glycogen. The liver also uses the pathway of glycolysis to convert glucose to pyruvate, which provides carbon for the synthesis of fatty acids. Glycerol 3-phosphate, produced from glycolytic intermediates, combines with fatty acids to form triacylglycerols, which are secreted into the blood in very-low-density lipoprotein (VLDL; explained further in Chapter 31). During fasting, the liver releases glucose into the blood, so that glucose-dependent tissues do not suffer from a lack of energy. Two mechanisms are involved in this process: glycogenolysis and gluconeogenesis.

Hormones, particularly insulin and glucagon, dictate whether glucose flows through glycolysis or whether the reactions are reversed and glucose is produced via gluconeogenesis.

II. Gluconeogenesis

Gluconeogenesis, the process by which glucose is synthesized from noncarbohydrate precursors, occurs mainly in the liver under fasting conditions. Under the more extreme conditions of starvation, the kidney cortex also may produce glucose. For the most part, the glucose produced by the kidney cortex is used by the kidney medulla, but some may enter the bloodstream.

Starting with pyruvate, most of the steps of gluconeogenesis are simply reversals of those of glycolysis (Fig. 28.3). In fact, these pathways differ at only three points. Enzymes involved in catalyzing these steps are regulated so that either glycolysis or gluconeogenesis predominates, depending on physiologic conditions.

 The measurement of ketones (acetoacetate and β-hydroxybutyrate; see Chapter 3) in the blood and urine can indicate the level of starvation or the presence of diabetic ketoacidosis (DKA). There are several methods to detect ketones. One is the use of reagent strips for urine (based on the reaction of sodium nitroprusside with acetoacetate), but this method does not detect the major blood ketone (β-hydroxybutyrate). A cyclic enzymatic method has been developed to overcome this, in which blood or plasma samples are incubated with acetoacetate decarboxylase, which removes all acetoacetate from the sample (converting it to acetone and carbon dioxide). Once this has been accomplished, β-hydroxybutyrate dehydrogenase is then incubated with the sample, along with thionicotinamide adenine dinucleotide (thio-NAD$^+$). The thio-NAD$^+$ is converted to thio-NADH, generating a colored product and acetoacetate. Thio-NADH absorbs light at 405 nm, in the visible range, as compared to NADH, which absorbs at 340 nm, in the ultraviolet range. The use of thio-NAD$^+$ allows clinical laboratory instrumentation to be used. The acetoacetate is then recycled back to β-hydroxybutyrate, in which NADH is converted to NAD$^+$. The β-hydroxybutyrate produced is then cycled back to acetoacetate, generating more thio-NADH. The cycling enhances the sensitivity of the assay. Once equilibrium is reached, one can calculate, from the change in absorbance per minute, the concentration of the β-hydroxybutyrate in the sample.

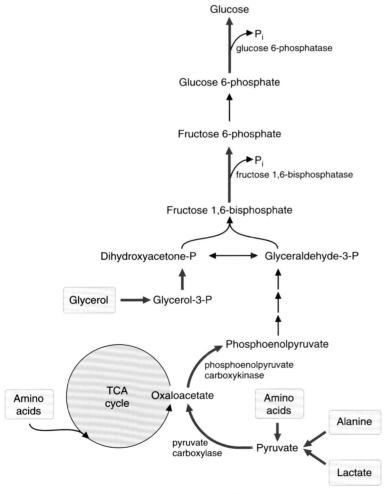

FIGURE 28.3 Key reactions of gluconeogenesis. The precursors are amino acids (particularly alanine), lactate, and glycerol. *Heavy red arrows* indicate steps that differ from those of glycolysis. *Dihydroxyacetone-P*, dihydroxyacetone phosphate; *Glyceraldehyde-3-P*, glyceraldehyde 3-phosphate; *Glycerol-3-P*, glycerol 3-phosphate; P_i, inorganic phosphate; *TCA*, tricarboxylic acid.

Comatose patients in DKA have the smell of acetone (a derivative of the ketone body acetoacetate) on their breath. In addition, DKA patients have deep, relatively rapid respirations typical of acidotic patients (Kussmaul respirations). These respirations result from an acidosis-induced stimulation of the respiratory center in the brain. More CO_2 is exhaled in an attempt to reduce the amount of acid in the body: $H^+ + HCO_3 \rightarrow H_2CO_3 \rightarrow H_2O + CO_2$ (exhaled). These signs are not observed in a hypoglycemic coma.

The severe hyperglycemia of DKA also causes osmotic diuresis (i.e., glucose entering the urine carries water with it), which, in turn, causes a contraction of blood volume. Volume depletion may be aggravated by vomiting, which is common in patients with DKA. DKA may cause dehydration (dry skin), low blood pressure, and a rapid heartbeat. These respiratory and hemodynamic alterations are not seen in patients with hypoglycemic coma. The flushed, wet skin of hypoglycemic coma is in contrast to the dry skin observed in DKA.

Most of the steps of gluconeogenesis use the same enzymes that catalyze the process of glycolysis. The flow of carbon, of course, is in the reverse direction. Three reaction sequences of gluconeogenesis differ from the corresponding steps of glycolysis. They involve the conversion of pyruvate to PEP and the reactions that remove phosphate from fructose 1,6-bisphosphate (fructose 1,6-bisP) to form fructose 6-phosphate (fructose 6-P) and from glucose 6-phosphate (glucose 6-P) to form glucose (see Fig. 28.3). The conversion of pyruvate to PEP is catalyzed during gluconeogenesis by a series of enzymes instead of the single enzyme used for glycolysis. The reactions that remove phosphate from fructose 1,6-bisP and from glucose 6-P each use single enzymes that differ from the corresponding enzymes of glycolysis. Although phosphate is added during glycolysis by kinases, which use adenosine triphosphate (ATP), it is removed during gluconeogenesis by phosphatases that release inorganic phosphate (P_i) via hydrolysis reactions.

A. Precursors for Gluconeogenesis

The three major carbon sources for gluconeogenesis in humans are lactate, glycerol, and amino acids, particularly alanine. Lactate is produced by anaerobic glycolysis in tissues such as exercising muscle or red blood cells as well as by adipocytes during the fed state. Glycerol is released from adipose stores of triacylglycerol, and amino acids come mainly from amino acid pools in muscle, where they may be obtained by degradation of muscle protein. Alanine, the major gluconeogenic amino acid, is produced in the muscle from other amino acids and from glucose (see Chapter 37). Because ethanol metabolism only gives rise to acetyl coenzyme A (acetyl-CoA), the carbons of ethanol cannot be used for gluconeogenesis.

B. Formation of Gluconeogenic Intermediates from Carbon Sources

The carbon sources for gluconeogenesis form pyruvate, intermediates of the tricarboxylic acid (TCA) cycle, or intermediates that are common to both glycolysis and gluconeogenesis.

Diabetes mellitus (DM) should be suspected if a venous plasma glucose level drawn regardless of when food was last eaten (a "random" sample of blood glucose) is "unequivocally elevated" (i.e., >200 mg/dL), particularly in a patient who manifests the classic signs and symptoms of chronic hyperglycemia (polydipsia, polyuria, blurred vision, headaches, rapid weight loss, sometimes accompanied by nausea and vomiting). To confirm the diagnosis, the patient should fast overnight (10 to 16 hours), and the blood glucose measurement should be repeated. Values of <100 mg/dL are considered normal. Values ≥126 mg/dL are indicative of DM. The level of glycosylated hemoglobin (HbA_{1c}) also can be measured to make the diagnosis, and if >6.5%, it is diagnostic for DM. The levels of HbA_{1c} can also gauge the extent of hyperglycemia over the past 4 to 8 weeks and is used to guide treatment. Values of fasting blood glucose between 100 and 125 mg/dL are designated as impaired fasting glucose (IFG) (or prediabetes), and further testing should be performed to determine whether these individuals will eventually develop overt DM. Individuals with blood glucose levels in this range have been defined as having "prediabetes." The determination that fasting blood glucose levels of 126 mg/dL, or a percentage of glycosylated hemoglobin of >6.5%, is diagnostic for DM is based on data indicating that at these levels of glucose or glycosylated hemoglobin, patients begin to develop complications of DM, specifically retinopathy.

The renal tubular transport maximum in the average healthy subject is such that glucose will not appear in the urine until the blood glucose level is >180 mg/dL. As a result, reagent tapes (Tes-Tape or Dextrostix) designed to detect the presence of glucose in the urine are not sensitive enough to establish a diagnosis of early DM.

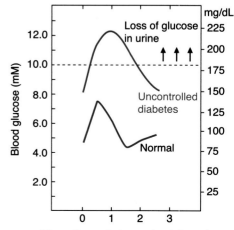

1. Lactate, Amino Acids, and Glycerol

Pyruvate is produced in the liver from the gluconeogenic precursors lactate and alanine. Lactate dehydrogenase oxidizes lactate to pyruvate, generating reduced nicotinamide adenine dinucleotide (NADH) (Fig. 28.4A), and alanine aminotransferase converts alanine to pyruvate (see Fig. 28.4B).

Although alanine is the major gluconeogenic amino acid, other amino acids, such as serine, serve as carbon sources for the synthesis of glucose because they also form pyruvate, the substrate for the initial step in the process. Some amino acids form intermediates of the TCA cycle (see Chapter 23), which can enter the gluconeogenic pathway.

The carbons of glycerol are gluconeogenic because they form *dihydroxyacetone phosphate* (DHAP), a glycolytic intermediate (see Fig. 28.4C).

2. Propionate

Fatty acids with an odd number of carbon atoms, which are obtained mainly from vegetables in the diet, produce propionyl coenzyme A (propionyl-CoA) from the three carbons at the ω-end of the chain (see Chapter 30). These carbons are relatively minor precursors of glucose in humans. Propionyl-CoA is converted to methylmalonyl coenzyme A (methylmalonyl-CoA), which is rearranged to form succinyl coenzyme A (succinyl-CoA), a four-carbon intermediate of the TCA cycle that can be used for gluconeogenesis. The remaining carbons of an odd-chain fatty acid form acetyl-CoA, from which no net synthesis of glucose occurs. In some species, propionate is a major source of carbon for gluconeogenesis. Ruminants can produce massive amounts of glucose from propionate. In cows, the cellulose in grass is converted to propionate by bacteria in the rumen. This substrate is then used to generate more than 5 lb of glucose each day by the process of gluconeogenesis.

β-Oxidation of fatty acids produces acetyl-CoA (see Chapter 30). Because the pyruvate dehydrogenase reaction is thermodynamically and kinetically irreversible, acetyl-CoA does not form pyruvate for gluconeogenesis. Therefore, if acetyl-CoA is to produce glucose, it must enter the TCA cycle and be converted to malate. For every two carbons of acetyl-CoA that are converted to malate, two carbons are

Glucocorticoids are naturally occurring steroid hormones. In humans, the major glucocorticoid is cortisol. Glucocorticoids are produced in the adrenal cortex in response to various types of stress (see Chapter 41). One of their actions is to stimulate the degradation of muscle protein. Thus, increased amounts of amino acids become available as substrates for gluconeogenesis. **Emma W.** noted muscle weakness, a result of the muscle-degrading action of the synthetic glucocorticoid prednisone, which she was taking for its anti-inflammatory effects.

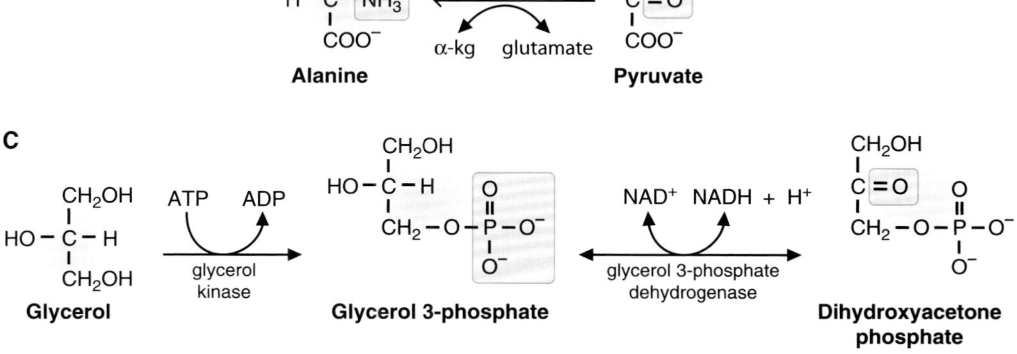

FIGURE 28.4 Metabolism of gluconeogenic precursors. **A.** Conversion of lactate to pyruvate. **B.** Conversion of alanine to pyruvate. In this reaction, alanine aminotransferase transfers the amino group of alanine to α-ketoglutarate to form glutamate. The coenzyme for this reaction, pyridoxal phosphate, accepts and donates the amino group. **C.** Conversion of glycerol to dihydroxyacetone phosphate. *α-kg*, α-ketoglutarate; *NAD*, nicotinamide adenine dinucleotide.

In a fatty acid with 19 carbons, how many carbons (and which ones) have the capability to form glucose?

released as CO_2: one in the reaction catalyzed by isocitrate dehydrogenase and the other in the reaction catalyzed by α-ketoglutarate dehydrogenase. Therefore, there is no *net* synthesis of glucose from acetyl-CoA.

C. Pathway of Gluconeogenesis

Gluconeogenesis occurs by a pathway that reverses many, but not all, of the steps of glycolysis.

1. Conversion of Pyruvate to Phosphoenolpyruvate

In glycolysis, PEP is converted to pyruvate by pyruvate kinase. In gluconeogenesis, a series of steps is required to accomplish the reversal of this reaction (Fig. 28.5). Pyruvate is carboxylated by pyruvate carboxylase to form oxaloacetate (OAA). This enzyme, which requires biotin, is the catalyst of an anaplerotic (refilling) reaction

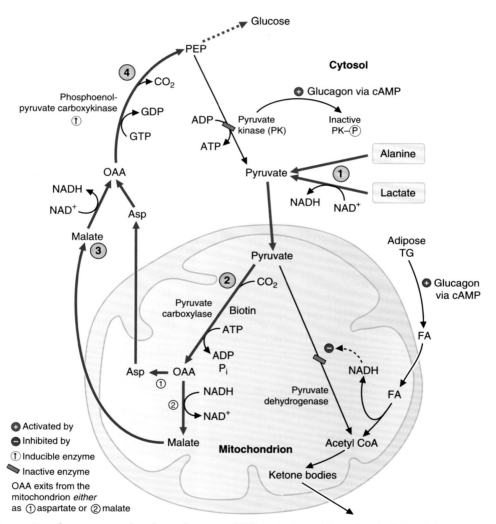

FIGURE 28.5 Conversion of pyruvate to phosphoenolpyruvate (PEP) in the liver. Follow the *shaded circled numbers* on the diagram, starting with the precursors alanine and lactate. The first step is the conversion of alanine and lactate to pyruvate. Pyruvate then enters the mitochondria and is converted to oxaloacetate (OAA) (*circle 2*) by pyruvate carboxylase. Pyruvate dehydrogenase has been inactivated by both the reduced nicotinamide adenine dinucleotide (NADH) and acetyl coenzyme A generated from fatty acid oxidation, which allows OAA production for gluconeogenesis. The OAA formed in the mitochondria is converted to either malate or aspartate to enter the cytoplasm via the malate/aspartate shuttle. In the cytoplasm, the malate or aspartate is converted back into OAA (*circle 3*), and phosphoenolpyruvate carboxykinase converts it to PEP (*circle 4*). The PEP formed is not converted to pyruvate because pyruvate kinase has been inactivated by phosphorylation by the cyclic adenosine monophosphate (cAMP)-dependent protein kinase under these conditions. The *white circled numbers* are alternative routes for exit of carbon from the mitochondrion using the malate/aspartate shuttle. *Acetyl CoA*, acetyl coenzyme A; *ADP*, adenosine diphosphate; *ATP*, adenosine triphosphate; *FA*, fatty acid; *GDP*, guanosine diphosphate; *GTP*, guanosine triphosphate; *Pᵢ*, inorganic phosphate; *PK*, pyruvate kinase; *TG*, triacylglycerol.

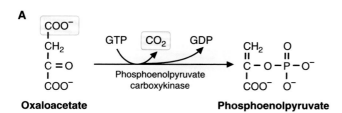

FIGURE 28.6 Conversion of pyruvate to oxaloacetate. *ADP*, adenosine diphosphate; *ATP*, adenosine triphosphate; *P*$_i$, inorganic phosphate.

of the TCA cycle (see Chapter 23). In gluconeogenesis, this reaction replenishes the OAA that is used for the synthesis of glucose (Fig. 28.6).

The CO_2 that was added to pyruvate to form OAA is released in the reaction catalyzed by phosphoenolpyruvate carboxykinase (PEPCK), which generates PEP (Fig. 28.7A). For this reaction, guanosine triphosphate (GTP) provides a source of energy as well as the phosphate group of PEP. Pyruvate carboxylase is found in mitochondria. In various species, PEPCK is located either in the cytosol or in mitochondria, or it is distributed between these two compartments. In humans, the enzyme is distributed about equally in each compartment.

OAA, generated from pyruvate by pyruvate carboxylase or from amino acids that form intermediates of the TCA cycle, does not readily cross the mitochondrial membrane. It is either decarboxylated to form PEP by the mitochondrial PEPCK or it is converted to malate or aspartate (see Fig. 28.7B and C). The conversion of OAA to malate requires NADH. PEP, malate, and aspartate can be transported into the cytosol.

After malate or aspartate traverses the mitochondrial membrane (acting as a carrier of OAA) and enters the cytosol, it is reconverted to OAA by reversal of the reactions given previously (see Fig. 28.7B and C). The conversion of malate to OAA generates NADH. Whether OAA is transported across the mitochondrial membrane as malate or aspartate depends on the need for reducing equivalents in the cytosol. NADH is required to reduce 1,3-bisphosphoglycerate to glyceraldehyde 3-phosphate (glyceraldehyde 3-P) during gluconeogenesis.

OAA, produced from malate or aspartate in the cytosol, is converted to PEP by the cytosolic PEPCK (see Fig. 28.7A).

Excessive ethanol metabolism blocks the production of gluconeogenic precursors. Cells have limited amounts of NAD, which exists either as NAD$^+$ or as NADH. As the levels of NADH rise, those of NAD$^+$ fall, and the ratio of the concentrations of NADH and NAD$^+$ ([NADH]/[NAD$^+$]) increases. In the presence of ethanol, which is very rapidly oxidized in the liver, the [NADH]/[NAD$^+$] ratio is much higher than it is in the normal fasting liver (see Chapter 33). High levels of NADH drive the lactate dehydrogenase reaction toward lactate. Therefore, lactate cannot enter the gluconeogenic pathway, and pyruvate that is generated from alanine is converted to lactate. Because glycerol is oxidized by NAD$^+$ during its conversion to DHAP, the conversion of glycerol to glucose is also inhibited when NADH levels are elevated. Consequently, the major precursors lactate, alanine, and glycerol are not used for gluconeogenesis under conditions in which alcohol metabolism is high.

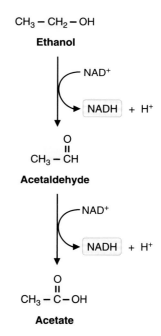

A.

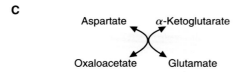

FIGURE 28.7 Generation of phosphoenolpyruvate (PEP) from gluconeogenic precursors. **A.** Conversion of oxaloacetate to PEP, using PEP carboxykinase. **B.** Interconversion of oxaloacetate and malate. **C.** Transamination of aspartate to form oxaloacetate. Note that the cytosolic reaction is the reverse of the mitochondrial reaction as shown in Figure 28.5. *GDP*, guanosine diphosphate; *GTP*, guanosine triphosphate; *NAD*, nicotinamide adenine dinucleotide.

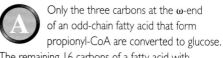

Only the three carbons at the ω-end of an odd-chain fatty acid that form propionyl-CoA are converted to glucose. The remaining 16 carbons of a fatty acid with 19 carbons form acetyl-CoA, which does not form any net glucose.

2. Conversion of Phosphoenolpyruvate to Fructose 1,6-Bisphosphate

The remaining steps of gluconeogenesis occur in the cytosol (Fig. 28.8). Starting with PEP as a substrate, the steps of glycolysis are reversed to form glyceraldehyde 3-P. For every two molecules of glyceraldehyde 3-P that are formed, one is converted to DHAP. These two triose phosphates, DHAP and glyceraldehyde 3-P, condense to form fructose 1,6-bisP by a reversal of the aldolase reaction. Because glycerol forms DHAP, it enters the gluconeogenic pathway at this level.

3. Conversion of Fructose 1,6-Bisphosphate to Fructose 6-Phosphate

The enzyme fructose 1,6-bisphosphatase releases inorganic phosphate from fructose 1,6-bisP to form fructose 6-P. This is not a reversal of the phosphofructokinase-1 (PFK-1) reaction; ATP is not produced when the phosphate is removed from the 1-position of fructose 1,6-bisP because that is a low-energy phosphate bond.

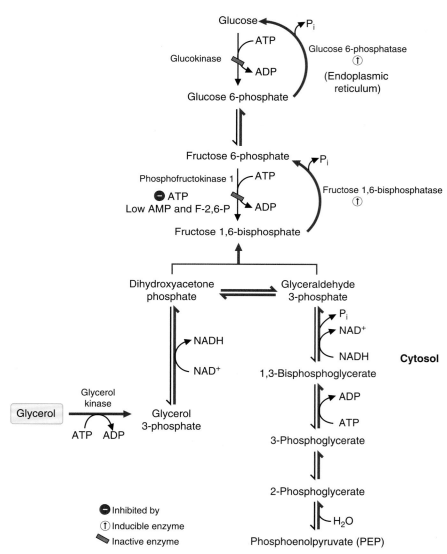

FIGURE 28.8 Conversion of phosphoenolpyruvate and glycerol to glucose. Gluconeogenic reactions are indicated by the *red arrows*. Glucokinase is inactive because of the low levels of glucose in the cell (below the K_m for glucokinase), whereas phosphofructokinase-1 (PFK-1) is inactive because of the low concentration of the allosteric activators adenosine monophosphate (AMP) and fructose 2,6-bisphosphate, coupled to high concentrations of adenosine triphosphate (ATP), an allosteric inhibitor. *ADP*, adenosine diphosphate; *F-2,6-P*, fructose 2,6-bisphosphate; *NAD*, nicotinamide adenine dinucleotide; P_i, inorganic phosphate.

Rather, inorganic phosphate is released in this hydrolysis reaction. In the next reaction of gluconeogenesis, fructose 6-P is converted to glucose 6-P by the same isomerase used in glycolysis (phosphoglucoisomerase).

4. Conversion of Glucose 6-Phosphate to Glucose

Glucose 6-phosphatase hydrolyzes P_i from glucose 6-P, and free glucose is released into the blood. As with fructose 1,6-bisphosphatase, this is not a reversal of the glucokinase reaction because the phosphate bond in glucose 6-P is a low-energy bond, and ATP is not generated at this step.

Glucose 6-phosphatase is located in the membrane of the endoplasmic reticulum. It is used not only in gluconeogenesis but also to produce blood glucose from the breakdown of liver glycogen.

D. Regulation of Gluconeogenesis

Although gluconeogenesis occurs during fasting, it is also stimulated during prolonged exercise, by a high-protein diet, and under conditions of stress. The factors that promote the overall flow of carbon from pyruvate to glucose include the availability of substrate and changes in the activity or amount of certain key enzymes of glycolysis and gluconeogenesis.

1. Availability of Substrate

Gluconeogenesis is stimulated by the flow of its major substrates (glycerol, lactate, and amino acids) from peripheral tissues to the liver. Glycerol is released from adipose tissue whenever the levels of insulin are low and the levels of glucagon or the "stress" hormones, epinephrine and cortisol (a glucocorticoid), are elevated in the blood (see Chapter 19). Lactate is produced by muscle during exercise and by red blood cells. Amino acids are released from muscle whenever insulin is low or when cortisol is elevated. Amino acids are also available for gluconeogenesis when the dietary intake of protein is high and intake of carbohydrate is low.

2. Activity or Amount of Key Enzymes

Three sequences in the pathway of gluconeogenesis are regulated:

1. Pyruvate → PEP
2. Fructose 1,6-bisP → fructose 6-P
3. Glucose 6-P → glucose

These steps correspond to those in glycolysis that are catalyzed by regulatory enzymes. The enzymes involved in these steps of gluconeogenesis differ from those that catalyze the reverse reactions in glycolysis. The net flow of carbon, whether from glucose to pyruvate (glycolysis) or from pyruvate to glucose (gluconeogenesis), depends on the relative activity or amount of these glycolytic or gluconeogenic enzymes (Fig. 28.9 and Table 28.1).

3. Conversion of Pyruvate to Phosphoenolpyruvate

Pyruvate, a key substrate for gluconeogenesis, is derived from lactate and amino acids, particularly alanine. Pyruvate is not converted to acetyl-CoA under conditions that favor gluconeogenesis because pyruvate dehydrogenase is relatively inactive. Instead, pyruvate is converted to OAA by pyruvate carboxylase. Subsequently, OAA is converted to PEP by PEPCK. The following is a description of activity states of enzymes under which PEP will be used to form glucose rather than pyruvate.

- **Pyruvate dehydrogenase is inactive.** Under conditions of fasting, insulin levels are low and glucagon levels are elevated. Consequently, fatty acids and glycerol are released from the triacylglycerol stores of adipose tissue. Fatty acids travel to the liver, where they undergo β-oxidation, producing acetyl-CoA, NADH, and ATP (see Chapter 31). As a consequence, the concentration of adenosine diphosphate (ADP) decreases. These changes result in the

Al M. had not eaten for 3 days, so he had no dietary source of glucose and his liver glycogen stores were essentially depleted. He was solely dependent on gluconeogenesis to maintain his blood glucose levels. One of the consequences of ethanol ingestion and the subsequent rise in NADH levels is that the major carbon sources for gluconeogenesis cannot readily be converted to glucose (the high NADH/NAD^+ ratio favors lactate formation from pyruvate, malate formation from OAA, and glycerol 3-P formation from DHAP). Intermediates of the TCA cycle derived from amino acids are converted to malate, which enters the cytosol and is converted to OAA, which proceeds through gluconeogenesis to form glucose. When excessive amounts of ethanol are ingested, elevated NADH levels inhibit the conversion of malate to OAA in the cytosol. During his alcoholic binges, **Al M.** became hypoglycemic. His blood glucose level was 28 mg/dL.

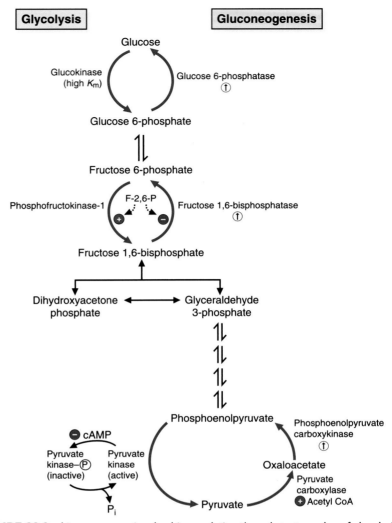

FIGURE 28.9 Liver enzymes involved in regulating the substrate cycles of glycolysis and gluconeogenesis. *Heavy arrows* indicate the three substrate cycles. *Acetyl CoA*, acetyl coenzyme A; *cAMP*, cyclic adenosine monophosphate; *F-2,6-P*, fructose 2,6-bisphosphate; P_i, inorganic phosphate. ⊕, activated by; ⊖, inhibited by; ⓣ, inducible enzyme.

phosphorylation of pyruvate dehydrogenase to the inactive form. Therefore, pyruvate is not converted to acetyl-CoA (see Chapter 30).

- **Pyruvate carboxylase is active.** Acetyl-CoA, which is produced by oxidation of fatty acids, activates pyruvate carboxylase. Therefore, pyruvate, derived from lactate or alanine, is converted to OAA. Acetyl-CoA levels, then, reciprocally regulate pyruvate dehydrogenase and pyruvate carboxylase. High levels of acetyl-CoA inhibit pyruvate dehydrogenase while activating pyruvate carboxylase.

- **Phosphoenolpyruvate carboxykinase is induced.** OAA produces PEP in a reaction catalyzed by PEPCK. Cytosolic PEPCK is an inducible enzyme, which means that the quantity of the enzyme in the cell increases because of increased transcription of its gene and increased translation of its messenger RNA (mRNA). The major inducer is cyclic adenosine monophosphate (cAMP), which is increased by hormones that activate adenylate cyclase. Adenylate cyclase produces cAMP from ATP. Glucagon is the hormone that causes cAMP to rise during fasting, whereas epinephrine acts during exercise or stress. cAMP activates protein kinase A, which phosphorylates a set of specific transcription factors (cAMP response element–binding protein

TABLE 28.1 Regulation of Enzymes of Glycolysis and Gluconeogenesis in Liver

ENZYME	MECHANISM
A. Glycolytic Enzymes	
Pyruvate kinase	Activated by F-1,6-BP
	Inhibited by ATP, alanine
	Inhibited by phosphorylation (glucagon and epinephrine lead to an increase in cAMP levels, which activates protein kinase A)
Phosphofructokinase-1	Activated by F-2,6-BP, AMP
	Inhibited by ATP, citrate
Glucokinase	High K_m for glucose
	Induced by insulin
B. Gluconeogenic Enzymes	
Pyruvate carboxylase	Activated by acetyl-CoA
PEPCK	Induced (increase in gene transcription) by glucagon, epinephrine, glucocorticoids
	Repressed (decrease in gene transcription) by insulin
Glucose 6-phosphatase	Induced (increase in gene transcription) during fasting
Fructose 1,6-bisphosphatase	Inhibited by F-2,6-BP, AMP
	Induced (increase in gene transcription) during fasting

F-1,6-BP, fructose 1,6-bisphosphate; F-2,6-BP, fructose 2,6-bisphosphate; ATP, adenosine triphosphate; cAMP, cyclic adenosine monophosphate; AMP, adenosine monophosphate; acetyl-CoA, acetyl coenzyme A; PEPCK, phosphoenolpyruvate carboxykinase.

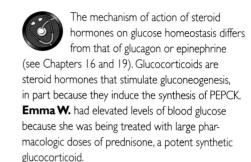

The mechanism of action of steroid hormones on glucose homeostasis differs from that of glucagon or epinephrine (see Chapters 16 and 19). Glucocorticoids are steroid hormones that stimulate gluconeogenesis, in part because they induce the synthesis of PEPCK. **Emma W.** had elevated levels of blood glucose because she was being treated with large pharmacologic doses of prednisone, a potent synthetic glucocorticoid.

[CREB]) that stimulate transcription of the *PEPCK* gene (see Chapter 16 and Fig. 16.17). Increased synthesis of mRNA for PEPCK results in increased synthesis of the enzyme. Cortisol, the major human glucocorticoid, also induces PEPCK but through a different regulatory site on the *PEPCK* promoter.

- **Pyruvate kinase is inactive.** When glucagon is elevated, liver pyruvate kinase is phosphorylated and inactivated by a mechanism that involves cAMP and protein kinase A. Therefore, PEP is not reconverted to pyruvate. Rather, it continues along the pathway of gluconeogenesis. If PEP were reconverted to pyruvate, these substrates would simply cycle, causing a net loss of energy with no net generation of useful products. The inactivation of pyruvate kinase prevents such futile cycling and promotes the net synthesis of glucose.

4. Conversion of Fructose 1,6-Bisphosphate to Fructose 6-Phosphate

The carbons of PEP reverse the steps of glycolysis, forming fructose 1,6-bisP. Fructose 1,6-bisphosphatase acts on this bisphosphate to release inorganic phosphate and produce fructose 6-P. A futile substrate cycle is prevented at this step because, under conditions that favor gluconeogenesis, the concentrations of the compounds that activate the glycolytic enzyme PFK-1 are low. These same compounds, fructose 2,6-bisphosphate (fructose 2,6-bisP; whose levels are regulated by insulin and glucagon) and AMP, are allosteric inhibitors of fructose 1,6-bisphosphatase. When the concentrations of these allosteric effectors are low, PFK-1 is less active, fructose 1,6-bisphosphatase is more active, and the net flow of carbon is toward fructose 6-P and, thus, toward glucose. The synthesis of fructose 1,6-bisphosphatase is also induced during fasting.

5. Conversion of Glucose 6-Phosphate to Glucose

Glucose 6-phosphatase catalyzes the conversion of glucose 6-P to glucose, which is released from the liver cell (Fig. 28.10). The glycolytic enzyme glucokinase, which catalyzes the reverse reaction, is relatively inactive during gluconeogenesis. Glucokinase, which has a high $S_{0.5}$ (K_m) for glucose (see Chapter 9, Fig. 9.4), is not very active during fasting because the blood glucose level is lower (~5 mM) than the $S_{0.5}$ of the enzyme.

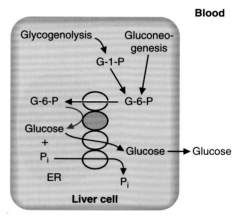

○ Transport proteins
● Glucose 6-phosphatase

FIGURE 28.10 Location and function of glucose 6-phosphatase. Glucose 6-phosphate travels on a transporter into the endoplasmic reticulum (ER), where it is hydrolyzed by glucose 6-phosphatase to glucose and inorganic phosphate (P_i). These products travel back to the cytosol on transporters. *G-1-P*, glucose 1-phosphate; *G-6-P*, glucose 6-phosphate.

Glucokinase is also an inducible enzyme. The concentration of the enzyme increases in the fed state, when blood glucose and insulin levels are elevated, and decreases in the fasting state, when glucose and insulin are low.

E. Energy Is Required for the Synthesis of Glucose

During the gluconeogenic reactions, 6 mol of high-energy phosphate bonds are cleaved. Two moles of pyruvate are required for the synthesis of 1 mol of glucose. As 2 mol of pyruvate are carboxylated by pyruvate carboxylase, 2 mol of ATP are hydrolyzed. PEPCK requires 2 mol of GTP (the equivalent of 2 mol of ATP) to convert 2 mol of OAA to 2 mol of PEP. An additional 2 mol of ATP are used when 2 mol of 3-phosphoglycerate are phosphorylated, forming 2 mol of 1,3-bisphosphoglycerate. Energy in the form of reducing equivalents (NADH) is also required for the conversion of 1,3-bisphosphoglycerate to glyceraldehyde 3-P. Under fasting conditions, the energy required for gluconeogenesis is obtained from β-oxidation of fatty acids. Defects in fatty acid oxidation can lead to hypoglycemia in part because of reduced fatty acid–derived energy production within the liver.

III. Changes in Blood Glucose Levels after a Meal

After a high-carbohydrate meal, blood glucose rises from a fasting level of approximately 80 to 100 mg/dL (~5 mM) to a level of approximately 120 to 140 mg/dL (8 mM) within a period of 30 minutes to 1 hour (Fig. 28.11). The concentration of glucose in the blood then begins to decrease, returning to the fasting range by approximately 2 hours after the meal (see also Chapter 19).

Blood glucose levels increase as dietary glucose is digested and absorbed. The values go no higher than approximately 140 mg/dL in a normal, healthy person because tissues take up glucose from the blood, storing it for subsequent use and oxidizing it for energy. After the meal is digested and absorbed, blood glucose levels decline because cells continue to metabolize glucose.

If blood glucose levels continued to rise after a meal, the high concentration of glucose would cause the release of water from tissues as a result of the osmotic effect of glucose. Tissues would become dehydrated, and their function would be affected. If hyperglycemia becomes severe, a hyperosmolar coma could result from dehydration of the brain.

Conversely, if blood glucose levels continued to drop after a meal, tissues that depend on glucose would suffer from a lack of energy. If blood glucose levels dropped abruptly, the brain would not be able to produce an adequate amount of ATP. Light-headedness and dizziness would result, followed by drowsiness and, eventually, coma. Red blood cells would not be able to produce enough ATP to maintain the integrity of their membranes. Hemolysis of these cells would decrease the transport of oxygen to the tissues of the body. Eventually, all tissues that rely on oxygen for energy production would fail to perform their normal functions. If the problem were severe enough, death could result.

Devastating consequences of glucose excess or insufficiency are normally avoided because the body is able to regulate its blood glucose levels. As the concentration of blood glucose approaches the normal fasting range of 80 to 100 mg/dL roughly 2 hours after a meal, the process of glycogenolysis is activated in the liver. Liver glycogen is the primary source of blood glucose during the first few hours of fasting. Subsequently, gluconeogenesis begins to play a role as an additional source of blood glucose. The carbon for gluconeogenesis, a process that occurs in the liver, is supplied by other tissues. Exercising muscle and red blood cells provide lactate through glycolysis, muscle also provides amino acids by degradation of protein, and glycerol is released from adipose tissue as triacylglycerol stores are mobilized.

Even during a prolonged fast, blood glucose levels do not decrease dramatically. After 5 to 6 weeks of starvation, blood glucose levels decrease to only approximately 65 mg/dL (Table 28.2).

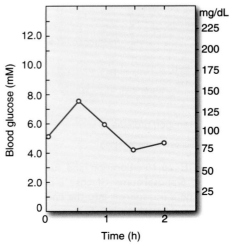

FIGURE 28.11 Blood glucose concentrations at various times after a meal.

TABLE 28.2	**Blood Glucose Levels at Various Stages of Fasting**
STAGE OF FASTING	**GLUCOSE (mg/dL)**
Glucose, 700 g/d IV	100
Fasting, 12 h	80
Starvation, 3 d	70
Starvation, 5–6 wk	65

IV, intravenous.

Source: Ruderman NB, Aoki TT, Cahill GF Jr. Gluconeogenesis and its disorders in man. In: Hanson RW, Mehlman MA, eds. *Gluconeogenesis: Its Regulation in Mammalian Species.* New York, NY: John Wiley & Sons; 1976:517.

A. Blood Glucose Levels in the Fed State

The major factors involved in regulating blood glucose levels are the blood glucose concentration itself and hormones, particularly insulin and glucagon.

As blood glucose levels rise after a meal, the increased glucose concentration stimulates the β-cells of the pancreas to release insulin (Fig. 28.12). Certain amino acids, particularly arginine and leucine, also stimulate insulin release from the pancreas.

Blood levels of glucagon, which is secreted by the α-cells of the pancreas, may increase or decrease, depending on the content of the meal. Glucagon levels decrease in response to a high-carbohydrate meal, but they increase in response to a high-protein meal. After a typical mixed meal containing carbohydrate, protein, and fat, glucagon levels remain relatively constant, whereas insulin levels increase.

1. Fate of Dietary Glucose in the Liver

After a meal, the liver oxidizes glucose to meet its immediate energy needs. Any excess glucose is converted to stored fuels. Glycogen is synthesized and stored in the liver, and glucose is converted to fatty acids and to the glycerol moiety that reacts with the fatty acids to produce triacylglycerols. These triacylglycerols are packaged in VLDL (see Chapter 29) and transported to adipose tissue, where the fatty acids are stored in adipose triacylglycerols. The VLDL can also deliver triglycerides (fatty acids) to the muscle for immediate oxidation, if required.

Regulatory mechanisms control the conversion of glucose to stored fuels. As the concentration of glucose increases in the hepatic portal vein, the concentration of glucose in the liver may increase from the fasting level of 80 to 100 mg/dL ($\sim$5 mM) to a concentration of 180 to 360 mg/dL (10 to 20 mM). Consequently, the velocity of the glucokinase reaction increases because this enzyme has a high $S_{0.5}$ (K_m) for glucose (see Fig. 9.4). Glucokinase is also induced by a high-carbohydrate diet; the quantity of the enzyme increases in response to elevated insulin levels.

Insulin promotes the storage of glucose as glycogen by countering the effects of glucagon-stimulated phosphorylation. The response to insulin activates the phosphatases that dephosphorylate glycogen synthase (which leads to glycogen synthase activation) and glycogen phosphorylase (which leads to inhibition of the enzyme) (Fig. 28.13A). Insulin also promotes the synthesis of the triacylglycerols that are released from the liver into the blood as VLDL. The regulatory mechanisms for this process are described in Chapter 31.

2. Fate of Dietary Glucose in Peripheral Tissues

Almost every cell in the body oxidizes glucose for energy. Certain critical tissues, particularly the brain, other nervous system tissues, and red blood cells, depend especially on glucose for their energy supply. The brain requires approximately 150 g of glucose per day. In addition, approximately 40 g of glucose per day is required by other glucose-dependent tissues. Furthermore, all tissues require glucose for the pentose phosphate pathway, and many tissues use glucose for synthesis of glycoproteins and other carbohydrate-containing compounds.

When **Dianne A.** inadvertently injected insulin without eating, she caused an acute reduction in her blood glucose levels 1 to 2 hours later. Had she been awake, she would have first experienced symptoms caused by hypoglycemia-induced hyperactivity of her sympathetic nervous system (e.g., sweating, tremulousness, palpitations). Eventually, as her hypoglycemia became more profound, she would have experienced symptoms of *neuroglycopenia* (inadequate glucose supply to the brain), such as confusion, speech disturbances, emotional instability, possible seizure activity, and, finally, coma.

Ann R., who is recovering from anorexia nervosa and whose intake of glucose and of glucose precursors has been severely restricted, has not developed any of these manifestations. Her lack of hypoglycemic symptoms can be explained by the very gradual reduction of her blood glucose levels as a consequence of near-starvation and her ability to maintain blood glucose levels within an acceptable fasting range through hepatic gluconeogenesis. In addition, lipolysis of adipose triacylglycerols produces fatty acids, which are used as fuel and converted to ketone bodies by the liver. The oxidation of fatty acids and ketone bodies by the brain and muscle reduces the need for blood glucose.

In **Dianne A.'s** case, the excessive dose of insulin inhibited lipolysis and ketone body synthesis, so these alternative fuels were not available to spare blood glucose. The rapidity with which hypoglycemia was induced could not be compensated for quickly enough by hepatic glycogenolysis and gluconeogenesis, which are inhibited by the insulin, and hypoglycemia ensued.

An immediate fingerstick revealed that Dianne's capillary blood glucose level was <20 mg/dL. An intravenous infusion of a 50% solution of glucose was started, and her blood glucose level was determined frequently. When Di regained consciousness, the intravenous solution was eventually changed to 10% glucose. After 6 hours, her blood glucose levels stayed in the upper-normal range, and she was able to tolerate oral feedings. By the next morning, her previous diabetes treatment regimen could be reestablished. The reasons that she had developed hypoglycemic coma were explained to Di, and she was discharged to the care of her family doctor.

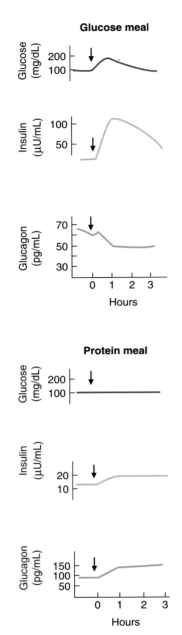

FIGURE 28.12 Blood glucose, insulin, and glucagon levels after a high-carbohydrate meal and after a high-protein meal. The meal occurred at the time indicated by the *down arrows*.

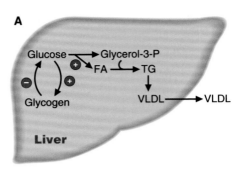

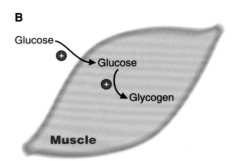

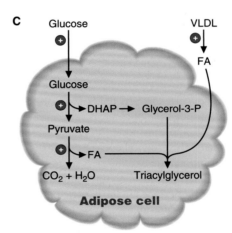

FIGURE 28.13 Glucose metabolism in various tissues. **A.** Effect of insulin on glycogen synthesis and degradation and on very-low-density lipoprotein (VLDL) synthesis in the liver. **B.** Glucose metabolism in resting muscle in the fed state. Transport of glucose into cells and synthesis of glycogen are stimulated by insulin. **C.** Glucose metabolism in adipose tissue in the fed state. *DHAP*, dihydroxyacetone phosphate; *FA*, fatty acids; *Glycerol-3-P*, glycerol 3-phosphate; *TG*, triacylglycerols; ⊕, stimulated by insulin; ⊖, inhibited by insulin.

Insulin stimulates the transport of glucose into adipose and muscle cells by promoting the recruitment of glucose transporters to the cell membrane (see Fig. 28.13C). Other tissues, such as the liver, brain, and red blood cells, have a different type of glucose transporter that is not as significantly affected by insulin.

In muscle, glycogen is synthesized after a meal by a mechanism similar to that in the liver (see Fig. 28.13B). Metabolic differences exist between these tissues (see Chapter 26), but, in essence, insulin stimulates glycogen synthesis in resting muscle as it does in the liver. A key difference between muscle and liver is that insulin greatly stimulates the transport of glucose into muscle cells but only slightly stimulates its transport into liver cells.

3. Return of Blood Glucose to Fasting Levels

After a meal has been digested and absorbed, blood glucose levels reach a peak and then begin to decline. The uptake of dietary glucose by cells, particularly those in the liver, muscle, and adipose tissue, lowers blood glucose levels. By 2 hours after a meal, blood glucose levels return to the normal fasting level of <100 mg/dL.

B. Blood Glucose Levels in the Fasting State

1. Changes in Insulin and Glucagon Levels

During fasting, as blood glucose levels decrease, insulin levels decrease and glucagon levels rise. These hormonal changes cause the liver to degrade glycogen by the process of glycogenolysis and to produce glucose by the process of gluconeogenesis so that blood glucose levels are maintained.

2. Stimulation of Glycogenolysis

Within a few hours after a high-carbohydrate meal, glucagon levels begin to rise. Glucagon binds to cell surface receptors and activates adenylate cyclase, causing cAMP levels in liver cells to rise (see Fig. 26.7). cAMP activates protein kinase A, which phosphorylates and inactivates glycogen synthase. Therefore, glycogen synthesis decreases.

At the same time, protein kinase A stimulates glycogen degradation by a two-step mechanism. Protein kinase A phosphorylates and activates phosphorylase kinase. This enzyme, in turn, phosphorylates and activates glycogen phosphorylase.

Glycogen phosphorylase catalyzes the phosphorolysis of glycogen, producing glucose 1-phosphate, which is converted to glucose 6-P. Dephosphorylation of glucose 6-P by glucose 6-phosphatase produces free glucose, which then enters the blood.

3. Stimulation of Gluconeogenesis

By 4 hours after a meal, the liver is supplying glucose to the blood not only by the process of glycogenolysis but also by the process of gluconeogenesis. Hormonal changes cause peripheral tissues to release precursors that provide carbon for gluconeogenesis, specifically lactate, amino acids, and glycerol.

Regulatory mechanisms promote the conversion of gluconeogenic precursors to glucose (Fig. 28.14). These mechanisms prevent the occurrence of potential futile cycles, which would continuously convert substrates to products while consuming energy but producing no useful result.

These regulatory mechanisms inactivate the glycolytic enzymes pyruvate kinase, PFK-1, and glucokinase during fasting and promote the flow of carbon to glucose via gluconeogenesis. These mechanisms operate at the three steps where glycolysis and gluconeogenesis differ:

1. Pyruvate (derived from lactate and alanine) is converted by the gluconeogenic pathway to PEP. PEP is not reconverted to pyruvate (a potentially futile cycle) because glucagon-stimulated phosphorylation inactivates pyruvate kinase. Therefore, PEP reverses the steps of glycolysis and forms fructose 1,6-bisP.
2. Fructose 1,6-bisP is converted to fructose 6-P by a bisphosphatase. Because the glycolytic enzyme PFK-1 is relatively inactive, mainly as a result of low fructose 2,6-bisP levels, fructose 6-P is not converted back to fructose 1,6-bisP, and a second potential futile cycle is avoided. The low fructose 2,6-bisP levels are attributable in part to the phosphorylation of phosphofructokinase-2 by protein kinase A, which has been activated in response to glucagon. Fructose 6-P is converted to glucose 6-P.
3. Glucose 6-P is dephosphorylated by glucose 6-phosphatase, forming free glucose. Because glucokinase has a high $S_{0.5}$ (K_m) for glucose, and glucose concentrations are relatively low in liver cells during fasting,

The pathophysiology leading to an elevation of blood glucose after a meal differs between patients with type 1 DM and those with type 2 DM. **Dianne A.**, who has type 1 disease, cannot secrete insulin adequately in response to a meal because of a defect in the β-cells of her pancreas. **Deborah S.**, however, has type 2 disease. In this form of the disorder, the cause of glucose intolerance is more complex, involving at least a delay in the release of relatively appropriate amounts of insulin after a meal combined with a degree of resistance to the actions of insulin in skeletal muscle and adipocytes. Excessive hepatic gluconeogenesis occurs even though blood glucose levels are elevated.

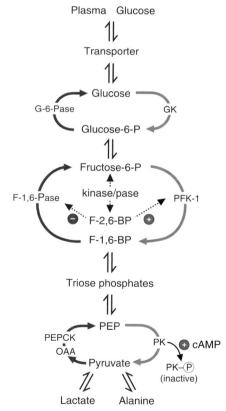

FIGURE 28.14 Regulation of gluconeogenesis (*red arrows*) in the liver. *cAMP*, cyclic adenosine monophosphate; *F-1,6-Pase*, fructose 1,6-bisphosphatase; *F-1,6-BP*, fructose 1,6-bisphosphate; *F-2,6-BP*, fructose 2,6-bisphosphate; *GK*, glucokinase; *G-6-Pase*, glucose 6-phosphatase; *OAA*, oxaloacetate; *PEPCK*, phosphoenolpyruvate carboxykinase; *PFK-1*, phosphofructokinase-1; *PK*, pyruvate kinase.

glucose is released into the blood. Therefore, the third potential futile cycle does not occur.

4. Enzymes that participate in gluconeogenesis, but not in glycolysis, are active under fasting conditions. Pyruvate carboxylase is activated by acetyl-CoA, derived from oxidation of fatty acids. PEPCK, fructose 1,6-bisphosphatase, and glucose 6-phosphatase are induced; that is, the quantity of the enzymes increases. Fructose 1,6-bisphosphatase is also active because levels of fructose 2,6-bisP, an inhibitor of the enzyme, are low.

4. Stimulation of Lipolysis

The hormonal changes that occur during fasting stimulate the breakdown of adipose triacylglycerols (see Chapters 3, 31, and 41). Consequently, fatty acids and glycerol are released into the blood (Fig. 28.15). Glycerol serves as a source of carbon for gluconeogenesis. Fatty acids become the major fuel of the body and are oxidized to CO_2 and H_2O by various tissues, which enables these tissues to decrease their use of glucose. Fatty acids are also oxidized to acetyl-CoA in the liver to provide energy for gluconeogenesis. In a prolonged fast, acetyl-CoA is converted to ketone bodies, which enter the blood and serve as an additional fuel source for the muscle and the brain.

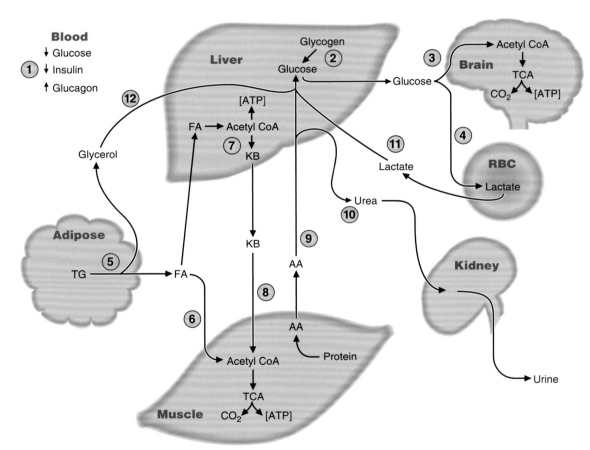

FIGURE 28.15 Tissue interrelationships during fasting. (*1*) Blood glucose levels drop, decreasing insulin and raising blood glucagon levels. (*2*) Glycogenolysis is induced in the liver to raise blood glucose levels. (*3*) The brain uses the glucose released by the liver, as do the red blood cells (RBCs) (*4*). (*5*) Adipose tissues are induced to release free fatty acids and glycerol from stored triglycerides. (*6*) The muscle and liver use fatty acids for energy. (*7*) The liver converts fatty acid–derived acetyl coenzyme A to ketone bodies for export, which the muscles (*8*) and brain can use for energy. (*9*) Protein turnover is induced in muscle, and amino acids leave the muscle and travel to the liver for use as gluconeogenic precursors. (*10*) The high rate of amino acid metabolism in the liver generates urea, which travels to the kidney for excretion. (*11*) RBCs produce lactate, which returns to the liver as a substrate for gluconeogenesis. (*12*) The glycerol released from adipose tissue is used by the liver for gluconeogenesis. *AA*, amino acids; *Acetyl CoA*, acetyl coenzyme A; *ATP*, adenosine triphosphate; *FA*, fatty acids; *KB*, ketone bodies; *TCA*, tricarboxylic acid; *TG*, triacylglycerols.

C. Blood Glucose Levels during Prolonged Fasting (Starvation)

During prolonged fasting, several changes occur in fuel use. These changes cause tissues to use less glucose than they use during a brief fast and to use predominantly fuels derived from adipose triacylglycerols (i.e., fatty acids and their derivatives, the ketone bodies). Therefore, blood glucose levels do not decrease drastically. In fact, even after 5 to 6 weeks of starvation, blood glucose levels are still in the range of 65 mg/dL (Fig. 28.16; see Table 28.2).

The major change that occurs in starvation is a dramatic elevation of blood ketone body levels after 3 to 5 days of fasting (see Fig. 28.16). At these levels, the brain and other nervous tissues begin to use ketone bodies, and consequently, they oxidize less glucose, requiring roughly one-third as much glucose (~40 g/day) as under normal dietary conditions. As a result of reduced glucose use, the rate of gluconeogenesis in the liver decreases, as does the production of urea (see Fig. 28.16). Because in this stage of starvation amino acids, obtained from the degradation of existing proteins, are the major gluconeogenic precursor, reducing glucose requirements in tissues reduces the rate of protein degradation and hence the rate of urea formation. Protein from muscle and other tissues is, therefore, spared because there is less need for amino acids for gluconeogenesis.

Body protein, particularly muscle protein, is not primarily a storage form of fuel in the same sense as glycogen or triacylglycerol; proteins have many functions besides fuel storage. For example, proteins function as enzymes, as structural proteins, and in muscle contraction. If tissue protein is degraded to too great an extent, body function can be severely compromised. If starvation continues and no other problems, such as infections, occur, a starving individual usually dies because of severe protein loss that causes malfunction of major organs such as the heart. Therefore, the increase in ketone body levels that results in the sparing of body protein allows individuals to survive for extended periods without ingesting food.

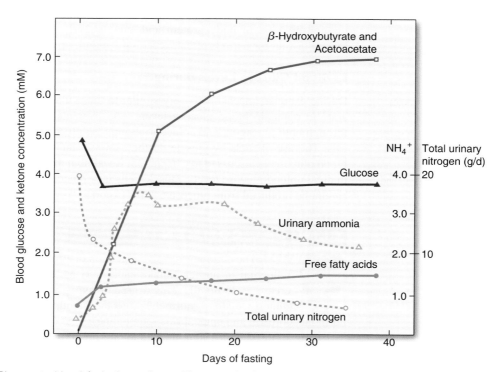

FIGURE 28.16   Changes in blood fuels during fasting. The units for fatty acids, glucose, and ketone bodies are millimolar (*on left*) and for urinary nitrogen and ammonia are grams per day (*on right*). (Modified from Linder MC, ed. *Nutritional Biochemistry and Metabolism with Clinical Applications.* 2nd ed. Norwalk, CT: Appleton & Lange; 1991:103. Copyright © 1991 Appleton & Lange.)

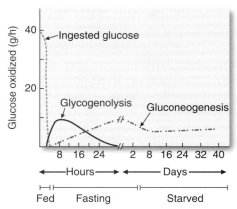

FIGURE 28.17 Sources of blood glucose in fed, fasting, and starved states. Note that the scale changes from hours to days. (From Ruderman NB, Aoki TT, Cahill GF Jr. In: Hanson RW, Mehlman MA, eds. *Gluconeogenesis: Its Regulation in Mammalian Species.* New York, NY: John Wiley & Sons; 1976:518. Copyright © 1976 John Wiley & Sons.)

D. Summary of Sources of Blood Glucose

Immediately after a meal, dietary carbohydrates serve as the major source of blood glucose (Fig. 28.17). As blood glucose levels return to the fasting range within 2 hours after a meal, glycogenolysis is stimulated and begins to supply glucose to the blood. Subsequently, glucose is also produced by gluconeogenesis.

During a 12-hour fast, glycogenolysis is the major source of blood glucose. Thus, it is the major pathway by which glucose is produced in the basal state (after a 12-hour fast). However, by approximately 16 hours of fasting, glycogenolysis and gluconeogenesis contribute equally to the maintenance of blood glucose.

By 30 hours after a meal, liver glycogen stores are substantially depleted. Subsequently, gluconeogenesis is the primary source of blood glucose.

The mechanisms that cause fats to be used as the major fuel and that allow blood glucose levels to be maintained during periods of food deprivation result in the conservation of body protein and, consequently, permit survival during prolonged fasting for periods often exceeding 1 month or more.

E. Blood Glucose Levels during Exercise

During exercise, mechanisms very similar to those that are used during fasting operate to maintain blood glucose levels. The liver maintains blood glucose levels through both glucagon- and epinephrine-induced glycogenolysis and gluconeogenesis. The use of fuels by muscle during exercise, including the uptake and use of blood glucose, is discussed in Chapter 45. Recall that muscle glycogen is not used to maintain blood glucose levels; muscle cells lack glucose 6-phosphatase, so glucose cannot be produced from glucose 6-P for export.

Otto S. is able to jog for 45 minutes before eating breakfast without developing symptoms of hypoglycemia, in spite of enhanced glucose use by skeletal muscle during exercise. He maintains his blood glucose level in an adequate range through hepatic glycogenolysis and gluconeogenesis.

CLINICAL COMMENTS

Al M. The chronic excessive ingestion of ethanol concurrent with a recent reduction in nutrient intake caused **Al M.'s** blood glucose level to decrease to 28 mg/dL. This degree of hypoglycemia caused the release of several "counterregulatory" hormones into the blood, including glucagon, growth hormone, cortisol, and epinephrine (adrenaline).

Some of the patient's signs and symptoms are primarily the result of an increase in adrenergic nervous system activity after a rapid decrease in blood glucose. The subsequent increase in epinephrine levels in the blood leads to tremulousness, excessive sweating, and rapid heart rate. Other manifestations arise when the brain has insufficient glucose, hence the term *neuroglycopenic symptoms*. Mr. M. was confused and combative, had slurred speech, and eventually had a grand mal seizure. If he was not treated quickly with intravenous glucose administration, Mr. M. might have lapsed into a coma. Permanent neurologic deficits and even death may result if severe hypoglycemia is not corrected in 6 to 10 hours.

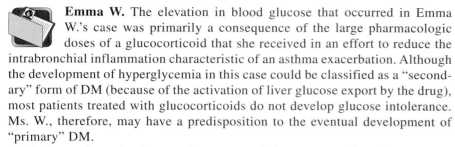 **Emma W.** The elevation in blood glucose that occurred in Emma W.'s case was primarily a consequence of the large pharmacologic doses of a glucocorticoid that she received in an effort to reduce the intrabronchial inflammation characteristic of an asthma exacerbation. Although the development of hyperglycemia in this case could be classified as a "secondary" form of DM (because of the activation of liver glucose export by the drug), most patients treated with glucocorticoids do not develop glucose intolerance. Ms. W., therefore, may have a predisposition to the eventual development of "primary" DM.

In hyperglycemia, increased amounts of glucose enter the urine, causing large amounts of water to be excreted. This "osmotic diuresis" is responsible for the increased volume of urine (polyuria) noted by the patient. Because of increased urinary water loss, the effective circulating blood volume is reduced. Therefore, less blood reaches volume-sensitive receptors in the central nervous system, which then trigger the sensation of thirst, causing increased drinking activity (polydipsia).

A diabetic diet and the tapering of her steroid dose over a period of several weeks gradually returned Ms. W.'s blood glucose level to the normal range.

Dianne A. and **Deborah S.** Chronically elevated levels of glucose in the blood may contribute to the development of the microvascular complications of DM, such as diabetic retinal damage, kidney damage, and nerve damage as well as macrovascular complications such as cerebrovascular, peripheral vascular, and coronary artery disease. The precise mechanism by which long-term hyperglycemia induces these vascular changes is not fully established.

One postulated mechanism proposes that nonenzymatic glycation (glycosylation) of proteins in vascular tissue alters the structure and functions of these proteins. A protein that is exposed to chronically increased levels of glucose will covalently bind glucose, a process called *glycation* or *glycosylation*. This process is not regulated by enzymes (see Chapter 9). These nonenzymatically glycated proteins slowly form cross-linked protein adducts (often called *advanced glycosylation end products*) within the microvasculature and macrovasculature.

By cross-linking vascular matrix proteins and plasma proteins, chronic hyperglycemia may cause narrowing of the luminal diameter of the microvessels in the retina (causing diabetic retinopathy), the renal glomeruli (causing diabetic nephropathy), and the microvessels supplying peripheral and autonomic nerve fibers (causing diabetic neuropathy). The same process has been postulated to accelerate atherosclerotic change in the macrovasculature, particularly in the brain (causing strokes), the coronary arteries (causing heart attacks), and the peripheral arteries (causing peripheral arterial insufficiency and possibly gangrene). The abnormal lipid metabolism associated with poorly controlled DM also may contribute to the accelerated atherosclerosis associated with this metabolic disorder (see Chapters 31 and 32).

The publication of the Diabetes Control and Complications Trial followed by the United Kingdom Prospective Diabetes Study were the first large human studies to show that maintaining long-term controlled blood glucose levels in patients with diabetes, such as **Dianne A.** and **Deborah S.** (who has type 2 diabetes), favorably affects the course of microvascular complications. More recent studies have confirmed this, and although it is thought that controlling blood sugar decreases macrovascular complications, this has been more difficult to demonstrate in human studies.

A

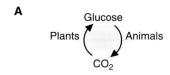

B

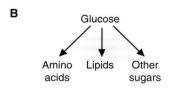

C

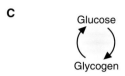

D

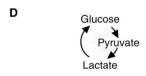

E

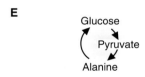

F

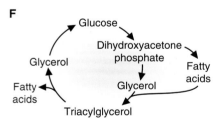

FIGURE 28.18 Recycling of glucose.

BIOCHEMICAL COMMENTS

Glucose Production. Plants are the ultimate source of Earth's supply of glucose. Plants produce glucose from atmospheric CO_2 by the process of photosynthesis (Fig. 28.18A). In contrast to plants, humans cannot synthesize glucose by the fixation of CO_2. Although we have a process called *gluconeogenesis*, the term may really be a misnomer. Glucose is not generated anew by gluconeogenesis; compounds produced from glucose are simply recycled to glucose. We obtain glucose from the plants, including bacteria, that we eat and, to some extent, from animals in our food supply. We use this glucose both as a fuel and as a source of carbon for the synthesis of fatty acids, amino acids, and other sugars (see Fig. 28.18B). We store glucose as glycogen, which, along with gluconeogenesis, provides glucose when needed for energy (see Fig. 28.18C).

Lactate, one of the carbon sources for gluconeogenesis, is actually produced from glucose by tissues that obtain energy by oxidizing glucose to pyruvate through glycolysis. The pyruvate is then reduced to lactate, released into the bloodstream, and reconverted to glucose by the process of gluconeogenesis in the liver. This process is known as the *Cori cycle* (Fig. 28.18D).

Carbons of alanine, another carbon source for gluconeogenesis, may be produced from glucose. In muscle, glucose is converted via glycolysis to pyruvate and transaminated to alanine. Alanine from muscle is recycled to glucose in the liver. This process is known as the *glucose–alanine cycle* (Fig. 28.18E). Glucose also may be used to produce nonessential amino acids other than alanine, which are subsequently reconverted to glucose in the liver by gluconeogenesis. Even the essential amino acids that we obtain from dietary proteins are synthesized in plants and bacteria using glucose as the major source of carbon. Therefore, all amino acids that are converted to glucose in humans, including the essential amino acids, were originally synthesized from glucose.

The production of glucose from glycerol, the third major source of carbon for gluconeogenesis, is also a recycling process. Glycerol is derived from glucose via the DHAP intermediate of glycolysis. Fatty acids are then esterified to the glycerol and stored as triacylglycerol. When these fatty acids are released from the triacylglycerol, the glycerol moiety can travel to the liver and be reconverted to glucose (see Fig. 28.18F).

KEY CONCEPTS

- The process of glucose production is termed gluconeogenesis. Gluconeogenesis occurs primarily in the liver.
- The major precursors for glucose production are lactate, glycerol, and amino acids.
- The gluconeogenic pathway uses the reversible reactions of glycolysis, plus additional reactions to bypass the irreversible steps.
  - Pyruvate carboxylase (pyruvate to oxaloacetate [OAA]) and phosphoenolpyruvate carboxykinase (PEPCK, OAA to phosphoenolpyruvate [PEP]) bypass the pyruvate kinase step.
  - Fructose 1,6-bisphosphatase (fructose 1,6-bisphosphate to fructose 6-phosphate) bypasses the phosphofructokinase-1 step.
  - Glucose 6-phosphatase (glucose 6-phosphate to glucose) bypasses the glucokinase step.
- Gluconeogenesis and glycogenolysis are carefully regulated so that blood glucose levels can be maintained at a constant level during fasting. The regulation of triglyceride metabolism is also linked to the regulation of blood glucose levels.
- Table 28.3 summarizes the diseases discussed in this chapter.

DISEASE OR DISORDER	ENVIRONMENTAL OR GENETIC	COMMENTS
Ethanol-induced hypoglycemia	Environmental	Ethanol, combined with poor nutrition, leads to hypoglycemia caused by excessive ethanol metabolism altering the NADH/NAD$^+$ ratio in the liver.
Asthma	Both	A treatment to reduce bronchoconstriction is inhalation/administration of glucocorticoids. Systemic treatments stimulate gluconeogenesis and can lead to hyperglycemia.
Insulin overdose	Environmental	Hypoglycemia as a result of insulin overdose caused by insulin stimulation of glucose transport into muscle and fat cells
Anorexia nervosa	Both	The use of ketone bodies as an alternative energy source during prolonged fasting preserves muscle protein because reduced levels of glucose are now required by the nervous system.
Weight loss	Environmental	Maintenance of blood glucose levels during dieting occurs because of glycogenolysis and gluconeogenesis.
Type I diabetes/ diabetic ketoacidosis	Environmental	Excessive production of ketone bodies in a person with type I diabetes whose insulin levels are too low, coupled with hyperglycemia; rarely observed in type 2 diabetes

TABLE 28.3 Diseases Discussed in Chapter 28

NAD, nicotinamide adenine dinucleotide.

REVIEW QUESTIONS—CHAPTER 28

1. A common intermediate in the conversion of glycerol and lactate to glucose is which one of the following?
   A. Pyruvate
   B. OAA
   C. Malate
   D. Glucose 6-phosphate
   E. PEP

2. A patient presented with a bacterial infection that produced an endotoxin that inhibits PEPCK. In this patient, then, under these conditions, glucose production from which one of the following precursors would be inhibited?
   A. Alanine
   B. Glycerol
   C. Even-chain-number fatty acids
   D. PEP
   E. Galactose

3. Which one of the following is most likely to occur in a normal individual after ingesting a high-carbohydrate meal?
   A. Only insulin levels decrease.
   B. Only insulin levels increase.
   C. Only glucagon levels increase.
   D. Both insulin and glucagon levels decrease.
   E. Both insulin and glucagon levels increase.

4. A patient arrives at the hospital in an ambulance. She is currently in a coma. Before lapsing into the coma, her symptoms included vomiting, dehydration, low blood pressure, and a rapid heartbeat. She also had relatively rapid respirations, resulting in more carbon dioxide being exhaled. These symptoms are consistent with which one of the following conditions?
   A. The patient lacks a pancreas.
   B. Ketoalkalosis
   C. Hypoglycemic coma
   D. DKA
   E. Insulin shock in a patient with diabetes

5. Assume that an individual had a glucagon-secreting pancreatic tumor (glucagonoma). Which one of the following is most likely to result from hyperglucagonemia?
   A. Weight loss
   B. Hypoglycemia
   C. Increased muscle protein synthesis
   D. Decreased lipolysis
   E. Increased liver glycolytic rate

6. A patient is rushed to the emergency department after a fainting episode. Blood glucose levels were extremely low; insulin levels were normal, but there was no detectable C-peptide. The cause of the fainting episode may be which one of the following?
   A. An insulin-producing tumor
   B. An overdose of insulin
   C. A glucagon-producing tumor
   D. An overdose of glucagon
   E. An overdose of epinephrine

7. A marathon runner reaches the last mile of the race but becomes dizzy, light-headed, and confused. These symptoms arise because of which one of the following?
   A. Enhanced induction of GLUT 4 transporters
   B. Reduced blood glucose levels for GLUT 2 transport
   C. Inhibition of GLUT 5 transporters
   D. Reduced blood glucose levels for GLUT 1 transport
   E. Lack of induction of GLUT 4 transporters

8. A patient went on a 3-day "cleansing" fast but did continue to consume water and vitamins. What is this patient's source of fuel to maintain blood glucose levels under these conditions?
   A. Fatty acids
   B. Glycerol
   C. Liver glycogen stores
   D. Muscle glycogen stores
   E. Ketone bodies

9. A patient with type 1 diabetes, who has forgotten to take insulin before a meal, will have difficulty assimilating blood glucose into which one of the following tissues?
   A. Brain
   B. Adipose
   C. Red blood cell
   D. Liver
   E. Intestine

10. A patient told her doctor that a friend told her that if she ate only carbohydrates and proteins and no fats, she would no longer store fats in adipose tissue. The doctor told the patient her friend was misinformed and then should further respond to this statement via which one of the following?
    A. Dietary glucose is converted into fatty acids but not glycerol by the liver.
    B. Dietary glucose is converted by the liver into fatty acids and glycerol.
    C. Dietary glucose is converted into glycerol but not fatty acids by the liver.
    D. Low-density lipoprotein transports the dietary converted products from the liver to the adipose tissue.
    E. Low-density lipoprotein transports the dietary converted products to the muscle tissue for oxidation.

ANSWERS

1. **The answer is D.** Glycerol is converted to glycerol 3-P, which is oxidized to form glyceraldehyde 3-P. The glyceraldehyde 3-P formed then follows the gluconeogenic pathway to glucose. Lactate is converted to pyruvate, which is then carboxylated to form OAA. The OAA is decarboxylated to form PEP and then run through gluconeogenesis to glucose. Because glycerol enters the gluconeogenic pathway at the glyceraldehyde 3-P step and lactate at the PEP step, the only compounds in common between these two starting points are the steps from glyceraldehyde 3-P to glucose. Of the choices listed in the question, only glucose 6-P is in that part of the pathway.

2. **The answer is A.** PEPCK converts OAA to PEP. In combination with pyruvate carboxylase, it is used to bypass the pyruvate kinase reaction. Thus, compounds that enter gluconeogenesis between PEP and OAA (such as lactate, alanine, or any TCA cycle intermediate) must use PEPCK to produce PEP. Glycerol enters gluconeogenesis as glyceraldehyde 3-P, bypassing the PEPCK step. Galactose is converted to glucose 1-phosphate, then glucose 6-P, also bypassing the PEPCK step. Even-chain fatty acids can only give rise to acetyl-CoA, which cannot be used to synthesize glucose.

3. **The answer is B.** High blood glucose levels signal the release of insulin from the pancreas; glucagon levels either stay the same or decrease slightly.

4. **The answer is D.** The hyperglycemia in an untreated diabetic creates osmotic diuresis, which means that excessive water is lost through urination. This can lead to a contraction of blood volume, leading to low blood pressure and a rapid heartbeat. It also leads to dehydration. The rapid respirations results from acidosis-induced stimulation of the respiratory center of the brain in order to reduce the amount of acid in the blood. Ketone bodies have accumulated, leading to DKA (thus, B is incorrect). A patient in a hypoglycemic coma (which can be caused by excessive insulin administration) does not exhibit dehydration, low blood pressure, or rapid respirations; in fact, the patient will sweat profusely as a result of epinephrine release (thus, C and E are incorrect). Answer A is incorrect because lack of a pancreas would be fatal.

5. **The answer is A.** The high levels of glucagon will antagonize the effects of insulin and will lead to hyperglycemia because glucagon stimulates glucose export from the liver by stimulating glycogenolysis and gluconeogenesis. Owing to the overriding effects of glucagon, blood glucose cannot enter muscle and fat cells, and fat oxidation is stimulated to provide energy for these tissues. This leads to a loss of stored triglyceride, which, in turn, leads to weight loss. Insulin is required to stimulate protein synthesis in muscles (glucagon does not have this effect), and glucagon

signals export of glucose from the liver, which means that the rate of glycolysis is suppressed in hepatic cells under these conditions. Glucagon also stimulates lipolysis in adipocytes to provide fatty acids as an energy source for muscle and liver.

6. **The answer is B.** The key to answering this question correctly relates to the absence of detectable C-peptide levels in the blood. An overproduction of insulin by the β-cells of the pancreas can lead to hypoglycemia severe enough to cause loss of consciousness, but because there was no detectable C-peptide in the blood, the loss of consciousness was most likely the result of the administration of exogenous insulin, which lacks the C-peptide (see Chapter 19). An overdose of glucagon (either through injection or from a glucagon-producing tumor), or epinephrine, would promote glucose release by the liver and not lead to hypoglycemia.

7. **The answer is D.** GLUT 1 is the carrier for glucose across the blood brain–barrier (as well as red blood cells). When blood glucose levels drop below the K_m for this transporter, then the nervous system does not receive sufficient glucose to keep functioning properly—hence, the signs of hypoglycemia. The GLUT 2 and GLUT 5 transporters are not responsible for glucose entry into the nervous system (the liver and pancreas use GLUT 2, whereas GLUT 5 primarily transports fructose, not glucose). GLUT 4 transporters are insulin-responsive transporters, expressed primarily in the muscle and fat cells. Altering the number of GLUT 4 transporters will not affect glucose entry into the nervous system.

8. **The answer is A.** During a fast, liver glycogen stores are exhausted after about 30 hours, so the only pathway through which the liver can produce glucose is via gluconeogenesis. Gluconeogenesis requires energy, which is provided by fatty acid oxidation. Glycerol is a substrate for gluconeogenesis, but it is not oxidized to provide energy for gluconeogenesis. Muscle glycogen stores can provide glucose 1-phosphate for use by the muscle, but the glucose produced from muscle glycogen cannot enter the blood to be used by any other tissue. The liver will produce ketone bodies from fatty acid oxidation, but the liver does not express the coenzyme A transferase needed to metabolize ketone bodies.

9. **The answer is B.** Insulin stimulates the transport of glucose into adipose and muscle cells by promoting the recruitment of GLUT 4 glucose transporters to the cell membrane. Liver, brain, intestine, and red blood cells have different types of glucose transporters that are not significantly affected by insulin.

10. **The answer is B.** The liver can convert dietary glucose into fatty acids and glycerol to produce triacetylglycerols, which are packaged into VLDL for transport to adipose tissue (for storage) or to the muscle for immediate oxidation if necessary. A low-fat diet, if excessive in overall calories, will lead to triglyceride formation and storage of the triglyceride in adipose tissue.

Lipid Metabolism

Most of the lipids found in the body fall into the categories of fatty acids and triacylglycerols; glycerophospholipids and sphingolipids; eicosanoids; cholesterol, bile salts, and steroid hormones; and fat-soluble vitamins. These lipids have very diverse chemical structures and functions. However, they are related by a common property: their relative insolubility in water.

Fatty acids are a major fuel in the body. After eating, we store excess fatty acids and carbohydrates that are not oxidized as fat (triacylglycerols) in adipose tissue. Between meals, these fatty acids are released and circulate in blood bound to albumin (Fig. V.1). In muscle, liver, and other tissues, fatty acids are oxidized to acetyl coenzyme A (acetyl-CoA) in the pathway of β-oxidation. Reduced nicotinamide adenine dinucleotide (NADH) and reduced flavin adenine dinucleotide (FAD[2H]) generated from β-oxidation are reoxidized by O_2 in the electron-transport chain, thereby generating adenosine triphosphate (ATP). Small amounts of certain fatty acids are oxidized through other pathways that convert them to either oxidizable fuels or urinary excretion products (e.g., peroxisomal β-oxidation).

Not all acetyl-CoA generated from β-oxidation enters the tricarboxylic acid (TCA) cycle. In the liver, acetyl-CoA generated from β-oxidation of fatty acids can also be converted to the ketone bodies acetoacetate and β-hydroxybutyrate. Ketone bodies are taken up by muscle and other tissues, which convert them back to acetyl-CoA for oxidation in the TCA cycle. They become a major fuel for the brain during prolonged fasting.

Glycerophospholipids and sphingolipids, which contain esterified fatty acids, are found in membranes and in blood lipoproteins at the interfaces between the lipid components of these structures and the surrounding water. These membrane lipids form hydrophobic barriers between subcellular compartments and between cellular constituents and the extracellular milieu. Polyunsaturated fatty acids containing 20 carbons form the eicosanoids, which regulate many cellular processes (Fig. V.2).

Cholesterol adds stability to the phospholipid bilayer of membranes. It serves as the precursor of the bile salts, detergentlike compounds that function in the process of lipid digestion and absorption (Fig. V.3). Cholesterol also serves as the precursor of the steroid hormones, which have many actions, including the regulation of metabolism, growth, and reproduction.

The fat-soluble vitamins are lipids that are involved in such varied functions as vision, growth, and differentiation (vitamin A); blood clotting (vitamin K); prevention of oxidative damage to cells (vitamin E); and calcium metabolism (vitamin D).

Triacylglycerols, the major dietary lipids, are digested in the lumen of the intestine (Fig. V.4). The initial digestive products, free fatty acids and 2-monoacylglycerol, are reconverted to triacylglycerols in intestinal epithelial cells, packaged in lipoproteins known as *chylomicrons* (so they can safely enter the circulation), and secreted into the lymph. Ultimately, chylomicrons enter the blood, serving as one of the major blood lipoproteins.

Very-low-density lipoprotein (VLDL) is produced in the liver, mainly from dietary carbohydrate. Lipogenesis is an insulin-stimulated process through which glucose is converted to fatty acids, which are subsequently esterified to glycerol to form the triacylglycerols that are packaged in VLDL and secreted from the liver. Thus, chylomicrons primarily transport dietary lipids, and VLDL transports endogenously synthesized lipids.

The triacylglycerols of chylomicrons and VLDL are digested by lipoprotein lipase (LPL), an enzyme found attached to capillary endothelial cells (see Fig. V.4).

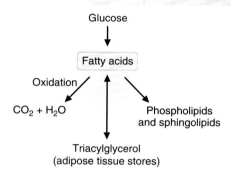

FIGURE V.1 Summary of fatty acid metabolism.

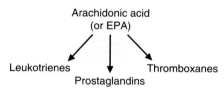

FIGURE V.2 Summary of eicosanoid synthesis. *EPA*, eicosapentaenoic acid.

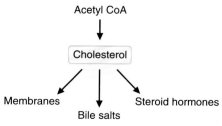

FIGURE V.3 Summary of cholesterol metabolism.

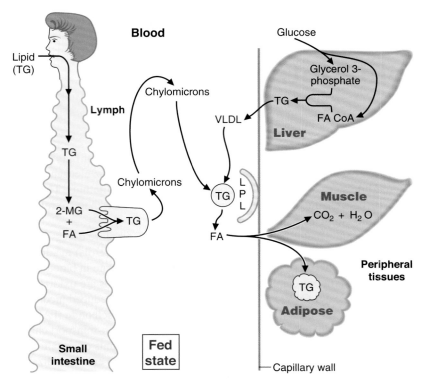

FIGURE V.4 Overview of triacylglycerol metabolism in the fed state. *CoA*, coenzyme A; *TG*, triacylglycerol; *2-MG*, 2-monoacylglycerol; *FA*, fatty acid; *VLDL*, very-low-density lipoprotein; *circled TG*, triacylglycerols of VLDL and chylomicrons; *LPL*, lipoprotein lipase.

The fatty acids that are released are taken up by muscle and many other tissues and are oxidized to CO_2 and water to produce energy. After a meal, these fatty acids are taken up by adipose tissue and stored as triacylglycerols.

LPL converts chylomicrons to chylomicron remnants and VLDL to intermediate-density lipoprotein (IDL). These products, which have a relatively low triacylglycerol content, are taken up by the liver by the process of endocytosis and degraded by lysosomal action. IDL may also be converted to low-density lipoprotein (LDL) by further digestion of triacylglycerol. Endocytosis of LDL occurs in peripheral tissues as well as the liver (Table V.1) and is the major means of cholesterol transport and delivery to peripheral tissues.

TABLE V.1   **Blood Lipoproteins**
Chylomicrons • Produced in intestinal epithelial cells from dietary fat • Carry triacylglycerol in blood
Very-low-density lipoprotein (VLDL) • Produced in liver, mainly from dietary carbohydrate • Carries triacylglycerol in blood
Intermediate-density lipoprotein (IDL) • Produced in blood (remnant of VLDL after triacylglycerol digestion) • Endocytosed by liver or converted to low-density lipoprotein
Low-density lipoprotein (LDL) • Produced in blood (remnant of IDL after triacylglycerol digestion; end product of VLDL) • Contains high concentration of cholesterol and cholesterol esters • Endocytosed by liver and peripheral tissues
High-density lipoprotein (HDL) • Produced in liver and intestine • Exchanges proteins and lipids with other lipoproteins • Functions in the return of cholesterol from peripheral tissues to the liver

The principal function of high-density lipoprotein (HDL) is to transport excess cholesterol obtained from peripheral tissues to the liver and to exchange proteins and lipids with chylomicrons and VLDL. The protein exchange converts "nascent" particles to "mature" particles.

During fasting, fatty acids and glycerol are released from adipose triacylglycerol stores (Fig. V.5). The glycerol travels to the liver and is used for gluconeogenesis. Only the liver contains glycerol kinase, which is required for glycerol metabolism. The fatty acids form complexes with albumin in the blood and are taken up by muscle, kidney, and other tissues, where ATP is generated by their oxidation to CO_2 and water. Liver also converts some of the carbon to ketone bodies, which are released into the blood. Ketone bodies are oxidized for energy in muscle, kidney, and other tissues during fasting, and in the brain during prolonged starvation.

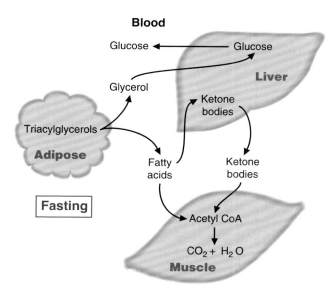

FIGURE V.5   Overview of triacylglycerol metabolism during fasting. *Acetyl CoA*, acetyl coenzyme A.

29

Digestion and Transport of Dietary Lipids

Triacylglycerols are the major fat in the human diet, consisting of three **fatty acids** esterified to a **glycerol** backbone. Limited digestion of these lipids occurs in the mouth (**lingual lipase**) and stomach (**gastric lipase**) because of the low solubility of the substrate. In the intestine, however, the fats are emulsified by **bile salts** that are released from the gallbladder. This increases the available surface area of the lipids for **pancreatic lipase and colipase** to bind and to digest the triglycerides. Degradation products are **free fatty acids** and **2-monoacylglycerol**. When partially digested food enters the intestine, the hormone **cholecystokinin** is secreted by the intestine, which signals the gallbladder to contract and release bile acids, and the pancreas to release digestive enzymes.

In addition to triacylglycerols, phospholipids, cholesterol, and cholesterol esters (cholesterol esterified to fatty acids) are present in the foods we eat. Phospholipids are hydrolyzed in the intestinal lumen by **phospholipase A2**, and cholesterol esters are hydrolyzed by **cholesterol esterase**. Both of these enzymes are secreted from the pancreas.

The products of enzymatic digestion (free fatty acids, glycerol, **lysophospholipids**, cholesterol) form **micelles** with bile acids in the intestinal lumen. The micelles interact with the enterocyte membrane and allow diffusion of the lipid-soluble components across the enterocyte membrane into the cell. The bile acids, however, do not enter the enterocyte at this time. They remain in the intestinal lumen, travel farther down, and are then reabsorbed and sent back to the liver by the **enterohepatic circulation**. This allows the bile salts to be used multiple times in fat digestion.

The intestinal epithelial cells resynthesize triacylglycerol from free fatty acids and 2-monacylglycerol and package them with a protein, **apolipoprotein B-48**, phospholipids, and cholesterol esters into a soluble **lipoprotein particle** known as a **chylomicron**. The chylomicrons are secreted into the **lymph** and eventually end up in the circulation, where they can distribute dietary lipids to all tissues of the body.

Once they are in the circulation, the newly released ("nascent") chylomicrons interact with another lipoprotein particle, **high-density lipoprotein (HDL)**, and acquire two **apolipoproteins** from HDL, **apolipoprotein CII (apoCII)** and **apolipoprotein E (apoE)**. This converts the nascent chylomicron to a "mature" chylomicron. The apoCII on the mature chylomicron activates the enzyme **lipoprotein lipase (LPL)**, which is located on the inner surface of the capillary endothelial cells of muscle and adipose tissue. The LPL digests the triglyceride in the chylomicron, producing free fatty acids and glycerol. The fatty acids enter the adjacent organs either for energy production (muscle) or fat storage (adipocyte). The glycerol that is released is metabolized in the liver.

As the chylomicron loses triglyceride, its density increases and it becomes a **chylomicron remnant**, which is taken up by the liver by receptors that recognize apoE. In the liver, the chylomicron remnant is degraded into its component parts for further disposition by the liver.

The lymph system is a network of vessels that surround interstitial cavities in the body. Cells secrete various compounds into the lymph, and the lymph vessels transport these fluids away from the interstitial spaces in the body tissues and into the bloodstream. In the case of the intestinal lymph system, the lymph enters the bloodstream through the thoracic duct. These vessels are designed so that under normal conditions, the contents of the blood cannot enter the lymphatic system. The lymph fluid is similar in composition to that of the blood but lacks the cells found in blood.

THE WAITING ROOM

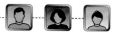

Will S. has had several episodes of mild back and lower extremity pain over the last year, probably caused by minor sickle cell crises. He then developed abdominal pain in the right upper quadrant. He states that the pain is not like his usual crisis pain. Intractable vomiting began 12 hours after the onset of these new symptoms, and he then went to the emergency department.

On physical examination, his body temperature is slightly elevated and his heart rate is rapid. The whites of his eyes (the sclerae) are slightly jaundiced (or icteric, a yellow discoloration caused by the accumulation of bilirubin pigment). He is exquisitely tender to pressure over his right upper abdomen.

The emergency department physician suspects that Will is not in sickle cell crisis but instead has acute cholecystitis (gallbladder inflammation). His hemoglobin level is low, at 7.6 mg/dL (reference range, 12 to 16 mg/dL), but is unchanged from his baseline 3 months earlier. His serum total bilirubin level is 2.3 mg/dL (reference range, 0.2 to 1.0 mg/dL), and his direct (conjugated) bilirubin level is 0.9 mg/dL (reference range, 0 to 0.2 mg/dL).

Intravenous fluids were started, he was not allowed to take anything by mouth, and symptomatic therapy was started for pain and nausea. He was sent for an ultrasonographic (ultrasound) study of his upper abdomen.

Al M. has continued to abuse alcohol and to eat poorly. After a particularly heavy intake of vodka, a steady severe pain began in his upper midabdomen. This pain spread to the left upper quadrant and eventually radiated to his midback. He began vomiting nonbloody material and was brought to the hospital emergency department with fever, a rapid heartbeat, and a mild reduction in blood pressure. On physical examination, he was dehydrated and tender to pressure over the upper abdomen. His vomitus and stool were both negative for occult blood.

Blood samples were sent to the laboratory for a variety of hematologic and chemical tests, including a measurement of serum lipase, one of the digestive enzymes that is normally secreted from the exocrine pancreas through the pancreatic ducts into the lumen of the small intestine.

I. Digestion of Triacylglycerols

Triacylglycerols are the major fat in the human diet because they are the major storage lipid in the plants and animals that constitute our food supply. Triacylglycerols contain a glycerol backbone to which three fatty acids are esterified (Fig. 29.1). The main route for digestion of triacylglycerols involves hydrolysis to fatty acids and 2-monoacylglycerol in the lumen of the intestine. However, the route depends to some extent on the chain length of the fatty acids. Lingual and gastric *lipases* are produced by cells at the back of the tongue and in the stomach, respectively. These lipases preferentially hydrolyze short- and medium-chain fatty acids (containing 12 or fewer carbon atoms) from dietary triacylglycerols. Therefore, they are most active in infants and young children who drink relatively large quantities of cow's milk, which contains triacylglycerols with a high percentage of short- and medium-chain fatty acids.

 Amylase is produced only in the salivary glands and the acinar cells of the pancreas, whereas lipase is produced only in the pancreas. An elevated serum amylase, coupled with an elevated lipase, was used to diagnose pancreatitis in the past, but only serum lipase is used currently. Serum lipase levels increase at the same rate as do serum amylase levels, but they stay elevated longer and are more specific for pancreatitis than are serum amylase levels. For example, salivary gland lesions, such as mumps, can also increase serum amylase levels. The assay for serum lipase is more difficult than that for amylase (and has been more difficult to automate for the clinical laboratory), but currently, several assays can be performed to determine lipase levels. Two such assays will be described here. The first involves incubating the serum sample with a known amount of triglyceride. The serum lipase will generate two free fatty acids and one 2-monoacylglycerol for each triglyceride. Monoacylglycerol lipase is then added (to convert the 2-monoacylglycerol to free glycerol), as is glycerol kinase (to convert glycerol to glycerol 3-phosphate) and glycerol 3-phosphate oxidase (which converts molecular oxygen and glycerol 3-phosphate to dihydroxyacetone phosphate and hydrogen peroxide). The H_2O_2 generated can be determined colorimetrically using an appropriate chromogen and horseradish peroxidase. The amount of glycerol produced is dependent on the lipase activity. A second assay for lipase is turbidimetric (based on light-scattering). The triglyceride sample does not easily go into solution; thus, when the assay is started, the solution is cloudy (turbid). As the lipase hydrolyzes the fatty acids from the triacylglycerol, the turbidity decreases, and this can be measured and compared to a standard curve generated with known lipase amounts.

 Currently, 38% of the calories (kilocalories) in the typical American diet come from fat. The content of fat in the diet increased from the early 1900s until the 1960s and then it decreased as we became aware of the unhealthy effects of a high-fat diet. According to current recommendations, fat should provide no more than 30% of the total calories of a healthy diet.

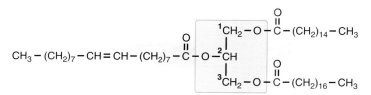

FIGURE 29.1 Structure of a triacylglycerol. The glycerol moiety is *highlighted*, and its carbons are *numbered*.

The mammary gland produces milk, which is the major source of nutrients for the breastfed human infant. The fatty acid composition of human milk varies, depending on the diet of the mother. However, long-chain fatty acids predominate, particularly palmitic, oleic, and linoleic acids. Although the amount of fat contained in human milk and cow's milk is similar, cow's milk contains more short- and medium-chain fatty acids and does not contain the long-chain polyunsaturated fatty acids found in human milk that are important in brain development.

Although the concentrations of pancreatic lipase and bile salts are low in the intestinal lumen of the newborn infant, the fat of human milk is still readily absorbed. This is true because lingual and gastric lipases produced by the infant partially compensate for the lower levels of pancreatic lipase. The human mammary gland also produces lipases that enter the milk. One of these lipases, which requires lower levels of bile salts than pancreatic lipase, is not inactivated by stomach acid and functions in the intestine for several hours.

A. Action of Bile Salts

Dietary fat leaves the stomach and enters the small intestine, where it is emulsified (suspended in small particles in the aqueous environment) by bile salts (Fig. 29.2). The bile salts are amphipathic compounds (containing both hydrophobic and hydrophilic components), synthesized in the liver (see Chapter 32 for the pathway) and secreted via the gallbladder into the intestinal lumen. The contraction of the gallbladder and secretion of pancreatic enzymes are stimulated by the gut hormone *cholecystokinin*, which is secreted by the intestinal cells when stomach contents enter the intestine. Bile salts act as detergents, binding to the globules of dietary fat as they are broken up by the peristaltic action of the intestinal muscle. This emulsified fat, which has an increased surface area compared with unemulsified fat, is attacked by digestive enzymes from the pancreas (Fig. 29.3).

B. Action of Pancreatic Lipase

The major enzyme that digests dietary triacylglycerols is a lipase produced in the pancreas. *Pancreatic lipase* is secreted along with another protein, *colipase*, in response to the release of cholecystokinin from the intestine. The peptide hormone *secretin* is also released by the small intestine in response to acidic materials (such as the partially digested materials from the stomach, which contains hydrochloric

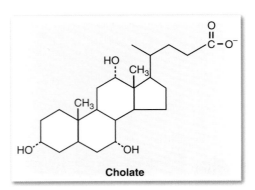

FIGURE 29.2 Structure of a bile salt. The bile salts are derived from cholesterol and retain the cholesterol ring structure. They differ from cholesterol in that the rings in bile salts contain more hydroxyl groups and a polar side chain and lack a C5–C6 double bond.

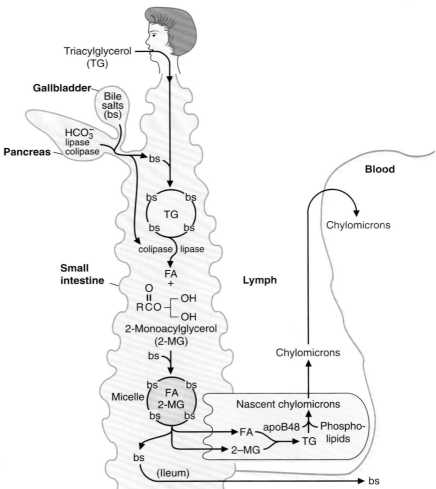

FIGURE 29.3 Digestion of triacylglycerols in the intestinal lumen. Prior to reaching the intestine, lingual lipase (mouth) and gastric lipase (stomach) have begun digestion of the triacylglycerol. *FA*, fatty acid.

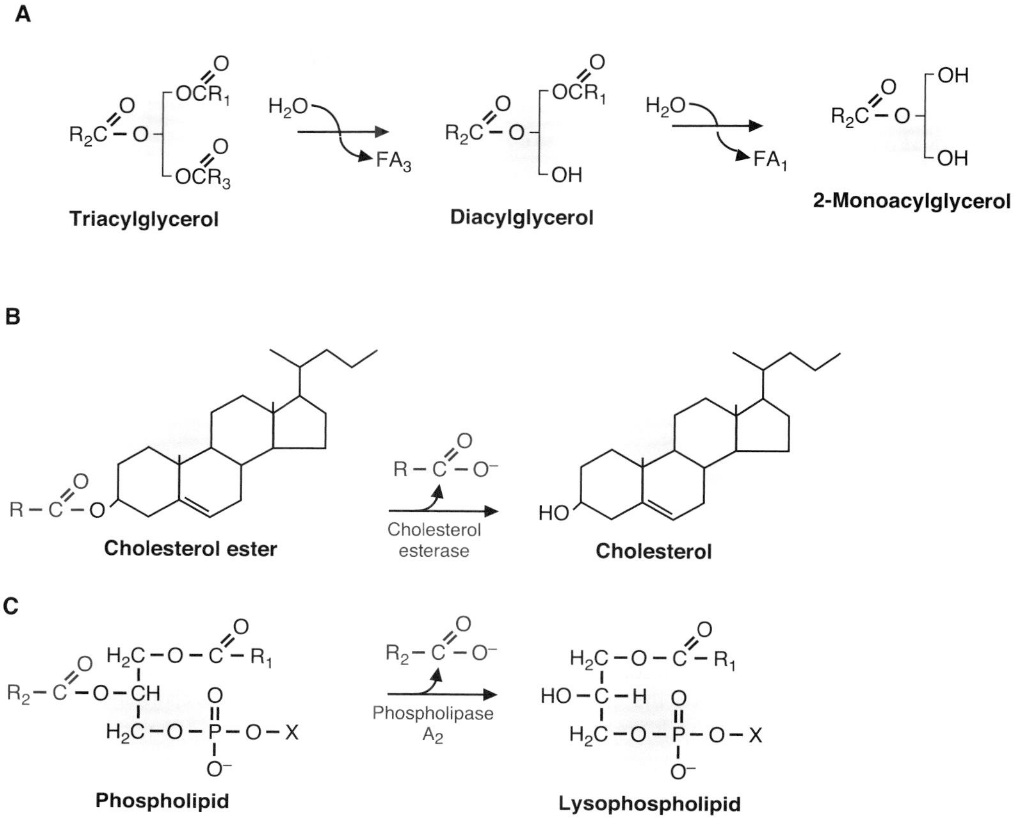

A

Triacylglycerol   **Diacylglycerol**   **2-Monoacylglycerol**

B

Cholesterol ester   Cholesterol
                              esterase   **Cholesterol**

C

Phospholipid   Phospholipase
                        A₂   **Lysophospholipid**

FIGURE 29.4   Action of pancreatic enzymes on fatty acid digestion. **A.** Action of pancreatic lipase. Fatty acids (FA) are cleaved from positions 1 and 3 of the triacylglycerol, and a monoacylglycerol with a fatty acid at position 2 is produced. **B.** Action of pancreatic cholesterol esterase. **C.** Action of phospholipase A2.

acid [HCl]) entering the duodenum. Secretin signals the liver, pancreas, and certain intestinal cells to secrete bicarbonate. Bicarbonate raises the pH of the contents of the intestinal lumen into a range (pH ~6) that is optimal for the action of all of the digestive enzymes of the intestine.

Bile salts inhibit pancreatic lipase activity by coating the substrate and not allowing the enzyme access to it. The colipase binds to the dietary fat and to the lipase, relieving the bile salt inhibition and allowing triglyceride to enter the active site of the lipase. This enhances lipase activity. Pancreatic lipase hydrolyzes fatty acids of all chain lengths from positions 1 and 3 of the glycerol moiety of the triacylglycerol, producing free fatty acids and 2-monoacylglycerol—that is, glycerol with a fatty acid esterified at position 2 (Fig. 29.4). The pancreas also produces *esterases* that remove fatty acids from compounds (such as cholesterol esters) and *phospholipase A₂* (which is released in its zymogen form and is activated by trypsin) that digests phospholipids to a free fatty acid and a lysophospholipid (see Fig. 29.4B and C).

II. Absorption of Dietary Lipids

The fatty acids and 2-monoacylglycerols produced by digestion are packaged into *micelles*, tiny microdroplets that are emulsified by bile salts (see Fig. 29.3). For bile salt micelles to form, the concentration of bile salts in the intestinal lumen must reach 5 to 15 mM (the critical micelle concentration [CMC]). Below this concentration, the bile salts are soluble; above it, micelles will form. Other dietary lipids, such as cholesterol, lysophospholipids, and fat-soluble vitamins, are also packaged in micelles. The micelles travel through a layer of water (the unstirred water layer) to

Al M.'s serum levels of pancreatic lipase were elevated—a finding consistent with a diagnosis of acute pancreatitis. The elevated level of this enzyme in the blood is the result of its escape from the inflamed exocrine cells of the pancreas into the surrounding pancreatic veins. The cause of the inflammatory pancreatic process in this case was related to the toxic effect of acute and chronic excessive alcohol ingestion.

In patients such as **Will S.** who have severe and recurrent episodes of increased red blood cell destruction (hemolytic anemia), greater than normal amounts of the red-cell pigment heme must be processed by the liver and spleen. In these organs, heme (derived from hemoglobin) is degraded to bilirubin, which is excreted by the liver in the bile.

If large quantities of bilirubin are presented to the liver as a consequence of acute hemolysis, the capacity of the liver to conjugate it—that is, convert it to the water-soluble bilirubin diglucuronide—can be overwhelmed. As a result, a greater percentage of the bilirubin entering the hepatic biliary ducts in patients with hemolysis is in the less water-soluble forms. In the gallbladder, these relatively insoluble particles tend to precipitate as gallstones that are rich in calcium bilirubinate. In some patients, one or more stones may leave the gallbladder through the cystic duct and enter the common bile duct. Most pass harmlessly into the small intestine and are later excreted in the stool. Larger stones, however, may become entrapped in the lumen of the cystic or common bile duct, where they cause varying degrees of obstruction to bile flow (cholestasis) with associated ductal spasm, producing pain. If adequate amounts of bile salts do not enter the intestinal lumen, dietary fats cannot readily be emulsified and digested.

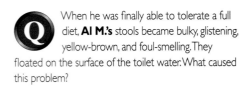

When he was finally able to tolerate a full diet, **Al M.'s** stools became bulky, glistening, yellow-brown, and foul-smelling. They floated on the surface of the toilet water. What caused this problem?

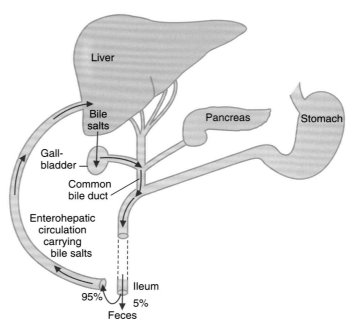

FIGURE 29.5 Recycling of bile salts. Bile salts are synthesized in the liver, stored in the gallbladder, secreted into the small intestine, resorbed in the ileum, and returned to the liver via the enterohepatic circulation. Under normal circumstances, 5% or less of luminal bile acids are excreted in the stool.

the microvilli on the surface of the intestinal epithelial cells, where the fatty acids, 2-monoacylglycerols, and other dietary lipids are absorbed, but the bile salts are left behind in the lumen of the gut.

The bile salts are extensively resorbed when they reach the ileum. Greater than 95% of the bile salts are recirculated, traveling through the enterohepatic circulation to the liver, which secretes them into the bile for storage in the gallbladder and ejection into the intestinal lumen during another digestive cycle (Fig. 29.5).

Short- and medium-chain fatty acids (C4 to C12) do not require bile salts for their absorption. They are absorbed directly into intestinal epithelial cells. Because they do not need to be packaged to increase their solubility, they enter the portal blood (rather than the lymph) and are transported to the liver bound to serum albumin.

III. Synthesis of Chylomicrons

Within the intestinal epithelial cells, the fatty acids and 2-monoacylglycerols are condensed by enzymatic reactions in the smooth endoplasmic reticulum (ER) to form triacylglycerols. The fatty acids are activated to fatty acyl coenzyme A (fatty acyl-CoA) by the same process used for activation of fatty acids before β-oxidation (see Chapter 30). A fatty acyl-CoA then reacts with 2-monoacylglycerol to form diacylglycerol, which reacts with another fatty acyl-CoA to form triacylglycerol (Fig. 29.6). The reactions for triacylglycerol synthesis in intestinal cells differ from those in liver and adipose cells in that 2-monoacylglycerol is an intermediate in triacylglycerol synthesis in intestinal cells, whereas phosphatidic acid is the necessary intermediate in other tissues.

Triacylglycerols, owing to their insolubility in water, are packaged in lipoprotein particles. If triacylglycerols entered the blood directly, they would coalesce, impeding blood flow. Intestinal cells package triacylglycerols together with proteins and phospholipids in *chylomicrons*, which are lipoprotein particles that do not readily coalesce in aqueous solutions (Fig. 29.7). Chylomicrons also contain

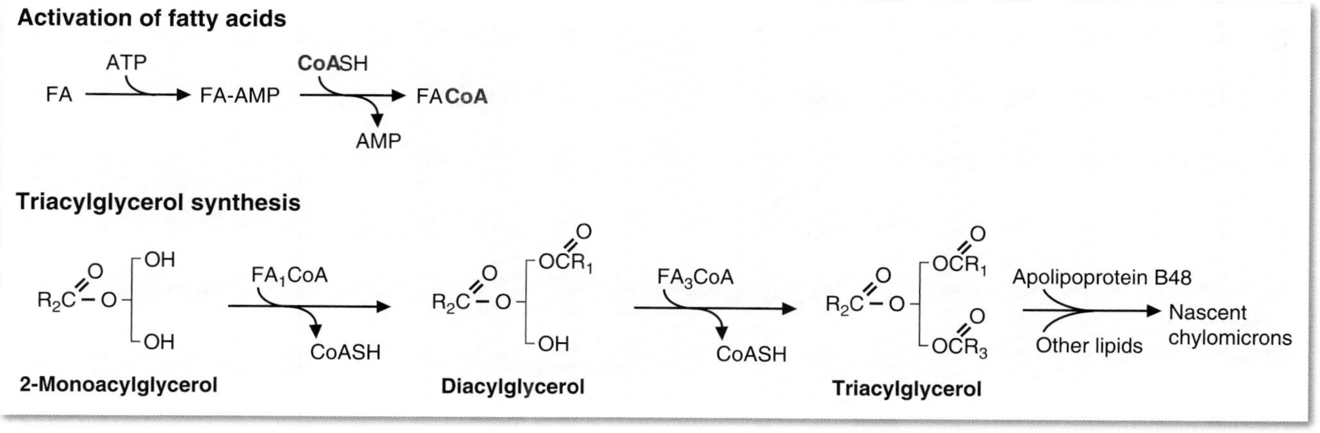

Activation of fatty acids

Triacylglycerol synthesis

FIGURE 29.6   Resynthesis of triacylglycerols in intestinal epithelial cells. Fatty acids (FA), produced by digestion, are activated in intestinal epithelial cells and then esterified to the 2-monoacylglycerol produced by digestion. The triacylglycerols are packaged in nascent chylomicrons and secreted into the lymph. *AMP*, adenosine monophosphate; *ATP*, adenosine triphosphate; *CoA*, coenzyme A.

cholesterol and fat-soluble vitamins, but their major component is triglyceride derived from the diet (Fig. 29.8). The protein constituents of the lipoproteins are known as *apolipoproteins*.

The major apolipoprotein associated with chylomicrons as they leave the intestinal cells is B-48. The B-48 apolipoprotein is structurally and genetically related to the B-100 apolipoprotein synthesized in the liver that serves as a major protein of another lipid carrier, *very-low-density lipoprotein* (VLDL). These two apolipoproteins are encoded by the same gene. In the intestine, the primary transcript of this gene undergoes RNA editing (Fig. 29.9, and see Chapter 15). A stop codon is generated that causes a protein to be produced in the intestine that is 48% of the size of the protein produced in the liver; hence, the designations *B-48* and *B-100*.

The protein component of the lipoproteins is synthesized on the rough ER. Lipids, which are synthesized in the smooth ER, are complexed with the proteins to form the chylomicrons.

Because the fat-soluble vitamins (A, D, E, and K) are absorbed from micelles along with the long-chain fatty acids and 2-monoacylglycerols, prolonged obstruction of the duct that carries exocrine secretions from the pancreas and the gallbladder into the intestine (via the common duct) could lead to a deficiency of these metabolically important substances.

Al M.'s stool changes are characteristic of steatorrhea (fat-laden stools caused by malabsorption of dietary fats), in this case caused by a lack of pancreatic secretions, particularly pancreatic lipase, which normally digests dietary fat. Steatorrhea also may be caused by insufficient production or secretion of bile salts. Therefore, **Will S.** might also develop this condition.

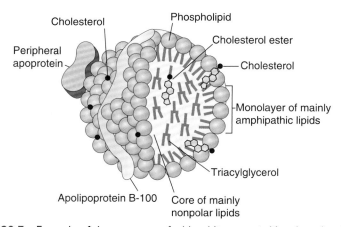

FIGURE 29.7   Example of the structure of a blood lipoprotein. Very-low-density lipoprotein (VLDL) is depicted. Lipoproteins contain phospholipids and proteins on the surface, with their hydrophilic regions interacting with water. Hydrophobic molecules are in the interior of the lipoprotein. The hydroxyl group of cholesterol is near the surface. In cholesterol esters, the hydroxyl group is esterified to a fatty acid. Cholesterol esters are found in the interior of lipoproteins and are synthesized by reaction of cholesterol with an activated fatty acid (see Chapter 32).

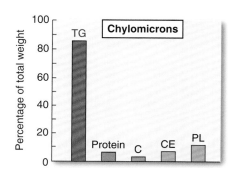

FIGURE 29.8   Composition of a typical chylomicron. Although the composition varies to some extent, the major component is triacylglycerol (TG). *C*, cholesterol; *CE*, cholesterol ester; *PL*, phospholipid.

Olestra is an artificial fat substitute designed to allow individuals to obtain the taste and food consistency of fat without the calories from fat. The structure of Olestra is shown below and consists of a sucrose molecule to which fatty acids are esterified to the hydroxyl groups.

Olestra = octa-acyl sucrose
R = fatty acyl group

The fatty acids attached to sucrose are resistant to hydrolysis by pancreatic lipase, so Olestra passes through the intestine intact and is eliminated in the feces. As a result, no useful calories can be obtained through the metabolism of Olestra, although in the mouth, the sucrose portion of the molecule imparts a sweet taste. In addition, because Olestra has the ability to pass through the digestive system unimpeded, it can also carry with it essential fat-soluble vitamins. Therefore, foods prepared with Olestra are supplemented with these vitamins. Unfortunately, the side effects of cramping and diarrhea decreased the popularity of Olestra as a food additive.

Because of their high triacylglycerol content, chylomicrons are the least dense of the blood lipoproteins. When blood is collected from patients with certain types of hyperlipoproteinemias (high concentrations of lipoproteins in the blood) in which chylomicron levels are elevated, and the blood is allowed to stand in the refrigerator overnight, the chylomicrons float to the top of the liquid and coalesce, forming a creamy layer.

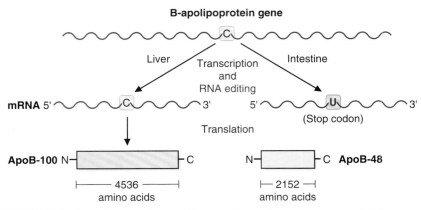

FIGURE 29.9 B apolipoprotein gene. The gene, located on chromosome 2, is transcribed and translated in liver to produce apoB-100, which is 4,536 amino acids in length (one of the longest single-polypeptide chains). In intestinal cells, RNA editing converts a cytosine (C) to a uracil (U) via deamination, producing a stop codon. Consequently, the B apolipoprotein of intestinal cells (apoB-48) contains only 2,152 amino acids. ApoB-48 is 48% of the size of apoB-100. *mRNA*, messenger RNA.

IV. Transport of Dietary Lipids in the Blood

By the process of exocytosis, nascent chylomicrons are secreted by the intestinal epithelial cells into the chyle of the lymphatic system and enter the blood through the thoracic duct. Nascent chylomicrons begin to enter the blood within 1 to 2 hours after the start of a meal; as the meal is digested and absorbed, they continue to enter the blood for many hours. Initially, the particles are called nascent (newborn) chylomicrons. As they accept proteins from *HDL* within the lymph and the blood, they become "mature" chylomicrons. HDL is the lipoprotein particle with the highest concentration of proteins, and lowest concentration of triacylglycerol (see Chapter 32 for further discussion of HDL and other lipoprotein particles found in the body).

HDL transfers proteins to the nascent chylomicrons, particularly apoE and apoCII (Fig. 29.10). ApoE is recognized by membrane receptors, particularly those on the surface of liver cells, allowing apoE-bearing lipoproteins to enter these cells by endocytosis for subsequent digestion by lysosomes. ApoCII acts as

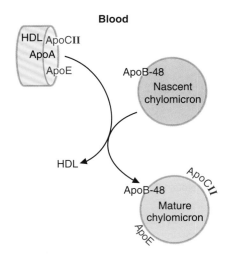

FIGURE 29.10 Transfer of proteins from high-density lipoprotein (HDL) to chylomicrons. Newly synthesized chylomicrons (nascent chylomicrons) mature as they receive apolipoproteins CII and E from HDL. HDL functions in the transfer of these apolipoproteins and also in transfer of cholesterol from peripheral tissues to the liver (see Table V.1 in the introduction to Section V).

an activator of *LPL*, the enzyme on capillary endothelial cells, primarily within muscle and adipose tissue, that digests the triacylglycerols of the chylomicrons and VLDL in the blood.

V. Fate of Chylomicrons

The triacylglycerols of the chylomicrons are digested by LPL attached to the proteoglycans in the basement membranes of endothelial cells that line the capillary walls (Fig. 29.11). LPL is produced by adipose cells, muscle cells (particularly cardiac muscle), and cells of the lactating mammary gland. The isozyme synthesized in adipose cells has a higher K_m than the isozyme synthesized in muscle cells. Therefore, adipose LPL is more active after a meal, when chylomicrons levels are elevated in the blood. Insulin stimulates the synthesis and secretion of adipose LPL, so that after a meal, when triglyceride levels increase in circulation, LPL has been upregulated (through insulin release) to facilitate the hydrolysis of fatty acids from the triglyceride.

The fatty acids released from triacylglycerols by LPL are not very soluble in water. They become soluble in blood by forming complexes with the protein albumin. The major fate of the fatty acids is storage as triacylglycerol in adipose tissue. However, these fatty acids also may be oxidized for energy in muscle and other tissues (see Fig. 29.11). The LPL in the capillaries of muscle cells has a lower K_m than adipose LPL. Thus, muscle cells can obtain fatty acids from blood lipoproteins whenever they are needed for energy, even if the concentration of the lipoproteins is low.

The glycerol released from chylomicron triacylglycerols by LPL may be used for triacylglycerol synthesis in the liver in the fed state.

The portion of a chylomicron that remains in the blood after LPL action is known as a *chylomicron remnant*. The remnant has lost many of the apoCII molecules bound to the mature chylomicron, which exposes apoE. This remnant binds to receptors on hepatocytes (the major cells of the liver), which recognize apoE, and is

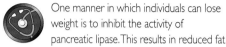 One manner in which individuals can lose weight is to inhibit the activity of pancreatic lipase. This results in reduced fat digestion and absorption and a reduced caloric yield from the diet. The drug orlistat is a chemically synthesized derivative of lipostatin, a natural lipase inhibitor found in certain bacteria. The drug works in the intestinal lumen and forms a covalent bond with the active-site serine residues of both gastric and pancreatic lipase, thereby inhibiting their activities. Nondigested triglycerides are not absorbed by the intestine and are eliminated in the feces. Under normal use of the drug, approximately 30% of dietary fat absorption is inhibited. Because excessive nondigested fat in the intestines can lead to gastrointestinal distress related to excessive intestinal gas formation, individuals who take this drug need to follow a diet with reduced daily intake of fat, which should be evenly distributed among the meals of the day.

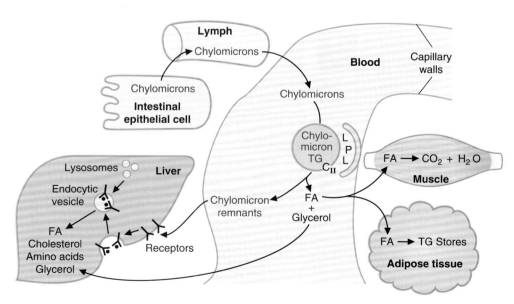

FIGURE 29.11 Fate of chylomicrons. Nascent chylomicrons are synthesized in intestinal epithelial cells, secreted into the lymph, pass into the blood, and become mature chylomicrons (see Fig. 29.10). On capillary walls in adipose tissue and muscle, lipoprotein lipase (LPL) activated by apoCII digests the triacylglycerols (TG) of chylomicrons to fatty acids and glycerol. Fatty acids (FA) are oxidized in muscle or stored in adipose cells as triacylglycerols. The remnants of the chylomicrons are taken up by the liver by receptor-mediated endocytosis (through recognition of apoE on the remnant). Lysosomal enzymes within the hepatocyte digest the remnants, releasing the products into the cytosol.

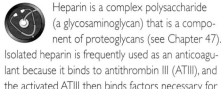

Heparin is a complex polysaccharide (a glycosaminoglycan) that is a component of proteoglycans (see Chapter 47). Isolated heparin is frequently used as an anticoagulant because it binds to antithrombin III (ATIII), and the activated ATIII then binds factors necessary for clotting and inhibits them from working. As LPL is bound to the capillary endothelium through binding to proteoglycans, heparin also can bind to LPL and dislodge it from the capillary wall. This leads to loss of LPL activity and an increase of triglyceride content in the blood.

taken up by the process of endocytosis. Lysosomes fuse with the endocytic vesicles, and the chylomicron remnants are degraded by lysosomal enzymes. The products of lysosomal digestion (e.g., fatty acids, amino acids, glycerol, cholesterol, phosphate) can be reused by the cell.

CLINICAL COMMENTS

Will S. The upper abdominal ultrasound study showed a large gallstone lodged in **Will S.'s** cystic duct, with dilation of this duct proximal to the stone. Intravenous fluids were continued, he was not allowed to take anything by mouth, antibiotics were started, and he was scheduled for a cholecystectomy.

Gallstones can also obstruct the common bile duct, which can cause bilirubin to flow back into the venous blood draining from the liver. As a consequence, serum bilirubin levels, particularly the direct (conjugated) fraction, increase. Tissues such as the sclerae of the eye take up this pigment, which causes them to become yellow (jaundiced, icteric). You can also see inflammation from a cystic duct obstruction and cholecystitis causing some obstruction of the common bile duct and mild elevation of bilirubin.

Al M. Alcohol excess may produce proteinaceous plugs in the small pancreatic ducts, causing back pressure injury and autodigestion of the pancreatic acini drained by these obstructed channels. This process causes one form of acute pancreatitis. **Al M.** had an episode of acute alcohol-induced pancreatitis superimposed on a more chronic alcohol-related inflammatory process in the pancreas—in other words, chronic pancreatitis. As a result of decreased secretion of pancreatic lipase through the pancreatic ducts and into the lumen of the small intestine, dietary fat was not absorbed at a normal rate, and steatorrhea (fat-rich stools) occurred. If abstinence from alcohol does not allow adequate recovery of the enzymatic secretory function of the pancreas, Mr. M. will have to take a commercial preparation of pancreatic enzymes with meals that contain even minimal amounts of fat.

BIOCHEMICAL COMMENTS

Microsomal Triglyceride Transfer Protein. The assembly of chylomicrons within the ER of the enterocyte requires the activity of *microsomal triglyceride transfer protein (MTP)*. The protein is a dimer of two nonidentical subunits. The smaller subunit (57 kDa) is protein disulfide isomerase (PDI; see Chapter 7, Section IX.A), whereas the larger subunit (97 kDa) contains the triglyceride transfer activity. MTP accelerates the transport of triglycerides, cholesterol esters, and phospholipids across membranes of subcellular organelles. The role of PDI in this complex is not known; the disulfide isomerase activity of this subunit is not needed for triglyceride transport to occur. The lack of triglyceride transfer activity leads to the disease *abetalipoproteinemia*. This disease affects both chylomicron assembly in the intestine and VLDL assembly in the liver. Both particles require a B apolipoprotein for their assembly (apoB-48 for chylomicrons, apoB-100 for VLDL), and MTP binds to the B apolipoproteins. For both chylomicron and VLDL assembly, a small apoB-containing particle is first produced within the lumen of the ER. The appropriate apoB is made on the rough ER and is inserted into the ER lumen during its synthesis (see Chapter 15, Section VIII). As the protein is being translated, lipid (a small amount of triglyceride) begins to associate with the protein, and the lipid association is catalyzed by MTP. This leads to the generation of small apoB–containing particles; these particles are not formed in patients with abetalipoproteinemia. Thus, it appears that MTP activity is necessary to transfer triacylglycerol formed within the ER to the apoB protein. The second stage of particle assembly is the fusion of the initial apoB particle with triacylglycerol droplets within the ER. The role of MTP in this second step is still

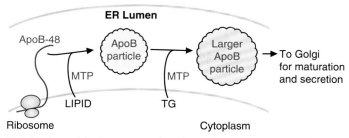

FIGURE 29.12 A model of microsomal triglyceride transfer protein (MTP) action. MTP is required to transfer lipid to apoB-48 as it is synthesized and to transfer lipid from the cytoplasm to the endoplasmic reticulum (ER) lumen. *TG*, triglyceride.

under investigation; it may be required for the transfer of triacylglycerol from the cytoplasm to the lumen of the ER to form this lipid droplet. These steps are illustrated in Figure 29.12.

The symptoms of abetalipoproteinemia include lipid malabsorption (and its accompanying symptoms such as steatorrhea and vomiting), which can result in caloric deficiencies and weight loss. Because lipid-soluble vitamin distribution occurs through chylomicron circulation, signs and symptoms of deficiencies in the lipid-soluble vitamins may be seen in these patients.

MTP inhibitors have been investigated and studied for their effect on circulating lipid and cholesterol levels. Although the inhibitors discovered to date are effective in lowering circulating lipid levels, they also initiate severe hepatic steatosis (fatty liver), an unacceptable complication which could lead to liver failure. The steatosis comes about by an accumulation of triglyceride in the liver owing to the inability to form VLDL and export the triglyceride from the liver. The accumulation of triglyceride within hepatocytes will eventually interfere with hepatic function and structure. Current research for MTP inhibitors is aimed toward reducing the severity of fat accumulation in the liver (e.g., by specifically targeting the intestinal MTP without affecting the hepatic MTP).

KEY CONCEPTS

- Triacylglycerols are the major fat source in the human diet.
- Lipases (lingual lipase in the saliva and gastric lipase in the stomach) perform limited digestion of triacylglycerol before food enters the intestine.
- As food enters the intestine, cholecystokinin is released, which signals the gallbladder to release bile acids and the exocrine pancreas to release digestive enzymes.
- Within the intestine, bile salts emulsify fats, which increase their accessibility to pancreatic lipase and colipase.
- Triacylglycerols are degraded to form free fatty acids and 2-monoacylgylcerol by pancreatic lipase and colipase.
- Dietary phospholipids are hydrolyzed by pancreatic phospholipase A2 in the intestine.
- Dietary cholesterol esters (cholesterol esterified to a fatty acid) are hydrolyzed by pancreatic cholesterol esterase in the intestine.
- Micelles, consisting of bile acids and the products of fat digestion, form within the intestinal lumen and interact with the enterocyte membrane. Lipid-soluble components diffuse from the micelle into the cell.
- Bile salts are resorbed farther down the intestinal tract and are returned to the liver by the enterohepatic circulation.
- The intestinal epithelial cells resynthesize triacylglycerol and package them into nascent chylomicrons for release into the circulation.

- Once they are in the circulation, the nascent chylomicrons interact with HDL particles and acquire two additional protein components, apoCII and apoE.
- ApoCII activates LPL on capillary endothelium of muscle and adipose tissue, which digests the triglycerides in the chylomicron. The fatty acids released from the chylomicron enter the muscle for energy production or the fat cell for storage. The glycerol released is metabolized only in the liver.
- As the chylomicron loses triglyceride, its density increases and it becomes a chylomicron remnant. Chylomicron remnants are removed from circulation by the liver through specific binding of the remnant to apoE receptors on the liver membrane.
- Once it is in the liver, the remnant is degraded and the lipids are recycled.
- Table 29.1 summarizes the diseases discussed in this chapter.

TABLE 29.1 Diseases Discussed in Chapter 29		
DISEASE OR DISORDER	**ENVIRONMENTAL OR GENETIC**	**COMMENTS**
Sickle cell disease	Genetic	Cholecystitis may result as a consequence of sickle cell disease, which is caused by increased red cell destruction in the spleen and an inability of the liver to conjugate all of the bilirubin resulting from heme degradation.
Alcoholism	Both	Pancreatitis may result from chronic alcohol abuse, leading to malabsorption problems within the intestine.
Abetalipoproteinemia	Genetic	Loss of microsomal triglyceride transfer protein activity, leading to an inability to produce both chylomicrons and very-low-density lipoprotein. Steatorrhea and fat-soluble vitamin deficiencies may result, as well as a deficiency in required dietary fatty acids.

REVIEW QUESTIONS—CHAPTER 29

1. Most of our dietary fats are incorporated into chylomicrons in the intestine. The most abundant component of chylomicrons is which one of the following?
   A. ApoB-48
   B. Triglyceride
   C. Phospholipid
   D. Cholesterol
   E. Cholesterol ester

2. In order for the lipids in chylomicrons to be used by the tissues of the body, the nascent chylomicrons need to be converted to mature chylomicrons. This conversion requires which one of the following?
   A. Bile salts
   B. 2-Monoacylglycerol
   C. LPL
   D. HDL
   E. Lymphatic system

3. Chylomicrons and VLDL contain similar and different apolipoproteins. The apolipoproteins B-48 and B-100 are similar with respect to which one of the following?
   A. They are synthesized from the same gene.
   B. They are derived by alternative spicing of the same heterogeneous nuclear RNA.

   C. ApoB-48 is a proteolytic product of apoB-100.
   D. Both are found in mature chylomicrons.
   E. Both are found in VLDL.

4. Bile salts must reach a particular concentration within the intestinal lumen before they are effective agents for lipid digestion. This is because of which one of the following?
   A. The bile salt concentration must be equal to the triglyceride concentration.
   B. The bile salt solubility in the lumen is a critical factor.
   C. The ability of bile salts to bind lipase is concentration-dependent.
   D. The bile salts cannot be reabsorbed in the ileum until they reach a certain concentration.
   E. The bile salts do not activate lipase until they reach a particular concentration.

5. Type III hyperlipidemia can be caused by a deficiency of apoE. Analysis of the serum of patients with this disorder would exhibit which one of the following?
   A. An absence of chylomicrons after eating
   B. Above-normal levels of VLDL after eating
   C. Normal triglyceride levels
   D. Elevated triglyceride levels
   E. Below-normal triglyceride levels

6. Pancreatitis can lead to a blockage of the pancreatic duct that, in turn, leads to steatorrhea. The steatorrhea is most likely caused by the absence of which one of the following?
   A. Trypsin
   B. Colipase
   C. Pepsin
   D. Cholesterol esterase
   E. Amylase

7. A patient has been taking an experimental drug to reduce weight. The drug leads to significant steatorrhea and some night-blindness. A potential target of this drug is which one of the following?
   A. LPL activity
   B. Albumin synthesis
   C. Glucagon release
   D. Insulin release
   E. Cholecystokinin release

8. A patient trying to lose weight is taking an over-the-counter "fat blocker" that supposedly blocks fat absorption from the gastrointestinal tract. If this supplement truly blocked fat absorption, for which vitamin below could the patient potentially develop a deficiency?
   A. K
   B. B_1
   C. B_3
   D. B_6
   E. C

9. The absence of which hormone listed would result in an inability to raise the pH of the partially digested food leaving the stomach, leading to an inability to digest lipids in the intestine?
   A. Pancreatic lipase
   B. Intestinal cholecystokinin
   C. Pancreatic cholecystokinin
   D. Intestinal secretin
   E. Pancreatic secretin

10. Short- and medium-chain fatty acids in the diet follow which one of the following digestive sequences?
    A. They are emulsified by bile acids.
    B. They are packaged in micelles.
    C. They enter the portal blood after intestinal absorption.
    D. They enter the lymph after intestinal absorption.
    E. They are formed by chylomicrons.

ANSWERS

1. **The answer is B.** Chylomicrons transport dietary lipids, and >80% of the chylomicron is triglyceride. All other components are present at <10%; hence, all other answers are incorrect.

2. **The answer is D.** HDL transfers apolipoproteins CII and E to nascent chylomicrons to convert them to mature chylomicrons. Bile salts are required to emulsify dietary lipid, 2-monacylglycerol is a digestion product of pancreatic lipase, lipoprotein lipase digests triglyceride from mature chylomicrons, and the lymphatic system delivers the nascent chylomicrons to the bloodstream.

3. **The answer is A.** Both apoB-48 and apoB-100 are derived from the same gene and from the same messenger RNA (there is no difference in splicing between the two; thus, B is incorrect). However, RNA editing introduces a stop codon in the message such that B_{48} stops protein synthesis approximately 48% along the message. Thus, proteolytic cleavage is not correct. B_{48} is found only in chylomicrons, and B_{100} is found only in VLDL particles.

4. **The answer is B.** The bile salts must be above their CMC in order to form micelles with the components of lipase digestion, fatty acids and 2-monoacylglycerol. In the absence of micelle formation, lipid absorption would not occur. The CMC is independent of triglyceride concentration (thus, A is incorrect). Bile salts do not bind or activate lipase (thus, C and E are incorrect). The absorption of bile salts in the ileum is not related to digestion (thus, D is incorrect).

5. **The answer is D.** Nascent chylomicrons would be synthesized, which can only acquire apoCII from HDL (thus, A is incorrect). The chylomicrons would be degraded in part by LPL, leading to chylomicron remnant formation. However, the chylomicron remnants would remain in circulation because of the lack of apoE (thus, B is incorrect). Because these remnant particles still contain a fair amount of triglyceride, serum triglyceride levels will be elevated (thus, C and E are incorrect).

6. **The answer is B.** Lipase and colipase together are required to digest triglycerides from the diet. Both are secreted by the exocrine pancreas through the pancreatic duct into the common duct and then into the intestine. If colipase cannot make its way into the intestine, lipase is relatively inactive, and triglyceride digestion will not occur. Thus, the triglycerides are eliminated via the feces, leading to steatorrhea. The simultaneous reduction in other pancreatic exocrine secretions leading to an inability to digest proteins (lack of trypsin; pepsin is found in the stomach), or cholesterol esters (cholesterol esterase), or starch (amylase) does not lead to steatorrhea because the triglycerides account for the majority of fat in the diet.

7. **The answer is E.** The patient, when taking the drug, is not digesting fat or absorbing fat-soluble vitamins (the night-blindness is caused by a lack of vitamin A). This can occur because of mutations in lipase or colipase, or an inability to release cholecystokinin. In the absence of cholecystokinin, the digestive enzymes from the pancreas (including lipase and colipase) will not be secreted to the intestine, nor will bile acids be secreted from the gallbladder to the intestine. This would lead to inefficient triglyceride digestion and to loss of triglyceride and lipid-soluble vitamins in the stools. Loss of LPL activity would lead to elevated triglyceride levels in the blood but not the stool. Loss of albumin synthesis would lead to problems in blood volume but would not lead to steatorrhea. Alterations in glucagon and insulin release do not affect triglyceride digestion in the intestine.

8. **The answer is A.** Of those listed, only vitamin K is a fat-soluble vitamin, and the fat-soluble vitamins are absorbed along with the lipids in the intestine. The other fat-soluble vitamins are D, E, and A. Vitamin B_1 is thiamin, B_3 is niacin, and B_6 is pyridoxamine. All of the B vitamins, and vitamin C, are water-soluble, so their absorption into the intestinal epithelial cells would not be blocked by this drug.

9. **The answer is D.** Intestinal cholecystokinin stimulates release of pancreatic lipase to digest triglyceride, along with other enzymes to digest carbohydrates and proteins. Intestinal secretin signals the liver, pancreas, and some intestinal cells to secrete bicarbonate. The pancreas does not produce cholecystokinin or secretin.

10. **The answer is C.** Short- and medium-chain fatty acids do not require bile salts for their absorption and therefore do not go into micelles or the lymph. They are absorbed directly into intestinal epithelial cells and enter the portal blood, where they bind to serum albumin.

Oxidation of Fatty Acids and Ketone Bodies

30

Fatty acids are a major fuel for humans and supply our energy needs between meals and during periods of increased demand, such as exercise. During overnight fasting, fatty acids become the major fuel for cardiac muscle, skeletal muscle, and liver. The liver converts fatty acids to ketone bodies (acetoacetate and β-hydroxybutyrate), which also serve as major fuels for tissues (e.g., the gut). The brain, which does not have a significant capacity for fatty acid oxidation, can use ketone bodies as a fuel during prolonged fasting.

The route of metabolism for a fatty acid depends somewhat on its chain length. Fatty acids are generally classified as **very-long-chain-length fatty acids** (>C20), **long-chain fatty acids** (C12 to C20), **medium-chain fatty acids** (C6 to C12), and **short-chain fatty acids** (C4).

ATP is generated from oxidation of fatty acids in the pathway of β-oxidation. Between meals and during overnight fasting, **long-chain fatty acids** are released from adipose tissue triacylglycerols. They circulate through blood bound to **albumin** (Fig. 30.1). In cells, they are converted to **fatty acyl coenzyme A** (**fatty acyl-CoA**) derivatives by **acyl-CoA synthetases**. The activated acyl group is transported into the mitochondrial matrix bound to **carnitine**, where fatty acyl-CoA is regenerated. In the pathway of **β-oxidation**, the fatty acyl group is sequentially oxidized to yield reduced flavin adenine dinucleotide (FAD[2H]), reduced nicotinamide adenine dinucleotide (NADH), and acetyl coenzyme A (acetyl-CoA). Subsequent oxidation of NADH and FAD(2H) in the electron-transport chain, and oxidation of acetyl-CoA to CO_2 in the tricarboxylic acid (TCA) cycle, generates adenosine triphosphate (ATP) from oxidative phosphorylation.

Many fatty acids have structures that require variations of this basic pattern. Long-chain fatty acids that are **unsaturated fatty acids** generally require additional isomerization and oxidation–reduction reactions to rearrange their double bonds during β-oxidation. Metabolism of water-soluble **medium-chain-length fatty acids** does not require carnitine and occurs only in the liver. **Odd-chain-length fatty acids** undergo β-oxidation to the terminal three-carbon propionyl coenzyme A (**propionyl-CoA**), which enters the TCA cycle as succinyl coenzyme A (succinyl-CoA).

Fatty acids that do not readily undergo mitochondrial β-oxidation are oxidized first by alternate routes that convert them to more suitable substrates or to urinary excretion products. **Excess fatty acids** may undergo microsomal **ω-oxidation**, which converts them to **dicarboxylic acids** that appear in urine. **Very-long-chain fatty acids** (both straight-chain and **branched fatty acids** such as phytanic acid) are whittled down to size in peroxisomes. **Peroxisomal α- and β-oxidation** generates hydrogen peroxide (H_2O_2), NADH, acetyl-CoA, or propionyl-CoA and a short- to medium-chain-length acyl-CoA. The acyl-CoA products are transferred to mitochondria to complete their metabolism.

In the liver, much of the acetyl-CoA generated from fatty acid oxidation is converted to the ketone bodies **acetoacetate** and **β-hydroxybutyrate**, which enter the blood (see Fig. 30.1). In other tissues, these ketone bodies are converted to acetyl-CoA, which is oxidized in the TCA cycle. The liver synthesizes ketone bodies but cannot use them as a fuel.

The **rate of fatty acid oxidation** is linked to the rate of NADH, FAD(2H), and acetyl-CoA oxidation and thus to the rate of oxidative phosphorylation and **ATP use**. Additional regulation occurs through **malonyl coenzyme A** (**malonyl-CoA**),

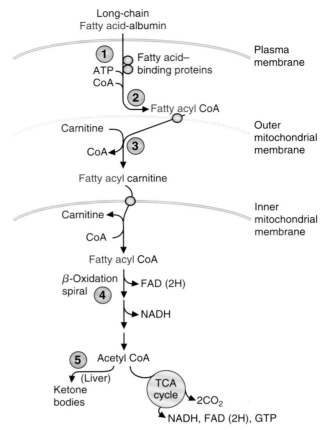

FIGURE 30.1 Overview of mitochondrial long-chain fatty acid metabolism. (*1*) Fatty acid–binding proteins transport fatty acids across the plasma membrane and bind them in the cytosol. (*2*) Fatty acyl coenzyme A (fatty acyl-CoA) synthetase activates fatty acids to fatty acyl-CoAs. (*3*) Carnitine transports the activated fatty acyl group into mitochondria. (*4*) β-Oxidation generates reduced nicotinamide adenine dinucleotide (NADH), reduced flavin adenine dinucleotide FAD(2H), and acetyl coenzyme A (acetyl-CoA). (*5*) In the liver, acetyl-CoA can be converted to ketone bodies. *ATP*, adenosine triphosphate; *CoA*, coenzyme A; *GTP*, guanosine triphosphate; *TCA*, tricarboxylic acid.

which inhibits mitochondrial entry of the fatty acylcarnitine derivatives. Fatty acids and ketone bodies are used as fuel when their level increases in the blood, which is determined by hormonal regulation of adipose tissue **lipolysis**.

THE WAITING ROOM

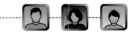

 Otto S. was disappointed that he did not place in his 5-km race and has decided that short-distance running is probably not right for him. After careful consideration, he decides to train for the marathon by running 12 miles three times per week. He is now 13 lb over his ideal weight, and he plans on losing this weight while studying for his pharmacology finals. He considers a variety of dietary supplements to increase his endurance and selects one that contains carnitine, coenzyme Q (CoQ), pantothenate, riboflavin, and creatine.

 Lola B. is a 16-year-old girl. Since age 14 months, she has experienced recurrent episodes of profound fatigue associated with vomiting and increased perspiration, which required hospitalization. These episodes occurred only if she fasted for >8 hours. Because her mother gave her food late at night and woke her early in the morning for breakfast, Lola's physical and mental development had progressed normally.

On the day of admission for this episode, Lola had missed breakfast, and by noon she was extremely fatigued, nauseated, and weak. She was unable to hold any food in her stomach and was rushed to the hospital, where an infusion of glucose was started intravenously. Her symptoms responded dramatically to this therapy.

Her initial serum glucose level was low, at 38 mg/dL (reference range for fasting serum glucose levels, 70 to 100 mg/dL). Her blood urea nitrogen (BUN) level was slightly elevated at 26 mg/dL (reference range, 8 to 25 mg/dL) because of vomiting, which led to a degree of dehydration. Her blood levels of liver transaminases were slightly elevated, although her liver was not palpably enlarged. Despite elevated levels of free fatty acids (4.3 mM) in the blood, which were later tested, blood ketone bodies were below normal.

 Dianne A., a 27-year-old woman with type 1 diabetes mellitus, had been admitted to the hospital in a ketoacidotic coma a year ago (see Chapter 4). She had been feeling drowsy and had been vomiting for 24 hours before that admission. At the time of admission, she was clinically dehydrated, her blood pressure was low, and her breathing was deep and rapid (Kussmaul breathing). Her pulse was rapid, and her breath had the odor of acetone. Her arterial blood pH was 7.08 (reference range, 7.36 to 7.44), and her blood ketone body levels were 15 mM (normal is ~0.2 mM for a person on a normal diet).

I. Fatty Acids as Fuels

The *fatty acids* oxidized as fuels are principally *long-chain fatty acids* released from adipose tissue triacylglycerol stores between meals, during overnight fasting, and during periods of increased fuel demand (e.g., during exercise). Adipose tissue triacylglycerols are derived from two sources; dietary lipids and triacylglycerols synthesized in the liver. The major fatty acids oxidized are the long-chain fatty acids, palmitate, oleate, and stearate, because they are highest in dietary lipids and are also synthesized in humans.

Between meals, a decreased insulin level and increased levels of insulin counterregulatory hormones (e.g., glucagon) activate lipolysis, and free fatty acids are transported to tissues bound to serum albumin. Within tissues, energy is derived from oxidation of fatty acids to acetyl-CoA in the pathway of *β-oxidation*. Most of the enzymes involved in fatty acid oxidation are present as two or three isoenzymes, which have different but overlapping specificities for the chain length of the fatty acid. Metabolism of *unsaturated fatty acids*, *odd-chain-length fatty acids*, and *medium-chain-length fatty acids* requires variations of this basic pattern. The *acetyl-CoA* produced from fatty acid oxidation is principally oxidized in the TCA cycle or converted to ketone bodies in the liver.

A. Characteristics of Fatty Acids Used as Fuels

Fat constitutes approximately 38% of the calories in the average North American diet. Of this, more than 95% of the calories are present as triacylglycerols (three fatty acids esterified to a glycerol backbone). During ingestion and absorption, dietary triacylglycerols are broken down into their constituents and then reassembled for transport to adipose tissue in chylomicrons (see Chapter 29). Thus, the fatty acid composition of adipose triacylglycerols varies with the type of food consumed.

The most common dietary fatty acids are the saturated long-chain fatty acids palmitate (C16) and stearate (C18), the monounsaturated fatty acid oleate (C18:1), and the polyunsaturated essential fatty acid linoleate (C18:2) (To review fatty acid nomenclature, consult Chapter 5.) Animal fat contains principally saturated and monounsaturated long-chain fatty acids, whereas vegetable oils contain linoleate and some longer chain and polyunsaturated fatty acids. They also contain smaller amounts of branched-chain and odd-chain-length fatty acids. Medium-chain-length fatty acids are present principally in dairy fat (e.g., milk, butter), maternal milk, and vegetable oils.

 The liver transaminases measured in the blood are aspartate aminotransferase (AST), which was previously designated serum glutamate-oxaloacetate transaminase (SGOT), and alanine aminotransferase (ALT), which was previously designated serum glutamate-pyruvate transaminase (SGPT). Elevation of these enzymes in the serum reflects damage to the liver cell plasma membrane. Transaminases catalyze the transfer of the nitrogen group of an amino acid to an acceptor α-keto acid. For AST, aspartate donates the nitrogen to α-ketoglutarate, forming oxaloacetate (the corresponding α-keto acid to aspartate) and glutamate. For ALT, alanine donates the nitrogen to α-ketoglutarate, forming pyruvate and glutamate. Transaminase activity is measured using a coupled reaction: Both oxaloacetate and pyruvate can be reduced by NADH to form, respectively, malate and lactate, in the presence of the appropriate secondary enzyme (malate dehydrogenase and lactate dehydrogenase). Thus, automated procedures that follow the loss of NADH in the reaction mix (by measuring the decrease in absorbance at 340 nm) can be used to measure the activity of AST and ALT in serum samples.

 During **Otto S.'s** distance running (a moderate-intensity exercise), decreases in insulin and increases in insulin counterregulatory hormones, such as epinephrine and norepinephrine, increase adipose tissue lipolysis. Thus, his muscles are being provided with a supply of fatty acids in the blood that they can use as a fuel.

 Lola B. developed symptoms during fasting, when adipose tissue lipolysis was elevated. Under these circumstances, muscle tissue, liver, and many other tissues are oxidizing fatty acids as a fuel. After overnight fasting, approximately 60% to 70% of our energy supply is derived from the oxidation of fatty acids.

Adipose tissue triacylglycerols also contain fatty acids synthesized in the liver, principally from excess calories ingested as glucose. The pathway of fatty acid synthesis generates palmitate, which can be elongated to form stearate or unsaturated to form oleate. These fatty acids are assembled into triacylglycerols and transported to adipose tissue as the lipoprotein very-low-density lipoprotein (VLDL).

B. Transport and Activation of Long-Chain Fatty Acids

Long-chain fatty acids are hydrophobic and, therefore, water-insoluble. In addition, they are toxic to cells because they can disrupt the hydrophobic bonding between amino acid side chains in proteins. Consequently, they are transported in the blood and in cells bound to proteins.

1. Cellular Uptake of Long-Chain Fatty Acids

During fasting and other conditions of metabolic need, long-chain fatty acids are released from adipose tissue triacylglycerols by lipases. They travel in the blood bound in the hydrophobic binding pocket of albumin, the major serum protein (see Fig. 30.1).

Fatty acids enter cells both by a saturable transport process and by diffusion through the lipid plasma membrane. A fatty acid–binding protein in the plasma membrane facilitates transport. An additional fatty acid–binding protein binds the fatty acid intracellularly and may facilitate its transport to the mitochondrion. The free fatty acid concentration in cells is, therefore, extremely low.

2. Activation of Long-Chain Fatty Acids

Fatty acids must be activated to acyl coenzyme A (acyl-CoA) derivatives before they can participate in β-oxidation and other metabolic pathways (Fig. 30.2). The process of activation involves an acyl-CoA synthetase (also called a *thiokinase*) that uses ATP energy to form the fatty acyl-CoA thioester bond. In this reaction, the β-bond of ATP is cleaved to form a fatty acyl adenosine monophosphate (AMP) intermediate and pyrophosphate (PP_i). Subsequent cleavage of PP_i helps to drive the reaction.

The acyl-CoA synthetase that activates long-chain fatty acids, 12 to 20 carbons in length, is present in three locations in the cell: the endoplasmic reticulum, outer

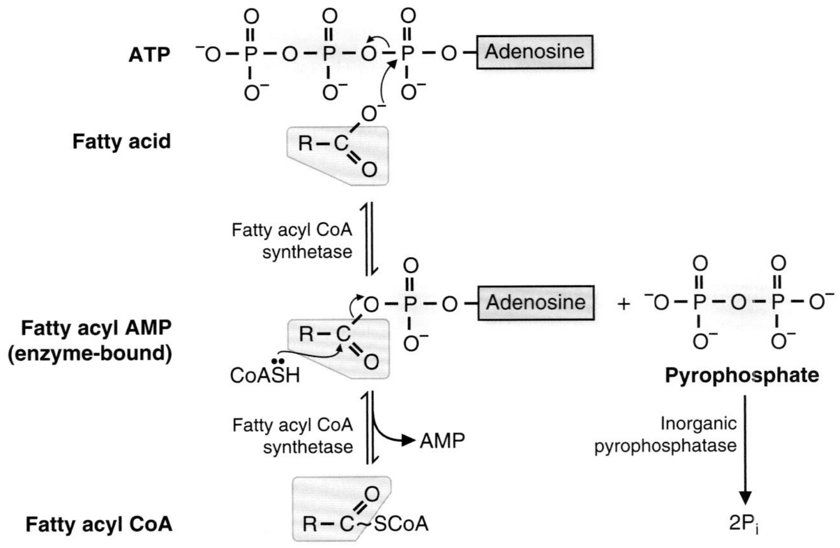

FIGURE 30.2 Activation of a fatty acid by a fatty acyl coenzyme A (acyl-CoA) synthetase. The fatty acid is activated by reacting with adenosine triphosphate (ATP) to form a high-energy fatty acyl adenosine monophosphate (AMP) and pyrophosphate. The AMP is then exchanged for coenzyme A (CoA). Pyrophosphate is cleaved by a pyrophosphatase. P_i, inorganic phosphate.

mitochondrial membranes, and peroxisomal membranes (Table 30.1). This enzyme has no activity toward C22 or longer fatty acids and little activity below C12. In contrast, the synthetase for activation of very-long-chain fatty acids is present in peroxisomes, and the medium-chain-length fatty acid–activating enzyme is present only in the mitochondrial matrix of liver and kidney cells.

3. Fates of Fatty Acyl Coenzyme A

Fatty acyl-CoA formation, like the phosphorylation of glucose, is a prerequisite to metabolism of the fatty acid in the cell (Fig. 30.3). The multiple locations of the long-chain acyl-CoA synthetase reflect the location of different metabolic routes

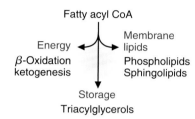

FIGURE 30.3 Major metabolic routes for long-chain fatty acyl coenzyme As (acyl-CoAs). Fatty acids are activated to acyl-CoA compounds for degradation in mitochondrial β-oxidation, or incorporation into triacylglycerols or membrane lipids. When β-oxidation is blocked through an inherited enzyme deficiency, or metabolic regulation, excess fatty acids are diverted into triacylglycerol synthesis.

TABLE 30.1 Chain-Length Specificity of Fatty Acid Activation and Oxidation Enzymes		
ENZYME	**CHAIN LENGTH**	**COMMENTS**
Acyl-CoA Synthetases		
Very-long-chain	14–26	Found only in peroxisomes
Long-chain	12–20	Enzyme present in membranes of endoplasmic reticulum, mitochondria, and peroxisomes to facilitate different metabolic routes of acyl-CoAs
Medium-chain	6–12	Exists as many variants, present only in mitochondrial matrix of kidney and liver; also involved in xenobiotic metabolism
Acetyl	2–4	Present in cytoplasm and possibly mitochondrial matrix
Acyltransferases		
CPTI	12–16	Although maximum activity is for fatty acids 12–16 carbons long, it also acts on many smaller acyl-CoA derivatives.
Medium-chain (carnitine octanoyltransferase)	6–12	Substrate is medium-chain acyl-CoA derivatives generated during peroxisomal oxidation.
Carnitine acetyltransferase	2	High level in skeletal muscle and heart to facilitate use of acetate as a fuel
Acyl-CoA dehydrogenases		
VLCAD	14–20	Present in inner mitochondrial membrane
LCAD	12–18	Members of same enzyme family, which also includes acyl-CoA dehydrogenases for carbon skeleton of branched-chain amino acids. Low expression of LCAD in humans; VLCAD is the predominant acyl-CoA dehydrogenase for long-chain fatty acids.
MCAD	4–12	
SCAD	4–6	
Other enzymes		
Enoyl-CoA hydratase, short-chain	>4	Also called crotonase. Activity decreases with increasing chain length.
L-3-Hydroxyacyl-CoA dehydrogenase, short-chain	4–16	Activity decreases with increasing chain length.
Acetoacetyl-CoA thiolase	4	Specific for acetoacetyl-CoA
Mitochondrial trifunctional protein	12–16	Complex of long-chain enoyl hydratase, L-3-hydroxyacyl-CoA dehydrogenase, and a thiolase with broad specificity; most active with longer chains

CoA, coenzyme A; CPT-1, carnitine palmitoyltransferase 1; VLCAD, very-long-chain acyl-CoA dehydrogenase; LCAD, long-chain acyl-CoA dehydrogenase; MCAD, medium-chain acyl-CoA dehydrogenase; SCAD, short-chain acyl-CoA dehydrogenase.

Several inherited diseases in the metabolism of carnitine or acylcarnitines have been described. These include defects in the following enzymes or systems: the transporter for carnitine uptake into muscle, CPTI, carnitine:acylcarnitine translocase, and CPTII. Classical CPTII deficiency, the most common of these diseases (although still very rare), is characterized by adolescent to adult onset of recurrent episodes of acute myoglobinuria, with muscle pain and weakness, precipitated by prolonged exercise or fasting. During these episodes, the patient is weak, and may be somewhat hypoglycemic with diminished ketosis (hypoketosis), but metabolic decompensation is not severe. Lipid deposits are found in skeletal muscles. Both creatine phosphokinase (CPK) and long-chain acylcarnitines are elevated in the blood. CPTII levels in fibroblasts are approximately 25% of normal. The residual CPTII activity probably accounts for the mild effect on liver metabolism. In contrast, when CPTII deficiency presents in infants, CPTII levels are <10% of normal, the hypoglycemia and hypoketosis are severe, hepatomegaly occurs from the triacylglycerol deposits, and cardiomyopathy is also present.

taken by fatty acyl-CoA derivatives in the cell (e.g., triacylglycerol and phospholipid synthesis in the endoplasmic reticulum, oxidation and plasmalogen synthesis in the peroxisome, and β-oxidation in mitochondria). In the liver and some other tissues, fatty acids that are not being used for energy generation are reincorporated (re-esterified) into triacylglycerols.

4. Transport of Long-Chain Fatty Acids into Mitochondria

Carnitine serves as the carrier that transports activated long-chain fatty acyl groups across the inner mitochondrial membrane (Fig. 30.4). Carnitine acyltransferases are able to reversibly transfer an activated fatty acyl group from coenzyme A (CoA) to the hydroxyl group of carnitine to form an acylcarnitine ester. The reaction is reversible, so the fatty acyl-CoA derivative can be regenerated from the carnitine ester.

Carnitine palmitoyltransferase I (CPTI; also called *carnitine acyltransferase I* [*CATI*]), the enzyme that transfers long-chain fatty acyl groups from CoA to carnitine, is located on the outer mitochondrial membrane (Fig. 30.5). Fatty acylcarnitine crosses the inner mitochondrial membrane with the aid of a translocase. The fatty acyl group is transferred back to CoA by a second enzyme, carnitine palmitoyltransferase II (CPTII [or CATII]). The carnitine released in this reaction returns to the cytosolic side of the mitochondrial membrane by the same translocase that brings fatty acylcarnitine to the matrix side. Long-chain fatty acyl-CoA, now located within the mitochondrial matrix, is a substrate for β-oxidation.

Carnitine is obtained from the diet or synthesized from the side chain of lysine by a pathway that begins in skeletal muscle, and is completed in the liver. The reactions use *S*-adenosylmethionine to donate methyl groups, and vitamin C (ascorbic acid) is also required for these reactions. Skeletal muscles have a high-affinity uptake system for carnitine, and most of the carnitine in the body is stored in skeletal muscle.

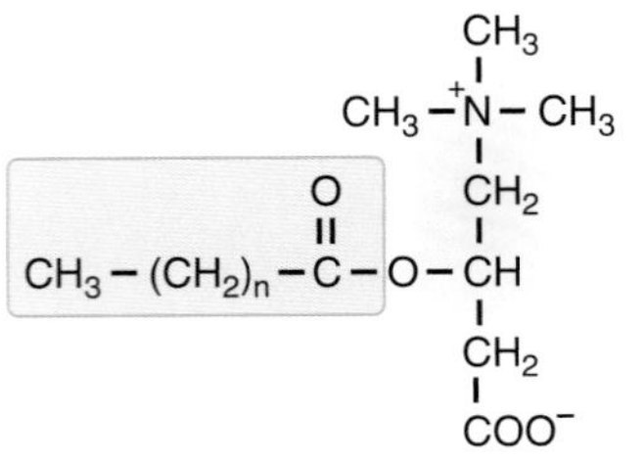

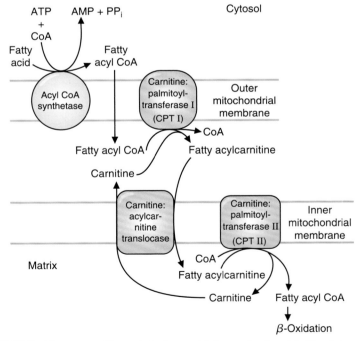

FIGURE 30.5 Transport of long-chain fatty acids into mitochondria. The fatty acyl coenzyme A (fatty acyl-CoA) crosses the outer mitochondrial membrane. Carnitine palmitoyltransferase I in the outer mitochondrial membrane transfers the fatty acyl group to carnitine and releases CoASH. The fatty acylcarnitine is translocated into the mitochondrial matrix as carnitine moves out. Carnitine palmitoyltransferase II on the inner mitochondrial membrane transfers the fatty acyl group back to CoASH, to form fatty acyl-CoA in the matrix. *AMP*, adenosine monophosphate; *ATP*, adenosine triphosphate; *CoA*, coenzyme A; *PP$_i$*, pyrophosphate.

Fatty acylcarnitine

FIGURE 30.4 Structure of fatty acylcarnitine. Carnitine palmitoyltransferases catalyze the reversible transfer of a long-chain fatty acyl group from the fatty acyl coenzyme A (fatty acyl-CoA) to the hydroxyl group of carnitine. The atoms in the *green box* originate from the fatty acyl-CoA.

C. β-Oxidation of Long-Chain Fatty Acids

The oxidation of fatty acids to acetyl-CoA in the β-oxidation spiral conserves energy as FAD(2H) and NADH. FAD(2H) and NADH are oxidized in the electron-transport chain, generating ATP from oxidative phosphorylation. Acetyl-CoA is oxidized in the TCA cycle or converted to ketone bodies.

I. The β-Oxidation Spiral

The fatty acid β-oxidation pathway sequentially cleaves the fatty acyl group into two-carbon acetyl-CoA units, beginning with the carboxyl end attached to CoA (Fig. 30.6). Before cleavage, the β-carbon is oxidized to a keto group in two reactions that generate NADH and FAD(2H); thus, the pathway is called *β-oxidation*. As each acetyl group is released, the cycle of β-oxidation and cleavage begins again, but each time, the fatty acyl group is two carbons shorter.

The β-oxidation pathway consists of four separate steps or reactions (Fig. 30.7).

1. In the first step, a double bond is formed between the β- and α-carbons by an acyl-CoA dehydrogenase that transfers electrons to FAD. The double bond is in the *trans* configuration (a Δ^2-*trans* double bond).
2. In the next step, an –OH from water is added to the β-carbon, and an –H from water is added to the α-carbon. The enzyme is called an *enoyl*

Otto S.'s power supplement contains carnitine. However, his body can synthesize enough carnitine to meet his needs, and his diet contains carnitine. Carnitine deficiency has been found only in infants fed a soy-based formula that was not supplemented with carnitine. His other supplements likewise probably provide no benefit but are designed to facilitate fatty acid oxidation during exercise. Riboflavin is the vitamin precursor of FAD, which is required for acyl-CoA dehydrogenases and electron-transfer flavoproteins (ETFs). CoQ is synthesized in the body, but it is the recipient in the electron-transport chain for electrons passed from complexes I and II and the ETFs. Some reports suggest that supplementation with pantothenate, the precursor of CoA, improves performance.

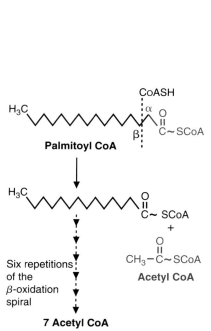

FIGURE 30.6 Overview of β-oxidation. Oxidation at the β-carbon is followed by cleavage of the α–β bond, releasing acetyl coenzyme A (acetyl-CoA) and a fatty acyl coenzyme A (fatty acyl-CoA) that is two carbons shorter than the original. The carbons cleaved to form acetyl-CoA are shown in *red*. Successive spirals of β-oxidation completely cleave an even-chain fatty acyl-CoA to acetyl-CoA. *CoA,* coenzyme A.

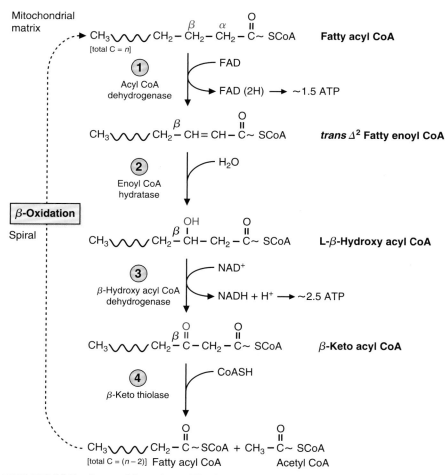

FIGURE 30.7 Steps of β-oxidation. The four steps are repeated until an even-chain fatty acid is completely converted to acetyl coenzyme A (acetyl CoA). The flavin adenine dinucleotide (FAD[2H]) and nicotinamide adenine dinucleotide (NADH) are reoxidized by the electron-transport chain, producing adenosine triphosphate (ATP). *CoA,* coenzyme A.

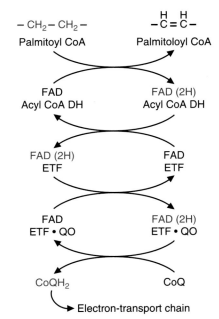

FIGURE 30.8 Transfer of electrons from acyl coenzyme A (acyl CoA) dehydrogenase to the electron-transport chain. A flavin adenine dinucleotide (FAD) is tightly bound to each protein in these three electron-transfer reactions. *CoA*, coenzyme A; *CoQ*, coenzyme Q; *DH*, dehydrogenase; *ETF*, electron-transfer flavoprotein; *ETF·QO*, electron-transfer flavoprotein–coenzyme Q oxidoreductase.

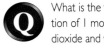

What is the total ATP yield for the oxidation of 1 mol of palmitic acid to carbon dioxide and water?

CoA hydratase (hydratases add the elements of water, and "-ene" in a name denotes a double bond).

3. In the third step of β-oxidation, the hydroxyl group on the β-carbon is oxidized to a ketone by a *hydroxyacyl-CoA dehydrogenase*. In this reaction, as in the conversion of most alcohols to ketones, the electrons are transferred to NAD⁺ to form NADH.

4. In the last reaction of the sequence, the bond between the β- and α-carbons is cleaved by a reaction that attaches CoASH to the β-carbon, and acetyl-CoA is released. This is a thiolytic reaction (*lysis* refers to breakage of the bond, and *thio* refers to the sulfur), catalyzed by enzymes called *β-ketothiolases*. The release of two carbons from the carboxyl end of the original fatty acyl-CoA produces acetyl-CoA and a fatty acyl-CoA that is two carbons shorter than the original. It is of interest to note that the β-oxidation spiral uses the same reaction types seen in the TCA cycle in the conversion of succinate to oxaloacetate.

The shortened fatty acyl-CoA repeats these four steps until all of its carbons are converted to acetyl-CoA. β-Oxidation is thus a spiral rather than a cycle. In the last spiral, cleavage of the four-carbon fatty acyl-CoA (butyryl coenzyme A [butyryl-CoA]) produces two molecules of acetyl-CoA. Thus, an even-chain fatty acid such as palmitoyl coenzyme A (palmitoyl-CoA), which has 16 carbons, is cleaved seven times, producing seven molecules of FAD(2H), seven of NADH, and eight of acetyl-CoA.

2. Energy Yield of β-Oxidation

Like the FAD in all flavoproteins, FAD(2H) bound to the acyl-CoA dehydrogenases is oxidized back to FAD without dissociating from the protein (Fig. 30.8). ETFs in the mitochondrial matrix accept electrons from the enzyme-bound FAD(2H) and transfer these electrons to *electron-transfer flavoprotein–CoQ oxidoreductase* (ETF-QO) in the inner mitochondrial membrane. ETF-QO, also a flavoprotein, transfers the electrons to CoQ in the electron-transport chain. Oxidative phosphorylation thus generates approximately 1.5 ATP for each FAD(2H) produced in the β-oxidation spiral.

The total energy yield from the oxidation of 1 mol of palmitoyl-CoA to 8 mol of acetyl-CoA is, therefore, 28 mol of ATP: 1.5 for each of the 7 FAD(2H), and 2.5 for each of the 7 NADH. To calculate the energy yield from oxidation of 1 mol of palmitate, two ATP need to be subtracted from the total because two high-energy phosphate bonds are cleaved when palmitate is activated to palmitoyl-CoA.

3. Chain-Length Specificity in β-Oxidation

The four reactions of β-oxidation are catalyzed by sets of enzymes that are each specific for fatty acids with different chain lengths (see Table 30.1). The acyl-CoA dehydrogenases, which catalyze the first step of the pathway, are part of an enzyme family that, in mammals, has three different ranges of specificity. The subsequent steps of the spiral use enzymes that are specific for long- or short-chain enoyl coenzyme As (enoyl-CoAs). Although these enzymes are structurally distinct, their specificities overlap to some extent. As the fatty acyl chains are shortened by consecutive cleavage of two carbon units, they are transferred from enzymes that act on longer chains to those that act on shorter chains. Medium- or short-chain fatty acyl-CoA that may be formed from dietary fatty acids, or transferred from peroxisomes, enters the spiral at the enzyme that is most active for fatty acids of its chain length.

4. Oxidation of Unsaturated Fatty Acids

Approximately one-half of the fatty acids in the human diet are unsaturated, containing *cis* double bonds, with oleate (C18:1, Δ^9) and linoleate (18:2, $\Delta^{9,12}$) being the most common. In β-oxidation of saturated fatty acids, a *trans* double bond is created between the second and third (α and β) carbons. For unsaturated fatty acids to undergo the β-oxidation spiral, their *cis* double bonds must be isomerized to *trans* double bonds that will end up between the second and third carbons during β-oxidation, or the double bond must be reduced. The process is illustrated for the polyunsaturated fatty acid linoleate in Figure 30.9. Linoleate is obtained from the diet and cannot be synthesized by humans; thus, it is considered an essential fatty acid. Therefore, only that portion of linoleate that is not needed for other processes will be oxidized. Linoleate undergoes β-oxidation until one double bond is between carbons 3 and 4 near the carboxyl end of the fatty acyl chain and the other is between carbons 6 and 7. An isomerase moves the double bond from the 3,4-position so that it is *trans* and in the 2,3-position, and β-oxidation continues. When a conjugated

After reviewing **Lola B.'s** previous hospital records, a specialist suspected that Lola's medical problems were caused by a disorder in fatty acid metabolism. A battery of tests showed that Lola's blood contained elevated levels of several partially oxidized medium-chain fatty acids, such as octanoic acid (8:0) and 4-decenoic acid (10:1, Δ^4). A urine specimen showed an increase in organic acid metabolites of medium-chain fatty acids containing 6 to 10 carbons, including medium-chain acylcarnitine derivatives. The profile of acylcarnitine species in the urine was characteristic of a genetically determined medium-chain acyl-CoA dehydrogenase (MCAD) deficiency. In this disease, long-chain fatty acids are metabolized by β-oxidation to a medium-chain-length acyl-CoA, such as octanoyl coenzyme A. Because further oxidation of this compound is blocked in MCAD deficiency, the medium-chain acyl group is transferred back to carnitine. These acylcarnitines are water-soluble and appear in blood and urine. The specific enzyme deficiency was demonstrated in cultured fibroblasts from Lola's skin as well as in her circulating monocytic leukocytes.

In LCAD deficiency, fatty acylcarnitines accumulate in the blood. Those containing 14 carbons predominate. However, these do not appear in the urine.

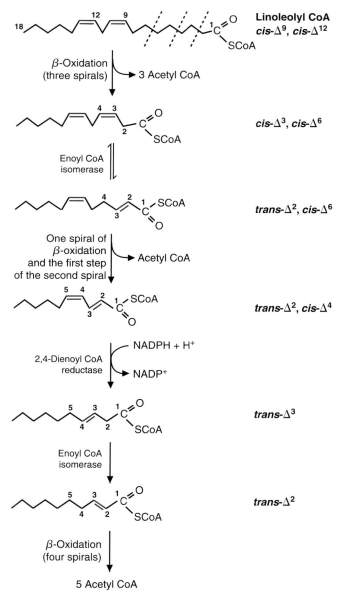

FIGURE 30.9 Oxidation of linoleate. After three spirals of β-oxidation (*dashed lines*), there is now a 3,4-*cis* double bond and a 6,7-*cis* double bond. The 3,4-*cis* double bond is isomerized to a 2,3-*trans* double bond, which is in the proper configuration for the normal enzymes to act. One spiral of β-oxidation occurs, plus the first step of a second spiral. A reductase that uses reduced nicotinamide adenine dinucleotide phosphate (NADPH) now converts these two double bonds (between carbons 2 and 3 and between carbons 4 and 5) to one double bond between carbons 3 and 4 in a *trans* configuration. The isomerase (which can act on double bonds that are in either the *cis* or the *trans* configuration) moves this double bond to the 2,3-*trans* position, and β-oxidation can resume. *CoA*, coenzyme A.

Palmitic acid is 16 carbons long, with no double bonds, so it requires seven oxidation spirals to be completely converted to acetyl-CoA. After seven spirals, there are 7 FAD(2H), 7 NADH, and 8 acetyl-CoA. Each NADH yields 2.5 ATP, each FAD(2H) yields 1.5 ATP, and each acetyl-CoA yields 10 ATP as it is processed through the TCA cycle. This then yields $17.5 + 10.5 + 80 = 108$ ATP. However, activation of palmitic acid to palmitoyl-CoA requires two high-energy bonds, so the net yield is $108 - 2$, or 106 mol of ATP.

The unripe fruit of the ackee tree produces a toxin, hypoglycin, which causes a condition known as *Jamaican vomiting sickness.* The victims of the toxin are usually unwary children who eat this unripe fruit and develop a severe hypoglycemia, which is often fatal.

Although hypoglycin causes hypoglycemia, it acts by inhibiting an acyl-CoA dehydrogenase involved in β-oxidation that has specificity for short- and medium-chain fatty acids. Because more glucose must be oxidized to compensate for the decreased ability of fatty acids to serve as fuel, blood glucose levels may fall to extremely low levels. Fatty acid levels, however, rise because of decreased β-oxidation. As a result of the increased fatty acid levels, ω-oxidation increases, and dicarboxylic acids are excreted in the urine. The diminished capacity to oxidize fatty acids in liver mitochondria results in decreased levels of acetyl-CoA, the substrate for ketone body synthesis.

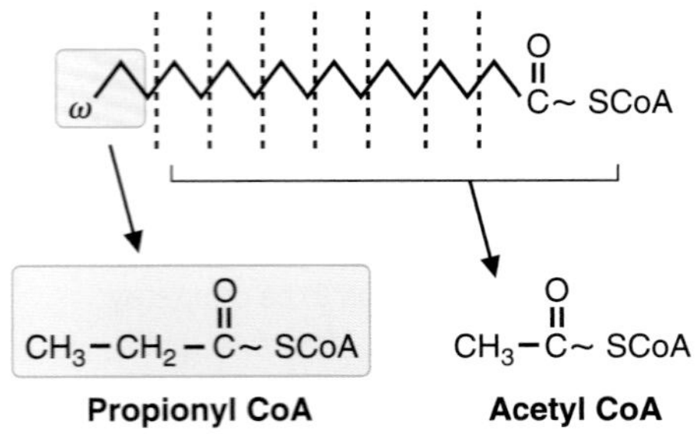

pair of double bonds is formed (two double bonds separated by one single bond) at positions 2 and 4, an NADPH-dependent reductase reduces the pair to one *trans* double bond at position 3. Then, isomerization and β-oxidation resume.

In oleate (C18:1, Δ^9), there is only one double bond between carbons 9 and 10. It is handled by an isomerization reaction similar to that shown for the double bond at position 9 of linoleate.

5. Odd-Chain-Length Fatty Acids

Fatty acids that contain an odd number of carbon atoms undergo β-oxidation, producing acetyl-CoA, until the last spiral, when five carbons remain in the fatty acyl-CoA. In this case, cleavage by thiolase produces acetyl-CoA and a three-carbon fatty acyl-CoA, propionyl coenzyme A (propionyl-CoA) (Fig. 30.10). Carboxylation of propionyl-CoA yields methylmalonyl coenzyme A (methylmalonyl-CoA), which is ultimately converted to succinyl-CoA in a vitamin B_{12}–dependent reaction (Fig. 30.11). Propionyl-CoA also arises from the oxidation of branched-chain amino acids.

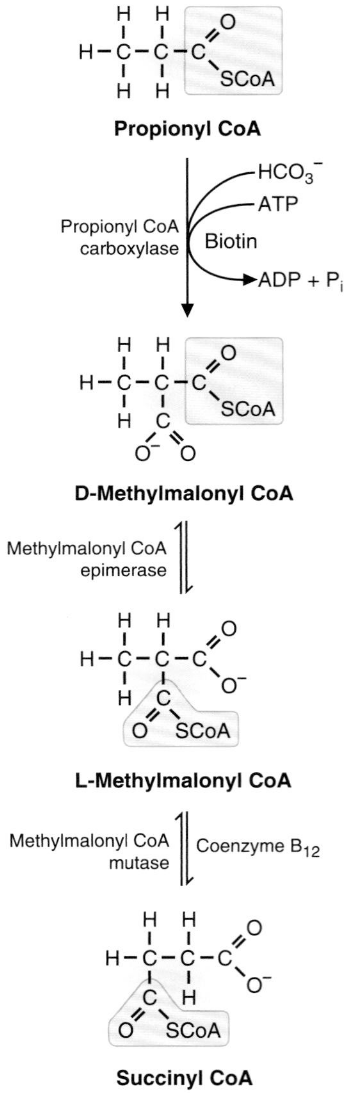

FIGURE 30.11 Conversion of propionyl coenzyme A (propionyl-CoA) to succinyl coenzyme A (succinyl-CoA). Succinyl-CoA, an intermediate of the tricarboxylic acid cycle, can form malate, which can be converted to glucose in the liver through the process of gluconeogenesis. Certain amino acids also form glucose by this route (see Chapter 37). *ADP,* adenosine diphosphate; *ATP,* adenosine triphosphate; *CoA,* coenzyme A; P_i, inorganic phosphate.

FIGURE 30.10 Formation of propionyl coenzyme A (propionyl-CoA) from odd-chain fatty acids. Successive spirals of β-oxidation cleave each of the bonds marked with *dashed lines,* producing acetyl coenzyme A (acetyl-CoA) except for the three carbons at the ω-end, which produce propionyl-CoA.

The propionyl-CoA–succinyl-CoA pathway is a major anaplerotic route for the TCA cycle and is used in the degradation of valine, isoleucine, and several other compounds. In the liver, this route provides precursors of oxaloacetate, which is converted to glucose. Thus, this small proportion of the odd-carbon-number fatty acid chain can be converted to glucose. In contrast, the acetyl-CoA formed from β-oxidation of even-chain-number fatty acids in the liver either enters the TCA cycle, where it is principally oxidized to CO_2, or it is converted to ketone bodies.

D. Oxidation of Medium-Chain-Length Fatty Acids

Dietary medium-chain-length fatty acids are more water-soluble than long-chain fatty acids and are not stored in adipose triacylglycerol. After a meal, they enter the blood and pass into the portal vein to the liver. In the liver, they enter the mitochondrial matrix by the monocarboxylate transporter and are activated to acyl-CoA derivatives in the mitochondrial matrix (see Fig. 30.1). Medium-chain-length acyl-CoAs, like long-chain acyl-CoAs, are oxidized to acetyl-CoA via the β-oxidation spiral. Medium-chain acyl-CoAs also can arise from the peroxisomal oxidation pathway.

The medium-chain-length acyl-CoA synthetase has a broad range of specificity for compounds of approximately the same size that contain a carboxyl group, such as drugs (salicylate, from aspirin metabolism, and valproate, which is used to treat epileptic seizures) or benzoate, a common component of plants. Once the drug CoA derivative is formed, the carboxyl group is conjugated with glycine to form a urinary excretion product. With certain disorders of fatty acid oxidation, medium- and short-chain fatty acylglycines may appear in the urine, together with acylcarnitines or dicarboxylic acids. Octanoylglycine, for example, will appear in the urine of a patient with MCAD deficiency.

E. Regulation of β-Oxidation

Fatty acids are used as fuels principally when they are released from adipose tissue triacylglycerols in response to hormones that signal fasting or increased demand. Many tissues, such as muscle and kidney, oxidize fatty acids completely to CO_2 and H_2O. In these tissues, the acetyl-CoA produced by β-oxidation enters the TCA cycle. The FAD(2H) and the NADH from β-oxidation and the TCA cycle are reoxidized by the electron-transport chain, and ATP is generated. The process of β-oxidation is regulated by the cells' requirements for energy (i.e., by the levels of ATP and NADH) because fatty acids cannot be oxidized any faster than NADH and FAD(2H) are reoxidized in the electron-transport chain.

Fatty acid oxidation also may be restricted by the mitochondrial CoASH pool size. Acetyl-CoASH units must enter the TCA cycle or another metabolic pathway to regenerate CoASH required for formation of the fatty acyl-CoA derivative from fatty acylcarnitine.

An additional type of regulation occurs at CPTI. CPTI is inhibited by malonyl coenzyme A (malonyl-CoA), which is synthesized in the cytosol of many tissues by acetyl-CoA carboxylase (Fig. 30.12). Acetyl-CoA carboxylase is regulated by several different mechanisms, some of which are tissue-dependent. In skeletal muscles and liver, it is inhibited when it is phosphorylated by the AMP-activated protein kinase (AMPK). Thus, during exercise, when AMP levels increase, AMPK is activated and phosphorylates acetyl-CoA carboxylase, which becomes inactive. Consequently, malonyl-CoA levels decrease, CPTI is activated, and the β-oxidation of fatty acids is able to restore ATP homeostasis and decrease AMP levels. In liver, in addition to the negative regulation by the AMPK, acetyl-CoA carboxylase is activated by insulin-dependent mechanisms leading to elevated cytoplasmic citrate, an allosteric activator, which promotes the conversion of malonyl-CoA to palmitate in the fatty acid synthesis pathway. Thus, in the liver, malonyl-CoA inhibition of CPTI prevents newly synthesized fatty acids from being oxidized.

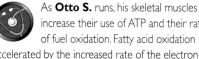
As **Otto S.** runs, his skeletal muscles increase their use of ATP and their rate of fuel oxidation. Fatty acid oxidation is accelerated by the increased rate of the electron-transport chain. As ATP is used and AMP increases, the AMPK acts to facilitate fuel use and maintain ATP homeostasis. Phosphorylation of acetyl-CoA carboxylase results in a decreased level of malonyl-CoA and increased activity of CPTI. At the same time, AMPK facilitates the recruitment of glucose transporters into the plasma membrane of skeletal muscle, thereby increasing the rate of glucose uptake. AMP and hormonal signals also increase the supply of glucose 6-P from glycogenolysis. Thus, his muscles are supplied with more fuel, and all the oxidative pathways are accelerated.

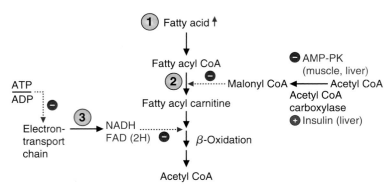

FIGURE 30.12 Regulation of β-oxidation. (*1*) Hormones control the supply of fatty acids in the blood. (*2*) Carnitine palmitoyltransferase I is inhibited by malonyl coenzyme A (malonyl-CoA), which is synthesized by acetyl coenzyme A (acetyl-CoA) carboxylase. *AMP-PK* is the AMP-activated protein kinase. (*3*) The rate of adenosine triphosphate (ATP) use controls the rate of the electron-transport chain, which regulates the oxidative enzymes of β-oxidation and the tricarboxylic acid cycle. *ADP*, adenosine diphosphate; *AMP*, adenosine monophosphate; *CoA*, coenzyme A; *FAD(2H)*, flavin adenine dinucleotide; *NADH*, reduced nicotinamide adenine dinucleotide.

β-Oxidation is strictly an aerobic pathway, dependent on oxygen, a good blood supply, and adequate levels of mitochondria. Tissues that lack mitochondria, such as red blood cells, cannot oxidize fatty acids by β-oxidation. Fatty acids also do not serve as a significant fuel for the brain. They are not used by adipocytes, whose function is to store triacylglycerols to provide a fuel for other tissues. Those tissues that do not use fatty acids as a fuel, or use them only to a limited extent, use ketone bodies instead.

II. Alternative Routes of Fatty Acid Oxidation

Fatty acids that are not readily oxidized by the enzymes of β-oxidation enter alternative pathways of oxidation, including peroxisomal β- and α-oxidation and microsomal ω-oxidation. The function of these pathways is to convert as much as possible of the unusual fatty acids to compounds that can be used as fuels or biosynthetic precursors and to convert the remainder to compounds that can be excreted in bile or urine. During prolonged fasting, fatty acids released from adipose triacylglycerols may enter the ω-oxidation or peroxisomal β-oxidation pathway, even though they have a normal composition. These pathways not only use fatty acids, they act on xenobiotic (a term used to cover all organic compounds that are foreign to an organism) carboxylic acids that are large hydrophobic molecules resembling fatty acids.

A. Peroxisomal Oxidation of Fatty Acids

A small proportion of our diet consists of very-long-chain fatty acids (20 or more carbons) or branched-chain fatty acids arising from degradative products of chlorophyll. Very-long-chain fatty acid synthesis also occurs within the body, especially in cells of the brain and nervous system, which incorporate them into the sphingolipids of myelin. These fatty acids are oxidized by *peroxisomal β- and α-oxidation pathways*, which are essentially chain-shortening pathways.

1. Very-Long-Chain Fatty Acids

Very-long-chain fatty acids of 24 to 26 carbons are oxidized exclusively in peroxisomes by a sequence of reactions similar to mitochondrial β-oxidation in that they generate acetyl-CoA and NADH. However, the peroxisomal oxidation of straight-chain fatty acids stops when the chain reaches 4 to 6 carbons in length. Some of the long-chain fatty acids also may be oxidized by this route.

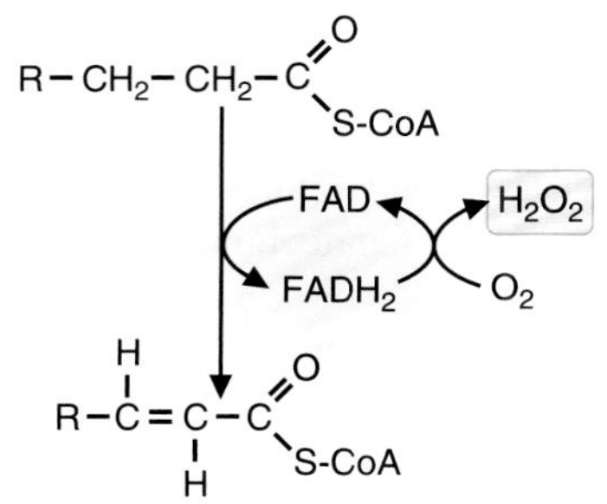

$$R - CH_2 - CH_2 - C\overset{\displaystyle O}{\underset{\displaystyle S\text{-}CoA}{}}$$

FAD ← | H_2O_2

FADH_2 → O_2

$$R - \overset{\displaystyle H}{\underset{\displaystyle }{C}} = \overset{\displaystyle }{\underset{\displaystyle H}{C}} - C\overset{\displaystyle O}{\underset{\displaystyle S\text{-}CoA}{}}$$

FIGURE 30.13   Oxidation of fatty acids in peroxisomes. The first step of β-oxidation is catalyzed by a flavin adenine dinucleotide (FAD)-containing oxidase. The electrons are transferred from FAD(2H) to O_2, which is reduced to hydrogen peroxide (H_2O_2). *CoA*, coenzyme A.

The long-chain fatty acyl-CoA synthetase is present in the peroxisomal membrane, and the acyl-CoA derivatives enter the peroxisome by a transporter that does not require carnitine. The first enzyme of peroxisomal β-oxidation is an oxidase, which donates electrons directly to molecular oxygen and produces hydrogen peroxide (H_2O_2) (Fig. 30.13). (In contrast, the first enzyme of mitochondrial β-oxidation is a dehydrogenase that contains FAD and transfers the electrons to the electron-transport chain via ETF.) Thus, the first enzyme of peroxisomal oxidation is not linked to energy production. The three remaining steps of β-oxidation are catalyzed by enoyl-CoA hydratase, hydroxyacyl-CoA dehydrogenase, and thiolase, enzymes with activities similar to those found in mitochondrial β-oxidation but coded for by different genes. Thus, one NADH and one acetyl-CoA are generated for each turn of the spiral. The peroxisomal β-oxidation spiral continues generating acetyl-CoA until a medium-chain acyl-CoA, which may be as short as butyryl-CoA, is produced (Fig. 30.14).

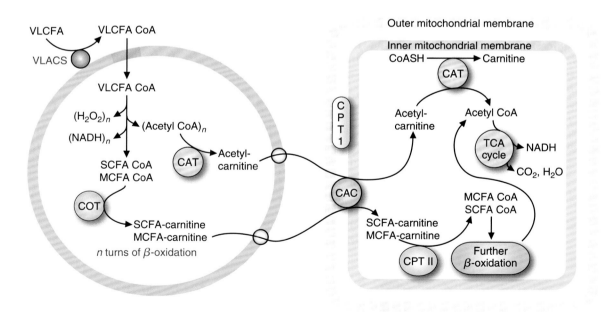

FIGURE 30.14   Chain shortening by peroxisomal β-oxidation. Very-long-chain fatty acyl coenzyme As (acyl-CoAs) and some long-chain fatty acyl-CoAs are oxidized in peroxisomes through *n* cycles of β-oxidation to the stage of a short- to medium-chain fatty acyl-CoA. These short- to medium-chain fatty acyl-CoAs are converted to carnitine derivatives by COT or CAT in the peroxisomes. In the mitochondria, short-chain fatty acylcarnitine is converted back to acyl-CoA derivatives by either CPTII or CAT. *VLCFA*, very-long-chain fatty acyl; *VLACS*, very-long-chain acyl-CoA synthetase; *MCFA*, medium-chain fatty acyl; *SCFA*, short-chain fatty acyl; *CAT*, carnitine acetyltransferase; *COT*, carnitine octanoyltransferase; *CAC*, carnitine:acylcarnitine carrier; *CPT1*, carnitine palmitoyltransferase I; *CPT2*, carnitine palmitoyltransferase II; *OMM*, outer mitochondrial membrane; *IMM*, inner mitochondrial membrane; *NADH*, reduced nicotinamide adenine dinucleotide.

Several inherited deficiencies of peroxisomal enzymes have been described. Zellweger syndrome, the most severe form of a group of related conditions called the *Zellweger spectrum disorder*, results from defective peroxisomal biogenesis. It leads to complex developmental and metabolic phenotypes that affect, principally, the liver and the brain. One of the metabolic characteristics of these diseases is an elevation of C26:0 and C26:1 fatty acid levels in plasma. Refsum disease is caused by a deficiency in a single peroxisomal enzyme, the phytanoyl coenzyme A hydroxylase that carries out α-oxidation of phytanic acid. Symptoms include retinitis pigmentosa, cerebellar ataxia, and chronic polyneuropathy. Because phytanic acid is obtained solely from the diet, placing patients on a low-phytanic acid diet has resulted in marked improvement.

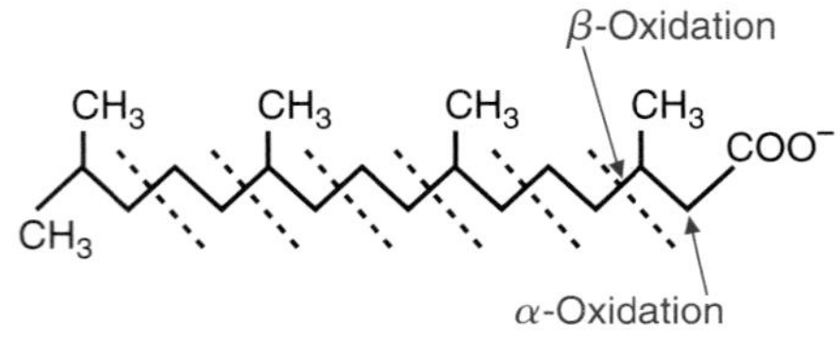

FIGURE 30.15 Oxidation of phytanic acid. A peroxisomal α-hydroxylase oxidizes the α-carbon, and its subsequent oxidation to a carboxyl group releases the carboxyl carbon as CO_2. Subsequent spirals of peroxisomal β-oxidation alternately release propionyl and acetyl coenzyme A. At a chain length of approximately eight carbons, the remaining branched fatty acid is transferred to mitochondria as a medium-chain carnitine derivative.

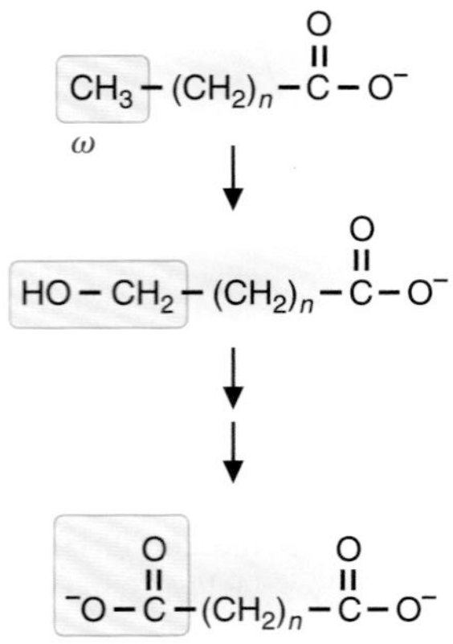

Within the peroxisome, the acetyl groups can be transferred from CoA to carnitine by an acetylcarnitine transferase, or they can enter the cytosol. A similar reaction converts medium-chain-length acyl-CoAs and the short-chain butyryl-CoA to acylcarnitine derivatives. These acylcarnitines diffuse from the peroxisome to the mitochondria, pass through the outer mitochondrial membrane, and are transported through the inner mitochondrial membrane via the carnitine translocase system. They are converted back to acyl-CoAs by carnitine acyltransferases appropriate for their chain length and enter the normal pathways for β-oxidation and acetyl-CoA metabolism. The electrons from NADH and acetyl-CoA can also pass from the peroxisome to the cytosol. The export of NADH-containing electrons occurs through use of a shuttle system similar to those described for NADH electron transfer into the mitochondria.

Peroxisomes are present in almost every cell type and contain many degradative enzymes, in addition to fatty acyl-CoA oxidase, that generate hydrogen peroxide. H_2O_2 can generate toxic free radicals. Thus, these enzymes are confined to peroxisomes, where the H_2O_2 can be neutralized by the free-radical defense enzyme catalase. Catalase converts H_2O_2 to water and O_2 (see Chapter 25).

2. Long-Chain Branched-Chain Fatty Acids

Two of the most common branched-chain fatty acids in the diet are phytanic acid and pristanic acid, which are degradation products of chlorophyll and thus are consumed in green vegetables. Animals do not synthesize branched-chain fatty acids. These two multimethylated fatty acids are oxidized in peroxisomes to the level of a branched C8 fatty acid, which is then transferred to mitochondria. The pathway thus is similar to that for the oxidation of straight very-long-chain fatty acids.

Phytanic acid, a multimethylated C20 fatty acid, is first oxidized to pristanic acid using the α-oxidation pathway (Fig. 30.15). Phytanic acid hydroxylase introduces a hydroxyl group on the α-carbon, which is then oxidized to a carboxyl group with release of the original carboxyl group as CO_2. By shortening the fatty acid by one carbon, the methyl groups will appear on the α-carbon rather than the β-carbon during the β-oxidation spiral and can no longer interfere with oxidation of the β-carbon. Peroxisomal β-oxidation thus can proceed normally, releasing propionyl-CoA and acetyl-CoA with alternate turns of the spiral. When a medium-chain length of approximately eight carbons is reached, the fatty acid is transferred to the mitochondrion as a carnitine derivative, and β-oxidation is resumed.

B. ω-Oxidation of Fatty Acids

Fatty acids also may be oxidized at the ω-carbon of the chain (the terminal methyl group) by enzymes in the endoplasmic reticulum (Fig. 30.16). The ω-methyl group is first oxidized to an alcohol by an enzyme that uses cytochrome P450, molecular oxygen, and NADPH. Dehydrogenases convert the alcohol group to a carboxylic acid. The dicarboxylic acids produced by ω-oxidation can undergo β-oxidation, forming compounds with 6 to 10 carbons that are water-soluble. Such compounds may then enter the blood, be oxidized as medium-chain fatty acids, or be excreted in urine as medium-chain dicarboxylic acids.

Normally, ω-oxidation is a minor process. However, in conditions that interfere with β-oxidation (such as carnitine deficiency or deficiency in an enzyme of β-oxidation), ω-oxidation produces dicarboxylic acids in increased amounts. These dicarboxylic acids are excreted in the urine.

Lola B. was excreting dicarboxylic acids in her urine, particularly adipic acid (which has six carbons) and suberic acid (which has eight carbons):

$$^-OOC-CH_2-CH_2-CH_2-CH_2-COO^-$$ Adipic acid
$$^-OOC-CH_2-CH_2-CH_2-CH_2-CH_2-CH_2-COO^-$$ Suberic acid

Octanoylglycine was also found in the urine.

FIGURE 30.16 ω-Oxidation of fatty acids converts them to dicarboxylic acids.

The pathways of peroxisomal α- and β-oxidation, and microsomal ω-oxidation, are not feedback-regulated. These pathways function to decrease levels of water-insoluble fatty acids or of xenobiotic compounds with a fatty acid–like structure that would become toxic to cells at high concentrations. Thus, their rate is regulated by the availability of substrate.

III. Metabolism of Ketone Bodies

Overall, fatty acids released from adipose triacylglycerols serve as the major fuel for the body during fasting. These fatty acids are completely oxidized to CO_2 and H_2O by some tissues. In the liver, much of the acetyl-CoA generated from β-oxidation of fatty acids is used for synthesis of the ketone bodies acetoacetate and β-hydroxybutyrate, which enter the blood. In skeletal muscles and other tissues, these ketone bodies are converted back to acetyl-CoA, which is oxidized in the TCA cycle with generation of ATP. An alternate fate of acetoacetate in tissues is the formation of cytosolic acetyl-CoA.

A. Synthesis of Ketone Bodies

In the liver, ketone bodies are synthesized in the mitochondrial matrix from acetyl-CoA generated from fatty acid oxidation (Fig. 30.17). The thiolase reaction of fatty acid oxidation, which converts acetoacetyl-CoA to two molecules of acetyl-CoA, is a reversible reaction, although formation of acetoacetyl-CoA is not the favored direction. Therefore, when acetyl-CoA levels are high, this reaction can generate acetoacetyl-CoA for ketone body synthesis. The acetoacetyl-CoA will react with acetyl-CoA to produce 3-hydroxy-3-methylglutaryl coenzyme A (HMG-CoA). The enzyme that catalyzes this reaction is HMG-CoA synthase. In the next reaction of the pathway, HMG-CoA lyase catalyzes the cleavage of HMG-CoA to form acetyl-CoA and acetoacetate.

Acetoacetate can enter the blood directly or it can be reduced by β-hydroxybutyrate dehydrogenase to β-hydroxybutyrate, which enters the blood (see Fig. 30.17). This dehydrogenase reaction is readily reversible and interconverts these two ketone bodies, which exist in an equilibrium ratio determined by the $NADH/NAD^+$ ratio of the mitochondrial matrix. Under normal conditions, the ratio of β-hydroxybutyrate to acetoacetate in the blood is approximately 3:1.

An alternative fate of acetoacetate is spontaneous decarboxylation, a nonenzymatic reaction that cleaves acetoacetate into CO_2 and acetone (see Fig. 30.17). Because acetone is volatile, it is expired by the lungs. A small amount of acetone may be further metabolized in the body.

B. Oxidation of Ketone Bodies as Fuels

Acetoacetate and β-hydroxybutyrate can be oxidized as fuels in most tissues, including skeletal muscle, brain, certain cells of the kidney, and cells of the intestinal mucosa. Cells transport both acetoacetate and β-hydroxybutyrate from the circulating blood into the cytosol and into the mitochondrial matrix. Here, β-hydroxybutyrate is oxidized back to acetoacetate by β-hydroxybutyrate dehydrogenase. This reaction produces NADH. Subsequent steps convert acetoacetate to acetyl-CoA (Fig. 30.18).

In mitochondria, acetoacetate is activated to acetoacetyl-CoA by succinyl-CoA:acetoacetate-CoA transferase. As the name suggests, CoA is transferred from succinyl-CoA, a TCA-cycle intermediate, to acetoacetate. Although the liver produces ketone bodies, it does not use them because this thiotransferase enzyme is not present in sufficient quantity.

One molecule of acetoacetyl-CoA is cleaved to two molecules of acetyl-CoA by acetoacetyl-CoA thiolase, the same enzyme that is involved in β-oxidation. The principal fate of this acetyl-CoA is oxidation in the TCA cycle.

 Ketogenic diets, which are high-fat diets with a 3:1 ratio of lipid to carbohydrate, are being used to reduce the frequency of epileptic seizures in children with refractory seizures. The reason for its effectiveness in the treatment of epilepsy is not known. Ketogenic diets are also used to treat children with PDH deficiency. Ketone bodies can be used as a fuel by the brain in the absence of PDH. They also can provide a source of cytosolic acetyl-CoA for acetylcholine synthesis. They often contain medium-chain triglycerides, which induce ketosis more effectively than long-chain triglycerides.

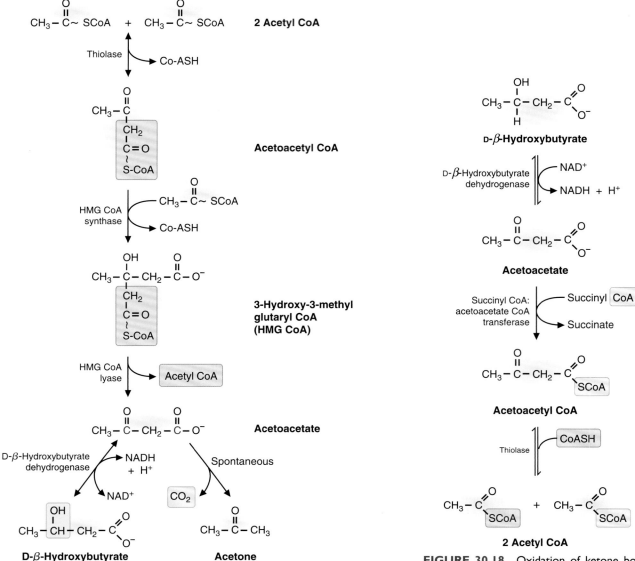

FIGURE 30.17 Synthesis of the ketone bodies acetoacetate, β-hydroxybutyrate, and acetone. The portion of 3-hydroxy-3-methylglutaryl coenzyme A (HMG-CoA) shown in the *tinted box* is released as acetyl coenzyme A (acetyl-CoA), and the remainder of the molecule forms acetoacetate. Acetoacetate is reduced to β-hydroxybutyrate or decarboxylated to acetone. Note that the dehydrogenase that interconverts acetoacetate and β-hydroxybutyrate is specific for the D-isomer. Thus, it differs from the dehydrogenases of β-oxidation, which act on 3-hydroxy acyl-CoA derivatives and is specific for the L-isomer. *CoA*, coenzyme A; *NAD*, nicotinamide adenine dinucleotide.

FIGURE 30.18 Oxidation of ketone bodies. β-Hydroxybutyrate is oxidized to acetoacetate, which is activated by accepting a coenzyme A (CoA) group from succinyl-CoA. Acetoacetyl-CoA is cleaved to two acetyl-CoA, which enter the tricarboxylic acid cycle and are oxidized. *CoA*, coenzyme A; *NAD*, nicotinamide adenine dinucleotide.

The energy yield from oxidation of acetoacetate is equivalent to the yield for oxidation of two molecules of acetyl-CoA in the TCA cycle (20 ATP) minus the energy for activation of acetoacetate (1 ATP). The energy of activation is calculated at one high-energy phosphate bond because succinyl-CoA is normally converted to succinate in the TCA cycle, with generation of one molecule of guanosine triphosphate (GTP) (the energy equivalent of ATP). However, when the high-energy thioester bond of succinyl-CoA is transferred to acetoacetate, succinate is produced without the generation of this GTP. Oxidation of β-hydroxybutyrate generates one additional NADH. Therefore, the net energy yield from 1 mol of β-hydroxybutyrate is approximately 21.5 mol of ATP.

C. Alternative Pathways of Ketone Body Metabolism

Although fatty acid oxidation is usually the major source of ketone bodies, they also can be generated from the catabolism of certain amino acids: leucine, isoleucine, lysine, tryptophan, phenylalanine, and tyrosine. These amino acids are called *ketogenic amino acids* because their carbon skeleton is catabolized to acetyl-CoA or acetoacetyl-CoA, which may enter the pathway of ketone body synthesis in liver. Leucine and isoleucine also form acetyl-CoA and acetoacetyl-CoA in other tissues as well as the liver.

Acetoacetate can be activated to acetoacetyl-CoA in the cytosol by an enzyme similar to the acyl-CoA synthetases. This acetoacetyl-CoA can be used directly in cholesterol synthesis. It also can be cleaved to two molecules of acetyl-CoA by a cytosolic thiolase. Cytosolic acetyl-CoA is required for processes such as acetylcholine synthesis in neuronal cells.

IV. The Role of Fatty Acids and Ketone Bodies in Fuel Homeostasis

Fatty acids are used as fuels whenever fatty acid levels are elevated in the blood (i.e., during fasting and starvation); because of a high-fat, low-carbohydrate diet; or during long-term low- to mild-intensity exercise. Under these conditions, a decrease in insulin and increased levels of glucagon, epinephrine, or other hormones stimulate adipose tissue lipolysis. Fatty acids begin to increase in the blood approximately 3 to 4 hours after a meal and progressively increase with time of fasting up to approximately 2 to 3 days (Fig. 30.19). In the liver, the rate of ketone body synthesis increases as the supply of fatty acids increases. However, the blood level of ketone bodies continues to increase, presumably because their use by skeletal muscles decreases.

After 2 to 3 days of starvation, ketone bodies rise to a level in the blood that enables them to enter brain cells, where they are oxidized, thereby reducing the amount of glucose required by the brain. During prolonged fasting, they may supply as much as two-thirds of the energy requirements of the brain. The reduction in glucose requirements spares skeletal muscle protein, which is a major source of amino acid precursors for hepatic glucose synthesis from gluconeogenesis.

 Children are more prone to ketosis than adults because their bodies enter the fasting state more rapidly. Their bodies use more energy per unit mass (because their ratio of muscle to adipose tissue is higher), and liver glycogen stores are depleted faster (the ratio of their brain mass to liver mass is higher). In children, blood ketone body levels reach 2 mM in 24 hours; in adults, it takes >3 days to reach this level. Mild pediatric infections that cause anorexia and vomiting are the most common causes of ketosis in children. Mild ketosis is observed in children after prolonged exercise, perhaps attributable to an abrupt decrease in muscular use of fatty acids liberated during exercise. The liver then oxidizes these fatty acids and produces ketone bodies.

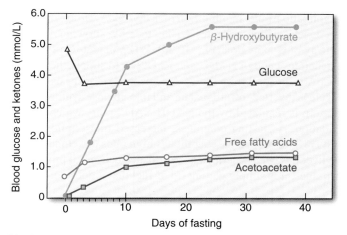

FIGURE 30.19 Levels of ketone bodies in the blood at various times during fasting. Glucose levels remain relatively constant, as do levels of fatty acids. Ketone body levels, however, increase markedly, rising to levels at which they can be used by the brain and other nervous tissue. (From Cahill GF Jr, Aoki TT. How metabolism affects clinical problems. *Med Times.* 1970;98:106.)

The level of total ketone bodies in **Dianne A.'s** blood greatly exceeds normal fasting levels and the mild ketosis produced during exercise. In a person on a normal mealtime schedule, total blood ketone bodies rarely exceed 0.2 mM. During prolonged fasting, they may rise to 4 to 5 mM. Levels >7 mM are considered evidence of ketoacidosis because the acid produced must reach this level to exceed the bicarbonate buffer system in the blood and compensatory respiration (Kussmaul respiration) (see Chapter 4).

A. Preferential Use of Fatty Acids

As fatty acid levels increase in the blood, they are used by skeletal muscles and certain other tissues in preference to glucose. Fatty acid oxidation generates NADH and FAD(2H) through both β-oxidation and the TCA cycle, resulting in relatively high NADH/NAD$^+$ ratios, acetyl-CoA concentrations, and ATP/adenosine diphosphate (ADP) or ATP/AMP levels. In skeletal muscles, AMPK (see Section I.E) adjusts the concentration of malonyl-CoA so that CPTI and β-oxidation operate at a rate that is able to sustain ATP homeostasis. With adequate levels of ATP obtained from fatty acid (or ketone body) oxidation, the rate of glycolysis is decreased. The activity of the regulatory enzymes in glycolysis and the TCA cycle (pyruvate dehydrogenase [PDH] and phosphofructokinase-1 [PFK-1]) are decreased by the changes in concentration of their allosteric regulators (concentrations of ADP, an activator of PDH, decrease; NADH and acetyl-CoA, inhibitors of PDH, increase under these conditions; and ATP and citrate, inhibitors of PFK-1, increase). As a consequence, glucose 6-phosphate (glucose 6-P) accumulates. Glucose 6-P inhibits hexokinase, thereby decreasing the uptake of glucose from the blood and its entry into glycolysis. In skeletal muscles, this pattern of fuel metabolism is facilitated by the decrease in insulin concentration (see Chapter 35). Preferential use of fatty acids does not, however, restrict the ability of glycolysis to respond to an increase in AMP or ADP levels, such as might occur during exercise or oxygen limitation.

B. Tissues that Use Ketone Bodies

Skeletal muscles, the heart, the liver, and many other tissues use fatty acids as their major fuel during fasting and under other conditions that increase fatty acids in the blood. However, several other tissues (or cell types), such as the brain, use ketone bodies to a greater extent. For example, cells of the intestinal mucosa, which transport fatty acids from the intestine to the blood, use ketone bodies and amino acids, rather than fatty acids, during starvation. Adipocytes, which store fatty acids in triacylglycerols, do not use fatty acids as a fuel during fasting but can use ketone bodies. Ketone bodies cross the placenta and can be used by the fetus. Almost all tissues and cell types, with the exception of liver and red blood cells, are able to use ketone bodies as fuel.

C. Regulation of Ketone Body Synthesis

Several events, in addition to the increased supply of fatty acids from adipose triacylglycerols, promote hepatic ketone body synthesis during fasting. The decreased insulin/glucagon ratio results in inhibition of acetyl-CoA carboxylase and decreased malonyl-CoA levels, which activates CPTI, thereby allowing fatty acyl-CoA to enter the pathway of β-oxidation (Fig. 30.20). When oxidation of fatty acyl-CoA to acetyl-CoA generates enough NADH and FAD(2H) to supply the ATP needs of the liver, acetyl-CoA is diverted from the TCA cycle into ketogenesis, and oxaloacetate in the TCA cycle is diverted toward malate and into glucose synthesis (gluconeogenesis). This pattern is regulated by the NADH/NAD$^+$ ratio, which is relatively high during β-oxidation. As fasting continues, increased transcription of the gene for mitochondrial HMG-CoA synthase facilitates high rates of ketone body production. Although the liver has been described as "altruistic" because it provides ketone bodies for other tissues, it is simply getting rid of fuel that it does not need.

Why can't red blood cells use ketone bodies for energy?

CLINICAL COMMENTS

Otto S. As Otto S. runs, he increases the rate at which his muscles oxidize all fuels. The increased rate of ATP use stimulates the electron-transport chain, which oxidizes NADH and FAD(2H) much faster, thereby increasing the rate at which fatty acids are oxidized. During exercise, he also uses muscle glycogen stores, which contribute glucose to glycolysis. In some of the fibers, the

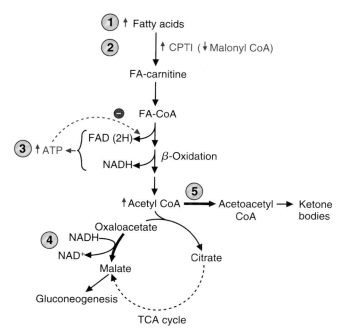

Red blood cells lack mitochondria, which is the site of ketone body use.

FIGURE 30.20   Regulation of ketone body synthesis. (*1*) The supply of fatty acids (FA) is increased. (*2*) The malonyl coenzyme A (malonyl-CoA) inhibition of carnitine palmitoyl-transferase I (CPTI) is lifted by inactivation of acetyl coenzyme A (acetyl-CoA) carboxylase. (*3*) β-Oxidation supplies reduced nicotinamide adenine dinucleotide (NADH) and reduced flavin adenine dinucleotide (FAD[2H]), which are used by the electron-transport chain for oxidative phosphorylation. As adenosine triphosphate (ATP) levels increase, less NADH is oxidized, and the NADH/NAD$^+$ ratio is increased. (*4*) Oxaloacetate is converted into malate because of the high NADH levels, and the malate enters the cytoplasm for gluconeogenesis. (*5*) Acetyl-CoA is diverted from the tricarboxylic acid (TCA) cycle into ketogenesis, in part because of low oxaloacetate levels, which reduces the rate of the citrate synthase reaction.

glucose is used anaerobically, thereby producing lactate. Some of the lactate will be used by his heart, and some will be taken up by the liver to be converted to glucose. As he trains, he increases his mitochondrial capacity, as well as his oxygen delivery, resulting in an increased ability to oxidize fatty acids and ketone bodies. As he runs, he increases fatty acid release from adipose tissue triacylglycerols. In the liver, fatty acids are being converted to ketone bodies, providing his muscles with another fuel. As a consequence, he experiences mild ketosis after his 12-mile run.

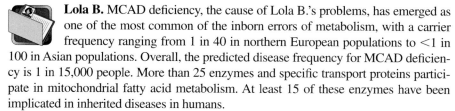

Lola B. MCAD deficiency, the cause of Lola B.'s problems, has emerged as one of the most common of the inborn errors of metabolism, with a carrier frequency ranging from 1 in 40 in northern European populations to <1 in 100 in Asian populations. Overall, the predicted disease frequency for MCAD deficiency is 1 in 15,000 people. More than 25 enzymes and specific transport proteins participate in mitochondrial fatty acid metabolism. At least 15 of these enzymes have been implicated in inherited diseases in humans.

MCAD deficiency is an autosomal-recessive disorder caused by the substitution of a T for an A at position 985 of the *MCAD* gene. This mutation causes a lysine to replace a glutamate residue in the protein, resulting in the production of an unstable dehydrogenase.

The most frequent manifestation of MCAD deficiency is intermittent hypoketotic hypoglycemia during fasting (low levels of ketone bodies and low levels of glucose in the blood). Fatty acids normally would be oxidized to CO_2 and H_2O under these conditions. In MCAD deficiency, however, fatty acids are oxidized only until they reach medium-chain length. As a result, the body must rely to a greater extent on oxidation of blood glucose to meet its energy needs.

Mitochondrial trifunctional protein (MTP) is located in the inner mitochondrial membrane and catalyzes the final three steps of long-chain fatty acid oxidation (the hydratase step, the L-3-hydroxyacyl-CoA dehydrogenase step, and the β-ketothiolase step). Deficiencies in MTP are rare (1 in 200,000 newborns), and the symptoms are quite diverse, depending on the nature of the mutation and the enzyme activity affected by the mutation. Overall, defects in MTP are often associated with significant mortality and morbidity. Because long-chain fatty acid oxidation is impaired, treatment of the disorder often uses dietary supplementation with medium-chain triacylglycerol, as no pharmacologic agents have yet to be developed to treat this disorder.

However, hepatic gluconeogenesis appears to be impaired in MCAD. Inhibition of gluconeogenesis may be caused by the lack of hepatic fatty acid oxidation to supply the energy required for gluconeogenesis, or by the accumulation of unoxidized fatty acid metabolites that inhibit gluconeogenic enzymes. As a consequence, liver glycogen stores are depleted more rapidly, and hypoglycemia results. The decrease in hepatic fatty acid oxidation results in less acetyl-CoA for ketone body synthesis, and consequently, a hypoketotic hypoglycemia develops.

Some of the symptoms once ascribed to hypoglycemia are now believed to be caused by the accumulation of toxic fatty acid intermediates, especially in patients with only mild reductions in blood glucose levels. **Lola B.'s** mild elevation in the blood of liver transaminases may reflect an infiltration of her liver cells with unoxidized medium-chain fatty acids.

The management of MCAD-deficient patients includes the intake of a relatively high-carbohydrate diet and the avoidance of prolonged fasting.

Dianne A. Dianne A., a 26-year-old woman with type 1 diabetes mellitus, was admitted to the hospital in diabetic ketoacidosis. In this complication of diabetes mellitus, an acute deficiency of insulin, coupled with a relative excess of glucagon, results in a rapid mobilization of fuel stores from muscle (amino acids) and adipose tissue (fatty acids). Some of the amino acids are converted to glucose, and fatty acids are converted to ketones (acetoacetate, β-hydroxybutyrate, and acetone). The high glucagon:insulin ratio promotes the hepatic production of ketones. In response to the metabolic "stress," the levels of insulin-antagonistic hormones, such as catecholamines, glucocorticoids, and growth hormone, are increased in the blood. The insulin deficiency further reduces the peripheral use of glucose and ketones. As a result of this interrelated dysmetabolism, plasma glucose levels can reach 500 mg/dL (27.8 mmol/L) or more (normal fasting levels are 70 to 100 mg/dL, or 3.9 to 5.5 mmol/L), and plasma ketones rise to levels of 8 to 15 mmol/L or more (normal is in the range of 0.2 to 2 mmol/L, depending on the fed state of the individual).

The increased glucose presented to the renal glomeruli induces an osmotic diuresis, which further depletes intravascular volume, further reducing the renal excretion of hydrogen ions and glucose. As a result, the metabolic acidosis worsens, and the hyperosmolarity of the blood increases, at times exceeding 330 mOsm/kg (normal is in the range of 285 to 295 mOsm/kg). The severity of the hyperosmolar state correlates closely with the degree of central nervous system dysfunction and may end in coma and even death if left untreated.

BIOCHEMICAL COMMENTS

Acetylation and Regulation of Fatty Acid Oxidation. Previously, in Chapter 16, acetylation of histones was described as a mechanism of regulating gene expression. Histone acetyltransferases (HATs) would catalyze histone acetylation on lysine side chains, leading to histone dissociation from the DNA. This freed the DNA to bind factors important for transcription to occur. Recent work has indicated that acetylation of very-long-chain acyl-CoA dehydrogenase (VLCAD) regulates the activity of the enzyme, and offers more complexity to the regulation of fatty acid oxidation. Acetylation of VLCAD reduces enzymatic activity, whereas deacetylation will restore activity.

A family of proteins known as the *sirtuins* are NAD^+-dependent protein deacetylases. There are seven forms in humans, designated SIRT1 through SIRT7, all of which affect certain areas of metabolism. The sirtuins catalyze the reaction shown in Figure 30.21, in which NAD^+ is split into nicotinamide and 2-*O*-acetyl ADP-ribose, and the protein target is deacetylated (the acetate group is transferred from the target to the 2'-hydroxy group of the ribose attached to the nicotinamide in NAD^+).

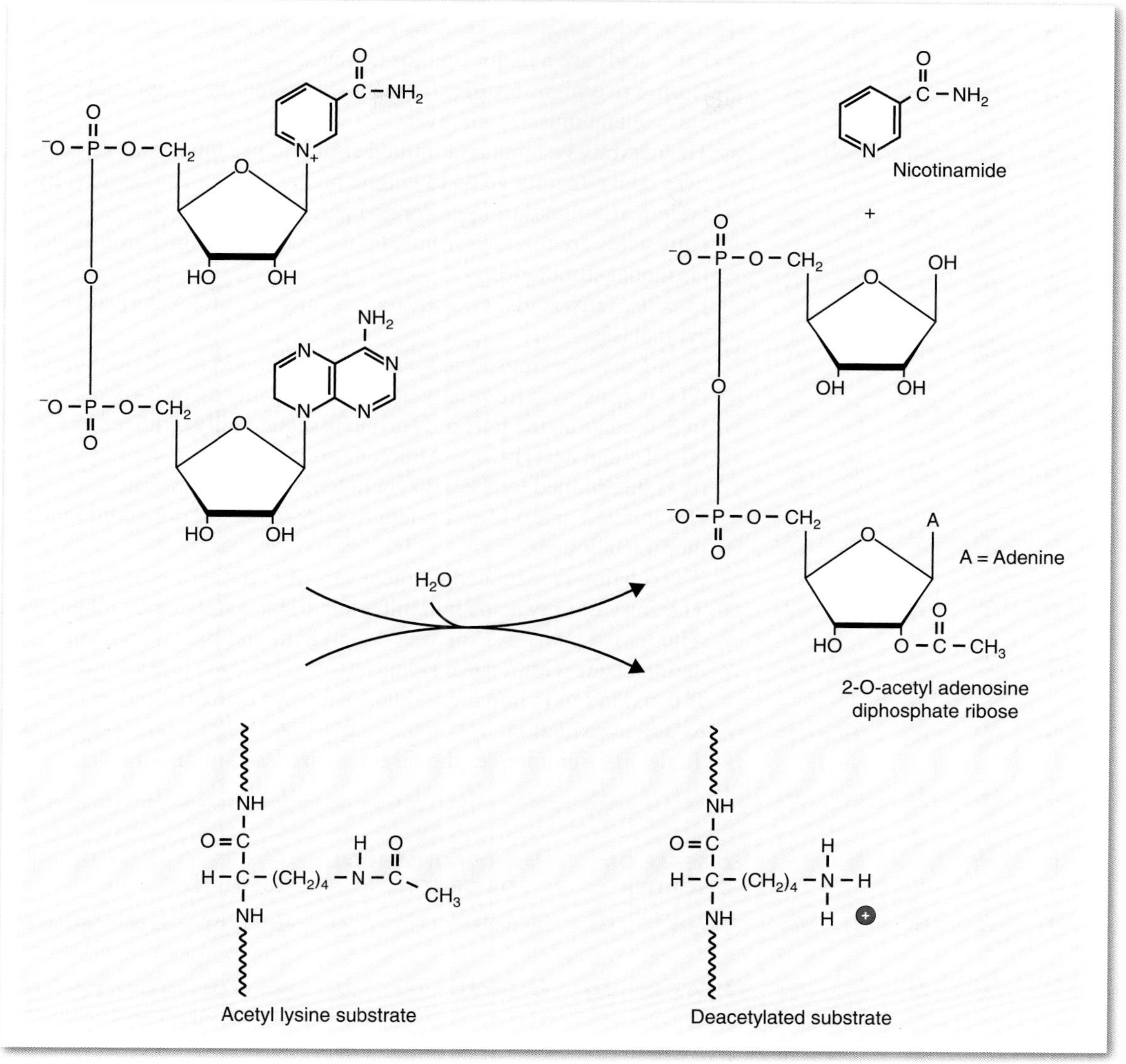

FIGURE 30.21 Generalized sirtuin reaction.

SIRT3 is localized to the mitochondrial matrix, and recent evidence indicates that it is a key regulator for fatty acid oxidation within the mitochondria. Using mice as a model system (which use LCAD, an enzyme present only at very low levels in human tissues), it was demonstrated that SIRT3 expression is upregulated during fasting in the liver. A primary target of SIRT3 deacetylation activity is LCAD, which is hyperacetylated on lysine-42. When hyperacetylated, LCAD activity is reduced. As LCAD will initiate fatty acid oxidation, regulating LCAD activity will regulate overall use of long-chain fatty acids by liver mitochondria. Fasting will upregulate the sirtuins, leading to activation of LCAD and increased fatty acid oxidation by the liver. Mice lacking SIRT3 activity were deficient in fatty acid oxidation during fasting conditions, accumulating long-chain intermediates and triglyceride in the liver. Human VLCAD (the predominant form in humans, as opposed to LCAD in mice) was also demonstrated to be acetylated, and SIRT3 would deacetylate the enzyme in a test tube.

The recent finding of acetylation as a regulatory tool for fatty acid oxidation provides another avenue for complex regulation between various aspects of metabolism, and it provides fertile ground for further research in this area.

KEY CONCEPTS

- Fatty acids are a major fuel for humans.
- During overnight fasting, fatty acids become the major fuel for cardiac muscle, skeletal muscle, and liver.
- The nervous system has a limited ability to use fatty acids directly as fuel. The liver converts fatty acids to ketone bodies, which can be used by the nervous system as a fuel during prolonged periods of fasting.
- Fatty acids are released from adipose tissue triacylglycerols under appropriate hormonal stimulation.
- In cells, fatty acids are activated to fatty acyl-CoA derivatives by acyl-CoA synthetases.
- Acyl-CoAs are transported into the mitochondria for oxidation via carnitine.
- ATP is generated from fatty acids by the pathway of β-oxidation.
- In β-oxidation, the fatty acyl group is sequentially oxidized to yield FAD(2H), NADH, and acetyl-CoA. Although the reactions are similar, enzyme specificity is determined by the acyl chain length of the substrate.
- Unsaturated and odd-chain-length fatty acids require additional reactions for their metabolism.
- β-Oxidation is regulated by the levels of FAD(2H), NADH, and acetyl-CoA.
- The entry of fatty acids into mitochondria is regulated by malonyl-CoA levels.
- Alternative pathways for very-long-chain and branched-chain fatty acid oxidation occur within peroxisomes.
- If β-oxidation is impaired, other pathways of oxidation will be used, such as α- and ω-oxidation.
- Table 30.2 summarizes the diseases discussed in this chapter.

TABLE 30.2 Diseases Discussed in Chapter 30		
DISEASE OR DISORDER	**ENVIRONMENTAL OR GENETIC**	**COMMENTS**
Obesity	Both	The contribution of fatty acids to overall energy metabolism and energy storage
MCAD deficiency	Genetic	Lack of medium-chain acyl-CoA dehydrogenase activity, leading to hypoglycemia and reduced ketone body formation under fasting conditions
Type 1 diabetes	Both	Ketoacidosis; overproduction of ketone bodies owing to lack of insulin and metabolic dysregulation in the liver
Carnitine deficiency	Both	A primary carnitine deficiency is the lack of a membrane transporter for carnitine; a secondary carnitine deficiency is the result of other metabolic disorders.
Zellweger syndrome	Genetic	A defect in peroxisome biogenesis, leading to a lack of peroxisomes and the inability to synthesize plasmalogens or oxidize very-long-chain fatty acids
MTP deficiency	Genetic	A lack of mitochondrial trifunctional protein, leading to hypoglycemia, lethargy, hypoketonemia, and liver problems
Jamaican vomiting disorder	Environmental	Inhibition of an acyl-CoA dehydrogenase activity by hypoglycin; can lead to death from severe hypoglycemia.

acyl-CoA, acyl coenzyme A; MCAD, medium-chain acyl-CoA dehydrogenase; MTP, mitochondrial trifunctional protein.

1. A lack of the enzyme ETF:QO may lead to death because of which one of the following reasons?
    A. The energy yield from glucose use is dramatically reduced.
    B. The energy yield from alcohol use is dramatically reduced.
    C. The energy yield from ketone body use is dramatically reduced.
    D. The energy yield from fatty acid use is dramatically reduced.
    E. The energy yield from glycogen use is dramatically reduced.

2. The ATP yield from the complete oxidation of 1 mol of a C18:0 fatty acid to carbon dioxide and water would be closest to which one of the following?
    A. 105
    B. 115
    C. 120
    D. 125
    E. 130

3. Which one of the following sets of reactions best describes the oxidation of fatty acids?
    A. Oxidation, hydration, oxidation, carbon–carbon bond breaking
    B. Oxidation, dehydration, oxidation, carbon–carbon bond breaking
    C. Oxidation, hydration, reduction, carbon–carbon bond breaking
    D. Oxidation, dehydration, reduction, oxidation, carbon–carbon bond breaking
    E. Reduction, hydration, oxidation, carbon–carbon bond breaking

4. Elevated levels of ketone bodies can be found in the blood of people with untreated type 1 diabetes and individuals on severe diets. A major difference in the laboratory findings of metabolites in the blood of each type of individual (type 1 diabetes vs. the diet) would be which of the following?
    A. Glucose levels
    B. Free fatty acid levels
    C. Lactate levels
    D. Six- and eight-carbon dicarboxylic acid levels
    E. Carnitine levels

5. In which one of the following time spans will fatty acids be the major source of fuel for the tissues of the body?
    A. Immediately after breakfast
    B. Minutes after a snack
    C. Immediately after dinner
    D. While running the first mile of a marathon
    E. While running the last mile of a marathon

6. If your patient has classic carnitine palmitoyltransferase II deficiency, which one of the following laboratory test results would you expect to observe?
    A. Elevated blood acylcarnitine levels
    B. Elevated ketone bodies in the blood
    C. Elevated blood glucose levels
    D. Low CPK blood levels
    E. Reduced blood fatty acid levels

7. A 6-month-old infant is brought to your office because of frequent crying episodes, lethargy, and poor eating. These symptoms were especially noticeable after the child had had an ear infection, at which time he did not eat well. The parents stated that this situation has happened before, but they found if they fed the child frequently, the lethargic episodes could be reduced in number. The results of blood work indicated that the child was hypoglycemic and hypoketotic. Six to eight carbon-chain dicarboxylic acids and acylcarnitine derivatives were found in the urine of the child as well. Based on your understanding of fatty acid metabolism, which enzyme would you expect to be defective in this child?
    A. CPTI
    B. CPTII
    C. LCAD
    D. MCAD
    E. Carnitine:acylcarnitine translocase

8. Vitamin B_{12} is a requirement in the complete oxidation of which of one the following fatty acids?
    A. Short-chain
    B. Medium-chain
    C. Long-chain
    D. Very-long-chain
    E. Odd-chain-length

9. A patient with diabetes in ketoacidosis has a specific odor to the breath. Which one of the following compounds is responsible for this odor?
    A. Acetoacetate
    B. β-Hydroxybutyrate
    C. Acetone
    D. Acetyl-CoA
    E. CO_2

10. A newborn child has been determined to be unable to oxidize phytanic acid and is placed on a diet containing very low levels of this unusual fatty acid. The organelle most likely to contain the defective enzyme, or be altered in this disorder, is which one of the following?
    A. Endoplasmic reticulum
    B. Golgi apparatus
    C. Lysosome
    D. Mitochondria
    E. Peroxisome

ANSWERS

1. **The answer is D.** The ETF:QO is required to transfer the electrons from the FAD(2H) of the acyl-CoA dehydrogenase to CoQ. When the oxidoreductase is missing, the electrons cannot be transferred, and the acyl-CoA dehydrogenase cannot continue to oxidize fatty acids because it contains a reduced cofactor instead of an oxidized cofactor. During times of fasting, when fatty acids are the primary energy source, no energy will be forthcoming, gluconeogenesis is shut down, and death may result. The lack of this enzyme does not affect the other pathways listed as potential answers.

2. **The answer is C.** An 18-carbon saturated fatty acid would require eight spirals of fatty acid oxidation, which yields 8 NADH, 8 FAD(2H), and 9 acetyl-CoA. As each NADH gives rise to 2.5 ATP, and each FAD(2H) gives rise to 1.5 ATP, the reduced cofactors will give rise to 32 ATP. Each acetyl-CoA gives rise to 10 ATP, for a total of 90 ATP. This then yields 122 ATP, but we must subtract 2 ATP for the activation step, at which two high-energy bonds are expended. Thus, the net yield is 120 ATPs for each molecule of fatty acid oxidized.

3. **The answer is A.** Fatty acid oxidation is initiated by the acyl-CoA dehydrogenase (an oxidation step), followed by hydration of the double bond formed in the first step, followed by the hydroxyacyl-CoA dehydrogenase step (another oxidation), and then attack of the β-carbonyl by CoA, breaking a carbon–carbon bond (the thiolase step).

4. **The answer is A.** People with type 1 diabetes exhibit high blood glucose levels caused by the lack of insulin and the inability of peripheral tissues to effectively transport glucose from the blood into the tissue. Individuals on diets would have low blood glucose levels because the majority of energy is being derived from fat and ketone body production. The level of free fatty acids in the blood would be elevated under both conditions owing to the high glucagon-to-insulin ratio. Lactate levels are low under both conditions because glycolysis does not need to act rapidly to provide energy. Six- and eight-carbon dicarboxylic acids in the serum are indicative of a problem in oxidizing fatty acids (MCAD deficiency), which does not apply under these conditions. Carnitine levels in the blood would be expected to be low in both individuals because the tissues require the carnitine for fatty acid oxidation, which is a primary energy source for each type of individual.

5. **The answer is E.** Fatty acids are the major fuel for the body during prolonged exercise and fasting. Answers A, B, and C are incorrect because glucose would be the major fuel after eating. Answer D is incorrect because, at the start of exercise, muscle glycogen and gluconeogenesis are being used as the major source of fuel.

6. **The answer is A.** A defect in CPTII activity would lead to fatty acids being added to carnitine (via CPTI) but not being able to have the carnitine removed. This would lead to a buildup of acylcarnitine levels in the blood. This would also lead to an inability to oxidize fatty acids or synthesize ketone bodies. Because of the lack of energy for gluconeogenesis (owing to reduced fatty acid oxidation), blood glucose levels would be low. The buildup of acylcarnitine in muscle will damage the muscle and release creatine phosphokinase into circulation, leading to increased levels of creatine phosphokinase. The lack of carnitine to accept fatty acids would lead to an accumulation of free fatty acids in the blood.

7. **The answer is D.** The lack of energy from fatty acid oxidation resulted in an inability to synthesize sufficient glucose for the circulation, resulting in the lethargy. Eating frequently maintained blood glucose levels such that the brain could function, and the symptoms were alleviated. As medium-chain fatty acids could not be metabolized further by β-oxidation, ω-oxidation is used and dicarboxylic acids accumulate. Because short-chain dicarboxylic fatty acids are found in the urine, some fatty acid metabolism is occurring, but it cannot go to completion. Even if CPTI, CPTII, or carnitine:acylcarnitine translocase were partially defective, once a fatty acid was transported into the mitochondria, it would be able to be oxidized to completion, and the short-chain dicarboxylic acids would not be observed. Because the observed dicarboxylic acids are short-chain, LCAD activity is normal.

8. **The answer is E.** Fatty acids that contain an odd number of carbons produce propionyl-CoA, a three-carbon fatty acyl-CoA in the final spiral of β-oxidation. This is ultimately converted to succinyl-CoA in a vitamin B_{12}-dependent reaction. Propionyl-CoA also arises from the oxidation of branched-chain amino acids. Vitamin B_{12} is not needed for the complete oxidation of fatty acids with an even number of carbons (saturated or unsaturated).

9. **The answer is C.** Acetoacetate and β-hydroxybutyrate are the ketone bodies produced by the liver. Acetoacetate can be converted to acetone and CO_2. Because acetone is volatile, it is expired by the lungs. In ketoacidosis, increased production of acetone gives the classic odor to the breath.

10. **The answer is E.** The child most likely has a peroxisomal biogenesis disorder such that functional peroxisomes are not produced. The first step of phytanic acid oxidation occurs in the peroxisomes, and lacking either the peroxisomes or phytanic acid oxidase activity can lead to an accumulation of phytanic acid in the blood.

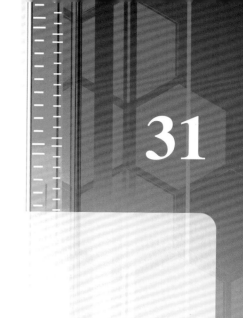

Synthesis of Fatty Acids, Triacylglycerols, and the Major Membrane Lipids

Fatty acids are synthesized mainly in the liver in humans, with dietary glucose serving as the major source of carbon. Glucose is converted through glycolysis to pyruvate, which enters the mitochondrion and forms both acetyl coenzyme A (acetyl-CoA) and oxaloacetate (OAA) (Fig. 31.1). These two compounds condense, forming citrate. Citrate is transported to the **cytosol**, where it is cleaved to form acetyl-CoA, the source of carbon for the reactions that occur on the **fatty acid synthase complex**. The key regulatory enzyme for the process, **acetyl-CoA carboxylase**, produces malonyl coenzyme A (**malonyl-CoA**) from acetyl-CoA.

The growing fatty acid chain, attached to the fatty acid synthase complex in the cytosol, is elongated by the sequential addition of two-carbon units provided by malonyl-CoA. Reduced nicotinamide adenine dinucleotide (**NADPH**), produced by the **pentose phosphate pathway** and **malic enzyme**, provides **reducing equivalents**. When the growing fatty acid chain is 16 carbons in length, it is released as **palmitate**. After activation to a coenzyme A (CoA) derivative, palmitate can be elongated and desaturated to produce a series of fatty acids.

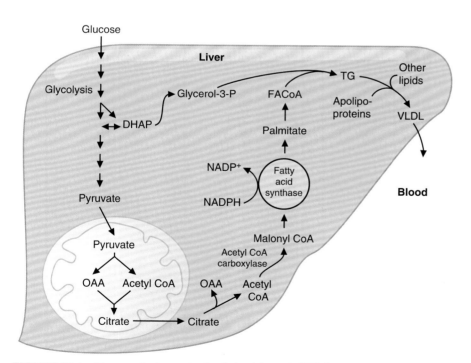

FIGURE 31.1 Lipogenesis, the synthesis of triacylglycerols (TG) from glucose. In humans, the synthesis of fatty acids from glucose occurs mainly in the liver. Fatty acids (FA) are converted to TG, packaged in very-low-density lipoprotein (VLDL), and secreted into the blood. *CoA*, coenzyme A; *DHAP*, dihydroxyacetone phosphate; *FACoA*, fatty acyl coenzyme A; *Glycerol 3-P*, glycerol 3-phosphate; *NADP*, nicotinamide adenine dinucleotide phosphate; *OAA*, oxaloacetate.

Eicosanoids are derived from polyunsaturated fatty acids containing 20 carbon atoms, which are found in cell membranes esterified to membrane phospholipids. Arachidonic acid, derived from the diet or synthesized from linoleate, is the compound from which most eicosanoids are produced in the body. Compounds that serve as signals for eicosanoid production bind to cell membrane receptors and activate phospholipases that cleave the polyunsaturated fatty acids from cell membrane phospholipids.

Fatty acids, produced in cells or obtained from the diet, are used by various tissues for the synthesis of **triacylglycerols** (the major storage form of fuel) and the **glycerophospholipids** and **sphingolipids** (the major components of cell membranes).

In the liver, triacylglycerols are produced from fatty acyl coenzyme A (fatty acyl-CoA) and glycerol 3-phosphate (glycerol 3-P). **Phosphatidic acid** serves as an intermediate in this pathway. The triacylglycerols are not stored in the liver but rather packaged with apolipoproteins and other lipids in **very-low-density lipoprotein (VLDL)** and secreted into the blood (see Fig. 31.1).

In the capillaries of various tissues (particularly adipose tissue, muscle, and the lactating mammary gland), **lipoprotein lipase (LPL)** digests the triacylglycerols of VLDL, forming **fatty acids** and **glycerol** (Fig. 31.2). The glycerol travels to the liver, where it is used. Some of the fatty acids are oxidized by muscle and other tissues. After a meal, however, most of the fatty acids are converted to triacylglycerols in **adipose cells**, where they are **stored**. These fatty acids are released during fasting and serve as the predominant fuel for the body.

Glycerophospholipids are also synthesized from fatty acyl-CoA, which forms esters with glycerol 3-P, producing phosphatidic acid. Various head groups are added to carbon 3 of the glycerol 3-P moiety of phosphatidic acid, generating amphipathic compounds such as **phosphatidylcholine, phosphatidylinositol,** and **cardiolipin** (Fig. 31.3A). In the formation of **plasmalogens** and **platelet-activating factor (PAF)**, a long-chain fatty alcohol forms an **ether** with carbon 1, replacing the fatty acyl ester (see Fig. 31.3B). Cleavage of phospholipids is catalyzed by **phospholipases** found in cell membranes, lysosomes, and pancreatic juice.

Sphingolipids, which are prevalent in membranes and the myelin sheath of the central nervous system, are built on **serine** rather than glycerol. In the synthesis of

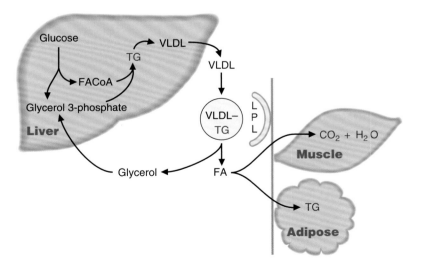

FIGURE 31.2 Fate of very-low-density lipoprotein (VLDL) triacylglycerol (TG). The TG of VLDL, produced in the liver, is digested by lipoprotein lipase (LPL) present on the endothelial cells lining the capillaries in adipose and skeletal muscle tissue. Fatty acids are released and either oxidized in the muscle or stored in adipose tissue as TG. Glycerol is used by the liver because hepatocytes contain glycerol kinase. *CoA,* coenzyme A; *FA,* fatty acid (or fatty acyl group); *FACoA,* fatty acyl coenzyme A.

A

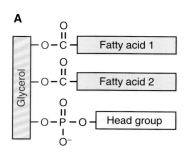

B

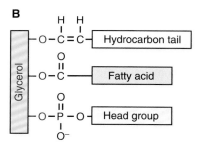

FIGURE 31.3   A. General structure of a glycerophospholipid. The fatty acids are joined by ester bonds to the glycerol moiety. Various combinations of fatty acids may be present. The fatty acid at carbon 2 of the glycerol is usually unsaturated. The head group is the group attached to the phosphate on position 3 of the glycerol moiety. The most common head group is choline, but ethanolamine, serine, inositol, or phosphatidylglycerol also may be present. The phosphate group is negatively charged, and the head group may carry a positive charge (choline and ethanolamine) or both a positive and a negative charge (serine). The inositol may be phosphorylated and thus negatively charged. **B.** General structure of a plasmalogen. Carbon 1 of glycerol is joined to a long-chain fatty alcohol by an ether linkage. The fatty alcohol group has a double bond between carbons 1 and 2. The head group is usually ethanolamine or choline. **C.** General structures of the sphingolipids. The "backbone" is sphingosine rather than glycerol. Ceramide is sphingosine with a fatty acid joined to its amino group by an amide linkage. Sphingomyelin contains phosphocholine, whereas glycolipids **(D)** contain carbohydrate groups.

C

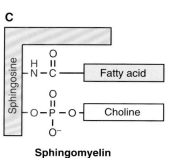

Sphingomyelin

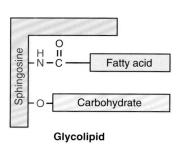

Glycolipid

sphingolipids, serine and palmitoyl-CoA condense, forming a compound that is related to **sphingosine**. Reduction of this compound, followed by addition of a second fatty acid in amide linkage, produces **ceramide**. Carbohydrate groups attach to ceramide, forming **glycolipids** such as the **cerebrosides**, **globosides**, and **gangliosides** (see Fig. 31.3D). The addition of **phosphocholine** to ceramide produces **sphingomyelin** (see Fig. 31.3C). These sphingolipids are degraded by lysosomal enzymes.

THE WAITING ROOM -----------------------------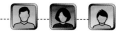

Emma W. has done well with regard to her respiratory function since her earlier hospitalization for an acute asthma exacerbation (see Chapter 28). She has been maintained on two puffs of triamcinolone acetonide, a potent inhaled corticosteroid, two times per day, and has not required systemic steroids for months. The glucose intolerance precipitated by high intravenous and oral doses of the synthetic glucocorticoid prednisone during her earlier hospitalization resolved after this drug was discontinued. She has come to her doctor now because she is

The dietitian did a careful analysis of **Percy V.'s** diet, which was indeed low in fat, adequate in protein, but excessive in carbohydrates, especially refined sugars. Percy's total caloric intake averaged about 430 kilocalories (kcal) per day in excess of his isocaloric requirements. This excess carbohydrate was being converted to fats, accounting for Percy's weight gain. A new diet with a total caloric content that would prevent further gain in weight was prescribed.

Cholesterol determinations in serum use a sequence of enzyme-coupled reactions. Cholesteryl esterase is used to release the fatty acids esterified to circulating cholesterol, producing free cholesterol. The second enzyme in the sequence, cholesterol oxidase, oxidizes cholesterol and reduces oxygen to form hydrogen peroxide. Horseradish peroxidase is then used to catalyze the conversion of a colorless dye to a colored dye, via an oxidation–reduction reaction using the electrons from hydrogen peroxide. The intensity of the color obtained is directly proportional to the level of cholesterol in the sample.

concerned that the low-grade fever and cough she has developed over the last 36 hours may trigger another asthma exacerbation.

Percy V.'s mental depression slowly responded to antidepressant medication, to the therapy sessions with his psychiatrist, and to frequent visits from an old high school sweetheart whose husband had died several years earlier. While he was hospitalized for malnutrition, Mr. V.'s appetite returned. By the time of discharge, he had gained back 8 of the 22 lb he had lost and weighed 131 lb.

During the next few months, Mr. V. developed a craving for "sweet foods" such as the candy he bought and shared with his new friend. After 6 months of this high-carbohydrate courtship, Percy had gained another 22 lb and now weighed 153 lb, 8 lb more than he weighed when his depression began. He became concerned about the possibility that he would soon be overweight and consulted his dietitian, explaining that he had faithfully followed his low-fat diet but had "gone overboard" with carbohydrates. He asked whether it was possible to become fat without eating fat.

Cora N.'s hypertension and heart failure have been well controlled on medication, and she has lost 10 lb since she had her recent heart attack. Her fasting serum lipid profile before discharge from the hospital indicated a significantly elevated serum low-density lipoprotein (LDL) cholesterol level of 175 mg/dL, a serum triacylglycerol level of 280 mg/dL (reference range, 60 to 150 mg/dL), and a serum high-density lipoprotein (HDL) cholesterol level of 34 mg/dL (reference range, >50 mg/dL for healthy women). While she was still in the hospital, she was asked to obtain the most recent serum lipid profiles of her older brother and her younger sister, both of whom were experiencing chest pain. Her brother's profile showed normal triacylglycerols, moderately elevated LDL cholesterol, and significantly suppressed HDL cholesterol levels. Her sister's profile showed only hypertriglyceridemia (high blood triacylglycerols).

Christy L. was born 9 weeks prematurely. She appeared normal until about 30 minutes after delivery, when her respirations became rapid at 64 breaths per minute with audible respiratory grunting. The spaces between her ribs (intercostal spaces) retracted inward with each inspiration, and her lips and fingers became cyanotic from a lack of oxygen in her arterial blood. An arterial blood sample indicated a low partial pressure of oxygen (Po_2) and a slightly elevated partial pressure of carbon dioxide (Pco_2). The arterial pH was somewhat suppressed, in part from an accumulation of lactic acid secondary to the hypoxemia (a low level of oxygen in her blood). A chest radiograph showed a fine reticular granularity of the lung tissue, especially in the left lower lobe area. From these clinical data, a diagnosis of respiratory distress syndrome (RDS), also known as *hyaline membrane disease*, was made.

Christy was immediately transferred to the neonatal intensive care unit, where, with intensive respiration therapy, she slowly improved.

I. Fatty Acid Synthesis

Fatty acids are synthesized whenever an excess of calories is ingested. The major source of carbon for the synthesis of fatty acids is dietary carbohydrate. An excess of dietary protein also can result in an increase in fatty acid synthesis. In this case, the carbon source is amino acids that can be converted to acetyl-CoA or tricarboxylic acid (TCA) cycle intermediates (see Chapter 37). Fatty acid synthesis occurs primarily in the liver in humans, although it can also occur, to a lesser extent, in adipose tissue.

When an excess of dietary carbohydrate is consumed, glucose is converted to acetyl-CoA, which provides the two-carbon units that condense in a series of reactions on the fatty acid synthase complex, producing *palmitate* (see Fig. 31.1). Palmitate is then converted to other fatty acids. The fatty acid synthase complex is located in the cytosol and, therefore, it uses *cytosolic acetyl-CoA*.

A. Conversion of Glucose to Cytosolic Acetyl Coenzyme A

The pathway for the synthesis of cytosolic acetyl-CoA from glucose begins with glycolysis, which converts glucose to pyruvate in the cytosol (Fig. 31.4). Pyruvate enters mitochondria, where it is converted to acetyl-CoA by pyruvate dehydrogenase (PDH) and to OAA by pyruvate carboxylase. The pathway pyruvate follows is dictated by the acetyl-CoA levels in the mitochondria. When acetyl-CoA levels are high, PDH is inhibited and pyruvate carboxylase activity is stimulated. As OAA levels increase because of the activity of pyruvate carboxylase, OAA condenses with acetyl-CoA to form citrate. This condensation reduces the acetyl-CoA levels, which leads to the activation of PDH and inhibition of pyruvate carboxylase. Through such reciprocal regulation, citrate can be continuously synthesized and transported across the inner mitochondrial membrane. In the cytosol, citrate is cleaved by citrate lyase to re-form acetyl-CoA and OAA. This circuitous route is required because PDH, the enzyme that converts pyruvate to acetyl-CoA, is found only in mitochondria and because acetyl-CoA cannot directly cross the mitochondrial membrane.

Reduced nicotinic adenine dinucleotide phosphate (NADPH) is required for fatty acid synthesis and is generated by the pentose phosphate pathway (see Chapter 27) and from recycling of the OAA produced by citrate lyase (see Fig. 31.4). OAA is converted back to pyruvate in two steps: the reduction of OAA to malate by the NAD$^+$-dependent malate dehydrogenase and the oxidation and decarboxylation of malate to pyruvate by an NADP$^+$-dependent malate dehydrogenase (malic enzyme) (Fig. 31.5). The pyruvate formed by malic enzyme is reconverted to citrate. The NADPH that is generated by malic enzyme, along with the NADPH generated by glucose 6-phosphate dehydrogenase and gluconate 6-phosphate dehydrogenase in the pentose phosphate pathway, is used for the reduction reactions that occur on the fatty acid synthase complex.

The generation of cytosolic acetyl-CoA from pyruvate is stimulated by elevation of the insulin/glucagon ratio after a carbohydrate meal. Insulin activates PDH by stimulating the phosphatase that dephosphorylates the enzyme to an active form (see Chapter 23). The synthesis of malic enzyme, glucose 6-phosphate dehydrogenase, and citrate lyase is induced by the high insulin/glucagon ratio. The ability of citrate to accumulate, and to leave the mitochondrial matrix for the synthesis of fatty acids, is attributable to the allosteric inhibition of isocitrate dehydrogenase by high energy levels within the matrix under these conditions. The concerted regulation of glycolysis and fatty acid synthesis is described in Chapter 34.

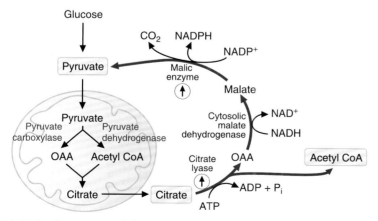

FIGURE 31.4 Conversion of glucose to cytosolic acetyl coenzyme A (acetyl CoA) and the fate of citrate in the cytosol. Citrate lyase is also called *citrate cleavage enzyme. ADP*, adenosine diphosphate; *ATP*, adenosine triphosphate; *NAD*, nicotinamide adenine dinucleotide; *OAA*, oxaloacetate; P_i, inorganic phosphate; ↑, inducible enzyme.

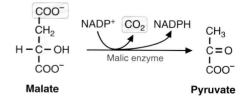

FIGURE 31.5 Reaction catalyzed by malic enzyme. This enzyme is also called the decarboxylating or nicotinamide adenine dinucleotide phosphate (NADP)-dependent malate dehydrogenase.

B. Conversion of Acetyl Coenzyme A to Malonyl Coenzyme A

Cytosolic acetyl-CoA is converted to *malonyl-CoA*, which serves as the immediate donor of the two-carbon units that are added to the growing fatty acid chain on the fatty acid synthase complex. To synthesize malonyl-CoA, *acetyl-CoA carboxylase* adds a carboxyl group to acetyl-CoA in a reaction that requires biotin and adenosine triphosphate (ATP) (Fig. 31.6).

Acetyl-CoA carboxylase is the rate-limiting enzyme of fatty acid synthesis. Its activity is regulated by phosphorylation, allosteric modification, and induction/repression of its synthesis (Fig. 31.7). Citrate allosterically activates acetyl-CoA carboxylase by causing the individual enzyme molecules (each composed of four subunits) to polymerize. Palmitoyl coenzyme A (palmitoyl-CoA), produced from palmitate (the end product of fatty acid synthase activity), inhibits acetyl-CoA carboxylase. Phosphorylation by the adenosine monophosphate (AMP)-activated protein kinase inhibits the enzyme in the fasting state when energy levels are low. Acetyl-CoA carboxylase is activated by dephosphorylation in the fed state when energy and insulin levels are high. A high insulin/glucagon ratio also results in induction of the synthesis of both acetyl-CoA carboxylase and the next enzyme in the pathway, fatty acid synthase.

C. Fatty Acid Synthase Complex

As an overview, *fatty acid synthase* sequentially adds two-carbon units from malonyl-CoA to the growing fatty acyl chain to form palmitate. After the addition of each two-carbon unit, the growing chain undergoes two reduction reactions that require NADPH.

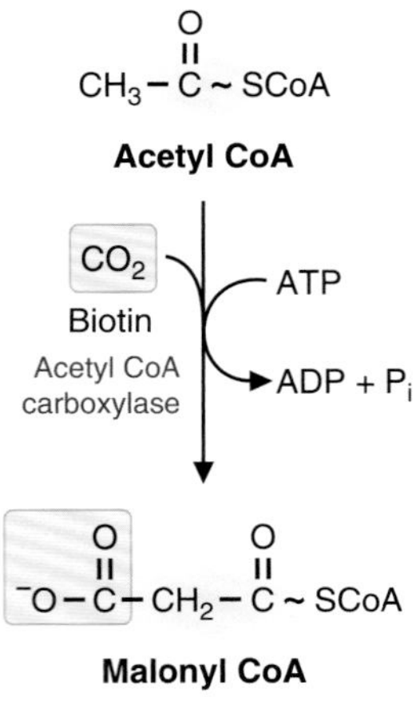

Q Why might certain enzymes use AMP as an allosteric regulator signifying low energy levels as opposed to ADP?

$$O$$
$$\parallel$$
$$CH_3 - C \sim SCoA$$

Acetyl CoA

CO_2 ⟶ ATP

Biotin

Acetyl CoA carboxylase ⟶ $ADP + P_i$

$$O \qquad\qquad O$$
$$\parallel \qquad\qquad \parallel$$
$$^-O - C - CH_2 - C \sim SCoA$$

Malonyl CoA

FIGURE 31.6 Reaction catalyzed by acetyl coenzyme A (acetyl-CoA) carboxylase. Initially, CO_2 is covalently attached to biotin, which is linked by an amide bond to the ε-amino group of a lysine residue of the enzyme. Hydrolysis of adenosine triphosphate (ATP) is required for the attachment of CO_2 to biotin. Subsequently, the CO_2 is transferred to acetyl-CoA to form malonyl coenzyme A. *ADP*, adenosine diphosphate; *CoA*, coenzyme A; *P_i*, inorganic phosphate.

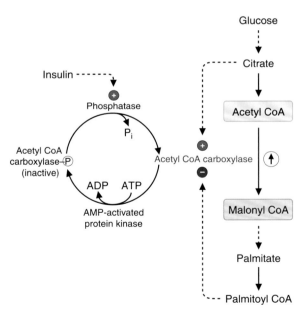

FIGURE 31.7 Regulation of acetyl coenzyme A (acetyl-CoA) carboxylase. This enzyme is regulated allosterically, both positively and negatively, by phosphorylation (Ⓟ) and dephosphorylation, and by diet-induced induction (↑). It is active in the dephosphorylated state when citrate causes it to polymerize. Dephosphorylation is catalyzed by an insulin-stimulated phosphatase. Low energy levels, via activation of the adenosine monophosphate (AMP)-activated protein kinase, cause the enzyme to be phosphorylated and inactivated. The ultimate product of fatty acid synthesis, palmitate, is converted to its coenzyme A (CoA) derivative, palmitoyl coenzyme A (palmitoyl-CoA), which inhibits the enzyme. A high-calorie diet increases the rate of transcription of the gene for acetyl-CoA carboxylase, whereas a low-calorie diet reduces transcription of this gene. *ADP*, adenosine diphosphate; *ATP*, adenosine triphosphate; *P_i*, inorganic phosphate.

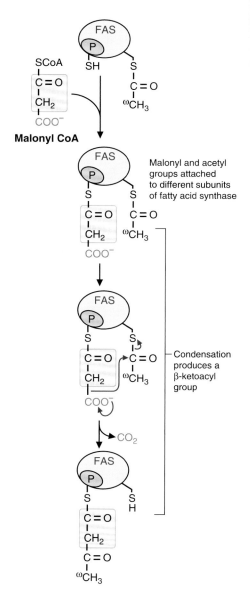

FIGURE 31.8 Addition of a two-carbon unit to an acetyl group on fatty acid synthase (FAS). The malonyl group attaches to the phosphopantetheinyl residue (P) of the acyl carrier protein (ACP) of the fatty acid synthase. The acetyl group, which is attached to a cysteinyl sulfhydryl group, condenses with the malonyl group. CO_2 is released, and a 3-ketoacyl group is formed. The carbon that eventually forms the ω-methyl group of palmitate is labeled ω (and originates from acetyl coenzyme A). *CoA,* coenzyme A; *Malonyl CoA,* malonyl coenzyme A.

The highly active adenylate kinase reaction, 2 ADP ⇔ AMP + ATP allows AMP to be a more sensitive indicator of low energy levels than ADP. Thus, as ADP levels increase, so do AMP levels. The ratio of [AMP]/[ATP] is proportional to the square of the [ADP]/[ATP] ratio. Thus, if the ratio of [ADP]/[ATP] increases 5-fold, the [AMP]/[ATP] may increase 25-fold. The alterations in the concentration of AMP, therefore, are a more sensitive indicator of low energy levels in the cell than alterations in the concentration of ADP.

Fatty acid synthase is a large enzyme composed of two identical subunits, which each have seven catalytic activities and an *acyl carrier protein (ACP)* segment in a continuous polypeptide chain. The ACP segment contains a phosphopantetheine residue that is derived from the cleavage of coenzyme A. The key feature of the ACP is that it contains a free sulfhydryl group (from the phosphopantetheine residue). The two dimers associate in a head-to-tail arrangement, so that the phosphopantetheinyl sulfhydryl group on one subunit and a cysteinyl sulfhydryl group on another subunit are closely aligned.

In the *initial step* of fatty acid synthesis, an acetyl moiety is transferred from acetyl-CoA to the ACP phosphopantetheinyl sulfhydryl group of one subunit and then to the cysteinyl sulfhydryl group of the other subunit. The malonyl moiety from malonyl-CoA then attaches to the ACP phosphopantetheinyl sulfhydryl group of the first subunit. The acetyl and malonyl moieties condense, with the release of the malonyl carboxyl group as CO_2. A four-carbon β-keto acyl chain is now attached to the ACP phosphopantetheinyl sulfhydryl group (Fig. 31.8).

A series of three reactions reduces the four-carbon keto group to an alcohol, then removes water to form a double bond, and lastly reduces the double bond (Fig. 31.9). NADPH provides the reducing equivalents for these reactions. The net result is that the original acetyl group is elongated by two carbons.

The four-carbon fatty acyl chain is then transferred to the cysteinyl sulfhydryl group and subsequently condenses with a malonyl group. This sequence of reactions is repeated until the chain is 16 carbons in length. At this point, hydrolysis occurs, and palmitate is released (Fig. 31.10).

Palmitate is elongated and desaturated to produce a series of fatty acids. In the liver, palmitate and other newly synthesized fatty acids are converted to triacylglycerols that are packaged into VLDL for secretion.

In the liver, the oxidation of newly synthesized fatty acids back to acetyl-CoA via the mitochondrial β-oxidation pathway is prevented by malonyl-CoA. *Carnitine palmitoyltransferase I,* the enzyme involved in the transport of long-chain fatty acids into mitochondria (see Chapter 30), is inhibited by malonyl-CoA (Fig. 31.11). Malonyl-CoA levels are elevated when acetyl-CoA carboxylase is activated, and thus, fatty acid oxidation is inhibited while fatty acid synthesis is proceeding. This inhibition prevents the occurrence of a futile cycle.

D. Elongation of Fatty Acids

After synthesis on the fatty acid synthase complex, palmitate is activated, forming palmitoyl-CoA. Palmitoyl-CoA and other activated long-chain fatty acids can be elongated, two carbons at a time, by a series of reactions that occur in the endoplasmic reticulum (Fig. 31.12). Malonyl-CoA serves as the donor of the two-carbon units, and NADPH provides the reducing equivalents. The series of elongation reactions resembles those of fatty acid synthesis except that the fatty acyl chain is attached to coenzyme A rather than to the phosphopantetheinyl residue of an ACP. The major elongation reaction that occurs in the body involves the conversion of palmityl-CoA (C16) to stearyl-CoA (C18). Very-long-chain fatty acids (C22 to C24) are also produced, particularly in the brain.

E. Desaturation of Fatty Acids

Desaturation of fatty acids involves a process that requires molecular oxygen (O_2), NADH, and cytochrome b_5. The reaction, which occurs in the endoplasmic

 Where does the methyl group of the first acetyl-CoA that binds to fatty acid synthase appear in palmitate, the final product?

The methyl group of acetyl-CoA becomes the ω-carbon (the terminal methyl group) of palmitate. Each new two-carbon unit is added to the carboxyl end of the growing fatty acyl chain (see Fig. 31.8).

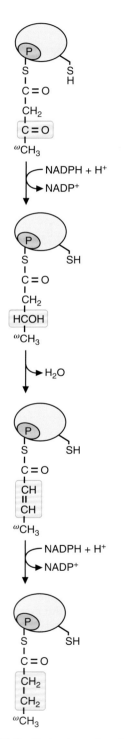

FIGURE 31.9 Reduction of a β-ketoacyl group on the fatty acid synthase complex. Reduced nicotinamide adenine dinucleotide phosphate (NADPH) is the reducing agent.

reticulum, results in the oxidation of both the fatty acid and NADH (Fig. 31.13). The most common desaturation reactions involve the placement of a double bond between carbons 9 and 10 in the conversion of palmitic acid to palmitoleic acid (16:1, Δ^9) and the conversion of stearic acid to oleic acid (18:1, Δ^9). Other positions that can be desaturated in humans include carbons 5 and 6.

Polyunsaturated fatty acids with double bonds three carbons from the methyl end (ω3 fatty acids) and six carbons from the methyl end (ω6 fatty acids) are required for the synthesis of eicosanoids (see Section II of this chapter). Because humans cannot synthesize these fatty acids de novo (i.e., from glucose via palmitate), they must be present in the diet or the diet must contain other fatty acids that can be converted to these fatty acids. We obtain ω6 and ω3 polyunsaturated fatty acids mainly from dietary plant oils that contain the ω6 fatty acid linoleic acid (18:2, $\Delta^{9,12}$) and the ω3 fatty acid α-linolenic acid (18:3, $\Delta^{9,12,15}$). Linoleic and linolenic acids are thus considered essential fatty acids for the human diet. In the body, linoleic acid can be converted by elongation and desaturation reactions to arachidonic acid (20:4, $\Delta^{5,8,11,14}$), which is used for the synthesis of the major class of human prostaglandins and other eicosanoids (Fig. 31.14). Elongation and desaturation of α-linolenic acid produces eicosapentaenoic acid (EPA; 20:5, $\Delta^{5,8,11,14,17}$), which is the precursor of a different class of eicosanoids (see Section II).

Plants are able to introduce double bonds into fatty acids in the region between C10 and the ω-end and, therefore, can synthesize ω3 and ω6 polyunsaturated fatty acids. Fish oils also contain ω3 and ω6 fatty acids, particularly EPA (ω3, 20:5, $\Delta^{5,8,11,14,17}$) and docosahexaenoic acid (ω3, 22:6, $\Delta^{4,7,10,13,16,19}$). The fish obtain these fatty acids by eating phytoplankton (plants that float in water).

Arachidonic acid is listed in some textbooks as an essential fatty acid. Although it is an ω6 fatty acid, it is not essential in the diet if linoleic acid is present because arachidonic acid can be synthesized from dietary linoleic acid (see Fig. 31.14).

The essential fatty acid linoleic acid is required in the diet for at least three reasons: (1) It serves as a precursor of arachidonic acid from which eicosanoids are produced. (2) It covalently binds another fatty acid attached to cerebrosides in the skin, forming an unusual lipid (acylglucosylceramide) that helps to make the skin impermeable to water. This function of linoleic acid may help to explain the red, scaly dermatitis and other skin problems associated with a dietary deficiency of essential fatty acids. (3) It is the precursor of important neuronal fatty acids.

II. Synthesis of the Eicosanoids

Eicosanoids (eicosa is the Greek word for the number 20) are biologically active lipids derived from 20-carbon fatty acids. They consist primarily of the prostaglandins, thromboxanes, and leukotrienes. These lipids are the most potent regulators of cellular function in nature and are produced by almost every cell in the body. They act mainly as "local" hormones, affecting the cells that produce them or neighboring cells of a different type.

Eicosanoids participate in many processes in the body, particularly the *inflammatory response* that occurs after *infection* or *injury*. The inflammatory response is the sum of the body's efforts to destroy invading organisms and to repair damage. It includes control of bleeding through the formation of blood clots. In the process of protecting the body from a variety of insults, the inflammatory response can produce *symptoms* such as *pain*, *swelling*, and *fever*. An exaggerated or inappropriate expression of the normal inflammatory response may occur in individuals who have *allergic* or *hypersensitivity* reactions.

In addition to participating in the inflammatory response, eicosanoids also regulate *smooth muscle contraction* (particularly in the intestine and uterus). They increase *water* and *sodium excretion* by the kidney and are involved in *regulating blood pressure*. They frequently serve as modulators; some eicosanoids stimulate and others inhibit the same process. For example, some serve as constrictors and others as dilators of blood vessels. They are also involved in regulating *bronchoconstriction* and *bronchodilation*.

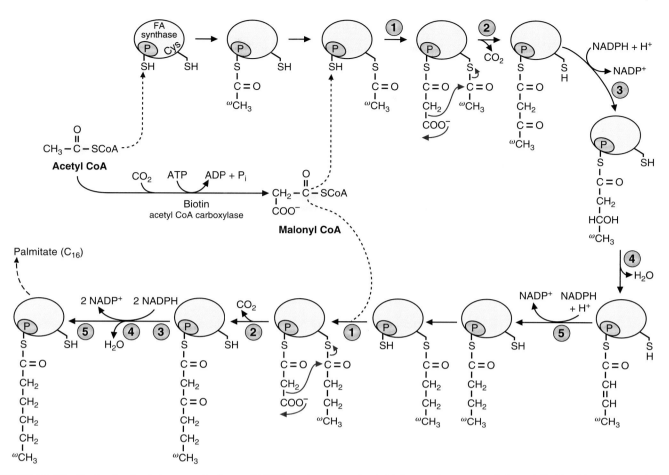

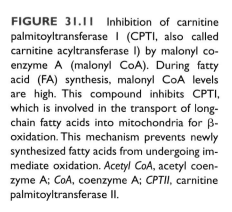

FIGURE 31.10 Synthesis of palmitate on the fatty acid (FA) synthase complex. Initially, acetyl coenzyme A (acetyl CoA) adds to the synthase. It provides the ω-methyl group of palmitate. Malonyl coenzyme A (malonyl CoA) provides the two-carbon units that are added to the growing fatty acyl chain. The addition and reduction steps are repeated until palmitate is produced. (1) Transfer of the malonyl group to the phosphopantetheinyl residue. (2) Condensation of the malonyl and fatty acyl groups. (3) Reduction of the β-ketoacyl group. (4) Dehydration. (5) Reduction of the double bond. P, a phosphopantetheinyl group attached to the fatty acid synthase complex; Cys-SH, a cysteinyl residue on a different subunit of the fatty acid synthase; ADP, adenosine diphosphate; ATP, adenosine triphosphate; NADP, nicotinamide adenine dinucleotide phosphate; P$_i$, inorganic phosphate.

FIGURE 31.11 Inhibition of carnitine palmitoyltransferase I (CPTI, also called carnitine acyltransferase I) by malonyl coenzyme A (malonyl CoA). During fatty acid (FA) synthesis, malonyl CoA levels are high. This compound inhibits CPTI, which is involved in the transport of long-chain fatty acids into mitochondria for β-oxidation. This mechanism prevents newly synthesized fatty acids from undergoing immediate oxidation. Acetyl CoA, acetyl coenzyme A; CoA, coenzyme A; CPTII, carnitine palmitoyltransferase II.

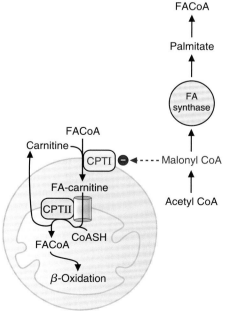

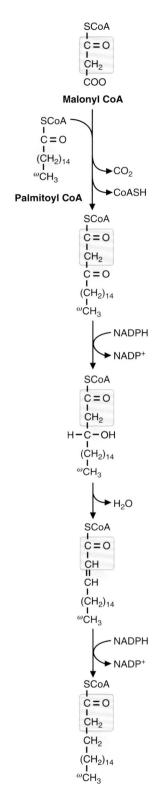

FIGURE 31.12 Elongation of long-chain fatty acids in the endoplasmic reticulum. The example shown is palmitoyl coenzyme A (palmitoyl CoA) being extended to stearoyl coenzyme A (stearoyl CoA). *CoA*, coenzyme A; *Malonyl CoA*, malonyl coenzyme A; *NADP*, nicotinamide adenine dinucleotide phosphate.

A. Source of the Eicosanoids

The most abundant, and therefore the most common, precursor of the eicosanoids is arachidonic acid (C20:4, $\Delta^{5,8,11,14}$), a polyunsaturated fatty acid with 20 carbons and four double bonds. Because arachidonic acid cannot be synthesized in the body (it is an ω6 fatty acid), the diet must contain arachidonic acid or other fatty acids from which arachidonic acid can be produced (such as linoleic acid, found in plant oils). An overview of eicosanoid biosynthesis is shown in Fig. 31.15.

The arachidonic acid present in membrane phospholipids is released from the lipid bilayer as a consequence of the activation of membrane-bound phospholipase A2 or C (see Fig. 31.15). This activation occurs when a variety of stimuli (agonists), such as histamine or the cytokines interact with a specific plasma membrane receptor on the target cell surface. Phospholipase A2 is specific for the sn-2 position of phosphoacylglycerols, the site of attachment of arachidonic acid to the glycerol moiety. Phospholipase C, conversely, hydrolyzes phosphorylated inositol from the inositol glycerophospholipids, generating a diacylglycerol (DAG) containing arachidonic acid. This arachidonic acid is subsequently released by the action of other lipases.

B. Pathways for Eicosanoid Synthesis

After arachidonic acid is released into the cytosol, it is converted to eicosanoids by a variety of enzymes with activities that vary among tissues. This variation explains why some cells, such as those in the vascular endothelium, synthesize prostaglandins E_2 and I_2 (PGE_2 and PGI_2), whereas cells such as platelets synthesize primarily thromboxane A_2 (TXA_2) and 12-hydroxyeicosatetraenoic acid (12-HETE).

Three major pathways for the metabolism of arachidonic acid occur in various tissues (Fig. 31.16). The first of these, the cyclooxygenase pathway, leads to the synthesis of prostaglandins and thromboxanes. The second, the lipoxygenase pathway, yields the leukotrienes, HETEs, and lipoxins. The third pathway, catalyzed by the cytochrome P450 system, is responsible for the synthesis of the epoxides, HETEs, and diHETEs. Only the *cyclooxygenase pathway* will be discussed further in this text. Information about the other pathways can be found in the online supplement to the text.

C. Cyclooxygenase Pathway: Synthesis of the Prostaglandins and Thromboxanes

1. Structures of the Prostaglandins

Prostaglandins are fatty acids containing 20 carbon atoms, including an internal 5-carbon ring. In addition to this ring, each of the biologically active prostaglandins has a hydroxyl group at carbon 15, a double bond between carbons 13 and 14, and various substituents on the ring.

The nomenclature for the prostaglandins (PGs) involves the assignment of a capital letter (PGE), an Arabic numeral subscript (PGE_1), and, for the PGF family, a Greek letter subscript (e.g., $PGF_{2\alpha}$). The capital letter, in this case "F," refers to the ring substituents shown in Figure 31.17.

The subscript that follows the capital letter (PGF_1) refers to the PG series 1, 2, or 3 determined by the number of unsaturated bonds present in the linear portion of the hydrocarbon chain. It does not include double bonds in the internal ring. Prostaglandins of the 1-series have one double bond (between carbons 13 and 14). The 2-series has two double bonds (between carbons 13 and 14, and 5 and 6), and the 3-series has three double bonds (between carbons 13 and 14, 5 and 6, and 17 and 18). The double bonds between carbons 13 and 14 are *trans*; the others are *cis*. The precursor for the 1-series of prostaglandins is *cis* $\Delta^{8,11,14}$ eicosatrienoic acid; for the 2-series, it is arachidonic acid; for the 3-series, it is *cis* $\Delta^{5,8,11,14,17}$ EPA.

The Greek letter subscript, found only in the F series, refers to the position of the hydroxyl group at carbon 9. This hydroxyl group primarily exists in the α-position, where it lies below the plane of the ring, as does the hydroxyl group at carbon 11.

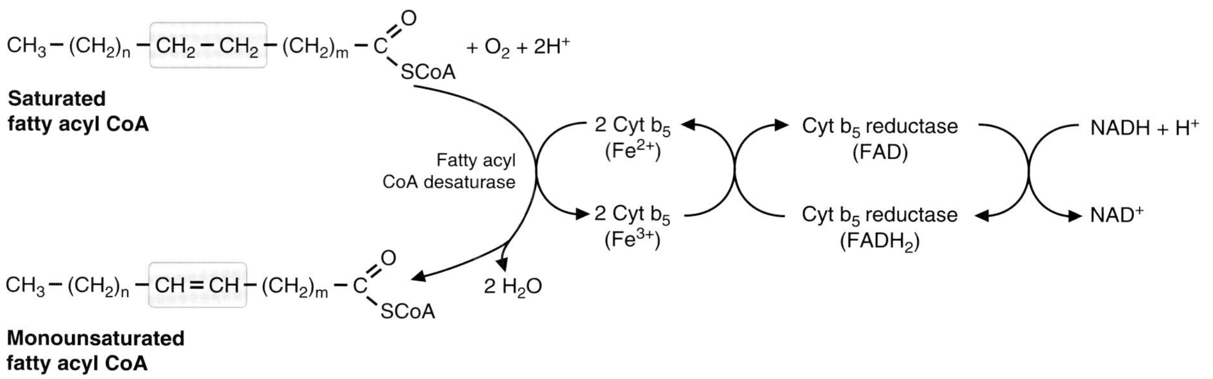

$$CH_3 - (CH_2)_n - \boxed{CH_2 - CH_2} - (CH_2)_m - C\overset{\displaystyle O}{\underset{\displaystyle SCoA}{\big\langle}} + O_2 + 2H^+$$

**Saturated
fatty acyl CoA**

Fatty acyl
CoA desaturase

2 Cyt b_5
(Fe^{2+})

2 Cyt b_5
(Fe^{3+})

Cyt b_5 reductase
(FAD)

Cyt b_5 reductase
($FADH_2$)

NADH + H⁺

NAD⁺

2 H_2O

$$CH_3 - (CH_2)_n - \boxed{CH = CH} - (CH_2)_m - C\overset{\displaystyle O}{\underset{\displaystyle SCoA}{\big\langle}}$$

**Monounsaturated
fatty acyl CoA**

FIGURE 31.13 Desaturation of fatty acids. The process occurs in the endoplasmic reticulum and uses molecular oxygen. Both the fatty acid and reduced nicotinamide adenine dinucleotide (NADH) are oxidized. Human desaturases cannot introduce double bonds between carbon 9 and the methyl end, and are limited to positions 5, 6, and 9. Therefore, m is ≤ 7. *CoA*, coenzyme A; *Cyt*, cytochrome; *FAD*, flavin adenine dinucleotide; *Fatty acyl CoA*, fatty acyl coenzyme A.

2. Structure of the Thromboxanes

The *thromboxanes*, derived from arachidonic acid via the cyclooxygenase pathway, closely resemble the prostaglandins in structure except that they contain a six-membered ring that includes an oxygen atom (see Fig. 31.15). The most common thromboxane, TXA_2, contains an additional oxygen atom attached both to carbon 9 and carbon 11 of the ring. The thromboxanes were named for their action in producing blood clots (thrombi).

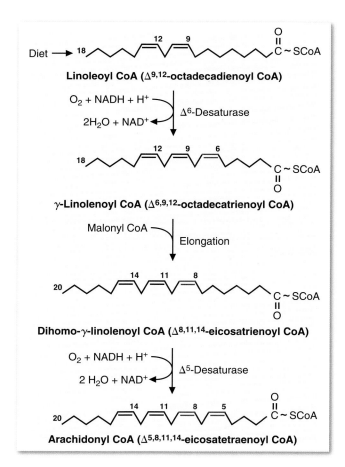

FIGURE 31.14 Conversion of linoleic acid to arachidonic acid. Dietary linoleic acid (as linoleoyl coenzyme A [linoleoyl CoA]) is desaturated at carbon 6, elongated by two carbons, and then desaturated at carbon 5 to produce arachidonyl coenzyme A (arachidonyl CoA). *CoA*, coenzyme A; *NAD*, nicotinamide adenine dinucleotide.

M The measurement of prostaglandin levels, in plasma or urine, is best done by radioimmunoassay (see Chapter 41, "Biochemical Comments"). Antibodies specific for each prostaglandin, or thromboxane form, are commercially available, and through competition with a standard amount of antigen, one can determine the concentration of the metabolite in the biologic fluid. Recently, a more sensitive technique has been developed, which can assay prostaglandin levels as low as 40 pg/mL. This technique is called *fluorescent polarization immunoassay* (FPIA). The method is based on the properties of small fluorescent molecules. Molecules that fluoresce absorb light at a particular wavelength and will emit light of a lower wavelength (the fluorescence). If one excites a small fluorophore with polarized light, the fluorescence will be polarized if the molecule rotates slowly; if the molecule rotates rapidly, the emitted light will not be polarized. If, then, the fluorophore is bound to a much larger molecule, such as an antibody, its rotation would be greatly diminished, and the fluorescent signal emitted will be highly polarized. One can, therefore, measure the polarization of the emitted light as a function of how much fluorescent standard is bound to the antibody. So for these assays, a known amount of a fluorescent prostaglandin is incubated with the samples; if the sample contains nonfluorescent prostaglandin, it will compete for binding with the fluorescent prostaglandin, relegating some fluorescent prostaglandin to being nonbound. When the excitation light hits the sample, the amount of polarization will decrease in proportion to the amount of fluorescent prostaglandin displaced from the antibody. Through use of a standard curve, one can then calculate the level of prostaglandin in the sample to very low levels.

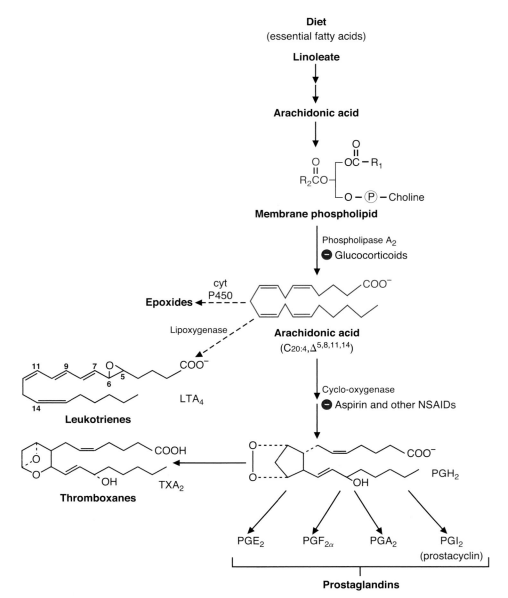

FIGURE 31.15 Overview of eicosanoid metabolism. Eicosanoids are produced from fatty acids released from membrane phospholipids. In humans, arachidonic acid is the major precursor of the eicosanoids, which include the prostaglandins (PG), leukotrienes (LT), and thromboxanes (TX). ⊖, inhibits; *cyt*, cytochrome; *NSAID*, nonsteroidal antiinflammatory drug.

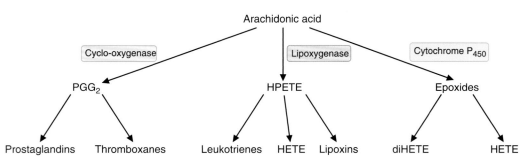

FIGURE 31.16 Pathways for the metabolism of arachidonic acid. *PG*, prostaglandin; *diHETE*, dihydroxyeicosatetraenoic acid; *HETE*, hydroxyeicosatetraenoic acid; *HPETE*, hydroperoxyeicosatetraenoic acid.

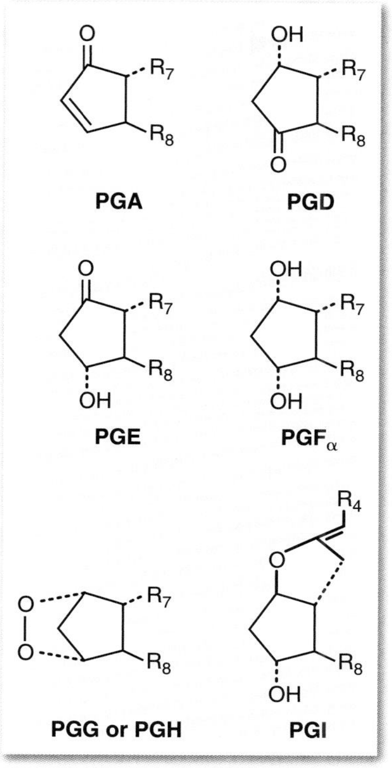

FIGURE 31.17 Ring substituents of the prostaglandins (PG). The letter after PG denotes the configuration of the ring and its substituents. R_4, R_7, and R_8 represent the nonring portions of the molecule. R_4 contains four carbons (including the carboxyl group). R_7 and R_8 contain seven and eight carbons, respectively. Note that the prostacyclins (PGI) contain two rings.

3. Biosynthesis of the Prostaglandins and Thromboxanes

Only the biosynthesis of those prostaglandins derived from arachidonic acid (e.g., the 2-series, such as PGE_2, PGI_2, TXA_2) is described because those derived from eicosatrienoic acid (the 1-series) or from EPA (the 3-series) are present in very small amounts in humans on a normal diet.

The biochemical reactions that lead to the synthesis of prostaglandins and thromboxanes are illustrated in Figure 31.18. The initial step, which is catalyzed by a cyclooxygenase, forms the five-membered ring and adds four atoms of oxygen (two between carbons 9 and 11, and two at carbon 15) to form the unstable endoperoxide, PGG_2. The hydroperoxy group at carbon 15 is quickly reduced to a hydroxyl group by a peroxidase to form another endoperoxide, PGH_2.

The next step is tissue-specific (see Fig. 31.18). Depending on the type of cell involved, PGH_2 may be reduced to PGE_2 or PGD_2 by specific enzymes (PGE synthase and PGD synthase). PGE_2 may be further reduced by PGE 9-ketoreductase to form $PGF_{2\alpha}$. $PGF_{2\alpha}$ also may be formed directly from PGH_2 by the action of an endoperoxide reductase. Some of the major functions of the prostaglandins are listed in Table 31.1.

PGH_2 may be converted to the thromboxane TXA_2, a reaction catalyzed by TXA synthase (see Fig. 31.18). This enzyme is present in high concentration in platelets. In the vascular endothelium, however, PGH_2 is converted to the prostaglandin PGI_2 (prostacyclin) by PGI synthase (see Fig. 31.18). TXA_2 and PGI_2 have important antagonistic biologic effects on vasomotor and smooth muscle tone and on platelet aggregation. Some of the known functions of the thromboxanes are listed in Table 31.2.

In the 1990s, the cyclooxygenase enzyme was found to exist as two distinct isoforms designated COX-1 and COX-2. COX-1 is regarded as a constitutive form of the enzyme, is widely expressed in almost all tissues, is the only form expressed in mature platelets, and is involved in the production of prostaglandins and

The predominant eicosanoid in platelets is TXA_2, a potent vasoconstrictor and a stimulator of platelet aggregation. The latter action initiates thrombus formation at sites of vascular injury as well as in the vicinity of a ruptured atherosclerotic plaque in the lumen of vessels such as the coronary arteries. Such thrombi may cause sudden total occlusion of the vascular lumen, causing acute ischemic damage to tissues distal to the block (i.e., acute myocardial infarction).

Aspirin, by covalently acetylating the active site of cyclooxygenase, blocks the production of TXA_2 from its major precursor, arachidonic acid. By causing this mild hemostatic defect, low-dose aspirin has been shown to be effective in prevention of acute myocardial infarction. For **Ivan A.** (who has symptoms of coronary heart disease), aspirin is used to prevent a first heart attack (primary prevention). For **Anne J.** and **Cora N.** (who already have had heart attacks), aspirin is used in the hope of preventing a second heart attack (secondary prevention).

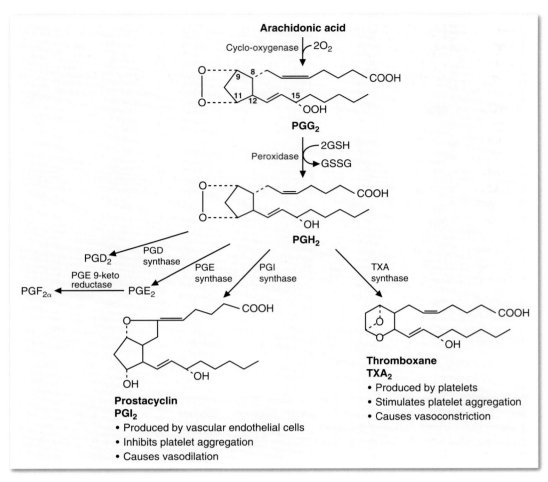

FIGURE 31.18   Formation of prostaglandins (including the prostacyclin PGI$_2$) and thromboxane TXA$_2$ from arachidonic acid. The conversion of arachidonic acid to PGH$_2$ is catalyzed by a membrane-bound enzyme, prostaglandin endoperoxide synthase, which has cyclooxygenase and peroxidase activities. The reducing agent is glutathione (GSH), which is oxidized to form a disulfide between the two glutathione molecules (GSSG).

thromboxanes for "normal" physiologic functions. COX-2 is an inducible form of the enzyme regulated by a variety of cytokines and growth factors. COX-2 messenger RNA (mRNA) and protein levels are usually low in most healthy tissue but are expressed at high levels in inflamed tissue.

Because of the importance of prostaglandins in mediating the inflammatory response, drugs that block prostaglandin production should provide relief from pain.

TABLE 31.1 Some Functions of the Prostaglandins	
PGI$_2$, PGE$_2$, PGD$_2$	**PGF$_{2\alpha}$**
Increases	Increases
Vasodilation	Vasoconstriction
cAMP	Bronchoconstriction
Decreases	Smooth muscle contraction
Platelet aggregation	
Leukocyte aggregation	
IL-1^a and IL-2	
T-cell proliferation	
Lymphocyte migration	

cAMP, cyclic adenosine monophosphate; PG, prostaglandin.
^{a}IL, interleukin, a cytokine that augments the activity of many cells in the immune system.

TABLE 31.2   Some Functions of Thromboxane A₂

Increases

Vasoconstriction

Platelet aggregation

Lymphocyte proliferation

Bronchoconstriction

The cyclooxygenase enzyme is inhibited by all nonsteroidal antiinflammatory drugs (NSAIDs) such as aspirin (acetylsalicylic acid). Aspirin transfers an acetyl group to the enzyme, irreversibly inactivating it (Fig. 31.19). Other NSAIDs (e.g., ibuprofen, naproxen) act as reversible inhibitors of cyclooxygenase. Ibuprofen is the major ingredient in popular over-the-counter NSAIDs such as Motrin and Advil (see Fig. 31.19). Although they have some relative selectivity for inhibiting either COX-1 or COX-2, NSAIDs block the activity of both isoforms. These findings provided the impetus for the development of selective COX-2 inhibitors, which act as potent antiinflammatory agents by inhibiting COX-2 activity, but with less gastrointestinal and antiplatelet side effects than commonly associated with NSAID use. These adverse effects of NSAIDs are thought to be caused by COX-1 inhibition. An example of a selective COX-2 inhibitor is celecoxib (Celebrex). Some properties of COX-1 and COX-2 are indicated in Table 31.3.

4. Inactivation of the Prostaglandins and Thromboxanes

Prostaglandins and thromboxanes are rapidly inactivated. Their half-lives ($t_{1/2}$) range from seconds to minutes. The prostaglandins are inactivated by oxidation of the 15-hydroxy group, critical for their activity, to a ketone. The double-bond at carbon 13 is reduced. Subsequently, both β- and ω-oxidation of the nonring portions occur, producing dicarboxylic acids that are excreted in the urine. Active TXA₂ is rapidly metabolized to TXB₂ by cleavage of the oxygen bridge between carbons 9 and 11 to form two hydroxyl groups. TXB₂ has no biologic activity.

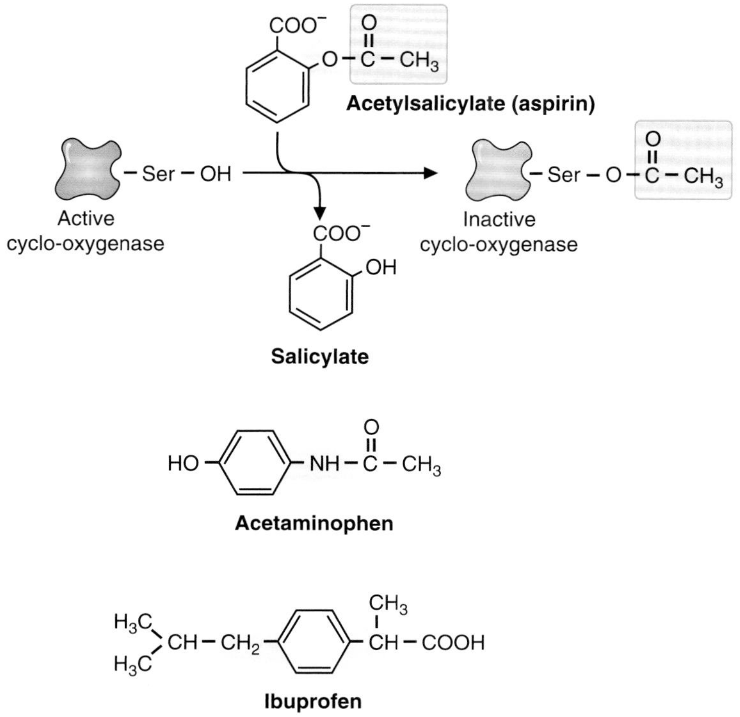

Diets that include cold-water fish (e.g., salmon, mackerel, brook trout, herring), with a high content of polyunsaturated fatty acids, EPA, and docosahexaenoic acid (DHA), result in a high content of these fatty acids in membrane phospholipids. It has been suggested that such diets are effective in preventing heart disease, in part because they lead to formation of more TXA₃ relative to TXA₂. TXA₃ is less effective in stimulating platelet aggregation than its counterpart in the 2-series, TXA₂.

Although the COX-2 inhibitors did relieve the development of gastrointestinal ulcers in patients taking NSAIDs, further studies indicated that specific COX-2 inhibitors may have a negative effect on cardiovascular function. Vioxx was withdrawn from the market by its manufacturer because of these negative patient studies. It has been postulated that long-term use of COX-2 inhibitors alter the balance of prostacyclin (antithrombotic, PGI₂) and thromboxane (prothrombotic) because platelets, the major source of the thromboxanes, do not express COX-2 and thromboxane synthesis is not reduced with COX-2 inhibitors (see Figure 31.18 and Table 31.3). This will tilt the balance of the eicosanoids synthesized toward a thrombotic pathway. The COX-2 inhibitors that remain on the market must be used with caution, because they are contraindicated in patients with ischemic heart disease or stroke.

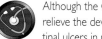

FIGURE 31.19 Action of aspirin and other nonsteroidal antiinflammatory drugs.

TABLE 31.3 Properties of COX-1 and COX-2

	COX-1	COX-2
Primary function	Platelet aggregation, stomach cytoprotection	Inflammation, hyperalgesia
Response to:		
Nonsteroidal antiinflammatory drugs	Decreased activity	Decreased activity
Steroids	No effect	Decreased synthesis and activity
COX-2 inhibitor	No effect	Decreased activity

Data adapted from Patrono and Baigent (see References) indicate that low-dose aspirin (50 to 100 mg/day) reduces platelet thromboxane A_2 (TXA_2) levels by 97%, with no effect on whole-body prostaglandin I_2 (PGI_2), thereby leading to cardioprotection. High-dose aspirin (650 to 1,300 mg/day), in addition to reducing TXA_2 levels, also reduced PGI_2 levels by 60% to 80%. COX-2 specific inhibitors, at high levels, had no effect on TXA_2 levels but reduced whole-body PGI_2 levels by 60% to 80%, leading to an increased risk of myocardial infarction.

D. Mechanism of Action of the Eicosanoids

The eicosanoids have a wide variety of physiologic effects, which are generally initiated through interaction of the eicosanoid with a specific receptor on the plasma membrane of a target cell (Table 31.4). This eicosanoid-receptor binding either activates the adenylate cyclase-cAMP-protein kinase A (PKA) system (PGE, PGD, and PGI series) or causes an increase in the level of calcium in the cytosol of target cells ($PGF_{2\alpha}$, TXA_2, the endoperoxides, and the leukotrienes).

In some systems, the eicosanoids appear to modulate the degree of activation of adenylate cyclase in response to other stimuli. In these instances, the eicosanoid may bind to a regulatory subunit of the guanosine triphosphate (GTP)-binding proteins (G-proteins) within the plasma membrane of the target cell (see Chapter 11). If the eicosanoid binds to the stimulatory subunit, the effect of the stimulus is amplified. Conversely, if the eicosanoid binds to the inhibitory subunit, the cellular response to the stimulus is reduced. Through these influences on the activation of adenylate cyclase, eicosanoids contribute to the regulation of cell function.

Some of the biologic effects of certain eicosanoids occur as a result of a paracrine or autocrine action. One paracrine action is the contraction of vascular smooth muscle cells caused by TXA_2 released from circulating platelets (vasoconstriction).

TABLE 31.4 Prostaglandin and Thromboxane Receptors

RECEPTOR	TYPE OF LIGAND	G-PROTEIN-COUPLED	cAMP RESPONSE	CALCIUM RESPONSE
DP	PGD series	Yes	Increase	Increase
CRTH2	PGD series	Yes	Decrease	Increase
EP1	PGE series	Yes	None	Increase
EP2	PGE series	Yes	Increase	None
EP3	PGE series	Yes	Decrease	None
EP4	PGE series	Yes	Increase	None
FP	PGF series	Yes	None	Increase
IP	PGI series	Yes	Increase or decrease[a]	None
TP	Thromboxane A	Yes	Increase or decrease[b]	Increase

cAMP, cyclic adenosine monophosphate; PG, prostaglandin.
[a]Depends on a modification of the C terminus of the receptor.
[b]Depends on cell type responding to the ligand.

An autocrine action of eicosanoids is exemplified by platelet aggregation induced by TXA_2 produced by the platelets themselves.

The eicosanoids influence the cellular function of almost every tissue of the body. Certain organ systems are affected to a greater degree than others.

III. Synthesis of Triacylglycerols and VLDL Particles

In liver and adipose tissue, *triacylglycerols* are produced by a pathway that contains a phosphatidic acid intermediate (Fig. 31.20). Phosphatidic acid is also the precursor of the glycerolipids found in cell membranes and the blood lipoproteins.

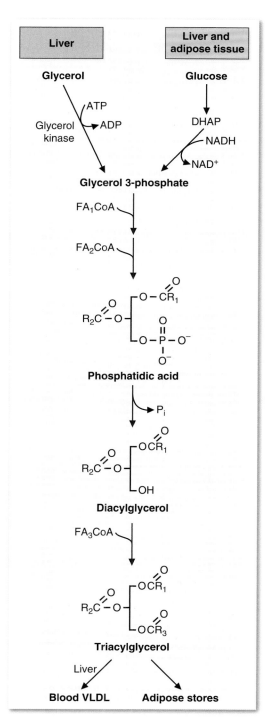

FIGURE 31.20 Synthesis of triacylglycerol in liver and adipose tissue. Glycerol 3-phosphate is produced from glucose in both tissues. It is also produced from glycerol in liver, but not in adipose tissue, which lacks glycerol kinase. The steps from glycerol 3-phosphate are the same in the two tissues. *FA*, fatty acyl group; *CoA*, coenzyme A; *ADP*, adenosine diphosphate; *ATP*, adenosine triphosphate; *DHAP*, dihydroxyacetone phosphate; *NAD*, nicotinamide adenine dinucleotide; *VLDL*, very-low-density lipoprotein (VLDL).

 Although our knowledge of the spectrum of biologic actions of the endogenous eicosanoids is incomplete, several actions are well enough established to allow their application in a variety of clinical situations or diseases. For example, drugs that are analogs of PGE_1 and PGE_2 suppress gastric ulceration, in part by inhibiting secretion of hydrochloric acid in the mucosal cells of the stomach. Analogs of PGE_1 are used in the treatment of sexual impotence. Men with certain forms of sexual impotence can self-inject this agent into the corpus cavernosum of the penis to induce immediate but temporary penile tumescence. The erection lasts for 1 to 3 hours. The stimulatory action of PGE_2 and $PGF_{2\alpha}$ on uterine muscle contraction has led to the use of these prostaglandins to induce labor and to control postpartum bleeding. PGE_1 is also used as palliative therapy in neonates with congenital heart defects to maintain patency of the ductus arteriosus until surgery can be performed. Analogs of PGI_2 have been shown to be effective in the treatment of primary pulmonary hypertension.

The gene for glycerol kinase is located on the X-chromosome, close to the *DMD* gene (which codes for dystrophin) and the *NROB1* gene, which codes for a protein designated as DAX1. DAX1 is critical for the development of the adrenal glands, pituitary, hypothalamus, and gonads. Complex glycerol kinase deficiency results from a contiguous deletion of the X-chromosome, which deletes all or part of the glycerol kinase gene along with the *NROB1* gene and/or the *DMD* gene. The patient exhibits adrenal insufficiency, hyperglycerolemia, and, if the *DMD* gene is deleted, Duchenne's muscular dystrophy.

Abetalipoproteinemia, which is caused by a lack of MTP (see Chapter 29) activity, results in an inability to assemble both chylomicrons in the intestine and VLDL particles in the liver.

Q Why do some people with alcoholism have high VLDL levels?

The sources of glycerol 3-P, which provides the glycerol moiety for triacylglycerol synthesis, differ in liver and adipose tissue. In liver, glycerol 3-P is produced from the phosphorylation of glycerol by glycerol kinase or from the reduction of dihydroxyacetone phosphate (DHAP) derived from glycolysis. White adipose tissue lacks glycerol kinase and can produce glycerol 3-P only from glucose via DHAP. Thus, adipose tissue can store fatty acids only when glycolysis is activated; that is, in the fed state.

In both adipose tissue and liver, triacylglycerols are produced by a pathway in which glycerol 3-P reacts with fatty acyl-CoA to form phosphatidic acid. Dephosphorylation of phosphatidic acid produces DAG. Another fatty acyl-CoA reacts with the DAG to form a triacylglycerol (see Fig. 31.20).

The triacylglycerol, which is produced in the smooth endoplasmic reticulum of the liver, is packaged with cholesterol, phospholipids, and proteins (synthesized in the rough endoplasmic reticulum) to form VLDL (Fig. 31.21, see Fig. 29.7). The microsomal triglyceride transfer protein (MTP), which is required for chylomicron assembly, is also required for VLDL assembly. The major protein of VLDL is apolipoprotein B-100 (apoB-100). There is one long apoB-100 molecule wound through the surface of each VLDL particle. ApoB-100 is encoded by the same gene as the apoB-48 of chylomicrons, but it is a longer protein (see Fig. 29.9). In intestinal cells, RNA editing produces a stop codon in the mRNA produced by the gene and a protein which is 48% the size of apoB-100 (apoB-48; see Figure 29.9).

VLDL is processed in the Golgi complex and secreted into the blood by the liver (Figs. 31.22 and 31.23). The fatty acid residues of the triacylglycerols ultimately are stored in the triacylglycerols of adipose cells. Note that, in comparison to chylomicrons (see Chapter 29), VLDL particles are more dense, as they contain a lower percentage of triglyceride (and hence more protein) than do the chylomicrons. Similar to chylomicrons, VLDL particles are first synthesized in a nascent form, and on entering the circulation, they acquire apolipoproteins CII and E from HDL particles to become mature VLDL particles.

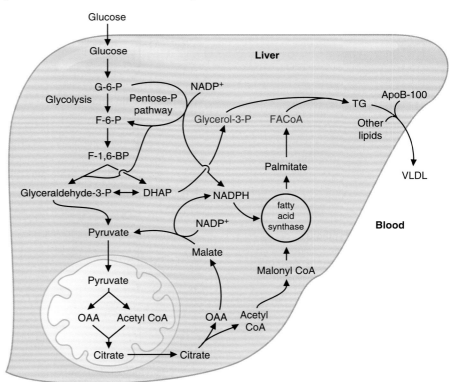

FIGURE 31.22 Synthesis of very-low-density lipoprotein (VLDL) from glucose in the liver. *G-6-P*, glucose 6-phosphate; *F-6-P*, fructose 6-phosphate; *F-1,6-BP*, fructose 1,6-bisphosphate; *FA*, fatty acyl group; *TG*, triacylglycerol; *DHAP*, dihydroxyacetone phosphate; *NAD*, nicotinamide adenine dinucleotide; *OAA*, oxaloacetate; *NADP*, nicotinamide adenine dinucleotide phosphate.

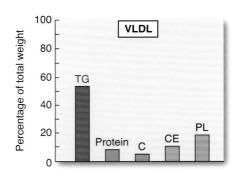

FIGURE 31.21 Composition of a typical very-low-density lipoprotein (VLDL) particle. The major component is triacylglycerol (TG). *C*, cholesterol; *CE*, cholesterol ester; *PL*, phospholipid.

The fact that several different abnormal lipoprotein profiles were found in **Cora N.** and her siblings, and that each had evidence of coronary artery disease, suggests that Cora has familial combined hyperlipidemia (FCH). This diagnostic impression is further supported by the finding that Cora's profile of lipid abnormalities appeared to change somewhat from one determination to the next, a characteristic of FCH. This hereditary disorder of lipid metabolism is believed to be quite common, with an estimated prevalence of about 1 per 100 population.

The mechanisms for FCH are incompletely understood but may involve, in part, a genetically determined increase in the production of apoB-100. As a result, packaging of VLDL is increased, and blood VLDL levels may be elevated. Depending on the efficiency of lipolysis of VLDL by LPL, VLDL levels may be normal and LDL levels may be elevated, or both VLDL and LDL levels may be high. In addition, the phenotypic expression of FCH in any given family member may be determined by the degree of associated obesity, the diet, the use of specific drugs, or other factors that change over time. Furthermore, FCH may be a multigenic trait, and even though the disease appears as an autosomal-dominant trait in pedigree analysis, no genes have yet been definitively linked to this condition.

In alcoholism, NADH levels in the liver are elevated (see Chapter 28). High levels of NADH inhibit the oxidation of fatty acids. Therefore, fatty acids, mobilized from adipose tissue, are re-esterified to glycerol 3-P in the liver, forming triacylglycerols, which are packaged into VLDL and secreted into the blood. Elevated VLDL is frequently associated with chronic alcoholism. As alcohol-induced liver disease progresses, the ability to secrete the triacylglycerols is diminished, resulting in a fatty liver.

IV. Fate of the VLDL Triglyceride

LPL, which is attached to the basement membrane proteoglycans of capillary endothelial cells, cleaves the triacylglycerols in both VLDL and chylomicrons, forming fatty acids and glycerol. Apolipoprotein CII, which these lipoproteins obtain from HDL, activates LPL. The low K_m of the muscle LPL isozyme permits muscle to use the fatty acids of chylomicrons and VLDL as a source of fuel even when the blood concentration of these lipoproteins is very low. The LPL isozyme in adipose tissue has a high K_m and is most active after a meal, when blood levels of chylomicrons and VLDL are elevated. The fate of the VLDL particle after triglyceride has been removed by LPL is the generation of an intermediate-density lipoprotein (IDL) particle, which can further lose triglyceride to become an LDL particle. The fate of the IDL and LDL particles is discussed in Chapter 32.

V. Storage of Triacylglycerols in Adipose Tissue

After a meal, the triacylglycerol stores of adipose tissue increase (Fig. 31.24). Adipose cells synthesize LPL and secrete it into the capillaries of adipose tissue when the insulin/glucagon ratio is elevated. This enzyme digests the triacylglycerols of both chylomicrons and VLDL. The fatty acids enter adipose cells and are activated, forming fatty acyl-CoA, which reacts with glycerol 3-P to form triacylglycerol by the same pathway used in the liver (see Fig. 31.20). Because adipose tissue lacks glycerol kinase and cannot use the glycerol produced by LPL, the glycerol travels through the blood to the liver, which uses it for the synthesis of triacylglycerol. In adipose cells, under fed conditions, glycerol 3-P is derived from glucose.

In addition to stimulating the synthesis and release of LPL, insulin stimulates glucose metabolism in adipose cells. Insulin leads to the activation of the glycolytic enzyme phosphofructokinase-1 by activation of the kinase activity of phosphofructokinase-2, which increases fructose 2,6-bisphosphate levels. Insulin also stimulates the dephosphorylation of PDH, so that the pyruvate produced by glycolysis can be oxidized in the TCA cycle. Furthermore, insulin stimulates the conversion of glucose to fatty acids in adipose cells, although the liver is the major site of fatty acid synthesis in humans.

Fatty acids for VLDL synthesis in the liver may be obtained from the blood or they may be synthesized from glucose. In a healthy individual, the major source of the fatty acids of VLDL triacylglycerol is excess dietary glucose. In individuals with diabetes mellitus, fatty acids mobilized from adipose triacylglycerols in excess of the oxidative capacity of tissues are a major source of the fatty acids re-esterified in liver to VLDL triacylglycerol. These individuals frequently have elevated levels of blood triacylglycerols.

Because the fatty acids of adipose triacylglycerols come both from chylomicrons and VLDL, we produce our major fat stores both from dietary fat (which produces chylomicrons) and dietary sugar (which produces VLDL). An excess of dietary protein also can be used to produce the fatty acids for VLDL synthesis. The dietitian carefully explained to **Percy V.** that we can become fat from eating excess fat, excess sugar, or excess protein.

VI. Release of Fatty Acids from Adipose Triacylglycerols

During fasting, the decrease of insulin and the increase of glucagon cause cAMP levels to rise in adipose cells, stimulating lipolysis (Fig. 31.25). PKA phosphorylates hormone-sensitive lipase (HSL) to produce a more active form of the enzyme. Adipose triglyceride lipase (ATGL) is the rate-limiting enzyme of triglyceride degradation, and it catalyzes the conversion of triglyceride to diglyceride plus a free fatty acid. Activated HSL coverts diglyceride to monoacylglycerol plus a free fatty acid, and monoglyceride lipase converts monoacylglycerol to free glycerol and a free fatty acid.

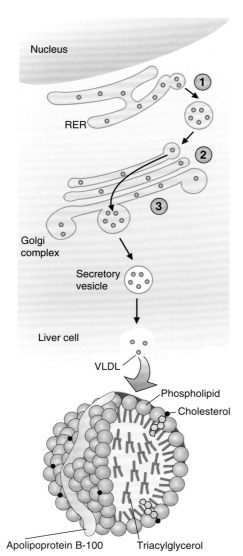

FIGURE 31.23 Synthesis, processing, and secretion of very-low-density lipoprotein (VLDL). Proteins synthesized on the rough endoplasmic reticulum (RER) (*circle 1*) are packaged with triacylglycerols in the endoplasmic reticulum and Golgi complex to form VLDL (*circle 2*). VLDL are transported to the cell membrane in secretory vesicles (*circle 3*) and secreted by exocytosis. *Red circles* represent VLDL particles. An enlarged VLDL particle is depicted at the bottom of the figure.

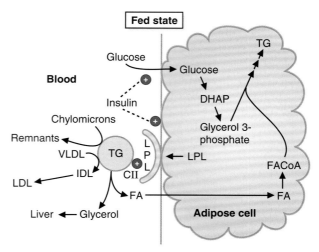

FIGURE 31.24 Conversion of the fatty acid (FA) from the triacylglycerols (TG) of chylomicrons and very-low-density lipoprotein (VLDL) to the TG stored in adipose cells. Note that insulin stimulates both the transport of glucose into adipose cells and the synthesis and secretion of lipoprotein lipase (LPL) from the cells. Glucose provides the glycerol 3-phosphate for TG synthesis. Apolipoprotein CII activates LPL. *DHAP*, dihydroxyacetone phosphate; *LDL*, low-density lipoprotein; *IDL*, intermediate-density lipoprotein.

ATGL is regulated, in part, by a protein designated as comparative gene identification-58 (CGI-58). In the basal state, CGI-58 is complexed with perilipin 1 (PLIN1), and ATGL activity is low. When PKA is activated, PLIN1 is phosphorylated, releasing bound CGI-58, which binds to ATGL to activate it. Perilipins are proteins that bind to triacylglycerol droplets and regulate their ability to be degraded. The end result, after PKA activation, is that fatty acids and glycerol are released into the blood. Simultaneously, to regulate the amount of fatty acids released into circulation, triglyceride synthesis occurs along with glyceroneogenesis (see a further explanation of glyceroneogenesis in

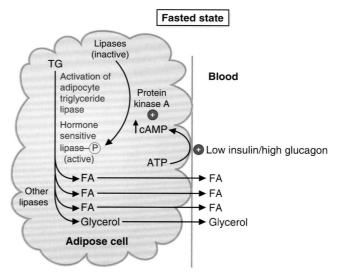

FIGURE 31.25 Mobilization of adipose triacylglycerol (TG). In the fasted state, when insulin levels are low and glucagon is elevated, intracellular cyclic adenosine monophosphate (cAMP) increases and activates protein kinase A, which phosphorylates both perilipin 1 and hormone-sensitive lipase (HSL). Phosphorylated perilipin-1 dissociates from CGI-58, which then binds to adipocyte triglyceride lipase (ATGL), activating the lipase. Phosphorylated HSL is active and participates in the breakdown of adipose TG. Re-esterification of fatty acids does occur, along with the synthesis of glycerol 3-phosphate, in the fasted state, in order to regulate the release of fatty acids from the adipocyte. *ATP*, adenosine triphosphate; *FA*, fatty acid.

the online supplement). *Glyceroneogenesis* refers to the adipocyte resynthesizing triglyceride from newly synthesized glycerol 3-P (derived from amino acids or lactate) and free fatty acids, as a mechanism to reduce fatty acid export from the adipocyte.

The fatty acids, which travel in the blood complexed with albumin, enter cells of muscle and other tissues, where they are oxidized to CO_2 and water to produce energy. During prolonged fasting, acetyl-CoA produced by β-oxidation of fatty acids in the liver is converted to ketone bodies, which are released into the blood. The glycerol derived from lipolysis in adipose cells is used by the liver during fasting as a source of carbon for gluconeogenesis.

Q In some cases of hyperlipidemia, LPL is defective. If a blood lipid profile is performed on patients with an LPL deficiency, which lipids will be elevated?

VII. Metabolism of Glycerophospholipids and Sphingolipids

Fatty acids, obtained from the diet or synthesized from glucose, are the precursors of *glycerophospholipids* and of *sphingolipids* (Fig. 31.26). These lipids are major components of cellular membranes. Glycerophospholipids are also components of blood lipoproteins, bile, and lung surfactant. They are the source of the polyunsaturated fatty acids, particularly arachidonic acid, that serve as precursors of the eicosanoids. *Ether glycerophospholipids* differ from other glycerophospholipids in that the alkyl or alkenyl chain (an alkyl chain with a double bond) is joined to carbon 1 of the glycerol moiety by an ether rather than an ester bond. Examples of ether lipids are the plasmalogens and platelet-activating factor (PAF). Sphingolipids are particularly important in forming the myelin sheath surrounding nerves in the central nervous system, and in signal transduction.

In glycerolipids and ether glycerolipids, glycerol serves as the backbone to which fatty acids and other substituents are attached. Sphingosine, derived from serine, provides the backbone for sphingolipids.

A. Synthesis of Phospholipids Containing Glycerol

1. Glycerophospholipids

The initial steps in the synthesis of glycerophospholipids are similar to those of triacylglycerol synthesis. Glycerol 3-P reacts with two activated fatty acids to form

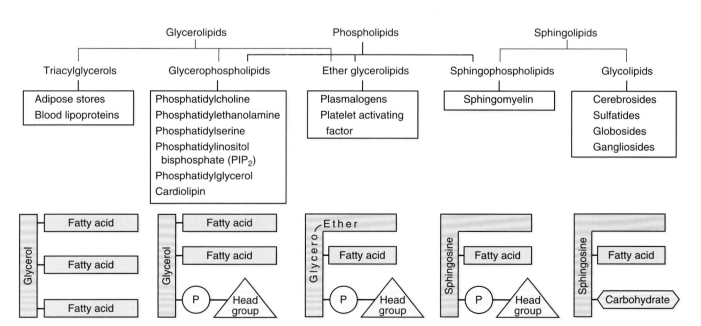

FIGURE 31.26 Types of glycerolipids and sphingolipids. Glycerolipids contain glycerol, and sphingolipids contain sphingosine. The category of phospholipids overlaps both glycerolipids and sphingolipids. The head groups include choline, ethanolamine, serine, inositol, glycerol, and phosphatidylglycerol. The carbohydrates are monosaccharides (which may be sulfated), oligosaccharides, and oligosaccharides with branches of *N*-acetylneuraminic acid. *P*, phosphate.

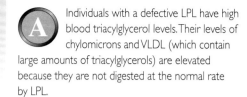

Individuals with a defective LPL have high blood triacylglycerol levels. Their levels of chylomicrons and VLDL (which contain large amounts of triacylglycerols) are elevated because they are not digested at the normal rate by LPL.

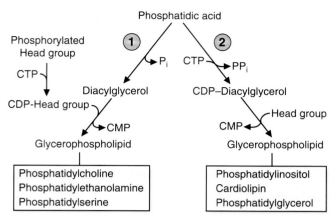

FIGURE 31.27 Strategies for addition of the head group to form glycerophospholipids. In both cases, cytidine triphosphate (CTP) is used to drive the reaction. *CDP*, cytidine diphosphate; *CMP*, cytidine monophosphate; P_i, inorganic phosphate; PP_i, pyrophosphate.

phosphatidic acid. Two different mechanisms are then used to add a head group to the molecule (Fig. 31.27). A head group is a chemical group, such as choline or serine, attached to the phosphate on carbon 3 of a glycerol moiety that contains hydrophobic groups, usually fatty acids, at positions 1 and 2. Head groups are hydrophilic, either charged or polar. The head groups all contain a free hydroxyl group, which is used to link to the phosphate on carbon 3 of the glycerol backbone.

In the first mechanism, phosphatidic acid is cleaved by a phosphatase to form DAG. DAG then reacts with an activated head group. In the synthesis of phosphatidylcholine, the head group choline is activated by combining with cytidine triphosphate (CTP) to form cytidine diphosphate (CDP)-choline (Fig. 31.28). Phosphocholine is then transferred to carbon 3 of DAG, and cytidine monophosphate (CMP) is released. Phosphatidylethanolamine is produced by a similar reaction involving CDP-ethanolamine.

Various types of interconversions occur among these phospholipids (see Fig. 31.28). Phosphatidylserine is produced by a reaction in which the ethanolamine moiety of phosphatidylethanolamine is exchanged for serine. Phosphatidylserine can be converted back to phosphatidylethanolamine by a decarboxylation reaction. Phosphatidylethanolamine can be methylated to form phosphatidylcholine (see Chapter 38).

In the second mechanism for the synthesis of glycerolipids, phosphatidic acid reacts with CTP to form CDP-DAG (Fig. 31.29). This compound can react with phosphatidylglycerol (which itself is formed from the condensation of CDP-DAG and glycerol 3-P) to produce cardiolipin or with inositol to produce phosphatidylinositol. Cardiolipin is a component of the inner mitochondrial membrane. Phosphatidylinositol can be phosphorylated to form phosphatidylinositol 4,5-bisphosphate (PIP_2), which is a component of cell membranes. In response to signals such as the binding of hormones to membrane receptors, PIP_2 can be cleaved to form the second messengers diacylglycerol and inositol trisphosphate (see Chapter 11).

2. Ether Glycerolipids

The ether glycerolipids are synthesized from the glycolytic intermediate DHAP. A fatty acyl-CoA reacts with carbon 1 of DHAP, forming an ester (Fig. 31.30). This fatty acyl group is exchanged for a fatty alcohol, produced by reduction of a fatty acid. Thus, the ether linkage is formed. Then, the keto group on carbon 2 of the DHAP moiety is reduced and esterified to a fatty acid. Addition of the head group proceeds by a series of reactions analogous to those for synthesis of phosphatidylcholine. Formation of a double bond between carbons 1 and 2 of the alkyl group

Phosphatidylcholine (lecithin) is not required in the diet because it can be synthesized in the body. The components of phosphatidylcholine (including choline) all can be produced, as shown in Figure 31.28. A pathway for de novo choline synthesis from glucose exists, but the rate of synthesis is inadequate to provide for the necessary amounts of choline. Thus, choline has been classified as an essential nutrient, with an adequate intake (AI) of 425 mg/day in women and 550 mg/day in men.

Because choline is widely distributed in the food supply, primarily in phosphatidylcholine (lecithin), deficiencies have not been observed in humans on a normal diet. Deficiencies may occur, however, in patients on total parenteral nutrition (TPN); that is, supported solely by intravenous feeding. The fatty livers that have been observed in these patients probably result from a decreased ability to synthesize phospholipids for VLDL formation.

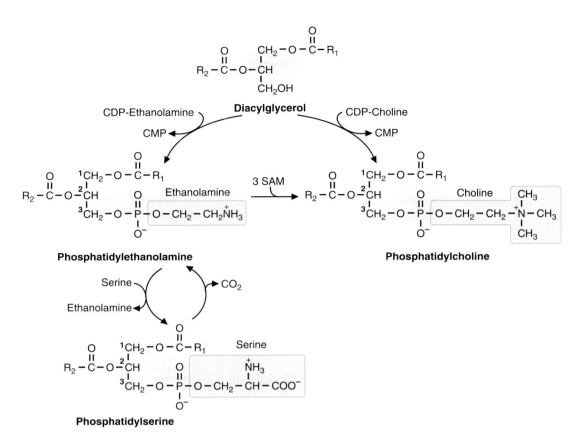

FIGURE 31.28 Synthesis of phosphatidylcholine, phosphatidylethanolamine, and phosphatidylserine. The multiple pathways reflect the importance of phospholipids in membrane structure. For example, phosphatidylcholine (PC) can be synthesized from dietary choline when it is available. If choline is not available, PC can be made from dietary carbohydrate, although the amount synthesized is inadequate to prevent choline deficiency. *SAM* is S-adenosylmethionine, a methyl group donor for many biochemical reactions (see Chapter 38). *CDP*, cytidine diphosphate; *CMP*, cytidine monophosphate.

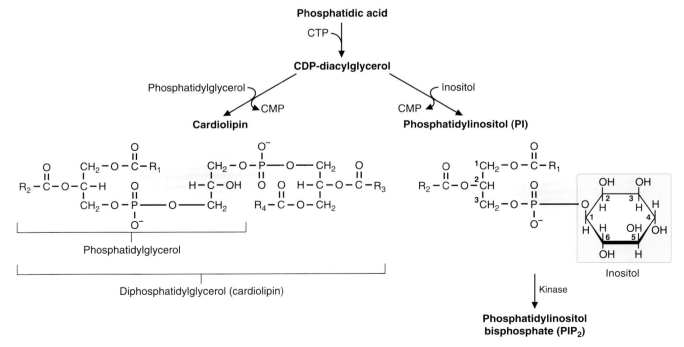

FIGURE 31.29 Synthesis of cardiolipin and phosphatidylinositol. *CDP*, cytidine diphosphate; *CMP*, cytidine monophosphate; *CTP*, cytidine triphosphate.

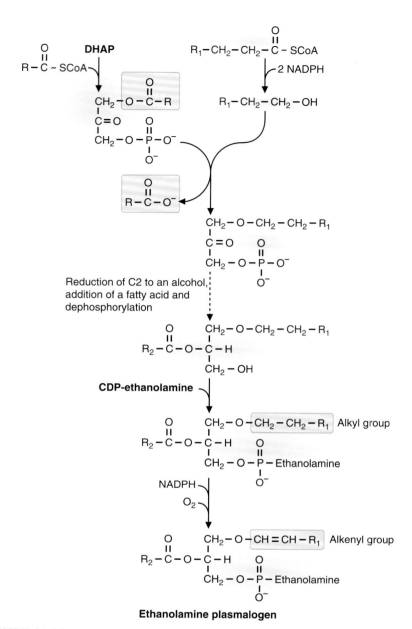

FIGURE 31.30 Synthesis of a plasmalogen. *CDP,* cytidine diphosphate; *DHAP,* dihydroxyacetone phosphate; *NADPH,* reduced nicotinamide adenine dinucleotide phosphate; *CoA,* coenzyme A.

produces a plasmalogen. Ethanolamine plasmalogen is found in myelin and choline plasmalogen in heart muscle. PAF is similar to choline plasmalogen except that an acetyl group replaces the fatty acyl group at carbon 2 of the glycerol moiety, and the alkyl group on carbon 1 is saturated. PAF is released from phagocytic blood cells in response to various stimuli. It causes platelet aggregation, edema, and hypotension, and it is involved in the allergic response. Plasmalogen synthesis occurs within peroxisomes, and, in individuals with Zellweger syndrome (a defect in peroxisome biogenesis), plasmalogen synthesis is compromised. If it is severe enough, this syndrome leads to death at an early age.

B. Degradation of Glycerophospholipids

Phospholipases located in cell membranes or in lysosomes degrade glycerophospholipids. Phospholipase A1 removes the fatty acyl group on carbon 1 of the glycerol

The RDS of a premature infant such as **Christy L.** is, in part, related to a deficiency in the synthesis of a substance known as *lung surfactant*. The major constituents of surfactant are dipalmitoylphosphatidylcholine, phosphatidylglycerol, apolipoproteins (surfactant proteins: Sp-A,B,C), and cholesterol.

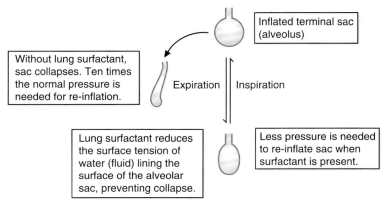

Dipalmitoylphosphatidylcholine,
the major component of lung surfactant

These components of lung surfactant normally contribute to a reduction in the surface tension within the air spaces (alveoli) of the lung, preventing their collapse. The premature infant has not yet begun to produce adequate amounts of lung surfactant.

Inflated terminal sac (alveolus)

Without lung surfactant, sac collapses. Ten times the normal pressure is needed for re-inflation.

Expiration | Inspiration

Lung surfactant reduces the surface tension of water (fluid) lining the surface of the alveolar sac, preventing collapse.

Less pressure is needed to re-inflate sac when surfactant is present.

The effect of lung surfactant

moiety, and phospholipase A2 removes the fatty acid on carbon 2 (Fig. 31.31). The C2 fatty acid in cell membrane phospholipids is usually an unsaturated fatty acid, which is frequently arachidonic acid. It is removed in response to signals for the synthesis of eicosanoids. The bond joining carbon 3 of the glycerol moiety to phosphate is cleaved by phospholipase C. Hormonal stimuli activate phospholipase C, which hydrolyzes PIP$_2$ to produce the second messengers DAG and inositol

Phospholipase A$_1$

^{1}CH$_2$—O—C

^{2}CH—O—C

^{3}CH$_2$

Phospholipase A$_2$

Phospholipase C

O=P—O—Head group

Phospholipase D

FIGURE 31.31 Bonds cleaved by phospholipases.

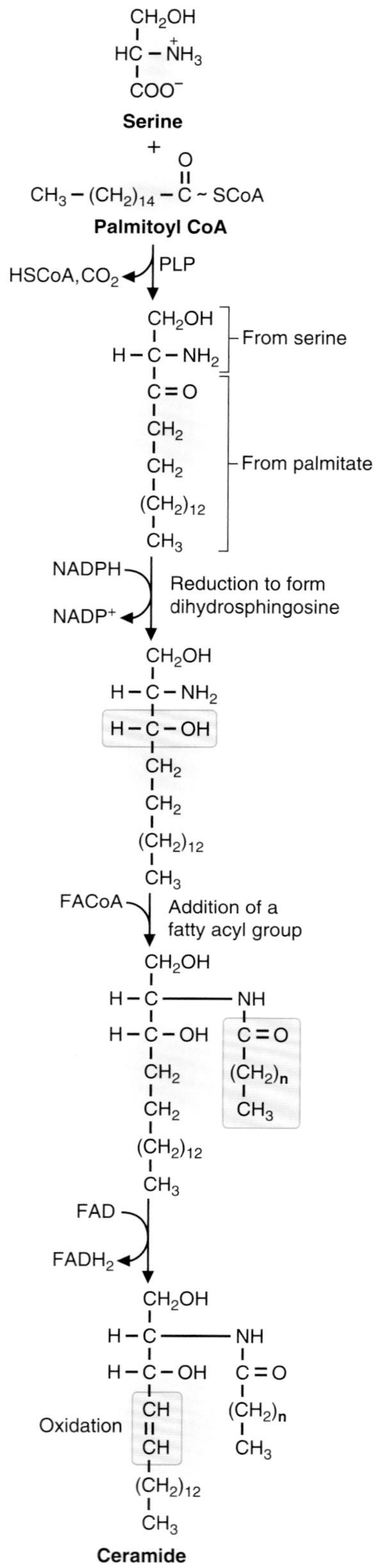

FIGURE 31.32 Synthesis of ceramide. The changes that occur in each reaction are highlighted. *PLP,* pyridoxal phosphate; *FAD,* flavin adenine dinucleotide; *NADP,* nicotinamide adenine dinucleotide phosphate; *CoA,* coenzyme A; *FA,* fatty acid.

trisphosphate (IP$_3$). The bond between the phosphate and the head group is cleaved by phospholipase D, producing phosphatidic acid and the free alcohol of the head group.

Phospholipase A2 provides the major repair mechanism for membrane lipids damaged by oxidative free-radical reactions. Arachidonic acid, which is a polyunsaturated fatty acid, can be peroxidatively cleaved in free-radical reactions to malondialdehyde and other products. Phospholipase A2 recognizes the distortion of membrane structure caused by the partially degraded fatty acid and removes it. Acyltransferases then add back a new arachidonic acid molecule.

C. Sphingolipids

Sphingolipids serve in intercellular communication and as the antigenic determinants of the ABO blood groups. Some are used as receptors by viruses and bacterial toxins, although it is unlikely that this was the purpose for which they originally evolved. Before the functions of the sphingolipids were elucidated, these compounds appeared to be inscrutable riddles. They were, therefore, named for the Sphinx of Thebes, who killed passersby that could not solve her riddle.

The synthesis of sphingolipids begins with the formation of ceramide (Fig. 31.32). Serine and palmitoyl-CoA condense to form a product that is reduced. A very-long-chain fatty acid (usually containing 22 carbons) forms an amide with the amino group, a double bond is generated, and ceramide is formed.

Ceramide reacts with phosphatidylcholine to form sphingomyelin, a component of the myelin sheath (Fig. 31.33) and the only sphingosine-based phospholipid. Ceramide also reacts with uridine diphosphate (UDP)-sugars to form cerebrosides (which contain a single monosaccharide, usually galactose or glucose). Galactocerebroside may react with 3′-phosphoadenosine 5′-phosphosulfate ([PAPS] an active sulfate donor; Fig. 31.34) to form sulfatides, the major sulfolipids of the brain.

Additional sugars may be added to ceramide to form globosides, and gangliosides are produced by the addition of *N*-acetylneuraminic acid (NANA) as branches from the oligosaccharide chains (see Fig. 31.33 and Chapter 27).

Sphingolipids are degraded by lysosomal enzymes (see Table 27.5). Deficiencies of these enzymes result in a group of lysosomal storage diseases known as the *sphingolipidoses,* or the *gangliosidoses.*

VIII. The Adipocyte as an Endocrine Organ

It has become increasingly apparent in recent years that adipose tissue does more than just store triglyceride; it is also an active endocrine organ that secretes a variety of factors to regulate both glucose and fat metabolism. Two of the best-characterized factors are leptin and adiponectin.

A. Leptin

Leptin was initially discovered in an obese mouse model as a circulating factor that, when added to a genetically obese mouse (ob/ob), resulted in a loss of weight. Leptin binds to a receptor that is linked to JAK (see Chapter 11), so leptin's signal is transmitted by variations in the activity of the STAT transcription factors. Leptin is released from adipocytes as their triglyceride levels increase and binds to receptors in the hypothalamus, which leads to the release of neuropeptides that signal a cessation of eating (anorexigenic factors). Giving leptin to leptin-deficient patients will result in a weight loss, but administering leptin to obese patients does not have the same effect. It is believed that the lack of a leptin effect is the result of the development of leptin resistance in many obese patients. Leptin resistance could result from the constant stimulation of the leptin receptors in obese individuals, leading to receptor desensitization. Another possibility is leptin-induced synthesis of factors that

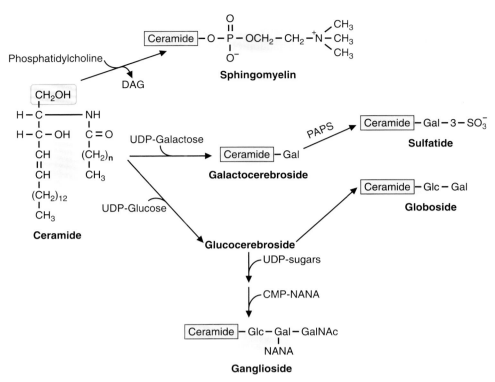

FIGURE 31.33 Synthesis of sphingolipids from ceramide. Phosphocholine or sugars add to the hydroxymethyl group of ceramide (*yellow box*) to form sphingomyelins, cerebrosides, sulfatides, globosides, and gangliosides. The ganglioside shown in the figure is GM_2. *Gal*, galactose; *Glc*, glucose; *GalNAc*, N-acetylgalactosamine; *NANA*, N-acetylneuraminic acid; *PAPS*, 3'-phosphoadenosine 5'-phosphosulfate; *CMP*, cytidine monophosphate; *UDP*, uridine diphosphate; *DAG*, diacylglycerol.

block leptin-induced signal transduction. As an example, leptin induces the synthesis of suppressor of cytokine signaling-3 (SOCS3), a factor that antagonizes STAT activation. Long-term leptin stimulation may lead to constant expression of SOCS3, which would result in a diminished cellular response to leptin.

B. Adiponectin

Adiponectin is the most abundantly secreted hormone from the adipocyte. Unlike leptin, adiponectin secretion is reduced as the adipocyte gets larger. The reduced secretion of adiponectin may be linked to the development of insulin resistance in obesity (reduced cellular responses to insulin; see the "Biochemical Comments" for a further discussion of insulin resistance). Adiponectin will bind to either of two receptors (AdipoR1 and AdipoR2), which initiates a signal transduction cascade resulting in the activation of the AMP-activated protein kinase (AMPK) and activation of the nuclear transcription factor peroxisome proliferator-activated receptor α (PPARα).

Within the muscle, activation of AMPK leads to enhanced fatty acid oxidation and glucose uptake. Within the liver, activation of AMPK also leads to enhanced fatty acid oxidation as opposed to synthesis. AMPK activation in liver and muscle then lead to a reduction of blood glucose levels and free fatty acids. Recall that as the adipocytes increase in size, less adiponectin is released; so, as obesity occurs, it is more difficult for circulating fatty acids and glucose to be used by the tissues. This contributes, in part, to the elevated glucose and fat levels seen in the circulation of obese patients (the insulin-resistance syndrome).

Activation of PPARα (see Chapter 44 for more details) leads to enhanced fatty acid oxidation by the liver and muscle. PPARα is the target of the fibrate group of

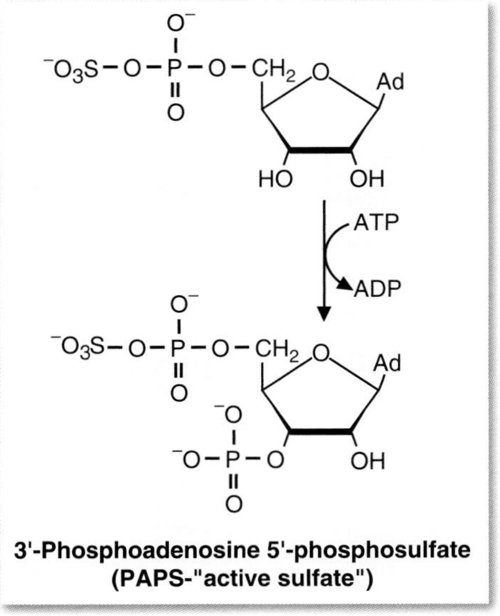

3'-Phosphoadenosine 5'-phosphosulfate (PAPS-"active sulfate")

FIGURE 31.34 The synthesis of 3'-phosphoadenosine 5'-phosphosulfate (PAPS), an active sulfate donor. PAPS donates sulfate groups to cerebrosides to form sulfatides and is also involved in glycosaminoglycan biosynthesis (see Chapter 47). *Ad*, adenine; *ADP*, adenosine diphosphate; *ATP*, adenosine triphosphate.

lipid-lowering drugs. PPARα activation leads to increased transcription of genes involved in fatty acid transport, energy uncoupling, and fatty acid oxidation (for further information on the action of fibrates, see the "Biochemical Comments" in Chapter 33).

The thiazolidinedione group of antidiabetic drugs (such as pioglitazone) is used to control type 2 diabetes. These drugs bind to and activate PPARγ in adipose tissues and lead, in part, to increased adiponectin synthesis and release, which aids in reducing circulating fat and glucose levels.

CLINICAL COMMENTS

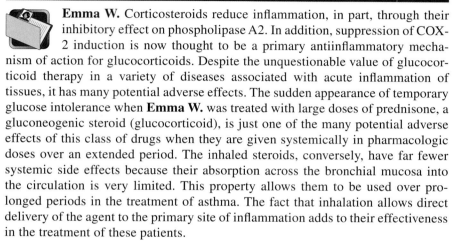

Emma W. Corticosteroids reduce inflammation, in part, through their inhibitory effect on phospholipase A2. In addition, suppression of COX-2 induction is now thought to be a primary antiinflammatory mechanism of action for glucocorticoids. Despite the unquestionable value of glucocorticoid therapy in a variety of diseases associated with acute inflammation of tissues, it has many potential adverse effects. The sudden appearance of temporary glucose intolerance when **Emma W.** was treated with large doses of prednisone, a gluconeogenic steroid (glucocorticoid), is just one of the many potential adverse effects of this class of drugs when they are given systemically in pharmacologic doses over an extended period. The inhaled steroids, conversely, have far fewer systemic side effects because their absorption across the bronchial mucosa into the circulation is very limited. This property allows them to be used over prolonged periods in the treatment of asthma. The fact that inhalation allows direct delivery of the agent to the primary site of inflammation adds to their effectiveness in the treatment of these patients.

Percy V. If Percy V. had continued to eat a hypercaloric diet rich in carbohydrates, he would have become obese. In an effort to define obesity, it has been agreed internationally that the ratio of the patient's body weight in kilograms to his or her height in meters squared (W/H^2) is the most useful and reproducible measure. This ratio is referred to as the body mass index (BMI). Normal men and women fall into the range of 18.5 to 25. Percy's current value is 21.3 and rising.

It is estimated that >30% of adults in the United States have a BMI >30, with >60% exhibiting a BMI >25. For individuals with a BMI >27, which is quite close to a weight 20% above the "ideal" or desirable weight, an attempt at weight loss should be strongly advised. The idea that obesity is a benign condition unless it is accompanied by other risk factors for cardiovascular disease is disputed by several long-term, properly controlled prospective studies. These studies show that obesity is an independent risk factor not only for heart attacks and strokes, but for the development of insulin resistance, type 2 diabetes mellitus, hypertension, and gallbladder disease.

Percy did not want to become overweight and decided to follow his new diet faithfully.

Cora N. Because Cora N.'s lipid profile indicated an elevation in both serum triacylglycerols and LDL cholesterol, she was classified as having a combined hyperlipidemia. The dissimilarities in the lipid profiles of Cora and her two siblings, both of whom were experiencing anginal chest pain, are characteristic of the multigenic syndrome referred to as *familial combined hyperlipidemia* (FCH).

Approximately 1% of the North American population has FCH. It is the most common cause of coronary artery disease in the United States. In contrast to patients with familial hypercholesterolemia (FH), patients with FCH do not have fatty deposits within the skin or tendons (xanthomas) (see Chapter 32). In FCH, coronary artery disease usually appears by the fifth decade of life.

Treatment of FCH includes restriction of dietary fat. Patients who do not respond adequately to dietary therapy are treated with antilipidemic drugs. Selection of the appropriate antilipidemic drugs depends on the specific phenotypic expression of the patients' multigenic disease as manifest by their particular serum lipid profile. In Cora's case, a decrease in both serum triacylglycerols and LDL cholesterol must be achieved.

Because Cora has known coronary artery disease, she was prescribed a high-dose statin (atorvastatin). Treatment of hypercholesterolemia is based on overall risk of cardiovascular disease. Nicotinic acid (niacin) could also potentially be used to treat patients with hyperlipidemia because these agents have the potential to lower serum triacylglycerol levels and cause a reciprocal rise in serum HDL cholesterol levels as well as lowering serum total and LDL cholesterol levels. The mechanisms suggested for niacin's triacylglycerol-lowering action include enhancement of the action of LPL, inhibition of lipolysis in adipose tissue, and a decrease in esterification of triacylglycerols in the liver (see Chapter 32, Table 32.6). The mechanism by which niacin lowers the serum total and LDL cholesterol levels is related to the decrease in hepatic production of VLDL. When the level of VLDL in the circulation decreases, the production of its daughter particles, IDL and LDL, also decreases. Niacin's side effects of flushing and itching are often found to be intolerable.

Statins, such as atorvastatin, inhibit cholesterol synthesis by inhibiting the activity of hydroxymethylglutaryl coenzyme A (HMG-CoA) reductase, the rate-limiting enzyme in the pathway (see Chapter 32). After 3 months of therapy, atorvastatin decreased Cora's LDL cholesterol from a pretreatment level of 175 mg/dL to 122 mg/dL. Her fasting serum triacylglycerol concentration was decreased from a pretreatment level of 280 mg/dL to 178 mg/dL.

Cora was also told to take 81 mg of aspirin every day. In the presence of aspirin, cyclooxygenase is irreversibly inactivated by acetylation. New cyclooxygenase molecules are not produced in platelets because platelets have no nuclei and, therefore, cannot synthesize new mRNA. Thus, the inhibition of cyclooxygenase by aspirin persists for the lifespan of the platelet (7 to 10 days). When aspirin is taken daily at doses between 81 and 325 mg, new platelets are affected as they are generated. Higher doses do not improve efficacy but do increase side effects, such as gastrointestinal bleeding and easy bruisability.

Patients with established or suspected atherosclerotic coronary disease, such as **Anne J.**, **Cora N.**, and **Ivan A.**, benefit from the action of low-dose aspirin (~81 mg/day), which produces a mild defect in hemostasis. This action of aspirin helps to prevent thrombus formation in the area of an atherosclerotic plaque at critical sites in the vascular tree.

 Christy L. suffered from RDS, which is a major cause of death in the newborn. RDS is preventable if prematurity can be avoided by appropriate management of high-risk pregnancy and labor. Before delivery, the obstetrician must attempt to predict and possibly treat pulmonary prematurity in utero. For example, estimation of fetal head circumference by ultrasonography, monitoring for fetal arterial oxygen saturation, and determination of the ratio of the concentrations of phosphatidylcholine (lecithin) and that of sphingomyelin in the amniotic fluid may help to identify premature infants who are predisposed to RDS (Fig. 31.35).

The administration of synthetic corticosteroids to women at risk of preterm birth can reduce the incidence or mortality of RDS by stimulating fetal synthesis of lung surfactant. They are given to women who are between 24 and 34 weeks pregnant and at risk of delivering within 7 days.

The administration of one dose of surfactant into the trachea of the premature infant immediately after birth, for babies with very poor respiratory function, can improve morbidity and mortality. In Christy's case, intensive therapy allowed her to survive this acute respiratory complication of prematurity.

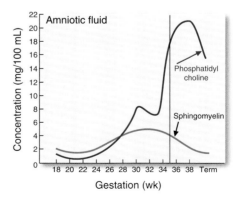

FIGURE 31.35 Comparison of phosphatidylcholine and sphingomyelin in amniotic fluid. Phosphatidylcholine is the major lipid in lung surfactant. The concentration of phosphatidylcholine relative to sphingomyelin rises at 35 weeks of gestation, indicating pulmonary maturity.

BIOCHEMICAL COMMENTS

 Metabolic Syndrome. Obesity is a relatively modern problem brought about by an excess of nutrients and reduced physical activity. As individuals become obese, adipocyte function, in terms of its biochemical and endocrine roles, is altered. Adiponectin levels fall, and with it, reduced fatty acid oxidation occurs in tissues. The release of free fatty acids is also increased in large adipocytes, presumably because of the high concentration of substrate (triglyceride), even if HSL is not activated. This is coupled with a deficiency of perilipins in obese individuals. Perilipins are adipocyte phosphoproteins that bind to triacylglycerol droplets and regulate the accessibility of the triglyceride to the lipases. A decrease in perilipin synthesis leads to an enhanced basal rate of lipolysis.

Fat cells begin to proliferate early in life, starting in the third trimester of gestation. Proliferation essentially ceases before puberty, and thereafter, fat cells change mainly in size. However, some increase in the number of fat cells can occur in adulthood if preadipocytes are induced to proliferate by growth factors and changes in the nutritional state. Weight reduction results in a decrease in the size of fat cells rather than a decrease in number. After weight loss, the amount of LPL, an enzyme involved in the transfer of fatty acids from blood triacylglycerols to the triacylglycerol stores of adipocytes, increases. In addition, the amount of mRNA for LPL also increases. All of these factors suggest that individuals who become obese, particularly those who do so early in life, will have difficulty losing weight and maintaining a lower body adipose mass.

Signals that initiate or inhibit feeding are extremely complex and include psychological and hormonal factors as well as neurotransmitter activity. These signals are integrated and relayed through the hypothalamus. Destruction of specific regions of the hypothalamus can lead to overeating and obesity or to anorexia and weight loss. Overeating and obesity are associated with damage to the ventromedial or the paraventricular nucleus, whereas weight loss and anorexia are related to damage to more lateral hypothalamic regions. Compounds that act as satiety signals have been identified in brain tissue and include leptin and glucagonlike peptide-1 (GLP-1). Appetite suppressors developed from compounds such as these may be used in the future for the treatment of obesity.

Increased circulating levels of nonesterified (or free) fatty acids (NEFA) are observed in obesity and are associated with insulin resistance. Insulin resistance is also a hallmark of type 2 diabetes. There are several theories as to why increased NEFA promote insulin resistance. One will be presented here, along with the effects of NEFA on insulin release from the pancreas. As NEFA levels in the circulation rise, muscle begins to use predominantly NEFA as an energy source. This reduces muscle glucose metabolism, as a result of the buildup of acetyl-CoA in the mitochondria, export of citrate to the cytoplasm, and inhibition of phosphofructokinase-1. Because glucose is not being metabolized, its uptake by muscle is reduced. Because muscle is the predominant tissue that takes up glucose in response to insulin, impaired glucose uptake (resulting from fat oxidation) is manifest as a sign of insulin resistance. NEFA are also postulated to interfere with pancreatic β-cell secretion of insulin, further contributing to insulin resistance (see the following for more on this topic).

Obesity, insulin resistance, and altered blood lipid levels are the start of a syndrome known as *metabolic syndrome*. The metabolic syndrome commonly is diagnosed mostly based on criteria from the International Diabetes Federation (IDF) Task Force on Epidemiology and Prevention and the American Heart Association/National Heart, Lung, and Blood Institute (AHA/NHLBI). For a diagnosis of metabolic syndrome, at least three of the following components should be evident:

- Increased waist circumference: 40 inches or more for men, 35 inches or more for woman
- Elevated triglycerides ($\geq$150 mg/dL)
- Reduced HDL ($<$40 mg/dL for men, $<$50 mg/dL for women)
- Elevated blood pressure ($\geq$130/85 mm Hg)
- Elevated fasting glucose ($\geq$100 mg/dL)

Individuals with metabolic syndrome are at increased risk for type 2 diabetes and cardiovascular disease. Treatment, in addition to lifestyle changes to reduce weight, increase exercise, and change diet, will be discussed further in Chapter 32.

A characteristic of the metabolic syndrome is insulin resistance. Part of this resistance is caused by altered insulin release from the β-cells of the pancreas under hyperlipidemic conditions. To understand how this occurs, it is necessary to revisit normal glucose-stimulated insulin secretion (see Fig. 19.11).

Glucose is metabolized in the pancreatic β-cell to generate ATP, which closes ATP-sensitive K^+ channels, which leads to a membrane depolarization, which activates voltage-gated Ca^{2+} channels in the membrane. The corresponding increase in intracellular calcium levels leads to stimulation of the exocytosis of insulin-containing vesicles. However, the process is more complicated than this and is coupled to pyruvate cycling within the β-cell and the generation of NADPH. The exact role of NADPH in stimulating insulin release has not yet been elucidated.

Islet cells express pyruvate carboxylase but very low levels of phosphoenolpyruvate carboxykinase. As seen in Figure 31.36, NADPH is generated in the cytosol of the islet cells by malic enzyme and the cytosolic isozyme of isocitrate dehydrogenase, which uses $NADP^+$ instead of NAD^+ as the mitochondrial enzyme does.

Thus, under normal conditions, glucose is metabolized to pyruvate, and the pyruvate enters the mitochondria. Some of the pyruvate is converted to acetyl-CoA to generate energy; some of the pyruvate is converted to OAA. The OAA generated can be converted to malate and exported to the cytoplasm, where it is recycled to pyruvate by malic enzyme, generating NADPH. Alternatively, the OAA and acetyl-CoA generated within the mitochondria can condense and form citrate, isocitrate, and α-ketoglutarate, all of which can leave the mitochondria and enter the cytosol. Cytosolic isocitrate is oxidized to α-ketoglutarate, generating NADPH. Cytosolic citrate is split by citrate lyase to acetyl-CoA and OAA, and the OAA is reduced to malate and cycled to pyruvate, generating more NADPH. The cytosolic acetyl-CoA is used for limited fatty acid production in the islet cell. The elevated cytosolic NADPH then aids, in an unknown manner, in the release of insulin from the β-cell.

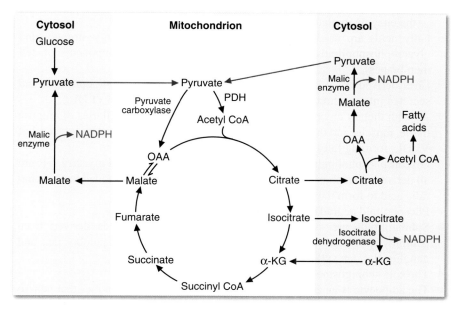

FIGURE 31.36 Generation of reduced nicotinamide adenine dinucleotide phosphate (NADPH) via pyruvate cycling in islet cells in response to glucose. Details are provided in the text. α-KG, α-ketoglutarate; *Acetyl CoA*, acetyl coenzyme A; *DHAP*, dihydroxyacetone phosphate; *OAA*, oxaloacetate; (Adapted from Muoio DM, Newgard CB. Obesity-related derangements in metabolic regulation. *Annu Rev Biochem*. 2006;75:367–401.)

So what goes wrong when β-cells are chronically exposed to high levels of NEFA in the circulation? The β-cell begins to oxidize the fatty acids, which dramatically raises the acetyl-CoA levels in the β-cell mitochondria. This leads to the activation of pyruvate carboxylase and enhanced pyruvate cycling, with significant increases in resting NADPH levels. This, then, leads to blunted increases in NADPH levels when glucose levels increase, as pyruvate cycling is already maximal because of the activation of pyruvate carboxylase. Thus, the β-cell releases less insulin in response to the increase in blood glucose levels, thereby contributing further to hyperglycemia that was initiated by the resistance to insulin's action in peripheral tissues.

KEY CONCEPTS

- Fatty acids are synthesized mainly in the liver, primarily from glucose.
- Glucose is converted to pyruvate via glycolysis, which enters the mitochondrion and forms both acetyl-CoA and OAA, which then forms citrate.
- The newly synthesized citrate is transported to the cytosol, where it is cleaved to form acetyl-CoA, which is the source of carbons for fatty acid biosynthesis.
- Two enzymes, acetyl-CoA carboxylase (the key regulatory step) and fatty acid synthase, produce palmitic acid (16 carbons, no double bonds) from acetyl-CoA. After activation to palmitoyl-CoA, the fatty acid can be elongated or desaturated (adding double bonds) by enzymes in the endoplasmic reticulum.
  - The eicosanoids (prostaglandins, thromboxanes and leukotrienes) are potent regulators of cellular function (such as the inflammatory response, smooth muscle contraction, blood pressure regulation, and bronchoconstriction and bronchodilation) and are derived from polyunsaturated fatty acids containing 20 carbon atoms.
  - The prostaglandins and thromboxanes require cyclooxygenase activity to be synthesized, whereas the leukotrienes require lipoxygenase activity.
  - Cyclooxygenase is the target of nonsteroidal antiinflammatory drugs (NSAIDs), including aspirin, which covalently acetylates and inactivates the enzyme in platelets.
- Fatty acids are used to produce triacylglycerols (for energy storage) and glycerophospholipids and sphingolipids (for structural components of cell membranes).
- Liver-derived triacylglycerol is packaged with various apolipoproteins and secreted into the circulation as very-low-density lipoprotein (VLDL).
- As with dietary chylomicrons, lipoprotein lipase in the capillaries of adipose tissue, muscle, and the lactating mammary gland digests the triacylglycerol of VLDL, forming fatty acids and glycerol.
- Glycerophospholipids, synthesized from fatty acyl-CoA and glycerol 3-P, are all derived from phosphatidic acid. Various head groups are added to phosphatidic acid to form the mature glycerophospholipids.
- Phospholipid degradation is catalyzed by phospholipases.
- Sphingolipids are synthesized from sphingosine, which is derived from palmitoyl-CoA and serine. Glycolipids, such as cerebrosides, globosides, and gangliosides, are sphingolipids.
- The sole sphingosine-based phospholipid is sphingomyelin.
- The adipocyte is an active endocrine organ, producing adipokines that help to regulate appetite and adipocyte size.
- *Metabolic syndrome* refers to a clustering of a variety of metabolic abnormalities that together dramatically increase the risk of type 2 diabetes and cardiovascular disease.
- Diseases discussed in the chapter are summarized in Table 31.5.

TABLE 31.5 Diseases Discussed in Chapter 31

DISEASE OR DISORDER	ENVIRONMENTAL OR GENETIC	COMMENTS
Obesity	Both	Weight gain will occur because of excessive calorie consumption: fat can be derived from carbohydrates, protein, and triglyceride in the diet.
Heart disease, familial combined hyperlipidemia (FCH)	Both	FCH, leading to elevated cholesterol and triglyceride levels in the serum. Levels of lipid in the blood, and symptoms displayed by patients, will vary from patient to patient.
Respiratory distress syndrome of the newborn	Both	Inability of lungs to properly expand and contract owing to lack of surfactant, a complex mixture of lipids and apolipoproteins
Abetalipoproteinemia	Genetic	Lack of microsomal triglyceride transport protein, leading to reduced production of VLDL and chylomicrons within the liver, and intestine, respectively
Cardiovascular disease (protection against future myocardial infarctions)	Environmental	NSAIDs, such as aspirin, are used to block prostaglandin production via inhibition of cyclooxygenase. Low-dose aspirin provides potential protective effects for those with cardiovascular disease.
Asthma	Environmental	The use of inhalants, containing corticosteroids, can control and reduce inflammation by inhibiting the recruitment of leukocytes and monocytes into affected areas. They also lead to a decrease in the synthesis of prostaglandins and leukotrienes.

VLDL, very-low-density lipoprotein; NSAIDs, nonsteroidal antiinflammatory drugs.

REVIEW QUESTIONS—CHAPTER 31

1. Which one of the following is involved in the synthesis of triacylglycerols in adipose tissue?
   A. Fatty acids obtained from chylomicrons and VLDL
   B. Glycerol 3-P derived from blood glycerol
   C. 2-Monoacylglycerol as an obligatory intermediate
   D. LPL to catalyze the formation of ester bonds
   E. Acetoacetyl-CoA as an obligatory intermediate

2. A molecule of palmitic acid, attached to carbon 1 of the glycerol moiety of a triacylglycerol, is ingested and digested. The fatty acid is stored in a fat cell and, ultimately, is oxidized to carbon dioxide and water in a muscle cell. Choose the molecular complex in which the palmitate residue is carried from the lumen of the gut to the surface of the gut epithelial cell.
   A. VLDL
   B. Chylomicron
   C. Fatty acid–albumin complex
   D. Bile salt micelle
   E. LDL

3. A patient with hyperlipoproteinemia would be most likely to benefit from a low-carbohydrate diet if the lipoproteins that are elevated in blood are which of the following?
   A. Chylomicrons
   B. VLDL
   C. HDL
   D. LDL
   E. IDL

4. Patients with medium-chain acyl-CoA dehydrogenase (MCAD) deficiency exhibit fasting hypoglycemia for several reasons. In such patients, under fasting conditions, which one of the following enzymes may not be fully activated, thus leading to an inability to carry out gluconeogenesis?
   A. Glucose 6-phosphatase
   B. Pyruvate carboxylase
   C. Fructose 1,6-bisphosphatase
   D. Phosphoenolpyruvate carboxykinase
   E. Glyceraldehyde 3-phosphate dehydrogenase

5. Newly synthesized fatty acids are not immediately degraded because of which one of the following?
   A. Tissues that synthesize fatty acids do not contain the enzymes that degrade fatty acids.
   B. High NADPH levels inhibit β-oxidation.
   C. In the presence of insulin, the key fatty acid–degrading enzyme is not induced.
   D. Newly synthesized fatty acids cannot be converted to their CoA derivatives.
   E. Transport of fatty acids into mitochondria is inhibited under conditions in which fatty acids are being synthesized.

6. In humans, prostaglandins are derived primarily from which one of the following?
   A. Glucose
   B. Acetyl-CoA
   C. Arachidonic acid
   D. Oleic acid
   E. Leukotrienes

7. Individuals with a defect in glucose 6-phosphate dehydrogenase produce NADPH for the synthesis of fatty acids owing to the presence of which one of the following enzymes?
   A. Malic enzyme
   B. Fatty acid synthase
   C. Acetyl-CoA carboxylase
   D. C9-desaturase
   E. Citrate lyase

8. Which one of the following drugs leads to the covalent modification, and inactivation, of both the COX-1 and COX-2 enzymes?
   A. Aspirin
   B. Acetaminophen (Tylenol)
   C. Celecoxib (Celebrex)
   D. Rofecoxib (Vioxx)
   E. Ibuprofen (Advil)

9. Dietary fatty acids are precursors for sphingolipids. Of the following, which one is formed from sphingolipids?
   A. Lung surfactant
   B. Myelin sheath
   C. Bile
   D. Arachidonic acid
   E. Blood lipoproteins

10. Low-dose aspirin is used as a prevention of platelet aggregation and heart attacks, whereas high-dose aspirin is used as an antiinflammatory drug. Low-dose aspirin is used to block the formation of which eicosanoid?
    A. Prostaglandins
    B. Thromboxanes
    C. Leukotrienes
    D. Lysoxins
    E. Epoxides

ANSWERS

1. **The answer is A.** Fatty acids, cleaved from the triacylglycerols of blood lipoproteins by the action of LPL, are taken up by adipose cells and react with coenzyme A to form fatty acyl-CoA. Glucose is converted via DHAP to glycerol 3-P, which reacts with fatty acyl-CoA to form phosphatidic acid (adipose tissue lacks glycerol kinase, so it cannot use glycerol directly). After inorganic phosphate is released from phosphatidic acid, the resulting diacylglycerol reacts with another fatty acyl-CoA to form a triacylglycerol, which is stored in adipose cells (2-monoacylglycerol is an intermediate of triglyceride synthesis only in the intestine, not in adipose tissue).

2. **The answer is D.** The triacylglycerol is degraded by pancreatic lipase, which releases the fatty acids at positions 1 and 3. The fatty acids released are then transported to the cell surface in a bile salt micelle. The only exception are short-chain fatty acids (shorter than palmitic acid), which can diffuse to the cell surface and enter the intestinal cell in the absence of micelle formation.

3. **The answer is B.** Dietary carbohydrate is converted to lipid in the liver and exported via VLDL. Thus, a low-carbohydrate diet will reduce VLDL formation and reduce the hyperlipoproteinemia.

4. **The answer is B.** Pyruvate carboxylase is activated, within the mitochondria, by acetyl-CoA. High acetyl-CoA will also inhibit PDH, thereby allowing the pyruvate produced to be used for gluconeogenesis, and not energy production. In MCAD, fatty acids are not fully oxidized (thereby reducing the amount of energy available for gluconeogenesis), and acetyl-CoA levels do not reach a point at which pyruvate carboxylase can be fully activated, thereby reducing precursor levels available for gluconeogenesis. Glucose 6-phosphatase activity is not affected by acetyl-CoA levels, nor is phosphoenolpyruvate carboxykinase activity (which is regulated at a transcriptional level) or fructose 1,6-bisphosphatase activity (which is inhibited by fructose 2,6-bisphosphate). Glyceraldehyde 3-phosphate is not a regulated enzyme of glycolysis or gluconeogenesis.

5. **The answer is E.** When fatty acids are being synthesized, malonyl-CoA accumulates, which inhibits carnitine:palmitoyltransferase I. This blocks fatty acid entry into the mitochondrion for oxidation. Many tissues both synthesize and degrade fatty acids (such as liver and muscle; thus, A is incorrect). NADPH blocks the glucose 6-phosphate dehydrogenase reaction, but not fatty acid oxidation (thus, B is incorrect). Insulin has no effect on the synthesis of the enzymes involved in fatty acid degradation (unlike the effect of insulin on the induction of enzymes involved in fatty acid synthesis; thus, C is incorrect). Finally, newly synthesized fatty acids are converted to their CoA derivatives for elongation and desaturation (thus, E is incorrect).

6. **The answer is C.** Most prostaglandins are synthesized from arachidonic acid (cis-$\Delta^{5,8,11,14}$ C20:4), which is derived from the essential fatty acid linoleic acid (cis-$\Delta^{9,12}$ C18:2). Glucose, oleic acid, or acetyl-CoA cannot give rise to linoleic or arachidonic acid, as mammals cannot introduce double bonds six carbons from the ω-end of a fatty acid. Leukotrienes are also derived from arachidonic acid, but they are not precursors of prostaglandins; they follow a different pathway.

7. **The answer is A.** Fatty acid synthesis requires NADPH, which can be generated by the hexose monophosphate shunt pathway or by malic enzyme activity. In the absence of glucose 6-phosphate dehydrogenase activity, malic enzyme, along with a mitochondrial transhydrogenase, would provide the NADPH for fatty acid biosynthesis. Cytosolic isocitrate dehydrogenase can also produce NADPH under these conditions. Neither the fatty acid synthase, citrate lyase, C9-desaturase, or acetyl-CoA carboxylase generate NADPH.

8. **The answer is A.** Aspirin leads to the acetylation of COX-1 and COX-2, which inhibits the enzymes. Tylenol contains acetaminophen, which is a competitive inhibitor of both COX-1 and COX-2, but acetaminophen does not attach covalently to the enzymes. Advil contains ibuprofen, which is another competitive inhibitor of the COX enzymes. Vioxx and Celebrex contain inhibitors that are specific for COX-2, which is the form of cyclooxygenase that is induced during inflammation. Vioxx and Celebrex do not inhibit COX-1 activity.

9. **The answer is B.** Sphingolipids are important in signal transduction and the formation of myelin sheaths of the central nervous system. Glycerophospholipids are components of blood lipoproteins, bile, and lung surfactant. Arachidonic acid is a polyunsaturated fatty acid required for signal transduction, but it is not formed from a sphingolipid.

10. **The answer is B.** Aspirin irreversibly inhibits cyclooxygenase which produces prostaglandins and thromboxanes. Thromboxanes are in platelets and inhibition of their aggregation reduces clotting which can prevent a heart attack. Prostaglandins are involved in inflammation. Leukotrienes and lipoxins are produced by lipoxygenase and epoxides by a chromosome P450 system.

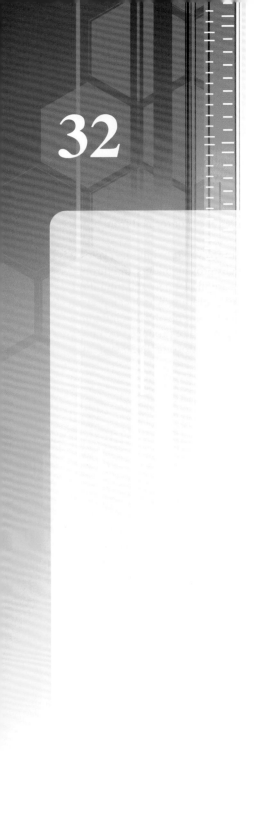

32

Cholesterol Absorption, Synthesis, Metabolism, and Fate

Cholesterol is one of the most well-recognized molecules in human biology, in part because of the direct relationship between its concentrations in blood and tissues and the development of **atherosclerotic vascular disease**. Cholesterol, which is transported in the blood in **lipoproteins** because of its absolute insolubility in water, serves as a **stabilizing component of cell membranes** and as a precursor of the **bile salts** and **steroid hormones**. Precursors of cholesterol are converted to **ubiquinone, dolichol**, and, in the skin, to **cholecalciferol, the active form of vitamin D**. As a **major component of blood lipoproteins**, cholesterol can appear in its free, unesterified form in the outer shell of these macromolecules and as cholesterol esters in the lipoprotein core.

Cholesterol is obtained from the diet or synthesized by a pathway that occurs in most cells of the body but to a greater extent in cells of the liver and intestine. The precursor for cholesterol synthesis is **acetyl coenzyme A (acetyl-CoA)**, which can be produced from glucose, fatty acids, or amino acids. Two molecules of acetyl-CoA form **acetoacetyl coenzyme A (acetoacetyl-CoA)**, which condenses with another molecule of acetyl-CoA to form **hydroxymethylglutaryl coenzyme A (HMG-CoA)**. Reduction of HMG-CoA produces **mevalonate**. This reaction, catalyzed by **HMG-CoA reductase**, is the major rate-limiting step of cholesterol synthesis. Mevalonate produces isoprene units that condense, eventually forming **squalene**. Cyclization of squalene produces the steroid ring system, and several subsequent reactions generate cholesterol. The adrenal cortex and the gonads also synthesize cholesterol in significant amounts and use it as a precursor for steroid hormone synthesis.

Cholesterol is packaged in **chylomicrons** in the intestine and in **very-low-density lipoprotein (VLDL)** in the liver. It is transported in the blood in these lipoprotein particles, which also transport triacylglycerols. As the triacylglycerols of the blood lipoproteins are digested by lipoprotein lipase (LPL), chylomicrons are converted to **chylomicron remnants**, and VLDL is converted to **intermediate-density lipoprotein (IDL)** and subsequently to **low-density lipoprotein (LDL)**. These products return to the liver, where they bind to receptors in cell membranes and are taken up by endocytosis and digested by lysosomal enzymes. LDL is also endocytosed by nonhepatic (peripheral) tissues. Cholesterol and other products of lysosomal digestion are released into the cellular pools. The liver uses this recycled cholesterol, and the cholesterol that is synthesized from acetyl-CoA, to produce VLDL and to synthesize bile salts.

Intracellular cholesterol obtained from blood lipoproteins decreases the synthesis of cholesterol within cells, stimulates the storage of cholesterol as cholesterol esters, and decreases the synthesis of **LDL receptors**. LDL receptors are found on the surface of the cells and bind various classes of lipoproteins before endocytosis.

Although **high-density lipoprotein (HDL)** contains triacylglycerols and cholesterol, its function is very different from that of the chylomicrons and VLDL, which transport triacylglycerols. HDL exchanges proteins and lipids with the other lipoproteins in the blood. HDL transfers **apolipoprotein E (apoE) and apolipoprotein CII (apoCII)** to chylomicrons and VLDL. After digestion of the VLDL triacylglycerols, apoE and apoCII are transferred back to HDL. In addition, HDL obtains cholesterol from other lipoproteins and from cell membranes and converts it to **cholesterol**

esters by the **lecithin–cholesterol acyltransferase** (**LCAT**) reaction. Then, HDL either directly transports cholesterol and cholesterol esters to the liver or transfers cholesterol esters to other lipoproteins via the **cholesterol ester transfer protein** (**CETP**). Ultimately, lipoprotein particles carry the cholesterol and cholesterol esters to the liver, where endocytosis and lysosomal digestion occur. Thus, **reverse cholesterol transport** (i.e., the return of cholesterol to the liver) is a major function of HDL.

Elevated levels of cholesterol in the blood are associated with the formation of **atherosclerotic plaques** that can occlude blood vessels, causing heart attacks and strokes. Although high levels of LDL cholesterol are especially atherogenic, high levels of HDL cholesterol are protective because HDL particles are involved in the process of removing cholesterol from tissues, such as the lining cells of vessels, and returning it to the liver.

Bile salts, which are produced in the liver from cholesterol obtained from the blood lipoproteins or synthesized from acetyl-CoA, are secreted into the bile. They are stored in the gallbladder and released into the intestine during a meal. The bile salts emulsify dietary triacylglycerols, thus aiding in digestion. The digestive products are absorbed by intestinal epithelial cells from bile salt micelles, tiny microdroplets that contain bile salts at their water interface. After the contents of the micelles are absorbed, most of the bile salts travel to the ileum, where they are resorbed and recycled by the liver. Less than 5% of the bile salts that enter the lumen of the small intestine are eventually excreted in the feces.

Although the fecal excretion of bile salts is relatively low, it is a major means by which the body disposes of the steroid nucleus of cholesterol. Because the ring structure of cholesterol cannot be degraded in the body, it is excreted mainly in the bile as free cholesterol and bile salts.

The steroid hormones, derived from cholesterol, include the adrenal cortical hormones (e.g., cortisol, aldosterone, and the adrenal sex steroids dehydroepiandrosterone [DHEA] and androstenedione) and the gonadal hormones (e.g., the ovarian and testicular sex steroids, such as testosterone and estrogen).

THE WAITING ROOM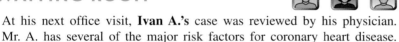

 At his next office visit, **Ivan A.'s** case was reviewed by his physician. Mr. A. has several of the major risk factors for coronary heart disease. These include a sedentary lifestyle, marked obesity, hypertension, hyperlipidemia, and early type 2 diabetes. Unfortunately, he has not been able to follow his doctor's advice with regard to a diabetic diet designed to effect a significant loss of weight, nor has he followed an aerobic exercise program. As a consequence, his weight has gone from 270 to 291 lb. After a 14-hour fast, his serum glucose is now 214 mg/dL (normal, <100 mg/dL), and his serum total cholesterol level is 314 mg/dL (according to recent guidelines, the LDL cholesterol value has an upper limit but not total cholesterol). His serum triacylglycerol level is 295 mg/dL (desired level is 150 mg/dL or less), and his serum HDL cholesterol is 24 mg/dL (desired level is ≥40 mg/dL for a man). His calculated serum LDL cholesterol level is 231 mg/dL (when LDL cholesterol is >190 mg/dL, treatment is strongly recommended to help prevent cardiovascular disease). Mr. A. exhibits sufficient criteria to be classified as having metabolic syndrome.

Anne J. was carefully followed by her physician after she survived her heart attack. Before she was discharged from the hospital, after a 14-hour fast, her serum triacylglycerol level was 158 mg/dL (slightly above the upper range of normal), and her HDL cholesterol level was low at 32 mg/dL (normal for women is ≥50 mg/dL). Her serum total cholesterol level was elevated at 420 mg/dL. From these values, her LDL cholesterol level was calculated to be 356 mg/dL (current guidelines recommend starting medications for her treatment because of her known cardiovascular disease) (Table 32.1).

 Until recently, the concentration of LDL cholesterol could only be directly determined by sophisticated laboratory techniques not available for routine clinical use. As a consequence, the LDL cholesterol concentration in the blood was derived indirectly by using the Friedewald formula: the sum of the HDL cholesterol level and the triacylglycerol (TG) level divided by 5 (which gives an estimate of the VLDL cholesterol level) subtracted from the total cholesterol level:

$$\text{LDL cholesterol} = \text{total cholesterol} - [\text{HDL cholesterol} + (\text{TG}/5)]$$

This equation yields inaccurate LDL cholesterol levels 15% to 20% of the time and fails completely when serum triacylglycerol levels exceed 400 mg/dL.

A recently developed test called *LDL direct* isolates LDL cholesterol by using a special immunoseparation reagent. Not only is this direct assay for LDL cholesterol more accurate than the indirect Friedewald calculation, it also is not affected by mildly to moderately elevated serum triacylglycerol levels and can be used for a patient who has not fasted. It does not require the expense of determining serum total cholesterol, HDL cholesterol, and triacylglycerol levels.

TABLE 32.1	The Four Major Statin Benefit Groups
PATIENT STATUS	**STATIN TREATMENT**
Patient exhibits clinical atherosclerotic cardio-vascular disease (ASCVD)[a]	If age ≤75 years, a high-intensity statin[b]; if >75 years, or not a candidate for a high-intensity statin, a moderate-intensity statin[c]
Patient with low-density lipoprotein (LDL) cholesterol ≥190 mg/dL; no ASCVD	High-intensity statin (moderate-intensity statin if not a candidate for high-intensity statin)
Patients with type 1 or 2 diabetes ages 40–75 years old with LDL cholesterol between 70 and 189 mg/dL, without ASCVD	Moderate-intensity statin; if the calculated 10-year ASCVD risk is ≥7.5%, a high-intensity statin
No clinical ASCVD or diabetes with LDL cholesterol between 70 and 189 mg/dL and an estimated 10-year ASCVD risk of ≥7.5%	Moderate- to high-intensity statin

[a]*Clinical disease* refers to acute coronary syndrome, or a history of heart attacks, stable or unstable angina, coronary or other arterial revascularization, stroke, transient ischemic attacks (TIAs), or peripheral arterial disease.

[b]A high-intensity statin is a daily dose of statin that lowers LDL cholesterol by approximately ≥50%.

[c]A moderate-intensity statin is a daily dose of statin that lowers LDL cholesterol by approximately 30% to 50%.

Data derived from Stone NJ, Robinson J, Lichtenstein AH, et al. 2013 ACC/AHA Guideline on the Treatment of Blood Cholesterol to Reduce Atherosclerotic Cardiovascular Risk in Adults: a report of the American College of Cardiology/American Heart Association Task Force on Practice Guidelines. *Circulation.* 2013; http://circ.ahajournals.org/content/early/2013/11/11/01.cir.0000437738.63853.7a.citation.

Both of Ms. J.'s younger brothers had "very high" serum cholesterol levels, and both had suffered heart attacks in their mid-40s. With this information, a tentative diagnosis of familial hypercholesterolemia, type IIA, was made, and the patient was started on a diet and medication as recommended by the American College of Cardiology and the American Heart Association Task Force (see online references). This task force recommends that decisions with regard to when dietary and drug therapy should be initiated are based on risk of cardiovascular disease (Table 32.2).

Ms. J. was also started on a high-intensity statin, atorvastatin, because she had already experienced a myocardial infarction.

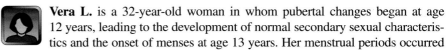 **Vera L.** is a 32-year-old woman in whom pubertal changes began at age 12 years, leading to the development of normal secondary sexual characteristics and the onset of menses at age 13 years. Her menstrual periods occurred on a monthly basis over the next 7 years, but the flow was scant. At age 20 years, she noted a gradual increase in her intermenstrual interval from her normal of 28 days to 32 to 38 days. The volume of her menstrual flow also gradually diminished. After 7 months, her menstrual periods ceased. She complained of increasing oiliness of her skin, the appearance of acnelike lesions on her face and upper back, and the appearance of short, dark terminal hairs on the mustache and sideburn areas of her face. The amount of extremity hair also increased, and she noticed a disturbing loss of hair from her scalp.

TABLE 32.2	Dietary Therapy for Elevated Blood Cholesterol
NUTRIENT[a]	
Saturated fat	5%–6%
Trans fat	Avoid
Calories	To achieve and maintain desirable body weight

[a]All values are percentage of total calories eaten daily.

Data from Stone NJ, Robinson J, Lichtenstein AH, et al. 2013 ACC/AHA Guideline on the Treatment of Blood Cholesterol to Reduce Atherosclerotic Cardiovascular Risk in Adults: a report of the American College of Cardiology/American Heart Association Task Force on Practice Guidelines. *J Am Coll Cardiol.* 2014;63:2889–2934.

I. Intestinal Absorption of Cholesterol

Cholesterol absorption by intestinal cells is a key regulatory point in human sterol metabolism because it ultimately determines what percentage of the 1,000 mg of biliary cholesterol produced by the liver each day and what percentage of the 300 mg of dietary cholesterol entering the gut per day is eventually absorbed into the blood. In normal subjects, approximately 55% of this intestinal pool enters the blood through the enterocyte each day. The details of cholesterol absorption from dietary sources is outlined in Chapter 30.

Although the absorption of cholesterol from the intestinal lumen is a diffusion-controlled process, there is also a mechanism to remove unwanted or excessive cholesterol and plant sterols from the enterocyte. The transport of sterols out of the enterocyte and into the gut lumen is related to the products of genes that code for the adenosine triphosphate (ATP)–binding cassette (ABC) protein family, specifically ABCG5 and ABCG8. These proteins couple ATP hydrolysis to the transport of unwanted or excessive cholesterol and plant sterols (phytosterols) from the enterocyte back into the gut lumen. Another member of the ABC family, ABCA1, is required for reverse cholesterol transport and the biogenesis of HDL. Cholesterol cannot be metabolized to CO_2 and water and is, therefore, eliminated from the body principally in the feces as unreabsorbed sterols and bile acids. ABC protein expression increases the amount of sterols present in the gut lumen, with the potential to increase elimination of the sterols into the feces. Patients with a condition known as *phytosterolemia* (a rare autosomal-recessive disease, also known as *sitosterolemia*) have a defect in the function of either ABCG5 or ABCG8 in the enterocytes, which leads to accumulation of cholesterol and phytosterols within these cells. These eventually reach the bloodstream, markedly elevating the level of cholesterol and phytosterol in the blood. This accounts for the increased cardiovascular morbidity in individuals with this disorder. From these genetic anomalies, it is clear that agents that either amplify the expression of the ABC proteins within enterocytes or that block cholesterol absorption from the lumen have therapeutic potential in the treatment of patients with hypercholesterolemia. Ezetimibe is a compound that, although structurally distinct from the sterols, lowers serum cholesterol levels by blocking cholesterol absorption by the enterocyte. The target of ezetimibe is the Niemann–Pick C1-like 1 protein (NPC1L1), which is believed to transport cholesterol into cells via an absorptive endocytotic mechanism involving the protein clathrin. The reduction of cholesterol absorption from the intestinal lumen has been shown to reduce blood levels of LDL cholesterol, particularly when used with a drug that also blocks endogenous cholesterol synthesis.

 What effect would be predicted for ezetimibe on endogenous cholesterol synthesis?

II. Cholesterol Synthesis

Cholesterol is an alicyclic compound whose basic structure contains four fused rings (Fig. 32.1). In its "free" form, the cholesterol molecule contains several modifications to the basic ring structure (see Fig. 32.1B). Of note is the hydroxyl group at C3. Approximately one-third of plasma cholesterol exists in the free (or unesterified) form. The remaining two-thirds exists as *cholesterol esters* in which a long-chain fatty acid (usually *linoleic* acid) is attached by ester linkage to the hydroxyl group at C3 of the A ring. Esterified cholesterol is more hydrophobic than free cholesterol because of this modification. The proportions of free and esterified cholesterol in the blood can be measured using methods such as high-performance liquid chromatography (HPLC).

The synthesis of cholesterol, like that of fatty acids, occurs in the cytoplasm and requires significant reducing power, which is supplied in the form of reduced nicotinamide adenine dinucleotide phosphate (NADPH). The NADPH is produced by the **hexose monophosphate** (HMP) shunt pathway. All 27 carbons are derived from one precursor, acetyl-CoA. Acetyl-CoA can be obtained from several sources, including the β-oxidation of fatty acids; the oxidation of ketogenic

A If less cholesterol is obtained from the diet, then cellular cholesterol synthesis would be upregulated. Thus, ezetimibe has a better chance of reducing whole-body cholesterol levels when endogenous cholesterol synthesis is also inhibited than in the absence of such inhibition.

Anne J.'s serum total and LDL cholesterol levels improved only modestly after 3 months on her revised diet and the statin. Three additional months on a more calorie-restricted heart-healthy diet, limited in saturated and trans fat, brought only a small weight loss, with little further improvement in her lab values.

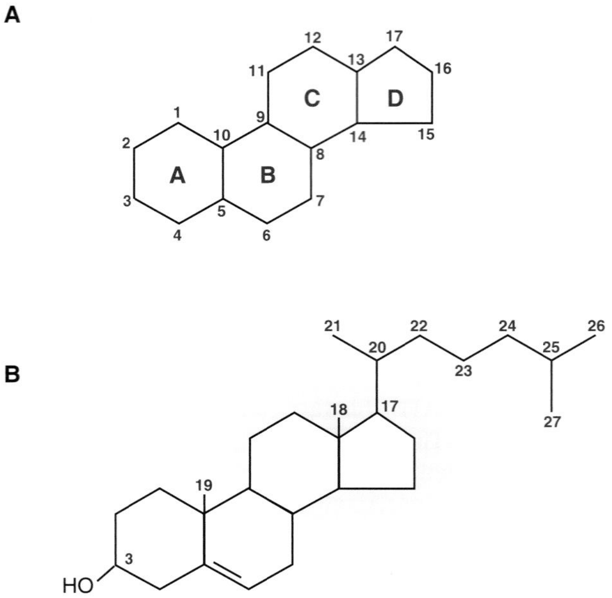

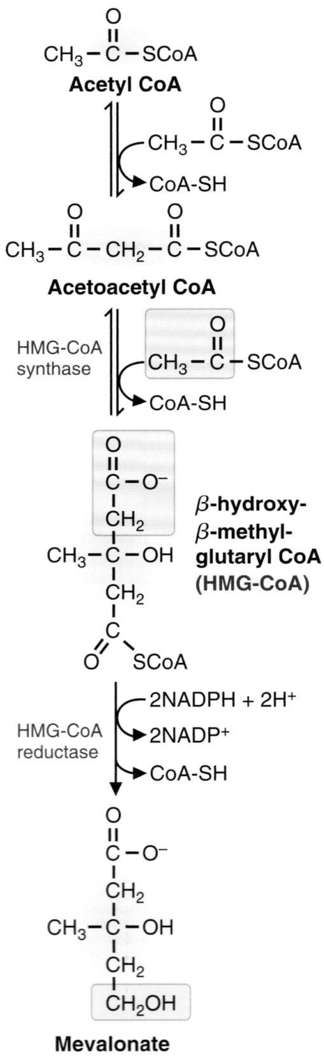

FIGURE 32.2 The conversion of three molecules of acetyl coenzyme A (acetyl-CoA) to mevalonic acid. *CoA*, coenzyme A; *HMG-CoA*, 3-hydroxymethylglutaryl coenzyme A; *acetoacetyl CoA*, acetoacetyl coenzyme A; *NADP*, nicotinamide adenine dinucleotide phosphate.

FIGURE 32.1   The steroid ring nucleus and cholesterol. **A.** The basic ring structure of sterols; the perhydrocyclopentanophenanthrene nucleus. Each ring is labeled *A, B, C,* or *D.* **B.** The structure of cholesterol.

amino acids, such as leucine and lysine; and the pyruvate dehydrogenase reaction. Energy is also required, which is provided by the hydrolysis of high-energy thioester bonds of acetyl-CoA and phosphoanhydride bonds of ATP. Cholesterol synthesis occurs in four stages.

A. Stage 1: Synthesis of Mevalonate from Acetyl-CoA

The first stage of cholesterol synthesis leads to the production of the intermediate mevalonate (Fig. 32.2). The synthesis of mevalonate is the committed, rate-limiting step in cholesterol formation. In this cytoplasmic pathway, two molecules of acetyl-CoA condense, forming acetoacetyl-CoA, which then condenses with a third molecule of acetyl-CoA to yield the 6-carbon compound 3-hydroxymethylglutaryl coenzyme A (HMG-CoA). The HMG-CoA synthase in this reaction is present in the cytosol and is distinct from the mitochondrial HMG-CoA synthase that catalyses HMG-CoA synthesis involved in production of ketone bodies. The committed step and major point of regulation of cholesterol synthesis in stage 1 involves reduction of HMG-CoA to mevalonate, a reaction that is catalyzed by HMG-CoA reductase, an enzyme embedded in the membrane of the endoplasmic reticulum (ER). HMG-CoA reductase contains eight membrane-spanning domains, and the amino-terminal domain, which faces the cytoplasm, contains the enzymatic activity. The reducing equivalents for this reaction are donated by two molecules of NADPH. The regulation of the activity of HMG-CoA reductase is controlled in multiple ways and is described in Section II.E.

B. Stage 2: Conversion of Mevalonate to Two Activated Isoprenes

In the second stage of cholesterol synthesis, three phosphate groups are transferred from three molecules of ATP to mevalonate (Fig. 32.3). The purpose of these phosphate transfers is to activate both carbon 5 and the hydroxyl group on carbon 3 for further reactions in which these groups will participate. The phosphate group attached to the C3 hydroxyl group of mevalonate in the 3-phospho-5-pyrophosphomevalonate intermediate is removed along with the carboxyl group on C1. This produces a double bond in the 5-carbon product Δ^3-isopentenyl pyrophosphate, the first of two

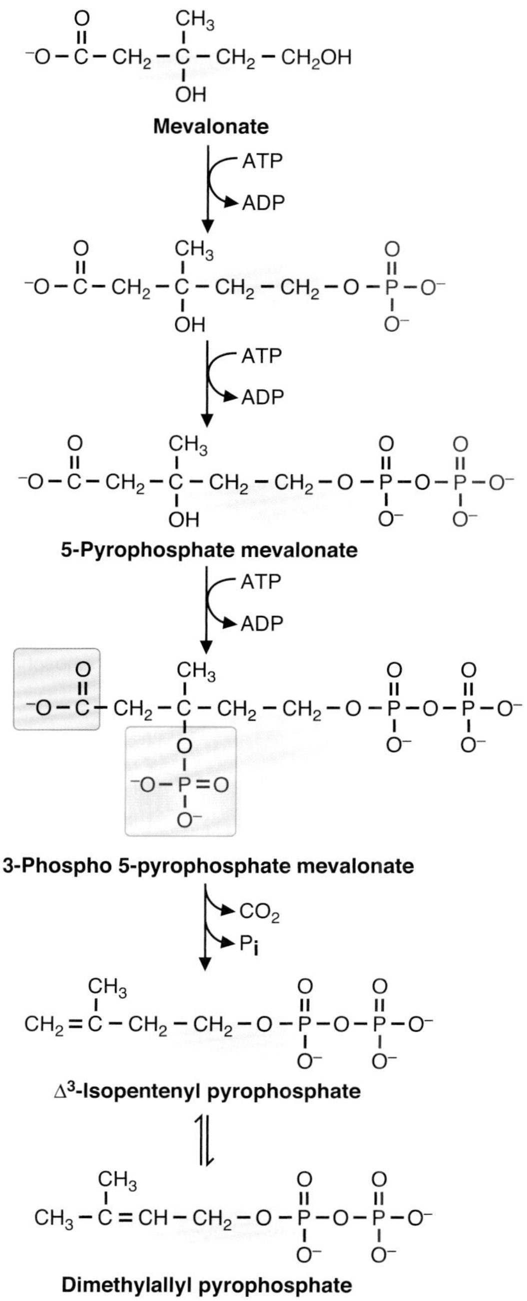

FIGURE 32.3 The formation of activated isoprene units (Δ^3-isopentenyl pyrophosphate and dimethylallyl pyrophosphate) from mevalonic acid. Note the large adenosine triphosphate (ATP) requirement for these steps. *ADP*, adenosine diphosphate; *P$_i$*, inorganic phosphate.

activated isoprenes that are necessary for the synthesis of cholesterol. The second activated isoprene is formed when Δ^3-isopentenyl pyrophosphate is isomerized to dimethylallyl pyrophosphate (see Fig. 32.3). Isoprenes, in addition to being used for cholesterol biosynthesis, are also used in the synthesis of coenzyme Q and dolichol.

C. Stage 3: Condensation of Six Activated Five-Carbon Isoprenes to Squalene

The next stage in the biosynthesis of cholesterol involves the head-to-tail condensation of isopentenyl pyrophosphate and dimethylallyl pyrophosphate. The *head* in

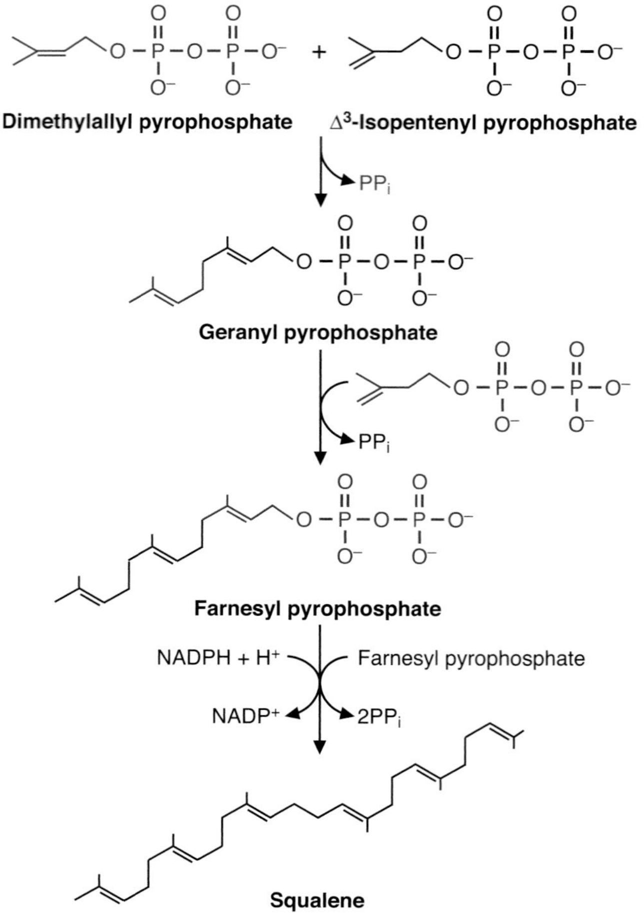

FIGURE 32.4 The formation of squalene from six isoprene units. The activation of the isoprene units drives their condensation to form geranyl pyrophosphate, farnesyl pyrophosphate, and squalene. *PP$_i$*, pyrophosphate; *NADP*, nicotinamide adenine dinucleotide phosphate.

this case refers to the end of the molecule to which pyrophosphate is linked. In this reaction, the pyrophosphate group of dimethylallyl pyrophosphate is displaced, and a 10-carbon chain, known as geranyl pyrophosphate, is generated (Fig. 32.4). Geranyl pyrophosphate then undergoes another head-to-tail condensation with isopentenyl pyrophosphate, resulting in the formation of the 15-carbon intermediate, farnesyl pyrophosphate. After this, two molecules of farnesyl pyrophosphate undergo a head-to-head fusion, and both pyrophosphate groups are removed to form squalene, a compound that was first isolated from the liver of sharks (genus *Squalus*). Squalene contains 30 carbons (24 in the main chain and 6 in the methyl group branches; see Fig. 32.4).

Geranyl pyrophosphate and farnesyl pyrophosphate are key components in cholesterol biosynthesis, and both farnesyl and geranyl groups can form covalent bonds with proteins, particularly the G-proteins and certain protooncogene products involved in signal transduction. These hydrophobic groups anchor the proteins in the cell membrane.

D. Stage 4: Conversion of Squalene to the Steroid Nucleus

The enzyme squalene monooxygenase adds a single oxygen atom from O_2 to the end of the squalene molecule, forming an epoxide. NADPH then reduces the other oxygen atom of O_2 to H_2O. The unsaturated carbons of the squalene 2,3-epoxide are aligned in a way that allows conversion of the linear squalene epoxide into a cyclic structure. The cyclization leads to the formation of lanosterol, a sterol with the four-ring structure characteristic of the steroid nucleus. A series of complex reactions, containing many steps and elucidated in the late 1950s, leads to the formation of cholesterol (Fig. 32.5).

E. Regulation of HMG-CoA Reductase

HMG-CoA reductase is the rate-limiting step of cholesterol biosynthesis and, as such, is highly regulated. It is also the target of the statins, which are cholesterol-lowering drugs. The regulation of the activity of HMG-CoA reductase is controlled in multiple ways, including transcriptional regulation, regulation of the amount of enzyme by proteolysis, and covalent modification.

1. Transcriptional Regulation

The rate of synthesis of HMG-CoA reductase messenger RNA (mRNA) is controlled by one of the family of sterol-regulatory element–binding proteins (SREBPs) (Fig. 32.6A). These transcription factors belong to the helix–loop–helix–leucine zipper (bHlH-Zip) family of transcription factors that directly activate the expression of >30 genes dedicated to the synthesis and uptake of cholesterol, fatty acids, triacylglycerols, and phospholipids as well as the production of the NADPH cofactors required to synthesize these molecules.

SREBPs specifically enhance transcription of the HMG-CoA reductase gene by binding to the sterol-regulatory element (SRE) upstream of the gene. When bound, the rate of transcription is increased. SREBPs, after synthesis, are integral proteins of the ER. The SREBP is bound to *SREBP cleavage-activating protein* (SCAP) in the ER membrane when cholesterol levels are high. When cholesterol levels drop, the sterol leaves its SCAP-binding site, and the SREBP:SCAP complex is transported to the Golgi apparatus. Within the Golgi, two proteolytic cleavages occur (via the site 1 [S1P] and site 2 [S2P] proteases), which release the *N*-terminal transcription factor domain from the Golgi membrane. Once released, the active amino-terminal component travels to the nucleus to bind to SREs. The soluble SREBPs are rapidly turned over and need to be continuously produced to stimulate reductase mRNA transcription effectively. When cytoplasmic sterol levels rise, the sterols bind to SCAP and prevent translocation of the complex to the Golgi, leading to a decrease in transcription of the reductase gene and thus to less reductase protein being produced.

2. Proteolytic Degradation of HMG-CoA Reductase

Rising levels of cholesterol and bile salts in cells that synthesize these molecules also may cause a change in the oligomerization state of the membrane domain of HMG-CoA reductase, rendering the enzyme more susceptible to proteolysis (see Fig. 32.6B). This, in turn, decreases its activity. The membrane domains of HMG-CoA reductase contain sterol-sensing regions, which are similar to those in SCAP.

3. Regulation by Covalent Modification

In addition to the inductive and repressive influences previously mentioned, the activity of the reductase is also regulated by phosphorylation and dephosphorylation (see Fig. 32.6C). Elevated glucagon levels increase phosphorylation of the enzyme, thereby inactivating it, whereas hyperinsulinemia increases the activity of the reductase by activating phosphatases, which dephosphorylate the reductase. Increased levels of intracellular sterols may also increase phosphorylation of HMG-CoA reductase, thereby reducing its activity as well (feedback suppression). Thyroid hormone also increases enzyme activity, whereas glucocorticoids decrease its activity. The enzyme that phosphorylates HMG-CoA reductase is the adenosine monophosphate (AMP)-activated protein kinase, which itself is regulated by phosphorylation by one of several AMP-activated protein kinase kinases (one of which is LKB1; see below). Thus, cholesterol synthesis decreases when ATP levels are low and increases when ATP levels are high, similar to what occurs with fatty acid synthesis (recall that

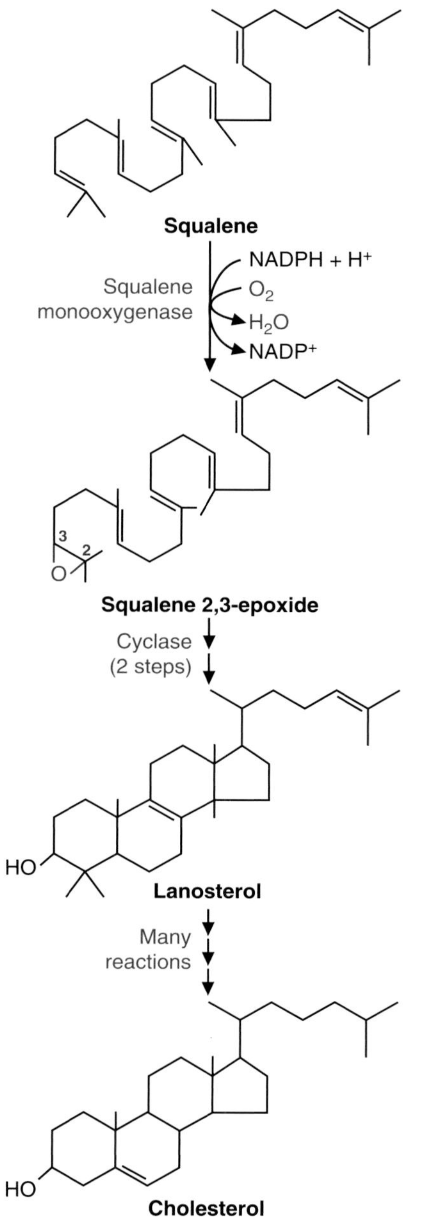

FIGURE 32.5 The conversion of squalene to cholesterol. Squalene is shown in a different conformation than in Figure 32.4 to indicate better how the cyclization reaction occurs. *NADP*, nicotinamide adenine dinucleotide phosphate.

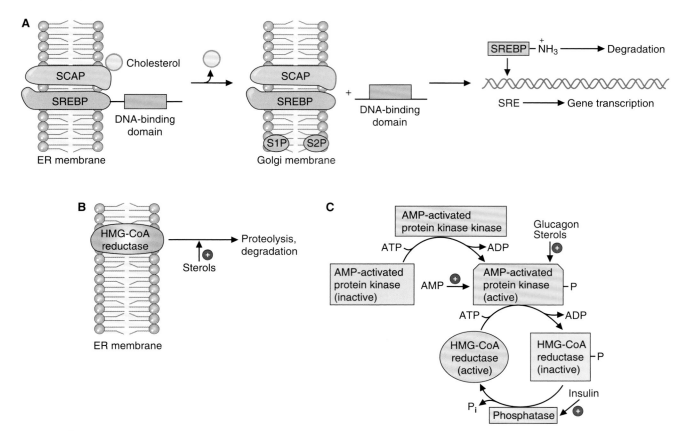

FIGURE 32.6 Regulation of 3-hydroxymethylglutaryl coenzyme A (HMG-CoA) reductase activity. See text for details. **A.** Transcriptional control. **B.** Regulation by proteolysis. **C.** Regulation by phosphorylation. *ADP*, adenosine diphosphate; *AMP*, adenosine monophosphate; *ATP*, adenosine triphosphate; *P_i*, inorganic phosphate; *SRE*, sterol-regulatory element; *SREBPs*, sterol-regulatory element–binding proteins; *ER*, endoplasmic reticulum; *SCAP*, SREBP cleavage-activating protein; *S1P*, site 1 protease; *S2P*, site 2 protease.

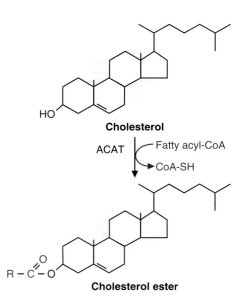

FIGURE 32.7 The acyl coenzyme A–cholesterol acyltransferase (ACAT) reaction, producing cholesterol esters. *CoA*, coenzyme A.

acetyl-CoA carboxylase is also phosphorylated and inhibited by the AMP-activated protein kinase). As has been seen during the discussion of cholesterol biosynthesis, large amounts of ATP are required to synthesize cholesterol, so low energy levels will lead to inhibition of the pathway.

III. Several Fates of Cholesterol

Almost all mammalian cells are capable of producing cholesterol. Most of the biosynthesis of cholesterol occurs within liver cells, although the gut, the adrenal cortex, and the gonads (as well as the placenta in pregnant women) also produce significant quantities of the sterol. A fraction of hepatic cholesterol is used for the synthesis of hepatic membranes, but the bulk of synthesized cholesterol is secreted from the hepatocyte as one of three moieties: cholesterol esters, biliary cholesterol (cholesterol found in the bile), or bile acids. Cholesterol ester production in the liver is catalyzed by acyl-CoA–cholesterol acyltransferase (ACAT). ACAT catalyzes the transfer of a fatty acid from coenzyme A to the hydroxyl group on carbon 3 of cholesterol (Fig. 32.7). The liver packages some of the very hydrophobic esterified cholesterol into the hollow core of lipoproteins, primarily VLDL. VLDL is secreted from the hepatocyte into the blood and transports the cholesterol esters (and triacylglycerols, phospholipids, apolipoproteins, etc.) to the tissues that require greater amounts of cholesterol than they can synthesize de novo. These tissues then use the cholesterol for the synthesis of membranes, for the formation of steroid hormones, and for the biosynthesis of vitamin D. The residual cholesterol esters not used in these ways are stored in the liver for later use.

The hepatic cholesterol pool also serves as a source of cholesterol for the synthesis of the relatively hydrophilic bile acids and their salts (see Section IV). These derivatives of cholesterol are very effective detergents because they contain both polar and nonpolar regions. They are introduced into the biliary ducts of the liver. They are stored and concentrated in the gallbladder and later discharged into the gut in response to the ingestion of food. They aid in the digestion of intraluminal lipids by forming micelles with them, which increases the surface area of lipids exposed to the digestive action of intraluminal lipases. Free cholesterol also enters the gut lumen via the biliary tract (~1,000 mg daily, which mixes with 300 mg of dietary cholesterol to form an intestinal pool, roughly 55% of which is resorbed by the enterocytes and enters the bloodstream daily). On a low-cholesterol diet, the liver synthesizes approximately 800 mg of cholesterol per day to replace bile salts and cholesterol lost from the enterohepatic circulation into the feces. Conversely, a greater intake of dietary cholesterol suppresses the rate of hepatic cholesterol synthesis (feedback repression).

IV. Synthesis of Bile Salts

A. Conversion of Cholesterol to Cholic Acid and Chenocholic Acid

Bile salts are synthesized in the liver from cholesterol by reactions that hydroxylate the steroid nucleus and cleave the side chain. In the first and rate-limiting reaction, an α-hydroxyl group is added to carbon 7 (on the α side of the B-ring). The activity of the 7α-hydroxylase that catalyzes this step is decreased by an increase in bile salt concentration (Fig. 32.8).

In subsequent steps, the double bond in the B-ring is reduced, and an additional hydroxylation may occur. Two different sets of compounds are produced. One set has α-hydroxyl groups at positions 3, 7, and 12 and produces the cholic acid series of bile salts. The other set has α-hydroxyl groups at positions 3 and 7 and produces the chenodeoxycholic acid series (also known as the chenocholic acid series; Fig. 32.9). Three carbons are removed from the side chain by an oxidation reaction. The remaining five-carbon fragment attached to the ring structure contains a carboxyl group (see Fig. 32.9).

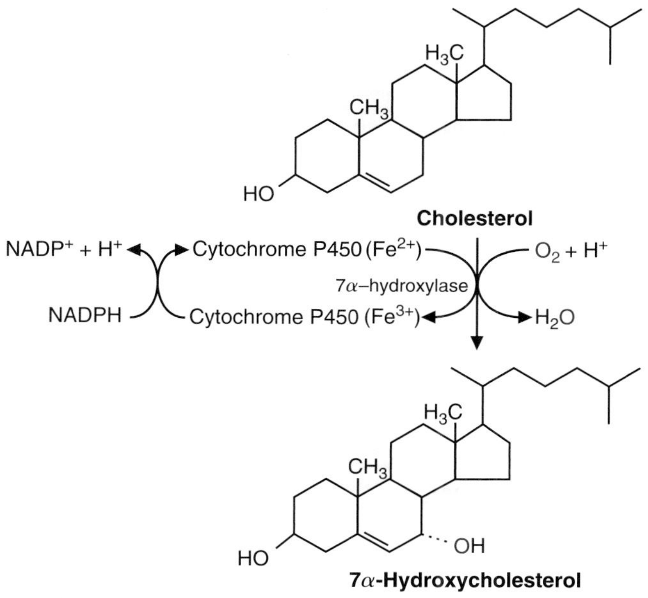

FIGURE 32.8 The reaction catalyzed by 7α-hydroxylase. An α-hydroxyl group is formed at position 7 of cholesterol. This reaction, which is inhibited by bile salts, is the rate-limiting step in bile salt synthesis. *NADP*, nicotinamide adenine dinucleotide phosphate.

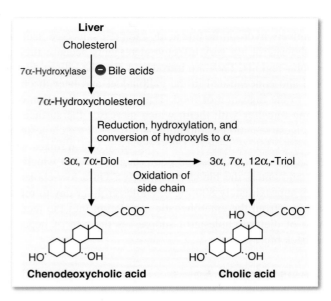

FIGURE 32.9 Synthesis of bile salts. Two sets of bile salts are generated; one with α-hydroxyl groups at positions 3 and 7 (the chenodeoxycholate series) and the other with α-hydroxyls at positions 3, 7, and 12 (the cholate series). Note how bile salt accumulation will inhibit the initial step of the pathway, catalyzed by 7α-hydroxylase.

The pK_a of the bile acids is approximately 6. Therefore, in the contents of the intestinal lumen, which normally have a pH of 6, approximately 50% of the molecules are present in the protonated form and 50% are ionized, which form bile salts. (The terms *bile acids* and *bile salts* are often used interchangeably, but *bile salts* actually refers to the ionized form of the molecules.)

B. Conjugation of Bile Salts

The carboxyl group at the end of the side chain of the bile salts is activated by a reaction that requires ATP and coenzyme A. The CoA derivatives can react with either glycine or taurine (which is derived from cysteine), forming amides that are known as conjugated bile salts (Fig. 32.10). In glycocholic acid and glycochenodeoxycholic acid, the bile acids are conjugated with glycine. These compounds have a pK_a of approximately 4, so compared to their unconjugated forms, a higher percentage of the molecules is present in the ionized form at the pH of the intestine. The taurine conjugates taurocholic acid and taurochenodeoxycholic acid have a pK_a of approximately 2. Therefore, compared with the glycoconjugates, an even greater percentage of the molecules of these conjugates is ionized in the lumen of the gut.

C. Fate of the Bile Salts

Bile salts are produced in the liver and secreted into the bile (Fig. 32.11). They are stored in the gallbladder and released into the intestine during a meal, where they serve as detergents that aid in the digestion of dietary lipids (see Chapter 29).

Intestinal bacteria deconjugate and dehydroxylate the bile salts, removing the glycine and taurine residues and the hydroxyl group at position 7. The bile salts that lack a hydroxyl group at position 7 are called *secondary bile salts*. The deconjugated and dehydroxylated bile salts are less soluble and, therefore, are less readily resorbed from the intestinal lumen than the bile salts that have not been subjected to bacterial action (Fig. 32.12). Lithocholic acid, a secondary bile salt that has a hydroxyl group only at position 3, is the least soluble bile salt. Its major fate is excretion.

Greater than 95% of the bile salts are resorbed in the ileum and return to the liver via the enterohepatic circulation (via the portal vein; see Fig. 32.11).

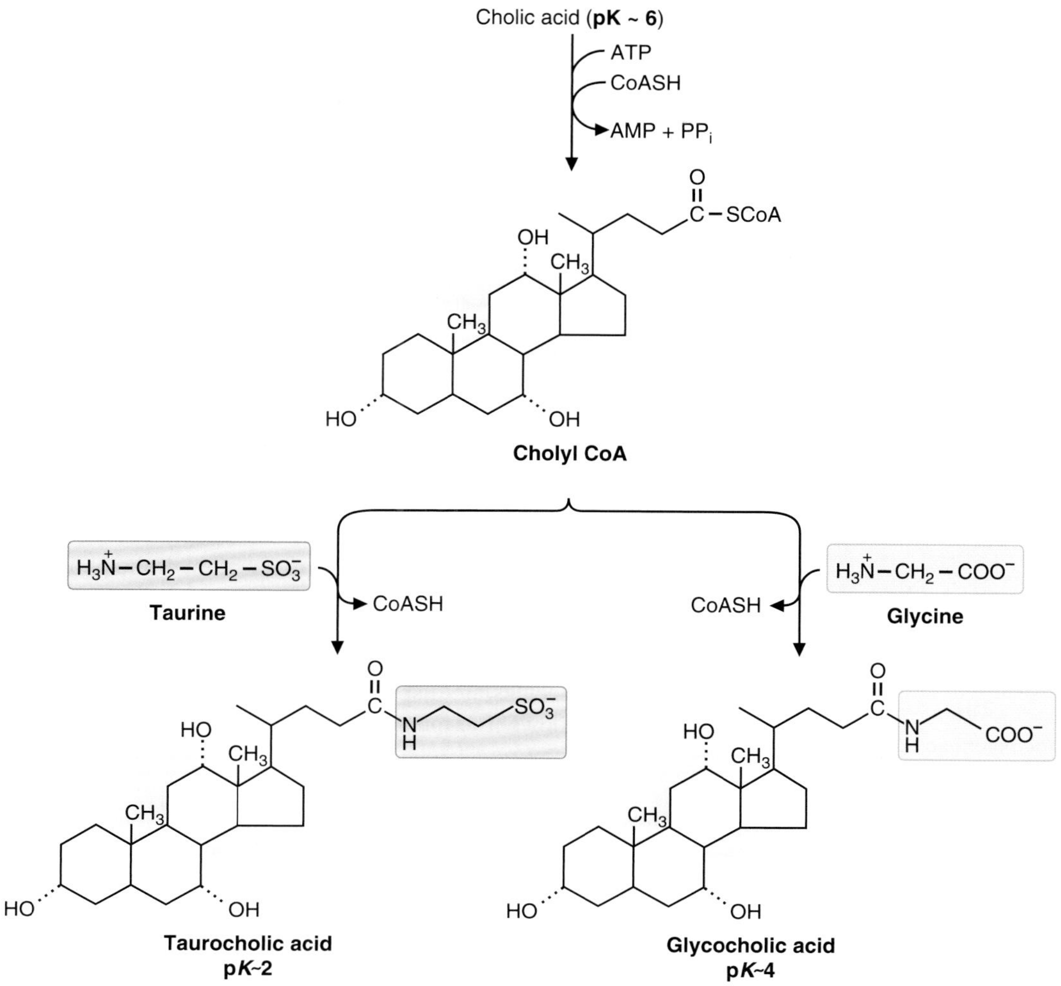

Cholic acid (**pK ~ 6**)

ATP
CoASH
AMP + PP$_i$

O
‖
C − SCoA

OH
CH$_3$

CH$_3$

HO︙ ︙OH

Cholyl CoA

H$_3$N$^+$ − CH$_2$ − CH$_2$ − SO$_3^-$

Taurine

CoASH

CoASH

H$_3$N$^+$ − CH$_2$ − COO$^-$

Glycine

O
‖
HO C

CH$_3$
N SO$_3^-$
H
CH$_3$

HO︙ ︙OH

Taurocholic acid
pK~2

O
‖
HO C

CH$_3$
N COO$^-$
H
CH$_3$

HO︙ ︙OH

Glycocholic acid
pK~4

FIGURE 32.10 Conjugation of bile salts. Conjugation lowers the pK$_a$ of the bile salts, making them better detergents; that is, they are more ionized in the contents of the intestinal lumen (pH ≈ 6) than are the unconjugated bile salts (pK$_a$ ≈ 6). The reactions are the same for the chenodeoxycholic acid series of bile salts. *ADP*, adenosine diphosphate; *AMP*, adenosine monophosphate; *ATP*, adenosine triphosphate; *PP$_i$*, pyrophosphate; *CoA*, coenzyme A.

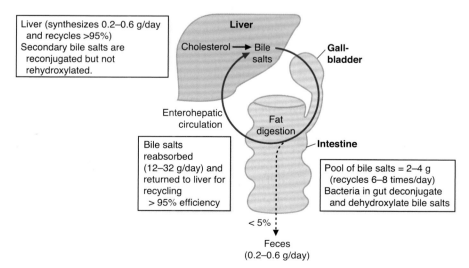

Liver (synthesizes 0.2–0.6 g/day
and recycles >95%)
Secondary bile salts are
reconjugated but not
rehydroxylated.

Liver

Cholesterol → Bile
salts

**Gall-
bladder**

Enterohepatic
circulation

Fat
digestion

Intestine

Bile salts
reabsorbed
(12–32 g/day) and
returned to liver for
recycling
> 95% efficiency

Pool of bile salts = 2–4 g
(recycles 6–8 times/day)
Bacteria in gut deconjugate
and dehydroxylate bile salts

< 5%

Feces
(0.2–0.6 g/day)

FIGURE 32.11 Overview of bile salt metabolism.

The secondary bile salts may be reconjugated in the liver, but they are not rehydroxylated. The bile salts are recycled by the liver, which secretes them into the bile. This enterohepatic recirculation of bile salts is extremely efficient. Less than 5% of the bile salts entering the gut are excreted in the feces each day. Because the steroid nucleus cannot be degraded in the body, the excretion of bile salts serves as a major route for removal of the steroid nucleus and thus of cholesterol from the body.

V. Transport of Cholesterol by the Blood Lipoproteins

Because they are hydrophobic and essentially insoluble in the water of the blood, cholesterol and cholesterol esters, like triacylglycerols and phospholipids, must be transported through the bloodstream packaged as *lipoproteins*. These macromolecules are water-soluble. Each lipoprotein particle is composed of a core of hydrophobic lipids such as cholesterol esters and triacylglycerols surrounded by a shell of polar lipids (the phospholipids), and a variety of apolipoproteins, which allows a hydration shell to form around the lipoprotein (see Fig. 29.7). This occurs when the positive charge of the nitrogen atom of the phospholipid (phosphatidylcholine, phosphatidylethanolamine, or phosphatidylserine) forms an ionic bond with the negatively charged hydroxyl ion of the environment. The surface bound apolipoproteins also increase the water solubility of the lipoprotein particle. Free cholesterol molecules are dispersed throughout the lipoprotein shell to stabilize it in a way that allows it to maintain its spherical shape. The major carriers of lipids are *chylomicrons* (see Chapter 29), *VLDL*, and *HDL*. Metabolism of VLDL leads to *IDL* and *LDL*. Metabolism of chylomicrons leads to formation of chylomicron remnants.

Through this carrier mechanism, lipids leave their tissue of origin, enter the bloodstream, and are transported to the tissues, where their components are either used in synthetic or oxidative process or stored for later use. The apolipoproteins ("apo" describes the protein within the shell of the particle in its lipid-free form) not only add to the hydrophilicity and structural stability of the particle, they have other functions as well: (1) They activate certain enzymes required for normal lipoprotein metabolism and (2) they act as ligands on the surface of the lipoprotein that target specific receptors on peripheral tissues that require lipoprotein delivery for their innate cellular functions.

Ten principal apolipoproteins have been characterized. Their tissue sources, molecular mass, distribution within lipoproteins, and metabolic functions are shown in Table 32.3.

The lipoproteins themselves are distributed among eight major classes. Some of their characteristics are shown in Table 32.4. Each class of lipoprotein has a specific function determined by its apolipoprotein content, its tissue of origin, and the proportion of the macromolecule made up of triacylglycerols, cholesterol esters, free cholesterol, and phospholipids (see Tables 32.3 and 32.4).

A. Chylomicrons

Chylomicrons are the largest of the lipoproteins and the least dense because of their rich triacylglycerol content. They are synthesized from dietary lipids (the exogenous lipoprotein pathway) within the epithelial cells of the small intestine and then secreted into the lymphatic vessels draining the gut (see Fig. 29.11). They enter the bloodstream via the left subclavian vein. The major apolipoproteins of chylomicrons are apolipoprotein B-48 (apoB-48), apoCII, and apoE (see Table 32.3). The apoCII activates LPL, an enzyme that projects into the lumen of capillaries in adipose tissue, cardiac muscle, skeletal muscle, and the acinar cells of mammary tissue. This activation allows LPL to hydrolyze the triacylglycerol of the chylomicrons, leading to the release of free fatty acids. The muscle cells then oxidize the fatty acids as fuel,

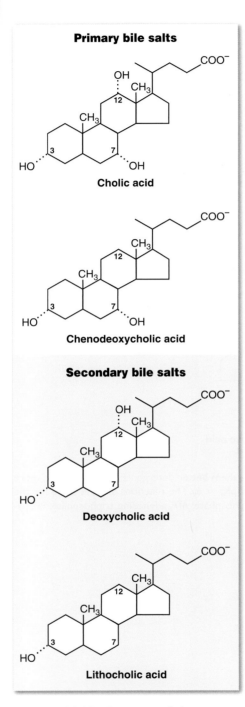

FIGURE 32.12 Structures of the primary and secondary bile salts. Primary bile salts form conjugates with taurine or glycine in the liver. After secretion into the intestine, they may be deconjugated and dehydroxylated by the bacterial flora, forming secondary bile salts. Note that dehydroxylation occurs at position 7, forming the deoxy family of bile salts. Dehydroxylation at position 12 also leads to excretion of the bile salt.

TABLE 32.3 **Characteristics of the Major Apolipoproteins**

APOLIPO-PROTEIN	PRIMARY TISSUE SOURCE	MOLECULAR MASS (DALTONS)	LIPOPROTEIN DISTRIBUTION	METABOLIC FUNCTION
ApoAI	Intestine, liver	28,016	HDL (chylomicrons)	Activates LCAT; structural component of HDL
ApoAII	Liver	17,414	HDL (chylomicrons)	Uncertain; may regulate transfer of apolipoproteins from HDL to other lipoprotein particles
ApoAIV	Intestine	46,465	HDL (chylomicrons)	Uncertain; may be involved in assembly of HDL and chylomicrons
ApoB-48	Intestine	264,000	Chylomicrons	Assembly and secretion of chylomicrons from small bowel
ApoB-100	Liver	540,000	VLDL, IDL, LDL	VLDL assembly and secretion; structural protein of VLDL, IDL, and LDL; ligand for LDL receptor
ApoCI	Liver	6,630	Chylomicrons, VLDL, IDL, HDL	Unknown; may inhibit hepatic uptake of chylomicron and VLDL remnants
ApoCII	Liver	8,900	Chylomicrons, VLDL, IDL, HDL	Cofactor activator of LPL
ApoCIII	Liver	8,800	Chylomicrons, VLDL, IDL, HDL	Inhibitor of LPL; may inhibit hepatic uptake of chylomicrons and VLDL remnants
ApoE	Liver	34,145	Chylomicron remnants, VLDL, IDL, HDL	Ligand for binding of several lipoproteins to the LDL receptor, to the LDL receptor-related protein (LRP) and possibly to a separate apoE receptor
Apo(a)	Liver		Lipoprotein "little" a (Lp[a])	Unknown; consists of apoB-100 linked by a disulfide bond to apolipoprotein(a)

HDL, high-density lipoprotein; LCAT, lecithin–cholesterol acyltransferase; VLDL, very-low-density lipoprotein; IDL, intermediate-density lipoprotein; LDL, low-density lipoprotein; LPL, lipoprotein lipase.

while the adipocytes and mammary cells store them as triacylglycerols (fat) or, in the case of the lactating breast, use them for milk formation. The partially hydrolyzed chylomicrons remaining in the bloodstream (the chylomicron remnants), now partly depleted of their core triacylglycerols, have lost their apoCII but still retain their apoE and apoB-48 proteins. Receptors in the plasma membranes of the liver cells bind to apoE on the surface of these remnants, allowing them to be taken up by the liver through a process of receptor-mediated endocytosis (see below).

TABLE 32.4 **Characteristics of the Major Lipoproteins**

| LIPOPROTEIN | DENSITY RANGE (g/mL) | PARTICLE DIAMETER (mm) RANGE | ELECTRO-PHORETIC MOBILITY | LIPID (%)[a] | | | FUNCTION |
				TG	CHOL	PL	
Chylomicrons	0.930	75–1,200	Origin	80–95	2–7	3–9	Deliver dietary lipids
Chylomicron remnants	0.930–1.006	30–80	Slow pre-β				Return dietary lipids to the liver
VLDL	0.930–1.006	30–80	Pre-β	55–80	5–15	10–20	Deliver endogenous lipids
IDL	1.006–1.019	25–35	Slow pre-β	20–50	20–40	15–25	Return endogenous lipids to the liver; precursor of LDL
LDL	1.019–1.063	18–25	β	5–15	40–50	20–25	Deliver cholesterol to cells
HDL$_2$	1.063–1.125	9–12	α	5–10	15–25	20–30	Reverse cholesterol transport
HDL$_3$	1.125–1.210	5–9	α				Reverse cholesterol transport
Lip(a)	1.050–1.120	25	Pre-β				

TG, triacylglycerols; Chol, the sum of free and esterified cholesterol; PL, phospholipid; VLDL, very-low-density lipoprotein; IDL, intermediate-density lipoprotein; LDL, low-density lipoprotein; HDL, high-density lipoprotein.
[a]The remaining percentage composition is composed of apolipoproteins.

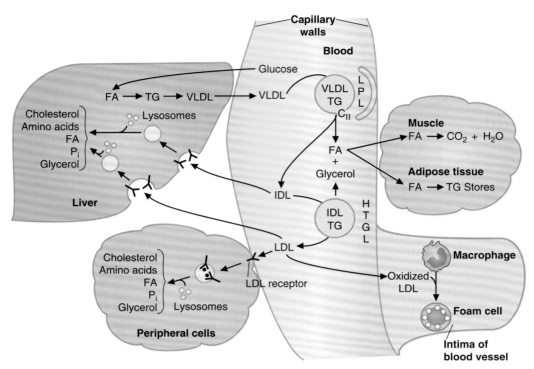

FIGURE 32.13 Fate of very-low-density lipoprotein (VLDL). VLDL triacylglycerol (TG) is degraded by lipoprotein lipase (LPL), forming intermediate-density lipoprotein (IDL). IDL can either be endocytosed by the liver through a receptor-mediated process or further digested, mainly by hepatic triacylglycerol lipase (HTGL), to form low-density lipoprotein (LDL). LDL may be endocytosed by receptor-mediated processes in the liver or in peripheral cells. LDL also may be oxidized and taken up by "scavenger" receptors on macrophages. The scavenger pathway plays a role in atherosclerosis. *FA*, fatty acids; *P_i*, inorganic phosphate.

B. Very-Low-Density Lipoprotein

If dietary intake of carbohydrates exceeds the immediate fuel requirements of the liver, the excess carbohydrates are converted to triacylglycerols, which, along with free and esterified cholesterol, phospholipids, and the major apolipoprotein apoB-100 (see Table 32.3), are packaged to form nascent VLDL. These particles are then secreted from the liver (the "endogenous" pathway of lipoprotein metabolism) into the bloodstream (Fig. 32.13), where they accept apoCII and apoE from circulating HDL particles. This then forms the mature VLDL particle. These particles are then transported from the hepatic veins to capillaries in skeletal and cardiac muscle and adipose tissue, as well as lactating mammary tissues, where LPL is activated by apoCII in the VLDL particles. The activated enzyme facilitates the hydrolysis of the triacylglycerol in VLDL, causing the release of fatty acids and glycerol from a portion of core triacylglycerols. These fatty acids are oxidized as fuel by muscle cells, used in the resynthesis of triacylglycerols in fat cells, and used for milk production in the lactating breast. As the VLDL particles are depleted of triacylglycerol, VLDL remnants are formed. Approximately 50% of these remnants are taken up from the blood by liver cells through the binding of VLDL apoE to the hepatocyte plasma membrane apoE receptor, followed by endocytic internalization of the VLDL remnant (similar to the fate of the chylomicron remnant).

C. Intermediate-Density Lipoprotein and Low-Density Lipoprotein

Approximately half of the VLDL remnants are not taken up by the liver but, instead, have additional core triacylglycerols removed to form IDL, a specialized class of VLDL remnants. With the removal of additional triacylglycerols from IDL through the action of hepatic triglyceride lipase within hepatic sinusoids, LDL is generated from IDL. As can be seen in Table 32.4, the LDL particles are rich in cholesterol and cholesterol esters. Approximately 60% of the LDL is transported back to the liver, where its apoB-100 binds to specific apoB-100 receptors in the liver cell plasma membranes, allowing particles to be endocytosed into the hepatocyte. The remaining 40% of LDL particles is carried to extrahepatic tissues such as adrenocortical and gonadal cells that also contain apoB-100 receptors, allowing them to internalize the LDL particles and use their cholesterol for the synthesis of steroid hormones. Some of the cholesterol of the internalized LDL is used for membrane synthesis and vitamin D synthesis as well. If an excess of LDL particles is present in the blood, this specific receptor-mediated uptake of LDL by hepatic and nonhepatic tissue becomes saturated. The "excess" LDL particles are now more readily available for nonspecific uptake of LDL by macrophages (scavenger cells) present near the endothelial cells of arteries. This exposure of vascular endothelial cells to high levels of LDL is believed to induce an inflammatory response by these cells, a process that has been suggested to initiate the complex cascade of atherosclerosis discussed below.

D. High-Density Lipoprotein

The fourth class of lipoproteins is HDL, which plays several roles in whole-body lipid metabolism.

1. Synthesis of HDL

HDL particles can be created by several mechanisms. The first is synthesis of nascent HDL by the liver and intestine as a relatively small molecule whose shell, like that of other lipoproteins, contains phospholipids, free cholesterol, and a variety of apolipoproteins, predominant among which are apoA1, apoAII, apoCI, and apoCII (see Table 32.3). Very low levels of triacylglycerols or cholesterol esters are found in the hollow core of this early, or nascent, version of HDL.

A second method for HDL generation is the budding of apolipoproteins from chylomicrons and VLDL particles as they are digested by LPL. The apolipoproteins (particularly apoAI) and shells can then accumulate more lipid, as described below.

A third method for HDL generation is free apoAI, which may be shed from other circulating lipoproteins. The apoAI acquires cholesterol and phospholipids from other lipoproteins and cell membranes, forming a nascent-like HDL particle within the circulation.

2. Maturation of Nascent HDL

In the process of maturation, the nascent HDL particles accumulate phospholipids and cholesterol from cells lining the blood vessels. As the central hollow core of nascent HDL progressively fills with cholesterol esters, HDL takes on a more globular shape to eventually form the mature HDL particle. The transfer of lipids to nascent HDL does not require enzymatic activity.

3. Reverse Cholesterol Transport

A major benefit of HDL particles derives from their ability to remove cholesterol from cholesterol-laden cells and to return the cholesterol to the liver, a process known as *reverse cholesterol transport*. This is particularly beneficial in vascular tissue; by reducing cellular cholesterol levels in the subintimal space, the likelihood that foam cells (lipid-laden macrophages that engulf oxidized LDL cholesterol and represent an early stage in the development of atherosclerotic plaque) will form within the blood vessel wall is reduced.

Reverse cholesterol transport requires a directional movement of cholesterol from the cell to the lipoprotein particle. Cells contain the protein ABCA1 (ATP-binding cassette protein 1) that uses ATP hydrolysis to move cholesterol from the inner leaflet of the membrane to the outer leaflet (similar to the efflux of phytosterols by ABCG5 and ABCG8; see Section I of this chapter). Once the cholesterol has

 Two genetically determined disorders, familial HDL deficiency and Tangier disease, result from mutations in the ATP-binding cassette 1 (ABCA1) protein. Cholesterol-depleted HDL cannot transport free cholesterol from cells that lack the ability to express this protein. As a consequence, HDL is rapidly degraded. These disorders have established a role for the ABCA1 protein in the regulation of HDL levels in the blood. In both disorders, early-onset coronary artery disease occurs, caused by the low levels of HDL.

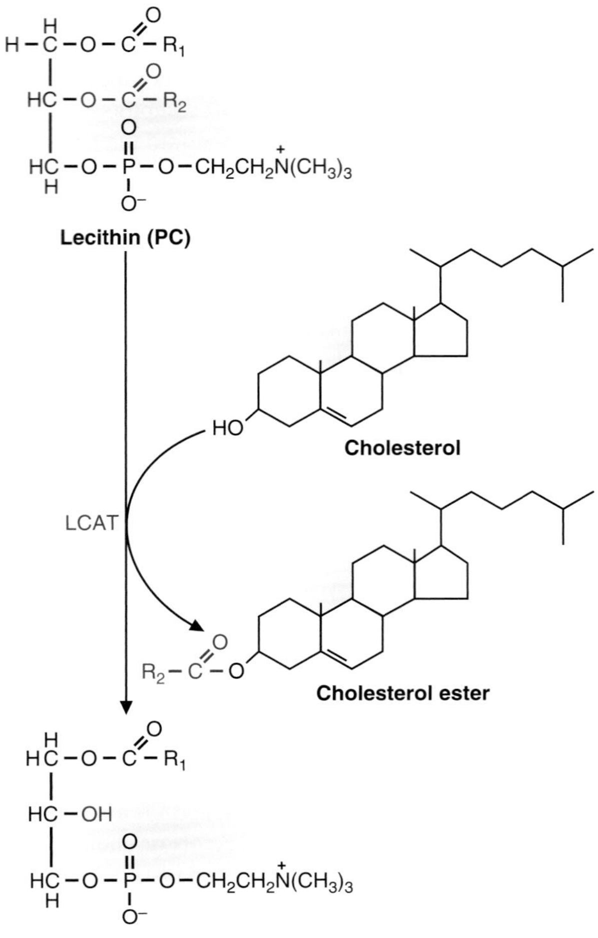

FIGURE 32.14 The reaction catalyzed by lecithin–cholesterol acyltransferase (LCAT). R_1, saturated fatty acid; R_2, unsaturated fatty acid.

reached the outer membrane leaflet, the HDL particle can accept it, but if the cholesterol is not modified within the HDL particle, the cholesterol can leave the particle by the same route that it entered. To trap the cholesterol within the HDL core, the HDL particle acquires the enzyme LCAT from the circulation (LCAT is synthesized and secreted by the liver). LCAT catalyzes the transfer of a fatty acid from the 2-position of lecithin (phosphatidylcholine) in the phospholipid shell of the particle to the 3-hydroxyl group of cholesterol, forming a cholesterol ester (Fig. 32.14). The cholesterol ester migrates to the core of the HDL particle and is no longer free to return to the cell.

Elevated levels of lipoprotein-associated cholesterol in the blood, particularly that associated with LDL and also the more triacylglycerol-rich lipoproteins, are associated with the formation of cholesterol-rich atheromatous plaque in the vessel wall, leading eventually to diffuse *atherosclerotic vascular disease* that can result in acute cardiovascular events such as myocardial infarction, stroke, or symptomatic peripheral vascular insufficiency. High levels of HDL in the blood, therefore, are believed to be vasculoprotective because these high levels increase the rate of reverse cholesterol transport "away" from the blood vessels and "toward" the liver ("out of harm's way").

4. Fate of HDL Cholesterol

Mature HDL particles can bind to specific receptors on hepatocytes (such as the apoE receptor), but the primary means of clearance of HDL from the blood is

Because **Anne J.** continued to experience intermittent chest pain in spite of good control of her hypertension and a 20-lb weight loss, her physician decided that in addition to seeing a cardiologist to further evaluate the chest pain, a second drug needed to be added to her regimen to further lower her blood LDL cholesterol level. Consequently, treatment with ezetimibe, a drug that blocks cholesterol absorption from the intestine, was added to complement the atorvastatin Anne was already taking.

through its uptake by the scavenger receptor SR-B1. This receptor is present on many cell types. It does not carry out endocytosis per se, but once the HDL particle is bound to the receptor, its cholesterol and cholesterol esters are transferred into the cells. When depleted of cholesterol and its esters, the HDL particle dissociates from the SR-B1 receptor and reenters the circulation. SR-B1 receptors can be upregulated in certain cell types that require cholesterol for biosynthetic purposes, such as the cells that produce the steroid hormones. The SR-B1 receptors are not downregulated when cholesterol levels are high.

5. HDL Interactions with Other Particles

In addition to its ability to pick up cholesterol from cell membranes, HDL also exchanges apolipoproteins and lipids with other lipoproteins in the blood. For example, HDL transfers apoE and apoCII to chylomicrons and to VLDL. The apoCII stimulates the degradation of the triacylglycerols of chylomicrons and VLDL by activating LPL (Fig. 32.15). After digestion of the chylomicrons and the VLDL triacylglycerols, apoE and apoCII are transferred back to HDL. When HDL obtains free cholesterol from cell membranes, the free cholesterol is esterified at the third carbon of the A-ring via the LCAT reaction (see Fig. 32.13). From this point, HDL either transports the free cholesterol and cholesterol esters directly to the liver, as described previously, or by CETP to circulating triacylglycerol-rich lipoproteins such as VLDL and VLDL remnants (see Fig. 32.15). In exchange, triacylglycerols from the latter lipoproteins are transferred to HDL (Fig. 32.16). The greater the concentration of triacylglycerol-rich lipoproteins in the blood, the greater will be the rate of these exchanges.

The CETP exchange pathway may explain the observation that whenever triacylglycerol-rich lipoproteins are present in the blood in high concentrations, the amount of cholesterol reaching the liver via cholesterol-enriched VLDL and VLDL remnants increases, coupled with a proportional reduction in the total amount of

 The CETP reaction, under conditions of high levels of triglyceride-rich lipoproteins, generates elevated levels of HDL$_3$, which are less atheroprotective than HDL$_2$. CETP inhibitors are currently being evaluated as a means of increasing HDL$_2$ levels, with limited success. Initial clinical trials of a promising drug was terminated early because of an increased incidence of cardiovascular events when the drug was given in combination with an inhibitor of HMG-CoA reductase. Different CETP inhibitors, however, are currently being examined as potential HDL$_2$ elevating agents.

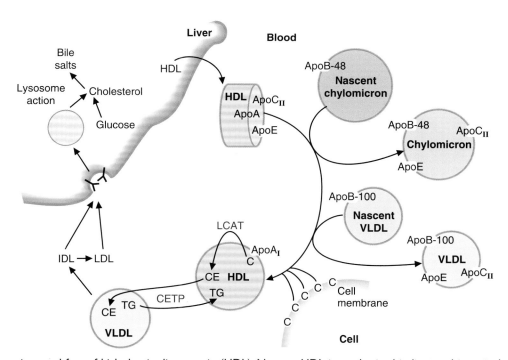

FIGURE 32.15 Functions and fate of high-density lipoprotein (HDL). Nascent HDL is synthesized in liver and intestinal cells. It exchanges proteins with chylomicrons and very-low-density lipoprotein (VLDL). HDL picks up cholesterol (C) from cell membranes. This cholesterol is converted to cholesterol ester (CE) by the lecithin–cholesterol acyltransferase (LCAT) reaction. HDL transfers CE to VLDL in exchange for triacylglycerol (TG). The cholesterol ester transfer protein (CETP) mediates this exchange. *apo*, apolipoprotein; *IDL*, intermediate-density lipoprotein; *LDL*, low-density lipoprotein.

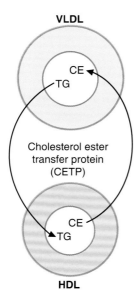

FIGURE 32.16 Function of cholesterol ester transfer protein (CETP). CETP transfers cholesterol esters (CE) from high-density lipoprotein (HDL) to very-low-density lipoprotein (VLDL) in exchange for triacylglycerol (TG).

cholesterol and cholesterol esters that are transferred directly to the liver via HDL. Mature HDL particles are designated as *HDL*$_3$; after reverse cholesterol transport and the accumulation of cholesterol esters, they become the atherogenic protective form, HDL$_2$. The CETP reaction then leads to the loss of cholesterol and gain of triacylglycerol, such that the particles become larger and eventually regenerate HDL$_3$ particles (see Table 32.4). Hepatic lipase can then remove triacylglycerol from HDL$_3$ particles to regenerate HDL$_2$ particles.

VI. Receptor-Mediated Endocytosis of Lipoproteins

As stated earlier, each lipoprotein particle contains specific apolipoproteins on its surface that act as ligands for specific plasma membrane receptors on target tissues such as the liver, the adrenal cortex, the gonads, and other cells that require one or more of the components of the lipoproteins. With the exception of the scavenger receptor SR-B1, the interaction of ligand and receptor initiates the process of endocytosis shown for LDL in Figure 32.17. The receptors for LDL, for example, are found in specific areas of the plasma membrane of the target cell for circulating lipoproteins. These are known as *coated pits*, and they contain a unique protein called *clathrin*. The plasma membrane in the vicinity of the receptor–LDL complex invaginates and fuses to form an endocytic vesicle. These vesicles then fuse with lysosomes, acidic subcellular vesicles that contain several degradative enzymes. The cholesterol esters of LDL are hydrolyzed to form free cholesterol, which is rapidly re-esterified through the action of ACAT. This rapid re-esterification is necessary to avoid the damaging effect of high levels of free cholesterol on cellular membranes.

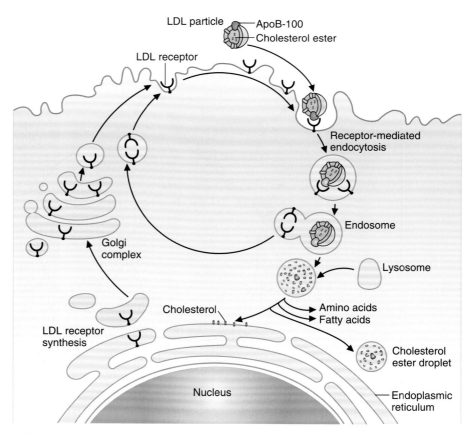

FIGURE 32.17 Cholesterol uptake by receptor-mediated endocytosis. *LDL*, low-density lipoprotein.

The newly esterified cholesterol contains primarily oleate or palmitoleate (monoun-saturated fatty acids), unlike those of the cholesterol esters in LDL, which are rich in linoleate, a polyunsaturated fatty acid.

As is true for the synthesis and activity of HMG-CoA reductase, the synthesis of the LDL receptor itself is subject to feedback inhibition by increasing levels of cholesterol within the cell. As cholesterol levels increase within a cell, synthesis of the LDL receptor is inhibited. When the intracellular levels of cholesterol decrease, both synthesis of cholesterol from acetyl-CoA and synthesis of the LDL receptor are stimulated. One probable mechanism for this feedback regulation involves one or more of the SREBPs described previously. These proteins or the cofactors that are required for the full expression of genes that code for the LDL receptor are also capable of sensing the concentration of sterols within the cell. When sterol levels are high, the process that leads to the binding of the SREBP to the SRE of these genes is suppressed (see Fig. 32.6A). The rate of synthesis from mRNA for the LDL re-ceptor is diminished under these circumstances. This, in turn, appropriately reduces the amount of cholesterol that can enter these cholesterol-rich cells by receptor-mediated endocytosis (downregulation of receptor synthesis). When the intracellular levels of cholesterol decrease, these processes are reversed, and cells act to increase their cholesterol levels. Both synthesis of cholesterol from acetyl-CoA and synthesis of LDL receptors are stimulated. An increased number of receptors (upregulation of receptor synthesis) results in an increased uptake of LDL cholesterol from the blood, with a subsequent reduction of LDL cholesterol levels. At the same time, the cellular cholesterol pool is replenished. The upregulation of LDL receptors forms the basis of the mechanism of statin drugs lowering blood LDL levels.

VII. Lipoprotein Receptors

The best-characterized lipoprotein receptor, the LDL receptor, specifically recog-nizes apoB-100 and apoE. Therefore, this receptor binds VLDL, IDL, and chylo-micron remnants in addition to LDL. The binding reaction is characterized by its saturability and occurs with high affinity and a narrow range of specificity. Other receptors, such as the LDL receptor–related proteins (LRP) and the macrophage scavenger receptor (notably types SR-A1 and SR-A2, which are located primarily near the endothelial surface of vascular endothelial cells) have broad specificity and bind many other ligands in addition to the blood lipoproteins.

A. The LDL Receptor

The *LDL receptor* has a mosaic structure encoded by a gene that was assem-bled by a process known as *exon shuffling*. The gene contains 18 exons and is >45 kilobases (kb) in length; it is located on the short arm of chromosome 19. The protein encoded by the gene is composed of six different regions (Fig. 32.18). The first region, at the amino terminus, contains the LDL-binding region, a cysteine-rich sequence of 40 residues. Acidic side chains in this region bind ionic calcium. When these side chains are protonated, calcium is released from its binding sites. This release leads to conformational changes that allow the LDL to dissociate from its receptor docking site. Disulfide bonds, formed from the cysteine resi-dues, have a stabilizing influence on the structural integrity of this portion of the receptor.

The second region of the receptor contains domains that are homologous with epidermal growth factor (EGF) as well as with a complex consisting of six repeats that resembles the blades of the transducin β-subunit, forming a propellerlike moiety.

The third region of the LDL receptor contains a chain of *N*-linked oligosac-charides, whereas the fourth region contains a domain that is rich in serine and threonine and contains *O*-linked sugars. This region may have a role in physically extending the receptor away from the membrane so that the LDL-binding region is accessible to the LDL molecule.

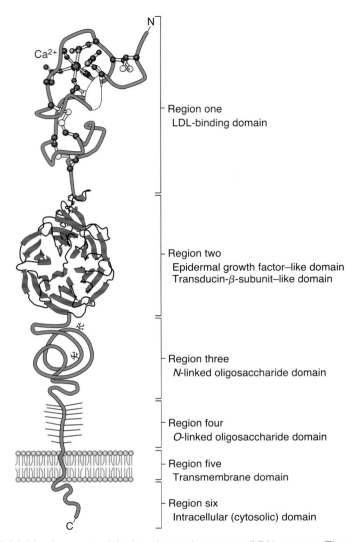

N

Ca²⁺

Region one
LDL-binding domain

Region two
Epidermal growth factor–like domain
Transducin-β-subunit–like domain

Region three
N-linked oligosaccharide domain

Region four
O-linked oligosaccharide domain

Region five
Transmembrane domain

Region six
Intracellular (cytosolic) domain

C

FIGURE 32.18   Structure of the low-density lipoprotein (LDL) receptor. The protein has six major regions, which are described in the text.

The fifth region contains 22 hydrophobic residues that constitute the membrane-spanning unit of the receptor, whereas the sixth region extends into the cytosol, where it regulates the interaction between the C-terminal domain of the LDL receptor and the clathrin-containing coated pit where the process of receptor-mediated endocytosis is initiated.

The number of LDL receptors, the binding of LDL to its receptors, and the postreceptor binding process can be diminished for a variety of reasons, all of which may lead to an accumulation of LDL cholesterol in the blood and premature atherosclerosis. These abnormalities can result from mutations in one (heterozygous—seen in approximately 1 in 500 people) or both (homozygous—seen in about 1 in 1 million people) of the alleles for the LDL receptor (*familial hypercholesterolemia*). Heterozygotes produce approximately half of the normal complement of LDL receptors, whereas the homozygotes produce almost no LDL receptor protein (receptor-negative familial hypercholesterolemia). The latter have serum total cholesterol levels in the range of 500 to 800 mg/dL.

The genetic mutations are mainly deletions, but insertions or duplications also occur as well as missense and nonsense mutations. Four classes of mutations have been identified. The first class involves "null" alleles that either direct the synthesis of no protein at all or a protein that cannot be precipitated by antibodies to the

LDL receptor. In the second class, the alleles encode proteins, but they cannot be transported to the cell surface. The third class of mutant alleles encodes proteins that reach the cell surface but cannot bind LDL normally. Finally, the fourth class encodes proteins that reach the surface and bind LDL but fail to cluster and internalize the LDL particles. The result of each of these mutations is that blood levels of LDL are elevated because cells cannot take up these particles at a normal rate.

B. LDL Receptor-Related Protein-1

The *LDL receptor-related protein-1* (LRP-1) is structurally related to the LDL receptor but recognizes a broader spectrum of ligands. LRP-1 is a member of a family of at least 8 proteins, all of which bind multiple ligands and have distinct roles in the cell. In addition to lipoproteins, LRP-1 binds the blood proteins α_2-macroglobulin (a protein that inhibits blood proteases) and tissue plasminogen activator (TPA) and its inhibitors. The LRP-1 receptor recognizes the apoE of lipoproteins and binds remnants produced by the digestion of the triacylglycerols of chylomicrons and VLDL by LPL. Thus, one of its functions is believed to be clearing these remnants from the blood. The LRP-1 receptor is abundant in the cell membranes of the liver, brain, and placenta. In contrast to the LDL receptor, synthesis of the LRP-1 receptor is not significantly affected by an increase in the intracellular concentration of cholesterol. However, insulin causes the number of these receptors on the cell surface to increase, consistent with the need to remove chylomicron remnants that otherwise would accumulate after eating a meal.

C. Macrophage Scavenger Receptor

Some cells, particularly the phagocytic macrophages, have nonspecific receptors known as *scavenger receptors* that bind various types of molecules, including oxidatively modified LDL particles. There are several different types of scavenger receptors. SR-B1 is used primarily for HDL binding, whereas the scavenger receptors expressed on macrophages are SR-A1 and SR-A2. Modification of LDL frequently involves oxidative damage, particularly of polyunsaturated fatty acyl groups (see Chapter 25). In contrast to the LDL receptors, the scavenger receptors are not subject to downregulation. The continued presence of scavenger receptors in the cell membrane allows the cells to take up oxidatively modified LDL long after intracellular cholesterol levels are elevated. When the macrophages become engorged with lipid, they are called *foam cells*. An accumulation of these foam cells in the subendothelial space of blood vessels form the earliest gross evidence of a developing atherosclerotic plaque known as a *fatty streak*.

The processes that cause oxidation of LDL involve superoxide radicals, nitric oxide, hydrogen peroxide, and other oxidants (see Chapter 25). Antioxidants, such as vitamin E, ascorbic acid (vitamin C), and carotenoids, may be involved in protecting LDL from oxidation.

VIII. Anatomic and Biochemical Aspects of Atherosclerosis

The normal artery is composed of three distinct layers (Fig. 32.19). That which is closest to the lumen of the vessel, the *intima*, is lined by a monolayer of endothelial cells that are bathed by the circulating blood. Just beneath these specialized cells lies the *subintimal extracellular matrix*, in which some vascular smooth muscle cells are embedded (the subintimal space). The middle layer, known as the *tunica media*, is separated from the intima by the *internal elastic lamina*. The tunica media contains lamellae of smooth muscle cells surrounded by an elastin- and collagen-rich matrix. The external elastic lamina forms the border between the tunica media and the outermost layer, the *adventitia*. This layer contains nerve fibers and mast cells. It is the origin of the vasa vasorum, which supplies blood to the outer two-thirds of the tunica media.

Anne J.'s blood lipid levels (in mg/dL) were as follows:

Triacylglycerol	158
Total cholesterol	420
HDL cholesterol	32
LDL cholesterol	356

She was diagnosed as having familial hypercholesterolemia (FH), type IIA, which is caused by genetic defects in the gene that encodes the LDL receptor (see Fig. 32.18). As a result of the receptor defect, LDL cannot readily be taken up by cells, and its concentration in the blood is elevated.

LDL particles contain a high percentage, by weight, of cholesterol and cholesterol esters, more than other blood lipoproteins. However, LDL triacylglycerol levels are low because LDL is produced by digestion of the triacylglycerols of VLDL and IDL. Therefore, individuals with type IIA hyperlipoproteinemia have very high blood cholesterol levels, but their levels of triacylglycerols may be in or near the normal range (see Table 32.4).

Ivan A.'s blood lipid levels were as follows:

Triacylglycerol	295
Total cholesterol	314
HDL cholesterol	24
LDL cholesterol	231

The elevated serum levels of LDL cholesterol found in patients such as **Ivan A.** who have type 2 diabetes mellitus is multifactorial. One of the mechanisms responsible for this increase involves the presence of chronically elevated levels of glucose in the blood of people with poorly controlled diabetes. This prolonged hyperglycemia increases the rate of nonenzymatic attachment of glucose to various proteins in the body, a process referred to as *glycation* or *glycosylation of proteins*.

Glycation may adversely affect the structure or the function of the protein involved. For example, glycation of the LDL receptor and of proteins in the LDL particle may interfere with the normal "fit" of LDL particles with their specific receptors. As a result, less circulating LDL is internalized into cells by receptor-mediated endocytosis, and the serum LDL cholesterol level rises. In addition, because Mr. A. is obese, he exhibits higher than normal levels of circulating free fatty acids, which the liver uses to increase the synthesis of VLDL, leading to hypertriglyceridemia.

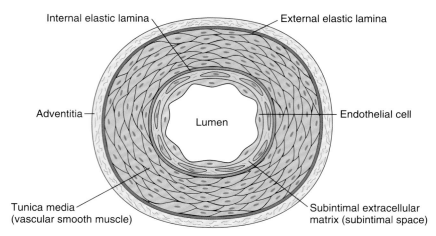

Internal elastic lamina

External elastic lamina

Adventitia

Lumen

Endothelial cell

Tunica media
(vascular smooth muscle)

Subintimal extracellular
matrix (subintimal space)

FIGURE 32.19 The different layers of the arterial wall.

In addition to nutrition therapy, aimed at reducing her blood cholesterol levels, **Anne J.** was treated with atorvastatin, an HMG-CoA reductase inhibitor. The HMG-CoA reductase inhibitors decrease the rate of synthesis of cholesterol in cells. As cellular cholesterol levels decrease, the synthesis of LDL receptors increases. As the number of receptors increase on the cell surface, the uptake of LDL is accelerated. Consequently, the blood level of LDL cholesterol decreases. Anne was also treated with ezetimibe, which blocks cholesterol absorption from the intestinal lumen but has not yet been shown to decrease cardiovascular risk.

HDL is considered to be the "good cholesterol" because it accepts free cholesterol from peripheral tissues, such as cells in the walls of blood vessels. This cholesterol is converted to cholesterol ester, part of which is transferred to VLDL by CETP, and returned to the liver by IDL and LDL. The remainder of the cholesterol is transferred directly as part of the HDL molecule to the liver. The liver reuses the cholesterol in the synthesis of VLDL, converts it to bile salts, or excretes it directly into the bile. HDL, therefore, tends to lower blood cholesterol levels. Lower blood cholesterol levels correlate with lower rates of death caused by atherosclerosis.

The initial step in the development of an atherosclerotic lesion within the wall of an artery is the formation of a *fatty streak*. The fatty streak represents an accumulation of lipid-laden macrophages or foam cells in the subintimal space. These fatty streaks are visible as a yellow-white linear streak that bulges slightly into the lumen of the vessel. These streaks are initiated when one or more known vascular risk factors for atherosclerosis, all of which have the potential to injure the vascular endothelial cells, reach a critical threshold at the site of future lesions. Examples of such risk factors include elevated intraarterial pressure (arterial hypertension); elevated circulating levels of various lipids such as LDL, chylomicron remnants, and VLDL remnants; low levels of circulating HDL; cigarette smoking; chronic elevations in blood glucose levels; high circulating levels of the vasoconstricting octapeptide angiotensin II; and others. The resulting insult to endothelial cells may trigger these cells to secrete adhesion molecules that bind to circulating monocytes and markedly slow their rate of movement past the endothelium. When these monocytic cells are slowed enough, they accumulate and have access to the physical spaces that exist between endothelial cells. This accumulation of monocytic cells resembles the classical inflammatory response to injury. These changes have led to the suggestion that atherosclerosis is, in fact, an inflammatory disorder and, therefore, is one that might be prevented or attenuated through the use of antiinflammatory agents. Two such agents, acetylsalicylic acid (aspirin) and HMG-CoA reductase inhibitors (statins), have been shown to suppress the inflammatory cascade, whereas statins also inhibit the action of HMG-CoA reductase.

The monocytic cells are transformed into macrophages that migrate through the spaces between endothelial cells. They enter the subintimal space under the influence of chemoattractant cytokines (e.g., chemokine macrophage chemoattractant protein I) secreted by vascular cells in response to exposure to oxidatively modified fatty acids within the lipoproteins.

These macrophages can replicate and exhibit augmented expression of receptors that recognize oxidatively modified lipoproteins. Unlike the classic LDL receptors on liver and many nonhepatic cells, these macrophage-bound receptors are high-capacity, low-specificity receptors (scavenger receptors). They bind to and internalize oxidatively modified fatty acids within LDLs to become subintimal foam cells as described previously. As these foam cells accumulate, they deform the overlying endothelium, causing microscopic separations between endothelial cells, exposing these foam cells and the underlying extracellular matrix to the blood. These exposed areas serve as sites for platelet adhesion and aggregation. Activated platelets secrete cytokines that perpetuate this process and increase the potential for thrombus (clot) formation locally. As the evolving plaque matures, a *fibrous cap* forms over its expanding "roof," which now bulges into the vascular

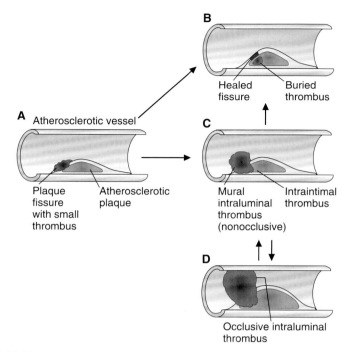

FIGURE 32.20 Evolution of an atherosclerotic plaque. Plaque capsule eroded near the "elbow" of plaque creating an early plaque fissure **(A)**, which may heal as plaque increases in size **(B)** or may grow as thrombus expands, having an intraluminal portion and an intraintimal portion **(C)**. If the fissure is not properly sealed, the thrombus may grow and completely occlude the vessel lumen **(D)**, causing an acute infarction of tissues downstream of the vessel occlusion.

In patients such as **Anne J.** and **Ivan A.**, who have elevated levels of VLDL or LDL, HDL levels are often low. These patients are predisposed to atherosclerosis and suffer from a high incidence of heart attacks and strokes.

Physical activity and estrogen administration both increase HDL levels. This is one of the reasons physical activity is often recommended to aid in the prevention or treatment of heart disease. Prior to menopause, the incidence of heart attacks is relatively low in women, but it rises after menopause and increases to the level found in men by the age of 65 or 70 years. Moderate consumption of ethanol (alcohol) has also been correlated with increased HDL levels. Recent studies suggest that the beneficial amount of ethanol may be quite low, about two small glasses of wine a day, and that beneficial effects ascribed to ethanol may result from other components of wine and alcoholic beverages. In spite of the evidence that postmenopausal hormone replacement therapy (HRT) decreases circulating levels of LDL and increases HDL levels, data from controlled trials show that HRT may actually increase the rate of atherosclerotic vascular disease in these women. As a result, the accepted indications for estrogen administration are now limited to intolerable "hot flashes" or vaginal dryness.

lumen, thereby partially occluding it. Vascular smooth muscle cells now migrate from the tunica media to the subintimal space and secrete additional plaque matrix material. The smooth muscle cells also secrete metalloproteinases that thin the fibrous cap near its "elbow" at the periphery of the plaque. This thinning progresses until the fibrous cap ruptures, allowing the plaque contents to physically contact the procoagulant elements present within the circulation. This leads to acute thrombus formation. If this thrombus completely occludes the remaining lumen of the vessel, an infarction of tissues distal to the occlusion (i.e., an acute myocardial infarction [AMI]) may occur (Fig. 32.20). Most plaques that rupture also contain focal areas of calcification, which appears to result from the induction of the same cluster of genes as those that promote the formation of bone. The inducers for this process include oxidized sterols as well as transforming growth factor β (TGF-β) derived from certain vascular cells.

Finally, high intraluminal shear forces develop in these thinning or eroded areas of the plaque's fibrous cap, inducing macrophages to secrete additional metalloproteinases that further degrade the arterial-fibrous cap matrix. This contributes further to plaque rupture and thrombus formation (see Fig. 32.20). The consequence is a macrovascular ischemic event such as an AMI or an acute cerebrovascular accident (CVA).

IX. Steroid Hormones

Cholesterol is the precursor of all five classes of *steroid hormones*: glucocorticoids, mineralocorticoids, androgens, estrogens, and progestogens. These hormones are synthesized in the adrenal cortex, ovaries, testes, and ovarian corpus luteum. Steroid hormones are transported through the blood from their sites of synthesis

Studies on LDL-receptor metabolism have recently identified a new potential drug target in order to increase LDL receptor expression on the cell surface. A protease with the cumbersome name of proprotein convertase subtilisin-like kexin type 9 (PCSK9) has been shown to regulate the levels of LDL receptor on the cell surface. PCSK9 does so by degrading the receptor, thereby reducing its expression on the cell surface. Humans with familial hypercholesterolemia have been identified with gain of function mutations in PCSK9; the protease is always active, reduces LDL receptor levels, and hypercholesterolemia results. Conversely, individuals have been identified with nonfunctional variants of PCSK9; their LDL levels are extremely low, and in population studies this group is much less likely to experience atherosclerotic disease than those with functional PCSK9. Recall that statins work, in part, by the activation of SREBP-2, which upregulates LDL receptor synthesis. SREBP-2 also upregulates PCSK9, which aids in regulating LDL receptor expression. Clinical trials using monoclonal antibodies directed against PCSK9, given in conjunction with a statin, showed a significant lowering of circulating LDL levels.

Lipoprotein(a) is essentially an LDL particle that is covalently bound to apolipoprotein(a). It is called *lipoprotein little a* to avoid confusion with the apolipoprotein A found in HDL. The structure of apolipoprotein(a) is very similar to that of plasminogen, a precursor of the protease plasmin that degrades fibrin, a major component of blood clots. Lipoprotein(a), however, cannot be converted to active plasmin. There are reports that high concentrations of lipoprotein(a) correlate with an increased risk of coronary artery disease, even in patients in whom the lipid profile is otherwise normal. The physiologic function of lipoprotein(a) remains elusive.

Vera L. consulted her gynecologist, who confirmed that her problems were probably the result of an excess production of androgens (virilization) and ordered blood and urine studies to determine whether Vera's adrenal cortices or her ovaries were causing her virilizing syndrome.

to their target organs, where, because of their hydrophobicity, they cross the cell membrane and bind to specific receptors in either the cytoplasm or the nucleus. The bound receptors then bind to DNA to regulate gene transcription (see Chapter 16, Section III.C.2, and Fig. 16.12). Because of their hydrophobicity, steroid hormones must be complexed with a serum protein. Serum albumin can act as a nonspecific carrier for the steroid hormones, but there are specific carriers as well. The cholesterol used for steroid hormone synthesis is either synthesized in the tissues from acetyl-CoA, extracted from intracellular cholesterol ester pools, or taken up by the cell in the form of cholesterol-containing lipoproteins (either internalized by the LDL receptor or absorbed by the SR-B1 receptor). In general, glucocorticoids and progestogens contain 21 carbons, androgens contain 19 carbons, and estrogens contain 18 carbons. The specific complement of enzymes present in the cells of an organ determines which hormones the organ can synthesize.

A. Overview of Steroid Hormone Synthesis

The biosynthesis of glucocorticoids and mineralocorticoids (in the adrenal cortex), and that of sex steroids (in the adrenal cortex and gonads), requires several distinct cytochrome P450 enzymes (see Chapter 25 and Table 32.5). These monooxygenases are involved in the transfer of electrons from NADPH through electron-transfer protein intermediates to molecular oxygen, which then oxidizes a variety of the ring carbons of cholesterol.

Cholesterol is converted to progesterone in the first two steps of the synthesis of all steroid hormones. Cytochrome $P450_{SCC}$ side-chain cleavage enzyme (previously referred to as *cholesterol desmolase* and classified as CYP11A) is located in the mitochondrial inner membrane and removes six carbons from the side chain of cholesterol, forming pregnenolone, which has 21 carbons (Fig. 32.21). The next step,

TABLE 32.5	**Overview of Steroid Hormones**		
STEROID GROUP	**SITE OF SYNTHESIS**	**SYNTHESIS STIMULATED BY**	**COMMENTS**
Glucocorticoids (Example: cortisol)	Adrenal cortex	Adrenal corticotrophic hormone	Requires a series of oxidative reactions
Mineralocorticoids (Example: aldosterone)	Adrenal cortex	Angiotensin I Angiotensin II Increased potassium concentration in the blood Reduced sodium concentration in the blood	Angiotensins are released in response to a reduction in extracellular fluid volume. Aldosterone stimulates sodium resorption in tissues, resulting in an increase in extracellular fluid volume and blood pressure
Androgens (Example: testosterone)	Leydig cells of testes Ovary	LH	In males, testosterone is converted to dihydrotestosterone, a higher affinity form of the hormone, in specific tissues.
Estrogens (Example: 17β-estradiol)	Ovarian follicle Corpus luteum	FSH	Estradiol inhibits the synthesis and secretion of FSH.
Progestogens (Example: progesterone)	Corpus luteum	LH	In combination with estradiol prepares the uterine endometrium for implantation of the fertilized ovum and acts as a differentiation factor in mammary gland development.

LH, luteinizing hormone; FSH, follicle-stimulating hormone.

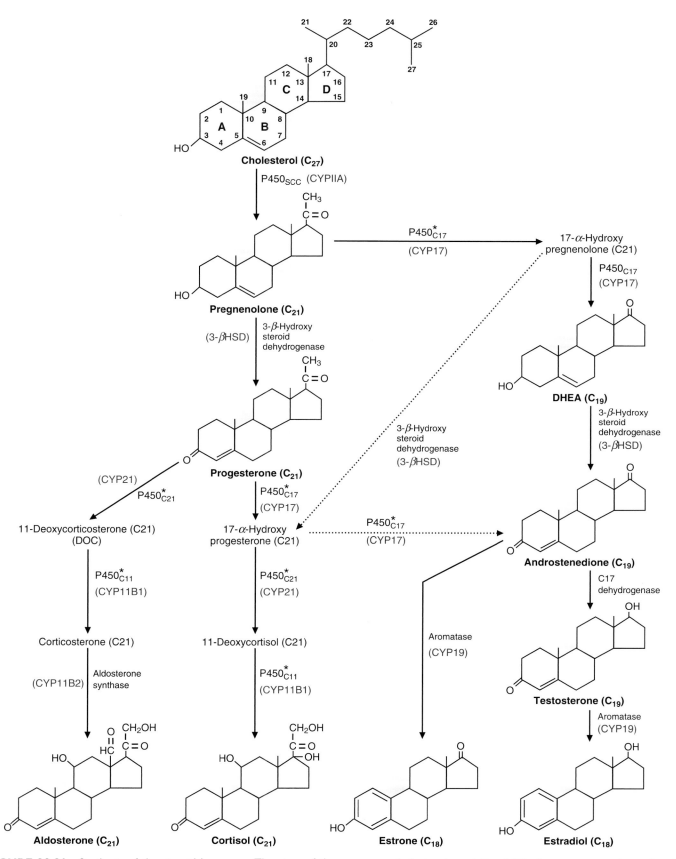

FIGURE 32.21 Synthesis of the steroid hormones. The rings of the precursor, cholesterol, are *lettered*. Dihydrotestosterone is produced from testosterone by reduction of the carbon–carbon double bond in ring A. The *dashed lines* indicate alternative pathways to the major pathways indicated. The *starred* enzymes are those that may be defective in congenital adrenal hyperplasia. *CYP*, a designation for a cytochrome P450 containing enzyme; *DHEA*, dehydroepiandrosterone.

the conversion of pregnenolone to progesterone, is catalyzed by 3β-hydroxysteroid dehydrogenase, an enzyme that is not a member of the cytochrome P450 family. Other steroid hormones are produced from progesterone by reactions that involve members of the P450 family. These include the mitochondrial enzyme cytochrome P450$_{C11}$ (CYP11B1), which catalyzes β-hydroxylation at carbon 11, and two ER enzymes, P450$_{C17}$ (17α-hydroxylation, CYP17) and P450$_{C21}$ (hydroxylation at carbon 21, CYP21). As the synthesis of the steroid hormones is discussed, notice how certain enzymes are used in more than one pathway. Defects in these enzymes lead to multiple abnormalities in steroid synthesis, which, in turn, results in a variety of abnormal phenotypes.

B. Synthesis of Cortisol

The adrenocortical biosynthetic pathway that leads to *cortisol* synthesis occurs in the middle layer of the adrenal cortex, known as the *zona fasciculata*. Free cholesterol is transported by an intracellular carrier protein to the inner mitochondrial membrane of cells (Fig. 32.22), where the side chain is cleaved to form pregnenolone. Pregnenolone returns to the cytosol, where it forms progesterone.

In the membrane of the ER, the enzyme P450$_{C17}$ (CYP17) catalyzes the hydroxylation of C17 of progesterone or pregnenolone and can also catalyze the cleavage

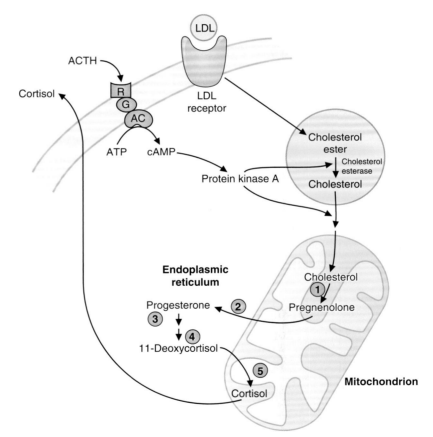

FIGURE 32.22 Cellular route for cortisol synthesis. Cholesterol is synthesized from acetyl coenzyme A or derived from low-density lipoprotein (LDL), which is endocytosed and digested by lysosomal enzymes. Cholesterol is stored in cells of the adrenal cortex as cholesterol esters. Adrenocorticotropic hormone (ACTH) signals the cell to convert cholesterol to cortisol and transmits its signal through a G-protein–coupled receptor that results in the activation of adenylate cyclase, and, ultimately, protein kinase A. (*1*) cholesterol desmolase (P450$_{SCC}$, involved in side-chain cleavage); (*2*) 3β-hydroxysteroid dehydrogenase; (*3*) 17α-hydroxylase (P450$_{C17}$); (*4*) 21-hydroxylase (P450$_{C21}$); (*5*) 11β-hydroxylase (P450$_{C11}$). *cAMP*, cyclic adenosine monophosphate; *ATP*, adenosine triphosphate.

of the two-carbon side chain of these compounds at C17 (a C17–C20 lyase activity), which forms androstenedione from 17α-hydroxyprogesterone. These two separate functions of the same enzyme allow further steroid synthesis to proceed along two separate pathways: The 17-hydroxylated steroids that retain their side chains are precursors of cortisol (C21), whereas those from which the side chain was cleaved (C19 steroids) are precursors of androgens (male sex hormones) and estrogens (female sex hormones).

In the pathway of cortisol synthesis, the 17-hydroxylation of progesterone yields 17α-hydroxyprogesterone, which, along with progesterone, is transported to the smooth ER. There, the membrane-bound $P450_{C21}$ (CYP21, 21α-hydroxylase) complex catalyzes the hydroxylation of C21 of 17α-hydroxyprogesterone to form 11-deoxycortisol and progesterone to form deoxycorticosterone (DOC), a precursor of the mineralocorticoid aldosterone (see Fig. 32.21).

The final step in cortisol synthesis requires transport of 11-deoxycortisol back to the inner membrane of the mitochondria, where $P450_{C11}$ (11β-hydroxylase, CYP11B1) catalyzes the β-hydroxylation of the substrate at carbon 21, in a reaction that requires molecular oxygen and electrons derived from NADPH, to form cortisol. The rate of biosynthesis of cortisol and other adrenal steroids depends on stimulation of the adrenal cortical cells by adrenocorticotropic hormone (ACTH).

C. Synthesis of Aldosterone

The synthesis of the potent mineralocorticoid *aldosterone* in the zona glomerulosa of the adrenal cortex also begins with the conversion of cholesterol to progesterone (see Figs. 32.21 and 32.22). Progesterone is then hydroxylated at C21, a reaction catalyzed by $P450_{C21}$ (CYP21), to yield 11-DOC. The $P450_{C11}$ (CYP11B1) enzyme system then catalyzes the reactions that convert DOC to corticosterone. The terminal steps in aldosterone synthesis, catalyzed by the P450 aldosterone system (CYP11B2), involve the oxidation of corticosterone to 18-hydroxycorticosterone, which is oxidized to aldosterone.

The primary stimulus for aldosterone production is the octapeptide angiotensin II, although hyperkalemia (greater than normal levels of potassium in the blood) or hyponatremia (less than normal levels of sodium in the blood) may stimulate aldosterone synthesis directly as well. ACTH has a permissive action in aldosterone production. It allows cells to respond optimally to their primary stimulus, angiotensin II.

D. Synthesis of the Adrenal Androgens

Adrenal androgen biosynthesis proceeds from cleavage of the two-carbon side chain of 17-hydroxypregnenolone at C17 to form the 19-carbon adrenal androgen DHEA and its sulfate derivative (DHEAS) in the zona reticularis of the adrenal cortex (see Fig. 32.21). These compounds, which are weak androgens, represent a significant percentage of the total steroid production by the normal adrenal cortex and are the major androgens synthesized in the adrenal gland.

Androstenedione, another weak adrenal androgen, is produced by oxidation of the β-hydroxy group to a carbonyl group by 3β-hydroxysteroid dehydrogenase. This androgen is converted to testosterone primarily in extraadrenal tissues. Although the adrenal cortex makes very little estrogen, the weak adrenal androgens may be converted to estrogens in the peripheral tissues, particularly in adipose tissue (Fig. 32.23).

E. Synthesis of Testosterone

Luteinizing hormone (LH) from the anterior pituitary stimulates the synthesis of testosterone and other androgens by the Leydig cells of the human testicle. In many ways, the pathways leading to androgen synthesis in the testicle are

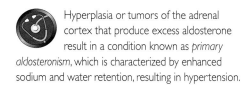

Hyperplasia or tumors of the adrenal cortex that produce excess aldosterone result in a condition known as *primary aldosteronism*, which is characterized by enhanced sodium and water retention, resulting in hypertension.

Although aldosterone is the major mineralocorticoid in humans, excessive production of a weaker mineralocorticoid, DOC, which occurs in patients with a deficiency of the 11-hydroxylase (the $P450_{C11}$ enzyme, CYP11B1), may lead to clinical signs and symptoms of mineralocorticoid excess even though aldosterone secretion is suppressed in these patients.

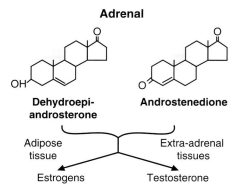

FIGURE 32.23 Adrenal androgens. These weak androgens are converted to testosterone or estrogens in other tissues.

Congenital adrenal hyperplasia (CAH) is a group of diseases caused by a genetically determined deficiency in a variety of enzymes required for cortisol synthesis. The most common deficiency is that of 21α-hydroxylase (CYP21), the activity of which is necessary to convert progesterone to 11-DOC and 17α-hydroxyprogesterone to 11-deoxycortisol. Thus, this deficiency reduces both aldosterone and cortisol production without affecting androgen production. If the enzyme deficiency is severe, the precursors for aldosterone and cortisol production are shunted to androgen synthesis, producing an overabundance of androgens, which leads to prenatal masculinization in females and postnatal virilization of males. Another enzyme deficiency in this group of diseases is that of 11β-hydroxylase (CYP11B1), which results in the accumulation of 11-DOC. An excess of this mineralocorticoid leads to hypertension (through binding of 11-DOC to the aldosterone receptor). In this form of CAH, 11-deoxycortisol also accumulates, but its biologic activity is minimal, and no specific clinical signs and symptoms result. The androgen pathway is unaffected, and the increased ACTH levels may increase the levels of adrenal androgens in the blood. A third possible enzyme deficiency is that of 17α-hydroxylase (CYP17). A defect in 17α-hydroxylase leads to aldosterone excess and hypertension; however, because adrenal androgen synthesis requires this enzyme, no virilization occurs in these patients.

Biologically, the most potent circulating androgen is testosterone. Approximately 50% of the testosterone in the blood in a normal woman is produced equally in the ovaries and in the adrenal cortices. The remaining half is derived from ovarian and adrenal androstenedione, which, after secretion into the blood, is converted to testosterone in adipose tissue, muscle, liver, and skin. The adrenal cortex, however, is the major source of the relatively weak androgen DHEA. The serum concentration of its stable metabolite, DHEAS, is used as a measure of adrenal androgen production in hyperandrogenic patients with diffuse excessive growth of secondary sexual hair (e.g., facial hair as well as that in the axillae, the suprapubic area, the chest, and the upper extremities).

Q The results of the blood tests on **Vera L.** showed that her level of testosterone was normal but that her serum DHEAS level was significantly elevated. Which tissue was the most likely source of the androgens that caused Vera's hirsutism (a male pattern of secondary sexual hair growth)?

similar to those described for the adrenal cortex. In the human testicle, the predominant pathway leading to testosterone synthesis is through pregnenolone to 17α-hydroxypregnenolone to DHEA (the Δ^5 pathway), and then from DHEA to androstenedione, and from androstenedione to testosterone (see Fig. 32.21). As for all steroids, the rate-limiting step in testosterone production is the conversion of cholesterol to pregnenolone. LH controls the rate of side-chain cleavage from cholesterol at carbon 21 to form pregnenolone and thus regulates the rate of testosterone synthesis. In its target cells, the double bond in ring A of testosterone is reduced through the action of 5α-reductase, forming the active hormone dihydrotestosterone (DHT).

F. Synthesis of Estrogens and Progesterone

Ovarian production of *estrogens*, *progestogens* (compounds related to progesterone), and *androgens* requires the activity of the cytochrome P450 family of oxidative enzymes used for the synthesis of other steroid hormones. Ovarian estrogens are C18 steroids with a phenolic hydroxyl group at C3 and either a hydroxyl group (estradiol) or a ketone group (estrone) at C17. Although the major steroid-producing compartments of the ovary (the granulosa cell, the theca cell, the stromal cell, and the cells of the corpus luteum) have all of the enzyme systems required for the synthesis of multiple steroids, the granulosa cells secrete primarily estrogens, the thecal and stromal cells secrete primarily androgens, and the cells of the corpus luteum secrete primarily progesterone.

The ovarian granulosa cell, in response to stimulation by follicle-stimulating hormone (FSH) from the anterior pituitary gland and through the catalytic activity of P450 aromatase (CYP19), converts testosterone to estradiol, the predominant and most potent of the ovarian estrogens (see Fig. 32.21). Similarly, androstenedione is converted to estrone in the ovary, although the major site of estrone production from androstenedione occurs in extraovarian tissues, principally skeletal muscle and adipose tissue.

G. Vitamin D Synthesis

Vitamin D is unique in that it can be either obtained from the diet (as vitamin D_2 or D_3) or synthesized from a cholesterol precursor, a process that requires reactions in the skin, liver, and kidney. The calciferols, including several forms of vitamin D, are a family of steroids that affect calcium homeostasis (Fig. 32.24). Cholecalciferol (vitamin D_3) requires ultraviolet light for its production from 7-dehydrocholesterol, which is present in cutaneous tissues (skin) in animals and available from ergosterol in plants. This irradiation cleaves the carbon–carbon bond at C9–C10, opening the B-ring to form cholecalciferol, an inactive precursor of 1,25-$(OH)_2$-cholecalciferol (calcitriol). Calcitriol is the most potent biologically active form of vitamin D (see Fig. 32.24).

The formation of calcitriol from cholecalciferol begins in the liver and ends in the kidney, where the pathway is regulated. In this activation process, carbon 25 of vitamin D_2 or D_3 is hydroxylated in the microsomes of the liver to form 25-hydroxycholecalciferol (calcidiol). Calcidiol circulates to the kidney bound to vitamin D–binding globulin (transcalciferin). In the proximal convoluted tubule of the kidney, a mixed-function oxidase, which requires molecular O_2 and NADPH as cofactors, hydroxylates carbon 1 on the A-ring to form calcitriol. This step is tightly regulated and is the rate-limiting step in the production of the active hormone. The release of parathyroid hormone from the parathyroid gland results in activation of this last step of active hormone formation.

1,25-$(OH)_2D_3$ (calcitriol) is approximately 100 times more potent than 25-(OH) D_3 in its actions, yet 25-$(OH)D_3$ is present in the blood in a concentration that may be 100 times greater, which suggests that it may play some role in calcium and phosphorus homeostasis.

The biologically active forms of vitamin D are sterol hormones and, like other steroids, diffuse passively through the plasma membrane. In the intestine, bone, and kidney, the sterol then moves into the nucleus and binds to specific vitamin D_3 receptors. This complex activates genes that encode proteins mediating the action of active vitamin D_3. In the intestinal mucosal cell, for example, transcription of genes that encode calcium-transporting proteins are activated. These proteins are capable of carrying Ca^{2+} (and phosphorus) absorbed from the gut lumen across the cell, making it available for eventual passage into the circulation.

CLINICAL COMMENTS

 Anne J. is typical of patients with essentially normal serum triacylglycerol levels and elevated serum total cholesterol levels that are repeatedly in the upper 1% of the general population (e.g., 325 to 500 mg/dL). When similar lipid abnormalities are present in other family members in a pattern of autosomal-dominant inheritance and no secondary causes for these lipid alterations (e.g., hypothyroidism) are present, the entity referred to as *familial hypercholesterolemia* (FH), *type IIA*, is the most likely cause of this hereditary dyslipidemia.

FH is a genetic disorder caused by an abnormality in one or more alleles responsible for the formation or the functional integrity of high-affinity LDL receptors on the plasma membrane of cells that normally initiate the internalization of circulating LDL and other blood lipoproteins. Heterozygotes for FH (1 in 500 of the population) have roughly one-half of the normal complement or functional capacity of such receptors, whereas homozygotes (1 in 1 million of the population) have essentially no functional LDL receptors. The rare patient with the homozygous form of FH has a more extreme elevation of serum total and LDL cholesterol than does the heterozygote and, as a result, has a more profound predisposition to premature coronary artery disease.

Chronic hypercholesterolemia not only may cause the deposition of lipid within vascular tissues leading to atherosclerosis but also may cause the deposition of lipid within the skin and eye. When this occurs in the medial aspect of the upper and lower eyelids, it is referred to as *xanthelasma*. Similar deposits known as *xanthomas* may occur in the iris of the eye (arcus lipidalis) as well as the tendons of the hands ("knuckle pads") and Achilles tendons.

Although therapy aimed at inserting competent LDL receptor genes into the cells of patients with homozygous FH is being designed for the future, the current approach in the treatment of heterozygotes is to attempt to increase the rate of synthesis of LDL receptors in cells pharmacologically.

In addition to a HMG-CoA inhibitor, **Anne J.** was treated with ezetimibe, to achieve the recommended decrease in her LDL. Ezetimibe blocks cholesterol absorption in the intestine, causing a portion of the dietary cholesterol to be carried into the feces rather than packaged into chylomicrons. This reduces the levels of chylomicron-based cholesterol and cholesterol delivered to the liver by chylomicron remnants.

HMG-CoA reductase inhibitors, such as atorvastatin, which Anne is also taking, stimulate the synthesis of additional LDL receptors by inhibiting HMG-CoA reductase, the rate-limiting enzyme for cholesterol synthesis. The subsequent decline in the intracellular free cholesterol pool stimulates the synthesis of additional LDL receptors. These additional receptors reduce circulating LDL cholesterol levels by increasing receptor-mediated endocytosis of LDL particles.

A combination of strict dietary and dual pharmacologic therapy, aimed at decreasing the cholesterol levels of the body, is usually quite effective in correcting the lipid abnormality and, hopefully, the associated risk of atherosclerotic cardiovascular disease in patients with heterozygous FH.

 Ivan A. LDL cholesterol is the primary target of cholesterol-lowering therapy because both epidemiologic and experimental evidence strongly suggest a benefit of lowering serum LDL cholesterol in the prevention of

 Vera L.'s hirsutism was most likely the result of a problem in her adrenal cortex that caused excessive production of DHEA.

 Rickets is a disorder of young children caused by a deficiency of vitamin D. Low levels of calcium and phosphorus in the blood are associated with skeletal deformities in these children.

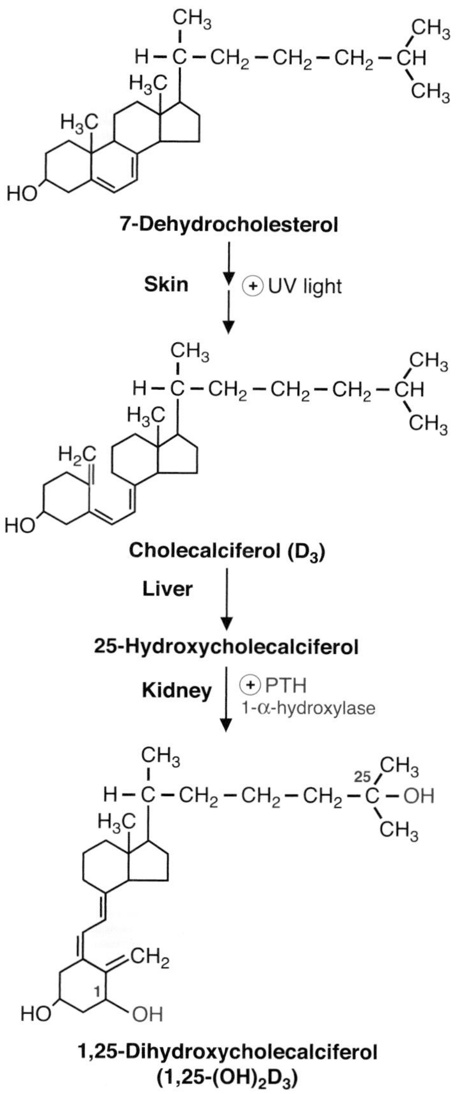

7-Dehydrocholesterol

Skin ↓ ⊕ UV light

Cholecalciferol (D₃)

Liver ↓

25-Hydroxycholecalciferol

Kidney ↓ ⊕PTH 1-α-hydroxylase

1,25-Dihydroxycholecalciferol (1,25-(OH)₂D₃)

FIGURE 32.24 Synthesis of active vitamin D. 1,25-(OH)₂D₃ is produced from 7-dehydrocholesterol, a precursor of cholesterol. In the skin, ultraviolet (UV) light produces cholecalciferol, which is hydroxylated at the 25-position in the liver and the 1-position in the kidney to form the active hormone. *PTH*, parathyroid hormone.

Anne J. was treated with a statin (atorvastatin) and ezetimibe. Ezetimibe reduces the percentage of absorption of free cholesterol present in the lumen of the gut and hence the amount of cholesterol available to the enterocyte to package into chylomicrons. This, in turn, reduces the amount of cholesterol returning to the liver in chylomicron remnants. The net result is a reduction in the cholesterol pool in hepatocytes. The latter induces the synthesis of an increased number of LDL receptors by the liver cells. As a consequence, the capacity of the liver to increase hepatic uptake of LDL from the circulation leads to a decrease in serum LDL levels. Despite this decrease in LDL levels, the drug has not been shown to decrease cardiovascular events in patients.

atherosclerotic cardiovascular disease. Similar evidence for raising subnormal levels of serum HDL cholesterol is less conclusive but adequate to support such efforts, particularly in high-risk patients, such as Ivan A., who have multiple cardiovascular risk factors.

So far, Mr. A. has failed in his attempts to reach his diet and physical activity goals. His LDL cholesterol level is 231 mg/dL. Based on his cardiovascular risk, he is a candidate for drug treatment. He should be given a high-intensity HMG-CoA reductase inhibitor. A low daily dose of aspirin (81 mg) could also be prescribed (see Chapter 31). It is important to gain early control of Mr. A.'s metabolic syndrome before the effects of insulin resistance can no longer be reversed. Various lipid-lowering agents are summarized in Table 32.6.

Vera L. Vera L. was born with a normal female genotype and phenotype, had normal female sexual development, spontaneous onset of puberty, and regular, although somewhat scanty, menses until the age of 20 years. At that point, she developed secondary amenorrhea (cessation of menses) and evidence of male hormone excess with early virilization (masculinization).

The differential diagnosis included an ovarian versus an adrenocortical source of the excess androgenic steroids. A screening test to determine whether the adrenal cortex or the ovary is the source of excess male hormone involves measuring the concentration of DHEAS in the patient's plasma because the adrenal cortex makes most of the DHEA and the ovary makes little or none. Vera's plasma DHEAS level was moderately elevated, identifying her adrenal cortices as the likely source of her virilizing syndrome.

If the excess production of androgens is not the result of an adrenal tumor, but rather the result of a defect in the pathway for cortisol production, the simple treatment is to administer glucocorticoids by mouth. The rationale for such treatment can be better understood by reviewing Figure 32.21. If **Vera L.** has a genetically determined partial deficiency in the $P450_{C11}$ enzyme system needed to convert 11-deoxycortisol to cortisol, her blood cortisol levels would fall. By virtue of the normal positive feedback mechanism, a subnormal level of cortisol in the blood would induce the anterior pituitary to make more ACTH. The latter would

TABLE 32.6 Mechanism(s) of Action and Efficacy of Lipid-Lowering Agents

AGENT	MECHANISM OF ACTION	PERCENTAGE CHANGE IN SERUM LIPID LEVEL (MONOTHERAPY)			
		TOTAL CHOLESTEROL	LDL CHOLESTEROL	HDL CHOLESTEROL	TRIACYLGLYCEROLS
Statins	Inhibits HMG-CoA reductase activity	↓ 15–60	↓ 20–60	↑ 5–15	↓ 10–40
Bile acid resins	Increase fecal excretion of bile salts	↓ 15–20	↓ 10–25	↑ 3–5	Variable, depending on pretreatment level of triacylglycerols (may increase)
Niacin	Activates LPL; reduces hepatic production of VLDL; reduces catabolism of HDL	↓ 22–25	↓ 10–25	↑ 15–35	↓ 20–50
Fibrates	Antagonizes the transcription factor PPARα, causing an increase in LPL activity, a decrease in apolipoprotein CIII production, and an increase in apolipoprotein AI production	↓ 12–15	Variable, depending on pretreatment levels of other lipids	↑ 5–15	↓ 20–50
Ezetimibe	Reduces intestinal absorption of free cholesterol from the gut lumen	↓ 10–15	↓ 15–20	↑ 1–3	↓ 5–8 if triacylglycerols are high pretreatment

HMG-CoA, 3-hydroxymethylglutaryl coenzyme A; LPL, lipoprotein lipase; LDL, low-density lipoprotein; HDL, high-density lipoprotein; triacylglycerols, triglycerides; PPAR, peroxisome proliferator-activated receptor.

Source: Adapted from Third report of the National Cholesterol Education Progran (NCEP) expert panel on detection, evaluation, and treatment of high blood cholesterol in adults (Adult Treatment Panel III) final report. *Circulation.* 2002;106:3143–3257.

not only stimulate the cortisol pathway to increase cortisol synthesis to normal but, in the process, would also induce increased production of adrenal androgens such as DHEA and DHEAS. The increased levels of the adrenal androgens (although relatively weak androgens) would cause varying degrees of virilization, depending on the severity of the enzyme deficiency. The administration of a glucocorticoid by mouth would suppress the high level of secretion of ACTH from the anterior pituitary gland that occurs in response to the reduced levels of cortisol secreted from the adrenal cortex. Treatment with prednisone (a synthetic glucocorticoid), therefore, will prevent the ACTH-induced overproduction of adrenal androgens. However, when ACTH secretion returns to normal, endogenous cortisol synthesis falls below normal. The administered prednisone brings the net glucocorticoid activity in the blood back to physiologic levels. Vera's adrenal androgen levels in the blood returned to normal after several weeks of therapy with prednisone (a synthetic glucocorticoid). As a result, her menses eventually resumed and her virilizing features slowly resolved.

Because Vera's symptoms began in adult life, her genetically determined adrenal hyperplasia is referred to as a *nonclassic* or *atypical* form of the disorder. A more severe enzyme deficiency leads to the "classic" disease, which is associated with excessive fetal adrenal androgen production in utero and manifests at birth, often with ambiguous external genitalia and virilizing features in the female neonate.

BIOCHEMICAL COMMENTS

 Drugs used to treat certain aspects of the metabolic syndrome improve insulin sensitivity and regulate lipid levels through modulation of the pathways discussed in Chapters 29 through 32. These drugs work by modifying the regulatory pathways that have been discussed so far with regard to carbohydrate and lipid metabolism.

 Metformin. Metformin has been used for more than 30 years as a treatment for type 2 diabetes. Metformin reduces blood glucose levels by inhibiting hepatic gluconeogenesis, which is active in these patients because of the liver's resistance to the effects of insulin. Metformin also reduces lipid synthesis in the liver, which aids in modulating blood lipid levels in these patients.

Metformin accomplishes its effects by activating the AMP-activated protein kinase (AMPK). It does so through activation of an upstream protein kinase, LKB1, via an unknown mechanism. As has been discussed previously, AMPK, when active, phosphorylates and reduces the activity of acetyl-CoA carboxylase (required for fatty acid synthesis) and HMG-CoA reductase (reducing the biosynthesis of cholesterol). Activation of AMPK also activates glucose uptake by the muscle (see Chapter 45), which is significant for reducing circulating blood glucose levels.

The activation of AMPK also leads to a cascade of transcriptional regulation that reduces the liver's ability to undergo both gluconeogenesis and lipogenesis. Activated AMPK phosphorylates a coactivator of the CREB transcription factor named *t*ransducer *of r*egulated *C*REB activity 2 (TORC2) (Fig. 32.25). When TORC2 is phosphorylated, it is sequestered in the cytoplasm, and CREB becomes very inefficient at transcribing a gene that is required to upregulate genes that code for the enzymes involved in gluconeogenesis. This important transcriptional coactivator is named peroxisome proliferator-activated receptor-γ coactivator 1α (PGC1α). PGC1α participates in the transcriptional activation of key gluconeogenic enzymes, such as glucose 6-phosphatase and phosphoenolpyruvate carboxykinase (PEPCK). Thus, in the presence of metformin, hepatic gluconeogenesis is reduced and muscle uptake of blood glucose is enhanced, leading to stabilization of blood glucose levels. The physiologic regulators of LKB1 have yet to be identified.

Activation of AMPK also inhibits liver lipogenesis. In addition to phosphorylating and inhibiting acetyl-CoA carboxylase activity (which reduces malonyl-CoA

 The LKB1 protein is a tumor suppressor; loss of LKB1 activity leads to Peutz-Jeghers syndrome (PJS). PJS exhibits the early development of hamartomatous polyps (benign polyps) in the gastrointestinal tract and an increased incidence of carcinomas at a relatively young age. LKB1 regulates the activity of 14 kinases that include, and are similar to, the AMPK. Loss of the normal regulation of these kinases, because of the absence of LKB1 activity, significantly contributes to tumor formation.

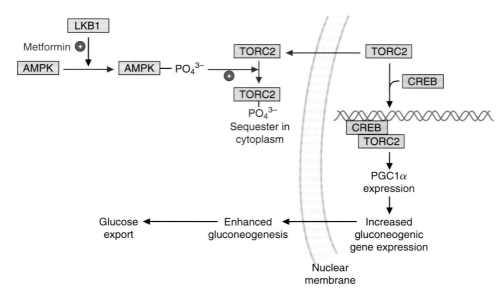

FIGURE 32.25 Action of metformin on gluconeogenesis. Under normal conditions, increases of hepatic cyclic adenosine monophosphate (cAMP) levels (e.g., in response to glucagon) activate cAMP response element–binding protein (CREB), which, in combination with transducer of regulated CREB activity 2 (TORC2), leads to increased transcription of genes required for gluconeogenesis. Under conditions of insulin resistance this pathway remains stimulated, even in the presence of insulin. Metformin stimulates the activation of AMP-activated protein kinase (AMPK), which phosphorylates TORC2 and sequesters it in the cytoplasm, thereby decreasing synthesis of gluconeogenic enzymes and reducing hepatic output of glucose. The abbreviations used are defined in the text. *PGC1α*, peroxisome proliferator-activated receptor-γ coactivator 1α.

levels, leading to reduced fatty acid synthesis and enhanced fatty acid oxidation), AMPK activity decreases the transcription of key lipogenic enzymes, including fatty acid synthase and acetyl-CoA carboxylase. The reduced transcriptional activity is mediated via an AMPK inhibition of the transcription of SREBP-1, which in addition to regulating the transcription of HMG-CoA reductase, also regulates the transcription of other lipogenic enzymes. The AMPK is discussed in more detail in the "Biochemical Comments" section of Chapter 34.

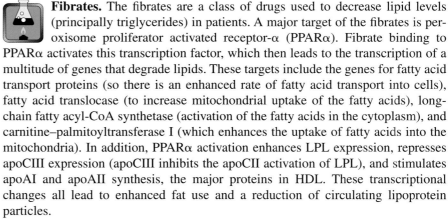

Fibrates. The fibrates are a class of drugs used to decrease lipid levels (principally triglycerides) in patients. A major target of the fibrates is peroxisome proliferator activated receptor-α (PPARα). Fibrate binding to PPARα activates this transcription factor, which then leads to the transcription of a multitude of genes that degrade lipids. These targets include the genes for fatty acid transport proteins (so there is an enhanced rate of fatty acid transport into cells), fatty acid translocase (to increase mitochondrial uptake of the fatty acids), long-chain fatty acyl-CoA synthetase (activation of the fatty acids in the cytoplasm), and carnitine–palmitoyltransferase I (which enhances the uptake of fatty acids into the mitochondria). In addition, PPARα activation enhances LPL expression, represses apoCIII expression (apoCIII inhibits the apoCII activation of LPL), and stimulates apoAI and apoAII synthesis, the major proteins in HDL. These transcriptional changes all lead to enhanced fat use and a reduction of circulating lipoprotein particles.

Thiazolidinediones. A third class of drugs used for the treatment of insulin resistance and type 2 diabetes mellitus is the thiazolidinediones (TZDs), which activate the PPARγ class of transcription factors. PPARγ is expressed primarily in adipose tissue. This transcription factor is responsible for activating the transcription of adiponectin (see Chapter 31, Section VIII.B), leading to increased circulating adiponectin levels. The increase in adiponectin reduces the fat content of the liver and enhances insulin sensitivity via an AMPK-dependent pathway. Thiazolidinediones also lead to a reduction in plasma free fatty acid levels, which leads to enhanced insulin sensitivity (see the "Biochemical Comments" in Chapter 31).

KEY CONCEPTS

- Cholesterol regulates membrane fluidity and is a precursor of bile salts, steroid hormones (such as estrogen and testosterone), and vitamin D.
- Cholesterol, because of its hydrophobic nature, is transported in the blood as a component of lipoproteins.
- Within the lipoproteins, cholesterol can appear in its unesterified form in the outer shell of the particle or as cholesterol esters in the core of the particle.
- De novo cholesterol synthesis requires acetyl-CoA as a precursor, which is initially converted to HMG-CoA. The cholesterol synthesized in this way is packaged, along with triglyceride, into VLDL in the liver and then released into circulation.
- The conversion of HMG-CoA to mevalonic acid, catalyzed by HMG-CoA reductase, is the regulated and rate-limiting step of cholesterol biosynthesis.
- In the circulation, the triglycerides in VLDL are digested by lipoprotein lipase, which converts the particle to IDL and then to LDL.
- IDL and LDL bind specifically to receptors on the liver cell, are internalized, and the particle components are recycled.
- A third lipoprotein particle, HDL, functions to transfer apolipoprotein E and apolipoprotein CII to nascent chylomicrons and nascent VLDL.
- HDL also participates in reverse cholesterol transport, the movement of cholesterol from cell membranes to the HDL particle, which returns the cholesterol to the liver.
- Atherosclerotic plaques are associated with elevated levels of blood cholesterol levels. High levels of LDL are more strongly associated with the generation of atherosclerotic plaques, whereas high levels of HDL are protective because of their participation in reverse cholesterol transport.
- Bile salts are required for fat emulsification and micelle formation in the small intestine.
- Bile salts are recycled via the enterohepatic circulation, forming the secondary bile acids in the process.
- The steroid hormones are derived from cholesterol, which is converted to pregnenolone, which is the precursor for the mineralocorticoids (such as aldosterone), the glucocorticoids (such as cortisol), and the sex steroids (such as testosterone and estrogen).
- Lipid-lowering drugs act on a variety of targets within liver, intestine, and adipocytes.
- Diseases discussed in this chapter are summarized in Table 32.7.

TABLE 32.7   Diseases Discussed in Chapter 32

DISEASE OR DISORDER	ENVIRONMENTAL OR GENETIC	COMMENTS
Hypercholesterolemia	Both	Defined by elevated levels of cholesterol in the blood, often leading to coronary artery disease
Familial hypercholesterolemia, type II	Genetic	Defect in low-density lipoprotein receptor, leading to elevated cholesterol levels and premature death from coronary artery disease
Virilization	Both	Excessive release of androgenic steroids, owing to a variety of causes
Congenital adrenal hyperplasia (CAH)	Genetic	CAH is a constellation of disorders caused by mutations in enzymes required for cortisol synthesis. One potential consequence is excessive androgen synthesis, which may lead to prenatal masculinization of females. The different symptoms observed between patients are caused by different enzyme deficiencies in the patients.
Rickets	Environmental	Owing to a lack of vitamin D, calcium metabolism is altered, leading to skeletal deformities.

1. The statins are the major class of medications used to lower elevated serum cholesterol by initially inhibiting the major rate-limiting step of cholesterol synthesis. Which metabolite of the pathway would accumulate under conditions of taking a statin?
   A. Acetoacetyl-CoA
   B. HMG-CoA
   C. Mevalonate
   D. Squalene
   E. Steroid ring

2. Cholesterol, and its precursors and products, have a variety of functions within cells. Which one statement correctly describes a function of a cholesterol precursor, cholesterol itself, or a product derived from cholesterol?
   A. Cholesterol is hydrophilic.
   B. Steroid hormones are precursors of cholesterol.
   C. Precursors of cholesterol can be converted to vitamin D.
   D. Cholesterol can appear in its free unesterified form in the core of lipoprotein particles.
   E. Malonyl-CoA is the major precursor of cholesterol synthesis.

3. A new patient is being evaluated for cardiovascular disease. The values for his lipid panel are a total cholesterol of 400 mg/dL, an HDL reading of 35 mg/dL, and a triglyceride reading of 200 mg/dL. What would be his calculated LDL cholesterol reading?
   A. 165
   B. 193
   C. 205
   D. 325
   E. 365

4. Which one of the following apolipoproteins acts as a cofactor activator of the enzyme LPL?
   A. ApoCIII
   B. ApoCII
   C. ApoB-100
   D. ApoB-48s
   E. ApoE

5. Which one of the following sequences places the lipoproteins in the order of most dense to least dense?
   A. HDL/VLDL/chylomicrons/LDL
   B. HDL/LDL/VLDL/chylomicrons
   C. LDL/chylomicrons/HDL/VLDL
   D. VLDL/chylomicrons/LDL/HDL
   E. LDL/chylomicrons/VLDL/HDL

6. Which one of the following would you expect to observe in a patient lacking microsomal triglyceride transfer protein (MTP) after eating a normal diet, in which each meal consisted of 30% fat?
   A. Constipation
   B. Elevated chylomicrons
   C. Steatorrhea
   D. Elevated VLDL
   E. Elevated IDL

7. Patients with elevated serum LDL levels (>120 mg/dL) are first encouraged to reduce these levels through a combination of diet and exercise. If this fails, they are often prescribed statins. The key for statin treatment reducing circulating cholesterol levels is which one of the following?
   A. Reduced synthesis of chylomicrons
   B. Increased activity of LPL
   C. Reduced synthesis of HDL
   D. Upregulation of LDL receptors
   E. Increased activity of CETP

8. A consequence of abetalipoproteinemia is a fatty liver (hepatic steatosis). This occurs because of which one of the following?
   A. Inability to produce VLDL
   B. Inability to produce chylomicrons
   C. Inability to produce HDL
   D. Inability to produce triglyceride
   E. Inability to produce LPL

9. Hormones are typically synthesized in one type of tissue, often in response to the release of a stimulatory hormone. Which one of the following correctly matches a hormone with its stimulatory hormone and its site of synthesis?
   A. Cortisol, ACTH, adrenal cortex
   B. Aldosterone, ACTH, adrenal cortex
   C. Testosterone, FSH, Leydig cells
   D. Estrogen, LH, ovarian follicle
   E. Progesterone, LH, ovarian follicle

10. Because the steroid nucleus cannot be degraded by the human body, excretion of bile salts in stool serves as a major route of removal of steroids from the body. Which one of the following must occur to bile salts in order for bile salts to be excreted in the stool?
    A. Intestinal bacteria deconjugate bile salts.
    B. Intestinal bacteria conjugate bile salts.
    C. ATP and coenzyme Q conjugate bile salts.
    D. ATP and coenzyme A deconjugate bile salts.
    E. Enterohepatic circulation occurs at 100% efficiency.

ANSWERS

1. **The answer is B.** The statins inhibit the enzyme HMG-CoA reductase, which reduces HMG-CoA to mevalonic acid. Therefore, HMG-CoA would be the metabolite that accumulates. The pathway is initiated with acetyl-CoA, which then forms acetoacetyl-CoA and then HMG-CoA. The HMG-CoA is reduced to mevalonic acid, which is then converted to isoprene units, to farnesyl units, geranyl units, and finally to squalene, which is converted to cholesterol.

2. **The answer is C.** Cholesterol is absolutely insoluble in water (it is very hydrophobic). It is a precursor of both the bile acids and the steroid hormones. Precursors of cholesterol are converted to ubiquinone, dolichol, and cholecalciferol (the active form of vitamin D). Cholesterol can appear unesterified in the outer shell of lipoproteins but as cholesterol esters in the core of such particles. Malonyl-CoA is the precursor of fatty acids; acetyl-CoA is the precursor for all the cholesterol carbons.

3. **The answer is D.** Total cholesterol is equal to the lipoproteins that carry it because cholesterol cannot freely float in blood serum. The total cholesterol would then be composed of the cholesterol content of HDL, VLDL, and LDL. Under fasting conditions, taking the triglyceride concentration and dividing it by 5 can estimate the cholesterol content of VLDL. Thus, for this patient, the HDL is 35 mg/dL, and the VLDL is 40 mg/dL. The total cholesterol is 400 mg/dL, indicating that the calculated LDL cholesterol is $400 - 75$, or 325 mg/dL.

4. **The answer is B.** ApoCIII appears to inhibit the activation of LPL. ApoE acts as a ligand in binding several lipoproteins to the LDL receptor, the LRP, and possibly to a separate apoE receptor. ApoB-48 is required for the normal assembly and secretion of chylomicrons from the small bowel, whereas apoB-100 is required in the liver for the assembly and secretion of VLDL. ApoCII is the activator of LPL.

5. **The answer is B.** Because chylomicrons contain the most triacylglycerol, they are the least dense of the blood lipoproteins. Because VLDL contains more protein, it is denser than chylomicrons. Because LDL is produced by degradation of the triacylglycerol in VLDL, LDL is denser than VLDL. HDL is the densest of the blood lipoproteins. It has the most protein and the least triacylglycerol.

6. **The answer is C.** MTP is required for the synthesis of nascent chylomicrons and VLDL. In the intestine, the lack of MTP activity leads to an accumulation of lipid in the intestinal epithelial, such that further lipid is not transported in from the lumen. This leads to elevated lipid content in the stools, which is manifest as steatorrhea. As MTP is also needed for VLDL production, VLDL levels will drop, as will IDL and LDL levels, because they are derived from VLDL.

7. **The answer is D.** Statins directly inhibit HMG-CoA reductase, thereby reducing endogenous cholesterol synthesis in the tissues. As the cell becomes "starved" for cholesterol, the LDL receptors are upregulated (increased in number on the cell surface) such that more circulating cholesterol can be taken up by the cells, thereby satisfying the cell's need for cholesterol while lowering serum cholesterol levels. In the absence of functional LDL receptors (homozygous familial hypercholesterolemia IIA and IIB), statins are ineffective in significantly reducing circulating LDL cholesterol levels. Statins do not reduce the synthesis of chylomicrons or HDL, nor do they alter the activity of LPL or CETP.

8. **The answer is A.** Abetalipoproteinemia is caused by a mutation in MTP (the microsomal triglyceride transfer protein) such that neither chylomicrons (in the intestine) or VLDL (in the liver) are produced. Thus, as the liver produces triglyceride from dietary carbohydrate, the triglyceride cannot be exported and accumulates within the liver. The triglyceride will eventually interfere with hepatic function and structure, leading to liver failure if untreated. The inability to produce chylomicrons would not affect liver function (the intestinal cells would become lipid-laden, but that does not lead to hepatic steatosis). A defect in MTP does not affect LPL production or secretion, nor does it affect triglyceride production. HDL synthesis also is not affected by the loss of MTP.

9. **The answer is A.** Cortisol is produced by the middle layer of the adrenal cortex as a result of stimulation by ACTH. Aldosterone is produced by the outer layer of the adrenal cortex in response to stimulation by angiotensin II. Testosterone is produced by the Leydig cells of the testes and in the ovary in response to LH. Estrogen is produced by the ovarian follicle and corpus luteum in response to FSH. Progesterone is produced by the corpus luteum in response to LH.

10. **The answer is A.** Bile salts are conjugated in the liver by a reaction that requires ATP and glycine or taurine such that a form of the bile salt is created in which the pK_a of the terminal carboxylate group is reduced as compared to the native bile salt. This allows for a higher percentage of the ionized form of the bile salt in the intestine (which is approximately at pH 6.0), which greatly aids in the emulsification and digestion of the dietary fats. As the bile salts travel through the intestine, bacteria deconjugate and dehydroxylate the steroids, making them less soluble and less readily reabsorbed into the enterohepatic circulation. Consequently, a percentage of the modified bile salts are lost in the stool. If the enterohepatic circulation operated at 100% efficiency, no bile acids would be lost to the stool and this route for elimination of the steroid nucleus would not exist. Coenzyme Q has no role in conjugating or deconjugating bile salts.

33 Metabolism of Ethanol

Ethanol is a **dietary fuel** that is metabolized to acetate principally in the liver, with the generation of reduced nicotinamide adenine dinucleotide (NADH). The principal route for metabolism of ethanol is through hepatic **alcohol dehydrogenases**, which oxidize ethanol to **acetaldehyde** in the cytosol (Fig. 33.1). Acetaldehyde is further oxidized by **acetaldehyde dehydrogenases** to **acetate**, principally in **mitochondria**. Acetaldehyde, which is toxic, also may enter the blood. **NADH** produced by these reactions is used for adenosine triphosphate (ATP) generation through oxidative phosphorylation. Most of the acetate enters the blood and is taken up by skeletal muscles and other tissues, where it is activated to **acetyl coenzyme A** (**acetyl-CoA**) and is oxidized in the tricarboxylic acid (TCA) cycle.

Approximately 10% to 20% of ingested ethanol is oxidized through a microsomal ethanol-oxidizing system (**MEOS**), comprising **cytochrome P450** enzymes in the endoplasmic reticulum (especially **CYP2E1**). CYP2E1 has a high K_m for ethanol and is inducible by ethanol. Therefore, the proportion of ethanol metabolized through this route is greater at high ethanol concentrations and greater after chronic consumption of ethanol.

Acute effects of alcohol ingestion arise principally from the generation of NADH, which greatly increases the **NADH/NAD$^+$** ratio of the liver. As a consequence, **fatty acid oxidation is inhibited**, and **ketogenesis** may occur. The elevated **NADH/NAD$^+$** ratio may also cause **lactic acidosis** and inhibit **gluconeogenesis**.

Ethanol metabolism may result in **alcohol-induced liver disease**, including **hepatic steatosis** (fatty liver), **alcohol-induced hepatitis**, and **cirrhosis**. The principal toxic products of ethanol metabolism include **acetaldehyde** and **free radicals**. Acetaldehyde forms **adducts** with proteins and other compounds. The **hydroxyethyl radical** produced by the MEOS and other radicals produced during inflammation cause irreversible damage to the liver. Many other tissues are adversely affected by ethanol, acetaldehyde, or by the consequences of **hepatic dysmetabolism** and injury. **Genetic polymorphisms** in the enzymes of ethanol metabolism may be responsible for individual variations in the development of alcoholism or the development of liver cirrhosis.

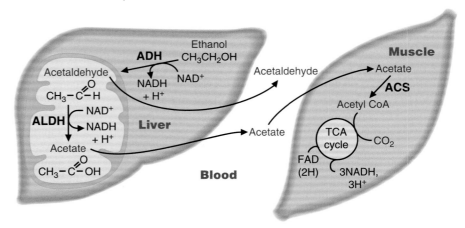

FIGURE 33.1   The major route for metabolism of ethanol and use of acetate by the muscle. *Acetyl CoA*, acetyl coenzyme A; *ADH*, alcohol dehydrogenase; *ALDH*, acetaldehyde dehydrogenase; *ACS*, acetyl coenzyme A synthetase; *NAD*, nicotinamide adenine dinucleotide; *FAD*, flavin adenine dinucleotide; *TCA*, tricarboxylic acid.

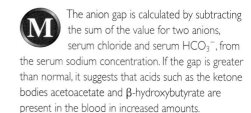

THE WAITING ROOM

 A dietary history for **Ivan A.** showed that he had continued his habit of drinking scotch and soda each evening while watching TV, but he did not add the ethanol calories to his dietary intake. He justifies this calculation on the basis of a comment he heard on a radio program that calories from alcohol ingestion "don't count" because they are empty calories that do not cause weight gain.

 Al M. was found lying semiconscious at the bottom of the stairs by his landlady when she returned from an overnight visit with friends. His face had multiple bruises and his right forearm was grotesquely angulated. Nonbloody dried vomitus stained his clothing. Mr. M. was rushed by ambulance to the emergency department at the nearest hospital. In addition to multiple bruises and the compound fracture of his right forearm, he had deep and rapid (Kussmaul) respirations and was moderately dehydrated.

Initial laboratory studies showed a relatively large anion gap of 34 mmol/L (reference range, 9 to 15 mmol/L). An arterial blood gas analysis (which measures pH in addition to the levels of dissolved O_2 and CO_2) confirmed the presence of a metabolic acidosis. Mr. M.'s blood alcohol level was only slightly elevated. His serum glucose was 68 mg/dL (low normal).

 Jean T., a 46-year-old commercial artist, recently lost her job because of absenteeism. Her husband of 24 years had left her 10 months earlier. She complains of loss of appetite, fatigue, muscle weakness, and emotional depression. She has had occasional pain in the area of her liver, at times accompanied by nausea and vomiting.

On physical examination, the physician notes tenderness to light percussion over her liver, and her abdomen is mildly distended. There is a suggestion of mild jaundice (yellow discoloration of her skin and mucus membranes). No obvious neurologic or cognitive abnormalities are present.

After detecting a hint of alcohol on Jean's breath, the physician questions Jean about her drinking. Jean admits that for the last 5 or 6 years, she has been drinking gin on a daily basis (~4 to 5 drinks, or 68 to 85 g of ethanol) and eating infrequently. Laboratory tests showed that her serum ethanol level on the initial office visit was 245 mg/dL (0.245%); values >150 mg/dL (0.15%) are indicative of inebriation.

I. Ethanol Metabolism

Ethanol is a small molecule that is both lipid- and water-soluble. It is therefore readily absorbed from the intestine by passive diffusion. A small percentage of ingested ethanol (0% to 5%) enters the gastric mucosal cells of the upper gastrointestinal (GI) tract (tongue, mouth, esophagus, and stomach), where it is metabolized. The remainder enters the blood. Of this, 85% to 98% is metabolized in the liver, and only 2% to 10% is excreted through the lungs or kidneys.

The major route of ethanol metabolism in the liver is through liver *alcohol dehydrogenase* (ADH), a cytosolic enzyme that oxidizes ethanol to acetaldehyde with reduction of NAD^+ to NADH (Fig. 33.2). If it is not removed by metabolism, acetaldehyde exerts toxic actions in the liver and can enter the blood and exert toxic effects in other tissues.

Approximately 90% of the acetaldehyde that is generated is further metabolized to acetate in the liver. The major enzyme involved is a low K_m mitochondrial acetaldehyde dehydrogenase (ALDH), which oxidizes acetaldehyde to acetate with generation of NADH (see Fig. 33.2). Acetate, which has no toxic effects, may be activated to acetyl coenzyme A (acetyl-CoA) in the liver (where it can enter either the TCA cycle or the pathway for fatty acid synthesis). However, most of the acetate that is generated enters the blood and is activated to acetyl-CoA in skeletal muscles

 The anion gap is calculated by subtracting the sum of the value for two anions, serum chloride and serum HCO_3^-, from the serum sodium concentration. If the gap is greater than normal, it suggests that acids such as the ketone bodies acetoacetate and β-hydroxybutyrate are present in the blood in increased amounts.

Jaundice is a yellow discoloration involving the sclerae (the "whites" of the eyes) and skin. It is caused by the deposition of bilirubin, a yellow degradation product of heme. Bilirubin accumulates in the blood under conditions of liver injury, bile duct obstruction, and excessive degradation of heme.

Jean T.'s admitted ethanol consumption exceeds the definition of moderate drinking. Moderate drinking is now defined as not more than two drinks per day for men but only one drink per day for women. A drink is defined as 12 oz of regular beer, 5 oz of wine, or 1.5 oz distilled spirits (80-proof).

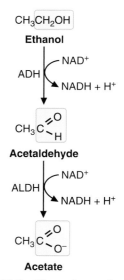

FIGURE 33.2 The pathway of ethanol metabolism. *ADH*, alcohol dehydrogenase; *ALDH*, acetaldehyde dehydrogenase; *NAD*, nicotinamide adenine dinucleotide.

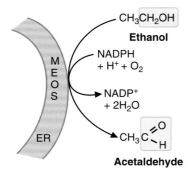

FIGURE 33.3 The reaction catalyzed by the microsomal ethanol-oxidizing system (MEOS; which includes CYP2E1) in the endoplasmic reticulum (ER). *NADP*, nicotinamide adenine dinucleotide phosphate.

and other tissues (see Fig. 33.1). Acetate is generally considered nontoxic and is a normal constituent of the diet.

The other principal route of ethanol oxidation in the liver is the *MEOS*, which also oxidizes ethanol to acetaldehyde (Fig. 33.3). The principal microsomal enzyme involved is a cytochrome P450 mixed-function oxidase isozyme (CYP2E1), which uses NADPH as an additional electron donor and O_2 as an electron acceptor. This route accounts for only 10% to 20% of ethanol oxidation in a moderate drinker.

Each of the enzymes involved in ethanol metabolism (ADH, ALDH, and CYP2E1) exists as a family of isoenzymes. Individual variations in the quantity of these isoenzymes influence several factors, such as the rate of ethanol clearance from the blood, the degree of inebriation exhibited by an individual, and differences in individual susceptibility to the development of alcohol-induced liver disease.

A. Alcohol Dehydrogenase

ADH exists as a family of isoenzymes with varying specificity for chain length of the alcohol substrate (Table 33.1). Ethanol is a small molecule that does not exhibit much in the way of unique structural characteristics and, at high concentrations, is nonspecifically metabolized by many members of the ADH family. The alcohol dehydrogenases that exhibit the highest specificity for ethanol are members of the ADH1 family. Humans have six genes for this family of alcohol dehydrogenases, each of which exists as allelic variants (polymorphisms).

The ADH1 family members are present in high quantities in the liver, representing approximately 3% of all soluble protein. These alcohol dehydrogenases, commonly referred to collectively as *liver ADH*, have a low K_m for ethanol between 0.02 and 5 mM (high affinities). Thus, the liver is the major site of ethanol metabolism and the major site at which the toxic metabolite acetaldehyde is generated.

Although the ADH4 and ADH2 enzymes make minor contributions to ethanol metabolism, they may contribute to its toxic effects. Ethanol concentrations can be quite high in the upper GI tract (e.g., beer is ~0.8 M ethanol), and acetaldehyde generated here by ADH4 enzymes (gastric ADH) might contribute to the risk for cancer associated with heavy drinking. ADH2 genes are expressed primarily in the liver and at lower levels in the lower GI tract.

TABLE 33.1	Major Isozymes of Medium-Chain-Length Alcohol Dehydrogenases		
GENE	**SUBUNIT**	**TISSUE DISTRIBUTION**	**PROPERTIES**
ADH1A *ADH1B* *ADH1C*	α β γ	Most abundant in liver and adrenal glands. Much lower levels in kidney, lung, colon, small intestine, eye, ovary, blood vessels. None in brain or heart.	K_m of 0.02 to 5 mM for ethanol. Active only with ethanol. High tissue capacity.
ADH2	π	Primarily liver, lower levels in GI tract	K_m of 23 mM for ethanol
ADH3	χ	Ubiquitously expressed, but at higher levels in liver. The only isozyme present in germinal cells.	Relatively inactive toward ethanol (K_m = 3,400 mM). Active mainly toward long-chain alcohols and ω-OH fatty acids.
ADH4	σ	Present in highest levels in upper GI tract, gingiva and mouth, esophagus, down to the stomach. Not present in liver.	K_m of 58 mM. It is the most active of medium-chain alcohol dehydrogenases toward the substrate retinal.

GI, gastrointestinal.

Genes for ADH5 and ADH6 have also been identified. ADH5 does not metabolize ethanol but is active on long-chain alcohols. The function of ADH6 is still speculative.

The human has at least seven, and possibly more, genes that code for specific isoenzymes of medium-chain-length alcohol dehydrogenases, the major enzyme responsible for the oxidation of ethanol to acetaldehyde in the human. These different alcohol dehydrogenases have an approximately 60% to 70% identity and are assumed to have arisen from a common ancestral gene similar to the ADH3 isoenzyme many millions of years ago. The ADH1 alcohol dehydrogenases (ADH1A, ADH1B, and ADH1C) are all present in high concentration in the liver, and they have relatively high affinity and capacity for ethanol at low concentrations. (These properties are quantitatively reflected by their low K_m, a parameter discussed in Chapter 9.) They have a 90% to 94% sequence identity and are able to form both homo- and heterodimers among themselves (e.g., ββ or βγ). However, none of the ADH1s can form dimers with an ADH subunit from subunits of ADH2, -3, or -4. The three genes for class I alcohol dehydrogenases are arranged in tandem, head to tail, on chromosome 4. The genes for the other classes of ADH are also on chromosome 4 in nearby locations.

B. Acetaldehyde Dehydrogenases

Acetaldehyde is oxidized to acetate, with the generation of NADH, by acetaldehyde dehydrogenases (see Fig. 33.2). More than 80% of acetaldehyde oxidation in the human liver is normally catalyzed by mitochondrial ALDH (ALDH2), which has a high affinity for acetaldehyde ($K_m = 0.2$ μM) and is highly specific. However, individuals with a common allelic variant of *ALDH2* (designated as *ALDH2*2*) have a greatly decreased capacity for acetaldehyde metabolism because of an increased K_m (46 μM) and a decreased V_{max} (0.017 U/mg vs. 0.60 U/mg).

Most of the remainder of acetaldehyde oxidation occurs through a cytosolic ALDH (ALDH1). Additional aldehyde dehydrogenases act on a variety of organic alcohols, toxins, and pollutants.

The accumulation of acetaldehyde causes nausea and vomiting, and, therefore, inactive acetaldehyde dehydrogenases are associated with a distaste for alcoholic beverages and protection against alcoholism. In one of the common allelic variants of ALDH2 (*ALDH2*2*), a single substitution increases the K_m for acetaldehyde 230-fold (lowers the affinity) and decreases the V_{max} 35-fold, resulting in a very inactive enzyme. Homozygosity for the *ALDH2*2* allele affords absolute protection against alcoholism; no individual with this genotype has been found among alcoholics. Alcoholics are frequently treated with ALDH inhibitors (e.g., disulfiram) to help them abstain from alcohol intake. Unfortunately, alcoholics who continue to drink while taking this drug are exposed to the toxic effects of elevated acetaldehyde levels.

C. Fate of Acetate

Metabolism of acetate requires activation to acetyl-CoA by acetyl-CoA synthetase in a reaction similar to that catalyzed by fatty acyl coenzyme A (fatty acyl-CoA) synthetases (Fig. 33.4). In liver, the principal isoform of acetyl-CoA synthetase (ACSI) is a cytosolic enzyme that generates acetyl-CoA for the cytosolic pathways of cholesterol and fatty acid synthesis. Acetate entry into these pathways is under regulatory control by mechanisms involving cholesterol or insulin. Thus, most of the acetate generated enters the blood.

Acetate is taken up and oxidized by other tissues, notably heart and skeletal muscle, which have a high concentration of the mitochondrial acetyl-CoA synthetase isoform (ACSII). This enzyme is present in the mitochondrial matrix. It, therefore, generates acetyl-CoA that can enter the TCA cycle directly and be oxidized to CO_2.

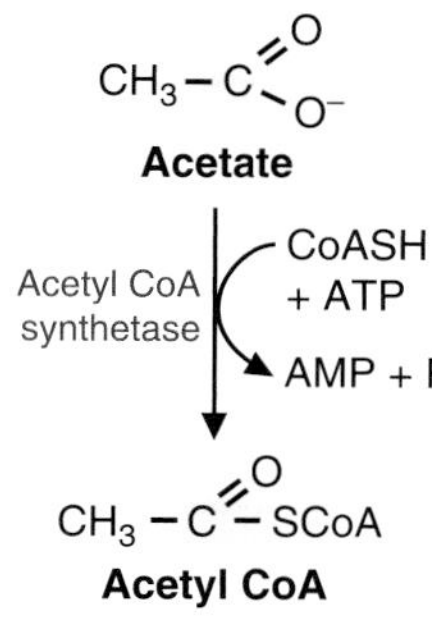

D. The Microsomal Ethanol-Oxidizing System

Ethanol is also oxidized to acetaldehyde in the liver by the MEOS, which comprises members of the cytochrome P450 superfamily of enzymes. Ethanol and NADPH

FIGURE 33.4 The activation of acetate to acetyl coenzyme A (acetyl-CoA). *AMP*, adenosine monophosphate; *ATP*, adenosine triphosphate; *CoA*, coenzyme A; *PP$_i$*, pyrophosphate.

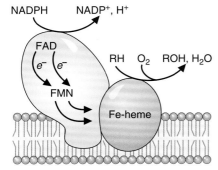

FIGURE 33.5 General structure of cytochrome P450 enzymes. O_2 binds to the P450 Fe-heme in the active site and is activated to a reactive form by accepting electrons (e^-). The electrons are donated by the cytochrome P450 reductase, which contains a flavin adenine dinucleotide (FAD) plus a flavin mononucleotide (FMN) or Fe–S center to facilitate the transfer of single electrons from NADPH to O_2. The P450 enzymes involved in steroidogenesis have a somewhat different structure. For CYP2E1, *RH* is ethanol (CH_3CH_2OH) and *ROH* is acetaldehyde (CH_3CHO). *NADP*, nicotinamide adenine dinucleotide phosphate.

ADH1A and ADH1C are present as functional polymorphisms that differ in their properties. Genetic polymorphisms for ADH partially account for the observed differences in ethanol elimination rates among various individuals or populations. Although susceptibility to alcoholism is a complex function of genetics and socioeconomic factors, possession of the ADH1B*2 allele, which encodes a relatively fast ADH (high V_{max}), is associated with a decreased susceptibility to alcoholism—presumably because of nausea and flushing caused by acetaldehyde accumulation (because the *ALDH* gene cannot keep up with the amount of acetaldehyde produced). This particular allele has a relatively high frequency in the East Asian population and a low frequency among white Europeans. In contrast, the ADH1B*1/1B*1 genotype (homozygous for allele 1 of the ADH1B gene) is a risk factor for the development of Wernicke-Korsakoff syndrome, a neuropsychiatric syndrome that is commonly associated with alcoholism.

both donate electrons in the reaction, which reduces O_2 to H_2O (Fig. 33.5). The cytochrome P450 enzymes all have two major catalytic protein components: an electron-donating reductase system that transfers electrons from NADPH (cytochrome P450 reductase) and a cytochrome P450. The cytochrome P450 protein contains the binding sites for O_2 and the substrate (e.g., ethanol) and carries out the reaction. The enzymes are present in the endoplasmic reticulum, which on isolation from disrupted cells forms a membrane fraction after centrifugation that was formerly called *microsomes* by biochemists.

1. CYP2E1

The MEOS is part of the superfamily of cytochrome P450 enzymes, all of which catalyze similar oxidative reactions. Within the superfamily, at least 10 distinct gene families are found in mammals. More than 100 different cytochrome P450 isozymes exist within these 10 gene families. Each isoenzyme has a distinct classification according to its structural relationship with other isoenzymes. The isoenzyme that has the highest activity toward ethanol is called *CYP2E1*. *CYP* represents cytochrome P450. In CYP2E1, the *2* refers to the gene family (isozymes with >40% amino acid sequence identity), the *E* to the subfamily (isozymes with >55% sequence identity), and the *1* refers to the individual enzymes within this subfamily. A great deal of overlapping specificity exists among the various P450 isoenzymes, and ethanol is also oxidized by several other P450 isoenzymes. *MEOS* refers to the combined ethanol-oxidizing activity of all the P450 enzymes.

CYP2E1 has a much higher K_m for ethanol than the ADH1 family members (11 mM [51 mg/dL] compared with 0.02 to 5 mM [0.09 to 22.5 mg/dL]). Thus, a greater proportion of ingested ethanol is metabolized through CYP2E1 at high levels of ethanol consumption than at low levels.

2. Induction of P450 Enzymes

The P450 enzymes are inducible both by their most specific substrate and by substrates for some of the other cytochrome P450 enzymes. Chronic consumption of ethanol increases hepatic CYP2E1 levels approximately 5- to 10-fold. However, it also causes a twofold to fourfold increase in some of the other P450s from the same subfamily, from different subfamilies, and even from different gene families. The endoplasmic reticulum undergoes proliferation, with a general increase in the content of microsomal enzymes, including those that are not involved directly in ethanol metabolism.

The increase in CYP2E1 with ethanol consumption occurs through transcriptional, posttranscriptional, and posttranslational regulation. Increased levels of mRNA, resulting from induction of gene transcription or stabilization of message, are found in patients who are actively drinking. The protein is also stabilized against degradation. In general, the mechanism for induction of P450 enzymes by their substrates occurs through the binding of the substrate (or related compound) to an intracellular receptor protein, followed by binding of the activated receptor to a response element in the target gene. Ethanol induction of CYP2E1 appears to act via stabilization of the protein and protection against degradation (an increased half-life for the synthesized protein).

Although induction of CYP2E1 increases ethanol clearance from the blood, it has negative consequences. Acetaldehyde may be produced faster than it can be metabolized by acetaldehyde dehydrogenases, thereby increasing the risk of hepatic injury. An increased amount of acetaldehyde can enter the blood and can damage other tissues. In addition, cytochrome P450 enzymes are capable of generating free radicals, which also may lead to increased hepatic injury and cirrhosis (see Chapter 25).

Overlapping specificity in the catalytic activity of P450 enzymes and in their inducers is responsible for several types of drug interactions. For example, phenobarbital, a barbiturate long used as a sleeping pill or for treatment of epilepsy, is converted to an inactive metabolite by cytochrome P450 monooxygenases CYP2B1 and CYP2B2. After treatment with phenobarbital, CYP2B2 is increased 50- to 100-fold. Individuals who take phenobarbital for prolonged periods develop a drug tolerance as CYP2B2 is induced, and the drug is metabolized to an inactive metabolite more rapidly. Consequently, these individuals use progressively higher doses of phenobarbital.

Ethanol is an inhibitor of the phenobarbital-oxidizing P450 system. When large amounts of ethanol are consumed, the inactivation of phenobarbital is directly or indirectly inhibited. Therefore, when high doses of phenobarbital and ethanol are consumed at the same time, toxic levels of the barbiturate can accumulate in the blood.

As blood ethanol concentration rises above 18 mM (the legal intoxication limit is now defined as 0.08% in most states of the United States, which is ~18 mM), the brain and central nervous system are affected. Induction of CYP2E1 increases the rate of ethanol clearance from the blood, thereby contributing to increased alcohol tolerance. However, the apparent ability of a chronic alcoholic to drink without appearing inebriated is partly a learned behavior.

E. Variations in the Pattern of Ethanol Metabolism

The routes and rates of ethanol oxidation vary from individual to individual. Differences in ethanol metabolism may influence whether an individual becomes a chronic alcoholic, develops alcohol-induced liver disease, or develops other diseases associated with increased alcohol consumption (e.g., hepatocarcinogenesis, lung cancer, breast cancer). Factors that determine the rate and route of ethanol oxidation in individuals include:

- Genotype—Polymorphic forms of alcohol dehydrogenases and acetaldehyde dehydrogenases can greatly affect the rate of ethanol oxidation and the accumulation of acetaldehyde. CYP2E1 activity may vary as much as 20-fold among individuals partly because of differences in the inducibility of different allelic variants.
- Drinking history—The level of gastric ADH decreases and CYP2E1 increases with the progression from a naïve, to a moderate, and to a heavy and chronic consumer of alcohol.
- Gender—Blood levels of ethanol after consuming a drink are normally higher for women than for men, partly because of lower levels of gastric ADH activity in women. After chronic consumption of ethanol, gastric ADH decreases in both men and women, but the gender differences become even greater. Gender differences in blood alcohol levels also occur because women are normally smaller. Furthermore, in women, alcohol is distributed in a 12% smaller water space because a woman's body composition consists of more fat and less water than that of a man.
- Quantity—The amount of ethanol an individual consumes over a short period of time determines its metabolic route. Small amounts of ethanol are metabolized most efficiently through the low-K_m pathway of *ADH1* genes and *ALDH2* genes. Little accumulation of NADH occurs to inhibit ethanol metabolism via these dehydrogenases. However, when higher amounts of ethanol are consumed within a short period, a disproportionately greater amount is metabolized through the MEOS. The MEOS, which has a much higher K_m for ethanol, functions principally at high concentrations of ethanol. A higher activity of the MEOS may be expected to correlate with a tendency to develop alcohol-induced liver disease because both acetaldehyde and free radical levels will be increased.

F. The Energy Yield of Ethanol Oxidation

The ATP yield from ethanol oxidation to acetate varies with the route of ethanol metabolism. If ethanol is oxidized by the major route of cytosolic ADH and mitochondrial ALDH, one cytosolic and one mitochondrial NADH are generated, with a maximum yield of 5 ATP. Oxidation of acetyl-CoA in the TCA cycle and the electron-transport chain leads to the generation of 10 high-energy

At **Ivan A.'s** low level of ethanol consumption, ethanol is oxidized to acetate via ADH and ALDH in the liver and the acetate is activated to acetyl-CoA and oxidized to CO_2 in skeletal muscle and other tissues. The overall energy yield of 13 ATP per ethanol molecule accounts for the caloric value of ethanol, approximately 7 kcal/g. However, chronic consumption of substantial amounts of alcohol does not have the effect on body weight expected from the caloric intake. This is partly attributable to induction of MEOS, resulting in a proportionately greater metabolism of ethanol through the MEOS with its lower energy yield (only ~8 ATP). In general, weight-loss diets recommend no, or low, alcohol consumption because ethanol calories are "empty" in the sense that alcoholic beverages are generally low in vitamins, essential amino acids, and other required nutrients but are not empty of calories.

phosphate bonds. However, activation of acetate to acetyl-CoA requires two high-energy phosphate bonds (one in the cleavage of ATP to adenosine monophosphate [AMP] + pyrophosphate and one in the cleavage of pyrophosphate to phosphate), which must be subtracted. Thus, the maximum total energy yield is 13 mol of ATP per mole of ethanol.

In contrast, oxidation of ethanol to acetaldehyde by CYP2E1 consumes energy in the form of NADPH, which is equivalent to 2.5 ATP. Thus, for every mole of ethanol metabolized by this route, only a maximum of 8.0 mol of ATP can be generated (10 ATP from acetyl-CoA oxidation through the TCA cycle, minus 2 for acetate activation; the NADH generated by ALDH is balanced by the loss of NADPH in the MEOS step).

II. Toxic Effects of Ethanol Metabolism

Alcohol-induced liver disease, a common and sometimes fatal consequence of chronic ethanol abuse, may manifest itself in three forms: fatty liver, alcohol-induced hepatitis, and cirrhosis. Each may occur alone, or they may be present in any combination in a given patient. Alcohol-induced cirrhosis is discovered in up to 9% of all autopsies performed in the United States, with a peak incidence in patients 40 to 55 years of age.

However, ethanol ingestion also has acute effects on liver metabolism, including inhibition of fatty acid oxidation and stimulation of triacylglycerol synthesis, leading to a fatty liver. It also can result in ketoacidosis or lactic acidosis and cause hypoglycemia or hyperglycemia, depending on the dietary state. These effects are considered reversible.

In contrast, acetaldehyde and free radicals generated from ethanol metabolism can result in alcohol-induced hepatitis, a condition in which the liver is inflamed and cells become necrotic and die. Diffuse damage to hepatocytes results in cirrhosis, characterized by fibrosis (scarring), disturbance of the normal architecture and blood flow, loss of liver function, and, ultimately, hepatic failure.

A. Acute Effects of Ethanol Arising from the Increased NADH/NAD$^+$ Ratio

Many of the acute effects of ethanol ingestion arise from the increased NADH/NAD$^+$ ratio in the liver (Fig. 33.6). At lower levels of ethanol intake, the rate of ethanol oxidation is regulated by the supply of ethanol (usually determined by how much ethanol we consume) and the rate at which NADH is reoxidized in the electron-transport chain. NADH is not a very effective product inhibitor of ADH or ALDH, and there is no other feedback regulation by ATP, adenosine diphosphate (ADP), or AMP. As a consequence, NADH generated in the cytosol and mitochondria tends to accumulate, increasing the NADH/NAD$^+$ ratio to high levels (see Fig. 33.6, circle 1). The increase is even greater as the mitochondria become damaged from acetaldehyde or free-radical injury.

1. Changes in Fatty Acid Metabolism

The high NADH/NAD$^+$ ratio generated from ethanol oxidation inhibits the oxidation of fatty acids, which accumulate in the liver (see Fig. 33.6, circles 2 and 3) These fatty acids are re-esterified into triacylglycerols by combining with glycerol 3-phosphate (glycerol 3-P). The increased NADH/NAD$^+$ ratio increases the availability of glycerol-3-P by promoting its synthesis from intermediates of glycolysis. The triacylglycerols are incorporated into very-low-density lipoproteins (VLDLs), which accumulate in the liver and enter the blood, resulting in an ethanol-induced hyperlipidemia.

Although just a few drinks may result in hepatic fat accumulation, chronic consumption of alcohol greatly enhances the development of a fatty liver. Reesterification

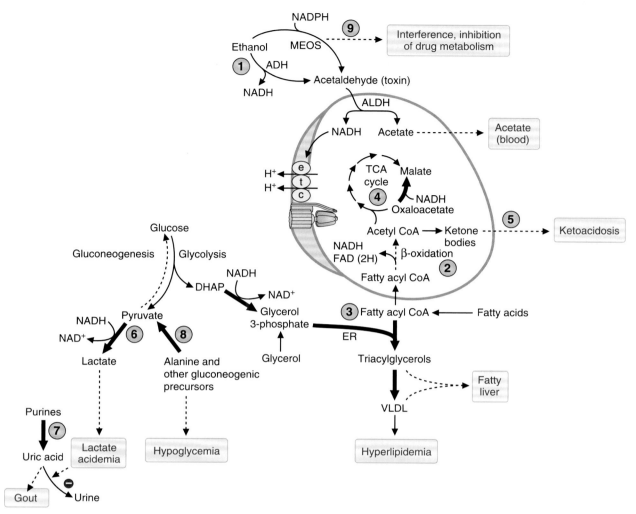

FIGURE 33.6 Acute effects of ethanol metabolism on lipid metabolism in the liver. (*1*) Metabolism of ethanol generates a high NADH/NAD$^+$ ratio. (*2*) The high NADH/NAD$^+$ ratio inhibits fatty acid oxidation and the tricarboxylic acid (TCA) cycle, resulting in accumulation of fatty acids. (*3*) Fatty acids are re-esterified to glycerol 3-phosphate by acyltransferases in the endoplasmic reticulum (ER). Glycerol 3-phosphate levels are increased because a high NADH/NAD$^+$ ratio favors its formation from dihydroxyacetone phosphate (DHAP; an intermediate of glycolysis). Ethanol-stimulated increases of ER enzymes also favors triacylglycerol formation. (*4*) NADH generated from ethanol oxidation can meet the requirements of the cell for adenosine triphosphate (ATP) generation from oxidative phosphorylation. Thus, acetyl coenzyme A (acetyl-CoA) oxidation in the TCA cycle is inhibited. (*5*) The high NADH/NAD$^+$ ratio shifts oxaloacetate toward malate, and acetyl-CoA is directed into ketone-body synthesis. Options (*6*) through (*8*) are discussed in the text. *NAD*, nicotinamide adenine dinucleotide; *VLDL*, very-low-density lipoprotein; *MEOS*, microsomal ethanol-oxidizing system; *ADH*, alcohol dehydrogenase; *ALDH*, acetaldehyde dehydrogenase; *FAD*, flavin adenine dinucleotide; *etc*, electron-transport chain.

of fatty acids into triacylglycerols by fatty acyl-CoA transferases in the endoplasmic reticulum is enhanced (see Fig. 33.6). Because the transferases are microsomal enzymes, they are induced by ethanol consumption just as the MEOS is induced. The result is a fatty liver (hepatic steatosis).

The source of the fatty acids can be dietary fat, fatty acids synthesized in the liver, or fatty acids released from adipose tissue stores. Adipose tissue lipolysis increases after ethanol consumption possibly because of a release of epinephrine.

2. Alcohol-Induced Ketoacidosis

Fatty acids that are oxidized are converted to acetyl-CoA and subsequently to ketone bodies (acetoacetate and β-hydroxybutyrate). Enough NADH is generated

Al M.'s admitting physician suspected an alcohol-induced ketoacidosis superimposed on a starvation ketoacidosis. Tests showed that Al's plasma β-hydroxybutyrate level was 40 times the upper limit of normal and, if measured, would show his plasma free fatty acid level was elevated. The increased NADH/NAD$^+$ ratio from ethanol consumption inhibited the TCA cycle and shifted acetyl-CoA from fatty acid oxidation into the pathway of ketone-body synthesis. The presence of the ketone bodies helped to explain the large anion gap measured when Mr. M. entered the hospital.

from oxidation of ethanol and fatty acids that there is no need to oxidize acetyl-CoA in the TCA cycle. The very high NADH/NAD$^+$ ratio shifts the oxaloacetate in the TCA cycle to malate, leaving the oxaloacetate levels too low for citrate synthase to synthesize citrate (see Fig. 33.6, circle 4). The acetyl-CoA enters the pathway for ketone body synthesis instead of the TCA cycle.

Although ketone bodies are being produced at a high rate, their metabolism in other tissues is restricted by the supply of acetate, which is the preferred fuel. Thus, the blood concentration of ketone bodies may be much higher than is found under normal fasting conditions.

3. Lactic Acidosis, Hyperuricemia, and Hypoglycemia

Another consequence of the very high NADH/NAD$^+$ ratio is that the balance in the lactate dehydrogenase reaction is shifted toward lactate, resulting in a lactic acidosis (see Fig. 33.6, circle 6). The elevation of blood lactate may decrease excretion of uric acid (see Fig. 33.6, circle 7) by the kidney. Consequently, patients with gout (which results from precipitated uric acid crystals in the joints) are advised not to drink excessive amounts of ethanol. Increased degradation of purines also may contribute to hyperuricemia.

The increased NADH/NAD$^+$ ratio also can cause hypoglycemia in a fasting individual who has been drinking and is dependent on gluconeogenesis to maintain blood glucose levels (Fig. 33.6, circles 6 and 8). Alanine and lactate are major gluconeogenic precursors that enter gluconeogenesis as pyruvate. The high NADH/NAD$^+$ ratio shifts the lactate dehydrogenase equilibrium to lactate, so that pyruvate formed from alanine is converted to lactate and cannot enter gluconeogenesis. The high NADH/NAD$^+$ ratio also prevents other major gluconeogenic precursors, such as oxaloacetate and glycerol, from entering the gluconeogenic pathway.

In contrast, ethanol consumption with a meal may result in a transient hyperglycemia, possibly because the high NADH/NAD$^+$ ratio inhibits glycolysis at the glyceraldehyde 3-phosphate dehydrogenase step.

B. Acetaldehyde Toxicity

Many of the toxic effects of chronic ethanol consumption result from accumulation of acetaldehyde, which is produced from ethanol by both alcohol dehydrogenases and the MEOS. Acetaldehyde accumulates in the liver and is released into the blood after heavy doses of ethanol (Fig. 33.7). It is highly reactive and binds covalently to amino groups, sulfhydryl groups, nucleotides, and phospholipids to form "adducts."

1. Acetaldehyde and Alcohol-Induced Hepatitis

One of the results of acetaldehyde-adduct formation with amino acids is a general decrease in hepatic protein synthesis (see Fig. 33.7, circle 1). Calmodulin, ribonuclease, and tubulin are some of the proteins affected. Proteins in the heart and other tissues also may be affected by acetaldehyde that appears in the blood.

As a consequence of forming acetaldehyde adducts of tubulin, there is a diminished secretion of serum proteins and VLDL from the liver. The liver synthesizes many blood proteins, including serum albumin, blood coagulation factors, and transport proteins for vitamins, steroids, and iron. These proteins accumulate in the liver, together with lipid. The accumulation of proteins results in an influx of water (see Fig. 33.7, circle 6) within the hepatocytes and a swelling of the liver that contributes to portal hypertension and a disruption of hepatic architecture.

2. Acetaldehyde and Free-Radical Damage

Acetaldehyde-adduct formation enhances free-radical damage. Acetaldehyde binds directly to glutathione and diminishes its ability to protect against H_2O_2 and prevent lipid peroxidation (see Fig. 33.7, circle 2). It also binds to free-radical defense enzymes.

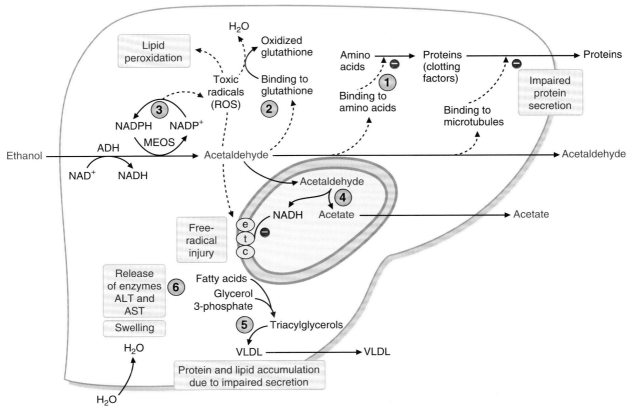

FIGURE 33.7 The development of alcohol-induced hepatitis. (*1*) Acetaldehyde-adduct formation decreases protein synthesis and impairs protein secretion. (*2*) Free-radical injury results partly from acetaldehyde-adduct formation with glutathione. (*3*) Induction of the microsomal ethanol-oxidizing system (MEOS) increases formation of free radicals, which leads to lipid peroxidation and cell damage. (*4*) Mitochondrial damage inhibits the electron-transport chain, which decreases acetaldehyde oxidation. (*5*) Microtubule damage increases very-low-density lipoprotein (VLDL) and protein accumulation. (*6*) Cell damage leads to release of the hepatic enzymes alanine aminotransferase (ALT) and aspartate aminotransferase (AST). *ADH*, alcohol dehydrogenase; *NAD*, nicotinamide adenine dinucleotide; *ROS*, reactive oxygen species; *etc*, electron-transport chain.

Damage to mitochondria from acetaldehyde and free radicals perpetuates a cycle of toxicity (see Fig. 33.7, circles 3 and 4). With chronic consumption of ethanol, mitochondria become damaged, the rate of electron transport is inhibited, and oxidative phosphorylation tends to become uncoupled. Fatty acid oxidation is decreased even further, thereby enhancing lipid accumulation (see Fig. 33.7, circle 5). The mitochondrial changes further impair mitochondrial acetaldehyde oxidation, thereby initiating a cycle of progressively increasing acetaldehyde damage.

C. Ethanol and Free-Radical Formation

Increased oxidative stress in the liver during chronic ethanol intoxication arises from increased production of free radicals, principally by CYP2E1. Flavin adenine dinucleotide (FAD) and flavin mononucleotide (FMN) in the reductase and heme in the cytochrome P450 system transfer single electrons, thus operating through a mechanism that can generate free radicals. The hydroxyethyl radical (CH$_3$CH$_2$O•) is produced during ethanol metabolism and can be released as a free radical. Induction of CYP2E1, as well as other cytochrome P450 enzymes, can increase the generation of free radicals from drug metabolism and from the activation of toxins and carcinogens (see Fig. 33.7, circle 3). These effects are enhanced by acetaldehyde-adduct damage.

Phospholipids, the major lipid in cellular membranes, are a primary target of peroxidation caused by free-radical release. Peroxidation of lipids in the inner mitochondrial membrane may contribute to the inhibition of electron transport and

 The noncaloric effect of heavy and chronic ethanol ingestion that led **Ivan A.** to believe ethanol has no calories may be partly attributable to uncoupling of oxidative phosphorylation. The hepatic mitochondria from tissues of chronic alcoholics may be partially uncoupled and unable to maintain the transmembrane proton gradient necessary for normal rates of ATP synthesis. Consequently, a greater proportion of the energy in ethanol is converted to heat. Metabolic disturbances such as the loss of ketone bodies in urine, or futile cycling of glucose, also might contribute to a diminished energy value for ethanol.

Because of the possibility of mild alcoholic hepatitis and perhaps chronic alcohol-induced cirrhosis, the physician ordered liver function studies on **Jean T.** The tests indicated an ALT level of 46 U/L (reference range, 5 to 30 U/L) and an AST level of 98 U/L (reference range, 10 to 30 U/L). The concentration of these enzymes is high in hepatocytes. When hepatocellular membranes are damaged in any way, these enzymes are released into the blood. Jean's serum alkaline phosphatase level was 195 U/L (reference range, 56 to 155 U/L for an adult female). The serum total bilirubin level was 2.4 mg/dL (reference range, 0.2 to 1.0 mg/L). These tests show impaired capacity for normal liver function. Her blood hemoglobin and hematocrit levels were slightly below the normal range, consistent with a toxic effect of ethanol on red blood cell production by bone marrow. Serum folate and vitamin B_{12} levels were also slightly suppressed. Folate is dependent on the liver for its activation and recovery from the enterohepatic circulation. Vitamin B_{12} is dependent on the liver for synthesis of its blood carrier proteins. Thus, **Jean T.** shows many of the consequences of hepatic damage.

uncoupling of mitochondria, leading to inflammation and cellular necrosis. Induction of CYP2E1 and other P450 cytochromes also increases formation of other radicals and the activation of hepatocarcinogens.

D. Hepatic Cirrhosis and Loss of Liver Function

Liver injury is irreversible at the stage that hepatic cirrhosis develops. Initially, the liver may be enlarged, full of fat, and crossed with collagen fibers (fibrosis) and may have nodules of regenerating hepatocytes ballooning between the fibers. As liver function is lost, the liver becomes shrunken (Laennec cirrhosis). During the development of cirrhosis, many of the normal metabolic functions of the liver are lost, including biosynthetic and detoxification pathways. Synthesis of blood proteins, including blood coagulation factors and serum albumin, is decreased. The capacity to incorporate amino groups into urea is decreased, resulting in the accumulation of toxic levels of ammonia in the blood. Conjugation and excretion of the yellow pigment bilirubin (a product of heme degradation) is diminished, and bilirubin accumulates in the blood. It is deposited in many tissues, including the skin and sclerae of the eyes, causing the patient to become visibly yellow. Such a patient is said to be jaundiced.

CLINICAL COMMENTS

When ethanol consumption is low (<15% of the calories in the diet), it is used efficiently to produce ATP, thereby contributing to **Ivan A.'s** weight gain. However, in individuals with chronic consumption of large amounts of ethanol, the caloric content of ethanol is not converted to ATP as effectively. Some of the factors that may contribute to this decreased efficiency include mitochondrial damage (inhibition of oxidative phosphorylation and uncoupling) resulting in the loss of calories as heat, increased recycling of metabolites such as ketone bodies, and inhibition of the normal pathways of fatty acid and glucose oxidation. In addition, heavier drinkers metabolize an increased amount of alcohol through the MEOS, which generates less ATP.

Al M. Al M. was suffering from acute effects of high ethanol ingestion in the absence of food intake. Both heavy ethanol consumption and low caloric intake increase adipose tissue lipolysis and elevate blood fatty acids. As a consequence of his elevated hepatic NADH/NAD$^+$ ratio, acetyl-CoA produced from fatty acid oxidation was diverted from the TCA cycle into the pathway of ketone-body synthesis. Because his skeletal muscles were using acetate as a fuel, ketone-body use was diminished, resulting in ketoacidosis. Al's moderately low blood glucose level also suggests that his high hepatic NADH level prevented pyruvate and glycerol from entering the gluconeogenic pathway. Pyruvate is diverted to lactate, which may have contributed to his metabolic acidosis and anion gap, along with the ketone bodies.

Rehydration with intravenous fluids containing glucose, thiamin, and potassium was initiated. Al's initial potassium level was low, possibly secondary to vomiting. Thiamin is given in case there is thiamin deficiency. An orthopedic surgeon was consulted regarding the compound fracture of his right forearm.

Jean T. Jean T.'s signs and symptoms, as well as her laboratory profile, were consistent with the presence of mild reversible alcohol-induced hepatocellular inflammation (alcohol-induced hepatitis) superimposed on a degree of irreversible scarring of liver tissues, known as *chronic alcoholic (Laennec) cirrhosis* of the liver. The chronic inflammatory process associated with long-term ethanol abuse in patients such as **Jean T.** is accompanied by increases in the levels of serum alanine aminotransferase (ALT) and aspartate aminotransferase (AST). Her elevated bilirubin and alkaline phosphatase levels in the blood were consistent with hepatic damage. Her values for ALT and AST were significantly below those seen in acute viral hepatitis. In addition, the ratio of the absolute values for serum

TABLE 33.2 Hepatic Injury

STAGE OF INJURY	MAIN FEATURES
Fibrosis: increase of connective tissue	Accumulation of both fibrillar and basement membrane–like collagens Increase of laminin and fibronectin Thickening of connective tissue septae Capillary formation within the sinusoids
Sclerosis: aging of fibrotic tissue	Decrease of hyaluronic acid and heparan sulfate proteoglycans Increase of chondroitin sulfate proteoglycans Progressive fragmentation and disappearance of elastic fibers Distortion of sinusoidal architecture and parenchymal damage
Cirrhosis: end-stage process of liver fibrotic degeneration	Whole liver heavily distorted by thick bands of collagen surrounding nodules of hepatocytes with regenerative foci

ALT and AST often differ in the two diseases, tending to be >1 in acute viral hepatitis and <1 in chronic alcohol-induced cirrhosis. The reason for the difference in ratio of enzyme activities released is not fully understood, but a lower level of ALT in the serum may be attributable to an alcohol-induced deficiency of pyridoxal phosphate. In addition, serologic tests for viral hepatitis were nonreactive. Her serum folate and vitamin B$_{12}$ were also slightly suppressed, indicating impaired nutritional status.

Jean was strongly cautioned to abstain from alcohol immediately and to improve her nutritional status. In addition, she was referred to the hospital drug and alcohol rehabilitation unit for appropriate psychological therapy and supportive social counseling. The physician also arranged for a follow-up office visit in 2 weeks.

BIOCHEMICAL COMMENTS

Fibrosis in Chronic Alcohol-Induced Liver Disease. Fibrosis is the excessive accumulation of connective tissue in parenchymal organs. In the liver, it is a frequent event following a repeated or chronic insult of sufficient intensity (such as chronic ethanol intoxication or infection by a hepatitis virus) to trigger a "wound healing–like" reaction. Regardless of the insult, the events are similar: An overproduction of extracellular matrix components occurs, with the tendency to progress to sclerosis, accompanied by a degenerative alteration in the composition of matrix components (Table 33.2). Some individuals (<20% of those who chronically consume alcohol) go on to develop cirrhosis.

The development of hepatic fibrosis after ethanol consumption is related to stimulation of the mitogenic development of stellate (Ito) cells into myofibroblasts, and stimulation of the production of collagen type I and fibronectin by these cells. The stellate cells are perisinusoidal cells lodged in the space of Disse that produce extracellular matrix protein. Normally, the space of Disse contains basement membrane–like collagen (collagen type IV) and laminin. As the stellate cells are activated, they change from a resting cell filled with lipids and vitamin A to one that proliferates, loses its vitamin A content, and secretes large quantities of extracellular matrix components.

One of the initial events in the activation and proliferation of stellate cells is the activation of Kupffer cells, which are macrophages that reside in the liver sinusoids (Fig. 33.8). The Kupffer cells are probably activated by a product of the damaged hepatocytes, such as necrotic debris, iron, reactive oxygen species (ROS), acetaldehyde, or aldehyde products of lipid peroxidation. Kupffer cells also may produce acetaldehyde from ethanol internally through their own MEOS pathway.

In liver fibrosis, disruption of the normal liver architecture, including sinusoids, impairs blood from the portal vein. Increased portal vein pressure (portal hypertension) causes capillaries to anastomose (to meet and unite or run into each other) and form thin-walled dilated esophageal venous conduits known as *esophageal varices*. When these burst, there is hemorrhaging into the GI tract. The bleeding can be very profuse because of the high venous pressure within these varices in addition to the adverse effect of impaired hepatic function on the production of blood-clotting proteins.

Although the full spectrum of alcohol-induced liver disease may be present in a well-nourished individual, the presence of nutritional deficiencies enhances the progression of the disease. Ethanol creates nutritional deficiencies in several different ways. The ingestion of ethanol reduces the GI absorption of foods that contain essential nutrients, including vitamins, essential fatty acids, and essential amino acids. For example, ethanol interferes with absorption of folate, thiamin, and other nutrients. Secondary malabsorption can occur through GI complications, pancreatic insufficiency, and impaired hepatic metabolism or impaired hepatic storage of nutrients such as vitamin A. Changes in the level of transport proteins produced by the liver also strongly affect nutrient status.

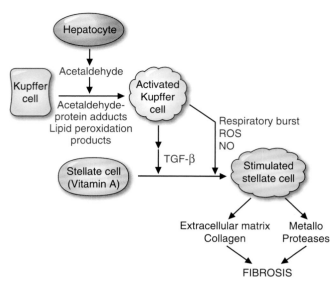

FIGURE 33.8 Proposed model for the development of hepatic fibrosis involving hepatocytes, Kupffer cells, and stellate (Ito) cells. *ROS*, reactive oxygen species; *NO*, nitric oxide: *TGF-β₁*, transforming growth factor β₁.

Activated Kupffer cells produce several products that contribute to activation of stellate cells. They generate additional ROS through NADPH oxidase during the oxidative burst and reactive nitrogen–oxygen species (RNOS) through inducible nitric oxide (NO) synthase (see Chapter 25). In addition, they secrete an impressive array of growth factors, such as cytokines, chemokines, prostaglandins, and other reactive molecules. The cytokine transforming growth factor β_1 (TGF-β_1), produced by both Kupffer cells and sinusoidal endothelial cells, is a major player in the activation of stellate cells. Once they are activated, the stellate cells produce collagen and proteases, leading to an enhanced fibrotic network within the liver. Stellate cells may also be partially activated by hepatocyte release of ROS and acetaldehyde directly, with the involvement of Kupffer cells.

Recent evidence also indicates that chronic alcohol usage can disrupt gene regulation within the liver, through modification of the activity of sirtuin1 (see "Biochemical Comments" in Chapter 30). Sirtuin 1 (SIRT-1) is a histone deacetylase that uses NAD^+ as a substrate (see Fig. 30.21), producing nicotinamide and acetyl-ADP-ribose. Deacylation of appropriate targets leads to alterations in gene expression. Ethanol will lead to a downregulation of SIRT-1 activity. Ethanol may lead to reduced SIRT-1 activity through an increase in the NADH/NAD^+ ratio in the liver, thereby reducing the level of substrate (NAD^+) required for SIRT-1 activity.

Interestingly, it also appears that a reduction in SIRT-1 activity leads to a reduction in AMP-activated protein kinase activity (AMPK). Under normal conditions, SIRT-1 deacetylates LBK1, activating it, which phosphorylates and activates the AMPK. AMPK (see "Biochemical Comments" in Chapter 34) phosphorylates and inhibits acetyl-CoA carboxylase, resulting in reduced production of malonyl coenzyme A (malonyl-CoA). Malonyl-CoA is an inhibitor of carnitine palmitoyltransferase I (CPTI), so reduced levels of malonyl-CoA lead to increased activity of CPTI and increased levels of fatty acid oxidation. Ethanol-induced inhibition of SIRT-1 will lead to inhibition of hepatic AMPK (because of LBK1 remaining inactive), thereby activating acetyl-CoA carboxylase, producing malonyl-CoA, and blocking fatty acid oxidation in the liver. This will result in the fatty acid and triglyceride synthesis in the liver, leading to the development of alcoholic fatty liver disease.

KEY CONCEPTS

- Ethanol metabolism occurs primarily in the liver, via a two-step oxidation sequence to acetate plus NADH.
- Acetate is activated to acetyl-CoA for energy generation by most tissues of the body.
- The ALD family of enzymes catalyzes the first step of alcohol oxidation. The ALDH family of enzymes catalyzes the second step of the pathway.
- When ethanol levels are high, the microsomal ethanol-oxidizing system (MEOS), consisting of CYP2E1, is induced.
- Acute effects of ethanol ingestion are caused by the elevated NADH/NAD$^+$ ratio, which leads to
  - Inhibition of fatty acid oxidation
  - Ketogenesis
  - Hyperlipidemia
  - Inhibition of gluconeogenesis
  - Lactic acidosis
  - Hyperuricemia
- Chronic effects of ethanol ingestion include
  - Hepatic steatosis (fatty acid accumulation within the liver)
  - Hepatitis
  - Fibrosis (excessive collagen production within the liver)
  - Cirrhosis (eventual liver death)
- The chronic effects of ethanol are caused by acetaldehyde and ROS production during ethanol metabolism.
- The diseases discussed in this chapter are summarized in Table 33.3.

TABLE 33.3 **Diseases Discussed in Chapter 33**

DISEASE OR DISORDER	ENVIRONMENTAL OR GENETIC	COMMENTS
Obesity	Both	Ethanol is a nutrient, and its caloric content can contribute to obesity.
Alcoholism	Both	Alcohol addiction (alcoholism) may occur, leading to damage of internal organs by acetaldehyde production.
Jaundice	Environmental	Altered liver function leads to a reduced ability to conjugate and solubilize bilirubin, which leads to bilirubin deposition in the eyes and skin, giving them a yellow pallor (jaundice). This is an indication of liver disease.
Liver fibrosis	Environmental	Excessive damage to liver, often caused by alcohol metabolism, particularly acetaldehyde accumulation, leading to extensive collagen secretion and loss of liver function.

REVIEW QUESTIONS—CHAPTER 33

1. The fate of acetate, the product of ethanol metabolism, is which one of the following?
   A. It is taken up by other tissues and activated to acetyl-CoA.
   B. It is toxic to the tissues of the body and can lead to hepatic necrosis.
   C. It is excreted in bile.
   D. It enters the TCA cycle directly to be oxidized.
   E. It is converted into NADH by ADH.

2. Which one of the following would be expected to occur after acute alcohol ingestion?
   A. Activation of fatty acid oxidation
   B. Lactic acidosis
   C. Inhibition of ketogenesis
   D. An increase in the NAD$^+$/NADH ratio
   E. An increase in gluconeogenesis

3. A chronic alcoholic is in treatment for alcohol abuse. The drug disulfiram is prescribed for the patient. This drug deters the consumption of alcohol by which one of the following mechanisms?
   A. Inhibiting the absorption of ethanol so that an individual cannot become intoxicated, regardless of how much he or she drinks
   B. Inhibiting the conversion of ethanol to acetaldehyde, which cause the excretion of unmetabolized ethanol
   C. Blocking the conversion of acetaldehyde to acetate, which causes the accumulation of acetaldehyde
   D. Activating the excessive metabolism of ethanol to acetate, which causes inebriation with consumption of a small amount of alcohol
   E. Preventing the excretion of acetate, which causes nausea and vomiting

4. Induction of CYP2E1 would result in which of the following?
   A. A decreased clearance of ethanol from the blood
   B. A decrease in the rate of acetaldehyde production
   C. A low possibility of the generation of free radicals
   D. Protection from hepatic damage
   E. An increase of one's alcohol tolerance level

5. Which one of the following consequences of chronic alcohol consumption is irreversible?
   A. Inhibition of fatty acid oxidation
   B. Activation of triacylglycerol synthesis
   C. Ketoacidosis
   D. Lactic acidosis
   E. Liver cirrhosis

6. A chronic alcoholic, on a binge, is severely hypoglycemic. Under these conditions, gluconeogenic precursors are trapped and cannot progress to form glucose. Which one of the following is such a trapped intermediate?
   A. Glycerol
   B. Dihydroxyacetone phosphate
   C. Glyceraldehyde 3-phosphate
   D. Glycerol 3-phosphate
   E. Pyruvate

7. Your patient is a chronic alcoholic who is frequently malnourished and is exhibiting symptoms of a vitamin deficiency because of chronic alcohol consumption. This patient would most likely have trouble catalyzing which one of the following reactions because of the vitamin deficiency?
   A. Sedoheptulose 7-phosphate + glyceraldehyde 3-phosphate → erythrose 4-phosphate + fructose 6-phosphate
   B. Ribose 5-phosphate + xylulose 5-phosphate → sedoheptulose 7-phosphate + glyceraldehyde 3-phosphate
   C. Glucose 6-phosphate + 2 $NADP^+$ → CO_2 + ribulose 5-phosphate + 2 NADPH
   D. Isocitrate + NAD^+ → CO_2 + α-ketoglutarate + NADH
   E. Oxaloacetate + guanosine triphosphate → phosphoenolpyruvate + CO_2 + guanosine diphosphate

8. The enzymes that metabolize ethanol exist as a variety of isozymes in the general population. A slow-activity isozyme of which enzyme is most likely responsible for an individual to exhibit a very low tolerance to alcohol, leading to the individual rarely drinking?
   A. Acetyl-CoA synthetase
   B. MEOS
   C. Acetyl-CoA carboxylase
   D. ADH
   E. ALDH

9. What would be an outcome if a person had a defect in which the metabolites of ethanol could not enter the mitochondria?
   A. Acetate would accumulate, which is toxic.
   B. Acetaldehyde would accumulate, which is toxic.
   C. Acetate would be activated by tissues to acetyl-CoA.
   D. Acetaldehyde would be activated by tissues to acetyl-CoA.
   E. The MEOS would not function.

10. The possibility of ROS being generated during ethanol metabolism occurs via which one of the following enzyme systems?
    A. MEOS
    B. ADH
    C. ALDH
    D. Acetyl-CoA Synthetase
    E. Citrate synthase

ANSWERS

1. **The answer is A.** Acetate is converted to acetyl-CoA by other tissues so that it can enter the TCA cycle to generate ATP. Answer B is incorrect because acetaldehyde, not acetate, is toxic to cells. Answer C is incorrect because acetate is excreted by the lung and kidney and not in the bile. Answer D is incorrect because acetate cannot enter the TCA cycle directly. It must be converted to acetyl-CoA first. Answer E is incorrect because alcohol dehydrogenase converts ethanol into acetaldehyde. It does not convert acetate into NADH.

2. **The answer is B.** There is an increase in the NADH/NAD^+ ratio because NADH is produced by the conversion of ethanol to acetate (thus, D is incorrect). The increased ratio of NADH/NAD^+ favors the conversion of gluconeogenic precursors (such as pyruvate and oxaloacetate) to their reduced counterparts (lactate and malate, respectively) in order to generate NAD^+ for ethanol metabolism. This reduces the concentration of gluconeogenic precursors and slows down gluconeogenesis (thus, E is incorrect) and can lead to lactic acidosis.

Answer A is incorrect because the increase of NADH inhibits fatty acid oxidation. Answer C is incorrect because ketogenesis increases as a result of the increase of NADH and acetyl-CoA in the mitochondria. NADH inhibits key enzymes of the TCA cycle, thereby diverting acetyl-CoA from the TCA cycle and toward ketone-body synthesis.

3. **The answer is C.** Disulfiram blocks the conversion of acetaldehyde to acetate (the reaction catalyzed by ALDH). The accumulation of acetaldehyde is toxic and causes vomiting and nausea. Answers A and B are incorrect because disulfiram would not interfere with the absorption of ethanol or the first step of its metabolism. Answer D is incorrect because an ALDH inhibitor (such as disulfiram) would inhibit the conversion of ethanol to acetate, not increase the rate of the conversion. Answer E is incorrect because disulfiram does not interfere with the excretion of acetate, nor does acetate accumulation lead to nausea and vomiting.

4. **The answer is E.** An increase in the concentration of CYP2E1 (the MEOS system) would result in an increase of ethanol metabolism and clearance from the blood (thus, A is incorrect). An increased rate of acetaldehyde production would result (thus, B is incorrect). The increase in CYP2E1 would cause an increase in the probability of producing free radicals (thus, C is incorrect). Answer D is incorrect because hepatic damage would be more likely to occur because there is an increase of free-radical production. Answer E is correct because the increased clearance rate of ethanol from the blood results in a higher alcohol tolerance level.

5. **The answer is E.** Liver cirrhosis is irreversible. It is an end-stage process of liver fibrosis. Answers A, B, C, and D are all consequences of liver disease, but they are all reversible. Therefore, E is the only answer that is correct.

6. **The answer is D.** The gluconeogenic precursors are lactate, glycerol, and amino acids (primarily alanine) from muscle protein degradation. Under the conditions of high alcohol intake for extended periods, the NADH/NAD$^+$ ratio is very high owing to alcohol being converted to acetaldehyde and then acetic acid. Gluconeogenesis is impaired because of the high levels of NADH present. Lactate cannot be converted to pyruvate (the reaction requires NAD$^+$, which is present in very low levels). Alanine can be converted to pyruvate, which is converted to oxaloacetate via pyruvate carboxylase, but the oxaloacetate is trapped and cannot be converted to malate owing to the low NAD$^+$ levels as well. Glycerol metabolism requires first, phosphorylation to glycerol 3-P, and then oxidation of carbon 2 to form dihydroxyacetone phosphate, an NAD$^+$-requiring reaction. Thus, when NAD$^+$ levels are low, glycerol 3-P, lactate, and oxaloacetate will all be trapped and cannot efficiently progress through the gluconeogenic pathway.

7. **The answer is B.** The patient is likely to be thiamin-deficient, which is a required factor for oxidative decarboxylation reactions (pyruvate dehydrogenase and α-ketoglutarate dehydrogenase) and transketolase. Ethanol interferes with the absorption of thiamin from the digestive tract. The reaction of ribose 5-phosphate with xylulose 5-phosphate to produce sedoheptulose 7-phosphate and glyceraldehyde 3-phosphate is catalyzed by transketolase. The conversion of sedoheptulose 7-phosphate and glyceraldehyde 3-phosphate to erythrose 4-phosphate and fructose 6-phosphate is a three-carbon transfer catalyzed by transaldolase, which does not require an exogenous vitamin for activity. The conversion of glucose 6-phosphate to ribulose 5-phosphate is catalyzed by glucose 6-phosphate dehydrogenase, which requires niacin as a cofactor but not thiamin. Isocitrate dehydrogenase, which requires niacin (but not thiamin), catalyzes the conversion of isocitrate to α-ketoglutarate. Phosphoenolpyruvate (PEP) carboxykinase catalyzes the conversion of oxaloacetate to PEP and does not require a vitamin cofactor.

8. **The answer is E.** An isozyme of ALDH has a dramatically increased K_m (>200-fold) and a 10-fold reduced V_{max}. In such individuals, acetaldehyde, the toxic component of alcohol ingestion, accumulates to a large extent, leading to the individual having a very low tolerance for alcohol. A slow-acting ADH would not lead to a low tolerance to alcohol because acetaldehyde accumulation (the toxic intermediate of alcohol metabolism) would be slowed such that the acetaldehyde produced can be safely metabolized without any side effects. Acetate, once produced, is not toxic, so a slow-acting acetyl-CoA synthetase (which uses acetate as a substrate) would not lead to the accumulation of a toxic intermediate. MEOS is used as an alternative ethanol-oxidizing system when ethanol levels are high. A slow-acting MEOS would reduce the production of acetaldehyde, which is the toxic intermediate of alcohol metabolism. This would not lead to a low level of tolerance to alcohol. Acetyl-CoA carboxylase is not involved in ethanol metabolism (the acetyl-CoA formed would be used for energy). Acetyl-CoA carboxylase is needed for fatty acid synthesis, and if its activity were low, fatty acid production would be reduced, but it would have no effect on the tolerance to alcohol.

9. **The answer is B.** The main route for metabolism of ethanol is through ADH in the cytosol producing acetaldehyde, which is the toxic intermediate of alcohol metabolism. Acetaldehyde is further oxidized in mitochondria to acetate, which is then activated by tissues to acetyl-CoA, which is oxidized in the TCA cycle. If entry of acetaldehyde into the mitochondria is blocked, then acetaldehyde accumulates and acetate is not formed. The MEOS is in the endoplasmic reticulum (cytosolic) and would continue to produce acetaldehyde and NADP$^+$.

10. **The answer is A.** The MEOS is induced by ethanol and uses a cytochrome P450 system to oxidize ethanol. The cytochrome P450 enzyme systems transfer a single electron at a time through an iron within a heme group in the cytochrome, and this is the step at which the electron may escape and convert oxygen to superoxide, thereby generating ROS. ADH and ALDH transfer hydride ions to NAD$^+$, and there is a very low probability of electrons escaping from those oxidation–reduction reactions. Acetyl-CoA synthetase does not catalyze an oxidation–reduction reaction (it catalyzes the conversion of acetate to acetyl-CoA), nor does citrate synthase (the formation of citrate from acetyl-CoA and oxaloacetate). The possibility of losing an electron during a reaction in which electrons are not being transferred is very low.

Integration of Carbohydrate and Lipid Metabolism

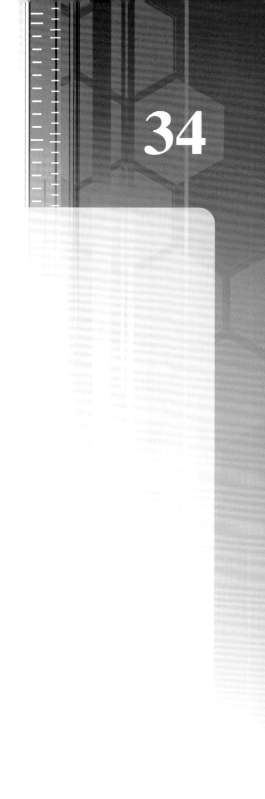

34

This chapter summarizes and integrates the major pathways for the use of carbohydrates and fats as fuels. We concentrate on reviewing the regulatory mechanisms that determine the flux of metabolites in the fed and fasting states, integrating the pathways that were described separately under carbohydrate and lipid metabolism. The next section of the book covers the mechanisms by which the pathways of nitrogen metabolism are coordinated with fat and carbohydrate metabolism.

For the species to survive, it is necessary for us to store excess food when we eat and to use these stores when we are fasting. Regulatory mechanisms direct compounds through the pathways of metabolism involved in the storage and use of fuels. These mechanisms are controlled by **hormones**, by the **concentration of available fuels**, and by the **energy needs** of the body.

Changes in hormone levels, in the concentration of fuels, and in energy requirements affect the activity of key enzymes in the major pathways of metabolism. Intracellular **enzymes** are generally regulated by **activation** and **inhibition**, by **phosphorylation** and **dephosphorylation** (or other covalent modifications), by **induction** and **repression** of synthesis, and by **degradation**. Activation and inhibition of enzymes cause immediate changes in metabolism. Phosphorylation and dephosphorylation of enzymes affect metabolism slightly less rapidly. Induction and repression of enzyme synthesis are much slower processes, usually affecting metabolic flux over a period of hours. Degradation of enzymes decreases the amount available to catalyze reactions.

The pathways of metabolism have **multiple control points** and **multiple regulators** at each control point. The function of these complex mechanisms is to produce a graded response to a stimulus and to provide sensitivity to multiple stimuli so that an exact balance is maintained between flux through a given step (or series of steps) and the need or use for the product. Pyruvate dehydrogenase (PDH) is an example of an enzyme that has multiple regulatory mechanisms. Regardless of insulin levels, the enzyme cannot become fully activated in the presence of products and absence of substrates.

The major hormones that regulate the pathways of fuel metabolism are **insulin** and **glucagon**. In liver, all effects of glucagon are reversed by insulin, and some of the pathways that insulin activates are inhibited by glucagon. Thus, the pathways of carbohydrate and lipid metabolism are generally regulated by changes in the **insulin/ glucagon ratio**.

Although **glycogen** is a critical storage form of fuel because blood glucose levels must be carefully maintained, adipose **triacylglycerols** are quantitatively the major fuel store in the human. After a meal, both dietary glucose and fat are stored in adipose tissue as triacylglycerol. This fuel is released during fasting, when it provides the main source of energy for the tissues of the body. The length of time we can survive without food depends mainly on the size of our bodies' fat stores.

THE WAITING ROOM

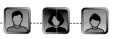

Within 2 months of her surgery to remove a benign insulin-secreting β-cell tumor of the pancreas, **Connie C.** (see Chapter 19) was again jogging lightly. She had lost the 8 lb that she had gained in the 6 weeks before her surgery. Because her hypoglycemic episodes were no longer occurring, she had no need to eat frequent carbohydrate snacks to prevent the adrenergic and neuroglycopenic symptoms that she had experienced when her tumor was secreting excessive amounts of insulin.

A few months after her last hospitalization, **Dianne A.** was once again brought to the hospital emergency department in diabetic ketoacidosis (DKA). Blood samples for glucose and electrolytes were drawn repeatedly during the first 24 hours. The hospital laboratory reported that the serum in each of these specimens appeared opalescent rather than having its normal clear or transparent appearance. This opalescence results from light-scattering caused by the presence of elevated levels of triacylglycerol-rich lipoproteins in the blood.

When **Deborah S.** initially presented (see Chapter 19) with type 2 diabetes mellitus at age 39, she was approximately 30 lb over her ideal weight. Her high serum glucose levels were accompanied by abnormalities in her 14-hour fasting lipid profile. Her serum total cholesterol, low-density lipoprotein (LDL) cholesterol, and triacylglycerol levels were elevated, and her serum high-density lipoprotein (HDL) cholesterol level was below the normal range.

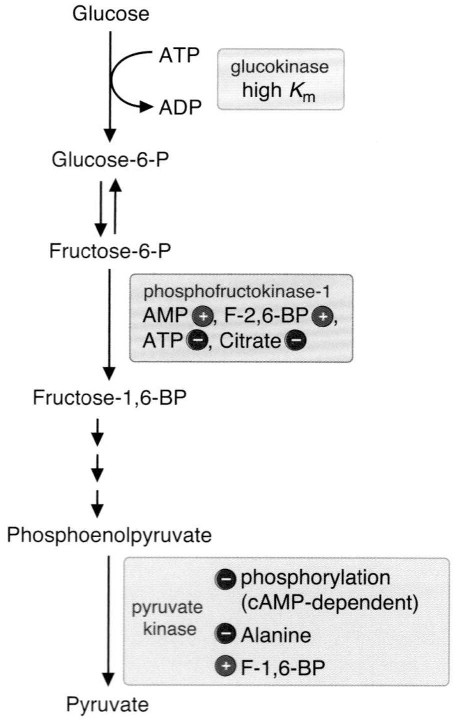

I. Regulation of Carbohydrate and Lipid Metabolism in the Fed State

A. Mechanisms that Affect Glycogen and Triacylglycerol Synthesis in Liver

After a meal, the liver synthesizes glycogen and triacylglycerol. The level of glycogen stored in the liver can increase from approximately 80 g after an overnight fast to a limit of approximately 200 to 300 g. Although the liver synthesizes triacylglycerol, it does not store this fuel but rather packages it in very-low-density lipoprotein (VLDL) and secretes it into the blood. The fatty acids of the VLDL triacylglycerols secreted from the liver are stored as adipose triacylglycerols. Adipose tissue has an almost infinite capacity to store fat, limited mainly by the ability of the heart to pump blood through the capillaries of the expanding adipose mass. Although we store fat throughout our bodies, it tends to accumulate in places where it does not interfere too much with our mobility: in the abdomen, hips, thighs, and buttocks.

Both the synthesis of liver glycogen and the conversion by the liver of dietary glucose to triacylglycerol (lipogenesis) are regulated by mechanisms involving key enzymes in these pathways.

1. Glucokinase

After a meal, glucose can be converted to glycogen or to triacylglycerol in the liver. For both processes, glucose is first converted to glucose 6-phosphate by glucokinase, a liver enzyme that has a high K_m for glucose (Fig. 34.1). Because of the enzyme's low affinity for glucose, this enzyme is most active in the fed state, when the concentration of glucose is particularly high because the hepatic portal vein carries digestive products directly from the intestine to the liver. Synthesis of glucokinase is also induced by insulin (which is elevated after a meal) and repressed by glucagon (which is elevated during fasting). In keeping with the liver's function in maintaining blood glucose levels, this system is set up such that the liver can metabolize glucose only when sugar levels are high and not when sugar levels are low.

FIGURE 34.1 Regulation of glucokinase, phosphofructokinase-1, and pyruvate kinase in the liver. *ADP*, adenosine diphosphate; *AMP*, adenosine monophosphate; *ATP*, adenosine triphosphate; *cAMP*, cyclic AMP; *Fructose 1,6-BP*, fructose 1,6-bisphosphate; *F-2,6-BP*, fructose 2,6-bisphosphate.

2. Glycogen Synthase

In the conversion of glucose 6-phosphate to glycogen, the key regulatory enzyme is glycogen synthase. This enzyme is activated by dephosphorylation, which occurs when insulin is elevated and glucagon is decreased (Fig. 34.2) and by the increased level of glucose.

3. Phosphofructokinase-1 and Pyruvate Kinase

For lipogenesis, glucose 6-phosphate is converted through glycolysis to pyruvate. Key enzymes that regulate this pathway in the liver are phosphofructokinase-1 (PFK-1) and pyruvate kinase. PFK-1 is allosterically activated in the fed state by fructose 2,6-bisphosphate and adenosine monophosphate (AMP) (see Fig. 34.1). Phosphofructokinase-2, the enzyme that produces the activator fructose 2,6-bisphosphate, is dephosphorylated and the kinase activity is active after a meal (see Chapter 22). Pyruvate kinase is also activated by dephosphorylation, which is stimulated by the increase of the insulin/glucagon ratio in the fed state (see Fig. 34.1).

4. Pyruvate Dehydrogenase and Pyruvate Carboxylase

The conversion of pyruvate to fatty acids requires a source of acetyl coenzyme A (acetyl-CoA) in the cytosol. Pyruvate can only be converted to acetyl-CoA in mitochondria, so it enters mitochondria and forms acetyl-CoA through the PDH reaction. This enzyme is dephosphorylated and most active when its supply of substrates and adenosine diphosphate (ADP) is high, its products are used, and insulin is present (see Fig. 23.15).

Pyruvate is also converted to oxaloacetate (OAA). The enzyme that catalyzes this reaction, pyruvate carboxylase, is activated by acetyl-CoA. Because acetyl-CoA cannot cross the mitochondrial membrane directly to form fatty acids in the cytosol, it condenses with OAA, producing citrate. The citrate that is not required for tricarboxylic acid (TCA) cycle activity crosses the membrane and enters the cytosol.

As fatty acids are produced under conditions of high energy, the high reduced nicotinamide adenine dinucleotide (NADH/NAD$^+$) ratio in the mitochondria inhibits isocitrate dehydrogenase, which leads to citrate accumulation within the mitochondrial matrix. As the citrate accumulates, it is transported out into the cytosol to donate carbons for fatty acid synthesis.

5. Citrate Lyase, Malic Enzyme, and Glucose 6-Phosphate Dehydrogenase

In the cytosol, citrate is cleaved by citrate lyase, an inducible enzyme, to form OAA and acetyl-CoA (Fig. 34.3). The acetyl-CoA is used for fatty acid biosynthesis and for cholesterol synthesis, pathways that are activated by insulin. OAA is recycled to pyruvate via cytosolic malate dehydrogenase and malic enzyme, which is inducible. Malic enzyme generates NADPH for the reactions of the fatty acid synthase complex. NADPH is also produced by the two enzymes of the pentose phosphate pathway (see Chapter 27), glucose 6-phosphate dehydrogenase and 6-phosphogluconate dehydrogenase. Glucose 6-phosphate dehydrogenase is also induced by insulin.

6. Acetyl Coenzyme A Carboxylase

Acetyl-CoA is converted to malonyl coenzyme A (malonyl-CoA), which provides the two-carbon units for elongation of the growing fatty acyl chain on the fatty acid synthase complex. Acetyl-CoA carboxylase, the enzyme that catalyzes the conversion of acetyl-CoA to malonyl-CoA, is controlled by three of the major mechanisms that regulate enzyme activity (Fig. 34.4). It is activated by citrate, which causes the enzyme to polymerize, and inhibited by long-chain fatty acyl coenzyme A (fatty acyl-CoA). A phosphatase stimulated by insulin activates the enzyme by dephosphorylation. The third means by which this enzyme is regulated is induction: The quantity of the enzyme increases in the fed state.

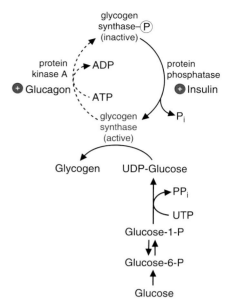

FIGURE 34.2 Regulation of glycogen synthase. This enzyme is phosphorylated by a series of kinases, which are initiated by the cyclic adenosine monophosphate (cAMP)-dependent protein kinase under fasting conditions. It is dephosphorylated and active after a meal, and glycogen is stored. *P*, phosphate; ⊕, activated by; *ADP*, adenosine diphosphate; *ATP*, adenosine triphosphate; *glucose 1-P*, glucose 1-phosphate; *glucose 6-P*, glucose 6-phosphate; *P$_i$*, inorganic phosphate; *PP$_i$*, pyrophosphate; *UDP*, uridine diphosphate; *UTP*, uridine triphosphate.

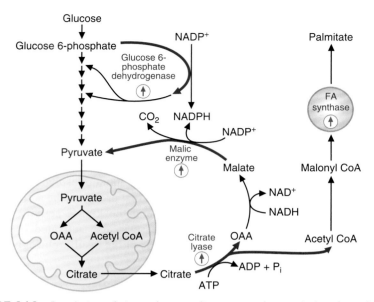

FIGURE 34.3 Regulation of citrate lyase, malic enzyme, glucose 6-phosphate dehydrogenase, and fatty acid synthase. Citrate lyase, which provides acetyl coenzyme A (acetyl-CoA) for fatty acid biosynthesis, the enzymes that provide NADPH (malic enzyme, glucose 6-phosphate dehydrogenase), as well as fatty acid synthase, are inducible ($\uparrow$). *ADP*, adenosine diphosphate; *ATP*, adenosine triphosphate; *FA*, fatty acid; *Malonyl CoA*, malonyl coenzyme A; *NAD*, nicotinamide adenine dinucleotide; *OAA*, oxaloacetate; *P_i*, inorganic phosphate.

Malonyl-CoA, the product of the acetyl-CoA carboxylase reaction, provides the carbons for the synthesis of palmitate on the fatty acid synthase complex. Malonyl-CoA also inhibits carnitine palmitoyltransferase I (CPTI, also known as *carnitine acyltransferase I*), the enzyme that prepares long-chain fatty acyl-CoA for transport into mitochondria (Fig. 34.5). In the fed state, when acetyl-CoA carboxylase is

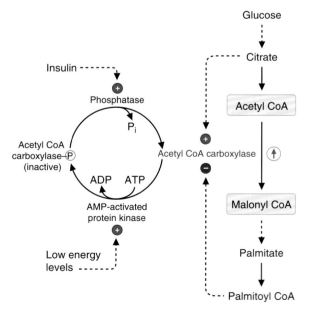

FIGURE 34.4 Regulation of acetyl coenzyme A carboxylase (ACC). ACC is regulated by activation and inhibition, by phosphorylation (mediated by the adenosine monophosphate [AMP]-activated protein kinase) and dephosphorylation (via an insulin-stimulated phosphatase), and by induction ($\uparrow$) and repression. It is active in the fed state. *ADP*, adenosine diphosphate; *ATP*, adenosine triphosphate; *Malonyl CoA*, malonyl coenzyme A; *Palmitoyl CoA*, palmitoyl coenzyme A; *P_i*, inorganic phosphate.

active and malonyl-CoA levels are elevated, newly synthesized fatty acids are converted to triacylglycerols for storage rather than being transported into mitochondria for oxidation and formation of ketone bodies.

7. Fatty Acid Synthase Complex

In a well-fed individual, the quantity of the fatty acid synthase complex is increased (see Fig. 34.3). The genes that produce this enzyme complex are induced by increases in the insulin/glucagon ratio. The amount of the complex increases slowly after a few days of a high-carbohydrate diet.

Glucose 6-phosphate dehydrogenase, which generates NADPH in the pentose phosphate pathway, and malic enzyme, which produces NADPH, are also induced by the increase of insulin.

The palmitate produced by the synthase complex is converted to palmityl-CoA and elongated and desaturated to form other fatty acyl-CoA molecules, which are converted to triacylglycerols. These triacylglycerols are packaged and secreted into the blood as VLDL.

B. Mechanisms that Affect the Fate of Chylomicrons and VLDL

The lipoprotein triacylglycerols in chylomicrons and VLDL are hydrolyzed to fatty acids and glycerol by lipoprotein lipase (LPL), an enzyme attached to endothelial cells of capillaries in muscle and adipose tissue. The enzyme found in muscle, particularly heart muscle, has a low K_m for these blood lipoproteins. Therefore, it acts even when these lipoproteins are present at very low concentrations in the blood. The fatty acids enter muscle cells and are oxidized for energy. The enzyme found in adipose tissue has a higher K_m and is most active after a meal when blood lipoprotein levels are elevated.

C. Mechanisms that Affect Triacylglycerol Storage in Adipose Tissue

Insulin stimulates adipose cells to synthesize and secrete LPL, which hydrolyzes the chylomicron and VLDL triacylglycerols. Apolipoprotein CII, donated to chylomicrons and VLDL by HDL activates LPL (Fig. 34.6).

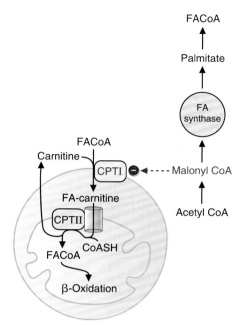

FIGURE 34.5 Inhibition of transport of fatty acids (FA) into mitochondria by malonyl coenzyme A (malonyl-CoA). In the fed state, malonyl-CoA (the substrate for fatty acid synthesis produced by acetyl coenzyme A [acetyl-CoA] carboxylase) is elevated. It inhibits carnitine palmitoyltransferase I (CPTI), preventing the transport of long-chain fatty acids into mitochondria. Therefore, substrate is not available for β-oxidation and ketone-body synthesis. *CoA*, coenzyme A; *CPTII*, carnitine palmitoyltransferase II.

 The measurement of triglycerides in blood samples is performed using a coupled assay. The sample is incubated with a lipase that converts the triglyceride to glycerol and three fatty acids. The glycerol is then converted to glycerol 3-phosphate (glycerol 3-P) by glycerol kinase and ATP, and the glycerol 3-P is then oxidized by a bacterial glycerol 3-P dehydrogenase to produce dihydroxyacetone phosphate and hydrogen peroxide. The hydrogen peroxide, in the presence of peroxidase, will oxidize a colorless substrate, which turns color when oxidized. Measurement of the color change is directly proportional to the amount of glycerol generated in the sample. Comparing values before and after lipase addition will also allow the free glycerol content in the blood to be determined.

 Dianne A. has type I diabetes mellitus, a disease associated with a severe deficiency or absence of insulin caused by destruction of the β-cells of the pancreas. One of the effects of insulin is to stimulate production of LPL. Because of low insulin levels, **Dianne A.** tends to have low levels of this enzyme. Hydrolysis of the triacylglycerols in chylomicrons and in VLDL is decreased, and hypertriglyceridemia results.

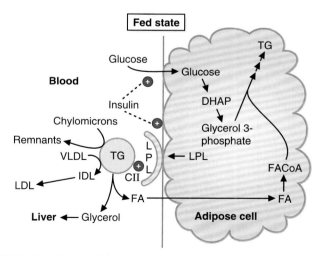

FIGURE 34.6 Regulation of the storage of triacylglycerols (TG) in adipose tissue. Insulin stimulates the secretion of lipoprotein lipase (LPL) from adipose cells and the transport of glucose into these cells. Apolipoprotein CII activates LPL. *CII*, apolipoprotein CII; *CoA*, coenzyme A; *DHAP*, dihydroxyacetone phosphate; *FA*, fatty acids; *HDL*, high-density lipoprotein; *IDL*, intermediate-density lipoprotein; *LDL*, low-density lipoprotein; *VLDL*, very-low-density lipoprotein.

Why does **Deborah S.** have a hypertriglyceridemia?

Twenty percent to 30% of patients with an insulinoma gain weight as part of their syndrome. **Connie C.** gained 8 lb in the 6 weeks before her surgery. Although she was primed by her high insulin levels both to store and to use fuel more efficiently, she would not have gained weight if she had not consumed more calories than she required for her daily energy expenditure during her illness (see Chapter 1). Connie consumed extra carbohydrate calories, mostly as hard candies and table sugar, to avoid the symptoms of hypoglycemia.

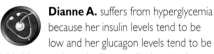

Dianne A. suffers from hyperglycemia because her insulin levels tend to be low and her glucagon levels tend to be high. Her muscle and adipose cells do not take up glucose at a normal rate, and she produces glucose by glycogenolysis and gluconeogenesis. As a result, her blood glucose levels are elevated. **Deborah S.** is in a similar metabolic state. However, in this case, she produces insulin but her tissues are resistant to its actions.

Insulin normally inhibits lipolysis by decreasing the lipolytic activity of adipocyte triglyceride lipase and HSL in the adipocyte. Individuals such as **Dianne A.**, who have a deficiency of insulin, have increased lipolysis and a subsequent increase in the concentration of free fatty acids in the blood. The liver, in turn, uses some of these fatty acids to synthesize triacylglycerols, which then are used in the hepatic production of VLDL. VLDL is not stored in the liver but is secreted into the blood, raising its serum concentration. Dianne also has low levels of LPL because of decreased insulin levels. Her hypertriglyceridemia is the result, therefore, of both overproduction of VLDL by the liver and decreased breakdown of VLDL triacylglycerol for storage in adipose cells.

The serum begins to appear cloudy when the triacylglycerol level reaches 200 mg/dL. As the triacylglycerol level increases still further, the degree of serum opalescence increases proportionately.

Fatty acids released from chylomicrons and VLDL by LPL are stored as triacylglycerols in adipose cells. The glycerol released by LPL is not used by adipose cells because they lack glycerol kinase. Glycerol can be used by liver cells, however, because these cells do contain glycerol kinase. In the fed state, liver cells convert glycerol to the glycerol moiety of the triacylglycerols of VLDL, which is secreted from the liver to distribute the newly synthesized triglycerides to the tissues.

Insulin causes the number of glucose transporters in adipose cell membranes to increase. Glucose enters these cells and is oxidized, producing energy and providing the glycerol 3-P moiety for triacylglycerol synthesis (via the dihydroxyacetone phosphate intermediate of glycolysis).

II. Regulation of Carbohydrate and Lipid Metabolism during Fasting

A. Mechanisms in Liver that Serve to Maintain Blood Glucose Levels

During fasting, the insulin/glucagon ratio decreases. Liver glycogen is degraded to produce blood glucose because enzymes of glycogen degradation are activated by cyclic AMP (cAMP)-directed phosphorylation (see Fig. 26.7). Glucagon stimulates adenylate cyclase to produce cAMP, which activates protein kinase A (PKA). PKA phosphorylates phosphorylase kinase, which then phosphorylates and activates glycogen phosphorylase. PKA also phosphorylates but, in this case, *in*activates glycogen synthase.

Gluconeogenesis is stimulated because the synthesis of phosphoenolpyruvate carboxykinase, fructose 1,6-bisphosphatase, and glucose 6-phosphatase is induced and because there is an increased availability of precursors. Fructose 1,6-bisphosphatase is also activated because the levels of its inhibitor, fructose 2,6-bisphosphate, are low (Fig. 34.7). During fasting, the activities of the corresponding enzymes of glycolysis are decreased.

Induction of enzyme synthesis requires activation of transcription factors. One of the factors that is activated is cAMP response element–binding protein (CREB). CREB is phosphorylated and activated by the cAMP-dependent protein kinase, which itself is activated upon glucagon or epinephrine stimulation. Other transcription factors are activated by cAMP, but the regulation of those factors by cAMP is not as well understood as it is for CREB.

B. Mechanisms that Affect Lipolysis in Adipose Tissue

During fasting, as blood insulin levels fall and glucagon levels rise, the level of cAMP rises in adipose cells. Consequently, PKA is activated which leads to the activation of both adipocyte triglyceride lipase and hormone-sensitive lipase (HSL; see Fig. 31.25). These activated lipases cleave fatty acids from triacylglycerols. Other hormones (e.g., epinephrine, adrenocorticotropic hormone [ACTH], growth hormone) also lead to the activation of these enzymes (see Chapter 41). The resynthesis of triglyceride (using regenerated glycerol 3-P) by the adipocyte regulates the rate of release of fatty acids during fasting.

C. Mechanisms that Affect Ketone Body Production by the Liver

As fatty acids are released from adipose tissue during fasting, they travel in the blood complexed with albumin. These fatty acids are oxidized by various tissues, particularly muscle. In the liver, fatty acids are transported into mitochondria because acetyl-CoA carboxylase is inactive, malonyl-CoA levels are low, and CPTI is active (see Fig. 34.5). Acetyl-CoA, produced by β-oxidation, is converted to ketone bodies. Ketone bodies are used as an energy source by many tissues (Table 34.1) to spare the use of glucose and the necessity of degrading muscle protein to provide the precursors for gluconeogenesis. The high levels of acetyl-CoA in the liver (derived

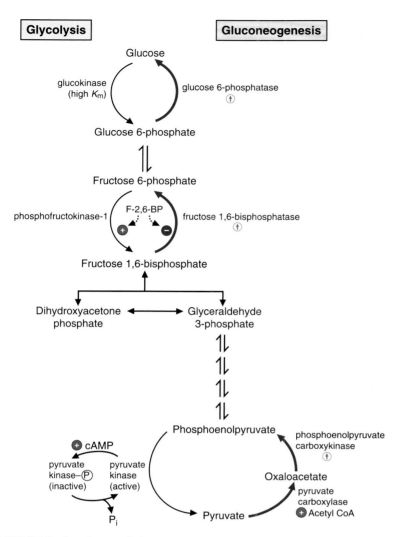

Deborah S. has type 2 diabetes mellitus. She produces insulin, but her adipose tissue is partially resistant to its actions. Therefore, her adipose tissue does not produce as much LPL as a normal person, which is one of the reasons why VLDL and chylomicrons remain elevated in her blood.

FIGURE 34.7 Regulation of gluconeogenesis (*red arrows*) and glycolysis (*black arrows*) during fasting. The gluconeogenic enzymes phosphoenolpyruvate carboxykinase, fructose 1,6-bisphosphatase, and glucose 6-phosphatase are induced ($\uparrow$). Fructose 1,6-bisphosphatase is also active because, during fasting, the level of its inhibitor, fructose 2,6-bisphosphate, is low. The corresponding enzymes of glycolysis are not very active during fasting. The rate of glucokinase is low because it has a high K_m for glucose and the glucose concentration is low. Phosphofructokinase-1 is not very active because the concentration of its activator fructose 2,6-bisphosphate is low. Pyruvate kinase is inactivated by cyclic adenosine monophosphate (cAMP)-mediated phosphorylation. *Acetyl CoA*, acetyl coenzyme A; *F-2,6-BP*, fructose 2,6-bisphosphate; P_i, inorganic phosphate.

TABLE 34.1	Fuel Use by Various Tissues during Starvation (Fasting)		
TISSUE	**GLUCOSE**	**FATTY ACIDS**	**KETONE BODIES**
Nervous system	++	−	++
Skeletal muscle	−	++	++
Heart muscle	−	++	++
Liver	−	++	−
Intestinal epithelial cells	−	−	++
Kidney	−	+	+

from fat oxidation) inhibit PDH (which prevents pyruvate from being converted to acetyl-CoA) and activate pyruvate carboxylase, which produces OAA for gluconeogenesis. The OAA does not condense with acetyl-CoA to form citrate for two reasons. The first is that under these conditions (a high rate of fat oxidation in the liver mitochondria), energy levels in the mitochondrial matrix are high; that is, there are high levels of NADH and ATP present. The high NADH level inhibits isocitrate dehydrogenase. As a result, citrate accumulates and inhibits citrate synthase from producing more citrate. The second reason that citrate synthesis is depressed is that the high $NADH/NAD^+$ ratio also diverts OAA into malate, such that the malate can exit the mitochondria (via the malate/aspartate shuttle) for use in gluconeogenesis.

D. Regulation of the Use of Glucose and Fatty Acids by Muscle

During exercise, the fuel that is used initially by muscle cells is muscle glycogen. As exercise continues and the blood supply to the tissue increases, glucose is taken up from the blood and oxidized. Liver glycogenolysis and gluconeogenesis replenish the blood glucose supply. However, as insulin levels drop, the concentration of the GLUT4 transporters in the membrane is reduced, thereby reducing glucose entry from the circulation into the muscle. However, muscle GLUT4 transporters are also induced by high AMP levels, through the action of the AMP-activated protein kinase (AMPK). Thus, if energy levels are low and the concentration of AMP increases, glucose can still be transported from the circulation into the muscle to provide energy. This will most frequently be the case during periods of exercise.

In addition, as fatty acids become available because of increased lipolysis of adipose triacylglycerols, the exercising muscle begins to oxidize fatty acids. β-Oxidation produces NADH and acetyl-CoA, which slow the flow of carbon from glucose through the reaction catalyzed by PDH (see Fig. 23.15). Thus, the oxidation of fatty acids provides a major portion of the increased demand for ATP generation and spares blood glucose.

III. The Importance of AMP and Fructose 2,6-Bisphosphate

The switch between catabolic and anabolic pathways is often regulated by the levels of AMP and fructose 2,6-bisphosphate in cells, particularly the liver. It is logical for AMP to be a critical regulator. Because a cell uses ATP in energy-requiring pathways, the levels of AMP accumulate more rapidly than that of ADP because of the adenylate kinase reaction (2 ADP → ATP and AMP). The rise in AMP levels then signals that more energy is required (usually through allosteric binding sites on enzymes and the activation of the AMPK), and the cell will switch to the activation of catabolic pathways. As AMP levels drop, and ATP levels rise, the anabolic pathways are activated to store the excess energy.

The levels of fructose 2,6-bisphosphate are also critical in regulating glycolysis versus gluconeogenesis in the liver. Under conditions of high blood glucose, and insulin release, fructose 2,6-bisphosphate levels are high because the PFK-2 kinase is in its activated state. The fructose 2,6-bisphosphate activates PFK-1 and inhibits fructose 1,6-bisphosphatase, thereby allowing glycolysis to proceed. When blood glucose levels are low and glucagon is released, PFK-2 is phosphorylated by the cAMP-dependent protein kinase and the kinase activity is inhibited (and the phosphatase activity is activated), thereby lowering fructose 2,6-bisphosphate levels and inhibiting glycolysis while favoring gluconeogenesis.

IV. General Summary

All of the material in this chapter was presented previously. However, because this information is so critical for understanding biochemistry in a way that will allow it to be used in interpreting clinical situations, it was summarized in this chapter. In addition, the information presented previously under carbohydrate metabolism has

Because **Dianne A.** produces very little insulin, she is prone to developing ketoacidosis. When insulin levels are low, adipocyte triglyceride lipase and HSL of adipose tissue are very active, resulting in increased lipolysis. The fatty acids that are released travel to the liver, where they are converted to the triacylglycerols of VLDL. They also undergo β-oxidation and conversion to ketone bodies. If Dianne does not take exogenous insulin or if her insulin levels decrease abruptly for some physiologic reason, she may develop DKA. In fact, she has had repeated bouts of DKA.

For reasons that are not as well understood, individuals with type 2 diabetes mellitus, such as **Deborah S.**, do not tend to develop DKA. One possible explanation is that the insulin resistance is tissue-specific; the insulin sensitivity of adipocytes may be greater than that of muscle and liver. It has been suggested that the level of insulin required to suppress lipolysis is only 10% that required to enhance glucose use by muscle and adipocyte. Such a tissue-specific sensitivity would lead to less fatty acids being released from adipocytes in type 2 diabetes than in type 1 diabetes, although in both cases, the release of fatty acids would be greater than that of an individual without the disease. If, however, a type II diabetic person has a precipitating event, such as the release of stress hormones (see Chapter 41), then ketoacidosis is more likely to be found as the stress hormones counteract the effects of insulin on the adipocyte.

been integrated with lipid metabolism. We have, for the most part, left out the role of allosteric modifiers and other regulatory mechanisms that finely coordinate these processes to an exquisite level. Because such details may be important for specific clinical situations, we hope this summary will serve as a framework to which the details can be fitted as students advance in their clinical studies.

Figure 34.8 is a comprehensive figure, and Tables 34.2 and 34.3 provide a list of the major regulatory enzymes of carbohydrate and lipid metabolism in the liver, an order to the events that occur, and the mechanisms by which they are controlled. This figure and tables should help students to integrate this mass of material.

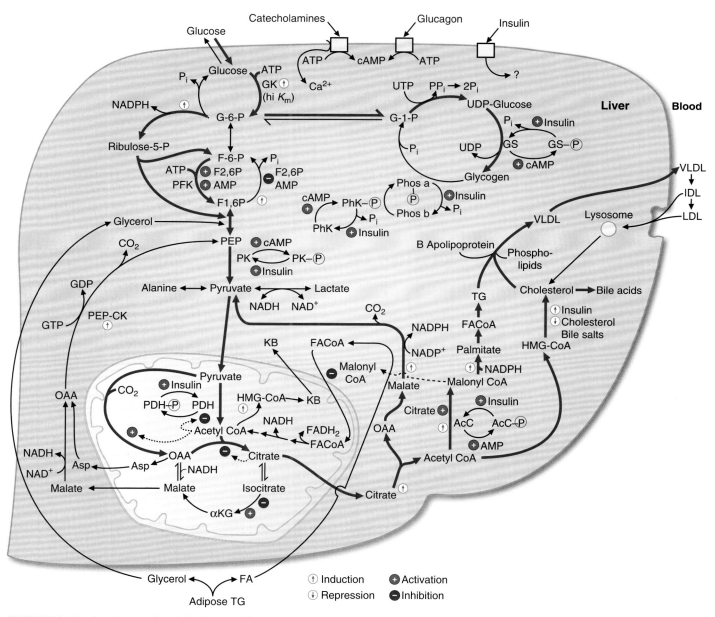

FIGURE 34.8 Regulation of carbohydrate and lipid metabolism in the liver. *Solid red arrows* indicate the flow of metabolites in the fed state. *Solid black arrows* indicate the flow during fasting. *AcC*, acetyl-CoA carboxylase; *αKG*, α-ketoglutarate; *ATP*, adenosine triphosphate; *cAMP*, cyclic adenosine monophosphate; *F1,6P*, fructose 1,6-bisphosphate; *F2,6BP*, fructose 2,6-bisphosphate; *F-6-P*, fructose 6-phosphate; *FA*, fatty acid or fatty acyl group; *FAD*, flavin adenine dinucleotide; *G-6-P*, glucose 6-phosphate; *GDP*, guanosine diphosphate; *GK*, glucokinase; *GS*, glycogen synthase; *GTP*, guanosine triphosphate; *HDL*, high-density lipoprotein; *HMG-CoA*, 3-hydroxy-3-methylglutaryl coenzyme A; *IDL*, intermediate-density lipoprotein; *LDL*, low-density lipoprotein; *NAD*, nicotinamide adenine dinucleotide; *OAA*, oxaloacetate; *circled P*, phosphate group; *PEP*, phosphoenolpyruvate; *PEPCK*, phosphoenolpyruvate carboxykinase; *PFK*, phosphofructokinase-1; *Phos*, glycogen phosphorylase; *PhK*, phosphorylase kinase; *P_i*, inorganic phosphate; *PK*, pyruvate kinase; *PP_i*, pyrophosphate; *TG*, triacylglycerol; *UDP*, uridine diphosphate; *UTP*, uridine triphosphate; *VLDL*, very-low-density lipoprotein.

TABLE 34.2	Flowchart of Changes in Liver Metabolism	
WHEN BLOOD SUGAR INCREASES	**WHEN BLOOD SUGAR DECREASES**
Insulin is released, which leads to the **dephosphorylation** of:	Glucagon is released, which leads to the **phosphorylation** of:
• PFK-2 (kinase activity now active)	• PFK-2 (phosphatase activity now active)
• Pyruvate kinase (now active)	• Pyruvate kinase (now inactive)
• Glycogen synthase (now active)	• Glycogen synthase (now inactive)
• Phosphorylase kinase (now inactive)	• Phosphorylase kinase (now active)
• Glycogen phosphorylase (now inactive)	• Glycogen phosphorylase (now active)
• Pyruvate dehydrogenase (now active)	• Pyruvate dehydrogenase (now inactive)
• Acetyl-CoA carboxylase (now active)	• Acetyl-CoA carboxylase (now inactive)
Which leads to **active**:	Which leads to **active**:
• Glycolysis	• Glycogenolysis
• Fatty acid synthesis	• Fatty acid oxidation
• Glycogen synthesis	• Gluconeogenesis

PFK-2, phosphofructokinase-2; Acetyl-CoA, acetyl-coenzyme A.

Now that many of the details of the pathways have been presented; it may be worthwhile to reread the first three chapters of this book. A student who understands biochemistry within the context of fuel metabolism is in a very good position to solve clinical problems that involve metabolic derangements.

CLINICAL COMMENTS

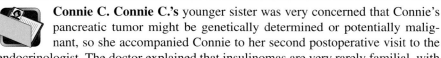

Connie C. Connie C.'s younger sister was very concerned that Connie's pancreatic tumor might be genetically determined or potentially malignant, so she accompanied Connie to her second postoperative visit to the endocrinologist. The doctor explained that insulinomas are very rarely familial, with around 10% of patients with insulinomas having a genetically determined syndrome known as *multiple endocrine neoplasia, type I*, or simply *MEN I*. This syndrome includes additional secretory neoplasms, which may occur in the anterior pituitary or the parathyroid glands. Connie's tumor showed no evidence of malignancy, and the histologic slides, although not always definitive, showed a benign-appearing process. The doctor was careful to explain, however, that close observation for recurrent hypoglycemia and for the signs and symptoms suggestive of other facets of MEN I would be necessary for the remainder of Connie's and her immediate family's life.

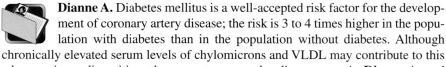

Dianne A. Diabetes mellitus is a well-accepted risk factor for the development of coronary artery disease; the risk is 3 to 4 times higher in the population with diabetes than in the population without diabetes. Although chronically elevated serum levels of chylomicrons and VLDL may contribute to this atherogenic predisposition, the premature vascular disease seen in **Dianne A.** and other patients with type 1 diabetes mellitus, as well as **Deborah S.** and other patients with type 2 diabetes mellitus, is also related to other abnormalities in lipid metabolism. Among these are the increase in glycation (nonenzymatic attachment of glucose molecules to proteins) of LDL apolipoproteins as well as glycation of the proteins of the LDL receptor, which occurs when serum glucose levels are chronically elevated. These glycations interfere with the normal interaction or "fit" of the circulating LDL particles with their specific receptors on cell membranes. As a consequence, the rate of uptake of circulating LDL by the normal target cells is diminished. The LDL particles, therefore, remain in the circulation and eventually bind nonspecifically to "scavenger" receptors located on macrophages adjacent to the endothelial surfaces of blood vessels, one of the early steps in the process of atherogenesis.

TABLE 34.3   Regulation of Liver Enzymes Involved in Glycogen, Blood Glucose, and Triacylglycerol Synthesis and Degradation

LIVER ENZYMES REGULATED BY ACTIVATION/INHIBITION

ENZYME	ACTIVATED BY	STATE IN WHICH ACTIVE
PFK-1	Fructose 2,6-bisP, AMP	Fed
Pyruvate carboxylase	Acetyl-CoA	Fed and fasting
Acetyl-CoA carboxylase	Citrate	Fed
CPTI	Loss of inhibitor (malonyl-CoA)	Fasting

LIVER ENZYMES REGULATED BY PHOSPHORYLATION/DEPHOSPHORYLATION

ENZYME	ACTIVE FORM	STATE IN WHICH ACTIVE
Glycogen synthase	Dephosphorylated	Fed
Phosphorylase kinase	Phosphorylated	Fasting
Glycogen phosphorylase	Phosphorylated	Fasting
PFK-2/fructose 2,6-bisphosphatase (acts as a kinase, increasing fructose 2,6-bisP levels)	Dephosphorylated	Fed
PFK-2/fructose 2,6-bisphosphatase (acts as a phosphatase, decreasing fructose 2,6-bisP levels)	Phosphorylated	Fasting
Pyruvate kinase	Dephosphorylated	Fed
Pyruvate dehydrogenase	Dephosphorylated	Fed
Acetyl-CoA carboxylase	Dephosphorylated	Fed

LIVER ENZYMES REGULATED BY INDUCTION/REPRESSION

ENZYME	STATE IN WHICH INDUCED	PROCESS AFFECTED
Glucokinase	Fed	Glucose → TG
Citrate lyase	Fed	Glucose → TG
Acetyl-CoA carboxylase	Fed	Glucose → TG
Fatty acid synthase	Fed	Glucose → TG
Malic enzyme	Fed	Production of NADPH
Glucose-6-P dehydrogenase	Fed	Production of NADPH
Glucose 6-phosphatase	Fasted	Production of blood glucose
Fructose 1,6-bisphosphatase	Fasted	Production of blood glucose
PEP carboxykinase	Fasted	Production of blood glucose

Acetyl-CoA, acetyl coenzyme A; AMP, adenosine monophosphate; CPTI, carnitine palmitoyltransferase I; fructose 2,6-bisP, fructose 2,6-bisphosphate; malonyl-CoA, malonyl coenzyme A; PEP, phosphoenolpyruvate; PFK-1, phosphofructokinase-1; PFK-2, phosphofructokinase-2; TG, triacylglycerol.

BIOCHEMICAL COMMENTS

AMP-Activated Protein Kinase. The AMPK is a pivotal regulatory molecule in the metabolism of carbohydrates and fats. The hepatic targets of AMPK include the following proteins:

- Acetyl-CoA carboxylase (phosphorylation reduces activity, leading to reduced fatty acid synthesis)
- Eukaryotic elongation factor 2 (eEF-2) kinase (this protein is activated when phosphorylated, and it will lead to a reduction in protein synthesis)
- Glycerol 3-P acyltransferase (GPAT) (phosphorylation reduces activity, leading to reduced triglyceride synthesis)
- 3-Hydroxy-3-methylglutaryl coenzyme A (HMG-CoA) reductase (phosphorylation reduces activity, leading to reduced cholesterol synthesis)
- Malonyl-CoA decarboxylase (MCD) (active when phosphorylated, reduces malonyl-CoA levels, allowing fatty acid oxidation to occur)
- Mammalian target of rapamycin (mTOR) (reduced activity when phosphorylated, leading to reduced protein synthesis)
- Tuberous sclerosis complex 2 (TSC2) (increased activity when phosphorylated, leading to reduced protein synthesis)
- TORC2 (the protein is sequestered in the cytoplasm when phosphorylated, leading to decreased expression [at the transcriptional level] of gluconeogenic enzymes)

The overall effect of AMPK activation is reduced fatty acid and triglyceride synthesis (via effects on acetyl-CoA carboxylase, GPAT, and MCD), reduced cholesterol synthesis (via inhibition of HMG-CoA reductase), and reduced protein synthesis (via effects on mTOR and TSC2). There is a concomitant increase in fatty acid oxidation to raise ATP levels. Because the processes described previously are all highly energy-dependent, it makes sense to turn them off when energy levels are low, as exemplified by increased AMP levels.

mTOR (rapamycin is a drug that is a potent immunosuppressant) is a protein kinase, which, when active, phosphorylates key proteins that regulate and initiate protein synthesis. AMPK phosphorylation of mTOR blocks the activation of mTOR. mTOR can be activated by TSC2 through a complex pathway involving the GTP-binding protein Rheb. The TSC complex (consisting of TSC1 and TSC2) acts as a GTPase-activating protein for Rheb. Rheb-GTP activates mTOR, whereas Rheb-GDP does not. Phosphorylation of TSC2 by the AMPK activates the GTPase-activating activity of TSC2, leading to Rheb-GDP formation, and reduced mTOR activity. The reduced mTOR activity leads to a reduction of protein synthesis.

mTOR also plays a critical role in transmitting the signal from the insulin receptor to an increase in protein synthesis within the cell. Insulin receptor activation leads to Akt activation (see Fig. 11.14). The protein kinase Akt (protein kinase B) will phosphorylate the TSC1/TSC2 complex and inactivate the GTPase-activating component of the complex. Under these conditions, then, Rheb-GTP will be long-lived, and mTOR will be active, leading to an enhancement of protein synthesis in the cell. The interaction of TSC1/TSC2, mTOR, and its regulatory kinases is depicted in Figure 34.9.

The AMPK can be activated in several ways, all of which depend on increased AMP levels within the cell. As the concentration of AMP increases, AMPK is activated by allosteric means, or by phosphorylation by LKB1 (see Chapter 32), or by phosphorylation by a calmodulin kinase kinase. AMPK is inactivated by dephosphorylation by protein phosphatases, or a decrease in AMP levels. Small changes in intracellular AMP levels can have profound effects on AMPK activity because of these multiple regulatory pathways.

AMPK is a heterotrimeric complex that consists of a catalytic subunit (α) and two regulatory subunits (β and γ). The allosteric activation of AMPK occurs via AMP binding to the α-subunit; the phosphorylation activation of AMPK occurs via threonine phosphorylation on the α-subunit. Different tissues express different isoforms of the α-, β-, and γ-subunits, giving rise to a wide variety of isozymes of AMPK in the different tissues.

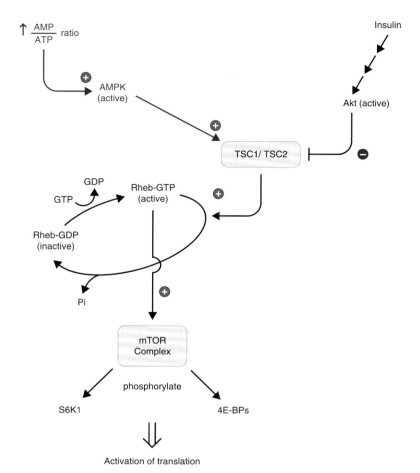

FIGURE 34.9 Central role of mTOR and the TSC1/TSC2 complex in regulating protein synthesis. The TSC1/TSC2 complex acts as a guanosine triphosphatase (GTPase)-activating protein for the G-protein Rheb. When active, Rheb-GTP activates the mTOR kinase, leading to phosphorylation events that promote protein synthesis (S6K1 and 4E-BPs are phosphorylated). AMP-activated protein kinase (AMPK) phosphorylation of the TSC1/TSC2 complex activates the complex such that the GTPase activity of Rheb is enhanced, leading to Rheb inactivation and loss of mTOR kinase activity. This will lead to a decrease in protein synthesis. Insulin binding to its receptor leads to the activation of the protein kinase Akt (see Fig. 11.14). Akt will phosphorylate the TSC1/TSC2 complex at sites distinct from AMPK, and which inhibits the GTPase-activating activity of the complex. This allows Rheb-GTP to be active for extended periods of time, activating mTOR, and increasing protein synthesis in the cell in response to insulin. *AMP*, adenosine monophosphate; *ATP*, adenosine triphosphate; *GDP*, guanosine diphosphate; *GTP*, guanosine triphosphate; *P$_i$*, inorganic phosphate.

KEY CONCEPTS

- Three key controlling elements determine whether a fuel is metabolized or stored: hormones, concentration of available fuels, and energy needs of the body.
- Key intracellular enzymes are generally regulated by allosteric activation and inhibition, by covalent modification, by transcriptional control, and by degradation.
- Regulation is complex in order to allow sensitivity and feedback to multiple stimuli so that an exact balance can be maintained between synthesis of a product and need for the product.

- The insulin/glucagon ratio is primarily responsible for the hormonal regulation of carbohydrate and lipid metabolism.
- The key enzymes of glycolysis, fatty acid synthesis, fatty acid degradation, glycogen synthesis, glycogenolysis, and gluconeogenesis are all regulated in a coordinated manner, allowing the appropriate pathways to be activated and inhibited without the creation of futile cycles.
- This chapter summarizes, in one package, all of the major regulatory events discussed in the previous 15 chapters.
- Diseases discussed in this chapter are summarized in Table 34.4.

TABLE 34.4 Diseases Discussed in Chapter 34		
DISEASE OR DISORDER	**ENVIRONMENTAL OR GENETIC**	**COMMENTS**
Insulinoma	Environmental (~10% genetic)	A tumor of the pancreas leading to excessive, episodic insulin secretion, usually coupled with weight gain to avoid hypoglycemia
Diabetic keto-acidosis (type I diabetes)	Environmental	Diabetic ketoacidosis (DKA) occurs because of an elevation of ketone-body levels owing to reduced levels of insulin in a type I diabetic person. DKA is not normally seen in type 2 diabetic persons because of only a partial resistance of adipocytes to circulating insulin.
Type 2 diabetes	Both	Reduced ability of tissues to respond to insulin, even though insulin is being produced. Different tissues may display a differential sensitivity to insulin, particularly fat cells as compared to muscle cells.

REVIEW QUESTIONS—CHAPTER 34

1. A 20-year-old woman with diabetes mellitus was admitted to the hospital in a semiconscious state with fever, nausea, and vomiting. Her breath smelled of acetone. A urine sample was strongly positive for ketone bodies. Which one of the following statements about this woman is correct?
   A. A blood glucose test will probably show that her blood glucose level is well below 80 mg/dL.
   B. An injection of insulin will decrease her ketone-body production.
   C. She should be given a glucose infusion so she will regain consciousness.
   D. Glucagon should be administered to stimulate glycogenolysis and gluconeogenesis in the liver.
   E. The acetone was produced by decarboxylation of the ketone body β-hydroxybutyrate.

2. A woman was told by her physician to go on a low-fat diet. She decided to continue to consume the same number of calories by increasing her carbohydrate intake while decreasing her fat intake. Which of the following blood lipoprotein levels would be decreased as a consequence of her diet?
   A. VLDL
   B. IDL
   C. HDL
   D. Chylomicrons
   E. HDL

3. Assume that an individual has been eating excess calories daily such that he will gain weight. Under which one of the following conditions will the person gain weight most rapidly?
   A. If all the excess calories are from carbohydrate
   B. If all the excess calories are from triacylglycerol
   C. If all the excess calories are split 50%/50% between carbohydrate and triacylglycerol
   D. If all the excess calories are split 25%/75% between carbohydrate and triacylglycerol
   E. It makes no difference what form the excess calories are in.

4. A chronic alcoholic has been admitted to the hospital because of a severe hypoglycemic episode brought about by excessive alcohol consumption for the past 5 days. A blood lipid analysis indicates much higher than expected VLDL levels. The elevated VLDL is attributable to which one of the following underlying causes?
   A. Alcohol-induced inhibition of LPL
   B. Elevated NADH levels in the liver
   C. Alcohol-induced transcription of the *apoB-100* gene
   D. NADH activation of phosphoenolpyruvate carboxykinase
   E. Acetaldehyde induction of enzymes on the endoplasmic reticulum

5. Certain patients with abetalipoproteinemia frequently have difficulty maintaining blood volume; their blood has trouble clotting. This symptom is attributable to which of the following?
   A. Inability to produce chylomicrons
   B. Inability to produce VLDL
   C. Inability to synthesize clotting factors
   D. Inability to synthesize fatty acids
   E. Inability to absorb short-chain fatty acids

6. Which one of the following schemes most accurately depicts the timeline of the metabolic processes of the liver after a carbohydrate meal is ingested followed by 3 hours of fasting?
   A. Glycolysis, glycogen synthesis, lipolysis, glycogenolysis, gluconeogenesis
   B. Glycogen synthesis, lipolysis, glycogenolysis, gluconeogenesis
   C. Glycolysis, lipolysis, glycogenolysis, gluconeogenesis, glycogen synthesis
   D. Glycogen synthesis, lipolysis, gluconeogenesis, glycolysis
   E. Glycogen synthesis, glycogenolysis, lipolysis, gluconeogenesis

7. A person with type 1 diabetes who has neglected to take insulin for 2 days, yet who ate normally, would exhibit elevated levels of circulating triglycerides because of which one of the following?
   A. Reduced synthesis of apolipoprotein CII
   B. Reduced release of LPL from muscle and fat cells
   C. Increased synthesis of LDL
   D. Reduced synthesis of chylomicrons
   E. Reduced synthesis of VLDL

8. Under conditions of a low insulin/glucagon ratio, which one of the following allosteric modifiers in muscle can lead to a stimulation of both glycolysis and fatty acid oxidation?
   A. ATP
   B. ADP
   C. AMP
   D. Acetyl-CoA
   E. Citrate

9. Which one of the following is a major difference between patients with diabetes mellitus types 1 and 2?
   A. In type 1, insulin levels are very low and insulin resistance is high.
   B. In type 2, insulin levels are very low and insulin resistance is high.
   C. In both types, the patient is usually at or below ideal body weight.
   D. In type 1, C-peptide levels are very low.
   E. In type 1, the patient is usually overweight.

10. A person is training for a half-marathon. After running 5 miles, which one of the following is providing most of the products for ATP generation in the muscles?
    A. Muscle glycogen
    B. Liver glycogen
    C. Blood glucose
    D. Ketone bodies
    E. Fatty acids

ANSWERS

1. **The answer is B.** The acetone on the woman's breath (which is produced by decarboxylation of acetoacetate; thus, E is incorrect) and the ketones in her urine indicate that she is in DKA. This is caused by low insulin levels, so her blood glucose levels are high because the glucose is not being taken up by the peripheral tissues (thus, A and C are incorrect). An insulin injection will reduce her blood glucose levels and decrease the release of fatty acids from adipose triglycerides. Consequently, ketone-body production will decrease. Glucagon injections would just exacerbate the woman's current condition (thus, D is incorrect).

2. **The answer is D.** Chylomicrons are blood lipoproteins produced from dietary fat. VLDL are produced mainly from dietary carbohydrate. Intermediate-density lipoprotein and LDL are produced from VLDL. HDL does not transport triacylglycerol to the tissues.

3. **The answer is B.** Consider the energy required to convert dietary carbohydrates to triacylglycerol. Some ATP is generated from glycolysis and the PDH reaction, but energy is also lost as the fatty acids are synthesized (the synthesis of each malonyl-CoA requires ATP, and the reduction

steps require two molecules of NADPH). Dietary fat, however, only requires activation and attachment to glycerol; the fatty acid chain does not need to be synthesized. Therefore, it requires less energy to package dietary fat into chylomicrons than it does to convert dietary carbohydrate into fatty acids for incorporation into VLDL. Thus, weight gain will be more rapid if all the excess calories are derived from fat as opposed to carbohydrates.

4. **The answer is B.** Metabolism of ethanol leads to production of NADH in the liver, which will inhibit fatty acid oxidation in the liver. Because the patient has not eaten for 5 days, the insulin/glucagon ratio is low, adipocyte triglyceride lipase and HSL are activated, and fatty acids are being released by the adipocyte and taken up by the muscle and liver. However, because the liver NADH levels are high as a result of ethanol metabolism, the fatty acids received from the adipocyte are repackaged into triacylglycerol (the high NADH promotes the conversion of dihydroxyacetone phosphate to glycerol 3-P as well) and secreted from the liver in the form of VLDL. None of the other answers is a correct statement.

5. **The answer is A.** The clotting problems are caused by a lack of vitamin K, a lipid-soluble vitamin. Vitamin K is absorbed from the diet in mixed micelles and packaged with chylomicrons for delivery to the other tissues. Individuals with abetalipoproteinemia lack the microsomal triglyceride transfer protein and cannot produce chylomicrons effectively, vitamin K deficiency can result. Such patients also cannot produce VLDL, but lipid-soluble vitamin distribution does not depend on VLDL particles, only on chylomicrons. The other answers are all incorrect statements.

6. **The answer is E.** After eating a high-carbohydrate meal, the excess carbohydrates in the liver are first stored as glycogen and then sent through glycolysis to generate pyruvate and then acetyl-CoA, for eventual fatty acid production. After time, as the blood glucose is used by tissues, its levels will drop, and glucagon will be released from the pancreas, which will stimulate glycogenolysis in the liver such that glucose can be exported to raise blood glucose levels. The glucagon release also stimulates lipolysis, and energy from fatty acid oxidation is used to produce glucose via gluconeogenesis.

7. **The answer is B.** Insulin is required for muscle and fat cells to synthesize and release LPL to bind to the capillary walls of the capillaries supplying these tissues with blood. In the absence of insulin, LPL levels would be reduced, and there would be a reduced rate of triglyceride removal from both chylomicrons and VLDL particles. Chylomicron synthesis would be normal on a normal diet. The problem is that the lipid is not leaving the chylomicron as rapidly as it normally would because of the reduced levels of LPL on the capillary walls. VLDL synthesis would actually increase, owing to fatty acid synthesis by the liver (because of the high levels of glucose in the blood), and because of excess fatty acids reaching the liver owing to increased lipolysis of triacylglycerol in the fat cell, as induced by the absence of insulin.

8. **The answer is C.** When blood glucose levels are low and the muscle requires energy, ATP is used and ADP is produced. Adenylate kinase catalyzes the conversion of two ADP to ATP and AMP, and an increase in AMP leads to the activation of the AMP-activated protein kinase. This kinase phosphorylates and inactivates acetyl-CoA carboxylase. This leads to lower levels of

malonyl-CoA, and a release of the inhibition of CPTI, such that fatty acid oxidation is enhanced because the fatty acids can enter the mitochondrial matrix to be oxidized. The increase in AMP levels also activates PFK-1, speeding up the glycolytic pathway. Citrate does not accumulate under conditions in which the insulin/glucagon ratio is low, and acetyl-CoA is not an allosteric modifier of any glycolytic enzyme.

9. **The answer is D.** In type 1 diabetes mellitus, the patient is producing low or no insulin, which means that C-peptide levels are very low or nondetectable. The patients are usually thin because low insulin does not promote adipose tissue storage of triacylglycerol. There is no insulin resistance in type 1 because the patients are not producing insulin. Insulin resistance at the cellular level primarily causes type 2 diabetes mellitus. Because of the resistance, insulin levels are generally elevated to attempt to overcome this resistance. With elevated insulin levels, adipose tissue storage of triacylglycerol is high and the patient is almost always overweight. There are exceptions to this general statement, and those are patients who have inherited a mutation leading to type 2 diabetes, such as maturity-onset diabetes of the young (MODY).

10. **The answer is E.** Initially, muscles use glucose from muscle glycogen, and fatty acids provided by the adipocyte. As the run continues, the levels of AMP increase in the muscle, which leads to activation of the AMP-activated protein kinase. This kinase leads to a reduction of malonyl-CoA levels in the muscle (by inhibiting, via phosphorylation, acetyl-CoA carboxylase and activating, via phosphorylation, MCD), which allows for fatty acid entrance into the mitochondria. The muscle does not contain sufficient glycogen to provide energy for the entire marathon, so a mixture of fatty acids and glucose (from glycogen) is used by the muscle for optimal performance. In an adult, there is no ketone-body production during the race. Blood glucose can be taken up by the muscle (the activation of the AMP-activated protein kinase stimulates the fusion of GLUT4 containing vesicles with the plasma membrane), but the runner will race at a pace that allows some of the blood glucose to be used by the nervous system, which requires that the muscles use fatty acids to generate energy.

Nitrogen Metabolism

Dietary proteins are the primary source of the nitrogen that is metabolized by the body (Fig. VI.1). Amino acids, produced by digestion of dietary proteins, are absorbed through intestinal epithelial cells and enter the blood. Various cells take up these amino acids, which enter the cellular pools. They are used for the synthesis of proteins and other nitrogen-containing compounds or they are oxidized for energy.

Protein synthesis, the translation of messenger RNA on ribosomes (see Chapter 15), is a dynamic process. Within the body, proteins are constantly being synthesized and degraded, partially draining and then refilling the cellular amino acid pools.

Compounds derived from amino acids include cellular proteins, hormones, neurotransmitters, creatine phosphate, the heme of hemoglobin and the cytochromes, the skin pigment melanin, and the purine and pyrimidine bases of nucleotides and nucleic acids. In fact, all of the nitrogen-containing compounds of the body are synthesized from amino acids. Many of these pathways are outlined in the following chapters.

In addition to serving as the precursors for the nitrogen-containing compounds of the body and as the building blocks for protein synthesis, amino acids are also a source of energy. Amino acids are either oxidized directly or the amino acid carbons are converted to glucose and then oxidized or stored as glycogen. The amino acid carbons may also be converted to fatty acids and stored as adipose triacylglycerols. Glycogen and triacylglycerols are oxidized during periods of fasting. The liver is the major site of amino acid oxidation. However, most tissues can oxidize the branched-chain amino acids (leucine, isoleucine, and valine).

Before the carbon skeletons of amino acids are oxidized, the nitrogen must be removed. Amino acid nitrogen forms ammonia, which is toxic to the body. In the liver, ammonia and the amino groups from amino acids are converted to urea, which is nontoxic, water-soluble, and readily excreted in the urine. The process by which urea is produced is known as the urea cycle. The liver is the organ responsible for producing urea. Branched-chain amino acids can be oxidized in many tissues, but the nitrogen must always travel to the liver for disposal.

Although urea is the major nitrogenous excretory product of the body, nitrogen is also excreted in other compounds (Table VI.1). Uric acid is the degradation product of the purine bases, creatinine is produced from creatine phosphate, and ammonia is released from glutamine, particularly by the kidney, where it helps to buffer the urine by reacting with protons to form ammonium ions (NH_4^+). These compounds are excreted mainly in the urine, but substantial amounts are also lost in the feces and through the skin. Small amounts of nitrogen-containing metabolites are formed from the degradation of neurotransmitters, hormones, and other specialized amino acid products and excreted in the urine. Some of these degradation products, such as bilirubin (formed from the degradation of heme), are excreted mainly in the feces.

Eleven of the 20 amino acids used to form proteins are synthesized in the body if an adequate amount is not present in the diet (Table VI.2). Ten of these amino acids can be produced from glucose; the 11th, tyrosine, is synthesized from the essential amino acid phenylalanine. It should be noted that cysteine, one of the

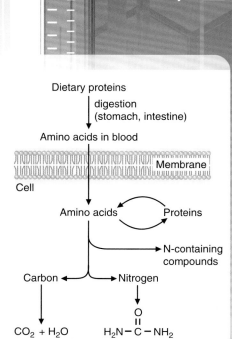

FIGURE VI.1 Summary of amino acid metabolism. Dietary proteins are digested to amino acids in the stomach and intestine, which are absorbed by the intestinal epithelium, transferred to the circulation, and taken up by cells. Amino acids are used to synthesize proteins and other nitrogen-containing compounds. The carbon skeletons of amino acids are also oxidized for energy, and the nitrogen is converted to urea and other nitrogenous excretory products.

 The healthy human adult is in nitrogen balance; in other words, the amount of nitrogen excreted each day (mainly in the urine) equals the amount consumed (mainly as dietary protein). Negative nitrogen balance occurs when the amount of nitrogen excreted is greater than the amount consumed, and positive nitrogen balance occurs when the amount excreted is less than that consumed (see Chapter 1).

TABLE VI.1	**Major Nitrogenous Urinary Excretory Products**	
AMOUNT EXCRETED IN URINE PER DAY[a]		
Urea[b]	12–20 g of urea nitrogen (12,000–20,000 mg)	
NH$_4^+$	140–1500 mg of ammonia nitrogen	
Creatinine	Men	14–26 mg/kg
	Women	11–20 mg/kg
Uric acid	250–750 mg	

[a]The amounts are expressed in the units that are generally reported by clinical laboratories. Note that the amounts for creatinine and uric acid are for the whole compound, whereas those for urea and ammonia are for the nitrogen content.

[b]Under normal circumstances, approximately 90% of the nitrogen excreted in the urine is in the form of urea. The exact amounts of each component vary, however, depending on dietary protein intake and physiologic state. For instance, NH$_4^+$ excretion increases during acidosis because the kidney secretes ammonia to bind protons in the urine.

TABLE VI.2	**Amino Acids Synthesized in the Body**[a]
FROM GLUCOSE	**FROM AN ESSENTIAL AMINO ACID**
Alanine	Tyrosine (from phenylalanine)
Arginine	
Asparagine	
Aspartate	
Cysteine[b]	
Glutamate	
Glutamine	
Glycine	
Proline	
Serine	

[a]These amino acids are called "nonessential" or "dispensable," terms that refer to dietary requirements. Of course, within the body, they are necessary. We cannot survive without them.

[b]Although the carbons of cysteine can be derived from glucose, its sulfur is obtained from the essential amino acid methionine.

TABLE VI.3	**Amino Acids Essential in the Diet**
Histidine	
Isoleucine	
Leucine	
Lysine	
Methionine	
Phenylalanine	
Threonine	
Tryptophan	
Valine	
Arginine (not required by adults, but required for growth)	

10 amino acids produced from glucose, obtains its sulfur atom from the essential amino acid methionine.

Nine amino acids are essential in the human. "Essential" means that the carbon skeleton cannot be synthesized, and therefore, these amino acids are required in the diet (Table VI.3). The essential amino acids are also called the "indispensable" amino acids. Arginine is essential during periods of growth; in adults, it is no longer considered essential.

After nitrogen is removed from amino acids, the carbon skeletons are oxidized (Fig. VI.2). Most of the carbons are converted to pyruvate, intermediates of the tricarboxylic acid (TCA) cycle, or to acetyl coenzyme A (acetyl-CoA). In the liver, particularly during fasting, these carbons may be converted to glucose or to ketone bodies and released into the blood. Other tissues then oxidize the glucose and ketone bodies. Ultimately, the carbons of the amino acids are converted to CO_2 and H_2O.

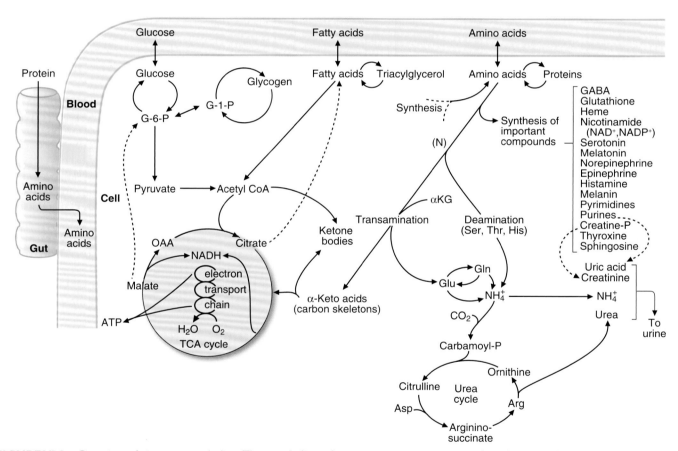

FIGURE VI.2 Overview of nitrogen metabolism. The metabolism of nitrogen-containing compounds is shown on the *right* and that of glucose and fatty acids is shown on the *left*. This figure shows a hypothetical composite cell. No single cell type has all of these pathways. Many of the pathways shown are described in the next few chapters. *Acetyl CoA*, acetyl coenzyme A; *ATP*, adenosine triphosphate; αKG, α-ketoglutarate; *OAA*, oxaloacetate; *G 6-P*, glucose 6-phosphate; *G 1-P*, glucose 1-phosphate; *TCA*, tricarboxylic acid.

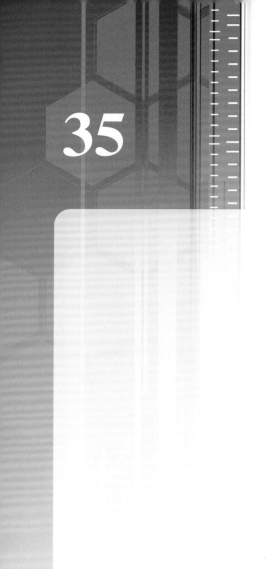

Protein Digestion and Amino Acid Absorption

Proteolytic enzymes (also called **proteases**) break down dietary proteins into their constituent amino acids in the **stomach** and the **intestine**. Many of these digestive proteases are synthesized as larger, inactive forms known as **zymogens**. After zymogens are secreted into the digestive tract, they are cleaved to produce the active proteases.

In the stomach, **pepsin** begins the digestion of proteins by hydrolyzing them to smaller polypeptides. The contents of the stomach pass into the small intestine, where enzymes produced by the exocrine pancreas act. The pancreatic proteases (**trypsin**, **chymotrypsin**, **elastase**, and the **carboxypeptidases**) cleave the polypeptides into oligopeptides and amino acids.

Further cleavage of the oligopeptides to amino acids is accomplished by enzymes produced by the intestinal epithelial cells. These enzymes include **aminopeptidases** located on the brush border and other peptidases located within the cells. Ultimately, the amino acids produced by protein digestion are absorbed through the **intestinal epithelial cells** and enter the **blood**.

A large number of overlapping transport systems exist for amino acids in cells. Some systems contain **facilitative transporters**, whereas others express **sodium-linked transporters**, which allow the **active transport** of amino acids into cells. Defects in amino acid transport can lead to disease.

Proteins are also continually synthesized and degraded (**turnover**) in cells. A wide variety of proteases in cells carry out this activity. **Lysosomal proteases** (**cathepsins**) degrade proteins that enter lysosomes. Cytoplasmic proteins targeted for turnover are covalently linked to the small protein **ubiquitin**, which then interacts with a large protein complex, the **proteasome**, to degrade the protein in an adenosine triphosphate (ATP)–dependent process. The amino acids released from proteins during turnover can then be used for the synthesis of new proteins or for energy generation.

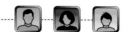

 Susan F., a young child with cystic fibrosis (see Chapter 17), has had repeated bouts of bronchitis/bronchiolitis caused by *Pseudomonas aeruginosa*. With each of these infections, her response to aerosolized antibiotics has been good. However, her malabsorption of food continues, resulting in foul-smelling, glistening, bulky stools. Her growth records show a slow decline. She is now in the 24th percentile for height and the 20th percentile for weight. She is often listless and irritable, and she tires easily. When her pediatrician discovered that her levels of the serum proteins albumin and prealbumin were low to low-normal (indicating protein malnutrition), Susan was given enteric-coated microspheres of pancreatic enzymes. Almost immediately, the character of Susan's stools became more normal and she began gaining weight. Over the next 6 months, her growth curves showed improvement, and she seemed brighter, more active, and less irritable.

 For the first few months after a painful episode of renal colic, during which he passed a kidney stone (see Chapter 6), **David K.** had faithfully maintained a high daily fluid intake and had taken the medication required to increase the pH of his urine. David had been diagnosed with cystinuria, a genetically determined amino acid substitution in the transport protein that normally reabsorbs cysteine, arginine, and lysine from the kidney lumen back into the renal tubular cells. Therefore, his urine contained high amounts of these amino acids. Cystine, which is less soluble than the other amino acids, precipitates in the urine to form renal stones (also known as *calculi*). The measures David was instructed to follow were necessary to increase the solubility of the large amounts of cystine present in his urine and thereby to prevent further formation of kidney stones. With time, however, he became increasingly complacent about his preventive program. After failing to take his medication for a month, he experienced another severe episode of renal colic with grossly bloody urine. Fortunately, he passed the stone spontaneously, after which he vowed to comply faithfully with his prescribed therapy.

His mother heard that some dietary amino acids were not absorbed in patients with cystinuria and asked whether any dietary changes would reduce David's chances of developing additional renal stones.

I. Protein Digestion

The digestion of proteins begins in the stomach and is completed in the intestine (Fig. 35.1). The enzymes that digest proteins are produced as inactive precursors (zymogens) that are larger than the active enzymes. The inactive zymogens are secreted from the cells in which they are synthesized and enter the lumen of the digestive tract, where they are cleaved to smaller forms that have proteolytic activity (Fig. 35.2). These active enzymes have different specificities; no single enzyme can completely digest a protein. However, by acting in concert, they can digest dietary proteins to amino acids and small peptides, which are cleaved by peptidases associated with intestinal epithelial cells.

A. Digestion in the Stomach

Pepsinogen is secreted by the chief cells of the stomach. The gastric parietal cells secrete hydrochloric acid (HCl). The acid in the stomach lumen alters the conformation of pepsinogen so that it can cleave itself, producing the active protease pepsin. Thus, the activation of pepsinogen is autocatalytic.

Dietary proteins are denatured by the acid in the stomach. This inactivates the proteins and partially unfolds them so that they are better substrates for proteases. However, at the low pH of the stomach, pepsin is not denatured and acts as an

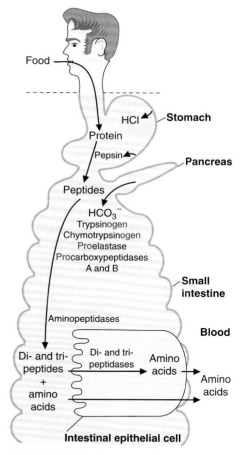

FIGURE 35.1 Digestion of proteins. The proteolytic enzymes—pepsin, trypsin, chymotrypsin, elastase, and the carboxypeptidases—are produced as zymogens (the *pro* and *ogen*, in *red*, accompanying the enzyme name) that are activated by cleavage after they enter the gastrointestinal lumen (see Fig. 35.2). Pepsinogen is produced within the stomach and is activated within the stomach (to pepsin) as the pH drops owing to hydrochloric acid (HCl) secretion.

Kwashiorkor, a common problem of children in Third World countries, is caused by a deficiency of protein in a diet that is adequate in calories. Children with kwashiorkor suffer from muscle wasting and decreased concentration of plasma proteins, particularly albumin. The result is an increase in interstitial fluid that causes edema and a distended abdomen, which makes the children appear "plump" (see Chapter 40). The muscle wasting is caused by the lack of essential amino acids in the diet; existing proteins must be broken down to produce these amino acids for new protein synthesis. These problems may be compounded by a decreased ability to produce digestive enzymes and new intestinal epithelial cells because of a decreased availability of amino acids for the synthesis of new proteins.

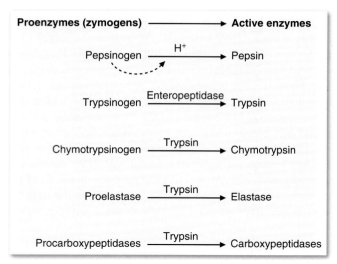

FIGURE 35.2 Activation of the gastric and pancreatic zymogens. Pepsinogen catalyzes its own cleavage as the pH of the stomach drops. Trypsinogen is cleaved by enteropeptidase in the intestine to form the active protease trypsin. Trypsin then plays a key role by catalyzing the cleavage and activation of the other pancreatic zymogens.

 Elastase is also found in neutrophils, which are white blood cells that engulf and destroy invading bacteria. Neutrophils frequently act in the lung, and elastase is sometimes released into the lung as the neutrophils work. In normal individuals, the released elastase is blocked from destroying lung cells by the action of circulating α_1-antitrypsin, a protease inhibitor that is synthesized and secreted by the liver. Certain individuals have a genetic mutation that leads to the production of an inactive α_1-antitrypsin protein (α_1-antitrypsin deficiency). The lack of this enzyme activity leads to the development of emphysema caused by proteolytic destruction of lung cells, which results in a reduction in the expansion/contraction capability of the lungs. Deficiency of α_1-antitrypsin can be measured using a dried blood spot. The blood is solubilized using a buffer and then various amounts of the blood sample are incubated with antibodies specific for α_1-antitrypsin. The antigen–antibody complexes formed will disperse light, and the extent of light-scattering is proportional to the concentration of α_1-antitrypsin in the solution. This procedure is known as *rate nephelometry*. Obtaining blood samples from a finger prick and allowing the blood to dry on a card enables rapid screening of individuals for this disorder.

endopeptidase, cleaving peptide bonds at various points within the protein chain. Although pepsin has fairly broad specificity, it tends to cleave peptide bonds in which the carboxyl group is provided by an aromatic or acidic amino acid (Fig. 35.3). Smaller peptides and some free amino acids are produced.

B. Digestion by Enzymes from the Pancreas

As the gastric contents empty into the intestine, they encounter the secretions from the exocrine pancreas. Recall that the exocrine pancreas secretes amylase for starch digestion, and lipase and colipase for dietary triacylglycerol digestion. Another pancreatic secretion is bicarbonate, which, in addition to neutralizing stomach acid, raises the pH so that the pancreatic proteases, which are also present in pancreatic secretions, can be active. As secreted, these pancreatic proteases are in the inactive proenzyme form (zymogens). Because the active forms of these enzymes can digest each other, it is important for their zymogen forms all to be activated within a short span of time. This is accomplished by the cleavage of trypsinogen to the active enzyme trypsin, which then cleaves the other pancreatic zymogens, producing their active forms (see Fig. 35.2).

The zymogen trypsinogen is cleaved to form trypsin by *enteropeptidase* (a protease, formerly called *enterokinase*) secreted by the brush-border cells of the small intestine. Trypsin catalyzes the cleavages that convert chymotrypsinogen to the active enzyme chymotrypsin, proelastase to elastase, and the procarboxypeptidases to the carboxypeptidases. Thus, trypsin plays a central role in digestion because it both cleaves dietary proteins and activates other digestive proteases produced by the pancreas.

Trypsin, chymotrypsin, and elastase are serine proteases (see Chapter 8) that act as endopeptidases. Trypsin is the most specific of these enzymes, cleaving peptide bonds in which the carboxyl (carbonyl) group is provided by lysine or arginine (see Fig. 35.3). Chymotrypsin is less specific but favors residues that contain hydrophobic amino acids. Elastase cleaves not only elastin (for which it was named) but also other proteins at bonds in which the carboxyl group is contributed by amino acid residues with small side chains (alanine, glycine, and serine). The actions of these pancreatic endopeptidases continue the digestion of dietary proteins begun by pepsin in the stomach.

The smaller peptides formed by the action of trypsin, chymotrypsin, and elastase are attacked by exopeptidases, which are proteases that cleave one amino acid at a time from the end of the chain. Procarboxypeptidases, zymogens produced by the pancreas, are converted by trypsin to the active carboxypeptidases. These exopeptidases remove amino acids from the carboxyl ends of peptide chains. Carboxypeptidase A preferentially releases hydrophobic amino acids, whereas carboxypeptidase B releases basic amino acids (arginine and lysine).

C. Digestion by Enzymes from Intestinal Cells

Exopeptidases produced by intestinal epithelial cells act within the brush border and also within the cell. Aminopeptidases, located on the brush border, cleave one amino acid at a time from the amino end of peptides. Intracellular peptidases act on small peptides that are absorbed by the cells.

The concerted action of the proteolytic enzymes produced by cells of the stomach, pancreas, and intestine cleaves dietary proteins to amino acids. The digestive enzymes digest themselves as well as dietary protein. They also digest the intestinal cells that are regularly sloughed off into the lumen. These cells are replaced by cells that mature from precursor cells in the duodenal crypts. The amount of protein that is digested and absorbed each day from digestive juices and cells released into the intestinal lumen may be equal to, or greater than, the amount of protein consumed in the diet (50 to 100 g).

II. Absorption of Amino Acids

Amino acids are absorbed from the intestinal lumen through secondary active Na^+-dependent transport systems and through facilitated diffusion.

A. Cotransport of Sodium Ions and Amino Acids

Amino acids are absorbed from the lumen of the small intestine principally by semispecific Na^+-dependent transport proteins in the luminal membrane of the intestinal cell brush border, similar to that already seen for carbohydrate transport (Fig. 35.4). The cotransport of Na^+ and the amino acid from the outside of the apical membrane to the inside of the cell is driven by the low intracellular Na^+ concentration.

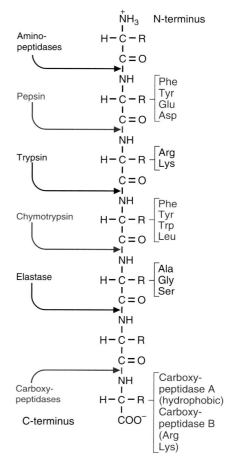

FIGURE 35.3 Action of the digestive proteases. Pepsin, trypsin, chymotrypsin, and elastase are endopeptidases; they hydrolyze peptide bonds within chains. The others are exopeptidases; aminopeptidases remove the amino acid at the N terminus and the carboxypeptidases remove the amino acid at the C terminus. For each proteolytic enzyme, the amino acid residues involved in the peptide bond that is cleaved are listed beside the R group to the *right* of the enzyme name.

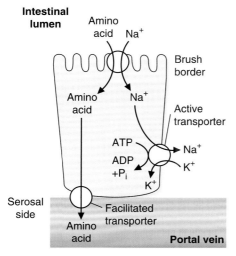

FIGURE 35.4 Transepithelial amino acid transport. Na^+-dependent carriers transport both Na^+ and an amino acid into the intestinal epithelial cell from the intestinal lumen. Na^+ is pumped out on the serosal side (across the basolateral membrane) in exchange for K^+ by the Na^+,K^+-ATPase. On the serosal side, the amino acid is carried by a facilitated transporter down its concentration gradient into the blood. This process is an example of secondary active transport. *ADP*, adenosine diphosphate; *ATP*, adenosine triphosphate; P_i, inorganic phosphate.

Patients with cystic fibrosis, such as **Susan F.**, have a genetically determined defect in the function of the chloride channels. In the pancreatic secretory ducts, which carry pancreatic enzymes into the lumen of the small intestine, this defect causes inspissation (drying and thickening) of pancreatic exocrine secretions, eventually leading to obstruction of these ducts. One result of this problem is the inability of pancreatic enzymes to enter the intestinal lumen to digest dietary proteins (as well as fats and carbohydrates).

The pancreas synthesizes and stores the zymogens in secretory granules. The pancreas also synthesizes a secretory trypsin inhibitor. The need for the inhibitor is to block any trypsin activity that may occur from accidental trypsinogen activation. If the inhibitor were not present, trypsinogen activation would lead to the activation of all of the zymogens in the pancreas, which would lead to the digestion of intracellular pancreatic proteins. Such episodes can lead to pancreatitis.

Hartnup disease is a genetically determined and relatively rare autosomal-recessive disorder. It is caused by a defect in the transport of neutral amino acids across both intestinal and renal epithelial cells (the amino acid transport system B^0, encoded by the gene *SLC6A19*, where *SLC* refers to the solute carrier family of transport proteins, of which there are 55, with a total of 362 different genes). The signs and symptoms are caused, in part, by a deficiency of essential amino acids (see "Clinical Comments"). *Cystinuria* (a defect in the amino acid transport system $B^{0,+}$, involving the genes *SLC7A9* and *SLC3A1*, because the transporter is a heteromeric complex) and Hartnup disease involve defects in two different transport proteins. In each case, the defect is present both in intestinal cells, causing malabsorption of the amino acids from the digestive products in the intestinal lumen, and in kidney tubular cells, causing a decreased resorption of these amino acids from the glomerular filtrate and an increased concentration of the amino acids in the urine.

Q Why do patients with cystinuria and Hartnup disease have hyperaminoaciduria without associated hyperaminoacidemia?

Low intracellular Na^+ results from the pumping of Na^+ out of the cell by a Na^+,K^+-adenosine triphosphatase (ATPase) on the serosal membrane. Thus, the primary transport mechanism is the creation of a sodium gradient; the secondary transport process is the coupling of amino acids to the influx of sodium. This mechanism allows the cells to concentrate amino acids from the intestinal lumen. The amino acids are then transported out of the cell into the interstitial fluid principally by facilitated transporters in the serosal membrane (see Fig. 35.4).

At least six different Na^+-dependent amino acid carriers are located in the apical brush-border membrane of the epithelial cells. These carriers have an overlapping specificity for different amino acids. One carrier preferentially transports neutral amino acids, another transports proline and hydroxyproline, a third preferentially transports acidic amino acids, and a fourth transports basic amino acids (lysine, arginine, the urea-cycle intermediate ornithine) and cystine (two cysteine residues linked by a disulfide bond). In addition to these Na^+-dependent carriers, some amino acids are transported across the luminal membrane by facilitated transport carriers. Most amino acids are transported by more than one transport system.

As with glucose transport, the Na^+-dependent carriers of the apical membrane of the intestinal epithelial cells are also present in the renal epithelium. However, different isozymes are present in the cell membranes of other tissues. Conversely, the facilitated transport carriers in the serosal membrane of the intestinal epithelia are similar to those found in other cell types in the body. During starvation, the intestinal epithelia, like these other cells, take up amino acids from the blood to use as an energy source. Thus, amino acid transport across the serosal membrane is bidirectional.

B. Transport of Amino Acids into Cells

Amino acids that enter the blood are transported across cell membranes of the various tissues principally by Na^+-dependent cotransporters and, to a lesser extent, by facilitated transporters (Table 35.1). In this respect, amino acid transport differs from glucose transport, which is Na^+-dependent transport in the intestinal and renal epithelium but facilitated transport in other cell types. The Na^+ dependence of amino acid transport in liver, muscle, and other tissues allows these cells to concentrate amino acids from the blood. These transport proteins have a different genetic basis, amino acid composition, and somewhat different specificity than those in the luminal membrane of intestinal epithelia. They also differ somewhat among tissues. For instance, the *N*-system for glutamine uptake is present in the liver but either is not present in other tissues or is present as an isoform with different properties. As with the epithelial cell transporters, there is also some overlap in specificity of the transport proteins, with most amino acids being transported by more than one carrier.

TABLE 35.1 A Partial Listing of Amino Acid Transport Systems[a]

SYSTEM NAME	SODIUM-DEPENDENT?	SPECIFICITY	TISSUES EXPRESSED
A	Yes	Small and polar neutral amino acids (Ala, Ser, Gln, Gly, Pro, Cys, Asn, His, Met)	Many
ASC	Yes	Small amino acids (Ala, Ser, Cys)	Many
N	Yes	Gln, Asn, His	Liver, basolateral membrane of kidney
L	No	Branched and aromatic amino acids (His, Met, Leu, Ile, Val, Phe, Tyr, Trp)	Many[b]
$B^{0,+}$	Yes	Basic amino acids	Intestine (brush border)[c] and kidney
B^0	Yes	Zwitterionic amino acids (monoamino, monocarboxylic acid amino acids)	Intestine and kidney[d]
X_{AG}^-	Yes	Anionic amino acids (Asp, Glu)	Intestine (brush border) and kidney
Imino	Yes	Pro, hydroxyproline, Gly	Intestine (brush border) and kidney

[a]Not all transport systems are listed.
[b]This transport system will be exploited in a treatment for phenylketonuria (PKU); see Chapter 37.
[c]This system is most likely defective in cystinuria.
[d]This system is most likely defective in Hartnup disease.

III. Protein Turnover and Replenishment of the Intracellular Amino Acid Pool

The amino acid pool within cells is generated both from dietary amino acids and from the degradation of existing proteins within the cell. All proteins within cells have a half-life ($t_{1/2}$), a time at which 50% of the protein that was synthesized at a particular time will have been degraded. Some proteins are inherently short-lived, with half-lives of 5 to 20 minutes. Other proteins are present for extended periods, with half-lives of many hours or even days. Thus, proteins are continuously being synthesized and degraded in the body, using a variety of enzyme systems to do so (Table 35.2). Examples of proteins that undergo extensive synthesis and degradation are hemoglobin, muscle proteins, digestive enzymes, and the proteins of cells sloughed off from the gastrointestinal tract. Hemoglobin is produced in reticulocytes and reconverted to amino acids by the phagocytic cells that remove mature red blood cells from the circulation on a daily basis. Muscle protein is degraded during periods of fasting, and the amino acids are used for gluconeogenesis. After ingestion of protein in the diet, muscle protein is resynthesized. Adults cannot increase the amount of muscle or other body proteins by eating an excess amount of protein. If dietary protein is consumed in excess of our needs, it is converted to glycogen and triacylglycerols, which are then stored.

A large amount of protein is recycled daily in the form of digestive enzymes, which are themselves degraded by digestive proteases. In addition, approximately one-fourth of the cells lining the walls of the gastrointestinal tract are lost each day and replaced by newly synthesized cells. As cells leave the gastrointestinal wall, their proteins and other components are digested by enzymes in the lumen of the gut, and the products are absorbed. Additionally, red blood cells have a lifespan of about 120 days. Every day, 3×10^{11} red blood cells die and are phagocytosed. The hemoglobin in these cells is degraded to amino acids by lysosomal proteases, and their amino acids are reused in the synthesis of new proteins. Only approximately 6% (~10 g) of the protein that enters the digestive tract (including dietary proteins, digestive enzymes, and the proteins in sloughed-off cells) is excreted in the feces each day. The remainder is recycled.

Proteins are also recycled within cells. The differences in amino acid composition of the various proteins of the body, the vast range in turnover times ($t_{1/2}$), and the recycling of amino acids are all important factors that help to determine the requirements for specific amino acids and total protein in the diet. The synthesis of many enzymes is induced in response to physiologic demand (such as fasting or feeding). These enzymes are continuously being degraded. Intracellular proteins

 Trace amounts of polypeptides pass into the blood. They may be transported through intestinal epithelial cells, probably by pinocytosis, or they may slip between the cells that line the gut wall. This process is particularly troublesome for premature infants, because it can lead to allergies caused by proteins in their food.

 Patients with cystinuria and Hartnup disease have defective transport proteins in both the intestine and the kidney. These patients do not absorb the affected amino acids at a normal rate from the digestive products in the intestinal lumen. They also do not readily resorb these amino acids from the glomerular filtrate into the blood. Therefore, they do not have hyperaminoacidemia (a high concentration in the blood). Normally, only a few percentage of the amino acids that enter the glomerular filtrate are excreted in the urine; most are resorbed. In these diseases, much larger amounts of the affected amino acids are excreted in the urine, resulting in hyperaminoaciduria.

 David K. and other patients with cystinuria have a genetically determined defect in the transport of cystine and the basic amino acids—lysine, arginine, and ornithine—across the brush-border membranes of cells in both their small intestine and renal tubules (system $B^{0,+}$). However, they do not appear to have any symptoms of amino acid deficiency, in part because the amino acids cysteine (which is oxidized in blood and urine to form the disulfide cystine) and arginine can be synthesized in the body (i.e., they are "nonessential" amino acids). Ornithine (an amino acid that is not found in proteins but serves as an intermediate of the urea cycle) can also be synthesized. The most serious problem for these patients is the insolubility of cystine, which can form kidney stones that may lodge in the ureter, causing genitourinary bleeding, obstruction of the ureters, and severe pain known as *renal colic*.

TABLE 35.2	Proteases Involved in Protein Turnover/Degradation	
CLASSIFICATION	**MECHANISM**	**ROLE**
Cathepsins	Cysteine proteases	Lysosomal enzymes
Caspases	Cysteine proteases, which cleave after aspartate	Apoptosis; activated from procaspases (see Chapter 18)
Matrix metalloproteinases	Require zinc for catalysis	Model extracellular matrix components; regulated by tissue inhibitors of matrix metalloproteinases (TIMPs)
Proteasome	Large complex that degrades ubiquitin-tagged proteins	Protein turnover
Serine proteases	Active-site serine in a catalytic triad with histidine and aspartic acid	Digestion and blood clotting; activated usually from zymogens (see Chapter 43)
Calpains	Calcium-dependent cysteine proteases	Many different cellular roles

are also damaged by oxidation and other modifications that limit their function. Mechanisms for intracellular degradation of unnecessary or damaged proteins involve lysosomes and the ubiquitin–proteasome system.

A. Lysosomal Protein Turnover

Lysosomes participate in the process of autophagy, in which intracellular components are surrounded by membranes that fuse with lysosomes, and endocytosis (see Chapter 10). *Autophagy* is a complex regulated process in which cytoplasm is sequestered into vesicles and delivered to the lysosomes. Within the lysosomes, the cathepsin family of proteases degrades the ingested proteins to individual amino acids. The recycled amino acids can then leave the lysosome and rejoin the intracellular amino acid pool. Although the details of how autophagy is induced are still being investigated, starvation of a cell is a trigger to induce this process. This will allow old proteins to be recycled and the newly released amino acids used for new protein synthesis, to enable the cell to survive starvation conditions. The mTOR kinase (see Chapter 34) plays a key role in regulating autophagy, as outlined in Figure 35.5.

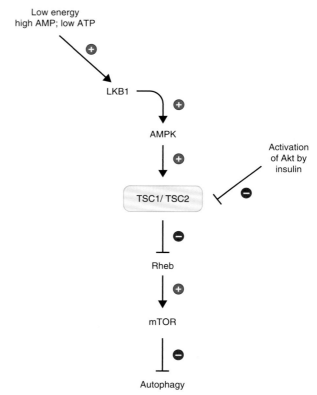

FIGURE 35.5 Overview of mTOR participation in autophagy. When active, the mTOR kinase will phosphorylate a protein crucial to the initiation of phagosome formation, which will inhibit autophagy. mTOR kinase is activated by Rheb-guanosine triphosphate (GTP). Under low-energy conditions (starvation) autophagy is favored as the adenosine monophosphate (AMP)-activated protein kinase (AMPK) is activated, which phosphorylates the TSC1/TSC2 complex, activating its Rheb-GTPase–activating activity. This leads to the inactivation of Rheb (Rheb-GTP is converted to the inactive Rheb-guanosine diphosphate [GDP]), which leads to the inactivation of mTOR. When inactive, mTOR does not block autophagy, and self-proteolysis is favored, as is an inhibition of protein synthesis. In the presence of growth factors, such as insulin, which activate the Akt kinase, Akt phosphorylates the TSC1/TSC2 complex at a site distinct from the AMPK site. The phosphorylation event by Akt leads to an inhibition of the TSC1/TSC2 Rheb-GTPase–activating activity, which allows Rheb to be active for extended periods of time. Active Rheb leads to activation of mTOR, and inhibition of autophagy, and activation of protein synthesis. *ATP*, adenosine triphosphate.

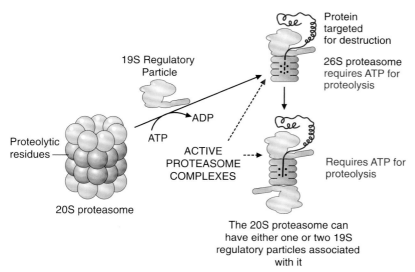

FIGURE 35.6 The proteasome and regulatory proteins. The regulatory particle (shown in this figure as the 19S regulator; others are PA28αβ1, PA28γ, and PA200) regulates the activity of this proteolytic complex by recruiting to the complex the substrates for proteolysis. The adenosine triphosphate (ATP) requirement is to unfold and denature the proteins targeted for destruction. *ADP*, adenosine diphosphate.

B. The Ubiquitin–Proteasome Pathway

Ubiquitin is a small protein (76 amino acids) that is highly conserved. Its amino acid sequence in yeast and humans differs by only three residues. Ubiquitin targets intracellular proteins for degradation by covalently binding to the ε-amino group of lysine residues. This is accomplished by a three-enzyme system that adds ubiquitin to proteins targeted for degradation. Often, the target protein is polyubiquitinylated, a process in which additional ubiquitin molecules are added to previous ubiquitin molecules, forming a long ubiquitin tail on the target protein. After polyubiquitinylation is complete, the targeted protein is released from the three-enzyme complex, and is directed to the proteasome, via a variety of mechanisms.

A protease complex, known as the *proteasome*, then degrades the targeted protein, releasing intact ubiquitin that can again mark other proteins for degradation (Fig. 35.6). The basic proteasome is a cylindrical 20S protein complex with multiple internal proteolytic sites. ATP hydrolysis is used both to unfold the tagged protein and to push the protein into the core of the cylinder. The complex is regulated by four different types of regulatory particles (cap complexes), which bind the ubiquinylated protein (a step that requires ATP) and deliver them to the complex. After the target protein is degraded, the ubiquitin is released intact and recycled. The resulting amino acids join the intracellular pool of free amino acids.

Many proteins that contain regions rich in the amino acids proline (P), glutamate (E), serine (S), and threonine (T) have short half-lives. These regions are known as *PEST sequences* based on the one-letter abbreviations used for these amino acids. Most of the proteins that contain PEST sequences are hydrolyzed by the ubiquitin–proteasome system.

CLINICAL COMMENTS

Susan F. Susan F.'s growth and weight curves were both subnormal until her pediatrician added pancreatic enzyme supplements to her treatment plan. These supplements digest dietary protein, releasing essential and other amino acids from the dietary protein, which are then absorbed by the epithelial cells of Susan's small intestine, through which they are transported into the blood.

A discernible improvement in Susan's body weight and growth curves was noted within months of starting this therapy.

Besides the proportions of essential amino acids present in various foods, the quality of a dietary protein is also determined by the rate at which it is digested and, in a more general way, by its capacity to contribute to the growth of the infant. In this regard, the proteins in foods of animal origin are more digestible than are those derived from plants. For example, the digestibility of proteins in eggs is approximately 97%; that of meats, poultry, and fish is 85% to 100%; and that from wheat, soybeans, and other legumes ranges from 75% to 90%.

The official daily dietary "protein requirement" accepted by the US and Canadian governments is 0.8 g of protein per kilogram of desirable body weight for adults (~56 g for an adult man and 44 g for an adult woman). On an average weight basis, the requirement per kilogram is much greater for infants and children. This fact underscores the importance of improving **Susan F.'s** protein digestion to optimize her potential for normal growth and development.

David K. In patients with cystinuria, such as **David K.**, the inability to normally absorb cystine and basic amino acids from the gut and the increased loss of these amino acids in the urine may be expected to cause a deficiency of these compounds in the blood. However, because three of these amino acids can be synthesized in the body (i.e., they are nonessential amino acids), their concentrations in the plasma remain normal, and clinical manifestations of a deficiency state do not develop. It is not clear why symptoms related to a lysine deficiency have not been observed.

In another disorder with a transport defect, which was first observed in the Hartnup family and bears their name, the intestinal and renal transport defect involves the neutral amino acids (monoamine, monocarboxylic acids), including several essential amino acids (isoleucine, leucine, phenylalanine, threonine, tryptophan, and valine) as well as certain nonessential amino acids (alanine, serine, and tyrosine). A reduction in the availability of these essential amino acids may be expected to cause a variety of clinical disorders. Yet, children with the Hartnup disorder identified by routine newborn urine screening almost always remain clinically normal.

However, some patients with the Hartnup biochemical phenotype eventually develop pellagralike manifestations, which usually include a photosensitivity rash, ataxia, and neuropsychiatric symptoms. Pellagra results from a dietary deficiency of the vitamin niacin or the essential amino acid tryptophan, which are both precursors for the nicotinamide moiety of nicotinamide adenine dinucleotide (NAD) and NADP. In asymptomatic patients, the transport abnormality may be incomplete and so subtle as to allow no phenotypic expression of Hartnup disease. These patients also may be capable of absorbing some small peptides that contain the neutral amino acids.

The only rational treatment for patients who have pellagralike symptoms is to administer niacin (nicotinic acid) in oral doses up to 300 mg/day. Although the rash, ataxia, and neuropsychiatric manifestations of niacin deficiency may disappear, the hyperaminoaciduria and intestinal transport defect do not respond to this therapy. In addition to niacin, a high-protein diet may benefit some patients.

BIOCHEMICAL COMMENTS

The γ-Glutamyl Cycle. The γ-glutamyl cycle is necessary for the synthesis of glutathione, a compound that protects cells from oxidative damage (see Chapter 25). When it was first discovered, the cycle was thought to be important in amino acid transport, but its involvement in such transport is now thought to be limited to salvage of cysteine. The enzymes of the cycle are present in many tissues, although certain tissues lack one or more of the enzymes of the cycle.

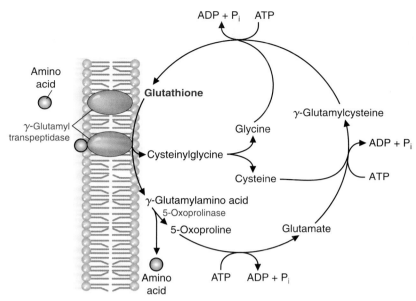

FIGURE 35.7 The γ-glutamyl cycle. In cells of the intestine and kidney, amino acids can be transported across the cell membrane by reacting with glutathione (γ-glutamyl-cysteinyl-glycine) to form a γ-glutamyl amino acid. The amino acid is released into the cell, and glutathione is resynthesized. However, the major role of this cycle is glutathione synthesis because many tissues lack the transpeptidase and 5-oxoprolinase activities. *ADP*, adenosine diphosphate; *ATP*, adenosine triphosphate; *P_i*, inorganic phosphate.

The entire cycle is presented in Figure 35.7. In this case, the extracellular amino acid reacts with glutathione (γ-glutamyl-cysteinyl-glycine) in a reaction catalyzed by a transpeptidase present in the cell membrane. A γ-glutamyl amino acid is formed, which travels across the cell membrane and releases the amino acid into the cell. The other products of these two reactions are reconverted to glutathione.

The reactions that convert glutamate to glutathione in the γ-glutamyl cycle are the same reactions as those required for the synthesis of glutathione. The enzymes for glutathione synthesis, but not the transpeptidase, are found in most tissues. The oxoprolinase is also missing from many tissues, so the major role of this pathway is one of glutathione synthesis from glutamate, cysteine, and glycine. The transpeptidase is the only protease in the cell that can break the γ-glutamyl linkage in glutathione. Glutathione is also involved in reducing compounds such as hydrogen peroxide (see Chapter 25). It also protects cells, particularly erythrocytes, from oxidative damage, through formation of oxidized glutathione, two glutathione residues connected by a disulfide bond (see Chapter 25).

KEY CONCEPTS

- Proteases (proteolytic enzymes) break down dietary proteins into peptides and then their constituent amino acids in the stomach and intestine.
- Pepsin initiates protein breakdown in the stomach.
- Upon entering the small intestine, inactive zymogens secreted from the pancreas are activated to continue protein digestion.
- Enzymes produced by the intestinal epithelial cells are also required to fully degrade proteins.
- The amino acids generated by proteolysis in the intestinal lumen are transported into the intestinal epithelial cells, from which they enter the circulation for use by the tissues.
- Transport systems for amino acids are similar to transport systems for monosaccharides; both facilitative and active transport systems exist.

- There are several overlapping transport systems for amino acids in cells.
- Protein degradation (turnover) occurs continuously in all cells.
- Proteins can be degraded by lysosomal enzymes (cathepsins).
- Proteins are also targeted for destruction by being covalently linked to the small protein ubiquitin.
- The ubiquitin-tagged proteins interact with the proteasome, a large complex that degrades proteins to small peptides in an ATP-dependent process.
- Amino acids released from proteins during turnover can be used for the synthesis of new proteins, for energy generation, or for gluconeogenesis.
- Diseases discussed in the chapter are summarized in Table 35.3.

TABLE 35.3	Diseases Discussed in Chapter 35	
DISEASE OR DISORDER	**GENETIC OR ENVIRONMENTAL**	**COMMENTS**
Cystic fibrosis	Genetic	Patients with cystic fibrosis often experience a blockage of the pancreatic duct, which necessitates oral ingestion of digestive enzymes for appropriate nutrient degradation and absorption.
Cystinuria	Genetic	A mutation in a membrane transport protein ($B^{0,+}$) for basic amino acids, including cystine, which is expressed in kidney and intestine. Kidney stones may develop because of this disorder.
Kwashiorkor	Environmental	Protein-calorie malnutrition (diet is adequate in calories but lacking in protein), leading to excessive protein degradation in the muscles, and edema
Hartnup disease	Genetic	A mutation in a membrane transport protein (B^0) for neutral amino acids, including tryptophan, which is expressed in both the kidney and intestine. Some patients may develop pellagralike symptoms, owing to the lack of tryptophan and inability to synthesize adequate amounts of $NAD(P)^+$.

REVIEW QUESTIONS—CHAPTER 35

1. An individual with a deficiency in the conversion of trypsinogen to trypsin would be expected to experience a more detrimental effect on protein digestion than an individual who was defective in any of the other digestive proteases. This is a result of which of the following?
   A. Trypsin has a greater and wider range of substrates on which to act.
   B. Trypsin activates pepsinogen, so digestion can begin in the stomach.
   C. Trypsin activates the other zymogens that are secreted by the pancreas.
   D. Trypsin activates enteropeptidase, which is needed to activate the other pancreatic zymogens.
   E. Trypsin inhibits intestinal motility, so the substrates can be hydrolyzed for longer periods.

2. An individual has been shown to have a deficiency in an intestinal epithelial cell amino acid transport system for leucine. However, the individual shows no symptoms of amino acid deficiency. This could be because of which of the following?
   A. The body synthesizes leucine to compensate for the transport defect.
   B. The kidney reabsorbs leucine and sends it to other tissues.

   C. There are multiple transport systems for leucine.
   D. Isoleucine takes the place of leucine in proteins.
   E. Leucine is not necessary for bulk protein synthesis.

3. Kwashiorkor can result from which one of the following?
   A. Consuming a calorie-deficient diet that is also deficient in protein
   B. Consuming a calorie-adequate diet that is deficient in carbohydrates
   C. Consuming a calorie-adequate diet that is deficient in fatty acids
   D. Consuming a calorie-adequate diet that is deficient in proteins
   E. Consuming a calorie-deficient diet that is primarily proteins

4. Which one of the following enzymes is activated through an autocatalytic process?
   A. Enteropeptidase
   B. Trypsinogen
   C. Pepsinogen
   D. Aminopeptidase
   E. Proelastase

5. Children with kwashiorkor usually have a fatty liver. This is the result of which one of the following?
   A. The high fat content of their diet
   B. The high carbohydrate content of their diet
   C. The high protein content of their diet
   D. The lack of substrates for gluconeogenesis in the liver
   E. The lack of substrates for protein synthesis in the liver
   F. The lack of substrates for glycogen synthesis in the liver

6. All of the nitrogen-containing compounds of the human body are synthesized from amino acids. Which one of the following statements about amino acid degradation is correct?
   A. Amino acid carbons can be stored only as glycogen.
   B. The liver is the only site of amino acid oxidation.
   C. The nitrogen of oxidized branched-chain amino acids must travel to the liver for disposal.
   D. The nitrogen of amino acids is always excreted as urea.
   E. The nitrogen of amino acids is only excreted by the kidney.

7. Proteases break down dietary proteins, and their release from the pancreas to the small intestine is often blocked in individuals with cystic fibrosis. Which one of the following is an example of a pancreatic protease?
   A. Pepsin
   B. Elastase
   C. Aminopeptidase
   D. Cathepsin
   E. Ubiquitin

8. A 38-year-old patient has developed chronic obstructive pulmonary disease (COPD) caused by an α_1-antitrypsin deficiency. Which one of the following correctly describes α_1-antitrypsin?
   A. It is synthesized by the lung.
   B. It is a protease enhancer.
   C. It enhances the action of trypsin in the lung.
   D. It blocks the action of elastase in the lung.
   E. It blocks the action of trypsin in the lung.

9. Proteolytic enzymes must be secreted as zymogens that are activated, or they would autodigest themselves and the organs that produce them. Trypsinogen, a zymogen, is cleaved to form trypsin by a protease that is secreted by which of one the following?
   A. Stomach
   B. Pancreas
   C. Colon
   D. Liver
   E. Small intestine

10. An adult patient is trying to increase his amount of muscle by ingesting protein-rich drinks daily without increasing his daily exercise routine. Which one of the following correctly describes a problem with this approach?
   A. Dietary proteins in excess of bodily needs pass unchanged and unabsorbed into the feces.
   B. Dietary proteins in excess of bodily needs pass unchanged in the urine.
   C. Dietary proteins in excess of bodily needs feed back and shut down pancreatic enzymes.
   D. Dietary proteins in excess of bodily needs are stored as amino acids in the liver.
   E. Dietary proteins in excess of bodily needs are converted to glycogen and triacylglycerols for storage.

ANSWERS

1. **The answer is C.** Trypsinogen, which is secreted by the intestine, is activated by enteropeptidase, a protein found in the intestine (thus, D is backward and incorrect). Once trypsin is formed, it activates all of the other zymogens secreted by the pancreas. Trypsin does not activate pepsinogen (thus, B is incorrect) because pepsinogen is found in the stomach and autocatalyzes its own activation when the pH drops as a result of acid secretion. Trypsin has no effect on intestinal motility (hence, E is incorrect) and also does not have a much broader base of substrates than any other protease (trypsin cleaves on the carboxyl side of basic side chains, lysine, and arginine; thus, A is incorrect).

2. **The answer is C.** Leucine can be transported by several different amino acid systems. Leucine is an essential amino acid, so the body cannot synthesize it (thus, A is incorrect). If the intestine cannot absorb leucine, then the kidneys do not have a chance to reabsorb it, so B is incorrect. Leucine and isoleucine have different structures and cannot substitute for each other in all positions within a protein (thus, D is incorrect). Leucine is an important component of proteins and is required for protein synthesis; hence, E is incorrect.

3. **The answer is D.** Kwashiorkor is a disease that results from eating a calorie-sufficient diet that lacks protein. None of the other answers is correct.

4. **The answer is C.** Pepsinogen, under acidic conditions, autocatalyzes its conversion to pepsin in the stomach. Both enteropeptidase and aminopeptidases are synthesized in active form by the intestine (thus, A and D are incorrect). Enteropeptidase activates trypsinogen (thus, B is incorrect), which then activates proelastase (thus, E is incorrect).

5. **The answer is E.** Because of the lack of protein in the diet, protein synthesis in the liver is impaired (lack of essential amino acids). The liver can still synthesize fatty acids from carbohydrate or fat sources, but very-low-density lipoprotein (VLDL) particles cannot be assembled because of the shortage of apolipoprotein B-100.

Thus, the fatty acids remain in the liver, leading to a fatty liver. None of the other answers explains this finding.

6. **The answer is C.** Branched-chain amino acids can be oxidized in many tissues, but the nitrogen must travel to the liver for disposal. The muscle is the primary site of branched-chain amino acid oxidation because of the high level of the branched-chain α-keto acid dehydrogenase in that tissue. Amino acid carbons can be oxidized directly, converted to glucose, and then oxidized or stored as glycogen, or they can be converted to fatty acids and stored as adipose triacylglycerols. Although urea is the major nitrogenous excretory product, nitrogen is also excreted in other compounds such as uric acid, creatinine, and ammonia. These compounds are excreted mostly in the urine, but substantial amounts are lost in feces and through the skin.

7. **The answer is B.** Pepsin is synthesized in the stomach. Trypsin, chymotrypsin, elastase, and carboxypeptidases are secreted from the pancreas into the small intestine. Aminopeptidases are found on the brush border of intestinal epithelial cells. Cathepsins degrade proteins that enter lysosomes. Ubiquitin is a small protein that is covalently linked to proteins targeted for turnover in the cytoplasm.

8. **The answer is D.** Elastase, found in neutrophils, can be released into the lung, where it causes proteolytic destruction of normal lung cells, leading to emphysema. α-Antitrypsin is a protease inhibitor synthesized in the liver and released into the circulation that blocks the action of elastase in the lung. Trypsin is not found in the lung. α-Antitrypsin was named owing to the fact that it will also inhibit trypsin activity, although that is not its physiologic function.

9. **The answer is E.** Trypsinogen is cleaved by the enzyme enteropeptidase, which is secreted by the brush-border cells of the small intestine. Trypsin then cleaves chymotrypsinogen, proelastase, and procarboxypeptidase to their active forms. Pepsinogen is essentially autocatalytic in the presence of acid and is found in the stomach. Pepsin does not activate zymogens in the small intestine.

10. **The answer is E.** Proteins are constantly being synthesized and degraded. Only about 6% of protein that enters the gastrointestinal tract is excreted in feces each day. The remainder is recycled. Excess proteins above dietary and metabolic needs are converted to glycogen and triacylglycerols for storage. The patient will gain weight as adipose tissue instead of increasing muscle mass.

Fate of Amino Acid Nitrogen: Urea Cycle

In comparison with carbohydrate and lipid metabolism, the metabolism of amino acids is complex. We must be concerned not only with the fate of the carbon atoms of the amino acids but also with the fate of the **nitrogen**. During their metabolism, amino acids travel in the blood from one tissue to another. Ultimately, most of the nitrogen is converted to **urea** in the **liver**, and the carbons are oxidized to CO_2 and H_2O by several tissues (Fig. 36.1).

After a meal that contains protein, amino acids released by digestion (see Chapter 35) pass from the gut through the hepatic portal vein to the liver (see Fig. 36.2A). In a normal diet containing 60 to 100 g of protein, most of the amino acids are used for the synthesis of proteins in the liver and in other tissues. Excess amino acids may be converted to glucose or triacylglycerol.

During fasting, muscle protein is cleaved to amino acids. Some of the amino acids are partially oxidized to produce energy (see Fig. 36.2B). Portions of these amino acids are converted to **alanine** and **glutamine**, which, along with other amino acids, are released into the blood. Glutamine is oxidized by various tissues, including the **lymphocytes**, **gut**, and **kidney**, which convert some of the carbons and nitrogen to alanine. Alanine and other amino acids travel to the liver, where the carbons are converted to glucose and ketone bodies and the nitrogen is converted to urea, which is excreted by the kidneys. Glucose, produced by gluconeogenesis, is subsequently oxidized to CO_2 and H_2O by many tissues, and ketone bodies are oxidized by tissues such as muscle and kidney.

Several enzymes are important in the process of interconverting amino acids and in removing nitrogen so that the carbon skeletons can be oxidized. These include **dehydratases, transaminases, glutamate dehydrogenase, glutaminase**, and **deaminases**.

The conversion of amino acid nitrogen to urea occurs mainly in the liver. Urea is formed in the urea cycle from NH_4^+, bicarbonate, and the nitrogen of **aspartate** (see Fig. 36.1). Initially, NH_4^+, bicarbonate, and adenosine triphosphate (ATP) react to produce **carbamoyl phosphate**, which reacts with **ornithine** to form **citrulline**. Aspartate then reacts with citrulline to form **argininosuccinate**, which releases **fumarate**, forming **arginine**. Finally, **arginase** cleaves arginine to release urea and regenerate ornithine. The cycle is regulated in a **feed-forward** manner, such that when amino acid degradation is occurring, the rate of the cycle is increased.

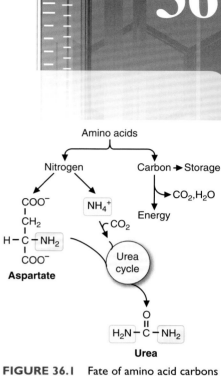

FIGURE 36.1   Fate of amino acid carbons and nitrogen. Amino acid carbon can be used either for energy storage (glycogen, fatty acids) or for energy. Amino acid nitrogen is used for urea synthesis. One nitrogen of urea comes from NH_4^+, the other from aspartate.

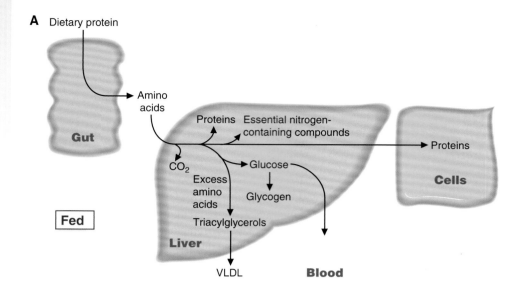

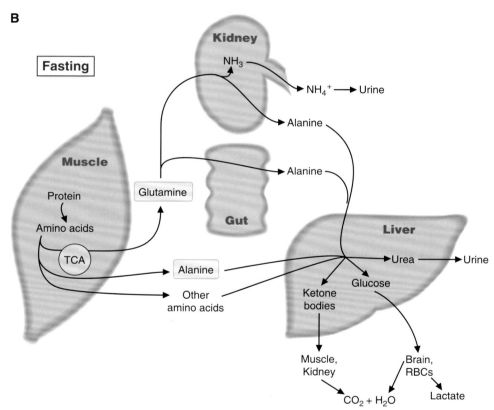

FIGURE 36.2 Roles of various tissues in amino acid metabolism. **A.** In the fed state, amino acids released by digestion of dietary proteins travel through the hepatic portal vein to the liver, where they are used for the synthesis of proteins, particularly the blood proteins, such as serum albumin. The carbon skeletons of excess amino acids are converted to glucose or to triacylglycerols. The latter are then packaged and secreted in very-low-density lipoprotein (VLDL). The glucose produced from amino acids in the fed state is stored as glycogen or released into the blood if blood glucose levels are low. Amino acids that pass through the liver are converted to proteins in cells of other tissues. **B.** During fasting, amino acids are released from muscle protein. Some enter the blood directly. Others are partially oxidized and the nitrogen stored in the form of alanine and glutamine, which enter the blood. In the kidney, glutamine releases ammonia into the urine and is converted to alanine and serine. In the cells of the gut, glutamine is converted to alanine. Alanine (the major gluconeogenic amino acid) and other amino acids enter the liver, where their nitrogen is converted to urea, which is excreted in the urine, and their carbons are converted to glucose and ketone bodies, which are oxidized by various tissues for energy. *RBCs*, red blood cells; *TCA*, tricarboxylic acid.

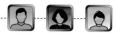

  Percy V. and his high school friend decided to take a Caribbean cruise, during which they sampled the cuisine of many of the islands on their itinerary. One month after their return to the United States, Percy complained of severe malaise, loss of appetite, nausea, vomiting, headache, and abdominal pain. He had a low-grade fever and noted a persistent and increasing pain in the area of his liver. His friend noted a yellow discoloration of the whites of Percy's eyes and skin. Percy's urine turned the color of iced tea, and his stool became a light clay color. His doctor found his liver to be enlarged and tender. Liver function tests were ordered.

Serologic testing for viral hepatitis types B and C were nonreactive, but tests for antibodies to antigens of the hepatitis A virus (anti-HAV) in the serum were positive for the immunoglobulin M type.

A diagnosis of acute viral hepatitis type A was made, probably contracted from virus-contaminated food Percy had eaten while on his cruise. His physician explained that there was no specific treatment for type A viral hepatitis but recommended symptomatic and supportive care and prevention of transmission to others by the fecal–oral route. Percy took acetaminophen three to four times a day for fever and headaches throughout his illness.

I. Fate of Amino Acid Nitrogen

A. Transamination Reactions

Transamination is the major process for removing nitrogen from amino acids. In most instances, the nitrogen is transferred as an amino group from the original amino acid to α-ketoglutarate, forming glutamate, whereas the original amino acid is converted to its corresponding α-keto acid (Fig. 36.3). For example, the amino acid aspartate can be transaminated to form its corresponding α-keto acid, oxaloacetate. In the process, the amino group is transferred to α-ketoglutarate, which is converted to its corresponding amino acid, glutamate.

All amino acids except lysine and threonine undergo transamination reactions. The enzymes that catalyze these reactions are known as *transaminases* or *aminotransferases*. For most of these reactions, α-ketoglutarate and glutamate serve as one of the α-keto acid–amino acid pairs. Pyridoxal phosphate (PLP; derived from vitamin B_6) is the required cofactor for these reactions.

Overall, in a transamination reaction, an amino group from one amino acid becomes the amino group of a second amino acid. Because these reactions are readily reversible, they can be used to remove nitrogen from amino acids or to transfer nitrogen to α-keto acids to form amino acids. Thus, they are involved both in amino acid degradation and in amino acid synthesis.

B. Removal of Amino Acid Nitrogen as Ammonia

Cells in the body and bacteria in the gut release the nitrogen of certain amino acids as ammonia or ammonium ion (NH_4^+) (Fig. 36.4). Because these two forms of nitrogen can be interconverted, the terms are sometimes used interchangeably. Ammonium ion releases a proton to form ammonia by a reaction with a pK_a of 9.3. Therefore, at physiologic pH, the equilibrium favors NH_4^+ by a factor of approximately 100/1 (see Chapter 4, the Henderson-Hasselbalch equation). However, it is important to note that NH_3 is also present in the body because this is the form that can cross cell membranes. For example, NH_3 passes into the urine from kidney tubule cells and decreases the acidity of the urine by binding protons, forming NH_4^+. Once the NH_4^+ is formed, the compound can no longer freely diffuse across membranes.

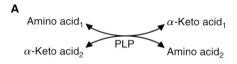

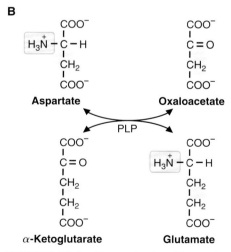

FIGURE 36.3 Transamination. The amino group from one amino acid is transferred to another. Pairs of amino acids and their corresponding α-keto acids are involved in these reactions. α-Ketoglutarate and glutamate are usually one of the pairs. The reactions, which are readily reversible, use pyridoxal phosphate (PLP) as a cofactor. The enzymes are called transaminases or aminotransferases. **A.** A generalized reaction. **B.** The aspartate transaminase reaction.

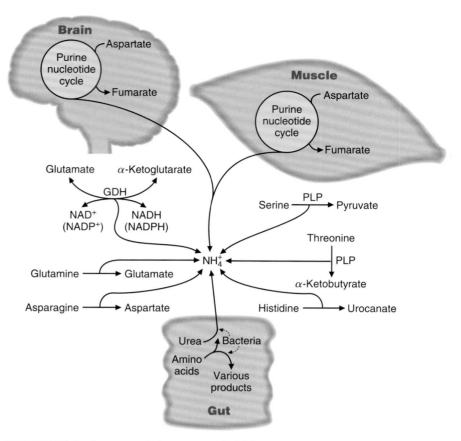

FIGURE 36.4 Summary of the sources of NH_4^+ for the urea cycle. All of the reactions are irreversible except that of glutamate dehydrogenase (GDH). Only the dehydratase reactions, which produce NH_4^+ from serine and threonine, require pyridoxal phosphate (PLP) as a cofactor. The reactions that are not shown occurring in the muscle or the gut can all occur in the liver, where the NH_4^+ generated can be converted to urea. The purine nucleotide cycle of the brain and muscle is described further in Chapter 39. *NAD*, nicotinamide adenine dinucleotide.

Glutamate is oxidatively deaminated by a reaction catalyzed by glutamate dehydrogenase that produces ammonium ion and α-ketoglutarate (Fig. 36.5). Either nicotinamide adenine dinucleotide (NAD^+) or $NADP^+$ can serve as the cofactor. This reaction, which occurs in the mitochondria of most cells, is readily reversible; it can incorporate ammonia into glutamate or release ammonia from glutamate. Glutamate can collect nitrogen from other amino acids as a consequence of transamination reactions and then release ammonia through the glutamate dehydrogenase reaction. This process provides one source of the ammonia that enters the

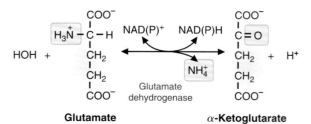

FIGURE 36.5 Reaction catalyzed by glutamate dehydrogenase. This reaction is readily reversible and can use either nicotinamide adenine dinucleotide (NAD^+) or $NADP^+$ as a cofactor. The oxygen on α-ketoglutarate is derived from H_2O.

urea cycle. Glutamate dehydrogenase is one of three mammalian enzymes that can "fix" ammonia into organic molecules. The other two are glutamine synthetase and carbamoyl phosphate synthetase I (CPSI).

In addition to glutamate, several amino acids release their nitrogen as NH_4^+ (see Fig. 36.4). Histidine may be directly deaminated to form NH_4^+ and urocanate. The deaminations of serine and threonine are dehydration reactions that require PLP and are catalyzed by serine dehydratase. Serine forms pyruvate, and threonine forms α-ketobutyrate. In both cases, NH_4^+ is released.

Glutamine and asparagine contain R-group amides that may be released as NH_4^+ by deamidation. Asparagine is deamidated by asparaginase, yielding aspartate and NH_4^+. Glutaminase acts on glutamine, forming glutamate and NH_4^+. The glutaminase reaction is particularly important in the kidney, where the ammonium ion produced is excreted directly into the urine, where it forms salts with metabolic acids, facilitating their removal in the urine.

In muscle and brain, but not in liver, the purine nucleotide cycle allows NH_4^+ to be released from amino acids (see Fig. 36.4). Nitrogen is collected by glutamate from other amino acids by means of transamination reactions. Glutamate then transfers its amino group to oxaloacetate to form aspartate, which supplies nitrogen to the purine nucleotide cycle (see Chapter 39). The reactions of the cycle release fumarate and NH_4^+. The ammonium ion formed can leave the muscle in the form of glutamine.

In summary, NH_4^+ that enters the urea cycle is produced in the body by deamination or deamidation of amino acids (see Fig. 36.4). A significant amount of NH_4^+ is also produced by bacteria that live in the lumen of the intestinal tract. This ammonium ion enters the hepatic portal vein and travels to the liver.

C. Role of Glutamate in the Metabolism of Amino Acid Nitrogen

Glutamate plays a pivotal role in the metabolism of amino acids. It is involved in both synthesis and degradation.

Glutamate provides nitrogen for amino acid synthesis (Fig. 36.6). In this process, glutamate obtains its nitrogen either from other amino acids by transamination reactions or from NH_4^+ by the glutamate dehydrogenase reaction. Transamination reactions then serve to transfer amino groups from glutamate to α-keto acids to produce their corresponding amino acids.

When amino acids are degraded and urea is formed, glutamate collects nitrogen from other amino acids by transamination reactions. Some of this nitrogen

 Percy V.'s laboratory studies showed that his serum alanine transaminase (ALT) level was 675 U/L (reference range, 5 to 30 U/L), and his serum aspartate transaminase (AST) level was 601 U/L (reference range, 10 to 30 U/L). His serum alkaline phosphatase level was 284 U/L (reference range, adult male = 40 to 125 U/L), and his serum total bilirubin was 9.6 mg/dL (reference range, 0.2 to 1.0 mg/dL). Bilirubin is a degradation product of heme, as described in Chapter 42.

Cellular enzymes such as AST, ALT, and alkaline phosphatase leak into the blood through the membranes of hepatic cells that have been damaged as a result of the inflammatory process. In acute viral hepatitis, the serum ALT level is often elevated to a greater extent than the serum AST level. Alkaline phosphatase, which is present on membranes between liver cells and the bile duct, is also elevated in the blood in acute viral hepatitis.

The rise in serum total bilirubin occurs as a result of the inability of the infected liver to conjugate bilirubin and of a partial or complete occlusion of the hepatic biliary drainage ducts caused by inflammatory swelling within the liver. In fulminant hepatic failure, the serum bilirubin level may exceed 20 mg/dL, a poor prognostic sign.

 Vitamin B_6 deficiency symptoms include dermatitis; a microcytic, hypochromic anemia; weakness; irritability; and, in some cases, seizures. Xanthurenic acid (a degradation product of tryptophan) and other compounds appear in the urine because of an inability to completely metabolize amino acids. A decreased ability to synthesize heme from glycine may cause the microcytic anemia (see Chapter 42), and decreased decarboxylation of amino acids to form neurotransmitters (see Chapter 46) may explain the convulsions. Although vitamin B_6 is required for a large number of reactions involved in amino acid metabolism, it is also required for the glycogen phosphorylase reaction (see Chapter 27).

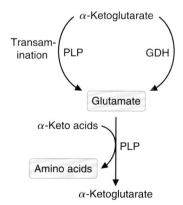

FIGURE 36.6 Role of glutamate in amino acid synthesis. Glutamate transfers nitrogen by means of transamination reactions to α-keto acids to form amino acids. This nitrogen is either obtained by glutamate from transamination of other amino acids or from NH_4^+ by means of the glutamate dehydrogenase (GDH) reaction. *PLP*, pyridoxal phosphate, the active form of vitamin B_6 (pyridoxine).

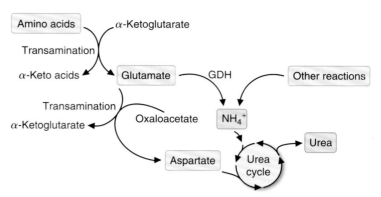

FIGURE 36.7 Role of glutamate in urea production. Glutamate collects nitrogen from other amino acids by transamination reactions. This nitrogen can be released as NH_4^+ by glutamate dehydrogenase (GDH). NH_4^+ is also produced by other reactions (see Fig. 36.4). NH_4^+ provides one of the nitrogens for urea synthesis. The other nitrogen comes from aspartate and is obtained from glutamate by transamination of oxaloacetate.

is released as ammonia by the glutamate dehydrogenase reaction, but much larger amounts of ammonia are produced from the other sources shown in Figure 36.4. NH_4^+ is one of the two forms in which nitrogen enters the urea cycle (Fig. 36.7).

The second form of nitrogen for urea synthesis is provided by aspartate (see Fig. 36.7). Glutamate can be the source of the nitrogen. Glutamate transfers its amino group to oxaloacetate, and aspartate and α-ketoglutarate are formed.

D. Role of Alanine and Glutamine in Transporting Amino Acid Nitrogen to the Liver

Protein turnover and amino acid degradation occur in all tissues; however, the urea-cycle enzymes are active primarily in the liver (the intestine expresses low levels of activity of these enzymes; see Chapter 40). Thus, a mechanism needs to be in place to transport amino acid nitrogen to the liver. Alanine and glutamine are the major carriers of nitrogen in the blood. Alanine is primarily exported by muscle. Because the muscle is metabolizing glucose through glycolysis, pyruvate is available in the muscle. The pyruvate is transaminated by glutamate to form alanine, which travels to the liver (Fig. 36.8). The glutamate is formed by transamination of an amino acid that is being degraded. Upon arriving at the liver, alanine is transaminated to pyruvate, and the nitrogen is used for urea synthesis. The pyruvate formed is used for gluconeogenesis and the

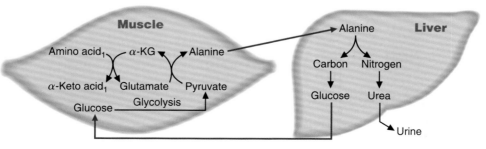

FIGURE 36.8 The glucose–alanine cycle. Within the muscle, amino acid degradation leads to the transfer of nitrogens to α-ketoglutarate (α-KG) and pyruvate. The alanine formed travels to the liver, where the carbons of alanine are used for gluconeogenesis and the alanine nitrogen is used for urea biosynthesis. This could occur during exercise, when the muscle uses bloodborne glucose (see Chapter 45).

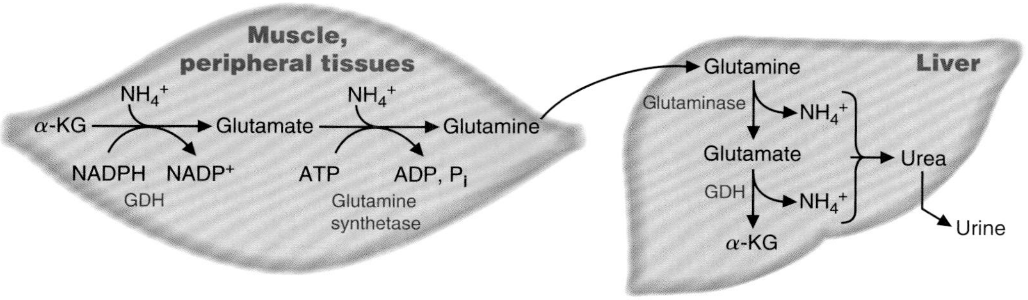

FIGURE 36.9 Synthesis of glutamine in peripheral tissues and its transport to the liver. Within the liver, glutaminase converts glutamine to glutamate. Note how α-ketoglutarate (α-KG) can accept two molecules of ammonia to form glutamine. *ADP*, adenosine diphosphate; *ATP*, adenosine triphosphate; *GDH*, glutamate dehydrogenase; *P$_i$*, inorganic phosphate.

glucose exported to the muscle for use as energy. This cycle of moving carbons and nitrogen between the muscle and liver is known as the **glucose–alanine cycle**.

Glutamine is synthesized from glutamate by the fixation of ammonia, requiring energy (ATP) and the enzyme glutamine synthetase (Fig. 36.9), which is a cytoplasmic enzyme found in all cells. In the liver, glutamine synthetase is located in cells surrounding the portal vein. Its major role is to convert any ammonia that has escaped from urea production into glutamine, so that free ammonia does not leave the liver and enter the circulation.

Under conditions of rapid amino acid degradation within a tissue, so that ammonia levels increase, the glutamate that has been formed from transamination reactions accepts another nitrogen molecule to form glutamine. The glutamine travels to the liver, kidney, or intestines, where glutaminase (see Fig. 36.9) will remove the amide nitrogen to form glutamate plus ammonia. In the kidney, the release of ammonia, and the formation of ammonium ion, serves to form salts with metabolic acids in the urine. In the intestine, the glutamine is used as a fuel (see Chapter 40). In the liver, the ammonia is used for urea biosynthesis.

II. Urea Cycle

The normal human adult is in nitrogen balance; that is, the amount of nitrogen ingested each day, mainly in the form of dietary protein, is equal to the amount of nitrogen excreted. The major nitrogenous excretory product is urea, which exits from the body in the urine. This innocuous compound, produced mainly in the liver by the urea cycle, serves as the disposal form of ammonia, which is toxic, particularly to the brain and central nervous system (CNS). Normally, little ammonia (or NH$_4^+$) is present in the blood. The concentration ranges between 30 and 60 μM. Ammonia is rapidly removed from the blood and converted to urea by the liver. Nitrogen travels in the blood mainly in amino acids, particularly alanine and glutamine. The urea cycle was proposed in 1932 by Hans Krebs and a medical student, Kurt Henseleit, based on their laboratory observations. It was originally called the *Krebs-Henseleit cycle*. Subsequently, Krebs used this concept of metabolic cycling to explain a second process that also bears his name, the Krebs (or tricarboxylic acid [TCA]) cycle.

A. Reactions of the Urea Cycle

Nitrogen enters the urea cycle as NH$_4^+$ and aspartate (Fig. 36.10). NH$_4^+$ forms carbamoyl phosphate, which reacts with ornithine to form citrulline. Ornithine is the compound that both initiates and is regenerated by the cycle (similar to oxaloacetate in the TCA cycle). Aspartate reacts with citrulline, eventually donating its nitrogen

Percy V.'s symptoms and laboratory abnormalities did not slowly subside over the next 6 weeks, as they usually do in uncomplicated viral hepatitis A infections. Instead, his serum total bilirubin, ALT, AST, and alkaline phosphatase levels increased further. His vomiting became intractable, and his friend noted jerking motions of his arms (asterixis), facial grimacing, restlessness, slowed mentation, and slight disorientation. He was admitted to the hospital with a diagnosis of hepatic failure with incipient hepatic encephalopathy (brain dysfunction caused by accumulation of various toxins in the blood), a rare complication of acute type A viral hepatitis alone. The possibility of a superimposed acute hepatic toxicity caused by the use of acetaminophen was considered.

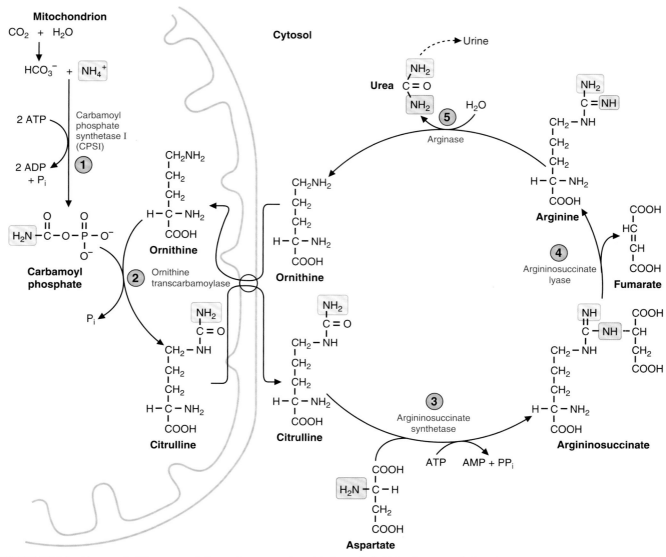

FIGURE 36.10 Urea cycle. The steps of the cycle are *numbered 1* through *5. ADP*, adenosine diphosphate; *AMP*, adenosine monophosphate; *ATP*, adenosine triphosphate; *P_i*, inorganic phosphate.

for urea formation. Arginine is formed in two successive steps. Cleavage of arginine by arginase releases urea and regenerates ornithine.

1. Synthesis of Carbamoyl Phosphate

In the first step of the urea cycle, NH_4^+, bicarbonate, and ATP react to form carbamoyl phosphate (see Fig. 36.10). The cleavage of two molecules of ATP is required to form the high-energy phosphate bond of carbamoyl phosphate. CPSI, the enzyme that catalyzes this first step of the urea cycle, is found mainly in mitochondria of the liver and intestine. The Roman numeral suggests that another carbamoyl phosphate synthetase exists, and indeed, CPSII, located in the cytosol, produces carbamoyl phosphate for pyrimidine biosynthesis, using nitrogen from glutamine (see Chapter 39).

2. Production of Arginine by the Urea Cycle

Carbamoyl phosphate reacts with ornithine to form citrulline (see Fig. 36.10). The high-energy phosphate bond of carbamoyl phosphate provides the energy required for this reaction, which occurs in mitochondria and is catalyzed by ornithine trans-carbamoylase (OTC). The product citrulline is transported across the mitochondrial membranes in exchange for cytoplasmic ornithine and enters the cytosol. The carrier for this transport reaction catalyzes an electroneutral exchange of the two compounds.

In the cytosol, citrulline reacts with aspartate, the second source of nitrogen for urea synthesis, to produce argininosuccinate (see Fig. 36.10). This reaction, catalyzed by argininosuccinate synthetase, is driven by the hydrolysis of ATP to adenosine monophosphate (AMP) and pyrophosphate. Aspartate is produced by transamination of oxaloacetate.

Argininosuccinate is cleaved by argininosuccinate lyase to form fumarate and arginine (see Fig. 36.10). Fumarate is produced from the carbons of argininosuc-cinate provided by aspartate. Fumarate is converted to malate (using cytoplasmic fumarase), which is used either for the synthesis of glucose by the gluconeogenic pathway or for the regeneration of oxaloacetate by cytoplasmic reactions similar to those observed in the TCA cycle (Fig. 36.11). The oxaloacetate that is formed is transaminated to generate the aspartate that carries nitrogen into the urea cycle. Thus, the carbons of fumarate can be recycled to aspartate.

3. Cleavage of Arginine to Produce Urea

Arginine, which contains nitrogens derived from NH_4^+ and aspartate, is cleaved by arginase, producing urea and regenerating ornithine (see Fig. 36.10). Urea is produced from the guanidinium group on the side chain of arginine. The portion of arginine originally derived from ornithine is reconverted to ornithine.

The reactions by which citrulline is converted to arginine and arginine is cleaved to produce urea occur in the cytosol. Ornithine, the other product of the arginase re-action, is transported into the mitochondrion in exchange for citrulline, where it can react with carbamoyl phosphate, initiating another round of the cycle.

B. Origin of Ornithine

Ornithine is an amino acid. However, it is not incorporated into proteins during the process of protein synthesis because no genetic codon exists for this amino acid. Although ornithine is normally regenerated by the urea cycle (as one of the products of the arginase reaction), ornithine also can be synthesized de novo if needed. The reaction is an unusual transamination reaction catalyzed by ornithine aminotransferase under specific conditions in the intestine (Fig. 36.12). The usual direction of this reaction is the formation of glutamate semialdehyde, which is the first step of the degradation pathway for ornithine.

When OTC is deficient, the carbamoyl phosphate that normally would enter the urea cycle accumulates and floods the pathway for pyrimidine biosynthesis. Carbamoyl phosphate, produced by a cytoplasmic enzyme (CPSII), is the precursor for pyrimidine synthesis. Under these conditions, excess orotic acid (orotate), an intermediate in pyrimidine biosynthesis, is excreted in the urine. It produces no ill effects but is indicative of a problem in the urea cycle.

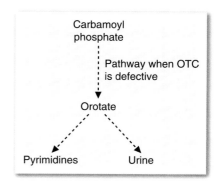

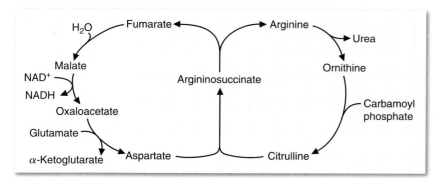

FIGURE 36.11 The Krebs bi-cycle, indicating the common steps between the tricar-boxylic acid (TCA) and urea cycles. All reactions shown occur in the cytoplasm except for the synthesis of citrulline, which occurs in the mitochondria. *NAD*, nicotinamide adenine dinucleotide.

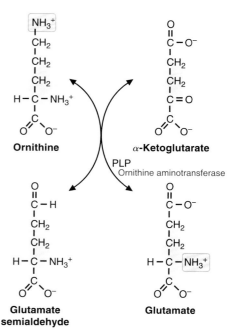

FIGURE 36.12 The ornithine aminotrans-ferase reaction. This is a reversible reaction that requires pyridoxal phosphate (PLP), which normally favors ornithine degradation.

The precise pathogenesis of the CNS signs and symptoms that accompany liver failure (hepatic encephalopathy) in patients such as **Percy V.** is not completely understood. These changes are, however, attributable in part to toxic materials that are derived from the metabolism of nitrogenous substrates by bacteria in the gut that circulate to the liver in the portal vein. These materials bypass their normal metabolism by the liver cells, however, because the acute inflammatory process of viral hepatitis severely limits the ability of liver cells to degrade these compounds to harmless metabolites. As a result, these toxins are shunted into the hepatic veins unaltered and eventually reach the brain through the systemic circulation ("portal–systemic encephalopathy").

NH_4^+ is one of the toxins that results from the degradation of urea or proteins by intestinal bacteria and is not metabolized by the infected liver. The subsequent elevation of ammonia concentrations in the fluid bathing the brain causes depletion of TCA-cycle intermediates and ATP in the CNS. α-Ketoglutarate, a TCA-cycle intermediate, combines with ammonia to form glutamate in a reaction catalyzed by glutamate dehydrogenase. Glutamate subsequently reacts with ammonia to form glutamine. This effectively reduces α-ketoglutarate levels in the mitochondria, thereby reducing the rate at which the TCA cycle can operate.

The absolute level of ammonia and its metabolites, such as glutamine, in the blood or cerebrospinal fluid in patients with hepatic encephalopathy correlates only roughly with the presence or severity of the neurologic signs and symptoms. γ-Aminobutyric acid (GABA), an important inhibitory neurotransmitter in the brain, is also produced in the gut lumen and is shunted into the systemic circulation in increased amounts in patients with hepatic failure. In addition, other compounds (such as aromatic amino acids, false neurotransmitters, and certain short-chain fatty acids) bypass liver metabolism and accumulate in the systemic circulation, adversely affecting CNS function. Their relative importance in the pathogenesis of hepatic encephalopathy remains to be determined.

C. Regulation of the Urea Cycle

The human liver has a vast capacity to convert amino acid nitrogen to urea, thereby preventing toxic effects from ammonia, which would otherwise accumulate. In general, the urea cycle is regulated by substrate availability; the higher the rate of ammonia production, the higher is the rate of urea formation. Regulation by substrate availability is a general characteristic of disposal pathways, such as the urea cycle, which remove toxic compounds from the body. This is a type of feed-forward regulation, in contrast to the feedback regulation characteristic of pathways that produce functional end products.

Two other types of regulation control the urea cycle: allosteric activation of CPSI by *N*-acetylglutamate (NAG) and induction and repression of the synthesis of urea-cycle enzymes. NAG is formed specifically to activate CPSI; it has no other known function in mammals. The synthesis of NAG from acetyl coenzyme A (acetyl-CoA) and glutamate is stimulated by arginine (Fig. 36.13). Thus, as arginine levels increase within the liver, two important reactions are stimulated. The first is the synthesis of NAG, which increases the rate at which carbamoyl phosphate is produced. The second is to produce more ornithine (via the arginase reaction) such that the cycle can operate more rapidly.

The induction of urea-cycle enzymes occurs in response to conditions that require increased protein metabolism, such as a high-protein diet or prolonged fasting. In both of these physiologic states, as amino acid carbon is converted to glucose, amino acid nitrogen is converted to urea. The induction of the synthesis of urea-cycle enzymes under these conditions occurs even though the uninduced enzyme levels are far in excess of the capacity required. The ability of a high-protein diet to increase urea-cycle enzyme levels is another type of feed-forward regulation.

D. Function of the Urea Cycle during Fasting

During fasting, the liver maintains blood glucose levels. Amino acids from muscle protein are a major carbon source for the production of glucose by the pathway of gluconeogenesis. As amino acid carbons are converted to glucose, the nitrogens are converted to urea. Thus, the urinary excretion of urea is high during fasting (Fig. 36.14).

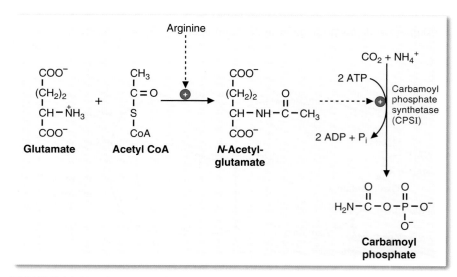

FIGURE 36.13 Activation of carbamoyl phosphate synthetase I (CPSI). Arginine stimulates the synthesis of *N*-acetylglutamate, which activates CPSI. *Acetyl CoA*, acetyl coenzyme A; *ADP*, adenosine diphosphate; *ATP*, adenosine triphosphate; *Pᵢ*, inorganic phosphate.

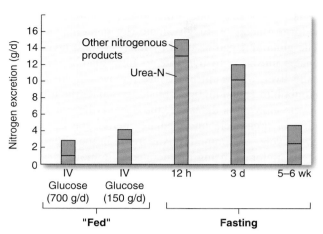

FIGURE 36.14 Nitrogen excretion during fasting. Human subjects were initially given intravenous (IV) glucose as indicated, then fasted. Total nitrogen excretion was measured as well as the nitrogen in urea (*brown area*). (Based on Ruderman NB, Aoki TT, Cahill GF Jr. Gluconeogenesis and its disorders in man. In: Hanson RW, Mehlman MA, eds. *Gluconeogenesis: Its Regulation in Mammalian Species*. New York, NY: John Wiley & Sons; 1976:518.)

 In addition to producing urea, the reactions of the urea cycle also serve as the pathway for the biosynthesis of arginine. Therefore, this amino acid is not required in the diet of the adult; however, it is required in the diet for growth. Urea is not cleaved by human enzymes. However, bacteria, including those in the human digestive tract, can cleave urea to ammonia and CO_2, using the enzyme urease. Urease is not produced by humans.

To some extent, humans excrete urea into the gut and saliva. Intestinal bacteria convert urea to ammonia. This ammonia, as well as ammonia produced by other bacterial reactions in the gut, is absorbed into the hepatic portal vein. It is normally extracted by the liver and converted to urea. Approximately one fourth of the total urea released by the liver each day is recycled by bacteria.

As fasting progresses, however, the brain begins to use ketone bodies, sparing blood glucose. Less muscle protein is cleaved to provide amino acids for gluconeogenesis, and decreased production of glucose from amino acids is accompanied by decreased production of urea (see Chapter 28).

The major amino acid substrate for gluconeogenesis is alanine, which is synthesized in peripheral tissues to act as a nitrogen carrier (see Fig. 36.8). Glucagon release, which is expected during fasting, stimulates alanine transport into the liver by activating the transcription of transport systems for alanine. Two molecules of alanine are required to generate one molecule of glucose. The nitrogen from the two molecules of alanine is converted to one molecule of urea (Fig. 36.15).

E. Disorders of the Urea Cycle

Disorders of the urea cycle are dangerous because of the accumulation of ammonia in the circulation. Ammonia is toxic to the nervous system, and its concentration in the body must be carefully controlled. Under normal conditions,

 Blood ammonia levels can be determined in several ways. One is to use an ammonia-specific electrode. Another is to use enzyme-coupled reactions that result in either a color change or an absorbance change. One enzyme-coupled system takes advantage of glutamate dehydrogenase. The unknown sample is incubated with glutamate dehydrogenase, α-ketoglutarate and NADPH. If ammonia is present, glutamate will be produced as will $NADP^+$. As NADPH is converted to $NADP^+$, the absorbance of light at 340 nm will decrease, and because one $NADP^+$ is formed per ammonia molecule used, the concentration of ammonia can be determined.

Blood urea nitrogen (BUN) is a measurement for the urea content of the blood. The key to measuring BUN is to split urea into carbon dioxide and two ammonia molecules by the bacterial enzyme urease. The ammonia levels are then determined as described previously or via a colorimetric assay based on pH indicator dyes. As ammonia is generated, it binds protons, forming ammonium ions, which raises the pH. The extent of the pH change will be proportional to the amount of ammonia generated. Once BUN is determined, the urea concentration can be determined (in milligrams per deciliter) by multiplying the nitrogen value by 2.14.

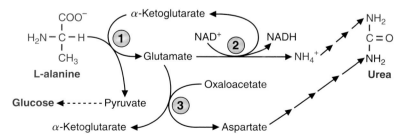

FIGURE 36.15 Conversion of alanine to glucose and urea. (*1*) Alanine, the key gluconeogenic amino acid, is transaminated to form pyruvate, which is converted to glucose. The nitrogen, now in glutamate, can be released as NH_4^+ (2) or transferred to oxaloacetate to form aspartate (3). NH_4^+ and aspartate enter the urea cycle, which produces urea. In summary, the carbons of alanine form glucose and the nitrogens form urea. Two molecules of alanine are required to produce one molecule of glucose and one molecule of urea. *NAD*, nicotinamide adenine dinucleotide.

free ammonia is rapidly fixed into either α-ketoglutarate (by glutamate dehydrogenase, to form glutamate) or glutamate (by glutamine synthetase, to form glutamine). The glutamine can be used by many tissues, including the liver; the glutamate donates nitrogens to pyruvate to form alanine, which travels to the liver. Within the liver, as the nitrogens are removed from their carriers, CPSI fixes the ammonia into carbamoyl phosphate to initiate the urea cycle. However, when a urea-cycle enzyme is defective, the cycle is interrupted, which leads to an accumulation of urea-cycle intermediates before the block. Because of the block in the urea cycle, glutamine levels increase in the circulation, and because α-ketoglutarate is no longer being regenerated by removal of nitrogen from glutamine, the α-ketoglutarate levels are too low to fix more free ammonia, leading to elevated ammonia levels in the blood. Therefore, defects in any urea-cycle enzyme lead to elevated glutamine and ammonia levels in the circulation. However, the extent of the elevation depends on which enzyme is defective; see question 1 at the end of this chapter.

Ammonia toxicity will lead to brain swelling, caused, in part, by an osmotic imbalance owing to high levels of both ammonia and glutamine in the astrocytes. As ammonia levels increase in the astrocytes, more glutamine is produced (via glutamine synthetase), which only exacerbates the osmotic imbalance. The ammonia levels inhibit glutaminase, leading to glutamine elevation. Additionally, high levels of glutamine alter the permeability of the mitochondrial membrane, leading to an opening of the mitochondrial permeability transition pore, which leads to cell death (see Chapter 24). Another toxic effect of ammonia is a lowering of glutamate levels (owing to the high activity of the glutamine synthetase reaction). Glutamate is a neurotransmitter, and glutamatergic neurotransmission, if impaired, causes brain dysfunction because glutamate is one of the excitatory neurotransmitters, and in the absence of glutamate neurotransmission, lethargy and reduced nervous system activity can result.

The most common urea-cycle defect is OTC deficiency, which is an X-linked disorder. This disorder occurs with a frequency of about 1 in 80,000 people.

The major clinical problem in treating patients with urea-cycle defects is reducing the effects of excessive blood ammonia on the nervous system. High ammonia levels can lead to irreversible neuronal damage and intellectual disability. So, how is hyperammonemia treated?

The key to treating patients with urea-cycle defects is to diagnose the disease early and then treat aggressively with compounds that can aid in nitrogen removal from the patient. Low-protein diets are essential to reduce the potential for excessive amino acid degradation. If the enzyme defect in the urea cycle comes after the synthesis of argininosuccinate, massive arginine supplementation has proved beneficial. Once argininosuccinate has been synthesized, the two nitrogen molecules destined for excretion have been incorporated into the substrate; the problem is that ornithine cannot be regenerated. If ornithine could be replenished to allow the cycle to continue, argininosuccinate could be used as the carrier for nitrogen excretion from the body. Thus, ingesting large levels of arginine leads to ornithine production by the arginase reaction, and nitrogen excretion via argininosuccinate in the urine can be enhanced.

Arginine therapy will not work for enzyme defects that exist in steps before the synthesis of argininosuccinate. For these disorders, drugs are used that form conjugates with amino acids. The conjugated amino acids are excreted, and the body then has to use its nitrogen to resynthesize the excreted amino acid. The two compounds most frequently used are benzoic acid and phenylbutyrate (the active component of phenylbutyrate is phenylacetate, its oxidation product. Phenylacetate has a bad odor, which makes it difficult to take orally). As indicated in Figure 36.16A, benzoic acid, after activation, reacts with glycine to form hippuric acid, which is excreted. As glycine is synthesized from serine, the body now uses nitrogens to synthesize

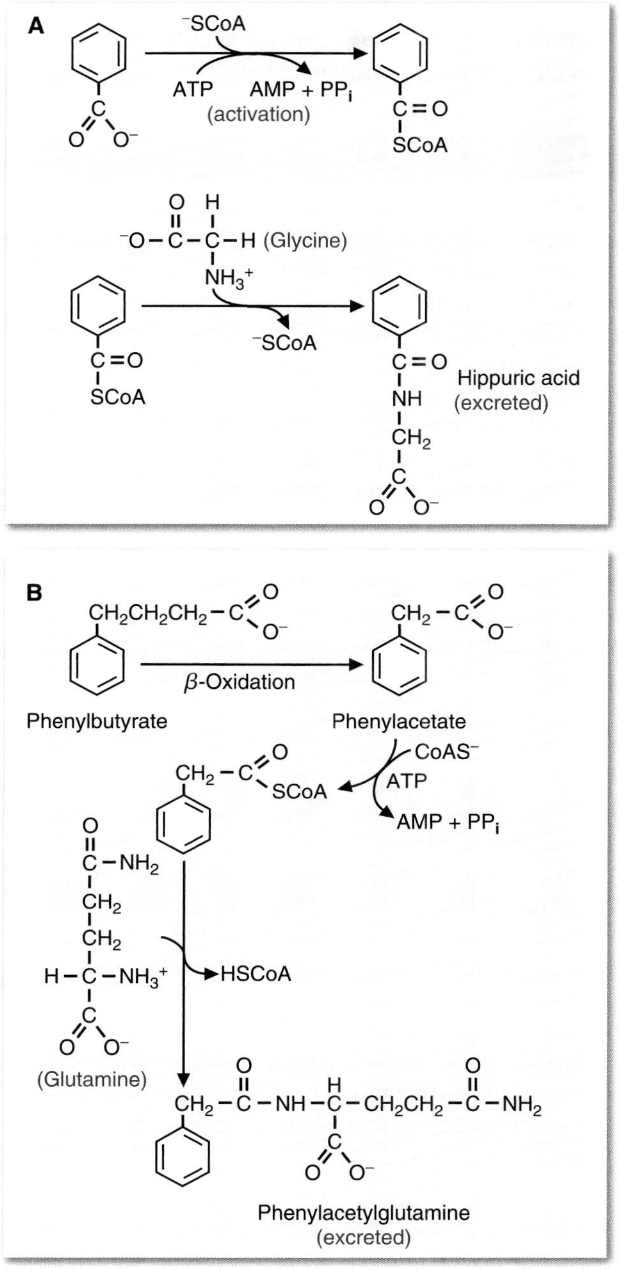

FIGURE 36.16   The metabolism of benzoic acid **(A)** and phenylbutyrate **(B)**, two agents used to reduce nitrogen levels in patients with urea-cycle defects. *CoA*, coenzyme A; *AMP*, adenosine monophosphate; *ATP*, adenosine triphosphate; *PP$_i$*, pyrophosphate.

serine, so more glycine can be produced. Phenylacetate (see Fig. 36.16B) forms a conjugate with glutamine, which is excreted. This conjugate removes two nitrogens per molecule and requires the body to resynthesize glutamine from glucose, thereby using another two nitrogen molecules.

Urea-cycle defects are excellent candidates for treatment by gene therapy. This is because the defect has to be repaired in only one cell type (in this case, the hepatocyte), which makes it easier to target the vector carrying the replacement gene. Preliminary gene therapy experiments had been carried out on individuals with OTC deficiency (the most common inherited defect of the urea cycle), but the experiments came to a halt when one of the patients died of a severe immunologic reaction to the vector used to deliver the gene. This incident led to a review and improvements of gene therapy protocols in the United States.

CLINICAL COMMENTS

Percy V. The two most serious complications of acute viral hepatitis found in patients such as **Percy V.** are massive hepatic necrosis leading to fulminant liver failure and the eventual development of chronic hepatitis. Both complications are rare in acute viral hepatitis type A, however, suggesting that acetaminophen toxicity may have contributed to Percy's otherwise unexpectedly severe hepatocellular dysfunction and early hepatic encephalopathy.

Fortunately, bed rest, rehydration, parenteral nutrition, and therapy directed at decreasing the production of toxins that result from bacterial degradation of nitrogenous substrates in the gut lumen (e.g., administration of lactulose, which reduces gut ammonia levels by a variety of mechanisms; the use of enemas and certain antibiotics, such as rifaximin, to decrease the intestinal flora; a low-protein diet) prevented Percy from progressing to the later stages of hepatic encephalopathy. As with most patients who survive an episode of fulminant hepatic failure, recovery to his previous state of health occurred over the next 3 months. Percy's liver function studies returned to normal, and a follow-up liver biopsy showed no histologic abnormalities.

BIOCHEMICAL COMMENTS

Pyridoxal Phosphate. PLP is a key coenzyme for amino acid metabolism. This cofactor participates in a wide variety of reactions involving amino acids, such as transamination, deamination, decarboxylation, β-elimination, racemization, and γ-elimination. The type of reaction that takes place is dictated by the amino acid substrate and the enzymes that catalyze the reaction.

All amino acid reactions that require PLP occur with the amino group of the amino acid bonded covalently to the aldehyde carbon of the coenzyme (Fig. 36.17). As an example of a mechanism through which PLP aids catalysis, Figure 36.18 indicates how a transamination reaction occurs. The other reaction types that require PLP follow similar mechanisms.

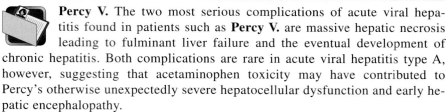

FIGURE 36.17 Pyridoxal phosphate (PLP) attached covalently to an amino acid substrate. The *arrows* indicate which bonds are broken for the various types of reactions in which PLP is involved. *X* and *Y* represent chemical leaving groups that may be present on the amino acid (such as the hydroxyl group on serine or threonine).

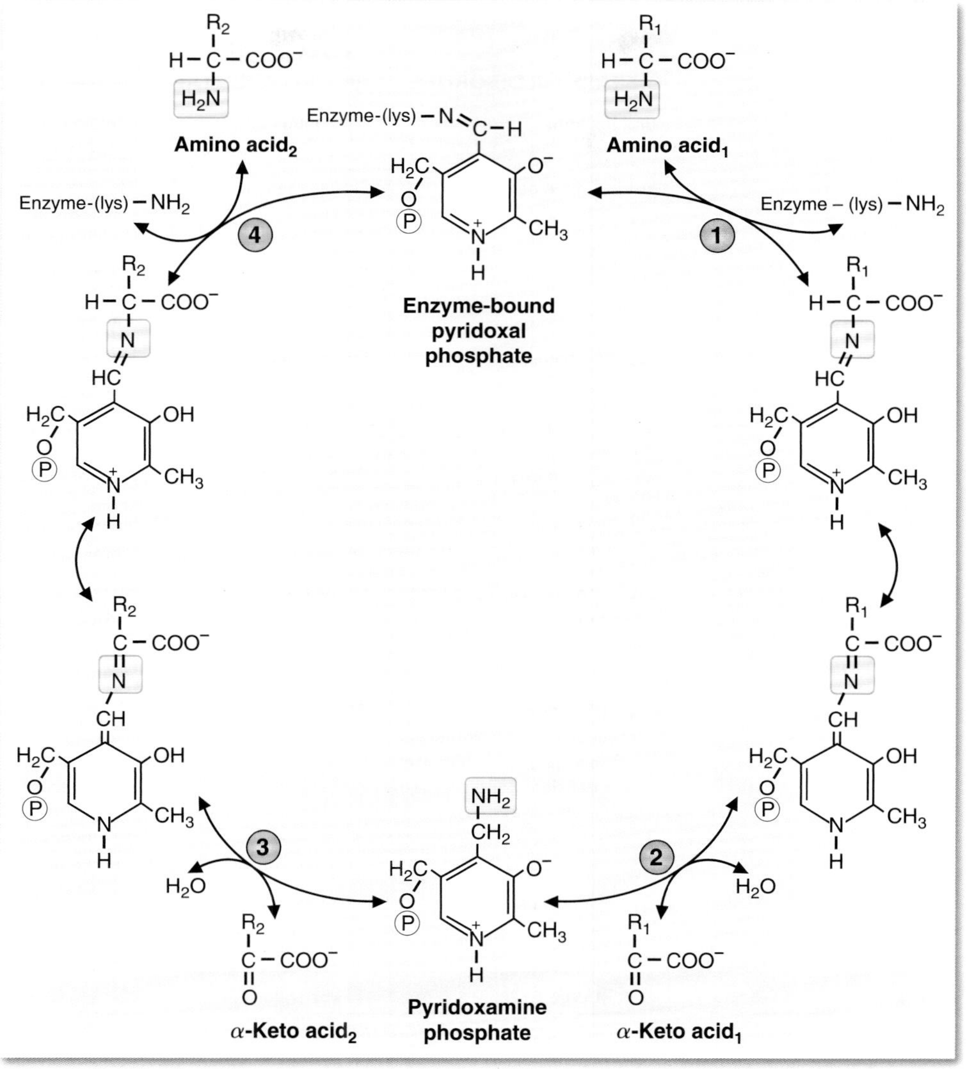

FIGURE 36.18 Function of pyridoxal phosphate (PLP) in transamination reactions. The order in which the reactions occur is 1 to 4. PLP (enzyme-bound) reacts with amino acid$_1$, forming a Schiff base (a carbon–nitrogen double bond). After a shift of the double bond, α-keto acid$_1$ is released through hydrolysis of the Schiff base, and pyridoxamine phosphate is produced. Pyridoxamine phosphate then forms a Schiff base with α-keto acid$_2$. After the double bond shifts, amino acid$_2$ is released through hydrolysis of the Schiff base, and enzyme-bound PLP is regenerated. The net result is that the amino group from amino acid$_1$ is transferred to α-keto acid$_2$.

KEY CONCEPTS

- Amino acid catabolism generates urea, which is a nontoxic carrier of nitrogen atoms.
- Urea synthesis occurs in the liver. The amino acids alanine and glutamine carry amino acid nitrogen from peripheral tissues to the liver.
- Key enzymes involved in nitrogen disposal are transaminases, glutamate dehydrogenase, and glutaminase.
- The urea cycle consists of four steps and incorporates a nitrogen from ammonia and one from aspartate into urea.
- Disorders of the urea cycle lead to hyperammonemia, a condition that is toxic to nervous system health and development.
- Diseases discussed in this chapter are summarized in Table 36.1.

DISEASE OR DISORDER	GENETIC OR ENVIRONMENTAL	COMMENTS
Viral hepatitis	Environmental	Infection of the liver by viral hepatitis may lead to liver failure.
Pyridoxamine deficiency	Environmental	The lack of vitamin B_6 affects many systems, such as heme synthesis, glycogen phosphorylase activity, and neurotransmitter synthesis, possibly leading to dementia, dermatitis, anemia, weakness, and convulsions.
Hepatic encephalopathy	Environmental	Liver failure leading to brain dysfunction, caused by the liver's inability to rid the body of toxins, including ammonia
Ammonia toxicity	Both	Ammonia accumulation interferes with energy production and neurotransmitter synthesis in the brain, altering brain function.
Ornithine transcarbamoylase deficiency	Genetic	Most common urea-cycle defect, leading to elevated blood ammonia and orotic acid levels, and will lead to mental impairment if not treated
CPSI deficiency, argininosuccinate synthetase deficiency, argininosuccinate lyase deficiency, and arginase deficiency	All genetic	Mutations in urea-cycle enzymes, leading to various degrees of hyperammonemia and inability to synthesize urea; can be distinguished by the type of urea-cycle intermediates that accumulate in the blood

TABLE 36.1   Diseases Discussed in Chapter 36

CPSI, carbamoyl phosphate synthetase I.

REVIEW QUESTIONS—CHAPTER 36

1. Deficiency diseases have been described that involve each of the five enzymes of the urea cycle. Clinical manifestations may appear in the neonatal period. Infants with defects in the first four enzymes usually appear normal at birth but after 24 hours progressively develop lethargy, hypothermia, and apnea. They have high blood ammonia levels, and the brain becomes swollen. One possible explanation for the swelling is the osmotic effect of the accumulation of glutamine in the brain produced by the reactions of ammonia with α-ketoglutarate and glutamate. Arginase deficiency is not as severe as deficiencies of the other urea-cycle enzymes.

   Given the following information about five newborn infants (identified as *I* through *V*) who appeared normal at birth but developed hyperammonemia after 24 hours, determine which urea-cycle enzyme might be defective in each case (for each infant, choose from the same five answers, A through E). All infants had low levels of BUN. (Normal citrulline levels are 10 to 20 μM.)

Infant	Urine Orotate	Blood Citrulline	Blood Arginine	Blood NH$_3$
I	Low	Low	Low	High
II	—	High ($>$1,000 μM)	Low	High
III	—	—	High	Moderately high
IV	High	Low	Low	High
V	—	High (200 μM)	Low	High

—, value not determined; low, below normal; high, above normal.

   A. CPSI
   B. OTC
   C. Argininosuccinate synthetase
   D. Argininosuccinate lyase
   E. Arginase

2. The nitrogens in urea are derived directly from which of the following compounds?
   A. Ornithine and carbamoyl phosphate
   B. Ornithine and aspartate
   C. Ornithine and glutamate
   D. Carbamoyl phosphate and aspartate
   E. Carbamoyl phosphate and glutamine
   F. Aspartate and glutamine

3. Which one of the following enzymes can fix ammonia into an organic molecule?
   A. Alanine–pyruvate aminotransferase
   B. Glutaminase
   C. Glutamate dehydrogenase
   D. Arginase
   E. Argininosuccinate synthetase

4. Under conditions of high rates of protein turnover, glutamine is used as a nitrogen carrier to deliver nitrogen to the liver for safe disposal as urea. The carbons of glutamine can then be used for gluconeogenesis, which would require which one of the following enzymes?
   A. Malate dehydrogenase
   B. Pyruvate dehydrogenase
   C. Pyruvate carboxylase
   D. Citrate synthase
   E. Pyruvate kinase

5. Drugs used to treat urea-cycle defects, such as sodium benzoate and phenylbutyrate, need to be activated once they enter cells. The activation of these drugs is very similar to which one of the following reactions?
   A. Formation of acetyl-CoA by pyruvate dehydrogenase
   B. Activation of glucose for the glycolytic pathway
   C. Activation of fatty acids
   D. Activation of glucose for glycogen synthesis
   E. Activation of isoprene units

6. Which one of the following food is highest in the vitamin needed to form the required cofactor of transamination reactions?
   A. Eggs
   B. Dairy products
   C. Citrus fruits
   D. Dark-green leafy vegetables
   E. Carrots

7. Release of amino acid nitrogen and NH_4^+ is an important step in generating precursors for the urea cycle. Which statement best describes this release of amino acid nitrogen as NH_4^+ from amino acids?
   A. NH_4^+ freely diffuses across membranes.
   B. Glutamate deamination by oxidation is readily reversible.
   C. Serine deamination to pyruvate is readily reversible.
   D. Glutamine deamination to glutamate is readily reversible.
   E. NH_3 cannot freely diffuse across membranes.

8. Under conditions of rapid amino acid degradation, ammonia levels increase and must be safely removed from the cells. Glutamate can accept a nitrogen in the form of ammonia to form glutamine. Which statement correctly describes what happens to the glutamine, and resulting ammonia and glutamate via the action of glutaminase, in various tissues?
   A. In the liver, glutamine becomes part of the glucose/alanine cycle.
   B. In the kidney, glutamate forms salts with metabolic acids in the urine.
   C. In the intestine, glutamine is used as a fuel.
   D. In the kidney, the glutamate is used for urea synthesis.
   E. In the intestine, glutamine becomes part of the glucose/alanine cycle.

9. The urea cycle is the major mechanism in the human body for removal of nitrogen. Which statement correctly describes steps of the urea cycle?
   A. Three high-energy phosphate bonds are used for one complete cycle.
   B. Citrulline is synthesized in the cytosol.
   C. Citrulline initiates and is regenerated by the cycle.
   D. Ornithine is generated in the mitochondria.
   E. Citrulline is exchanged for ornithine across the mitochondrial membrane in an electroneutral exchange.

10. During fasting, amino acids are a major carbon source for gluconeogenesis, and the nitrogens are converted to urea. Which one of the following correctly describes alanine, the major amino acid substrate of gluconeogenesis from the muscle?
    A. One molecule of alanine is converted to two molecules of glucose and two molecules of urea.
    B. One molecule of alanine is converted to one molecule of glucose and one molecule of urea.
    C. One molecule of alanine is converted to one molecule of glucose and two molecules of urea.
    D. Two molecules of alanine are required to generate one molecule of glucose and one molecule of urea.
    E. Two molecules of alanine are required to generate three molecules of glucose and three molecules of urea.

ANSWERS

1. **Infant I has a defect in CPSI (answer A), and infant IV has a defect in OTC (answer B).** Infants with high ammonia, low arginine, and low citrulline levels must have a defect in a urea-cycle enzyme before the step that produces citrulline; that is, CPSI or OTC. If CPSI is functional and carbamoyl phosphate is produced but cannot be metabolized further, more than the normal amount is diverted to the pathway for pyrimidine synthesis and the intermediate orotate appears in the urine. Therefore, infant I has a defect in CPSI (citrulline is low, and less than the normal amount of orotate is in the urine). Infant IV has an OTC defect; carbamoyl phosphate is produced, but it cannot be converted to citrulline, so citrulline is low and orotate is present in the urine.

Infants II and V have high levels of citrulline but low levels of arginine. **Therefore, they cannot produce arginine from citrulline.** Argininosuccinate synthetase or argininosuccinate lyase is defective. The very elevated citrulline levels in infant II suggest that the block is in argininosuccinate synthetase (answer C). In infant V, citrulline levels are more moderately elevated, suggesting that citrulline can be converted to argininosuccinate and that the defect is in argininosuccinate lyase (answer D). Thus, the accumulated intermediates of the urea cycle are distributed between argininosuccinate and citrulline (both of which can be excreted in the urine). The high levels of arginine and more moderate hyperammonemia in infant III suggest that, in this case, the defect is in arginase (answer E).

2. **The answer is D.** The nitrogens in urea are derived from carbamoyl phosphate and aspartate directly during one turn of the cycle. The nitrogen in the side chain of ornithine is never incorporated into urea because it stays with ornithine (thus, A, B, and C are incorrect). Glutamine does not donate a nitrogen directly during the urea cycle, so E and F are also incorrect.

3. **The answer is C.** Glutamate dehydrogenase fixes ammonia into α-ketoglutarate, generating glutamate, in a reversible reaction that also requires NAD(P)H. Alanine–pyruvate aminotransferase catalyzes the transfer of nitrogen from alanine to an α-keto acid acceptor but does not use ammonia as a substrate. Glutaminase converts glutamine to glutamate and ammonia, but the reaction is not reversible. Arginase splits arginine into urea and ornithine, and argininosuccinate synthetase forms argininosuccinate from citrulline and aspirate. The only other two enzymes that can fix ammonia into an organic compound are CPSI and glutamine synthetase.

4. **The answer is A.** Glutamine is converted to ammonia and glutamate in the cytoplasm (glutaminase) and then to α-ketoglutarate and ammonia in the mitochondria (glutamate dehydrogenase). The α-ketoglutarate goes around the TCA cycle to form malate, which is then exported from the mitochondria to the cytoplasm. In the cytoplasm, the malate is converted to oxaloacetate by malate dehydrogenase. The oxaloacetate is converted to phosphoenolpyruvate by phosphoenolpyruvate carboxykinase, and then the standard gluconeogenic pathway is followed to glucose production. Pyruvate dehydrogenase, pyruvate carboxylase, citrate synthase, and pyruvate kinase are not required for these conversions to occur.

5. **The answer is C.** The activation of fatty acids requires a two-step reaction. In the first, ATP donates AMP to form a covalent bond with the carboxylic acid of the fatty acid, releasing pyrophosphate. In the second step, coenzyme A (CoA) displaces the AMP, forming a fatty acyl CoA. This is the exact same reaction pathway for the activation of these drugs, and the pathway uses enzymes similar to those for fatty acid activation. Activation of glucose for the glycolytic pathway requires phosphorylation (not addition of CoA). Activation of glucose for glycogen synthesis requires formation of a nucleotide sugar, not involving CoA. Formation of an activated isoprene requires two subsequent phosphorylations to create a pyrophosphate derivative (e.g., isopentenyl pyrophosphate). The formation of acetyl-CoA, via pyruvate dehydrogenase, is an oxidative decarboxylation reaction, which is not similar to the fatty acid activation reactions or to those that activate the drugs used for treatment of urea-cycle disorders.

6. **The answer is A.** PLP is the required cofactor for transamination reactions and is derived from pyridoxine (vitamin B_6) found in chicken, fish, pork, eggs, noncitrus fruits, peanuts, and walnuts. Dairy products contain choline and vitamin D, citrus fruits contain vitamin C, carrots contain vitamin A, and leafy vegetables are rich in folate and vitamin K.

7. **The answer is B.** Glutamate deamination to α-ketoglutarate is readily reversible (via the enzyme glutamate dehydrogenase). The other deaminations listed are irreversible reactions (serine deamination requires vitamin B_6, and glutamine deamination is a simple hydrolysis reaction). NH_3 can freely diffuse across membranes, but once NH_4^+ is formed, it can no longer do so because of its charge.

8. **The answer is C.** In the intestine, glutamine is used as fuel. In the liver, glutamate can transaminate oxaloacetate to aspartate or release NH_4^+, both of which join the urea cycle. Alanine, not glutamate, is part of the glucose/alanine cycle. In the kidney, the ammonia formed with glutamate from glutamine forms salts with metabolic acids. Urea is formed in the liver and transported to the kidney.

9. **The answer is E.** Citrulline is synthesized in the mitochondria, and ornithine is regenerated in the cytosol. A transporter exchanges these two amino acids via an electroneutral exchange. Ornithine is the compound that both initiates and is regenerated by the cycle. Four high-energy phosphate bonds are used for one complete cycle—2 ATP to produce carbamoyl phosphate from NH_4^+, and two high-energy bonds (ATP to AMP) to form argininosuccinate from citrulline and aspartate.

10. **The answer is D.** Two molecules of alanine are required to generate one molecule of glucose and one molecule of urea. Glucose contains six carbons, and alanine only three carbons. Urea contains two nitrogen groups, and alanine only contains one nitrogen group. Thus, starting with two molecules of alanine, there are six carbons available for glucose production and two nitrogens available for urea synthesis.

37

Synthesis and Degradation of Amino Acids

Because each of the 20 common amino acids has a unique structure, their metabolic pathways differ. Despite this, some generalities do apply to both the synthesis and the degradation of all amino acids. These are summarized in the following sections. Because several amino acid pathways are clinically relevant, we present most of the diverse pathways that occur in humans. However, we will be as succinct as possible.

Important Coenzymes. **Pyridoxal phosphate** (derived from vitamin B_6) is the quintessential coenzyme of amino acid metabolism. In degradation, it is involved in the removal of amino groups, principally through **transamination reactions** and in donation of amino groups for various amino acid biosynthetic pathways. It is also required for certain reactions that involve the carbon skeleton of amino acids. **Tetrahydrofolate** (**FH_4**) is a coenzyme that is used to transfer one-carbon groups at various oxidation states. FH_4 is used in both amino acid degradation (e.g., serine and histidine) and biosynthesis (e.g., glycine). **Tetrahydrobiopterin** (**BH_4**) is a cofactor that is required for ring hydroxylation reactions (e.g., phenylalanine to tyrosine).

Synthesis of the Amino Acids. Eleven of the 20 common amino acids can be synthesized in the body (Fig. 37.1). The other nine are considered "**essential**" and must be obtained from the diet. Almost all of the amino acids that can be synthesized by humans are amino acids used for the synthesis of additional nitrogen-containing compounds. Examples include glycine, which is used for porphyrin and purine synthesis; glutamate, which is required for neurotransmitter synthesis; and aspartate, which is required for both purine and pyrimidine biosynthesis.

Nine of the 11 "**nonessential**" **amino acids** can be produced from glucose plus, of course, a source of nitrogen, such as another amino acid or ammonia. The other two nonessential amino acids, tyrosine and cysteine, require an essential amino acid for their synthesis (phenylalanine for tyrosine, methionine for cysteine). The carbons for cysteine synthesis come from glucose; the methionine donates only the sulfur.

The carbon skeletons of the 10 nonessential amino acids derived from glucose are produced from intermediates of **glycolysis** and the **tricarboxylic acid** (**TCA**) **cycle** (see Fig. 37.1). Four amino acids (**serine**, **glycine**, **cysteine**, and **alanine**) are produced from glucose through components of the **glycolytic pathway**. TCA-cycle intermediates (which can be produced from glucose) provide carbon for synthesis of the six remaining nonessential amino acids. α-Ketoglutarate is the precursor for the synthesis of glutamate, glutamine, proline, and arginine. Oxaloacetate provides carbon for the synthesis of aspartate and asparagine.

Regulation of the biosynthesis of individual amino acids can be quite complex, but the overriding feature is that the **pathways are feedback-regulated** such that as the **concentration of free amino acid increases**, a key biosynthetic **enzyme is allosterically or transcriptionally inhibited**. Amino acid levels, however, are always maintained at a level such that the aminoacyl-transfer RNA synthetases can remain active, and protein synthesis can continue.

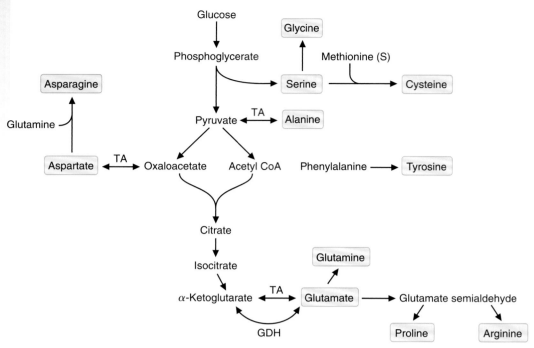

FIGURE 37.1 Overview of the synthesis of the nonessential amino acids. The carbons of 10 amino acids may be produced from glucose through intermediates of glycolysis or the tricarboxylic acid cycle. The 11th nonessential amino acid, tyrosine, is synthesized by hydroxylation of the essential amino acid phenylalanine. Only the sulfur of cysteine comes from the essential amino acid methionine; its carbons and nitrogen come from serine. Transamination (TA) reactions involve pyridoxal phosphate and another amino acid–α-keto acid pair. *Acetyl CoA*, acetyl coenzyme A; *GDH*, glutamate dehydrogenase.

Degradation of Amino Acids. The **degradation pathways** for amino acids are, in general, **distinct from biosynthetic pathways**. This allows for separate regulation of the anabolic and catabolic pathways. Because protein is a fuel, almost every amino acid has a degradative pathway that can generate NADH, which is used as an electron source for oxidative phosphorylation. However, the energy-generating pathway may involve direct oxidation, oxidation in the TCA cycle, conversion to glucose and then oxidation, or conversion to **ketone bodies**, which are then oxidized.

The fate of the carbons of the amino acids depends on the physiologic state of the individual and the tissue in which the degradation occurs. For example, in the liver during fasting, the carbon skeletons of the amino acids produce glucose, ketone bodies, and CO_2. In the fed state, the liver can convert intermediates of amino acid metabolism to glycogen and triacylglycerols. Thus, the **fate of the carbons of the amino acids parallels that of glucose and fatty acids**. The **liver** is the only tissue that has all of the pathways of amino acid synthesis and degradation.

As amino acids are degraded, their **carbons** are converted to (1) **CO_2**, (2) compounds that produce **glucose** in the liver (pyruvate and the TCA-cycle intermediates α-ketoglutarate, succinyl coenzyme A [succinyl-CoA], fumarate, and oxaloacetate), and (3) **ketone bodies** or their precursors (acetoacetate and acetyl coenzyme A [acetyl-CoA]) (Fig. 37.2). For simplicity, amino acids are considered to be **glucogenic** if their carbon skeletons can be converted to a precursor of glucose, and **ketogenic** if their carbon skeletons can be converted directly to acetyl-CoA or acetoacetate. Some amino acids contain carbons that produce a glucose precursor and other carbons that produce acetyl-CoA or acetoacetate. These amino acids are both glucogenic and ketogenic.

The amino acids that are synthesized from intermediates of glycolysis (**serine, alanine,** and **cysteine**) plus certain other amino acids (**threonine, glycine,**

A

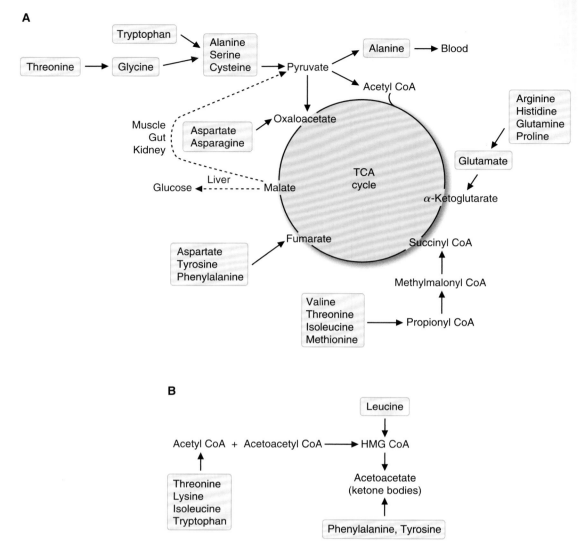

FIGURE 37.2 Degradation of amino acids. **A.** Amino acids that produce pyruvate or intermediates of the tricarboxylic acid (TCA) cycle. These amino acids are considered glucogenic because they can produce glucose in the liver. The fumarate group of amino acids produces cytoplasmic fumarate. Potential mechanisms whereby the cytoplasmic fumarate can be oxidized are presented in Section III.C.1. **B.** Amino acids that produce acetyl coenzyme A (acetyl CoA) or ketone bodies. These amino acids are considered ketogenic. *HMG CoA*, hydroxymethylglutaryl coenzyme A; *Methylmalonyl CoA*, methylmalonyl coenzyme A; *Propionyl CoA*, propionyl coenzyme A; *Succinyl CoA*, succinyl coenzyme A.

and **tryptophan**) produce **pyruvate** when they are degraded. The amino acids synthesized from TCA-cycle intermediates (**aspartate, asparagine, glutamate, glutamine, proline,** and **arginine**) are reconverted to these intermediates during degradation. **Histidine** is converted to **glutamate** and then to the TCA-cycle intermediate α-ketoglutarate. **Methionine, threonine, valine,** and **isoleucine** form **succinyl-CoA,** and **phenylalanine** (after conversion to **tyrosine**) forms **fumarate.** Because pyruvate and the TCA-cycle intermediates can produce glucose in the liver, these amino acids are glucogenic.

Some amino acids with carbons that produce glucose also contain other carbons that produce ketone bodies. **Tryptophan, isoleucine,** and **threonine** produce **acetyl-CoA,** and **phenylalanine** and **tyrosine** produce **acetoacetate.** These amino acids are both glucogenic and ketogenic.

Two of the essential amino acids (**lysine** and **leucine**) are strictly **ketogenic.** They do not produce glucose, only acetoacetate and acetyl-CoA.

All states have enacted legislation requiring that newborns be screened for various metabolic abnormalities, of which PKU is one. A common screening procedure is the Guthrie bacterial inhibition assay. In this assay, spores of the organism *Bacillus subtilis* are plated on an agar plate containing β_2-thienylalanine, an inhibitor of *B. subtilis* growth. The blood sample obtained from the infant (in the form of a dried blood spot on a filter disk) is placed on the agar plate. If the phenylalanine content of the blood is >2 to 4 mg/dL, the phenylalanine will counteract the effects of the β_2-thienylalanine, and bacterial growth will occur. An alternative assay is a microfluorometric determination of phenylalanine, via its incorporation into a ninhydrin–copper complex in the presence of the dipeptide l-leucyl-l-alanine. Positive results with either assay then require verification and actual measurement of phenylalanine levels, using either high-performance liquid chromatography (HPLC) separation of the components of the blood, or enzymatic and fluorometric assays.

 Petria Y., a 4-month-old female infant, emigrated from the Ukraine with her French mother and Russian father 1 month ago. She was normal at birth but in the last several weeks was less than normally attentive to her surroundings. Her psychomotor maturation seemed to be delayed, and a tremor of her extremities had recently appeared. When her mother found her having gross twitching movements in her crib, she brought the infant to the hospital emergency department. A pediatrician examined Petria and immediately noted a musty odor to the baby's wet diaper. A drop of her blood was obtained from a heel prick and used to perform a Guthrie bacterial inhibition assay using a special type of filter paper. This screening procedure was positive for the presence of an excess of phenylalanine in Petria's blood.

 Horace S., a 14-year-old boy, had a sudden weakness of the muscles of the left side of his face and of his left arm and leg. He was hospitalized with a tentative diagnosis of a cerebrovascular accident involving the right cerebral hemisphere.

Horace's past medical history included a downward partial dislocation of the lenses of both eyes, for which he had had a surgical procedure. He also has a slight intellectual disability requiring placement in a special education group.

Horace's left-sided neurologic deficits cleared within 3 days, but a computerized axial tomogram (CAT scan) showed changes consistent with a small infarct (a damaged area caused by a temporary or permanent loss of adequate arterial blood flow) in the right cerebral hemisphere. A neurologist noted that Horace had a slight waddling gait, which his mother said began several years earlier and was progressing with time. Further studies confirmed the decreased mineralization (decreased density) of the skeleton (called *osteopenia* if mild and *osteoporosis* if more severe) and high methionine and homocysteine but low cystine levels in the blood.

All of this information, plus the increased length of the long bones of Horace's extremities and a slight curvature of his spine (scoliosis), caused his physician to suspect that Horace might have an inborn error of metabolism.

I. The Role of Cofactors in Amino Acid Metabolism

Amino acid metabolism requires the participation of three important cofactors. Pyridoxal phosphate (PLP) is the quintessential coenzyme of amino acid metabolism (see "Biochemical Comments" in Chapter 36). It is required for the following types of reactions involving amino acids: transamination, deamination, decarboxylation, β-elimination, racemization, and γ-elimination. Almost all pathways involving amino acid metabolism will require PLP at one step of the pathway.

The coenzyme FH_4, which is derived from the vitamin folate, is required in certain amino acid pathways to either accept or donate a one-carbon group. The carbon can be in various states of oxidation. Chapter 38 describes the reactions of FH_4 in much more detail.

The coenzyme BH_4 is required for ring hydroxylations. The reactions involve molecular oxygen, and one atom of oxygen is incorporated into the product. The second is found in water (see Chapter 24). BH_4 is important for the synthesis of tyrosine and neurotransmitters (see Chapter 46).

II. Amino Acids Derived from Intermediates of Glycolysis

Four amino acids are synthesized from intermediates of glycolysis: serine, glycine, cysteine, and alanine. Serine, which produces glycine and cysteine, is synthesized from 3-phosphoglycerate, and alanine is formed by transamination of pyruvate, the product of glycolysis (Fig. 37.3). When these amino acids are degraded, their carbon atoms are converted to pyruvate or to intermediates of the glycolytic/gluconeogenic pathway and, therefore, can produce glucose or be oxidized to CO_2.

A. Serine

In the biosynthesis of serine from glucose, 3-phosphoglycerate is first oxidized to a 2-keto compound (3-phosphohydroxypyruvate), which is then transaminated to form phosphoserine (Fig. 37.4). Phosphoserine phosphatase removes the phosphate, forming serine. The major sites of serine synthesis are the liver and kidney.

Serine can be used by many tissues and is generally degraded by transamination to hydroxypyruvate, followed by reduction and phosphorylation to form 2-phosphoglycerate, an intermediate of glycolysis that forms phosphoenolpyruvate (PEP) and, subsequently, pyruvate. Serine also can undergo β-elimination of its hydroxyl group, catalyzed by serine dehydratase, to form pyruvate directly.

Regulatory mechanisms maintain serine levels in the body. When serine levels fall, serine synthesis is increased by induction of 3-phosphoglycerate dehydrogenase and by release of the feedback inhibition of phosphoserine phosphatase (caused by higher levels of serine). When serine levels rise, synthesis of serine decreases because synthesis of the dehydrogenase is repressed and the phosphatase is inhibited (see Fig. 37.4).

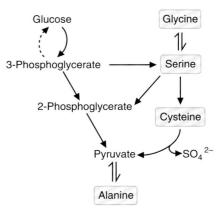

FIGURE 37.3 Amino acids derived from intermediates of glycolysis. These amino acids can be synthesized from glucose. Their carbons can be reconverted to glucose in the liver.

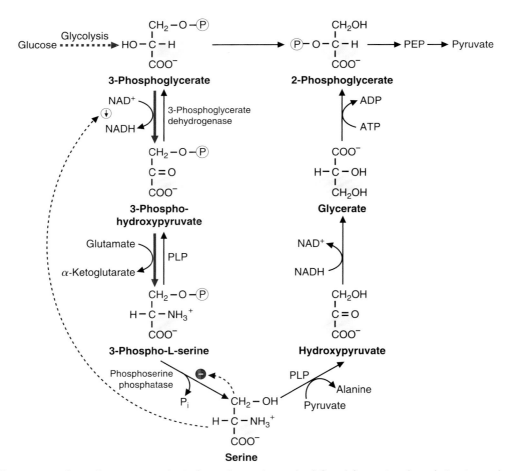

FIGURE 37.4 The major pathway for serine synthesis from glucose is on the *left* and for serine degradation is on the *right*. Serine levels are maintained because serine causes repression (↓) of 3-phosphoglycerate dehydrogenase synthesis. Serine also inhibits (⊖) phosphoserine phosphatase. *ADP*, adenosine diphosphate; *ATP*, adenosine triphosphate; *NAD*, nicotinamide adenine dinucleotide; *PEP*, phosphoenolpyruvate; P_i, inorganic phosphate; *PLP*, pyridoxal phosphate.

B. Glycine

Glycine can be synthesized from serine and, to a minor extent, threonine. The major route from serine is by a reversible reaction that involves FH_4 and PLP (Fig. 37.5). FH_4 is a coenzyme that transfers one-carbon groups at different levels of oxidation. It is derived from the vitamin folate and is discussed in more detail in Chapter 38. The minor pathway for glycine production involves threonine degradation (this is an aldolaselike reaction because threonine contains a hydroxyl group located two carbons from the carbonyl group).

The conversion of glycine to glyoxylate by the enzyme D-amino acid oxidase is a degradative pathway of glycine that is clinically relevant. Once glyoxylate is formed, it can be oxidized to oxalate, which is sparingly soluble and tends to precipitate in kidney tubules, leading to formation of kidney stones. Approximately 40% of oxalate formation in the liver comes from glycine metabolism. Dietary oxalate accumulation has been estimated to be a low contributor to excreted oxalate in the urine because of poor absorption of oxalate in the intestine.

Although glyoxylate can be transaminated back to glycine, this is not really considered a biosynthetic route for "new" glycine because the primary route for glyoxylate formation is from glycine oxidation.

Generation of energy from glycine occurs through a dehydrogenase (glycine cleavage enzyme) that oxidizes glycine to CO_2, ammonia, and a carbon that is donated to FH_4.

C. Cysteine

The carbons and nitrogen for cysteine synthesis are provided by serine, and the sulfur is provided by methionine (Fig. 37.6). Serine reacts with homocysteine (which is produced from methionine) to form cystathionine. This reaction is catalyzed by cystathionine β-synthase. Cleavage of cystathionine by cystathionase produces cysteine and α-ketobutyrate, which forms succinyl-CoA via propionyl-CoA. Both cystathionine β-synthase (β-elimination) and cystathionase (γ-elimination) require PLP.

Cysteine inhibits cystathionine β-synthase and, therefore, regulates its own production to adjust for the dietary supply of cysteine. Because cysteine derives its sulfur from the essential amino acid methionine, cysteine becomes essential if the

Oxalate, produced from glycine or obtained from the diet, forms precipitates with calcium. Kidney stones (renal calculi) are often composed of calcium oxalate. A lack of the transaminase that can convert glyoxylate to glycine (see Fig. 37.5) leads to the disease primary oxaluria type I (PH I). This disease has a consequence of renal failure attributable to excessive accumulation of calcium oxalate in the kidney.

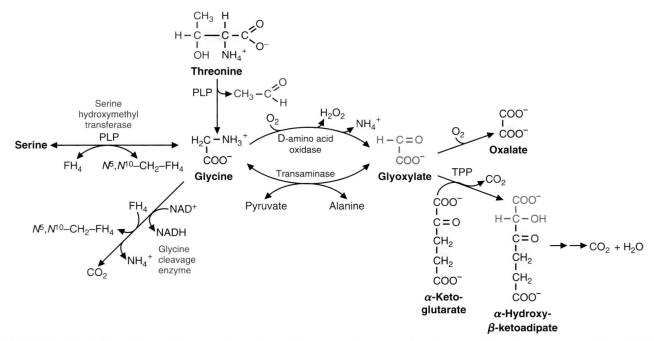

FIGURE 37.5 Metabolism of glycine. Glycine can be synthesized from serine (major route) or threonine. Glycine forms serine or CO_2 and NH_4^+ by reactions that require tetrahydrofolate (FH_4). Glycine also forms glyoxylate, which is converted to oxalate or to CO_2 and H_2O. N^5, N^{10}-CH_2–FH_4, N^5, N^{10}-methylene tetrahydrofolate (see Chapter 38); *NAD*, nicotinamide adenine dinucleotide; *PLP*, pyridoxal phosphate; *TPP*, thiamine pyrophosphate.

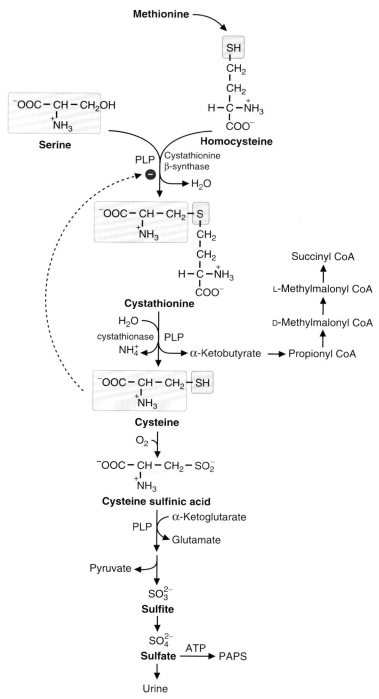

FIGURE 37.6 Synthesis and degradation of cysteine. Cysteine is synthesized from the carbons and nitrogen of serine and the sulfur of homocysteine (which is derived from methionine). During the degradation of cysteine, the sulfur is converted to sulfate and either excreted in the urine or converted to 3′-phosphoadenosine 5′-phosphosulfate (PAPS; the universal sulfate donor), and the carbons are converted to pyruvate. *ATP*, adenosine triphosphate; *Methylmalonyl CoA*, methylmalonyl coenzyme A; *Propionyl CoA*, propionyl coenzyme A; *PLP*, pyridoxal phosphate; *Succinyl CoA*, succinyl coenzyme A.

supply of methionine is inadequate for cysteine synthesis. Conversely, an adequate dietary source of cysteine "spares" methionine; that is, it decreases the amount that must be degraded to produce cysteine.

When cysteine is degraded, the nitrogen is converted to urea, the carbons to pyruvate, and the sulfur to sulfate, which has two potential fates (see Fig. 37.6;

 Cystathioninuria, the presence of cystathionine in the urine, is relatively common in premature infants. As they mature, cystathionase levels rise, and the levels of cystathionine in the urine decrease. In adults, a genetic deficiency of cystathionase causes cystathioninuria. Individuals with a genetically normal cystathionase can also develop cystathioninuria from a dietary deficiency of pyridoxine (vitamin B₆) because cystathionase requires the cofactor PLP. No characteristic clinical abnormalities have been observed in individuals with cystathionase deficiency, and it is probably a benign disorder.

Cystinuria and cystinosis are disorders involving two different transport proteins for cystine, the disulfide formed from two molecules of cysteine. Cystinuria is caused by a defect in the transport protein that carries cystine, lysine, arginine, and ornithine into intestinal epithelial cells and that permits resorption of these amino acids by renal tubular cells. Cystine, which is not very soluble in the urine, forms renal calculi (stones). **David K.**, a patient with cystinuria, developed cystine stones (see Chapter 35).

Cystinosis is a rare disorder caused by a defective carrier that normally transports cystine across the lysosomal membrane from lysosomal vesicles to the cytosol. Cystine accumulates in the lysosomes in many tissues and forms crystals, leading to a depletion of intracellular cysteine levels. Children with this disorder develop renal failure by 6 to 12 years of age, through a mechanism that has not yet been fully elucidated.

Homocysteine is oxidized to a disulfide, homocystine. To indicate that both forms are being considered, the term *homocyst(e)ine* is used.

Homocysteine

Homocysteine   Homocystine

Because a colorimetric screening test for urinary homocystine was positive, the doctor ordered several biochemical studies on **Horace S.'s** serum, which included tests for methionine, homocyst(e)ine (both free and protein-bound), cystine, vitamin B_{12}, and folate. The level of homocystine in a 24-hour urine collection was also measured.

The results were as follows: the serum methionine level was 980 μM (reference range, <30 μM); serum homocyst(e)ine (both free and protein-bound) was markedly elevated; cystine was not detected in the serum; the serum B_{12} and folate levels were normal. A 24-hour urine homocystine level was elevated.

Based on these measurements, **Horace S.'s** doctor concluded that he had homocystinuria caused by an enzyme deficiency. What was the rationale for this conclusion?

see also Chapter 40). Sulfate generation, in an aqueous medium, is essentially generating sulfuric acid, and both the acid and sulfate need to be disposed of in the urine. Sulfate is also used in most cells to generate an activated form of sulfate known as *PAPS* (3′-phosphoadenosine 5′-phosphosulfate), which is used as a sulfate donor in modifying carbohydrates or amino acids in various structures (glycosaminoglycans) and proteins in the body.

The conversion of methionine to homocysteine and homocysteine to cysteine is the major degradative route for these two amino acids. Because this is the only degradative route for homocysteine, vitamin B_6 deficiency or congenital cystathionine β-synthase deficiency can result in homocystinemia, which is associated with cardiovascular disease.

D. Alanine

Alanine is produced from pyruvate by a transamination reaction catalyzed by alanine aminotransaminase (ALT) and may be converted back to pyruvate by a reversal of the same reaction (see Fig. 37.3). Alanine is the major gluconeogenic amino acid because it is produced in many tissues for the transport of nitrogen to the liver.

III. Amino Acids Related to Tricarboxylic Acid–Cycle Intermediates

Two groups of amino acids are synthesized from TCA-cycle intermediates; one group from α-ketoglutarate and one from oxaloacetate (see Fig. 37.1). During degradation, four groups of amino acids are converted to the TCA-cycle intermediates α-ketoglutarate, oxaloacetate, succinyl coenzyme A (succinyl-CoA), and fumarate (see Fig. 37.2A).

A. Amino Acids Related through α-Ketoglutarate/Glutamate

1. Glutamate

The five carbons of glutamate are derived from α-ketoglutarate either by transamination or by the glutamate dehydrogenase reaction (see Chapter 36). Because α-ketoglutarate can be synthesized from glucose, all of the carbons of glutamate can be obtained from glucose (see Fig. 37.1). When glutamate is degraded, it is likewise converted back to α-ketoglutarate either by transamination or by glutamate dehydrogenase. In the liver, α-ketoglutarate leads to the formation of malate, which produces glucose via gluconeogenesis. Thus, glutamate can be derived from glucose and reconverted to glucose (Fig. 37.7).

Glutamate is used for the synthesis of several other amino acids (glutamine, proline, ornithine, and arginine) (see Fig. 37.7) and for providing the glutamyl moiety of glutathione (γ-glutamyl-cysteinyl-glycine; see "Biochemical Comments" in Chapter 35). Glutathione is an important antioxidant, as has been described previously (see Chapter 27).

2. Glutamine

Glutamine is produced from glutamate by glutamine synthetase, which adds NH_4^+ to the carboxyl group of the side chain, forming an amide (Fig. 37.8). This is one of only three human enzymes that can fix free ammonia into an organic molecule; the other two are glutamate dehydrogenase and carbamoyl phosphate synthetase I (see Chapter 36). Glutamine is reconverted to glutamate by a different enzyme, glutaminase, which is particularly important in the kidney. The ammonia it produces enters the urine and can be used as an expendable cation to aid in the excretion of metabolic acids ($NH_3 + H^+ \rightarrow NH_4^+$), as discussed in Chapter 36.

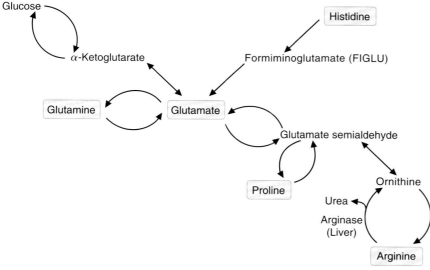

FIGURE 37.7 Amino acids related through glutamate. These amino acids contain carbons that can be reconverted to glutamate, which can be converted to glucose in the liver. All of these amino acids except histidine can be synthesized from glucose.

3. Proline

In the synthesis of proline, glutamate is first phosphorylated and then converted to glutamate 5-semialdehyde by reduction of the side-chain carboxyl group to an aldehyde (Fig. 37.9). This semialdehyde spontaneously cyclizes (forming an internal Schiff base between the aldehyde and the α-amino group). Reduction of this cyclic compound yields proline. Hydroxyproline is formed only after proline has been incorporated into collagen (see Chapter 47) by the prolyl hydroxylase system, which uses molecular oxygen, iron, α-ketoglutarate, and ascorbic acid (vitamin C).

Proline is converted back to glutamate semialdehyde, which is oxidized to form glutamate. The synthesis and degradation of proline use different enzymes even

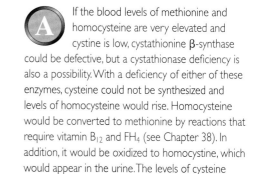

If the blood levels of methionine and homocysteine are very elevated and cystine is low, cystathionine β-synthase could be defective, but a cystathionase deficiency is also a possibility. With a deficiency of either of these enzymes, cysteine could not be synthesized and levels of homocysteine would rise. Homocysteine would be converted to methionine by reactions that require vitamin B_{12} and FH_4 (see Chapter 38). In addition, it would be oxidized to homocystine, which would appear in the urine. The levels of cysteine (measured as its oxidation product cystine) would be low. A measurement of serum cystathionine levels would help to distinguish between a cystathionase or cystathionine β-synthase deficiency.

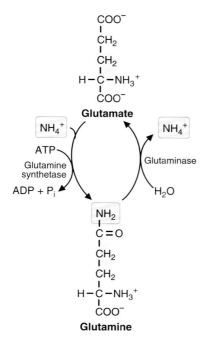

FIGURE 37.8 Synthesis and degradation of glutamine. Different enzymes catalyze the addition and the removal of the amide nitrogen of glutamine. *ADP*, adenosine diphosphate; *ATP*, adenosine triphosphate; P_i, inorganic phosphate.

FIGURE 37.9 Synthesis and degradation of proline. Reactions *1*, *3*, and *4* occur in mitochondria. Reaction *2* occurs in the cytosol. Synthesis and degradation involve different enzymes. The cyclization reaction (formation of a Schiff base) is nonenzymatic; that is, it is spontaneous. *ADP*, adenosine diphosphate; *ATP*, adenosine triphosphate; *FAD*, flavin adenine dinucleotide; *NAD*, nicotinamide adenine dinucleotide; P_i, inorganic phosphate.

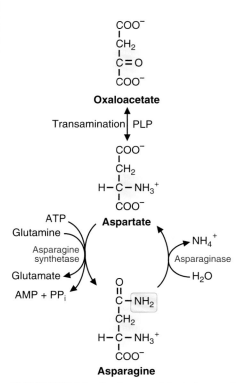

FIGURE 37.10 Synthesis and degradation of aspartate and asparagine. Note that the amide nitrogen of asparagine is derived from glutamine. (The amide nitrogen of glutamine comes from NH_4^+; see Fig. 37.8.) *AMP*, adenosine monophosphate; *ATP*, adenosine triphosphate; *PP_i*, pyrophosphate.

Certain types of tumor cells, particularly leukemic cells, require asparagine for their growth. Therefore, asparaginase has been used as an antitumor agent. It acts by converting asparagine to aspartate in the blood, decreasing the amount of asparagine available for tumor cell growth. Asparaginase has been used for >30 years to treat acute lymphoblastic leukemia.

though the intermediates are the same. Hydroxyproline, however, has an entirely different degradative pathway (not shown). The presence of the hydroxyl group in hydroxyproline allows an aldolaselike reaction to occur once the ring has been hydrolyzed, which is not possible with proline.

4. Arginine

Arginine is synthesized from glutamate via glutamate semialdehyde, which is transaminated to form ornithine, an intermediate of the urea cycle (see Fig. 36.12). This activity (ornithine aminotransferase) appears to be greatest in the epithelial cells of the small intestine (see Chapter 40). The reactions of the urea cycle then produce arginine. However, the quantities of arginine generated by the urea cycle are adequate only for the adult and are insufficient to support growth. Therefore, during periods of growth, arginine becomes an essential amino acid. It is important to realize that if arginine is used for protein synthesis, the levels of ornithine will drop, thereby slowing the urea cycle. This will stimulate the formation of ornithine from glutamate.

Arginine is cleaved by arginase to form urea and ornithine. If ornithine is present in amounts in excess of those required for the urea cycle, it is transaminated to glutamate semialdehyde, which is reduced to glutamate. The conversion of an aldehyde to a primary amine is a unique form of a transamination reaction and requires PLP.

5. Histidine

Although histidine cannot be synthesized in humans, five of its carbons form glutamate when it is degraded. In a series of steps, histidine is converted to formiminoglutamate (FIGLU). The subsequent reactions transfer one carbon of FIGLU to the FH_4 pool (see Chapter 38) and release NH_4^+ and glutamate.

B. Amino Acids Related to Oxaloacetate (Aspartate and Asparagine)

Aspartate is produced by transamination of oxaloacetate. This reaction is readily reversible, so aspartate can be reconverted to oxaloacetate (Fig. 37.10).

Asparagine is formed from aspartate by a reaction in which glutamine provides the nitrogen for formation of the amide group. Thus, this reaction differs from the synthesis of glutamine from glutamate, in which NH_4^+ provides the nitrogen. However, the reaction catalyzed by asparaginase, which hydrolyzes asparagine to NH_4^+ and aspartate, is analogous to the reaction catalyzed by glutaminase.

C. Amino Acids that Form Fumarate

1. Aspartate

Although the major route for aspartate degradation involves its conversion to oxaloacetate, carbons from aspartate can form fumarate in the urea cycle (see Chapter 36). This reaction generates cytosolic fumarate, which must be converted to malate (using cytoplasmic fumarase) for transport into the mitochondria for oxidative or anaplerotic purposes. An analogous sequence of reactions occurs in the purine nucleotide cycle. Aspartate reacts with inosine monophosphate (IMP) to form an intermediate (adenylosuccinate) that is then cleaved, forming adenosine monophosphate (AMP) and fumarate (see Chapter 39).

2. Phenylalanine and Tyrosine

Phenylalanine is converted to tyrosine by a hydroxylation reaction. Tyrosine, produced from phenylalanine or obtained from the diet, is oxidized, ultimately forming acetoacetate and fumarate. The oxidative steps required to reach this point are, surprisingly, not energy-generating. The conversion of fumarate to malate, followed by the action of malic enzyme, allows the carbons to be used for gluconeogenesis. The conversion of phenylalanine to tyrosine and the production of acetoacetate are considered further in Section IV of this chapter.

D. Amino Acids that Form Succinyl Coenzyme A

The essential amino acids methionine, valine, isoleucine, and threonine are degraded to form propionyl coenzyme A (propionyl-CoA). The conversion of propionyl-CoA to succinyl-CoA is common to their degradative pathways. Propionyl-CoA is also generated from the oxidation of odd-chain fatty acids.

Propionyl-CoA is carboxylated in a reaction that requires biotin and forms D-methylmalonyl coenzyme A (D-methylmalonyl-CoA). The D-methylmalonyl-CoA is racemized to L-methylmalonyl-CoA, which is rearranged in a vitamin B_{12}-requiring reaction to produce succinyl-CoA, a TCA-cycle intermediate (see Fig. 30.11).

I. Methionine

Methionine is converted to *S*-adenosylmethionine (SAM), which donates its methyl group to other compounds to form *S*-adenosylhomocysteine (SAH). SAH is then converted to homocysteine (Fig. 37.11). Methionine can be regenerated from homocysteine by a reaction that requires both FH_4 and vitamin B_{12} (a topic that is considered in more detail in Chapter 38). Alternatively, by reactions that require PLP, homocysteine can provide the sulfur needed for the synthesis of cysteine (see Fig. 37.6). Carbons of homocysteine are then metabolized to α-ketobutyrate, which undergoes oxidative decarboxylation to propionyl-CoA. The propionyl-CoA is then converted to succinyl-CoA (see Fig. 37.11).

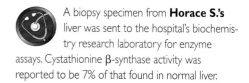

A biopsy specimen from **Horace S.'s** liver was sent to the hospital's biochemistry research laboratory for enzyme assays. Cystathionine β-synthase activity was reported to be 7% of that found in normal liver.

Homocystinuria is caused by deficiencies in the enzymes cystathionine β-synthase and cystathionase as well as by deficiencies of methyltetrahydrofolate (CH_3–FH_4) or of methyl-B_{12}. The deficiencies of CH_3–FH_4 or of methyl-B_{12} are either caused by an inadequate dietary intake of folate or vitamin B_{12} or by defective enzymes involved in joining methyl groups to FH_4, transferring methyl groups from FH_4 to vitamin B_{12}, or passing them from vitamin B_{12} to homocysteine to form methionine (see Chapter 38).

Is **Horace S.'s** homocystinuria caused by any of these problems?

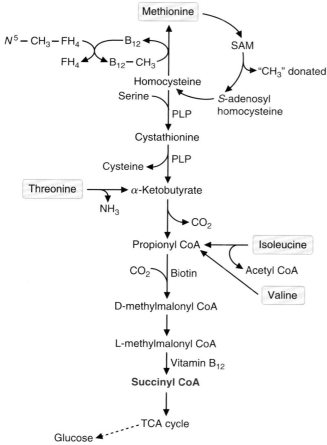

FIGURE 37.11 Conversion of methionine and other amino acids to succinyl coenzyme A (succinyl-CoA). The amino acids methionine, threonine, isoleucine, and valine, all of which form succinyl-CoA via methylmalonyl coenzyme A (methylmalonyl-CoA), are essential in the diet. The carbons of serine are converted to cysteine and do not form succinyl-CoA by this pathway. *Acetyl-CoA*, acetyl coenzyme A; *PLP*, pyridoxal phosphate; *Propionyl-CoA*, propionyl coenzyme A; *SAM*, *S*-adenosylmethionine; B_{12}–CH_3, methylcobalamin; N^5-CH_3–FH_4, N^5-methyltetrahydrofolate; *TCA*, tricarboxylic acid.

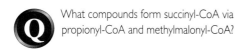

Horace S.'s methionine levels are elevated, and his vitamin B_{12} and folate levels are normal. Therefore, he does not have a deficiency of dietary folate or vitamin B_{12} or of the enzymes that transfer methyl groups from FH_4 to homocysteine to form methionine. In these cases, homocysteine levels are elevated but methionine levels are low.

Q What compounds form succinyl-CoA via propionyl-CoA and methylmalonyl-CoA?

2. Threonine

In humans, threonine is primarily degraded by a PLP-requiring dehydratase to ammonia and α-ketobutyrate, which subsequently undergoes oxidative decarboxylation to form propionyl-CoA, just as in the case of methionine (see Fig. 37.11).

3. Valine and Isoleucine

The branched-chain amino acids (valine, isoleucine, and leucine) are a universal fuel, and the degradation of these amino acids occurs at low levels in the mitochondria of most tissues, but the muscle carries out the highest level of branched-chain amino acid oxidation. The branched-chain amino acids make up almost 25% of the content of the average protein, so their use as fuel is quite significant. The degradative pathway for valine and isoleucine has two major functions: first, to generate energy; and second, to provide precursors to replenish TCA-cycle intermediates (anaplerosis). Both valine and isoleucine contain carbons that form succinyl-CoA. The initial step in the degradation of the branched-chain amino acids is a transamination reaction. Although the enzyme that catalyzes this reaction is present in most tissues, the level of activity varies from tissue to tissue. Its activity is particularly high in muscle, however. In the second step of the degradative pathway, the α-keto analogs of these amino acids undergo oxidative decarboxylation by the α-keto acid dehydrogenase complex in a reaction similar in its mechanism and cofactor requirements to pyruvate dehydrogenase and α-ketoglutarate dehydrogenase (see Chapter 23). As with the first enzyme of the pathway, the highest level of activity for this dehydrogenase is found in muscle tissue. Subsequently, the pathways for degradation of these amino acids follow parallel routes (Fig. 37.12). The steps are analogous to those for β-oxidation of fatty acids, so nicotinamide adenine dinucleotide (NADH) and flavin adenine dinucleotide (FAD[2H]) are generated for energy production.

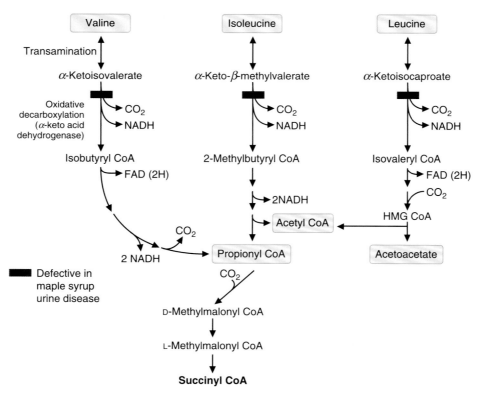

FIGURE 37.12 Degradation of the branched-chain amino acids. Valine forms propionyl coenzyme A (propionyl-CoA). Isoleucine forms propionyl-CoA and acetyl coenzyme A (acetyl-CoA). Leucine forms acetoacetate and acetyl-CoA. *HMG CoA*, hydroxymethylglutaryl coenzyme A; *Isobutyryl CoA*, isobutyryl coenzyme A; *Isovaleryl CoA*, isovaleryl coenzyme A; *Methylbutyryl CoA*, methylbutyryl coenzyme A; *Methylmalonyl CoA*, methylmalonyl coenzyme A; *FAD*, flavin adenine dinucleotide; *NADH*, reduced nicotinamide adenine dinucleotide; *Succinyl CoA*, succinyl coenzyme A.

Valine and isoleucine are converted to succinyl-CoA (see Fig. 37.11). Isoleucine also forms acetyl-CoA. Leucine, the third branched-chain amino acid, does not produce succinyl-CoA. It forms acetoacetate and acetyl-CoA and is strictly ketogenic.

IV. Amino Acids that Form Acetyl Coenzyme A and Acetoacetate

Seven amino acids produce acetyl-CoA or acetoacetate and, therefore, are categorized as ketogenic. Of these, isoleucine, threonine, and the aromatic amino acids (phenylalanine, tyrosine, and tryptophan) are converted to compounds that produce both glucose and acetyl-CoA or acetoacetate (Fig. 37.13). Leucine and lysine do not produce glucose; they produce acetyl-CoA and acetoacetate.

A. Phenylalanine and Tyrosine

Phenylalanine is converted to tyrosine, which undergoes oxidative degradation (Fig. 37.14). The last step in the pathway produces both fumarate and the ketone body acetoacetate. Deficiencies of different enzymes in the pathway result in phenylketonuria, tyrosinemia, and alkaptonuria.

Phenylalanine is hydroxylated to form tyrosine by a mixed-function oxidase, phenylalanine hydroxylase (PAH), which requires molecular oxygen and BH_4 (Fig. 37.15). The cofactor BH_4 is converted to quininoid dihydrobiopterin by this reaction. BH_4 is not synthesized from a vitamin; it can be synthesized in the body from guanosine triphosphate (GTP). However, as is the case with other cofactors, the body contains limited amounts. Therefore, dihydrobiopterin must be reconverted to BH_4 for the reaction to continue to produce tyrosine.

 In addition to methionine, threonine, isoleucine, and valine (see Fig. 37.11), the last three carbons at the ω-end of odd-chain fatty acids form succinyl-CoA by this route (see Chapter 30).

 Thiamin deficiency will lead to an accumulation of α-keto acids in the blood because of an inability of pyruvate dehydrogenase, α-ketoglutarate dehydrogenase, and branched-chain α-keto acid dehydrogenase to catalyze their reactions (see Chapter 8). **Al M.** had a thiamin deficiency resulting from his chronic alcoholism. His ketoacidosis resulted partly from the accumulation of these α-keto acids in his blood and partly from the accumulation of ketone bodies used for energy production. Beriberi is the disorder that results from thiamin deficiency.

In maple syrup urine disease, the branched-chain α-keto acid dehydrogenase that oxidatively decarboxylates the branched-chain amino acids is defective. As a result, the branched-chain amino acids and their α-keto analogs (produced by transamination) accumulate. They appear in the urine, giving it the odor of maple syrup or burnt sugar. The accumulation of α-keto analogs leads to neurologic complications. This condition is difficult to treat by dietary restriction, because abnormalities in the metabolism of three essential amino acids contribute to the disease.

 Alkaptonuria occurs when homogentisate, an intermediate in tyrosine metabolism, cannot be further oxidized because the next enzyme in the pathway, homogentisate oxidase, is defective. Homogentisate accumulates and autooxidizes, forming a dark pigment, which discolors the urine and stains the diapers of affected infants. Later in life, the chronic accumulation of this pigment in cartilage may cause arthritic joint pain.

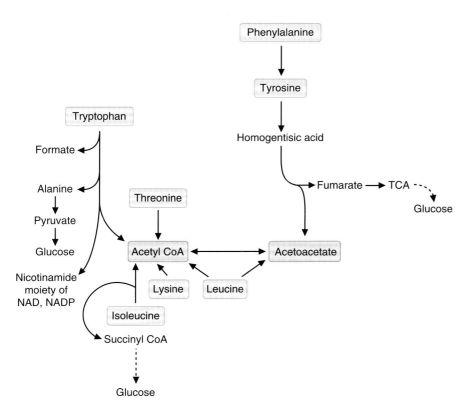

FIGURE 37.13 Ketogenic amino acids. Some of these amino acids (tryptophan, phenylalanine, and tyrosine) also contain carbons that can form glucose. Leucine and lysine are strictly ketogenic; they do not form glucose. *Acetyl-CoA*, acetyl coenzyme A; *NAD*, nicotinamide adenine dinucleotide; *Succinyl CoA*, succinyl coenzyme A; *TCA*, tricarboxylic acid.

Transient tyrosinemia is frequently observed in newborn infants, especially those that are premature. For the most part, the condition appears to be benign and dietary restriction of protein returns plasma tyrosine levels to normal. The biochemical defect is most likely a low level, attributable to immaturity, of 4-hydroxyphenylpyruvate dioxygenase. Because this enzyme requires ascorbate, ascorbate supplementation also aids in reducing circulating tyrosine levels.

Other types of tyrosinemia are related to specific enzyme defects (see Fig. 37.14). Tyrosinemia II is caused by a genetic deficiency of tyrosine aminotransferase (TAT) and may lead to lesions of the eye and skin as well as neurologic problems. Patients are treated with a low-tyrosine, low-phenylalanine diet.

Tyrosinemia I (also called *tyrosinosis*) is caused by a genetic deficiency of fumarylacetoacetate hydrolase. The acute form is associated with liver failure, a cabbagelike body odor, and death within the first year of life.

A small subset of patients with hyperphenylalaninemia show an appropriate reduction in plasma phenylalanine levels with dietary restriction of this amino acid; however, these patients can still develop progressive neurologic symptoms and seizures ("malignant" hyperphenylalaninemia). These infants exhibit normal PAH activity but have a deficiency in dihydropteridine reductase (DHPR), an enzyme required for the regeneration of BH$_4$, a cofactor of PAH (see Fig. 37.16). Less frequently, DHPR activity is normal but a defect in the biosynthesis of BH$_4$ exists. In either case, dietary therapy with administration of BH$_4$ corrects the hyperphenylalaninemia. However, BH$_4$ is also a cofactor for two other hydroxylations required in the synthesis of neurotransmitters in the brain: the hydroxylation of tryptophan to 5-hydroxytryptophan and of tyrosine to L-DOPA (see Chapter 46). Because BH$_4$ does not penetrate the central nervous system as well, patients also need replacement therapy for the neurotransmitters. However, patients will often still have neurologic deficits.

If the dietary levels of niacin and tryptophan are insufficient, the condition known as *pellagra* results. The symptoms of pellagra are dermatitis, diarrhea, dementia, and, finally, death. In addition, abnormal metabolism of tryptophan occurs in a vitamin B$_6$ deficiency. Kynurenine intermediates in tryptophan degradation cannot be cleaved because kynureninase requires PLP derived from vitamin B$_6$. Consequently, these intermediates enter a minor pathway for tryptophan metabolism that produces xanthurenic acid, which is excreted in the urine.

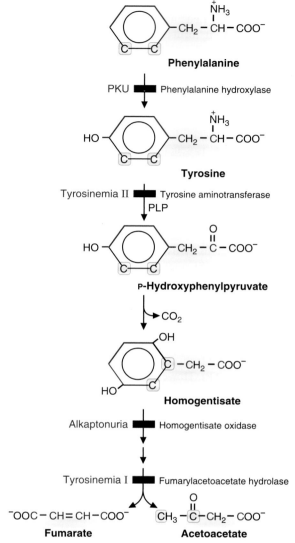

FIGURE 37.14 Degradation of phenylalanine and tyrosine. The carboxyl carbon forms CO$_2$, and the other carbons form fumarate or acetoacetate as indicated. Deficiencies of enzymes (*dark bars*) result in the indicated diseases. *PKU,* phenylketonuria; *PLP,* pyridoxal phosphate.

B. Tryptophan

Tryptophan is oxidized to produce alanine (from the nonring carbons), formate, and acetyl-CoA. Tryptophan is, therefore, both glucogenic and ketogenic (Fig. 37.16).

NAD$^+$ and NADP$^+$ can be produced from the ring structure of tryptophan. Therefore, tryptophan "spares" the dietary requirement for niacin. The higher the dietary levels of tryptophan, the lower are the levels of niacin required to prevent symptoms of deficiency.

C. Threonine, Isoleucine, Leucine, and Lysine

As discussed previously, the major route of threonine degradation in humans is by threonine dehydratase (see Section III.D.2). In a minor pathway, threonine degradation by threonine aldolase produces glycine and acetyl-CoA in the liver.

Isoleucine produces both succinyl-CoA and acetyl-CoA (see Section III.D.3).

Leucine is purely ketogenic and produces hydroxymethylglutaryl coenzyme A (HMG-CoA), which is cleaved to form acetyl-CoA and the ketone body acetoacetate (see Figs. 37.12 and 37.13). Most of the tissues in which it is oxidized can use ketone bodies, with the exception of the liver. As with valine and isoleucine, leucine is a universal fuel, with its primary metabolism occurring in muscle.

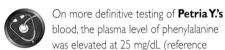

FIGURE 37.15 Hydroxylation of phenylalanine. Phenylalanine hydroxylase (PAH) is a mixed-function oxidase; that is, molecular oxygen (O_2) donates one atom to water and one to the product tyrosine. The cofactor tetrahydrobiopterin (BH_4) is oxidized to dihydrobiopterin (BH_2) and must be reduced back to BH_4 for PAH to continue forming tyrosine. BH_4 is synthesized in the body from guanosine triphosphate (GTP). The disorder phenylketonuria (PKU) results from deficiencies of PAH (the classic form), dihydropteridine reductase, or enzymes in the biosynthetic pathway for BH_4.

Lysine cannot be directly transaminated at either of its two amino groups. Lysine is degraded by a complex pathway in which saccharopine, α-ketoadipate, and crotonyl coenzyme A (crotonyl-CoA) are intermediates. During the degradation pathway, NADH and $FADH_2$ are generated for energy. Ultimately, lysine generates acetyl-CoA (see Fig. 37.13) and is strictly ketogenic.

On more definitive testing of **Petria Y.'s** blood, the plasma level of phenylalanine was elevated at 25 mg/dL (reference range, <1.2 mg/dL). Several phenyl ketones and other products of phenylalanine metabolism, which give the urine a characteristic odor, were found in significant quantities in the baby's urine.

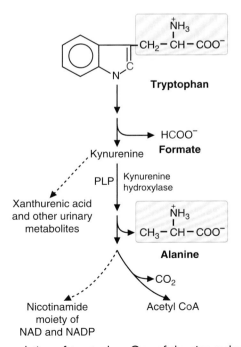

FIGURE 37.16 Degradation of tryptophan. One of the ring carbons (in *red*) produces formate. The nonring portion (indicated by the *box*) forms alanine. Kynurenine is an intermediate, which can be converted to several urinary excretion products (e.g., xanthurenate), degraded to CO_2 and acetyl coenzyme A (acetyl CoA), or converted to the nicotinamide moiety of nicotinamide adenine dinucleotide (NAD) and NADP, which also can be formed from the vitamin niacin. *PLP*, pyridoxal phosphate.

A liver biopsy was sent to the special chemistry research laboratory, where it was determined that the level of activity of PAH in Petria's liver was <1% of that found in normal infants. A diagnosis of "classic" PKU was made.

Until gene therapy allows substitution of the defective *PAH* gene with its normal counterpart in vivo, the mainstay of therapy in classic PKU is to maintain levels of phenylalanine in the blood between 3 and 12 mg/dL through dietary restriction of this essential amino acid.

CLINICAL COMMENTS

Petria Y. The overall incidence of phenylketonuria (PKU), leading to hyperphenylalaninemia, is approximately 1 per 10,000 births, with a wide geographic and ethnic variation. PKU occurs by autosomal-recessive transmission of a defective *PAH* gene, causing accumulation of phenylalanine in the blood that is well above the normal concentration in young children and adults (<1 to 2 mg/dL). In the newborn, the upper limit of normal is almost twice this value. Values >20 mg/dL are usually found in patients, such as Petria, with "classic" PKU.

Patients with classic PKU usually appear normal at birth. If the disease is not recognized and treated within the first month of life, the infant gradually develops varying degrees of irreversible intellectual disability (IQ scores frequently <50), delayed psychomotor maturation, tremors, seizures, eczema, and hyperactivity. The neurologic sequelae may result in part from the competitive interaction of phenylalanine with brain amino acid transport systems and inhibition of neurotransmitter synthesis. A successful dietary therapy for PKU includes a reduction in phenylalanine intake; in adults, this can include supplementation of the diet with large, neutral amino acids (such as tryptophan, tyrosine, histidine, and leucine). These large, neutral amino acids share a transport system (the L system) with phenylalanine and can overcome the high levels of phenylalanine in the blood, allowing the neurotransmitter precursors to enter the nervous system. If the disease is not recognized in time, the biochemical alterations lead to impaired myelin synthesis and delayed neuronal development, which result in the clinical picture in patients such as Petria. Because of the simplicity of the test for PKU (elevated phenylalanine levels in the blood), all newborns in the United States are required to have a PKU test at birth. Early detection of the disease can lead to early treatment, and if followed, the neurologic consequences of the disease can be avoided.

To restrict dietary levels of phenylalanine, special semisynthetic preparations (such as Lofenalac, Periflex, or PhenylAde) are used in the United States. Use of these preparations reduces dietary intake of phenylalanine to 250 to 500 mg/day while maintaining normal intake of all other dietary nutrients. Although it is generally agreed that scrupulous adherence to this regimen is mandatory for the first decade of life, less consensus exists regarding its indefinite use. Evidence suggests, however, that without lifelong compliance with dietary restriction of phenylalanine, even adults will develop at least neurologic sequelae of PKU. A pregnant woman with PKU must be particularly careful to maintain satisfactory plasma levels of phenylalanine throughout gestation to avoid the adverse effects of hyperphenylalaninemia on the fetus. The use of glycomacropeptide from whey is a promising development in PKU treatment. This protein, when pure, contains no phenylalanine but as isolated has a very low phenylalanine content (owing to contaminants) while providing adequate levels of the other amino acids. The use of glycomacropeptide in PKU diet preparation is expanding and provides alternatives to the dietary therapy not previously available.

Petria's parents were given thorough dietary instruction, which they followed carefully. Although her pediatrician was not optimistic, it was hoped that the damage done to her nervous system before dietary therapy was minimal and that her subsequent psychomotor development would allow her to lead a relatively normal life.

Horace S. The most characteristic biochemical features of the disorder that affects **Horace S.**, a cystathionine β-synthase deficiency, are the presence of an accumulation of both homocyst(e)ine and methionine in the blood. Because renal tubular reabsorption of methionine is highly efficient, this amino acid may not appear in the urine. Homocystine, the disulfide of homocysteine, is less efficiently reabsorbed, and amounts in excess of 1 mmol may be excreted in the urine each day.

In the type of homocystinuria in which the patient is deficient in cystathione β-synthase, the elevation in serum methionine levels is presumed to be the result of enhanced rates of conversion of homocysteine to methionine, caused by increased availability of homocysteine (see Fig. 37.11). In type II and type III homocystinuria, in which there is a deficiency in the synthesis of methylcobalamin and of N^5-methyltetrahydrofolate, respectively (both required for the methylation of homocysteine to form methionine), serum homocysteine levels are elevated but serum methionine levels are low (see Fig. 37.11).

Acute vascular events are common in these patients. Thrombi (blood clots) and emboli (clots that have broken off and traveled to a distant site in the vascular system) have been reported in almost every major artery and vein as well as in smaller vessels. These clots result in infarcts in vital organs such as the liver, the myocardium (heart muscle), the lungs, the kidneys, and many other tissues. Although increased serum levels of homocysteine have been implicated in enhanced platelet aggregation and damage to vascular endothelial cells (leading to clotting and accelerated atherosclerosis), no generally accepted mechanism for these vascular events has yet emerged.

Treatment is directed toward early reduction of the elevated levels of homocysteine and methionine in the blood. In addition to a diet that is low in methionine, very high oral doses of pyridoxine (vitamin B_6) have significantly decreased the plasma levels of homocysteine and methionine in some patients with cystathionine β-synthase deficiency. (Genetically determined "responders" to pyridoxine treatment make up ~50% of people with type I homocystinuria.) PLP serves as a cofactor for cystathionine β-synthase; however, the molecular properties of the defective enzyme that confer the responsiveness to vitamin B_6 therapy are not known.

The terms *hypermethioninemia*, *homocystinuria* (or *-emia*), and *cystathioninuria* (or *-emia*) designate biochemical abnormalities and are not specific clinical diseases. Each may be caused by more than one specific genetic defect. For example, at least seven distinct genetic alterations can cause increased excretion of homocystine in the urine. A deficiency of cystathionine β-synthase is the most common cause of homocystinuria; >600 such proven cases have been studied.

The pathologic findings that underlie the clinical features manifested by **Horace S.** are presumed (but not proved) to be the consequence of chronic elevations of homocysteine (and perhaps other compounds; e.g., methionine) in the blood and tissues. The zonular fibers that normally hold the lens of the eye in place become frayed and break, causing dislocation of the lens. The skeleton reveals a loss of bone density (i.e., osteoporosis), which may explain the curvature of the spine. The elongation of the long bones beyond their normal genetically determined length leads to tall stature.

Animal experiments suggest that increased concentrations of homocysteine and methionine in the brain may trap adenosine as SAH, diminishing adenosine levels. Because adenosine normally acts as a central nervous system depressant, its deficiency may be associated with a lowering of the seizure threshold as well as a reduction in cognitive function.

BIOCHEMICAL COMMENTS

Phenylketonuria. Many enzyme deficiency diseases have been discovered that affect the pathways of amino acid metabolism. These deficiency diseases have helped researchers to elucidate the pathways in humans, in whom experimental manipulation is, at best, unethical. These spontaneous mutations ("experiments" of nature), although devastating to patients, have resulted in an understanding of these diseases that now permit treatment of inborn errors of metabolism that were once considered to be untreatable.

Classic PKU is caused by mutations in the gene located on chromosome 12 that encodes the enzyme PAH. This enzyme normally catalyzes the hydroxylation of phenylalanine to tyrosine, the rate-limiting step in the major pathway by which phenylalanine is catabolized.

In early experiments, sequence analysis of mutant clones indicated a single base substitution in the gene, with a G-to-A transition at the canonical 5′ donor splice site of intron 12 and expression of a truncated unstable protein product. This protein lacked the C-terminal region, a structural change that yielded <1% of the normal activity of PAH.

Since these initial studies, DNA analysis has shown >100 mutations (missense, nonsense, insertions, and deletions) in the *PAH* gene, associated with PKU and non-PKU hyperphenylalaninemia. That PKU is a heterogeneous phenotype is supported by studies measuring PAH activity in needle biopsy samples taken from the livers of a large group of patients with varying degrees of hyperphenylalaninemia. PAH activity varied from <1% of normal in patients with classic PKU to up to 35% of normal in those with a non-PKU form of hyperphenylalaninemia (such as a defect in BH_4 production; see Chapter 46).

The genetic diseases affecting amino acid degradation that have been discussed in this chapter are summarized in Table 37.1. This is just a partial listing of disorders in amino acid metabolism; there are many others that are less common and were not discussed in this chapter.

TABLE 37.1	**Genetic Disorders of Amino Acid Metabolism**			
AMINO ACID DEGRADATION PATHWAY	**MISSING ENZYME**	**PRODUCT THAT ACCUMULATES**	**DISEASE**	**SYMPTOMS**
Phenylalanine	Phenylalanine hydroxylase	Phenylalanine	PKU (classic)	Intellectual disability
	Dihydropteridine reductase	Phenylalanine	PKU (nonclassic)	Intellectual disability
	Homogentisate oxidase	Homogentisic acid	Alkaptonuria	Black urine, arthritis
	Fumarylacetoacetate hydrolase	Fumarylacetoacetate	Tyrosinemia I	Liver failure, death early
Tyrosine	Tyrosine aminotransferase	Tyrosine	Tyrosinemia II	Neurologic defects
Methionine	Cystathionase	Cystathionine	Cystathioninuria	Benign
	Cystathionine β-synthase	Homocysteine	Homocysteinemia	Cardiovascular complications and neurologic problems
Glycine	Glycine transaminase	Glyoxylate	Primary oxaluria type I	Renal failure caused by stone formation
Branched-chain amino acids (leucine, isoleucine, valine)	Branched-chain α-keto acid dehydrogenase	α-Keto acids of the branched-chain amino acids	Maple syrup urine disease	Intellectual disability

PKU, phenylketonuria.

KEY CONCEPTS

- Humans can synthesize only 11 of the 20 amino acids required for protein synthesis; the other 9 are considered to be essential amino acids in the diet.
- Amino acid metabolism uses, to a large extent, the cofactors PLP, BH_4, and FH_4.
  - PLP is required primarily for transamination reactions.
  - BH_4 is required for ring hydroxylation reactions.
  - FH_4 is required for one-carbon metabolism and is discussed further in Chapter 38.
- The nonessential amino acids can be synthesized from glycolytic intermediates (serine, glycine, cysteine, and alanine), from TCA-cycle intermediates (aspartate, asparagine, glutamate, glutamine, proline, arginine, and ornithine), or from existing amino acids (tyrosine from phenylalanine).
- When amino acids are degraded, the nitrogen is converted to urea, and the carbon skeletons are classified as either glucogenic (a precursor of glucose) or ketogenic (a precursor of ketone bodies).
- Defects in amino acid degradation pathways can lead to disease.
  - Glycine degradation can lead to oxalate production, which may lead to one class of kidney stone formation.
  - Defects in methionine degradation can lead to hyperhomocysteinemia, which has been linked to blood clotting disorders and heart disease.
  - A defect in branched-chain amino acid degradation leads to maple syrup urine disease, which has severe neurologic consequences.
  - Defects in phenylalanine and tyrosine degradation lead to phenylketonuria (PKU), alkaptonuria, tyrosinemia I and II, and albinism.
- Table 37.2 summarizes, in a slightly different format than Table 37.1, the diseases discussed in this chapter.

TABLE 37.2 Diseases Discussed in Chapter 37

DISEASE OR DISORDER	ENVIRONMENTAL OR GENETIC	COMMENTS
Phenylketonuria (PKU)	Genetic	Classic PKU is caused by a defect in phenylalanine hydroxylase, whereas nonclassic PKU is caused by a defect in dihydropteridine reductase (or an inability to synthesize tetrahydrobiopterin). Both forms of PKU will lead to intellectual disability if treatment is not initiated at an early age.
Alkaptonuria	Genetic	Alkaptonuria is caused by a defect in homogentisate oxidase, leading to an accumulation of homogentisic acid. Arthritis may develop later in life.
Tyrosinemia	Genetic	Tyrosinemia type 1 is a defect in fumarylacetoacetate hydrolase, leading to liver failure and early death. Tyrosinemia type 2 is a defect in tyrosine aminotransferase, leading to neurologic defects.
Cystathioninuria	Genetic	Defect in cystathionase, leading to an accumulation of cystathionine. No major complications result from this mutation.
Homocysteinemia	Genetic	A defect in cystathionine β-synthase leads to accumulation of homocysteine, which can result in cardiac and neurologic complications in the patient.
Primary oxaluria type I	Genetic	Defect in glycine transaminase leading to oxalate accumulation, and renal failure caused by stone formation within the kidney.
Maple syrup urine disease	Genetic	A defect in the branched-chain α-keto acid dehydrogenase, leading to an accumulation of the α-keto acids of the branched-chain amino acids, resulting in intellectual disability.
Cystinosis	Genetic	A defect in the transport protein that carries cystine across lysosomal membranes. Cystine accumulates in lysosomes, interfering with and ultimately destroying their function.
Thiamin deficiency	Environmental	A thiamin deficiency leads to accumulation of α-keto acids since the enzymes that catalyze oxidative decarboxylation reactions will not function in the absence of this vitamin. This will interfere with energy production, and lead to a ketoacidosis.

REVIEW QUESTIONS—CHAPTER 37

1. If an individual has a vitamin B_6 deficiency, which one of the following amino acids could still be synthesized and be considered nonessential?
   A. Tyrosine
   B. Serine
   C. Alanine
   D. Cysteine
   E. Aspartate

2. The degradation of amino acids can be classified into families, which are named after the end product of the degradative pathway. Which one of the following is such an end product?
   A. Citrate
   B. Glyceraldehyde 3-phosphate
   C. Fructose 6-phosphate
   D. Malate
   E. Succinyl-CoA

3. A newborn infant has elevated levels of phenylalanine and phenylpyruvate in her blood. Which one of the following enzymes might be deficient in this baby?
   A. Phenylalanine dehydrogenase
   B. Phenylalanine oxidase
   C. Dihydropteridine reductase
   D. Tyrosine hydroxylase
   E. TH_4 synthase

4. PLP is required for which one of the following reaction pathways or individual reactions?
   A. Phenylalanine → tyrosine
   B. Methionine → cysteine + α-ketobutyrate
   C. Propionyl-CoA → succinyl-CoA
   D. Pyruvate → acetyl-CoA
   E. Glucose → glycogen

5. A folic acid deficiency would interfere with the synthesis of which one of the following amino acids from the indicated precursors?
   A. Aspartate from oxaloacetate and glutamate
   B. Glutamate from glucose and ammonia
   C. Glycine from glucose and alanine
   D. Proline from glutamate
   E. Serine from glucose and alanine

6. A newborn displayed symptoms of maple syrup urine disease but also displayed elevated levels of lactic acid in her blood (lactic acidosis). Assuming that this is an inherited disorder with a single gene mutation, which one of the following is a likely substrate for the mutated protein?
   A. α-Keto acids
   B. Amino acids
   C. Monosaccharides
   D. Nucleotides
   E. Nucleosides
   F. Dicarboxylic acids

7. A child was recently diagnosed with classic PKU. Part of the treatment plan for the child was supplementation with large doses of tryptophan, leucine, and tyrosine. The rationale for such treatment is which one of the following?
   A. To inhibit PAH activity
   B. To increase neurotransmitter synthesis
   C. To activate PAH activity

D. To stimulate protein synthesis
E. To inhibit protein synthesis
F. To decrease neurotransmitter biosynthesis

8. An individual has been diagnosed with Hartnup disease and is experiencing symptoms consistent with niacin deficiency. In this patient, which amino acid is no longer able to "spare" the dietary requirement for niacin?
   A. Alanine
   B. Tryptophan
   C. Glutamine
   D. Leucine
   E. Methionine

9. Amino acids are an important substrate for gluconeogenesis during fasting. Which one of the following is the major gluconeogenic amino acid received by the liver?
   A. Alanine
   B. Glycine
   C. Cysteine
   D. Pyruvate
   E. Tryptophan

10. Which amino acid is involved in producing glutathione, an important antioxidant?
   A. Glutamine
   B. Glutamate
   C. Proline
   D. Ornithine
   E. Arginine

ANSWERS

1. **The answer is A.** Tyrosine is derived from phenylalanine, which requires BH_4 but not vitamin B_6. Vitamin B_6 is required in the synthesis of serine (transamination), of alanine (another transamination), cysteine (β-elimination, β-addition, β-elimination), and aspartate (transamination).

2. **The answer is E.** The other end products are acetoacetate, acetyl-CoA, fumarate, oxaloacetate, α-ketoglutarate, and pyruvate.

3. **The answer is C.** The classic form of PKU, a deficiency of PAH, results in elevations of phenylalanine and phenylpyruvate. However, this enzyme is not a choice. In the nonclassic variant of PKU, there is a problem in either synthesizing or regenerating BH_4. The enzyme that converts BH_2 to BH_4 is dihydropteridine reductase.

4. **The answer is B.** The reaction pathway in which methionine goes to cysteine and α-ketobutyrate requires PLP at two steps, the cystathionine β-synthase reaction and the cystathionase reaction. Phenylalanine to tyrosine requires BH_4; propionyl-CoA to succinyl-CoA requires B_{12}; pyruvate to acetyl-CoA requires thiamin pyrophosphate, lipoic acid, NAD, FAD, and coenzyme A; and glucose to glycogen does not require a cofactor.

5. **The answer is C.** Folic acid is required for the conversion of serine to glycine, and the serine is produced from 3-phosphoglycerate and alanine. Folic acid is not needed to synthesize aspartate (from oxaloacetate by transamination), glutamate (from α-ketoglutarate by transamination), proline (from glutamate by a series of steps that do not require folic acid), or serine (from 3-phosphoglycerate, with no one-carbon metabolism needed).

6. **The answer is A.** Maple syrup urine disease is caused by a dysfunctional branched-chain α-keto acid dehydrogenase, such that the α-keto acids of all three branched-chain amino acids accumulate in the blood. The fact that lactic acidosis is also present (indicating high pyruvate and lactate levels) suggests that pyruvate dehydrogenase (the enzyme that converts pyruvate to acetyl-CoA) is also defective. The common link between the branched-chain α-keto acid dehydrogenase and pyruvate dehydrogenase is the E3 subunit of the enzymes, which are the same. The E3 subunit is the dihydrolipoyl dehydrogenase subunit, and it is present in all of the enzymes that catalyze oxidative decarboxylation reactions. Such reactions require, as substrates, α-keto acids. The reaction does not use as substrates amino acids, monosaccharides, nucleotides, nucleosides, or dicarboxylic acids.

7. **The answer is B.** A child with classic PKU has a deficiency in PAH, which blocks the conversion of the essential amino acid phenylalanine to tyrosine. This leads to phenylalanine accumulation in the blood, and

the high phenylalanine levels saturate the "L" amino acid transport system (for large, neutral amino acids) such that the nervous system is "starved" for tryptophan, leucine, and tyrosine. As tryptophan and tyrosine are precursors for neurotransmitter synthesis (serotonin and the catecholamines, respectively), neuronal dysfunction will occur. By saturating the system with large, neutral amino acids the tryptophan, leucine, and tyrosine can compete with the high phenylalanine levels to get into the nervous system, such that neurotransmitter synthesis can proceed. High levels of tryptophan, leucine, and tyrosine do not alter the activity of PAH, nor do they allosterically stimulate, or inhibit, protein synthesis.

8. **The answer is B.** The niacin requirement for the synthesis of NAD^+ and $NADP^+$ can be "spared" by the presence of tryptophan, which can be degraded and produce the nicotinamide component of these cofactors. In Hartnup disease, the neutral amino acid transporter is defective, leading to reduced uptake of tryptophan from the intestine. With less tryptophan available, the dietary requirement for niacin is increased. None of the other amino acids listed (alanine, glutamine, leucine, and methionine) as answers can produce the ring component of NAD^+ and $NADP^+$.

9. **The answer is A.** Pyruvate is not an amino acid. Alanine is produced from pyruvate in a reversible transamination reaction. Alanine is the major gluconeogenic amino acid because it is produced in multiple tissues as a transport mechanism for nitrogen to the liver. Once in the liver, the alanine is transaminated to pyruvate, which enters gluconeogenesis, and the nitrogen (now attached to glutamate) is used by the urea cycle for excretion of the nitrogen. Under conditions of starvation, glutamine is also a major nitrogen carrier in the blood (because of its ability to bind two nitrogen groups), but glutamine was not offered as an answer to this question. Glycine, cysteine, and tryptophan are not used as nitrogen carriers during fasting or any other conditions.

10. **The answer is B.** Glutathione is a tripeptide consisting of glutamate, cysteine, and glycine. The glutamate is linked to the cysteine via a peptide bond using the side-chain carboxylic acid of glutamate and the nitrogen group of cysteine. Glutamate is also used as a precursor for the synthesis of all the other amino acids listed as possible answers.

38

Tetrahydrofolate, Vitamin B$_{12}$, and S-Adenosylmethionine

Groups that contain a single carbon atom can be transferred from one compound to another. These carbon atoms may be in a number of different oxidation states. The most oxidized form, CO_2, is transferred by biotin. One-carbon groups at lower levels of oxidation than CO_2 are transferred by reactions involving tetrahydrofolate (FH$_4$), vitamin B$_{12}$, and S-adenosylmethionine (SAM).

Tetrahydrofolate. FH$_4$, which is produced from the vitamin **folate**, is the primary one-carbon carrier in the body. This vitamin obtains one-carbon units from serine, glycine, histidine, formaldehyde, and formate (Fig. 38.1). While these carbons are attached to FH$_4$, they can be either oxidized or reduced. As a result, folate can exist in a variety of chemical forms. Once a carbon has been reduced to the methyl level (methyl-FH$_4$), however, it cannot be reoxidized. Collectively, these one-carbon groups attached to their carrier FH$_4$ are known as the **one-carbon pool**. The term *folate* is used to represent a water-soluble B-complex vitamin that functions in transferring single-carbon groups at various stages of oxidation.

The one-carbon groups carried by FH$_4$ are used for many biosynthetic reactions. For example, one-carbon units are transferred to the pyrimidine base of deoxyuridine monophosphate (**dUMP**) to form deoxythymidine monophosphate (**dTMP**), to the amino acid **glycine** to form **serine**, to precursors of the purine bases to produce carbons C2 and C8 of the **purine ring**, and to **vitamin B$_{12}$**.

Vitamin B$_{12}$. Vitamin B$_{12}$ is involved in two reactions in the body. It participates in the rearrangement of the methyl group of L-methylmalonyl coenzyme A (L-methylmalonyl-CoA) to form succinyl coenzyme A (succinyl-CoA), and it transfers a methyl group, obtained from FH$_4$, to homocysteine, forming methionine.

S-Adenosylmethionine. SAM, produced from methionine and adenosine triphosphate (ATP), transfers the methyl group to precursors that form a number of compounds, including creatine, phosphatidylcholine, epinephrine, melatonin, methylated nucleotides, methylated histones, and methylated DNA.

Methionine metabolism is very dependent on both FH$_4$ and vitamin B$_{12}$. **Homocysteine** is derived from methionine metabolism and can be converted back into methionine by using both methyl-FH$_4$ and vitamin B$_{12}$. This is the only reaction in which methyl-FH$_4$ can donate the methyl group. If the enzyme that catalyzes this reaction is defective, or if vitamin B$_{12}$ or FH$_4$ levels are insufficient, homocysteine will accumulate. Elevated homocysteine levels have been linked to cardiovascular and neurologic disease. A vitamin B$_{12}$ deficiency can be brought about by the lack of **intrinsic factor**, a gastric protein required for the absorption of dietary B$_{12}$. A consequence of vitamin B$_{12}$ deficiency is the accumulation of methyl-FH$_4$ and a decrease in other folate derivatives. This is known as the **methyl-trap hypothesis**, in which, because of the B$_{12}$ deficiency, most of the carbons in the FH$_4$ pool are trapped in the methyl-FH$_4$ form, which is the most stable. The carbons cannot be released from the folate, because the one reaction in which they participate cannot occur because of the B$_{12}$ deficiency. This leads to a functional folate deficiency; even though total levels of folate are normal. A folate deficiency (whether

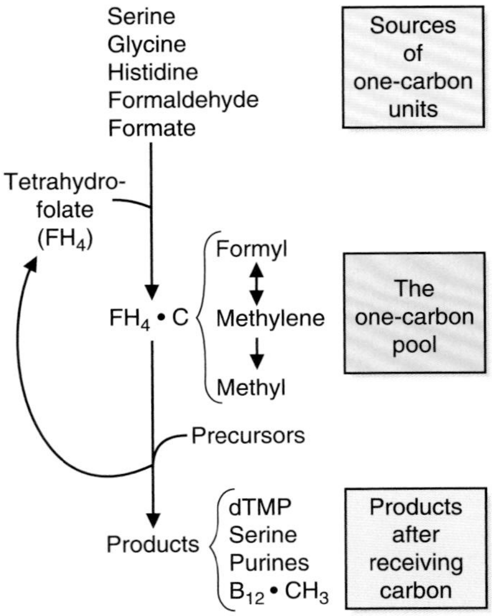

FIGURE 38.1 Overview of the one-carbon pool. *FH$_4$ • C* indicates tetrahydrofolate containing a one-carbon unit that is at the formyl, methylene, or methyl level of oxidation (see Fig. 38.3). The origin of the carbons is indicated, as are the final products after a one-carbon transfer. *dTMP*, deoxythymidine monophosphate.

functional or actual) leads to **megaloblastic anemia** caused by an inability of blood cell precursors to synthesize DNA and, therefore, to divide. This leads to large, partially replicated cells being released into the blood to attempt to replenish the cells that have died. Folate deficiencies also have been linked to an increased incidence of **neural tube defects**, such as spina bifida, in mothers who become pregnant while folate-deficient.

THE WAITING ROOM

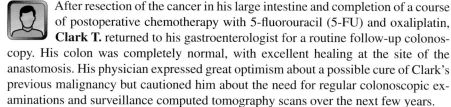

 After resection of the cancer in his large intestine and completion of a course of postoperative chemotherapy with 5-fluorouracil (5-FU) and oxaliplatin, **Clark T.** returned to his gastroenterologist for a routine follow-up colonoscopy. His colon was completely normal, with excellent healing at the site of the anastomosis. His physician expressed great optimism about a possible cure of Clark's previous malignancy but cautioned him about the need for regular colonoscopic examinations and surveillance computed tomography scans over the next few years.

 Beatrice T., a 75-year-old woman, went to see her physician because of numbness and tingling in her legs. A diet history indicated a normal and healthy diet, but Beatrice was not taking any supplemental vitamin pills. Laboratory results indicated a low level of serum B$_{12}$.

The initial laboratory profile, determined when **Jean T.** first presented to her physician with evidence of early alcohol-induced hepatitis, included a hematologic analysis that showed that Jean was anemic. Her hemoglobin was 11.0 g/dL (reference range, adult women = 12 to 16 g/dL). The erythrocyte (red blood cell) count was 3.6 million cells/mm^3 (reference range, adult woman = 4.0 to 5.2 million cells/mm^3). The average volume of her red blood cells (mean corpuscular volume [MCV]) was 108 fL (reference range, = 80 to 100 fL; 1 fL = 10^{-12} mL), and the hematology laboratory reported a striking variation in the size and shape of the red blood cells in a smear of her peripheral blood (see Chapter 42). The nuclei of the circulating granulocytic leukocytes had increased nuclear segmentation (polysegmented neutrophils). Because these findings are suggestive of a macrocytic anemia (in which blood cells are larger than normal), measurements of serum folate and vitamin B$_{12}$ (cobalamin) levels were ordered.

I. Tetrahydrofolate

A. Structure and Forms of Tetrahydrofolate

Folates exist in many chemical forms. The coenzyme form that functions in accepting one-carbon groups is FH$_4$ polyglutamate (Fig. 38.2), generally referred to as just *tetrahydrofolate* or *FH$_4$*. It has three major structural components: a bicyclic pteridine ring, *para*-aminobenzoic acid, and a polyglutamate tail consisting of several glutamate residues joined in amide linkage. The one-carbon group that is accepted by the coenzyme and then transferred to another compound is bound to N5, to N10, or both.

Different forms of folate may differ in the oxidation state of the one-carbon group, in the number of glutamate residues attached, or in the degree of oxidation of the pteridine ring. When the term "folate" or "folic acid" is applied to a specific chemical form, it is the most oxidized form of the pteridine ring (see Fig. 38.2). Folate is reduced to dihydrofolate (FH$_2$) and then to FH$_4$ by dihydrofolate reductase (DHFR) present in cells. Reduction is the favored direction of the reaction; therefore, most of the folate present in the body is present as the reduced coenzyme form, FH$_4$.

 The Schilling test, now a historic test, involves the patient ingesting radioactive ^{57}Co-labeled crystalline vitamin B$_{12}$, after which a 24-hour urine sample is collected. The radioactivity in the urine sample is compared with the input radioactivity, and the difference represents the amount of B$_{12}$ absorbed through the digestive tract. Such tests could distinguish whether the problem lies in removing B$_{12}$ from bound dietary proteins or if the deficiency is caused by a lack of intrinsic factor or other proteins involved in transporting B$_{12}$ throughout the body. Another method to determine if intrinsic factor activity is reduced is to determine the levels of anti–intrinsic factor antibodies in the blood. Autoantibodies toward intrinsic factor commonly develop in individuals with lack of intrinsic factor activity, and the levels of such antibodies can be determined in an enzyme-linked immunosorbent assay (ELISA) using recombinant human intrinsic factor bound to plastic wells as the antigen. The Schilling test has been replaced by a competitive binding luminescent assay. This new test has recently been criticized for being unreliable, particularly if a patient exhibits anti–intrinsic factor antibodies.

 Folate deficiencies occur frequently in chronic alcoholics. Several factors are involved: inadequate dietary intake of folate; direct damage to intestinal cells and brush-border enzymes, which interferes with absorption of dietary folate; a defect in the enterohepatic circulation, which reduces the absorption of folate; liver damage that causes decreased hepatic production of plasma proteins; and interference with kidney reabsorption of folate.

Hematopoietic precursor cells, when exposed to too little folate and/or vitamin B$_{12}$, show slowed cell division, but cytoplasmic development occurs at a normal rate. Hence, the megaloblastic cells tend to be large, with an increased ratio of RNA to DNA. Megaloblastic erythroid progenitors are usually destroyed in the bone marrow (although some reach the circulation). Thus, marrow cellularity is often increased, but production of red blood cells is decreased, a condition called *ineffective erythropoiesis*.

Therefore, Jean has megaloblastic anemia, characteristic of folate or B$_{12}$ deficiency.

Jean T.'s serum folic acid level was 3.1 ng/mL (reference range, 6 to 15 ng/mL), and her serum B_{12} level was 210 ng/L (reference range, 180 to 914 ng/L). Her serum iron level was normal. It was clear, therefore, that Jean's megaloblastic anemia was caused by a folate deficiency (although her B_{12} levels were in the low range of normal). The management of a pure folate deficiency in a patient with alcoholism includes cessation of alcohol intake and a diet that is rich in folate.

 Sulfa drugs, which are used to treat certain bacterial infections, are analogs of *para*-aminobenzoic acid. They prevent growth and cell division in bacteria by interfering with the synthesis of folate. Because we cannot synthesize folate, sulfa drugs do not affect human cells in this way.

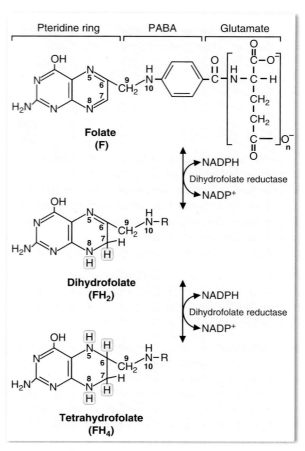

FIGURE 38.2 Reduction of folate to tetrahydrofolate (FH_4). The same enzyme, dihydrofolate reductase, catalyzes both reactions. Multiple glutamate residues are added within cells ($n \sim 5$). Plants can synthesize folate but humans cannot. Therefore, folate is a dietary requirement. *R* is the portion of the folate molecule shown to the right of N10. The different precursors of FH_4 are indicated in the figure. *NADP*, nicotinamide adenine dinucleotide phosphate; *PABA*, *para*-aminobenzoic acid.

B. The Vitamin Folate

Folates are synthesized in bacteria and higher plants and ingested in green leafy vegetables, fruits, and legumes in the diet. The vitamin was named for its presence in green leafy vegetables (foliage). Most of the dietary folate derived from natural food sources is present in the reduced coenzyme form. However, vitamin supplements and fortified foods contain principally the oxidized form of the pteridine ring.

As dietary folates pass into the proximal third of the small intestine, folate conjugases in the brush border of the lumen cleave off glutamate residues to produce the monoglutamate form of folate, which is then absorbed (see Fig. 38.2, upper structure, when $n = 1$). Within the intestinal cells, folate is converted principally to N^5-methyl-FH_4, which enters the portal vein and goes to the liver. Smaller amounts of other forms of folate also follow this route.

The liver, which stores half of the body's folate, takes up much of the folate from the portal circulation; uptake may be through active transport or receptor-mediated endocytosis. Within the liver, FH_4 is reconjugated to the polyglutamate form before being used in reactions. A small amount of the folate is partially degraded, and the components enter the urine. A relatively large portion of the folate enters the bile and is subsequently reabsorbed (very similar to the fate of bile salts in the enterohepatic circulation).

N^5-Methyl-FH_4, the major form of folate in the blood, is loosely bound to plasma proteins, particularly serum albumin.

 The current US Recommended Dietary Allowance (RDA) for folate equivalents is approximately 400 μg for adult men and women. In addition to being prevalent in green leafy vegetables, other good sources of this vitamin are liver, yeast, legumes, and some fruits. Protracted cooking of these foods, however, can destroy up to 90% of their folate content. A standard US diet provides 50 to 500 μg of absorbable folate each day. Folate deficiency in pregnant women, especially during the month before conception and the month after, increases the risk of neural tube defects, such as spina bifida, in the fetus. To reduce the potential risk of neural tube defects for women capable of becoming pregnant, the recommendation is to take 400 μg of folic acid daily in a multivitamin pill (some organizations recommend 400 to 800 μg daily). If the woman has a history of having a child with a neural tube defect, this amount is increased to 4,000 μg/day for the month before and the month after conception. Flour-containing products in the United States are now supplemented with folate to reduce the risk of neural tube defects in newborns.

C. Oxidation and Reduction of the One-Carbon Groups of Tetrahydrofolate

One-carbon groups transferred by FH$_4$ are attached to either N5 or N10, or they form a bridge between N5 and N10. The collection of one-carbon groups attached to FH$_4$ is known as the *one-carbon pool*. While they are attached to FH$_4$, these one-carbon units can be oxidized and reduced (Fig. 38.3). Thus, reactions that require a carbon

 Hereditary folate malabsorption is a rare disease caused by a mutation in a proton-coupled folate transporter (PCFT; gene *SLC46A1*). Loss of PCFT activity in the intestinal proximal jejunum and duodenum lead to systemic folate deficiency. Newborns begin to exhibit symptoms of folate deficiency after a few months of life, after the folate obtained from the mother has been excreted. The children develop anemia, diarrhea, and become immunocompromised (owing to the reduction in blood cell differentiation). High-dose oral folate can be used to treat the patients, because another folate transporter (the reduced folate carrier; gene *SLC19A1*) can absorb sufficient folate when folate is present at high concentrations.

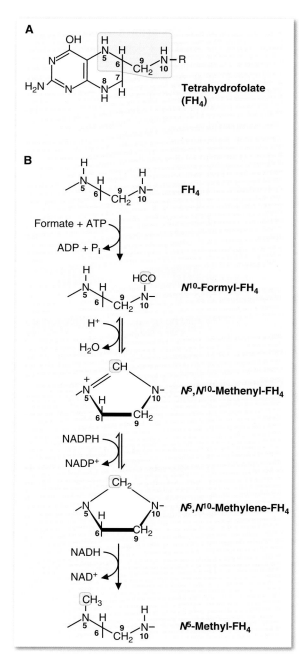

FIGURE 38.3   One-carbon units attached to tetrahydrofolate (FH$_4$). **A.** The active form of FH$_4$. *R* is the portion of the folate molecule shown to the right of N10. **B.** Interconversions of one-carbon units of FH$_4$. Only the portion of FH$_4$ from N5 to N10 is shown, which is indicated by the *green box* in **A**. After a formyl group forms a bridge between N5 and N10, two reductions can occur. Note that N^5-methyl-FH$_4$ cannot be reoxidized. The most oxidized form of FH$_4$ is at the *top* of the figure, whereas the most reduced form is at the *bottom*. *ADP*, adenosine diphosphate; *ATP*, adenosine triphosphate; *NAD*, nicotinamide adenine dinucleotide; *P$_i$*, inorganic phosphate.

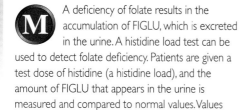

A deficiency of folate results in the accumulation of FIGLU, which is excreted in the urine. A histidine load test can be used to detect folate deficiency. Patients are given a test dose of histidine (a histidine load), and the amount of FIGLU that appears in the urine is measured and compared to normal values. Values greater than normal indicate folate deficiency.

The concentration of folate in serum can also be determined by a microbiologic test. Certain strains of bacteria require folate for growth, and if these bacteria are plated on a medium that lacks folate, they will not grow. Folate levels can be quantitated by preparing a standard curve using plates containing different levels of folate and determining the level of growth of the bacteria at that folate level. The unknown sample is then tested for bacterial growth and the extent of growth compared to the standard curve in order to determine the amount of folate in the unknown sample. Other tests for folate include measuring the binding of folate to certain proteins, and use of immunologic reagents that specifically bind to and identify folate.

FH$_4$ is required for the synthesis of dTMP and the purine bases used to produce the precursors for DNA replication. Therefore, FH$_4$ is required for cell division. Blockage of the synthesis of thymine and the purine bases, either by a dietary deficiency of folate or by drugs that interfere with folate metabolism, results in a decreased rate of cell division and growth.

in a particular oxidation state may use carbon from the one-carbon pool that was donated in a different oxidation state.

The individual steps for reduction of the one-carbon group are shown in Figure 38.3. The most oxidized form is N^{10}-formyl-FH$_4$. The most reduced form is N^5-methyl-FH$_4$. Once the methyl group is formed, it is not readily reoxidized back to N^5,N^{10}-methylene-FH$_4$, and thus, N^5-methyl-FH$_4$ tends to accumulate in the cell.

D. Sources of One-Carbon Groups Carried by Tetrahydrofolate

Carbon sources for the one-carbon pool include serine, glycine, formaldehyde, histidine, and formate (Fig. 38.4). These donors transfer the carbons to folate in different oxidation states. *Serine* is the major carbon source of one-carbon groups in the human. Its hydroxymethyl group is transferred to FH$_4$ in a reversible reaction, catalyzed by the enzyme serine hydroxymethyltransferase. This reaction produces glycine and N^5,N^{10}-methylene-FH$_4$. Because serine can be synthesized from *3-phosphoglycerate*, an intermediate of glycolysis, dietary carbohydrate can serve as a source of carbon for the one-carbon pool. The glycine that is produced may be further degraded by donation of a carbon to folate. Additional donors that form N^5,N^{10}-methylene-FH$_4$ are listed in Table 38.1.

Histidine and formate provide examples of compounds that donate carbon in different oxidation levels (see Fig. 38.4). Degradation of histidine produces formiminoglutamate (FIGLU), which reacts with FH$_4$ to donate a carbon and nitrogen (generating N^5-formimino-FH$_4$), thereby releasing glutamate. Formate, produced from tryptophan oxidation, can react with FH$_4$ and generate N^{10}-formyl-FH$_4$, the most oxidized folate derivative.

E. Recipients of One-Carbon Groups

The one-carbon groups on FH$_4$ may be oxidized or reduced (see Fig. 38.3) and then transferred to other compounds (see Fig. 38.4 and Table 38.1). Transfers of this sort are involved in the synthesis of glycine from serine, the synthesis of the base thymine required for DNA synthesis, the purine bases required for both DNA and RNA synthesis, and the transfer of methyl groups to vitamin B$_{12}$.

Because the conversion of serine to glycine is readily reversible, glycine can be converted to serine by drawing carbon from the one-carbon pool.

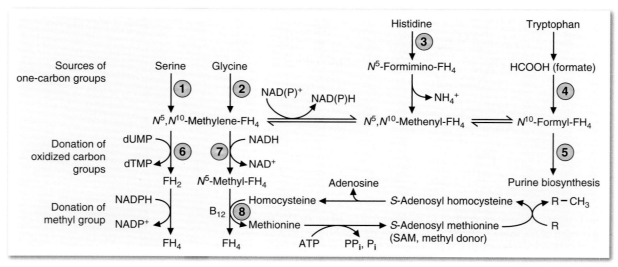

FIGURE 38.4 Sources of carbon (reactions 1 to 4) for the tetrahydrofolate (FH$_4$) pool and the recipients of carbon (reactions 5 to 8) from the pool. See Figure 38.3 to view the FH$_4$ derivatives involved in each reaction. *ATP*, adenosine triphosphate; *dTMP*, deoxythymidine monophosphate; *dUMP*, deoxyuridine monophosphate; *NAD*, nicotinamide adenine dinucleotide; *P$_i$*, inorganic phosphate; *PP$_i$*, pyrophosphate.

TABLE 38.1	One-Carbon Pool: Sources and Recipients of Carbon		
SOURCE[a]	**FORM OF ONE-CARBON DONOR PRODUCED**[b]	**RECIPIENT**	**FINAL PRODUCT**
Formate	N^{10}-Formyl-FH₄	Purine precursor	Purine (C2 and C8)
Serine	N^5,N^{10}-Methylene-FH₄	dUMP	dTMP
Glycine		Glycine	Serine
Formaldehyde			
N^5,N^{10}-Methylene-FH₄	N^5-Methyl-FH₄	Vitamin B₁₂	Methylcobalamin
Histidine	N^5-Formimino-FH₄ is converted to N^5,N^{10}-methenyl-FH₄.		
Choline	Betaine	Homocysteine	Methionine and dimethylglycine
Methionine	SAM	Glycine (there are many others; see Fig. 38.9B)	N-Methylglycine (sarcosine)

FH₄, tetrahydrofolate; dUMP, deoxyuridine monophosphate; dTMP, deoxythymidine monophosphate; SAM, S-adenosylmethionine

[a]The major source of carbon is serine.

[b]The carbon unit attached to FH₄ can be oxidized and reduced (see Fig. 38.3). At the methyl level, reoxidation does not occur.

The nucleotide dTMP is produced from dUMP by a reaction in which dUMP is methylated to form dTMP (Fig. 38.5). The source of carbon is N^5,N^{10}-methylene-FH₄. Two hydrogen atoms from FH₄ are used to reduce the donated carbon to the methyl level. Consequently, FH₂ is produced. Reduction of FH₂ by reduced nicotinamide adenine dinucleotide phosphate (NADPH) in a reaction catalyzed by DHFR regenerates FH₄. This is the only reaction involving FH₄ in which the folate group is oxidized as the one-carbon group is donated to the recipient. Recall that DHFR is also required to reduce the oxidized form of the vitamin, which is obtained from the diet (see Fig. 38.2). Thus, DHFR is essential for regenerating FH₄ both in the tissues and from the diet. These reactions contribute to the effect of folate deficiency on DNA synthesis because dTMP is required only for the synthesis of DNA.

Individuals with non-Hodgkin lymphoma receive several drugs to treat the tumor, including methotrexate. The structure of methotrexate is shown here.

Methotrexate

What compound does methotrexate resemble?

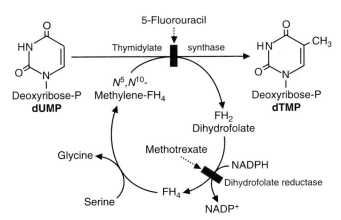

FIGURE 38.5 Transfer of a one-carbon unit from N^5,N^{10}-methylenetetrahydrofolate to deoxyuridine monophosphate (dUMP) to form deoxythymidine monophosphate (dTMP). Tetrahydrofolate (FH₄) is oxidized to dihydrofolate (FH₂) in this reaction. FH₂ is reduced to FH₄ by dihydrofolate reductase (DHFR), and FH₄ is converted to N^5,N^{10}-methylene-FH₄ using serine as a carbon donor. *Shaded bars* indicate the steps at which the antimetabolites 5-fluorouracil (5-FU), and methotrexate act. 5-FU inhibits thymidylate synthase. Methotrexate inhibits DHFR. *Deoxyribose-P*, deoxyribose phosphate; *NADP*, nicotinamide adenine dinucleotide phosphate.

Methotrexate has the same structure as folate except that it has an amino group on C4 and a methyl group on N10. Anticancer drugs such as methotrexate are folate analogs that act by inhibiting DHFR, thereby preventing the conversion of FH₂ to FH₄ (see Fig. 38.5). Thus, the cellular pools of FH₄ are not replenished, and reactions that require FH₄ cannot proceed.

A better understanding of the structure and function of the purine and pyrimidine bases and of folate metabolism led to the development of compounds having antimetabolic and antifolate action useful for treatment of neoplastic disease. For example, **Clark T.** was successfully treated for colon cancer with a combination of chemotherapy including 5-FU (see Chapter 12 and Fig. 38.5). 5-FU is a pyrimidine analog, which is converted in cells to the nucleotide fluorodeoxyuridylate (FdUMP). FdUMP causes a "thymineless death," especially for tumor cells that have a rapid turnover rate. It prevents the growth of cancer cells by blocking the thymidylate synthase reaction; that is, the conversion of dUMP to dTMP.

Jean T.'s megaloblastic anemia was treated in part with folate supplements (see Clinical Comments). Within 48 hours of the initiation of folate therapy, megaloblastic or "ineffective" erythropoiesis usually subsides, and effective erythropoiesis begins.

Megaloblastic anemia is caused by a decrease in the synthesis of thymine and the purine bases. These deficiencies lead to an inability of hematopoietic (and other) cells to synthesize DNA and, therefore, to divide. Their persistently thwarted attempts at normal DNA replication, DNA repair, and cell division produce abnormally large cells (called *megaloblasts*) with abundant cytoplasm capable of protein synthesis but with clumping and fragmentation of nuclear chromatin (see Chapter 42). Some of these large cells, although immature, are released early from the marrow in an attempt to compensate for the anemia. Thus, peripheral blood smears also contain megaloblasts. Many of the large immature cells, however, are destroyed in the marrow and never reach the circulation.

During the synthesis of the purine bases, carbons 2 and 8 are obtained from the one-carbon pool (see Chapter 39). N^{10}-Formyl-FH₄ provides both carbons. Folate deficiency would also hinder these reactions, contributing to an inability to replicate DNA because of the lack of precursors.

After the carbon group carried by FH₄ is reduced to the methyl level, it is transferred to vitamin B₁₂. This is the only reaction through which the methyl group can leave FH₄ (recall that the reaction that creates N^5-methyl-FH₄ is not reversible).

II. Vitamin B₁₂

A. Structure and Forms of Vitamin B₁₂

The structure of vitamin B₁₂ (also known as *cobalamin*) is complex (Fig. 38.6). It contains a corrin ring, which is similar to the porphyrin ring found in heme. The corrin ring differs from heme, however, in that two of the four pyrrole rings are joined directly rather than by a methylene bridge. Its most unusual feature is the presence of cobalt, coordinated with the corrin ring (similar to the iron coordinated with the porphyrin ring). This cobalt can form a bond with a carbon atom. In the body, it reacts with the carbon of a methyl group, forming methylcobalamin, or with

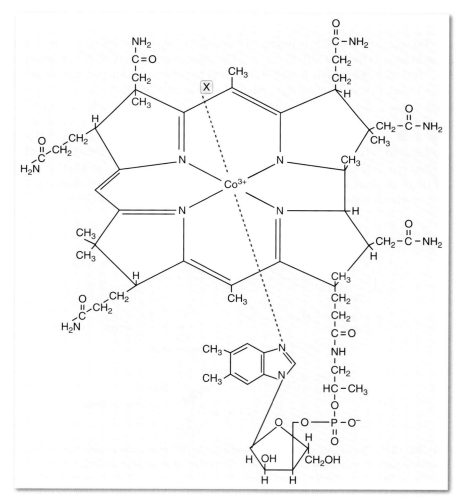

FIGURE 38.6 Vitamin B₁₂. When X is 5′-deoxyadenosine, the vitamin is deoxyadenosyl-cobalamin; when X is a methyl group, the vitamin is methylcobalamin; and when X is CN, the vitamin is cyanocobalamin (the commercial form found in vitamin tablets).

the 5'-carbon of 5'-deoxyadenosine, forming 5'-deoxyadenosylcobalamin (note that in this case the *deoxy* designation refers to the 5'-carbon, not the 2'-carbon as is the case in the sugar found in DNA). The form of B_{12} found in vitamin supplements is cyanocobalamin, in which a CN group is linked to the cobalt.

B. Absorption and Transport of Vitamin B_{12}

Although vitamin B_{12} is produced by bacteria, it cannot be synthesized by higher plants or animals. The major source of vitamin B_{12} is dietary meat, eggs, dairy products, fish, poultry, and seafood. The animals that serve as the source of these foods obtain B_{12} mainly from the bacteria in their food supply. The absorption of B_{12} from the diet is a complex process (Fig. 38.7).

Ingested B_{12} can exist in two forms, either free or bound to dietary proteins. If free, the B_{12} binds to proteins known as *R-binders* (haptocorrins, also known as *transcobalamin I*), which are secreted by the salivary glands and the gastric mucosa in either the saliva or the stomach. If the ingested B_{12} is bound to proteins, it must be released from the proteins by the action of digestive proteases in both the stomach and small intestine. Once the B_{12} is released from its bound protein, it binds to the haptocorrins. In the small intestine, the pancreatic proteases digest the haptocorrins, and the released B_{12} then binds to intrinsic factor, a glycoprotein secreted by the parietal cells of the stomach when food enters the stomach. The intrinsic factor–B_{12} complex attaches to specific receptors in the terminal segment of the small intestine known as the *ileum*, after which the complex is internalized.

The average daily diet in Western countries contains 5 to 30 μg of vitamin B_{12}, of which 1 to 5 μg is absorbed into the blood. (The RDA is 2.4 μg/day.) Total body content of this vitamin in an adult is approximately 2 to 5 mg, of which 1 mg is present in the liver. As a result, a dietary deficiency of B_{12} is uncommon and is observed only after a number of years on a diet that is deficient in this vitamin.

Despite **Jean T.'s** relatively malnourished state because of her chronic alcoholism, her serum cobalamin level was still within the low-to-normal range. If her undernourished state had continued, a cobalamin deficiency would eventually have developed.

Pernicious anemia, a deficiency of intrinsic factor, is a relatively common problem that is caused by malabsorption of dietary cobalamin. It may result from an inherited defect that leads to decreased ability of gastric parietal cells to synthesize intrinsic factor or from partial resection of the stomach or of the ileum. Production of intrinsic factor often declines with age and may be low in elderly individuals. An alternative circumstance that leads to the development of a vitamin B_{12} deficiency is pancreatic insufficiency or a high intestinal pH, which results from too little acid being produced by the stomach. Both of these conditions prevent the degradation of the R-binder–B_{12} complex; as a result, B_{12} is not released from the R-binder protein and, therefore, cannot bind to intrinsic factor. The protein receptor for the B_{12}–intrinsic factor complex is named *cubilin*, and the internalization of the B_{12}–intrinsic factor–cubilin complex requires the activity of a transmembrane protein named *amnionless*. Congenital malabsorption of B_{12} can also arise from inherited mutations in either *cubilin* or *amnionless*.

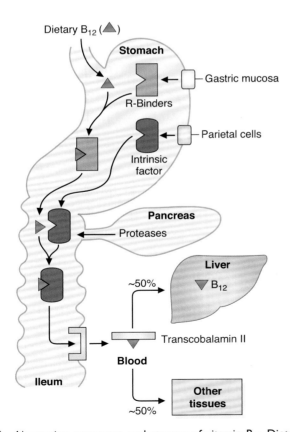

FIGURE 38.7 Absorption, transport, and storage of vitamin B_{12}. Dietary B_{12} binds to R-binders (haptocorrins) in the stomach and travels to the intestine, where the R-binders are destroyed by pancreatic proteases. The freed B_{12} then binds to intrinsic factor. B_{12} is absorbed in the ileum and carried by proteins named transcobalamins to the liver, where B_{12} is stored.

How should vitamin B_{12} be administered to a patient with pernicious anemia?

The B_{12} within the enterocyte complexes with transcobalamin II before it is released into the circulation. The transcobalamin II–B_{12} complex delivers B_{12} to the tissues, which contain specific receptors for this complex. The liver takes up approximately 50% of the vitamin B_{12}, and the remainder is transported to other tissues. The amount of the vitamin stored in the liver is large enough that 3 to 6 years pass before symptoms of a dietary deficiency occur.

C. Functions of Vitamin B_{12}

Vitamin B_{12} is involved in two reactions in the body: the transfer of a methyl group from N^5-methyl-FH$_4$ to homocysteine to form methionine and the rearrangement of L-methylmalonyl-CoA to form succinyl-CoA (Fig. 38.8).

FH$_4$ receives a one-carbon group from serine or from other sources. This carbon is reduced to the methyl level and transferred to vitamin B_{12}, forming methyl-B_{12} (or methylcobalamin). Methylcobalamin transfers the methyl group to homocysteine, which is converted to methionine by the enzyme methionine synthase. Methionine can then be activated to SAM to transfer the methyl group to other compounds (Fig. 38.9).

Vitamin B_{12} also participates in the conversion of L-methylmalonyl-CoA to succinyl-CoA. In this case, the active form of the coenzyme is 5′-deoxyadenosylcobalamin. This reaction is part of the metabolic route for the conversion of carbons from valine, isoleucine, threonine, and the last three carbons of odd-chain fatty acids, all of which form propionyl coenzyme A (propionyl-CoA), to the tricarboxylic acid (TCA)–cycle intermediate succinyl-CoA (see Chapter 37).

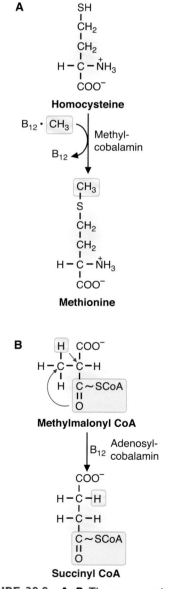

FIGURE 38.8 A, B. The two reactions involving vitamin B_{12} in humans. *CoA*, coenzyme A; *Methylmalonyl CoA*, methylmalonyl-coenzyme A; *Succinyl-CoA*, succinyl coenzyme A.

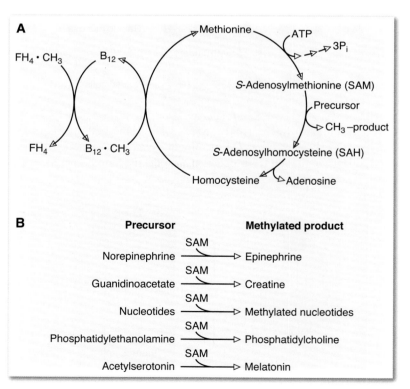

FIGURE 38.9 Relationships among tetrahydrofolate (FH$_4$), vitamin B_{12}, and S-adenosylmethionine (SAM). **A.** Overall scheme. **B.** Some specific reactions that require SAM. *ATP*, adenosine triphosphate; *P$_i$*, inorganic phosphate.

III. *S*-Adenosylmethionine

SAM participates in the synthesis of many compounds that contain methyl groups. It is used in reactions that add methyl groups to either oxygen or nitrogen atoms in the acceptor (contrast that to folate derivatives, which can add one-carbon groups to sulfur or to carbon). As examples, SAM is required for the conversion of phosphatidylethanolamine to phosphatidylcholine, guanidinoacetate to creatine, norepinephrine to epinephrine, acetylserotonin to melatonin, and nucleotides to methylated nucleotides (see Fig. 38.9B). It is also required for the inactivation of catecholamines and serotonin (see Chapter 46). More than 35 reactions in humans require methyl donation from SAM.

SAM is synthesized from methionine and ATP. As with the activation of vitamin B_{12}, ATP donates the adenosine. With the transfer of its methyl group, SAM forms *S*-adenosylhomocysteine (SAH), which is subsequently hydrolyzed to form homocysteine and adenosine.

Methionine, required for the synthesis of SAM, is obtained from the diet or produced from homocysteine, which accepts a methyl group from vitamin B_{12} (see Fig. 38.9A). Thus, the methyl group of methionine is regenerated. The portion of methionine that is essential in the diet is the homocysteine moiety. If we had an adequate dietary source of homocysteine, methionine would not be required in the diet. However, there is no good dietary source of homocysteine, whereas methionine is plentiful in the diet.

Homocysteine provides the sulfur atom for the synthesis of cysteine (see Chapter 37). In this case, homocysteine reacts with serine to form cystathionine, which is cleaved, yielding cysteine and α-ketobutyrate. The first reaction in this sequence is inhibited by cysteine. Thus, methionine, via homocysteine, is not used for cysteine synthesis unless the levels of cysteine in the body are lower than required for its metabolic functions. An adequate dietary supply of cysteine, therefore, can "spare" (or reduce) the dietary requirement for methionine.

IV. Relationships among Folate, Vitamin B₁₂, and *S*-Adenosylmethionine

A. The Methyl-Trap Hypothesis

If one analyzes the flow of carbon in the folate cycle, the equilibrium lies in the direction of the N^5-methyl-FH_4 form. This appears to be the most stable form of carbon attached to the vitamin. However, in only one reaction can the methyl group be removed from N^5-methyl-FH_4, and that is the methionine synthase reaction, which requires vitamin B_{12}. Thus, if vitamin B_{12} is deficient, or if the methionine synthase enzyme is defective, N^5-methyl-FH_4 accumulates. Eventually, most folate forms in the body become "trapped" in the N^5-methyl form. A functional folate deficiency results because the carbons cannot be removed from the folate. The appearance of a functional folate deficiency caused by a lack of vitamin B_{12} is known as the *methyl-trap hypothesis*, and its clinical implications are discussed in following sections.

B. Hyperhomocysteinemia

Elevated homocysteine levels have been linked to cardiovascular and neurologic disease. Homocysteine levels can accumulate in a number of ways, which are related to both folic acid and vitamin B_{12} metabolism. Homocysteine is derived from SAH, which arises when SAM donates a methyl group (Fig. 38.10). Because SAM is frequently donating methyl groups, there is constant production of SAH, which leads to constant production of homocysteine. Recall from Chapter 37 that homocysteine has two biochemical fates. The homocysteine produced can be either remethylated to methionine or condensed with serine to form cystathionine. There are two routes to methionine production. The major one is methylation by N^5-methyl-FH_4, which requires vitamin B_{12}.

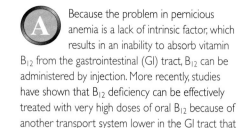

Because the problem in pernicious anemia is a lack of intrinsic factor, which results in an inability to absorb vitamin B_{12} from the gastrointestinal (GI) tract, B_{12} can be administered by injection. More recently, studies have shown that B_{12} deficiency can be effectively treated with very high doses of oral B_{12} because of another transport system lower in the GI tract that does not require intrinsic factor.

There are two major clinical manifestations of cobalamin (vitamin B_{12}) deficiency. One such presentation is hematopoietic (caused by the adverse effects of a B_{12} deficiency on folate metabolism) and the other is neurologic (caused by hypomethylation and myelin destabilization in the nervous system). The hemopoietic problems associated with a B_{12} deficiency are identical to those observed in a folate deficiency and, in fact, result from a folate deficiency secondary to (i.e., caused by) the B_{12} deficiency (i.e., the methyl-trap hypothesis). As the FH_4 pool is exhausted, deficiencies of the FH_4 derivatives needed for purine and dTMP biosynthesis develop, leading to the characteristic megaloblastic anemia.

The classical clinical presentation of the neurologic dysfunction associated with a B_{12} deficiency includes symmetric numbness and tingling of the feet (and less so the hands), diminishing vibratory and position sense, and progression to a spastic gait disturbance. The patient may develop dementia and depression. Rarely, they develop psychosis ("megaloblastic madness"). Other rare symptoms include blind spots that develop in the central portions of the visual fields, and alterations in gustatory (taste) and olfactory (smell) function. This is thought to be caused by two factors. The first is hypomethylation within the nervous system, brought about by an inability to recycle homocysteine to methionine and from there to SAM. The latter is the required methyl donor in these reactions. The nervous system lacks the betaine pathway of methionine regeneration (see Fig. 38.10) and is dependent on the B_{12} system for regenerating SAM. With a B_{12} deficiency, this pathway is inoperable in the nervous system, and DNA and histones are hypomethylated. The second factor is the accumulation of methylmalonic acid, which leads to myelin destabilization and loss of protection of the neurons. This occurs because of methylmalonyl-CoA being used in place of malonyl-CoA in fatty acid synthesis. This generates branched-chain fatty acids that are incorporated into phospholipids and eventually the myelin sheath.

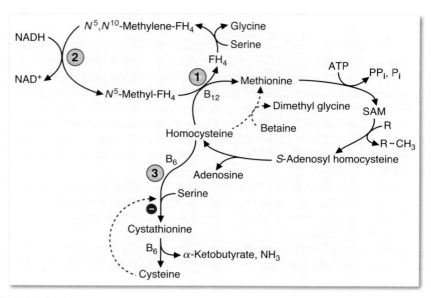

FIGURE 38.10 Reaction pathways that involve homocysteine. Defects in numbered enzymes (*1*, methionine synthase; *2*, N^5,N^{10}-methylenetetrahydrofolate reductase; *3*, cystathionine β-synthase) lead to elevated homocysteine. Recall that as cysteine accumulates, there is feedback inhibition on cystathionine β-synthase to stop further cysteine production. *ATP*, adenosine triphosphate; *FH₄*, tetrahydrofolate; *NAD*, nicotinamide adenine dinucleotide; *Pᵢ*, inorganic phosphate; *PPᵢ*, pyrophosphate; *SAM*, S-adenosylmethionine.

 Many health food stores now sell SAMe, a stabilized version of SAM. SAMe has been hypothesized to relieve depression because the synthesis of certain neurotransmitters requires methylation by SAM (see Chapter 46). This has led to the hypothesis that by increasing SAM levels in the nervous system, the biosynthesis of these neurotransmitters will be accelerated. This in turn might alleviate the feelings of depression. There have been reports in the literature indicating that this may occur, but its efficacy as an antidepressant must be confirmed. The major questions that must be addressed include the stability of SAMe in the digestive system and the level of uptake of SAMe by cells of the nervous system.

The liver also contains a second pathway in which betaine (derived from choline) can donate a methyl group to homocysteine to form methionine, but this is a minor pathway (see Section II of this chapter). The conversion of homocysteine to cystathionine requires pyridoxal phosphate (PLP). Thus, if an individual is deficient in vitamin B_{12}, the conversion of homocysteine to methionine by the major route is inhibited. This directs homocysteine to produce cystathionine, which eventually produces cysteine. As cysteine levels accumulate, the enzyme that makes cystathionine undergoes feedback inhibition, and that pathway is also inhibited (see Fig. 38.10). This, overall, leads to accumulation of homocysteine, which is released into the blood.

Homocysteine also accumulates in the blood if a mutation is present in the enzyme that converts N^5,N^{10}-methylene-FH₄ to N^5-methyl-FH₄. When this occurs, the levels of N^5-methyl-FH₄ are too low to allow homocysteine to be converted to methionine. The loss of this pathway, coupled with the feedback inhibition by cysteine on cystathionine formation, also leads to elevated homocysteine levels in the blood.

A third way in which serum homocysteine levels can be elevated is by a mutated cystathionine β-synthase or a deficiency in vitamin B_6, the required cofactor for that enzyme. These defects block the ability of homocysteine to be converted to cystathionine, and the homocysteine that does accumulate cannot all be accommodated by conversion to methionine. Thus, an accumulation of homocysteine results.

C. Neural Tube Defects

Folate deficiency during pregnancy has been associated with an increased risk of neural tube defects in the developing fetus. This risk is significantly reduced if women take folic acid supplements periconceptually. The link between folate deficiency and neural tube defects was first observed in women with hyperhomocysteinemia brought about by a thermolabile variant of N^5,N^{10}-methylene-FH₄ reductase. This form of the enzyme, which results from a single nucleotide change (C to T) in position 677 of the gene that encodes the protein, is less active at body temperature than at lower temperatures. This results in a reduced level of N^5-methyl-FH₄ being generated and, therefore, an increase in the levels of homocysteine. Along with the elevated homocysteine, the women were also folate-deficient. The folate deficiency and the subsequent inhibition of DNA synthesis leads to neural tube defects. The elevated homocysteine is one indication that such a deficit is present. These findings have led to the recommendation that women considering getting pregnant begin taking folate supplements before conception occurs and during pregnancy. The U.S. Department of Agriculture has, in fact, mandated that folate be added to flour-containing products in the United States.

D. Folate Deficiencies and DNA Synthesis

Folate deficiencies result in decreased availability of the deoxythymidine and purine nucleotides that serve as precursors for DNA synthesis. The decreased concentrations of these precursors affect not only the DNA synthesis that occurs during replication before cell division but also the DNA synthesis that occurs as a step in the processes that repair damaged DNA.

Decreased methylation of dUMP to form dTMP, a reaction that requires N^5, N^{10}-methylene-FH$_4$ as a coenzyme (see Fig. 38.5), leads to an increase in the intracellular dUTP/deoxythymidine triphosphate (dTTP) ratio. This ratio change causes a significant increase in the incorporation of uracil into DNA. Although much of this uracil can be removed by DNA-repair enzymes, the lack of available dTTP blocks the step of DNA repair that is catalyzed by DNA polymerase. The result is fragmentation of DNA as well as blockade of normal DNA replication.

These abnormal nuclear processes are responsible for the clumping and poly-segmentation seen in the nuclei of neutrophilic leukocytes in the bone marrow and in the peripheral blood of patients with megaloblastic anemia caused by a primary folate deficiency or one that is secondary to B$_{12}$ deficiency. The abnormalities in DNA synthesis and repair lead to an irreversible loss of the capacity for cell division and eventually to cell death.

V. Choline and One-Carbon Metabolism

Other compounds involved in one-carbon metabolism are derived from degradation products of choline. Choline, an essential component of certain phospholipids, is oxidized to form betaine aldehyde, which is further oxidized to betaine (trimethylglycine). In the liver, betaine can donate a methyl group to homocysteine to form methionine and dimethylglycine. This allows the liver to have two routes for homocysteine conversion to methionine. This is in contrast to the nervous system, which only expresses the primary B$_{12}$-requiring pathway. Under conditions in which SAM accumulates, glycine can be methylated to form sarcosine (N-methylglycine). This route of glycine metabolism is used when methionine levels are high and excess methionine needs to be metabolized (Fig. 38.11).

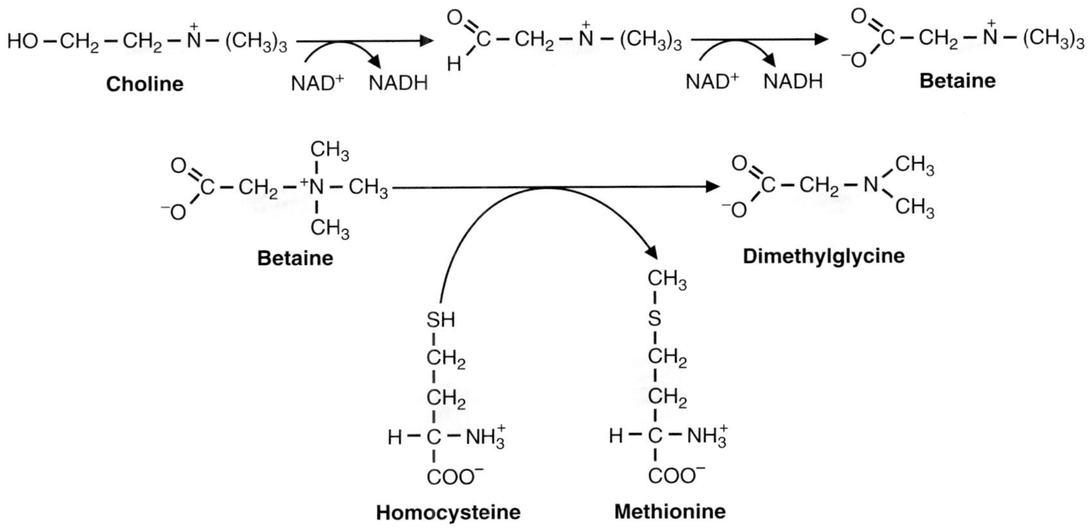

FIGURE 38.11 Choline and one-carbon metabolism. *NAD*, nicotinamide adenine dinucleotide.

CLINICAL COMMENTS

Jean T. Jean T. developed a folate deficiency and is on the verge of developing a cobalamin (vitamin B$_{12}$) deficiency as a consequence of prolonged, moderately severe malnutrition related to chronic alcoholism. Before folate therapy is started, the physician must ascertain that the megaloblastic anemia is not caused by a pure B$_{12}$ deficiency or a combined deficiency of folate and B$_{12}$.

If folate is given without cobalamin to a B$_{12}$-deficient patient, the drug only partially corrects the megaloblastic anemia because it will "bypass" the methyl-folate trap and provide adequate FH$_4$ coenzyme for the conversion of dUMP to dTMP and for a resurgence of purine synthesis. As a result, normal DNA synthesis, DNA repair, and cell division occur. However, the neurologic syndrome, resulting from hypomethylation in nervous tissue, and accumulation of methylmalonic acid, may progress unless the physician realizes that B$_{12}$ supplementation is required. In Jean's case, in which the serum B$_{12}$ concentration was borderline low and in which the dietary history supported the possibility of a B$_{12}$ deficiency, a combination of folate and B$_{12}$ supplements is required to avoid this potential therapeutic trap.

Clark T. Clark T. continued to do well and returned faithfully for his regular colonoscopic examinations.

Beatrice T. Beatrice T. was diagnosed with a decreased ability to absorb dietary B$_{12}$. One of the consequences of aging is a reduced acid production by the gastric mucosa (atrophic gastritis), which limits the ability of pepsin to work on dietary protein. Reduced pepsin efficiency then reduces the amount of bound B$_{12}$ released from dietary protein, as a result of which the B$_{12}$ is not available for absorption. Her condition can be treated by taking high-dose vitamin B$_{12}$ supplements orally.

BIOCHEMICAL COMMENTS

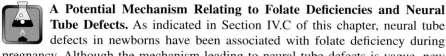

A Potential Mechanism Relating to Folate Deficiencies and Neural Tube Defects. As indicated in Section IV.C of this chapter, neural tube defects in newborns have been associated with folate deficiency during pregnancy. Although the mechanism leading to neural tube defects is vague, new research has indicated that the induction of micro RNAs (miRNAs) may play a role in altering the normal developmental pattern of neural tube closure.

Under conditions of a folate deficiency, hypomethylation occurs in the nervous system, affecting membrane phospholipid biosynthesis (such as phosphatidylcholine), myelin basic protein (see Chapter 46), and neurotransmitter biosynthesis (see Chapter 46). The reduced levels of neurotransmitters may interfere with normal gene expression during embryogenesis. DNA methylation is also reduced, owing to reduced SAM levels when folate is limiting. Hypomethylation is also the result of increased levels of SAH, which accumulates during a folate deficiency. SAH will inhibit DNA methyltransferase enzymes by tightly binding to the enzyme, and preventing the normal substrate, SAM, from binding to the enzyme. The enzymes affinity for SAH is higher than that of SAM, contributing to the hypomethylation observed.

miRNA genes are frequently in close proximity to CpG islands in DNA, and it has been predicted that alterations in cytosine methylation may be a means of regulating miRNA expression. Experimentally, a cell line in which two DNA methyltransferase genes were knocked out (inactivated) resulted in a significant reduction in global genomic methylation and the differential expression of 13 miRNAs (seven of those genes were overexpressed, whereas the other six displayed a reduction in expression). A similar result was obtained with another cell line that was placed in folate-deficient media; global hypomethylation and alterations in miRNA expression were observed.

As an example, miR-222 was identified as a potential miRNA that is upregulated under conditions of folate deprivation. A predicted target of miR-222 is the *DNMT-1* gene (a DNA methyltransferase), whose activity is critical for the maintenance of methylation patterns in DNA. Overexpression of miR-222 would reduce *DNMT-1* gene expression, thereby altering methylation patterns in the cell. A reduction of *DNMT-1* activity has been shown to increase the expression of a number of genes, including β-catenin (see Chapter 18). This will lead to enhanced cell proliferation and inhibition of differentiation in the nervous system (all leading to a failure to close the neural tube).

Studies such as those described previously are in their infancy but produce a promising start for unraveling the effects of DNA methylation, and miRNA expression, on cell growth and differentiation in the nervous system.

KEY CONCEPTS

- One-carbon groups at lower oxidation states than carbon dioxide (which is carried by biotin) are transferred by reactions that involve tetrahydrofolate (FH$_4$), vitamin B$_{12}$, and S-adenosylmethionine (SAM).
- FH$_4$ is produced from the vitamin folate and obtains one-carbon units from serine, glycine, histidine, formaldehyde, and formic acid.
- The carbon attached to FH$_4$ can be oxidized or reduced, thus producing several different forms of FH$_4$. However, once a carbon has been reduced to the methyl level, it cannot be reoxidized.
- The carbons attached to FH$_4$ are known collectively as the *one-carbon pool*.
- The carbons carried by folate are used in a limited number of biochemical reactions, but they are very important in forming deoxythymidine monophosphate (dTMP) and the purine rings.
- Vitamin B$_{12}$ participates in two reactions in the body: conversion of L-methylmalonyl-CoA to succinyl-CoA and conversion of homocysteine to methionine.
- SAM, formed from adenosine triphosphate (ATP) and methionine, transfers the methyl group to precursors of a variety of methylated compounds.
- Both vitamin B$_{12}$ and methyl-FH$_4$ are required in methionine metabolism; a deficiency of vitamin B$_{12}$ leads to overproduction and trapping of folate in the methyl form, leading to a functional folate deficiency. Such deficiencies can lead to
  - Megaloblastic anemia
  - Neural tube defects in newborns
- Diseases discussed in this chapter are summarized in Table 38.2.

TABLE 38.2 Diseases Discussed in Chapter 38		
DISEASE OR DISORDER	**ENVIRONMENTAL OR GENETIC**	**COMMENTS**
Colon cancer	Both	Colon cancer can be treated by drugs that block the action of thymidylate synthase, blocking DNA synthesis by reducing the supply of deoxythymidine triphosphate (dTTP).
Pernicious anemia	Both	Pernicious anemia is caused by the lack of intrinsic factor, which leads to a vitamin B$_{12}$ deficiency. The B$_{12}$ deficiency indirectly interferes with DNA synthesis. In cells of the erythroid lineage, cell size increases without cell division, leading to megaloblastic anemia.
Alcohol-induced megaloblastic anemia	Environmental	Alcohol-induced malnutrition, which can lead to folate and/or B$_{12}$ deficiencies. The folate and/or B$_{12}$ deficiency will lead to the development of megaloblastic anemia.
Neural tube defects	Both	A lack of folate derivatives leads to reduced methylation in the nervous system, altering gene expression and increasing the risk of neural tube defects.

REVIEW QUESTIONS—CHAPTER 38

1. Which one of the following reactions requires N^5,N^{10}-methylene-FH$_4$ as a carbon donor?
   A. Homocysteine to methionine
   B. Serine to glycine
   C. Betaine to dimethylglycine
   D. dUMP to dTMP
   E. The de novo biosynthesis of the purine ring

2. Propionic acid accumulation from amino acid degradation will result from a deficiency of which one of the following vitamins?
   A. Vitamin B_6
   B. Biotin
   C. Folic acid
   D. Vitamin B_1
   E. Vitamin B_2

3. A child with an acute otitis media (middle ear infection) is treated with a sulfa antibiotic. This medication interferes with the bacterial synthesis of which one of the following?
   A. Vitamin B_{12}
   B. SAM
   C. Folic acid
   D. Vitamin B_6
   E. Homocysteine

4. Which one of the following forms of FH$_4$ is required for the synthesis of methionine from homocysteine?
   A. N^5,N^{10}-Methylene-FH$_4$
   B. N^5-Methyl-FH$_4$
   C. N^5,N^{10}-Methenyl-FH$_4$
   D. N^{10}-Formyl-FH$_4$
   E. N^5-Formimino-FH$_4$

5. An alternative method to methylate homocysteine to form methionine is which one of the following?
   A. Using glycine and FH$_4$ as the methyl donor
   B. Using dimethylglycine as the methyl donor
   C. Using choline as the methyl donor
   D. Using sarcosine as the methyl donor
   E. Using betaine as the methyl donor

6. Both folic acid and B_{12} deficiencies will lead to the observation of hypomethylation in the nervous system. These two cofactors are most closely linked via which one of the following proteins?
   A. Transcobalamin II
   B. Methionine synthase

   C. Cystathionine β-synthase
   D. N^5,N^{10}-Methylene-FH$_4$ reductase
   E. DNA methyltransferase

7. A very strict vegan, who has not eaten animal products for over 5 years or taken exogenous vitamins, slowly develops tiredness and lethargy and also notes occasional tingling in the feet. An analysis of total folate indicated normal amounts. In which form would this folate most likely be found?
   A. N^5-Methyl-FH$_4$
   B. N^5,N^{10}-Methylene-FH$_4$
   C. N^{10}-Formyl-FH$_4$
   D. N^5-Formimino-FH$_4$
   E. N^5,N^{10}-Methenyl-FH$_4$

8. A patient presents to a clinic with symptoms of lethargy and tingling in the extremities. Bloodwork demonstrates a megaloblastic anemia. Measurement of which one of the following metabolites in the blood will aid in determining the cause of these symptoms in this patient?
   A. Lactic acid
   B. Pyruvic acid
   C. Methionine
   D. Methylmalonic acid
   E. Histidine

9. Which one of the following patients would be in danger of developing a vitamin B_{12} deficiency?
   A. A lacto–ovo vegetarian
   B. A patient with an inability to secrete gastrin
   C. A person who had his or her duodenum surgically removed
   D. A patient with Crohn's disease affecting the terminal ileum
   E. A patient with a biliary duct obstruction

10. Methotrexate is a medication that has been used as an anticancer drug and currently is used in treatment of psoriasis and rheumatoid arthritis. This folate analog directly inhibits which one of the following conversions?
    A. FH$_2$ to FH$_4$
    B. FH$_2$ to folate
    C. dUMP to dTMP
    D. Serine to glycine
    E. Homocysteine to methionine

ANSWERS

1. **The answer is D.** The homocysteine-to-methionine reaction requires N^5-methyl-FH$_4$; serine to glycine requires free FH$_4$ and generates N^5,N^{10}-methylene-FH$_4$; betaine donates a methyl group to homocysteine to form methionine without the participation of FH$_4$; and the purine ring requires N^{10}-formyl-FH$_4$ in its biosynthesis.

2. **The answer is B.** Propionic acid is derived from an accumulation of propionyl-CoA. The normal pathway

   for the degradation of propionyl-CoA is, first, a biotin-dependent carboxylation to D-methylmalonyl-CoA, racemization to L-methylmalonyl-CoA, and then the B_{12}-dependent rearrangement to succinyl-CoA.

3. **The answer is C.** Sulfa drugs are analogs of *para*-aminobenzoic acid and prevent growth and cell division in bacteria by interfering with the synthesis of folic acid (which is needed to produce FH$_4$). Humans cannot

synthesize folate de novo and must obtain folate from the diet. Because of this, the sulfa drugs do not affect human metabolism.

4. **The answer is B.** The only three forms of folate that transfer carbons are the N^5-methyl-FH$_4$ form, the N^5,N^{10}-methylene-FH$_4$ form, and the N^{10}-formyl form. None of the other forms participates in reactions in which the carbon is transferred. It is the N^5-methyl form that transfers the methyl group to form methionine from homocysteine.

5. **The answer is E.** Choline, derived from phosphatidylcholine, is converted to betaine (trimethylglycine). Betaine can donate a methyl group to homocysteine to form methionine plus dimethylglycine. Sarcosine is N-methylglycine, which is formed when excess SAM methylates glycine, but it is not used as a methyl donor in this reaction.

6. **The answer is B.** The conversion of homocysteine to methionine, catalyzed by methionine synthase, requires vitamin B$_{12}$ as a cofactor and N^5-methyl-FH$_4$ as a substrate. This is the only mammalian reaction in which N^5-methyl-FH$_4$ can donate its carbon. Once methionine is generated, it is converted to SAM, which acts as a methyl donor for neurotransmitter synthesis, myelin synthesis, phospholipid synthesis, and DNA modifications. Inability to catalyze the methionine synthase reaction, owing to either B$_{12}$ or folate deficiency, would lead to a reduction of SAM levels and hypomethylation in the nervous system. The liver does not exhibit hypomethylation because of the betaine pathway, in which betaine can donate a methyl group to homocysteine to form methionine, also forming dimethylglycine once betaine loses a methyl group. Transcobalamin II carries B$_{12}$ in the circulation and does not interact with folate. Cystathionine β-synthase catalyzes the conversion of homocysteine and serine to cystathionine and requires vitamin B$_6$ but not B$_{12}$ or folate. N^5,N^{10}-Methylene-FH$_4$ reductase converts N^5,N^{10}-methylene-FH$_4$ to N^5-methyl-FH$_4$ and requires NADH but not vitamin B$_{12}$. DNA methyltransferases require SAM to methylate cytosine residues in DNA, but folic acid is not required as a cofactor for that reaction.

7. **The answer is A.** The patient is suffering from a vitamin B$_{12}$ deficiency. Vitamin B$_{12}$ can only be obtained from meat and dairy products in the diet, and although the body may have a 2- to 3-year store of the vitamin, given the patient's diet and lack of vitamins, B$_{12}$ has become deficient. The tiredness and lethargy is owing to the development of megaloblastic anemia, and the tingling is caused by nervous system dysfunction owing to hypomethylation and methylmalonic acid in the nervous system. In the absence of vitamin B$_{12}$, folate will be trapped

as N^5-methyl-FH$_4$, because the methionine synthase reaction will be unable to proceed. Once N^5-methyl-FH$_4$ is formed, it cannot be converted back into the other folate forms. Because this is the most stable folate form, the other variants of folate will slowly be converted to this form and be trapped.

8. **The answer is D.** The megaloblastic anemia can be caused by a deficiency of either vitamin B$_{12}$ or folic acid. A B$_{12}$ deficiency will block two reactions, homocysteine to methionine and methylmalonyl-CoA to succinyl-CoA. A B$_{12}$ deficiency, therefore, will lead to elevated methylmalonic acid because the methylmalonyl-CoA produced cannot be metabolized further to succinyl-CoA. The lack of B$_{12}$ also traps folate as the N^5-methyl-FH$_4$ form (because the methyl group cannot be transferred to homocysteine), leading to a functional folate deficiency. The folate deficiency interferes with purine and thymidine synthesis, leading to an overall cessation of DNA synthesis in rapidly growing cells, such as reticulocytes. This leads to megaloblast development and ineffective erythropoiesis. If the patient had a folate deficiency, FIGLU would accumulate in the urine (a degradation product of histidine). Accumulation of lactate, or pyruvate, does not occur with B$_{12}$ or folate deficiencies. Methionine might accumulate (because of high homocysteine levels), but it usually stays fairly level and would not be diagnostic for determining between a B$_{12}$ or a folate deficiency. Histidine also would not accumulate, as FIGLU accumulates in a folate deficiency, and this would be used to distinguish between B$_{12}$ and folate deficiencies.

9. **The answer is D.** Lacto–ovo vegetarians eat eggs and dairy products. Eggs are a dietary source of vitamin B$_{12}$. Stomach intrinsic factor binds released B$_{12}$, but stomach gastrin has no role in B$_{12}$ absorption. Vitamin B$_{12}$ bound to intrinsic factor is absorbed in the terminal ileum, not the duodenum. The ileum is involved in Crohn's disease, which then interferes with B$_{12}$ absorption. Biliary duct obstruction would block bile acid release from the gallbladder into the intestine, which would interfere with absorption of dietary fat but not absorption of B$_{12}$, which is a water-soluble vitamin.

10. **The answer is A.** Methotrexate inhibits DHFR, which blocks the conversion of FH$_2$ to FH$_4$. The reduction of cellular pools of FH$_4$ would then indirectly affect reactions that require FH$_4$. 5-FU directly inhibits the conversion of dUMP to dTMP. The conversion of homocysteine to methionine requires vitamin B$_{12}$ and N^5-methyl-FH$_4$. The N^5-methyl-FH$_4$ levels will be low owing to the folate being trapped as FH$_2$ because of the direct inhibition of DHFR by methotrexate.

39

Purine and Pyrimidine Metabolism

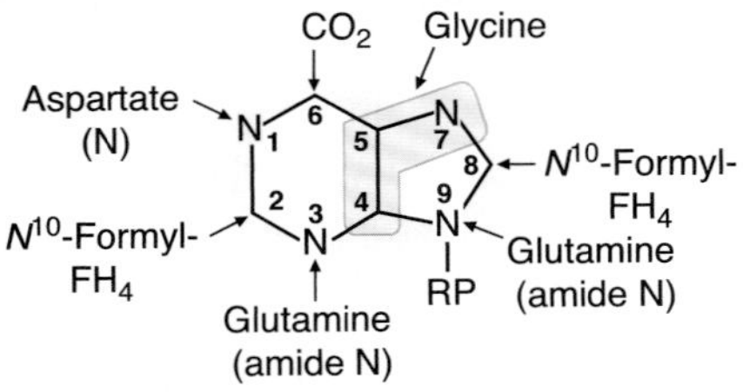

FIGURE 39.1 Origin of the atoms of the purine base. *FH₄*, tetrahydrofolate; *RP*, ribose 5'-phosphate.

Purines and pyrimidines are required for synthesizing **nucleotides** and **nucleic acids**. These molecules can be synthesized from scratch, **de novo**, or **salvaged** from existing bases. Dietary uptake of purine and pyrimidine bases is low because most of the ingested nucleic acids are metabolized by the intestinal epithelial cells.

The de novo pathway of purine synthesis is complex, consisting of 11 steps and requiring six molecules of adenosine triphosphate (ATP) for every purine synthesized. The precursors that donate components to produce purine nucleotides include **glycine, ribose 5-phosphate, glutamine, aspartate, carbon dioxide**, and N^{10}-**formyltetrahydrofolate** (Fig. 39.1). Purines are synthesized as **ribonucleotides**, with the initial purine synthesized being **inosine monophosphate** (**IMP**). Adenosine monophosphate (AMP) and guanosine monophosphate (GMP) are each derived from IMP in two-step reaction pathways.

The purine nucleotide salvage pathway allows free purine bases to be converted into nucleotides, nucleotides into nucleosides, and nucleosides into free bases. Enzymes included in this pathway are **AMP** and **adenosine deaminase** (**ADA**), **adenosine kinase, purine nucleoside phosphorylase, adenine phosphoribosyltransferase** (**APRT**), and **hypoxanthine–guanine phosphoribosyltransferase** (**HGPRT**). Mutations in several of these enzymes lead to serious diseases. Deficiencies in purine nucleoside phosphorylase and ADA lead to **immunodeficiency disorders**. A deficiency in HGPRT leads to **Lesch-Nyhan syndrome**. The **purine nucleotide cycle**, in which aspartate carbons are converted to fumarate to replenish tricarboxylic acid (TCA) cycle intermediates in working muscle, and the aspartate nitrogen is released as ammonia, uses components of the purine nucleotide salvage pathway.

Pyrimidine bases are first synthesized as the free base and then converted to a nucleotide. **Aspartate** and **carbamoyl phosphate** form all components of the pyrimidine ring. Ribose 5-phosphate, which is converted to **5'-phosphoribosyl 1'-pyrophosphate** (**PRPP**), is required to donate the sugar phosphate to form a nucleotide. The first pyrimidine nucleotide produced is **orotate monophosphate** (**OMP**). The OMP is converted to **uridine monophosphate** (**UMP**), which becomes the precursor for both **cytidine triphosphate** (**CTP**) and **deoxythymidine monophosphate** (**dTMP**) production.

The formation of deoxyribonucleotides requires **ribonucleotide reductase** activity, which catalyzes the reduction of ribose on nucleotide diphosphate substrates to 2'-deoxyribose. Substrates for the enzyme include adenosine diphosphate (ADP), guanosine diphosphate (GDP), cytidine diphosphate (CDP), and uridine diphosphate (UDP). Regulation of the enzyme is complex. There are two major allosteric sites. One controls the overall activity of the enzyme, whereas the other determines the substrate specificity of the enzyme. All deoxyribonucleotides are synthesized using this one enzyme.

The **regulation** of de novo purine nucleotide biosynthesis occurs at four points in the pathway. The enzymes **PRPP synthetase, amidophosphoribosyltransferase, IMP dehydrogenase**, and **adenylosuccinate synthetase** are regulated by allosteric modifiers because they occur at key branch points through the pathway. Pyrimidine synthesis is regulated at the first committed step, which is the synthesis of cytoplasmic carbamoyl phosphate, by the enzyme **carbamoyl phosphate synthetase II** (**CPSII**).

Purines, when degraded, cannot generate energy, nor can the purine ring be substantially modified. The end-product of purine ring degradation is **uric acid**, which is excreted in the urine. Uric acid has limited solubility, and if it were to accumulate, uric acid crystals would precipitate in tissues of the body that have a reduced temperature (such as the big toe). This condition of acute painful inflammation of specific soft tissues and joints is called **gout**. Pyrimidines, when degraded, however, give rise to water-soluble compounds such as urea, carbon dioxide, and water and do not lead to a disease state if pyrimidine catabolism is increased.

THE WAITING ROOM

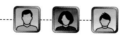

The initial acute inflammatory process that caused **Lotta T.** to experience a painful attack of gouty arthritis responded quickly to colchicine therapy (see Chapter 10). Several weeks after the inflammatory signs and symptoms in her right great toe subsided, Lotta was placed on allopurinol (while continuing colchicine), a drug that reduces uric acid synthesis. Her serum uric acid level gradually fell from a pretreatment level of 9.2 mg/dL into the normal range (2.5 to 8.0 mg/dL). She remained free of gouty symptoms when she returned to her physician for a follow-up office visit.

I. Purines and Pyrimidines

As has been seen in previous chapters, nucleotides serve numerous functions in different reaction pathways. For example, nucleotides are the activated precursors of DNA and RNA. Nucleotides form the structural moieties of many coenzymes (examples include nicotinamide adenine dinucleotide [NAD$^+$], flavin adenine dinucleotide [FAD], and coenzyme A). Nucleotides are critical elements in energy metabolism (ATP, guanosine triphosphate [GTP]). Nucleotide derivatives are frequently activated intermediates in many biosynthetic pathways. For example, UDP-glucose and CDP-diacylglycerol are precursors of glycogen and phosphoglycerides, respectively. *S*-Adenosylmethionine carries an activated methyl group. In addition, nucleotides act as second messengers in intracellular signaling (e.g., cyclic adenosine monophosphate [cAMP], cyclic guanosine monophosphate [cGMP]). Finally, nucleotides and nucleosides act as metabolic allosteric regulators. Think about all of the enzymes that have been studied that are regulated by levels of ATP, ADP, and AMP.

Dietary uptake of purine and pyrimidine bases is minimal. The diet contains nucleic acids, and the exocrine pancreas secretes deoxyribonuclease and ribonuclease, along with the proteolytic and lipolytic enzymes. This enables digested nucleic acids to be converted to nucleotides. The intestinal epithelial cells contain alkaline phosphatase activity, which converts nucleotides to nucleosides. Other enzymes within the epithelial cells tend to metabolize the nucleosides to uric acid (which is released into the circulation) or to salvage them for their own needs. Approximately 5% of ingested nucleotides make it into the circulation, either as the free base or as a nucleoside. Because of the minimal dietary uptake of these important molecules, de novo synthesis of purines and pyrimidines is required.

II. Purine Biosynthesis

The purine bases are produced de novo by pathways that use amino acids as precursors and produce nucleotides. Most de novo synthesis occurs in the liver (Fig. 39.2), and the nitrogenous bases and nucleosides are then transported to other tissues by red blood cells. The brain also synthesizes significant amounts of nucleotides. Because the de novo pathway requires at least six high-energy bonds per purine produced, a salvage pathway, which is used by many cell types, can convert free bases and nucleosides to nucleotides.

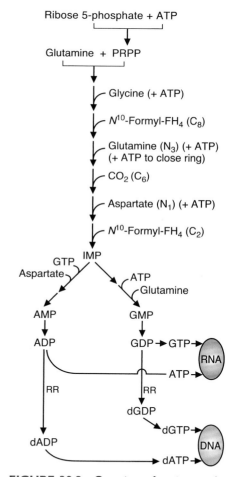

FIGURE 39.2 Overview of purine production, starting with glutamine, ribose 5-phosphate, and adenosine triphosphate (ATP). The steps that require ATP are also indicated in this figure. *ADP*, adenosine diphosphate; *AMP*, adenosine monophosphate; *dADP*, deoxyadenosine diphosphate; *dATP*, deoxyadenosine triphosphate; *dGDP*, deoxyguanosine diphosphate; *dGTP*, deoxyguanosine triphosphate; *FH$_4$*, tetrahydrofolate; *GMP*, guanosine monophosphate; *GTP*, guanosine triphosphate; *IMP*, inosine monophosphate; *PRPP*, 5-phosphoribosyl 1-pyrophosphate; *RR*, ribonucleotide reductase.

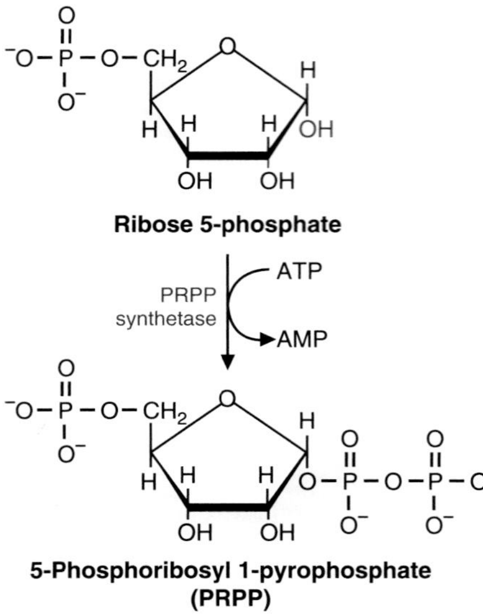

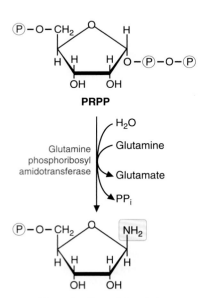

Ribose 5-phosphate

PRPP
synthetase

ATP

AMP

**5-Phosphoribosyl 1-pyrophosphate
(PRPP)**

FIGURE 39.3 Synthesis of 5-phosphoribosyl 1-pyrophosphate (PRPP). Ribose 5-phosphate is produced from glucose by the pentose phosphate pathway. *AMP*, adenosine monophosphate; *ATP*, adenosine triphosphate.

A. De Novo Synthesis of the Purine Nucleotides

1. Synthesis of Inosine Monophosphate

Because purines are built on a ribose base (see Fig. 39.2), an activated form of ribose is used to initiate the purine biosynthetic pathway. 5-Phosphoribosyl 1-pyrophosphate (PRPP) is the activated source of the ribose moiety. It is synthesized from ATP and ribose 5-phosphate (Fig. 39.3), which is produced from glucose through the pentose phosphate pathway (see Chapter 27). The enzyme that catalyzes this reaction, PRPP synthetase, is a regulated enzyme (see Section II.A.5); however, this step is not the committed step of purine biosynthesis. PRPP has many other uses, which are described as the chapter progresses.

In the first committed step of the purine biosynthetic pathway, PRPP reacts with glutamine to form 5′-phosphoribosyl 1′-amine (Fig. 39.4). This reaction, which produces nitrogen 9 of the purine ring, is catalyzed by glutamine phosphoribosylamidotransferase, a highly regulated enzyme.

In the next step of the pathway, the entire glycine molecule is added to the growing precursor. Glycine provides carbons 4 and 5 and nitrogen 7 of the purine ring (Fig. 39.5). This step requires energy in the form of ATP.

Subsequently, carbon 8 is provided by N^{10}-formyltetrahydrofolate (N^{10}-formyl-FH$_4$), nitrogen 3 by glutamine, carbon 6 by CO_2, nitrogen 1 by aspartate, and carbon 2 by N^{10}-formyl-FH$_4$ (see Fig. 39.1). Note that six high-energy bonds of ATP are required (starting with ribose 5-phosphate) to synthesize the first purine nucleotide, IMP. This nucleotide contains the base hypoxanthine joined by an N-glycosidic bond from nitrogen 9 of the purine ring to carbon 1 of the ribose (Fig. 39.6). Hypoxanthine is not found in DNA, but it is the precursor for the other purine bases. However, hypoxanthine is found in the anticodon of transfer RNA molecules (see Chapter 15) and is a critical component for allowing wobble base pairs to form.

2. Synthesis of Adenosine Monophosphate

IMP serves as the branch point from which both adenine and guanine nucleotides can be produced (see Fig. 39.2). AMP is derived from IMP in two steps (Fig. 39.7). In the first step, aspartate is added to IMP to form adenylosuccinate, a reaction similar to the one catalyzed by argininosuccinate synthetase in the urea cycle. Note that this reaction requires a high-energy bond, donated by GTP. Fumarate is then

PRPP

Glutamine
phosphoribosyl
amidotransferase

H$_2$O

Glutamine

Glutamate

PP$_i$

NH$_2$

5-Phosphoribosyl 1-amine

FIGURE 39.4 The first step in purine biosynthesis. The purine base is built on the ribose moiety. The availability of the substrate 5-phosphoribosyl 1-pyrophosphate (PRPP) is a major determinant of the rate of this reaction. *PP$_i$*, pyrophosphate.

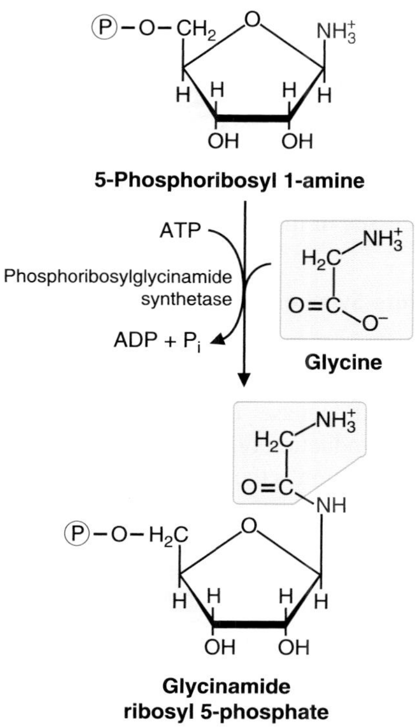

5-Phosphoribosyl 1-amine

FIGURE 39.5 Incorporation of glycine into the purine precursor. The adenosine triphosphate (ATP) is required for the condensation of the glycine carboxylic acid group with the 1′-amino group of phosphoribosyl 1-amine. *ADP*, adenosine diphosphate; *P*ᵢ, inorganic phosphate.

released from the adenylosuccinate by the enzyme adenylosuccinate lyase to form AMP. This is similar to the aspartate-to-fumarate conversion seen in the urea cycle (see Chapter 38). In both cases, aspartate donates a nitrogen to the product, whereas the carbons of aspartate are released as fumarate.

3. Synthesis of Guanosine Monophosphate

GMP is also synthesized from IMP in two steps (Fig. 39.8). In the first step, the hypoxanthine base is oxidized by IMP dehydrogenase to produce the base xanthine and the nucleotide xanthosine monophosphate (XMP). Glutamine then donates the amide nitrogen to XMP to form GMP in a reaction that is catalyzed by GMP synthetase. This second reaction requires energy, in the form of ATP.

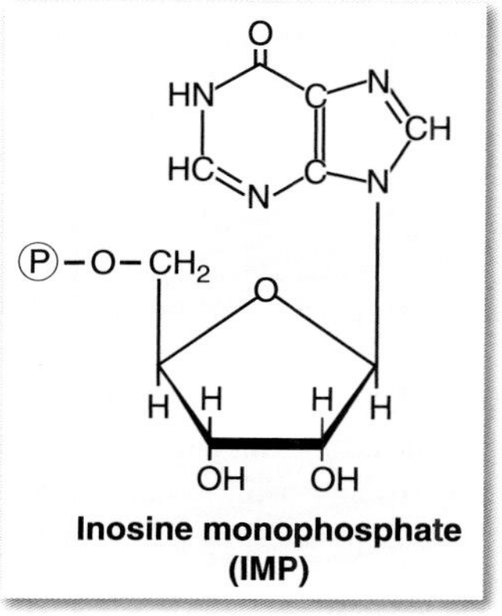

Inosine monophosphate (IMP)

FIGURE 39.6 Structure of inosine monophosphate (IMP). The base is hypoxanthine.

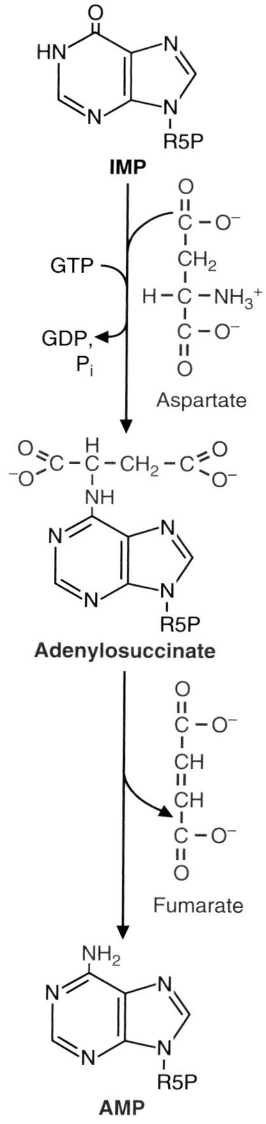

FIGURE 39.7 The conversion of inosine monophosphate (IMP) to adenosine monophosphate (AMP). Note that guanosine triphosphate (GTP) is required for the synthesis of AMP. The first enzyme is adenylosuccinate synthetase; the second enzyme is adenylosuccinate lyase. *GDP*, guanosine diphosphate; *P*ᵢ, inorganic phosphate; *R5P*, ribose 5-phosphate.

4. Phosphorylation of AMP and GMP

AMP and GMP can be phosphorylated to the diphosphate and triphosphate levels. The production of nucleoside diphosphates requires specific nucleoside monophosphate kinases, whereas the production of nucleoside triphosphates requires nucleoside diphosphate kinases, which are active with a wide range of nucleoside diphosphates. The purine nucleoside triphosphates are also used for energy-requiring processes in the cell and also as precursors for RNA synthesis (see Fig. 39.2).

5. Regulation of Purine Synthesis

Regulation of purine synthesis occurs at several sites (Fig. 39.9). Four key enzymes are regulated: PRPP synthetase, amidophosphoribosyltransferase, adenylosuccinate synthetase, and IMP dehydrogenase. The first two enzymes regulate IMP synthesis; the last two regulate the production of AMP and GMP, respectively.

A primary site of regulation is the synthesis of PRPP. PRPP synthetase is negatively affected by GDP and, at a distinct allosteric site, by ADP. Thus, the simultaneous binding of an oxypurine (e.g., GDP) and an aminopurine (e.g., ADP) can occur, with the result being a synergistic inhibition of the enzyme. This enzyme is not the committed step of purine biosynthesis; PRPP is also used in pyrimidine synthesis and both the purine and pyrimidine salvage pathways.

The committed step of purine synthesis is the formation of 5′-phosphoribosyl 1′-amine by glutamine phosphoribosylamidotransferase. This enzyme is strongly

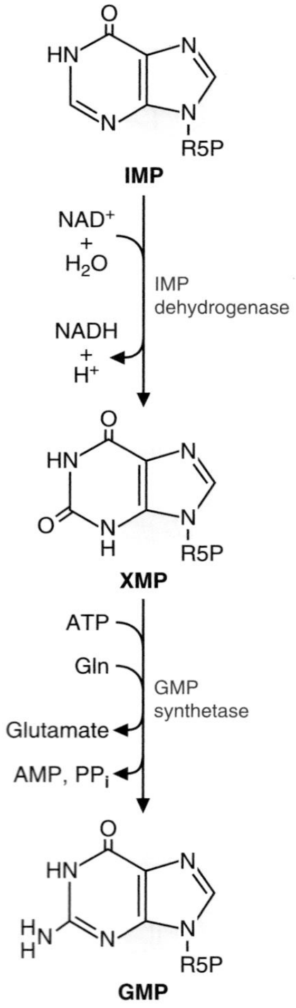

FIGURE 39.8 The conversion of inosine monophosphate (IMP) to guanosine monophosphate (GMP). Note that adenosine triphosphate (ATP) is required for the synthesis of GMP. *NAD*, nicotinamide adenine dinucleotide; *XMP*, xanthosine monophosphate; *AMP*, adenosine monophosphate; *PP$_i$*, pyrophosphate; *R5P*, ribose 5-phosphate.

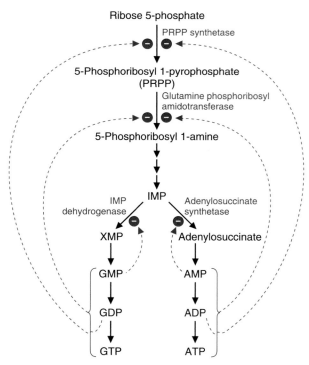

FIGURE 39.9 The regulation of purine synthesis. 5-phosphoribosyl 1-pyrophosphate (PRPP) synthetase has two distinct allosteric sites: one for adenosine diphosphate (ADP), the other for guanosine diphosphate (GDP). Glutamine phosphoribosylamidotransferase contains adenine nucleotide– and guanine nucleotide–binding sites; the monophosphates are the most important, although the diphosphates and triphosphates will also bind to and inhibit the enzyme. Adenylosuccinate synthetase is inhibited by adenosine monophosphate (AMP); inosine monophosphate (IMP) dehydrogenase is inhibited by guanosine monophosphate (GMP). *ATP*, adenosine triphosphate; *GTP*, guanosine triphosphate; *XMP*, xanthosine monophosphate.

inhibited by GMP and AMP (the end-products of the purine biosynthetic pathway). The enzyme is also inhibited by the corresponding nucleoside diphosphates and triphosphates, but under cellular conditions, these compounds probably do not play a central role in regulation. The active enzyme is a monomer of 133,000 Da but is converted to an inactive dimer (270,000 Da) by binding of the end-products. Cellular concentrations of PRPP and glutamine are usually below their K_m for glutamine phosphoribosylamidotransferase. Thus, any situation that leads to an increase in their concentration can lead to an increase in de novo purine biosynthesis.

The enzymes that convert IMP to XMP and adenylosuccinate are both regulated. GMP inhibits the activity of IMP dehydrogenase, and AMP inhibits adenylosuccinate synthetase. Note that the synthesis of AMP is dependent on GTP (of which GMP is a precursor), whereas the synthesis of GMP is dependent on ATP (which is made from AMP). This serves as a type of positive regulatory mechanism to balance the pools of these precursors. When the levels of ATP are high, GMP will be made; when the levels of GTP are high, AMP synthesis will take place. GMP and AMP act as negative effectors at these branch points, a classic example of feedback inhibition.

B. Purine Salvage Pathways

Most of the de novo synthesis of the bases of nucleotides occurs in the liver, and to some extent in the brain, neutrophils, and other cells of the immune system. Within the liver, nucleotides can be converted to nucleosides or free bases, which can be transported to other tissues via the red blood cells in the circulation. In addition, the small amounts of dietary bases or nucleosides that are absorbed also enter cells in this form. Thus, most cells can salvage these bases to generate nucleotides for RNA and DNA synthesis. For certain cell types, such as lymphocytes, the salvage of bases is the major form of nucleotide generation.

The overall picture of salvage is shown in Figure 39.10. The pathways allow free bases, nucleosides, and nucleotides to be easily interconverted. The major enzymes required are purine nucleoside phosphorylase, phosphoribosyltransferases, and deaminases.

Purine nucleoside phosphorylase catalyzes a phosphorolysis reaction of the N-glycosidic bond that attaches the base to the sugar moiety in the nucleosides guanosine and inosine (Fig. 39.11A). Thus, guanosine and inosine are converted to guanine and hypoxanthine, respectively, along with ribose 1-phosphate. The ribose 1-phosphate can be isomerized to ribose 5-phosphate, and the free bases then salvaged or degraded, depending on cellular needs.

The phosphoribosyltransferase enzymes catalyze the addition of a ribose 5-phosphate group from PRPP to a free base, generating a nucleotide and pyrophosphate (see Fig. 39.11B). Two enzymes do this for purine metabolism: APRT and HGPRT. The reactions they catalyze are the same, differing only in their substrate specificity.

Adenosine and AMP can be deaminated by ADA and AMP deaminase, respectively, to form inosine and IMP (see Fig. 39.10). Adenosine is also the only nucleoside to be directly phosphorylated to a nucleotide by adenosine kinase. Guanosine and inosine must be converted to free bases by purine nucleoside phosphorylase before they can be converted to nucleotides by HGPRT.

A portion of the salvage pathway that is important in muscle is the purine nucleotide cycle (Fig. 39.12). The net effect of these reactions is the deamination of aspartate to fumarate (as AMP is synthesized from IMP and then deaminated back to IMP by AMP deaminase). Under conditions in which the muscle must generate energy, the fumarate derived from the purine nucleotide cycle is used anaplerotically to replenish TCA-cycle intermediates and to allow the cycle to operate at high speed. Deficiencies in enzymes of this cycle lead to muscle fatigue during exercise.

A deficiency in purine nucleoside phosphorylase activity leads to an immune disorder in which T-cell immunity is compromised. B-Cell immunity, conversely, may be only slightly compromised or even normal. Children who lack this activity have recurrent infections, and more than half display neurologic complications. Symptoms of the disorder first appear at between 6 months and 4 years of age. It is an extremely rare autosomal-recessive disorder.

ADA activity is measured by coupling the deamination of adenosine (to inosine) with purine nucleoside phosphorylase, which will generate hypoxanthine and ribose 1-phosphate from inosine. The hypoxanthine generated then reacts with xanthine oxidase, generating uric acid and hydrogen peroxide. The hydrogen peroxide produced is then measured in the presence of peroxidase and a colorless dye. The oxidation of the colorless dye creates a colored dye, and the intensity of the color (which is directly proportional to the amount of inosine produced) can be determined spectrophotometrically.

Lesch-Nyhan syndrome is caused by a defective HGPRT (see Fig. 39.11B). In this condition, purine bases cannot be salvaged. Instead, they are degraded, forming excessive amounts of uric acid, leading to gout. Individuals with the severe form of this syndrome suffer from developmental delays and intellectual disabilities. They are also prone to self-injury, including biting and head banging.

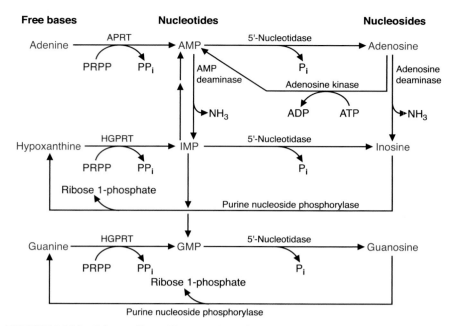

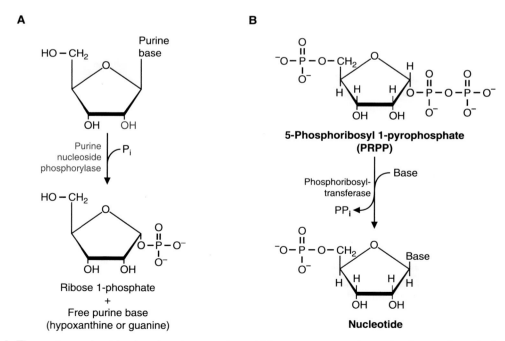

FIGURE 39.10 Salvage of bases. The purine bases hypoxanthine and guanine react with 5-phosphoribosyl 1-pyrophosphate (PRPP) to form the nucleotides inosine monophosphate (IMP) and guanosine monophosphate (GMP), respectively. The enzyme that catalyzes the reaction is hypoxanthine–guanine phosphoribosyltransferase (HGPRT). Adenine forms adenosine monophosphate (AMP) in a reaction that is catalyzed by adenine phosphoribosyltransferase (APRT). Nucleotides are converted to nucleosides by 5′-nucleotidase. Free bases are generated from nucleosides by purine nucleoside phosphorylase (although adenosine is not a substrate of this enzyme). Deamination of the base adenine occurs with AMP and adenosine deaminase. Of the purines, only adenosine can be phosphorylated directly back to a nucleotide, by adenosine kinase. *ADP*, adenosine diphosphate; *ATP*, adenosine triphosphate; *P$_i$*, inorganic phosphate; *PP$_i$*, pyrophosphate.

FIGURE 39.11 **A.** The purine nucleoside phosphorylase reaction, which converts guanosine or inosine to ribose 1-phosphate plus the free base guanine or hypoxanthine. **B.** The phosphoribosyltransferase reaction. Adenine phosphoribosyltransferase (APRT) uses the free base adenine; hypoxanthine–guanine phosphoribosyltransferase (HGPRT) can use either hypoxanthine or guanine as a substrate. *P$_i$*, inorganic phosphate; *PP$_i$*, pyrophosphate.

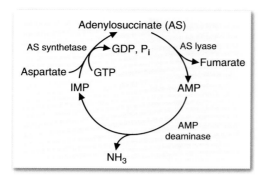

FIGURE 39.12 The purine nucleotide cycle. Using a combination of biosynthetic and salvage enzymes, the net effect is the conversion of aspartate to fumarate plus ammonia, with the fumarate playing an anaplerotic role in the muscle. *AMP*, adenosine monophosphate; *GDP*, guanosine diphosphate; *GTP*, guanosine triphosphate; *IMP*, inosine monophosphate; *P$_i$*, inorganic phosphate.

III. Synthesis of the Pyrimidine Nucleotides

A. De Novo Pathways

In the synthesis of the pyrimidine nucleotides, the base is synthesized first, and then it is attached to the ribose 5′-phosphate moiety (Fig. 39.13). The origin of the atoms of the ring (aspartate and carbamoyl phosphate, which is derived from carbon dioxide and glutamine) is shown in Figure 39.14. In the initial reaction of the pathway, glutamine combines with bicarbonate and ATP to form carbamoyl phosphate. This reaction is analogous to the first reaction of the urea cycle, except that it uses glutamine as the source of the nitrogen (rather than ammonia) and it occurs in the cytosol (rather than in mitochondria). The reaction is catalyzed by CPSII, which is the regulated step of the pathway. The analogous reaction in urea synthesis is catalyzed by carbamoyl phosphate synthetase I (CPSI), which is activated by *N*-acetylglutamate. The similarities and differences between these two carbamoyl phosphate synthetase enzymes are described in Table 39.1.

In the next step of pyrimidine biosynthesis, the entire aspartate molecule adds to carbamoyl phosphate in a reaction that is catalyzed by aspartate transcarbamoylase (Fig. 39.15). The molecule subsequently closes to produce a ring (catalyzed by dihydroorotase), which is oxidized to form orotic acid (or its anion, orotate) through the actions of dihydroorotate dehydrogenase. The enzyme orotate phosphoribosyltransferase catalyzes the transfer of ribose 5-phosphate from PRPP to orotate, producing orotidine 5′-phosphate, which is decarboxylated by orotidylic acid decarboxylase to form UMP (see Fig. 39.15). In mammals, the first three enzymes of the pathway (CPSII, aspartate transcarbamoylase, and dihydroorotase) are located on the same polypeptide, designated as *CAD*. The last two enzymes of the pathway are similarly located on a polypeptide known as *UMP synthase* (the orotate phosphoribosyltransferase and orotidylic acid decarboxylase activities).

UMP is phosphorylated to uridine triphosphate (UTP). An amino group, derived from the amide of glutamine, is added to carbon 4 to produce CTP by the enzyme CTP synthetase (this reaction cannot occur at the nucleotide monophosphate level). UTP and CTP are precursors for the synthesis of RNA (see Fig. 39.13). The synthesis of deoxythymidine triphosphate (dTTP) is described in Section IV.

B. Salvage of Pyrimidine Bases

Pyrimidine bases are normally salvaged by a two-step route. First, a relatively nonspecific pyrimidine nucleoside phosphorylase converts the pyrimidine bases to

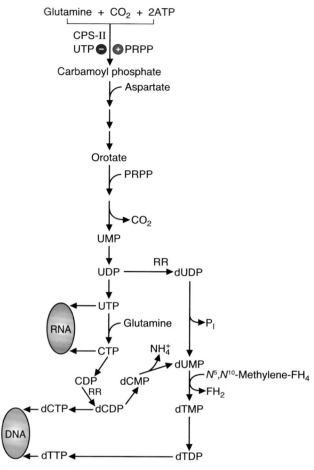

FIGURE 39.13 Synthesis of the pyrimidine bases. *ATP*, adenosine triphosphate; *CDP*, cytidine diphosphate; *CPS-II*, carbamoyl phosphate synthetase II; *CTP*, cytidine triphosphate; *dCDP*, deoxycytidine diphosphate; *dCMP*, deoxycytidine monophosphate; *dCTP*, deoxycytidine triphosphate; *dTDP*, deoxythymidine diphosphate; *dTMP*, deoxythymidine monophosphate; *dTTP*, deoxythymidine triphosphate; *dUDP*, deoxyuridine diphosphate; *dUMP*, deoxyuridine monophosphate; *FH₂*, dihydrofolate; *FH₄*, tetrahydrofolate; *Pᵢ*, inorganic phosphate; *PRPP*, 5-phosphoribosyl 1-pyrophosphate; *RR*, ribonucleotide reductase; *UDP*, uridine diphosphate; *UMP*, uridine monophosphate; *UTP*, uridine triphosphate; ⊕, stimulated by; ⊖, inhibited by.

their respective nucleosides (Fig. 39.16). Notice that the preferred direction for this reaction is the reverse phosphorylase reaction, in which phosphate is released and is not being used as a nucleophile to release the pyrimidine base from the nucleoside. The more specific nucleoside kinases then react with the nucleosides, forming nucleotides (Table 39.2). As with purines, further phosphorylation is carried out by increasingly more specific kinases. The nucleoside phosphorylase–nucleoside

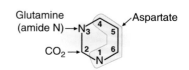

FIGURE 39.14 The origin of the atoms in the pyrimidine ring.

TABLE 39.1	Comparison of Carbamoyl Phosphate Synthetases (CPSI and CPSII)	
	CPSI	**CPSII**
Pathway	Urea cycle	Pyrimidine biosynthesis
Source of nitrogen	NH_4^+	Glutamine
Location	Mitochondria	Cytosol
Activator	*N*-Acetylglutamate	PRPP
Inhibitor	—	UTP

PRPP, 5-phosphoribosyl 1-pyrophosphate; UTP, uridine triphosphate.

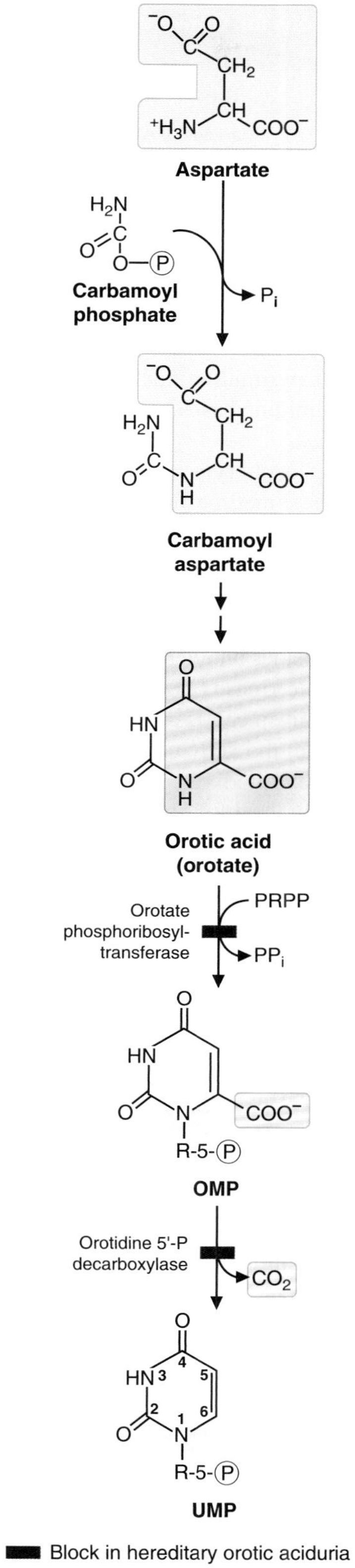

Aspartate

Carbamoyl phosphate

P_i

Carbamoyl aspartate

Orotic acid (orotate)

Orotate phosphoribosyltransferase

PRPP

PP_i

OMP

Orotidine 5'-P decarboxylase

CO_2

UMP

■ Block in hereditary orotic aciduria

FIGURE 39.15 Conversion of carbamoyl phosphate and aspartate to uridine monophosphate (UMP). The defective enzymes in hereditary orotic aciduria are indicated by the *dark bar*. OMP, orotate monophosphate; *Orotidine 5'-P*, orotidine 5'-phosphate; *P_i*, inorganic phosphate; *PP_i*, pyrophosphate; *PRPP*, 5-phosphoribosyl 1-pyrophosphate.

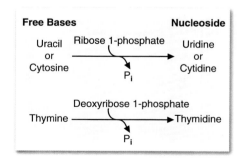

Free Bases   **Nucleoside**

Uracil or Cytosine — Ribose 1-phosphate / P_i → Uridine or Cytidine

Thymine — Deoxyribose 1-phosphate / P_i → Thymidine

FIGURE 39.16 Salvage reactions for pyrimidine nucleoside production. Thymine phosphorylase uses deoxyribose 1-phosphate as a substrate, so ribothymidine is rarely formed. *P_i*, inorganic phosphate.

TABLE 39.2 Salvage Reactions for Conversion of Pyrimidine Nucleosides to Nucleotides

ENZYME	REACTION
Uridine-cytidine kinase	Uridine + ATP → UMP + ADP
	Cytidine + ATP → CMP + ADP
Deoxythymidine kinase	Deoxythymidine + ATP → dTMP + ADP
Deoxycytidine kinase	Deoxycytidine + ATP → dCMP + ADP

ADP, adenosine diphosphate; ATP, adenosine triphosphate; CMP, cytidine monophosphate; dCMP, deoxycytidine monophosphate; dTMP, deoxythymidine monophosphate; UMP, uridine monophosphate.

In hereditary orotic aciduria, an extremely rare disorder, orotic acid is excreted in the urine because the enzymes that convert it to UMP, orotate phosphoribosyltransferase and orotidine 5′-phosphate decarboxylase, are defective (see Fig. 39.16). Pyrimidines cannot be synthesized and, therefore, normal growth does not occur. Oral administration of uridine is used to treat this condition. Uridine, which is converted to UMP, bypasses the metabolic block and provides the body with a source of pyrimidines because both CTP and dTMP can be produced from UMP.

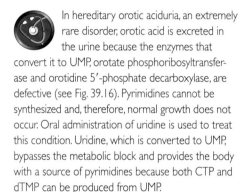

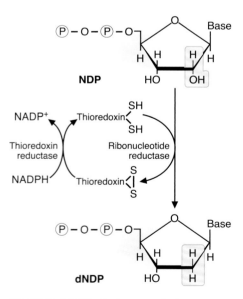

FIGURE 39.17 Reduction of ribose to deoxyribose. Reduction occurs at the nucleoside diphosphate level. A ribonucleoside diphosphate (NDP) is converted to a deoxyribonucleoside diphosphate (dNDP). Thioredoxin is oxidized to a disulfide, which must be reduced for the reaction to continue producing dNDP. *NADP*, nicotinamide adenine dinucleotide phosphate.

kinase route for synthesis of pyrimidine nucleoside monophosphates is relatively inefficient for salvage of pyrimidine bases because of the very low concentration of the bases in plasma and tissues.

Pyrimidine nucleoside phosphorylase can use all of the pyrimidines but has a preference for uracil and is sometimes called *uridine phosphorylase*. The phosphorylase uses cytosine fairly well but has an extremely low affinity for thymine; therefore, a ribonucleoside containing thymine is almost never made in vivo. A second phosphorylase, *thymine phosphorylase*, has a much higher affinity for thymine and adds a deoxyribose residue (see Fig. 39.16).

Of the various ribonucleosides and deoxyribonucleoside kinases, one that merits special mention is thymidine kinase (TK). This enzyme is allosterically inhibited by dTTP. Activity of TK in a given cell is closely related to the proliferative state of that cell. During the cell cycle, the activity of TK rises dramatically as cells enter S-phase, and in general, rapidly dividing cells have high levels of this enzyme. Radiolabeled thymidine is widely used for isotopic labeling of DNA; for example, in radioautographic investigations or to estimate rates of intracellular DNA synthesis.

C. Regulation of De Novo Pyrimidine Synthesis

The regulated step of pyrimidine synthesis in humans is CPSII. The enzyme is inhibited by UTP and activated by PRPP (see Fig. 39.13). Thus, as pyrimidines decrease in concentration (as indicated by UTP levels), CPSII is activated and pyrimidines are synthesized. The activity is also regulated by the cell cycle. As cells approach S-phase, CPSII becomes more sensitive to PRPP activation and less sensitive to UTP inhibition. At the end of S-phase, the inhibition by UTP is more pronounced and the activation by PRPP is reduced. These changes in the allosteric properties of CPSII are related to its phosphorylation state. Phosphorylation of the enzyme at a specific site by a mitogen-activated protein (MAP) kinase leads to a more easily activated enzyme. Phosphorylation at a second site by the cAMP-dependent protein kinase leads to a more easily inhibited enzyme.

IV. The Production of Deoxyribonucleotides

For DNA synthesis to occur, the ribose moiety must be reduced to deoxyribose (Fig. 39.17). This reduction occurs at the diphosphate level and is catalyzed by ribonucleotide reductase, which requires the protein thioredoxin. The deoxyribonucleoside diphosphates can be phosphorylated to the triphosphate level and used as precursors for DNA synthesis (see Figs. 39.2 and 39.13).

The regulation of ribonucleotide reductase is quite complex. The enzyme contains two allosteric sites, one controlling the activity of the enzyme and the other controlling the substrate specificity of the enzyme. ATP bound to the activity site activates the enzyme; deoxyadenosine triphosphate (dATP) bound to this site inhibits the enzyme. Substrate specificity is more complex. ATP bound to the substrate specificity site activates the reduction of pyrimidines (CDP and UDP), to form deoxycytidine diphosphate (dCDP) and deoxyuridine diphosphate (dUDP). The dUDP is

TABLE 39.3	**Effectors of Ribonucleotide Reductase Activity**	
PREFERRED SUBSTRATE	**EFFECTOR BOUND TO OVERALL ACTIVITY SITE**	**EFFECTOR BOUND TO SUBSTRATE SPECIFICITY SITE**
None	dATP	Any nucleotide
CDP	ATP	ATP or dATP
UDP	ATP	ATP or dATP
GDP	ATP	dTTP
ADP	ATP	dGTP

dATP, deoxyadenosine triphosphate; CDP, cytidine diphosphate; ATP, adenosine triphosphate; UDP, uridine diphosphate; GDP, guanosine diphosphate; dTTP, deoxythymidine triphosphate; ADP, adenosine diphosphate; dGTP, deoxyguanosine triphosphate.

not used for DNA synthesis; rather, it is used to produce dTMP (see the following text). Once dTMP is produced, it is phosphorylated to dTTP, which then binds to the substrate specificity site and induces the reduction of GDP. As deoxyguanosine triphosphate (dGTP) accumulates, it replaces dTTP in the substrate specificity site and allows ADP to be reduced to deoxyadenosine diphosphate (dADP). This leads to the accumulation of dATP, which inhibits the overall activity of the enzyme. These allosteric changes are summarized in Table 39.3.

dUDP can be dephosphorylated to form deoxyuridine monophosphate (dUMP), or, alternatively, deoxycytidine monophosphate (dCMP) can be deaminated to form dUMP. Methylene-FH$_4$ transfers a methyl group to dUMP to form dTMP (see Fig. 38.5). Phosphorylation reactions produce dTTP, a precursor for DNA synthesis and a regulator of ribonucleotide reductase.

V. Degradation of Purine and Pyrimidine Bases

A. Purine Bases

The degradation of the purine nucleotides (AMP and GMP) occurs mainly in the liver (Fig. 39.18). Salvage enzymes are used for most of these reactions. AMP is first deaminated to produce IMP (AMP deaminase). Then IMP and GMP are dephosphorylated (5′-nucleotidase), and the ribose is cleaved from the base by purine nucleoside phosphorylase. Hypoxanthine, the base produced by cleavage of IMP, is converted by xanthine oxidase to xanthine, and guanine is deaminated by the enzyme guanase to produce xanthine. The pathways for the degradation of adenine and guanine merge at this point. Xanthine is converted by xanthine oxidase to uric acid, which is excreted in the urine. Xanthine oxidase is a molybdenum-requiring enzyme that uses molecular oxygen and produces hydrogen peroxide (H$_2$O$_2$). Another form of xanthine oxidase uses nicotinamide adenine dinucleotide (NAD$^+$) as the electron acceptor (see Chapter 25).

Note how little energy is derived from the degradation of the purine ring. Thus, it is to the cell's advantage to recycle and salvage the ring, because it costs energy to produce and not much is obtained in return.

B. Pyrimidine Bases

The pyrimidine nucleotides are dephosphorylated, and the nucleosides are cleaved to produce ribose 1-phosphate and the free pyrimidine bases cytosine, uracil, and thymine. Cytosine is deaminated, forming uracil, which is converted to CO$_2$, NH$_4^+$, and β-alanine. Thymine is converted to CO$_2$, NH$_4^+$, and β-aminoisobutyrate. These products of pyrimidine degradation are excreted in the urine or converted to CO$_2$, H$_2$O, and NH$_4^+$ (which forms urea). They do not cause any problems for the body, in contrast to urate, which is produced from the purines and can precipitate, causing gout. As with the purine degradation pathway, little energy can be generated by pyrimidine degradation.

When ornithine transcarbamoylase is deficient (urea-cycle disorder), excess carbamoyl phosphate from the mitochondria leaks into the cytoplasm. The elevated levels of cytoplasmic carbamoyl phosphate lead to pyrimidine production, as the regulated step of the pathway, the reaction catalyzed by carbamoyl synthetase II, is being bypassed. Thus, orotic aciduria results.

Gout is caused by excessive uric acid levels in the blood and tissues. In studies to determine whether a person with gout has developed this problem because of overproduction of purine nucleotides or because of a decreased ability to excrete uric acid, an oral dose of a ^{15}N-labeled amino acid is sometimes used. Which amino acid would be most appropriate to use for this purpose?

Uric acid has a pK of 5.4. It is ionized in the body to form urate. Urate is not very soluble in an aqueous environment. The concentration of urate in normal human blood is very close to the solubility constant.

A The entire glycine molecule is incorporated into the precursor of the purine nucleotides. The nitrogen of this glycine also appears in uric acid, the product of purine degradation. ^{15}N-labeled glycine could be used, therefore, to determine whether purines are being overproduced.

Normally, as cells die, their purine nucleotides are degraded to hypoxanthine and xanthine, which are converted to uric acid by xanthine oxidase (see Fig. 39.18). Allopurinol (a structural analog of hypoxanthine) is a substrate for xanthine oxidase. It is converted to oxypurinol (also called *alloxanthine*), which remains tightly bound to the enzyme, preventing further catalytic activity (see Fig. 8.15). Thus, allopurinol is a suicide inhibitor. It reduces the production of uric acid and hence its concentration in the blood and tissues (e.g., the synovial lining of the joints in **Lotta T.'s** great toe). Xanthine and hypoxanthine accumulate, and urate levels decrease. Overall, the amount of purine being degraded is spread over three products rather than appearing in only one. Therefore, none of the compounds exceeds its solubility constant, precipitation does not occur, and the symptoms of gout gradually subside.

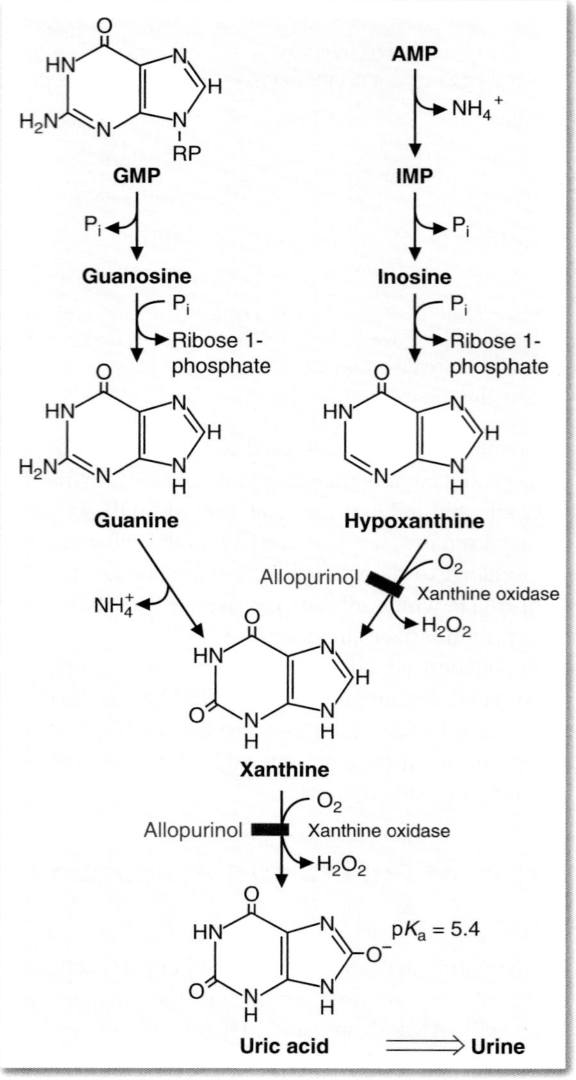

FIGURE 39.18 Degradation of the purine bases. The reactions inhibited by allopurinol are indicated. A second form of xanthine oxidase exists that uses nicotinamide adenine dinucleotide (NAD$^+$) instead of O$_2$ as the electron acceptor. *AMP*, adenosine monophosphate; *GMP*, guanosine monophosphate; *IMP*, inosine monophosphate; *P$_i$*, inorganic phosphate.

CLINICAL COMMENTS

Lotta T. Hyperuricemia in **Lotta T.'s** case arose as a consequence of overproduction of uric acid. Treatment with allopurinol not only inhibits xanthine oxidase, lowering the formation of uric acid with an increase in the excretion of hypoxanthine and xanthine, but also decreases the overall synthesis of purine nucleotides. Hypoxanthine and xanthine produced by purine degradation are often salvaged (i.e., converted to nucleotides) by reactions that require the consumption of PRPP. PRPP is a substrate for the glutamine phosphoribosylamidotransferase reaction that initiates purine biosynthesis. Because the normal cellular levels of PRPP and glutamine are below the K_m of the enzyme, changes in the level of either substrate can accelerate or reduce the rate of the reaction. Therefore, decreased levels of PRPP cause decreased synthesis of purine nucleotides.

BIOCHEMICAL COMMENTS

Adenosine Deaminase Deficiency. A deficiency in ADA activity leads to severe combined immunodeficiency disease (SCID). In the severe form of combined immunodeficiency, T-cells (which provide cell-based immunity; see Chapter 42) and B-cells (which produce antibodies) are both deficient, leaving the individual without a functional immune system. Children born with this disorder do not develop a mature thymus gland and suffer from many opportunistic infections because of their lack of a functional immune system. In order to avoid infection, which can be lethal, affected children must avoid exposure to infectious agents. Treatment with hematopoietic stem-cell transplantation or gene therapy is recommended. If neither is possible, administration of polyethylene glycol–modified ADA has been successful in treating the disorder. The question that remains, however, is that even though all the cells of the body lack ADA activity, why are the immune cells specifically targeted for destruction?

The specific immune disorder is not caused by any defect in purine salvage pathways because children with Lesch-Nyhan syndrome have a functional immune system, although there are other major problems in those children. This suggests that perhaps the accumulation of precursors to ADA lead to toxic effects. Three hypotheses have been proposed and are outlined below.

In the absence of ADA activity, both adenosine and deoxyadenosine accumulate. When deoxyadenosine accumulates, adenosine kinase can convert it to deoxyadenosine monophosphate. Other kinases then allow dATP to accumulate in the lymphocytes. Why specifically the lymphocytes? The other cells of the body secrete the deoxyadenosine they cannot use, and it accumulates in the circulation. Because the lymphocytes are present in the circulation, they tend to accumulate this compound more so than cells that are not constantly present in the blood. As dATP accumulates, ribonucleotide reductase becomes inhibited, and the cells can no longer produce deoxyribonucleotides for DNA synthesis. Thus, when cells are supposed to grow and differentiate in response to cytokines, they cannot, and they die.

A second hypothesis suggests that the accumulation of deoxyadenosine in lymphocytes leads to an inhibition of *S*-adenosylhomocysteine (SAH) hydrolase, the enzyme that converts SAH to homocysteine and adenosine. This leads to hypomethylation in the cell and to an accumulation of SAH. SAH accumulation has been linked to the triggering of apoptosis.

The third hypothesis suggested is that elevated adenosine levels lead to inappropriate activation of adenosine receptors. Adenosine is also a signaling molecule, and stimulation of the adenosine receptors results in activation of protein kinase A and elevated cAMP levels in thymocytes. Elevated levels of cAMP in these cells trigger both apoptosis and developmental arrest of the cell.

Although it is still not clear which potential mechanism best explains the arrested development of immune cells, it is clear that elevated levels of adenosine and deoxyadenosine are toxic.

Once nucleotide biosynthesis and salvage was understood at the pathway level, it was quickly realized that one way to inhibit cell proliferation would be to block purine or pyrimidine synthesis. Thus, drugs were developed that would interfere with a cell's ability to generate precursors for DNA synthesis, thereby inhibiting cell growth. This is particularly important for cancer cells, which have lost their normal growth-regulatory properties. Such drugs have been introduced previously with several different patients. **Clark T.** was treated with 5-fluorouracil, which inhibits thymidylate synthase (dUMP-to-TMP synthesis). **Charles F.** was treated with a combination of drugs (R-CHOP) for his leukemia. These drugs all interfere with DNA synthesis via a variety of mechanisms. Development of these drugs would not have been possible without an understanding of the biochemistry of both purine and pyrimidine salvage and synthesis and DNA replication. Such drugs also affect rapidly dividing normal cells, which brings about several of the side effects of chemotherapeutic regimens.

KEY CONCEPTS

- Purine and pyrimidine nucleotides can both be synthesized from scratch (de novo) or salvaged from existing bases.
- De novo purine synthesis is complex, requiring 11 steps and six molecules of adenosine triphosphate (ATP) for every purine synthesized. Purines are initially synthesized in the ribonucleotide form.
- The precursors for de novo purine synthesis are glycine, ribose 5-phosphate, glutamine, aspartate, carbon dioxide, and N^{10}-formyl-tetrahydrofolate (FH$_4$).
- The initial purine ribonucleotide synthesized is inosine monophosphate (IMP). Adenosine monophosphate (AMP) and guanosine monophosphate (GMP) are each derived from IMP.

- Because de novo purine synthesis requires a large amount of energy, purine nucleotide salvage pathways exist such that free purine bases can be converted to nucleotides.
- Mutations in purine salvage enzymes are associated with severe diseases, such as Lesch-Nyhan syndrome and severe combined immunodeficiency disease (SCID).
- Pyrimidine bases are initially synthesized as the free base and then converted to nucleotides.
- Aspartate and cytoplasmic carbamoyl phosphate are the precursors for pyrimidine ring synthesis.
- The initial pyrimidine nucleotide synthesized is orotate monophosphate, which is converted to uridine monophosphate (UMP). The other pyrimidine nucleotides are derived from a uracil-containing intermediate.
- Deoxyribonucleotides are derived by reduction of ribonucleotides, as catalyzed by ribonucleotide reductase. The regulation of ribonucleotide reductase is complex.
- Degradation of purine-containing nucleotides results in production of uric acid, which is eliminated in the urine. Elevated uric acid levels in the blood lead to gout.
- Diseases discussed in this chapter are summarized in Table 39.4.

TABLE 39.4 **Diseases Discussed in Chapter 39**

DISEASE OR DISORDER	ENVIRONMENTAL OR GENETIC	COMMENTS
Gout	Both	Painful joints due to the precipitation of uric acid in the blood
PNP (purine nucleoside phosphorylase) deficiency	Genetic	A defect in a purine salvage enzyme, leading to a loss of T-cell function, with near normal B-cell function and a partial immunodeficiency disease. Purine nucleosides will accumulate.
Lesch-Nyhan syndrome (lack of hypoxanthine–guanine phosphoribosyl-transferase activity)	Genetic	The loss of HGPRT activity leads to the accumulation of purines and uric acid, with intellectual disability and self-injury resulting in severe cases. Gout will also appear in these individuals.
Hereditary orotic aciduria	Genetic	A defect in UMP synthase, leading to orotic acid accumulation and growth retardation
Adenosine deaminase deficiency	Genetic	The loss of adenosine deaminase activity leads to severe combined immunodeficiency disease (SCID), with a loss of both T and B cell function. Deoxyadenosine (dA) and derivatives of dA accumulate in the blood and blood-based cells.
Cancer	Both	The use of drugs that interfere with DNA replication will destroy rapidly dividing cells at a faster rate than normal cells.

REVIEW QUESTIONS—CHAPTER 39

1. Similarities between CPSI and CPSII include which one of the following?
   A. Carbon source
   B. Intracellular location
   C. Nitrogen source
   D. Regulation by *N*-acetylglutamate
   E. Regulation by UMP

2. Gout can result from a reduction in activity of which one of the following enzymes?
   A. Glutamine phosphoribosylamidotransferase
   B. HGPRT
   C. Glucose 6-phosphate dehydrogenase
   D. PRPP synthetase
   E. Purine nucleoside phosphorylase

3. A 2-year-old boy is exhibiting developmental delay and has started to bite his lips and fingers. Orange-colored "sand" is found in his diapers. This child has an inability to metabolize which one of the following molecules?
   A. Uric acid
   B. Thymine
   C. Adenine
   D. Uracil
   E. Hypoxanthine

4. Allopurinol can be used to treat gout because of its ability to inhibit which one of the following reactions?
   A. AMP to XMP
   B. Xanthine to uric acid
   C. Inosine to hypoxanthine
   D. IMP to XMP
   E. XMP to GMP

5. The regulation of ribonucleotide reductase is quite complex. Assuming that an enzyme deficiency leads to highly elevated levels of dGTP, what effect would you predict on the reduction of ribonucleotides to deoxyribonucleotides under these conditions?
   A. Elevated levels of dCDP will be produced.
   B. The formation of dADP will be favored.
   C. AMP will begin to be reduced.
   D. Reduced thioredoxin will become rate-limiting, thereby reducing the activity of ribonucleotide reductase.
   E. dGTP will bind to the overall activity site and inhibit the functioning of the enzyme.

6. A patient with von Gierke's disease displays the symptoms of gout. This most likely occurs owing to the overproduction of which one of the following molecules?
   A. PRPP
   B. Aspartate
   C. Glucose
   D. NADPH
   E. UDP-glucose

7. A patient with ornithine transcarbamoylase deficiency exhibits orotic aciduria. This occurs owing to which one of the following?
   A. Activation of the regulated step of de novo pyrimidine biosynthesis
   B. Bypassing the regulated step of de novo pyrimidine biosynthesis
   C. Inhibition of the regulated step of de novo pyrimidine biosynthesis
   D. Activation of the CAD complex by carbamoyl phosphate
   E. Activation of the UMP synthase complex by carbamoyl phosphate

8. Purines and pyrimidines are necessary for the synthesis of DNA. Of the substances that donate atoms to the purine base and pyrimidine ring, which one of the following directly donates atoms to both the purine base and pyrimidine ring?
   A. CO_2
   B. Glycine
   C. Carbamoyl phosphate
   D. Aspartate
   E. Glutamine

9. Which one of the following statements is correct concerning purine and pyrimidine metabolism?
   A. Pyrimidines, when degraded, yield uric acid.
   B. Excess pyrimidine degradation can lead to gout.
   C. Purines cannot be degraded to generate energy.
   D. Purines degrade to CO_2 and water.
   E. An excess of urea leads to gout.

10. Allopurinol is used to treat gout. The drug is a suicide inhibitor that leads to a reduction in the amount of uric acid produced. Instead of accumulating uric acid, which other compound would accumulate in the presence of allopurinol?
    A. Hypoxanthine
    B. Ribose 1-phosphate
    C. IMP
    D. Guanine
    E. Adenine

ANSWERS

1. **The answer is A.** Both CPSI and CPSII use carbon dioxide as the carbon source in the production of carbamoyl phosphate. CPSI is located in the mitochondria, whereas CPSII is in the cytoplasm (thus, B is incorrect). CPSI can fix ammonia; CPSII requires glutamine as the nitrogen source (thus, C is incorrect). N-Acetylglutamate activates CPSI; CSPII is activated by PRPP (thus, D is incorrect). UMP inhibits CPSII but has no effect on CPSI (thus, E is also incorrect).

2. **The answer is B.** A lack of HGPRT activity (Lesch-Nyhan syndrome) leads to an accumulation of PRPP levels, which induces increased purine synthesis, leading to excessive levels of purines in the cells. The degradation of the extra purines leads to uric acid production and gout.

   A loss of either PRPP synthetase activity or glutamine phosphoribosylamidotransferase activity would lead to reduced purine synthesis and hypouricemia (thus, A and D are incorrect). A lack of glucose 6-phosphate dehydrogenase would hinder ribose 5-phosphate production and thus would not lead to excessive purine synthesis. A lack of purine nucleoside phosphorylase would hinder the salvage pathway, leading to an accumulation of nucleosides. Purine nucleoside phosphorylase activity is required to synthesize uric acid, so in the absence of this enzyme, less uric acid would be produced (thus, E is incorrect).

3. **The answer is E.** The child has Lesch-Nyhan syndrome, a deficiency of HGPRT activity. As such, hypoxanthine cannot be converted to IMP, and guanine cannot be converted

to GMP. One consequence of this is elevated uric acid levels, owing to an accumulation of hypoxanthine and guanine. Pyrimidine metabolism is not altered in Lesch-Nyhan patients, so thymine and uracil metabolism is normal. Adenine is converted to AMP by APRT, so a loss of HGPRT activity does not alter adenine metabolism.

4. **The answer is B.** Allopurinol inhibits the conversion of both hypoxanthine to xanthine and xanthine to uric acid. This occurs because both of those reactions are catalyzed by xanthine oxidase, the target of allopurinol. Answer A is incorrect because AMP is not converted directly to XMP (AMP, when degraded, is deaminated to form IMP, which loses its phosphate to become inosine, which undergoes phosphorolysis to generate hypoxanthine and ribose 1-phosphate). Answer C is incorrect because the inosine-to-hypoxanthine conversion, catalyzed by nucleoside phosphorylase, is not inhibited by allopurinol. Answer D is incorrect because the conversion of hypoxanthine to xanthine occurs at the free-base level, not at the nucleotide level. Answer E is incorrect because GMP is converted first to guanosine (loss of phosphate), the guanosine is converted to guanine and ribose 1-phosphate, and the guanine is then converted to xanthine by guanase.

5. **The answer is B.** If dGTP were to accumulate in cells, the dGTP would bind to the substrate specificity site of ribonucleotide reductase and direct the synthesis of dADP. This would lead to elevations of dATP levels, which would inhibit the activity of ribonucleotide reductase. The inhibition of ribonucleotide reductase leads to a cessation of cell proliferation, as the supply of deoxyribonucleotides for DNA synthesis becomes limiting. Answer A is incorrect because ATP would need to bind to the substrate specificity site to direct the synthesis of dCDP. That would not occur under these conditions of elevated dGTP levels. Answer C is incorrect because the enzyme works only on diphosphates; AMP would never be a substrate for this enzyme. Answer D is incorrect because the thioredoxin is always regenerated and does not become rate-limiting for the reductase reaction. Answer E is incorrect because dGTP does not bind to the activity site of the reductase; only ATP (activator) or dATP (inhibitor) is capable of binding to the activity site.

6. **The answer is A.** A patient with von Gierke's disease is lacking glucose 6-phosphatase activity, and glucose 6-phosphate cannot be converted to free glucose. Under conditions of gluconeogenesis, and glycogenolysis, in the liver glucose 6-phosphate will accumulate. The high glucose 6-phosphate levels will drive the hexose monophosphate (HMP) shunt pathway to produce additional ribose 5-phosphate, which will stimulate PRPP synthetase to produce more PRPP. The elevated PRPP leads to increased activity of amidophosphoribosyltransferase, producing more AMP and GMP. As the AMP and GMP are not required by the cell, they are degraded and produce uric acid, which accumulates, precipitates, and leads to the symptoms of a gout attack. Elevated levels of NADPH may occur owing to an increase in the oxidative steps of the HMP shunt, but this will not lead to an increase in uric acid production. Glucose levels will not increase because of the defect in glucose 6-phosphatase. UDP-glucose levels may increase, but if they do, glycogen synthesis will be stimulated and this will not affect uric acid production. Aspartate levels may increase (owing to increased protein turnover to provide substrates for gluconeogenesis) in patients with von Gierke's disease, but higher aspartate will not lead to uric acid production (because aspartate will not stimulate purine ring synthesis).

7. **The answer is B.** The regulated step of de novo pyrimidine synthesis is the CPSII step (CPSII uses the amide nitrogen of glutamine, the carbon and oxygen of carbon dioxide, and two high-energy bonds to produce carbamoyl phosphate). UTP will inhibit the activity of this enzyme, signifying high levels of pyrimidines in the cell. A patient with a lack of ornithine transcarbamolyase activity will accumulate carbamoyl phosphate in the mitochondria (as produced by CPSI). As the concentration of carbamoyl phosphate in the mitochondria increases, the molecule will escape from the mitochondria and enter the cytoplasm and be used for de novo pyrimidine synthesis. This is bypassing the regulated step of pyrimidine biosynthesis. It is not an activation of the regulated step or an inhibition of the regulated step of pyrimidine biosynthesis. CAD is not a regulated enzyme and neither is UMP synthase.

8. **The answer is D.** Aspartate and carbamoyl phosphate (generated from carbon dioxide and glutamine) form all of the components of the pyrimidine ring, whereas aspartate, CO_2, glycine, glutamine, and N^{10}-formyl-FH$_4$ all donate atoms to form the purine base. The direct donor of a carbon and nitrogen to pyrimidine ring biosynthesis is carbamoyl phosphate, not the glutamine and carbon dioxide required to synthesize the carbamoyl phosphate.

9. **The answer is C.** Purine degradation leads to uric acid formation and does not generate any energy. An excess of uric acid leads to gout (precipitation of the uric acid in joints). Pyrimidines are degraded to water-soluble compounds such as urea, CO_2, and water, although not much energy is obtained from pyrimidine degradation as well.

10. **The answer is A.** Allopurinol is a structural analog of hypoxanthine which reduces production of uric acid (by inhibition of the enzyme xanthine oxidase), allowing xanthine and hypoxanthine to accumulate as uric acid levels decrease. None of the other breakdown products will accumulate in the presence of allopurinol because the end-products are water-soluble and are removed from the body in the urine.

Intertissue Relationships in the Metabolism of Amino Acids

The body maintains a relatively large free amino acid pool in the blood, even during fasting. As a result, tissues have continuous access to individual amino acids for the synthesis of proteins and essential amino acid derivatives, such as neurotransmitters. The amino acid pool also provides the liver with **amino acid substrates** for **gluconeogenesis** and provides several other cell types with a source of **fuel**. The **free amino acid pool** is derived from **dietary amino acids** and the **turnover of proteins** in the body. During an **overnight fast** and during **hypercatabolic states**, **degradation** of labile **protein**, particularly that in **skeletal muscle**, is the major source of free amino acids.

The liver is the major site of amino acid metabolism in the body and the major site of **urea synthesis**. The liver is also the major site of amino acid degradation. Hepatocytes partially oxidize most amino acids, converting the carbon skeleton to glucose, ketone bodies, or CO_2. Because ammonia is toxic, the liver converts most of the nitrogen from amino acid degradation to urea, which is excreted in the urine. The nitrogen derived from amino acid catabolism in other tissues is transported to the liver as **alanine** or **glutamine** and converted to urea.

The **branched-chain amino acids** (BCAAs; valine, isoleucine, and leucine) are oxidized principally in **skeletal muscle** and other tissues and not in the liver. In skeletal muscle, the carbon skeletons and some of the nitrogen are converted to glutamine, which is released into the blood. The remainder of the nitrogen is incorporated into alanine, which is taken up by the liver and converted to urea and glucose.

The formation and release of glutamine from skeletal muscle and other tissues serves several functions. In the kidney, the NH_4^+ carried by glutamine is excreted into the urine. This process removes protons formed during fuel oxidation and helps to maintain the body's pH, especially during metabolic acidosis. **Glutamine** also provides a **fuel** for the **kidney** and **gut**. In rapidly dividing cells (e.g., lymphocytes and macrophages), glutamine is required as a fuel, as a nitrogen donor for biosynthetic reactions, and as a substrate for protein synthesis.

During conditions of **sepsis** (the presence of various pathogenic organisms, or their toxins, in the blood or tissues), **trauma**, **injury**, or **burns**, the body enters a **catabolic state** characterized by a **negative nitrogen balance** (Fig. 40.1). Increased net protein degradation in skeletal muscle increases the availability of glutamine and other amino acids for cell division and protein synthesis in cells involved in the immune response and wound healing. In these conditions, increased release of glucocorticoids from the adrenal cortex stimulates proteolysis.

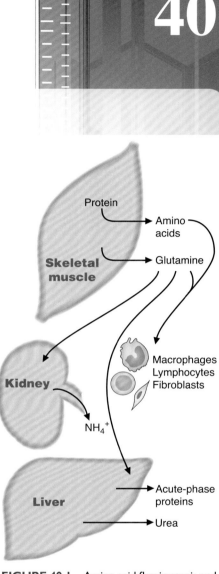

FIGURE 40.1 Amino acid flux in sepsis and trauma. In sepsis and traumatic injury, glutamine and other amino acids are released from skeletal muscle for uptake by tissues involved in the immune response and tissue repair, such as macrophages, lymphocytes, fibroblasts, and the liver. Nitrogen excretion as urea and NH_4^+ results in negative nitrogen balance.

Katherine B., a 62-year-old homeless woman, was found by a neighborhood child who heard Katherine's moans coming from an abandoned building. The child's mother called the police, who took Katherine to the hospital emergency department. The patient was semicomatose, incontinent of urine, and her clothes were stained with vomitus. She had a fever of 103°F, was trembling uncontrollably, appeared to be severely dehydrated, and had marked muscle wasting. Her heart rate was very rapid, and her blood pressure was low (85/46 mm Hg). Her abdomen was distended and without bowel sounds. She responded to moderate pressure on her abdomen with moaning and grimacing.

Blood was sent for a broad laboratory profile, and cultures of her urine and blood were taken. Intravenous saline with thiamine and folate, glucose, and parenteral broad-spectrum antibiotics were begun. Radiography performed after her vital signs were stabilized suggested a bowel perforation. These findings were compatible with a diagnosis of a ruptured viscus (e.g., an infected colonic diverticulum that perforated, allowing colonic bacteria to infect the tissues of the peritoneal cavity, causing peritonitis). Further studies confirmed that a diverticulum had ruptured, and appropriate surgery was performed. All of the blood cultures grew out *Escherichia coli*, indicating that Katherine also had a gram-negative infection of her blood (septicemia) that had been seeded by the proliferating organisms in her peritoneal cavity. Intensive fluid and electrolyte therapy and antibiotic coverage were continued. The medical team (surgeons, internists, and nutritionists) began developing a complex therapeutic plan to reverse Katherine's severely catabolic state.

I. Maintenance of the Free Amino Acid Pool in Blood

The body maintains a relatively large free amino acid pool in the blood, even in the absence of an intake of dietary protein. The large free amino acid pool ensures the continuous availability of individual amino acids to tissues for the synthesis of proteins, neurotransmitters, and other nitrogen-containing compounds (Fig. 40.2). In a normal, well-fed, healthy individual, approximately 300 to 600 g of body protein is degraded per day. At the same time, roughly 100 g of protein is consumed in the diet per day, which adds additional amino acids. From this pool, tissues use amino acids for the continuous synthesis of new proteins (300 to 600 g) to replace those degraded. The continuous turnover of proteins in the body makes the complete complement of amino acids available for the synthesis of new and different proteins, such as antibodies. Protein turnover allows shifts in the quantities of different proteins produced in tissues in response to changes in physiologic state and continuously removes modified or damaged proteins. It also provides a complete pool of specific amino acids that can be used as oxidizable substrates; precursors for gluconeogenesis and for heme, creatine phosphate, purine, pyrimidine, and neurotransmitter synthesis; for ammoniagenesis to maintain blood pH levels; and for numerous other functions.

The concentration of free amino acids in the blood is not nearly as rigidly controlled as blood glucose levels. The free amino acid pool in the blood is only a small part (0.5%) of the total amino acid pool in whole-body protein. Because of the large skeletal muscle mass, approximately 80% of the body's total protein is in skeletal muscle. Consequently, the concentration of individual amino acids in the blood is strongly affected by the rates of protein synthesis and degradation in skeletal muscle as well as the rate of uptake and use of individual amino acids for metabolism in liver and other tissues. For the most part, changes in the rate of protein synthesis and degradation take place over a span of hours.

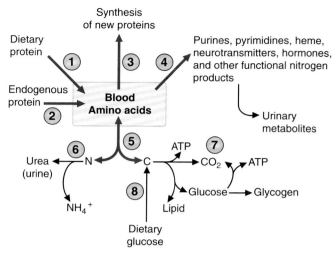

FIGURE 40.2   Maintenance of the blood amino acid pool. Dietary protein (*1*) and degradation of endogenous protein (*2*) provide a source of essential amino acids (those that cannot be synthesized in the human). (*3*) The synthesis of new protein is the major use of amino acids from the free amino acid pool. (*4*) Compounds synthesized from amino acid precursors are essential for physiologic functions. Many of these compounds are degraded to nitrogen-containing urinary metabolites and do not return to the free amino acid pool. (*5*) In tissues, the nitrogen is removed from amino acids by transamination and deamination reactions. (*6*) The nitrogen from amino acid degradation appears in the urine primarily as urea or NH_4^+, the ammonium ion. Ammonia excretion is necessary to maintain the pH of the blood. (*7*) Amino acids are used as fuels either directly or after being converted to glucose by gluconeogenesis. (*8*) Some amino acids can be synthesized in humans, provided that glucose and a nitrogen source are available. *ATP*, adenosine triphosphate.

A. Interorgan Flux of Amino Acids in the Postabsorptive State

The fasting state provides an example of the interorgan flux of amino acids necessary to maintain the free amino acid pool in the blood and supply tissues with their required amino acids (Fig. 40.3). During an overnight fast, protein synthesis in the liver and other tissues continues but at a diminished rate compared with the postprandial state. Net degradation of labile protein occurs in skeletal muscle (which contains the body's largest protein mass) and other tissues.

1. Release of Amino Acids from Skeletal Muscle during Fasting

The efflux of amino acids from skeletal muscle supports the essential amino acid pool in the blood (see Fig. 40.3). Skeletal muscle oxidizes the BCAAs (valine, leucine, isoleucine) to produce energy and glutamine. The amino groups of the BCAAs, and of aspartate and glutamate, are transferred out of skeletal muscle in alanine and glutamine. Alanine and glutamine account for approximately 50% of the total α-amino nitrogen released by skeletal muscle.

The release of amino acids from skeletal muscle is stimulated during an overnight fast by the decrease of insulin and increase of glucocorticoid (such as cortisol) levels in the blood (see Chapters 28 and 41). Insulin promotes the uptake of amino acids and the general synthesis of proteins. The mechanisms for the stimulation of protein synthesis in human skeletal muscle are not all known, but they probably include an activation of the A system for amino acid transport (a modest effect), a general effect on initiation of translation, and an inhibition of lysosomal proteolysis. The fall of blood insulin levels during an overnight fast results in net proteolysis and release of amino acids. As glucocorticoid release from the adrenal cortex increases, an induction of ubiquitin synthesis and increase of ubiquitin-dependent proteolysis also occur.

 What changes in hormone levels and fuel metabolism occur during an overnight fast?

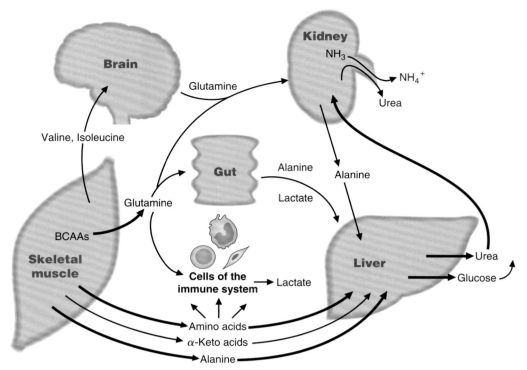

FIGURE 40.3 Interorgan amino acid exchange after an overnight fast. After an overnight fast (the postabsorptive state), the use of amino acids for protein synthesis, for fuels, and for the synthesis of essential functional compounds continues. The free amino acid pool is supported largely by net degradation of skeletal muscle protein. Glutamine and alanine serve as amino group carriers from skeletal muscle to other tissues. Glutamine brings NH_4^+ to the kidney for the excretion of protons and serves as a fuel for the kidney, gut, and cells of the immune system. Alanine transfers amino groups from skeletal muscle, the kidney, and the gut to the liver, where they are converted to urea for excretion. The brain continues to use amino acids for neurotransmitter synthesis.

A The hormonal changes that occur during an overnight fast include a decrease of blood insulin levels and an increase of glucagon relative to levels after a high-carbohydrate meal. Glucocorticoid levels also increase in the blood. These hormones coordinate the changes of fat, carbohydrate, and amino acid metabolism. Fatty acids are released from adipose triacylglycerols and are used as the major fuel by heart, skeletal muscle, liver, and other tissues. The liver converts some of the fatty acids to ketone bodies. Liver glycogen stores and gluconeogenesis maintain blood glucose levels for glucose-dependent tissues. The major precursors of gluconeogenesis include amino acids released from skeletal muscle, lactate, and glycerol.

2. Amino Acid Metabolism in Liver during Fasting

The major site of alanine uptake is the liver, which disposes of the amino nitrogen by incorporating it into urea (see Fig. 40.3). The liver also extracts free amino acids, α-keto acids, and some glutamine from the blood. Alanine and other amino acids are oxidized and their carbon skeletons are converted principally to glucose. Glucagon and glucocorticoids stimulate the uptake of amino acids into liver and increase gluconeogenesis and ureagenesis (Fig. 40.4). Alanine transport into the liver, in particular,

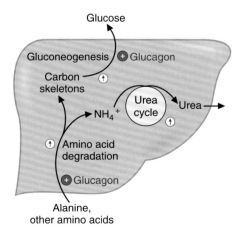

FIGURE 40.4 Hormonal regulation of hepatic amino acid metabolism in the postabsorptive state. Induction of urea cycle enzymes occurs both during fasting and after a high-protein meal. Because many individuals in the United States normally have a high-protein diet, the levels of urea-cycle enzymes may not fluctuate to any great extent. ⊕, glucagon-mediated activation of enzymes or proteins; ①, induction of enzyme synthesis mediated by glucagon and glucocorticoids.

is enhanced by glucagon. The induction of the synthesis of gluconeogenic enzymes by glucagon and glucocorticoids during the overnight fast correlates with an induction of many of the enzymes of amino acid degradation (e.g., tyrosine aminotransferase) and an induction of urea-cycle enzymes (see Chapter 36). Urea synthesis also increases because of the increased supply of NH_4^+ from amino acid degradation in the liver.

3. Metabolism of Amino Acids in Other Tissues during Fasting

Glucose, produced by the liver, is used for energy by the brain and other glucose-dependent tissues, such as erythrocytes. The muscle, under conditions of exercise, when the adenosine monophosphate (AMP)–activated protein kinase is active, also oxidizes some of this glucose to pyruvate, which is used for the carbon skeleton of alanine (the glucose–alanine cycle; see Chapter 36).

Glutamine is generated in skeletal muscle from the oxidation of BCAAs and by the lungs and brain for the removal of NH_4^+ formed from amino acid catabolism or entering from the blood. The kidney, the gut, and cells with rapid turnover rates, such as those of the immune system, are the major sites of glutamine uptake (see Fig. 40.3). Glutamine serves as a fuel for these tissues, as a nitrogen donor for purine synthesis, and as a substrate for ammoniagenesis in the kidney. Much of the unused nitrogen from glutamine is transferred to pyruvate to form alanine in these tissues. Alanine then carries the unused nitrogen back to the liver.

The brain is glucose-dependent but, like many cells in the body, can use BCAAs for energy. The BCAAs also provide a source of nitrogen for neurotransmitter synthesis during fasting. Other amino acids released from skeletal muscle protein degradation also serve as precursors of neurotransmitters.

B. Principles Governing Amino Acid Flux between Tissues

The pattern of interorgan flux of amino acids is strongly affected by conditions that change the supply of fuels (e.g., the overnight fast, a mixed meal, a high-protein meal) and by conditions that increase the demand for amino acids (metabolic acidosis, surgical stress, traumatic injury, burns, wound healing, and sepsis). The flux of amino acid carbon and nitrogen in these different conditions is dictated by several considerations:

1. Ammonia (NH_3) is toxic. Consequently, it is transported between tissues as alanine or glutamine. Alanine is the principal carrier of amino acid nitrogen from other tissues back to the liver, where the nitrogen is converted to urea and subsequently excreted into the urine by the kidneys. The amount of urea synthesized is proportional to the amount of amino acid carbon that is being oxidized as a fuel.

   The differences in amino acid metabolism between tissues are dictated by the types and amounts of different enzyme and transport proteins present in each tissue and the ability of each tissue to respond to different regulatory messages (hormones and neural signals).

2. The pool of glutamine in the blood serves several essential metabolic functions (Table 40.1). It provides ammonia for excretion of protons in the urine as NH_4^+. It serves as a fuel for the gut, the kidney, and the cells of the immune system. Glutamine is also required by the cells of the immune system and other rapidly dividing cells in which its amide group serves as the source of nitrogen for biosynthetic reactions. In the brain, the formation of glutamine from glutamate and NH_4^+ provides a means of removing ammonia and of transporting glutamate between different cell types within the brain. The use of the blood glutamine pool is prioritized. During metabolic acidosis, the kidney becomes the predominant site of glutamine uptake at the expense of glutamine use in other tissues. Conversely, during sepsis, in the absence of acidosis, cells involved in the immune response (macrophages, hepatocytes) become the preferential sites of glutamine uptake.

3. The BCAAs (valine, leucine, and isoleucine) form a significant portion of the composition of the average protein and can be converted to tricarboxylic acid (TCA) cycle intermediates and used as fuels by almost all tissues.

The body normally produces approximately 1 mmol of protons per kilogram of body weight per day. Nevertheless, the pH of the blood and extracellular fluid is normally maintained between 7.36 and 7.44. The narrow range is maintained principally by the bicarbonate (HCO_3^-), phosphate (HPO_4^-), and hemoglobin buffering systems, and by the excretion of an amount of acid equal to that produced. The excretion of protons by the kidney regenerates bicarbonate, which can be reclaimed from the glomerular filtrate.

The acids are produced from normal fuel metabolism. The major acid is carbonic acid, which is formed from water and CO_2 produced in the TCA cycle and other oxidative pathways. The oxidation of sulfur-containing amino acids (methionine and cysteine) ultimately produces sulfuric acid (H_2SO_4), which dissociates into $2H^+ + SO_4^{2-}$, and the protons and sulfate are excreted. The hydrolysis of phosphate esters produces the equivalent of phosphoric acid. What other acids produced during metabolism appear in the blood?

Katherine B. was in a severe stage of negative nitrogen balance on admission, which was caused by both her malnourished state and her intraabdominal infection complicated by sepsis. The physiologic response to advanced catabolic status includes a degradation of muscle protein with the release of amino acids into the blood. This release is coupled with an increased uptake of amino acids for acute-phase protein synthesis by the liver (systemic response) and other cells involved in the immune response to general and severe infection.

A Lactic acid is produced from glucose and amino acid metabolism. The ketone bodies (acetoacetate and β-hydroxybutyrate) produced during fatty acid oxidation are also acids. Many α-keto acids, formed from transamination reactions, are also found in the blood.

TABLE 40.1   Functions of Glutamine
Protein synthesis
Ammoniagenesis for proton excretion
Nitrogen donor for synthesis of:
Purines
Pyrimidines
Nicotinamide adenine dinucleotide (NAD$^+$)
Amino sugars
Asparagine
Other compounds
Glutamate donor for synthesis of:
Glutathione
γ-Aminobutyric acid (GABA)
Ornithine
Arginine
Proline
Other compounds

Valine and isoleucine are also the major precursors of glutamine. Except for the BCAAs and alanine, aspartate, and glutamate, the catabolism of amino acids occurs principally in the liver.

The ability to convert four-carbon intermediates of the TCA cycle to pyruvate is required for oxidation of both BCAAs and glutamine. This sequence of reactions requires phosphoenolpyruvate (PEP) carboxykinase or decarboxylating malate dehydrogenase (malic enzyme). Most tissues have one or both of these enzymes.

4. Amino acids are major gluconeogenic substrates, and most of the energy obtained from their oxidation is derived from oxidation of the glucose formed from their carbon skeletons. A much smaller percentage of amino acid carbon is converted to acetyl coenzyme A (acetyl-CoA) or to ketone bodies and oxidized. The use of amino acids for glucose synthesis for the brain and other glucose-requiring tissues is subject to the hormonal regulatory mechanisms of glucose homeostasis (see Chapters 28 and 34).

5. The relative rates of protein synthesis and degradation (protein turnover) determine the size of the free amino acid pools available for the synthesis of new proteins and for other essential functions. For example, the synthesis of new proteins to mount an immune response is supported by the net degradation of other proteins in the body.

II. Use of Amino Acids in Individual Tissues

Because tissues differ in their physiologic functions, they have different amino acid requirements and contribute differently to whole-body nitrogen metabolism. However, all tissues share a common requirement for essential amino acids for protein synthesis, and protein turnover is an ongoing process in all cells.

A. The Kidney

One of the primary roles of amino acid nitrogen is to provide ammonia in the kidney for the excretion of protons in the urine. NH_4^+ is released from glutamine by glutaminase and from glutamate by glutamate dehydrogenase, resulting in the formation of α-ketoglutarate (Fig. 40.5). α-Ketoglutarate is used as a fuel by the kidney and is

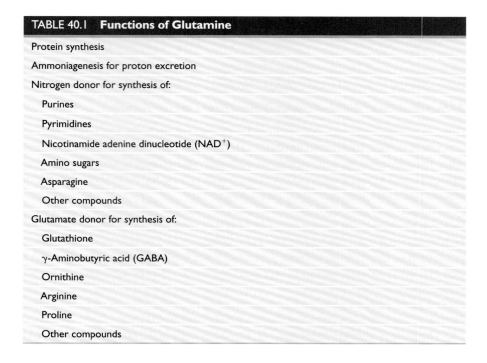

FIGURE 40.5 Renal glutamine metabolism. Renal tubule cells preferentially oxidize glutamine. During metabolic acidosis, it is the major fuel for the kidney. Conversion of glutamine to α-ketoglutarate generates NH_4^+. Ammonium ion excretion helps to buffer systemic acidemia.

TABLE 40.2	**Major Fuel Sources for the Kidney**		
	PERCENTAGE OF TOTAL CO$_2$ FORMED IN DIFFERENT PHYSIOLOGIC STATES		
FUEL	**NORMAL**	**ACIDOSIS**	**FASTED**
Lactate	45	20	15
Glucose^a	25	20	0
Fatty acids	15	20	60
Glutamine	15	40	25

^{a}Glucose used in the renal medulla is produced in the renal cortex.

oxidized to CO_2, converted to glucose for use in cells in the renal medulla, or converted to alanine to return ammonia to the liver for urea synthesis.

The rate of glutamine uptake from the blood and its use by the kidney depends principally on the amount of acid that must be excreted to maintain a normal pH in the blood. In metabolic acidosis, the excretion of NH_4^+ by the kidney increases severalfold. Because glutamine nitrogen provides approximately two-thirds of the NH_4^+ excreted by the kidney, glutamine uptake by the kidney also increases. Renal glutamine use for proton excretion takes precedence over the requirements of other tissues for glutamine.

Glutamine is used as a fuel by the kidney in the normal fed state and, to a greater extent, during fasting and metabolic acidosis (Table 40.2). The carbon skeleton forms α-ketoglutarate, which is oxidized to CO_2, converted to glucose, or released as the carbon skeleton of serine or alanine (Fig. 40.6). α-Ketoglutarate can be converted to oxaloacetate by TCA-cycle reactions, and oxaloacetate is converted to PEP by PEP carboxykinase. PEP can then be converted to pyruvate and subsequently to acetyl-CoA, alanine, serine, or glucose. The glucose is used principally by the cells of the renal medulla, which have a relatively high dependence on anaerobic glycolysis because of their lower oxygen supply and mitochondrial capacity. The lactate released from anaerobic glycolysis in these cells is taken up and oxidized in the renal cortical cells, which have a higher mitochondrial capacity and a greater blood supply.

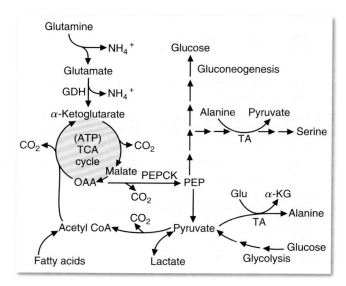

FIGURE 40.6 Metabolism of glutamine and other fuels in the kidney. To completely oxidize glutamate carbon to CO_2, it must enter the tricarboxylic acid (TCA) cycle as acetyl coenzyme A (acetyl-CoA). Carbon entering the TCA cycle as α-ketoglutarate (α-KG) exits as oxaloacetate and is converted to phosphoenolpyruvate (PEP) by PEP carboxykinase. PEP is converted to pyruvate, which may be oxidized to acetyl-CoA. PEP also can be converted to serine, glucose, or alanine. *ATP*, adenosine triphosphate; *GDH*, glutamate dehydrogenase; *OAA*, oxaloacetate; *PEPCK*, phosphoenolpyruvate carboxykinase; *TA*, transaminase.

B. Skeletal Muscle

Skeletal muscle, because of its large mass, is a major site of protein synthesis and degradation in humans. After a high-protein meal, insulin promotes the uptake of certain amino acids and stimulates net protein synthesis. The insulin stimulation of protein synthesis is dependent on an adequate supply of amino acids to undergo protein synthesis. During fasting and other catabolic states, a net degradation of skeletal muscle protein and release of amino acids occur (see Fig. 40.3). The net degradation of protein affects functional proteins, such as myosin, which are sacrificed to meet more urgent demands for amino acids in other tissues. During sepsis, degradation of skeletal muscle protein is stimulated by the glucocorticoid cortisol. The effect of cortisol is exerted through the activation of ubiquitin-dependent proteolysis. During fasting, the decrease of blood insulin levels and the increase of blood cortisol levels increase net protein degradation.

Skeletal muscle is a major site of glutamine synthesis, thereby satisfying the demand for glutamine during the postabsorptive state, during metabolic acidosis, and during septic stress and trauma. The carbon skeleton and nitrogen of glutamine are derived principally from the metabolism of BCAAs. Amino acid degradation in skeletal muscle is also accompanied by the formation of alanine, which transfers amino groups from skeletal muscle to the liver in the glucose–alanine cycle.

1. Oxidation of Branched-Chain Amino Acids in Skeletal Muscle

The BCAAs play a special role in muscle and most other tissues because they are the major amino acids that can be oxidized in tissues other than the liver. However, all tissues can interconvert amino acids and TCA-cycle intermediates through transaminase reactions; that is, alanine $\leftrightarrow$ pyruvate, aspartate $\leftrightarrow$ oxaloacetate, and α-ketoglutarate $\leftrightarrow$ glutamate. The first step of the pathway, transamination of the BCAAs to α-keto acids, occurs principally in brain, heart, kidney, and skeletal muscles. These tissues have a high content of BCAA transaminase relative to the low levels in liver. The α-keto acids of the BCAAs are then either released into the blood and taken up by liver, or oxidized to CO_2 or glutamine within the muscle or other tissue (Fig. 40.7). They can be oxidized by all tissues that contain mitochondria.

The oxidative pathways of the BCAAs convert the carbon skeleton to either succinyl coenzyme A (succinyl-CoA) or acetyl-CoA (see Chapter 37 and Fig. 40.7). The pathways generate reduced nicotinamide adenine dinucleotide (NADH) and reduced flavin adenine dinucleotide (FAD[2H]) for adenosine triphosphate (ATP) synthesis before the conversion of carbon into intermediates of the TCA cycle, thus providing the muscle with energy without loss of carbon as CO_2. Leucine is "ketogenic" in that it is converted to acetyl-CoA and acetoacetate. Skeletal muscle, adipocytes, and most other tissues are able to use these products and, therefore, oxidize leucine directly to CO_2. The portion of isoleucine that is converted to acetyl-CoA is also oxidized directly to CO_2. For the portion of valine and isoleucine that enters the TCA cycle as succinyl-CoA to be completely oxidized to CO_2, it must first be converted to acetyl-CoA. To form acetyl-CoA, succinyl-CoA is oxidized to malate in the TCA cycle, and malate is then converted to pyruvate by malic enzyme (malate + $NADP^+ \rightarrow$ pyruvate + NADPH + H^+) (see Fig. 40.7). Pyruvate can then be oxidized to acetyl-CoA. Alternatively, pyruvate can form alanine or lactate.

2. Conversion of Branched-Chain Amino Acids to Glutamine

The major route of valine and isoleucine catabolism in skeletal muscle is to enter the TCA cycle as succinyl-CoA and exit as α-ketoglutarate to provide the carbon skeleton for glutamine formation (see Fig. 40.7). Some of the glutamine and CO_2 that is formed from net protein degradation in skeletal muscle may also arise from the carbon skeletons of aspartate and glutamate. These amino acids are transaminated and become part of the pool of four-carbon intermediates of the TCA cycle.

Glutamine nitrogen is derived principally from the BCAAs (Fig. 40.8). The α-amino group arises from transamination reactions that form glutamate from α-ketoglutarate, and the amide nitrogen is formed from the addition of free ammonia to glutamate by glutamine synthetase. Free ammonia in skeletal muscle

---

Q When the carbon skeleton of alanine is derived from glucose, the efflux of alanine from skeletal muscle and its uptake by liver provide no net transfer of amino acid carbon to the liver for gluconeogenesis. However, some of the alanine carbon is derived from sources other than glucose. Which amino acids can provide carbon for alanine formation? (Hint: See Fig. 40.7.)

The purine nucleotide cycle is found in skeletal muscle and brain but is absent in liver and many other tissues. One of its functions in skeletal muscle is to respond to the rapid use of ATP during exercise. During exercise, the rapid hydrolysis of ATP increases AMP levels, resulting in an activation of AMP deaminase (see Fig. 40.9). As a consequence, the cellular concentration of IMP increases and ammonia is generated. IMP, like AMP, activates muscle glycogen phosphorylase during exercise (see Chapter 26). The ammonia that is generated may help to buffer the increased lactic acid production that occurs in skeletal muscles during strenuous exercise.

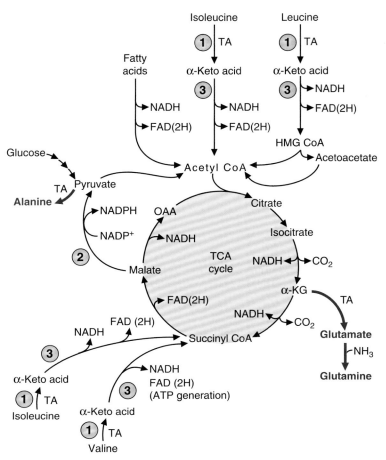

FIGURE 40.7 Metabolism of the carbon skeletons of branched-chain amino acids (BCAAs) in skeletal muscle. (*1*) The first step in the metabolism of BCAAs is transamination (TA). (*2*) Carbon from valine and isoleucine enters the tricarboxylic acid (TCA) cycle as succinyl coenzyme A (Succinyl CoA) and is converted to pyruvate by decarboxylating malate dehydrogenase (malic enzyme). (*3*) The oxidative pathways generate reduced nicotinamide adenine dinucleotide (NADH) and reduced flavin adenine dinucleotide (FAD[2H]) even before the carbon skeleton enters the TCA cycle. The rate-limiting enzyme in the oxidative pathways is the α-keto acid dehydrogenase complex. The carbon skeleton also can be converted to glutamate and alanine, shown in *red*. α-*KG*, α-ketoglutarate; *HMG CoA*, hydroxymethylglutaryl coenzyme A; *OAA*, oxaloacetate.

Some of the alanine released from skeletal muscle is derived directly from protein degradation. The carbon skeletons of valine, isoleucine, aspartate, and glutamate, which are converted to malate and oxaloacetate in the TCA cycle, can be converted to pyruvate and subsequently transaminated to alanine. The extent to which these amino acids contribute carbon to alanine efflux differs between different types of muscles in the human. These amino acids also may contribute to alanine efflux from the gut.

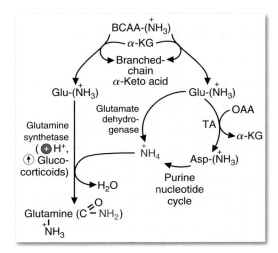

FIGURE 40.8 Formation of glutamine from the amino groups of branched-chain amino acids (BCAAs). The BCAAs are first transaminated with α-ketoglutarate to form glutamate and the branched-chain α-keto acids. The glutamate nitrogen can then follow either of two paths leading to glutamine formation. α-*KG*, α-ketoglutarate; *OAA*, oxaloacetate; *TA*, transamination.

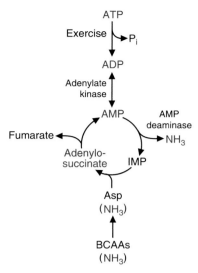

FIGURE 40.9 Purine nucleotide cycle. In skeletal muscle, the purine nucleotide cycle can convert the amino groups of the branched-chain amino acids (BCAAs) to NH₃, which is incorporated into glutamine. Compare this to Figure 39.12, in which the fumarate generated is used in an anaplerotic role in the muscle. *ADP*, adenosine diphosphate; *AMP*, adenosine monophosphate; *ATP*, adenosine triphosphate; *IMP*, inosine monophosphate; *Pi*, inorganic phosphate.

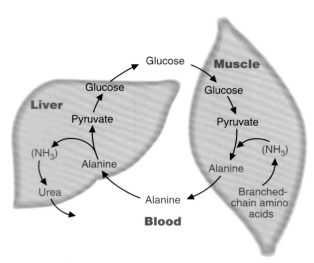

FIGURE 40.10 Glucose–alanine cycle. The pathway for transfer of the amino groups from branched-chain amino acids in skeletal muscle to urea in the liver is shown in *red*.

arises principally from the deamination of glutamate by glutamate dehydrogenase or from the purine nucleotide cycle.

In the purine nucleotide cycle (Fig. 40.9), the deamination of AMP to inosine monophosphate (IMP) releases NH_4^+. AMP is resynthesized with amino groups provided from aspartate. The aspartate amino groups can arise from the BCAAs through transamination reactions. The fumarate can be used to replenish TCA-cycle intermediates (see Fig. 39.12).

3. The Glucose–Alanine Cycle

The nitrogen arising from the oxidation of BCAAs in skeletal muscle can also be transferred back to the liver as alanine in the glucose–alanine cycle (Fig. 40.10; see also Fig. 36.8). The amino group of the BCAAs is first transferred to α-ketoglutarate to form glutamate and then transferred to pyruvate to form alanine by sequential transamination reactions. The pyruvate arises principally from glucose via the glycolytic pathway. The alanine released from skeletal muscle is taken up principally by the liver, where the amino group is incorporated into urea, and the carbon skeleton can be converted back to glucose through gluconeogenesis. Although the amount of alanine formed varies with dietary intake and physiologic state, the transport of nitrogen from skeletal muscle to liver as alanine occurs almost continuously throughout our daily fasting–feeding cycle.

C. The Gut

Amino acids are an important fuel for the intestinal mucosal cells after a protein-containing meal and in catabolic states such as fasting or surgical trauma (Fig. 40.11). During fasting, glutamine is one of the major amino acids used by the gut. The principal fates of glutamine carbon in the gut are oxidation to CO_2 and conversion to the carbon skeletons of lactate, citrulline, and ornithine. The gut also oxidizes BCAAs. Nitrogen derived from amino acid degradation is converted to citrulline, alanine, NH_4^+, and other compounds that are released into the blood and taken up by the liver. Although most of the carbon in this alanine is derived from glucose, the oxidation of glucose to CO_2 is not a major fuel pathway for the gut. Fatty acids are also not a significant source of fuel for the intestinal mucosal cells, although they do use ketone bodies.

Even though the liver is the organ that generates urea, the intestine also contains the enzymes for the urea cycle (including carbamoyl synthetase I). However, within the intestine, the V_{max} values for argininosuccinate synthetase and argininosuccinate lyase are very low, suggesting that the primary role of the urea-cycle enzymes in the

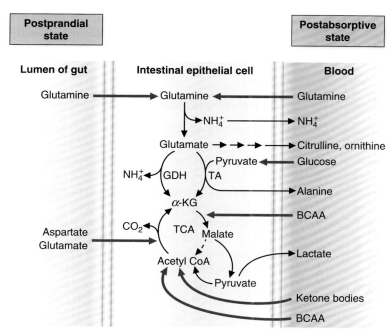

FIGURE 40.11   Amino acid metabolism in the gut. The pathways of glutamine metabolism in the gut are the same whether it is supplied by the diet (postprandial state) or from the blood (postabsorptive state). Cells of the gut also metabolize aspartate, glutamate, and branched-chain amino acids (BCAAs). Glucose is converted principally to the carbon skeleton of alanine. *Acetyl CoA*, acetyl coenzyme A; α-*KG*, α-ketoglutarate; *GDH*, glutamate dehydrogenase; *TA*, transaminase; *TCA*, tricarboxylic acid.

gut is to produce citrulline from the carbons of glutamine (glutamine → glutamate → glutamate semialdehyde → ornithine → citrulline). The citrulline is released in the circulation for use by the liver.

After a protein meal, dietary glutamine is a major fuel for the gut, and the products of glutamine metabolism are similar to those seen in the postabsorptive state. The gut also uses dietary aspartate and glutamate, which enter the TCA cycle. Colonocytes (the cells of the colon) also use short-chain fatty acids derived from bacterial action in the lumen.

The importance of the gut in whole-body nitrogen metabolism arises from the high rate of division and death of intestinal mucosal cells and the need to continuously provide these cells with amino acids to sustain the high rates of protein synthesis needed for cellular division. Not only are these cells important for the uptake of nutrients, they maintain a barrier against invading bacteria from the gut lumen and are, therefore, part of our passive defense system. As a result of these important functions, the intestinal mucosal cells are supplied with the amino acids required for protein synthesis and fuel oxidation at the expense of the more expendable skeletal muscle protein. However, glutamine use by the gut is diminished by metabolic acidosis compared with the postabsorptive or postprandial state. During metabolic acidosis, the uptake of glutamine by the kidney is increased and blood glutamine levels decrease. As a consequence, the gut takes up less glutamine.

D. The Liver

The liver is the major site of amino acid metabolism. It is the major site of amino acid catabolism and converts most of the carbon in amino acids to intermediates of the TCA cycle or the glycolytic pathway (which can be converted to glucose or oxidized to CO_2), or to acetyl-CoA and ketone bodies. The liver is also the major site for urea synthesis. It can take up both glutamine and alanine and convert the nitrogen to urea for disposal (see Chapter 36). Other pathways in the liver give it an unusually high amino acid requirement. The liver synthesizes plasma proteins, such as serum albumin, transferrin, and the proteins of the blood-coagulation cascade. It is a major site for the synthesis of nonessential amino acids, the conjugation of xenobiotic compounds with glycine, the synthesis of heme and purine nucleotides, and the synthesis of glutathione.

E. Brain and Nervous Tissue

1. The Amino Acid Pool and Neurotransmitter Synthesis

A major function of amino acid metabolism in neural tissue is the synthesis of neurotransmitters. More than 40 compounds are believed to function as neurotransmitters, and all of these contain nitrogen derived from precursor amino acids. They include amino acids, which are themselves neurotransmitters (e.g., glutamate, glycine); the catecholamines derived from tyrosine (dopamine, epinephrine, and norepinephrine); serotonin (derived from tryptophan); γ-aminobutyric acid (GABA; derived from glutamate); acetylcholine (derived from choline synthesized in the liver and acetyl-CoA); and many peptides. In general, neurotransmitters are formed in the presynaptic terminals of axons and stored in vesicles until they are released by a transient change in electrochemical potential along the axon. Subsequent catabolism of some of the neurotransmitters results in the formation of a urinary excretion product. The rapid metabolism of neurotransmitters requires the continuous availability of a precursor pool of amino acids for de novo neurotransmitter synthesis (see Chapter 46).

2. Metabolism of Glutamine in the Brain

The brain is a net glutamine producer owing principally to the presence of glutamine synthetase in astroglial cells, a supporting cell type of the brain (see Chapter 46). Glutamate and aspartate are synthesized in these cells, using amino groups donated by the BCAAs (principally valine) and TCA-cycle intermediates formed from glucose and from the carbon skeletons of BCAAs (Fig. 40.12). The glutamate is converted to glutamine by glutamine synthetase, which incorporates NH_4^+ released from deamination of amino acids and deamination of AMP in the purine nucleotide cycle in the brain. This glutamine may efflux from the brain, carrying excess NH_4^+ into the blood, or serve as a precursor of glutamate in neuronal cells.

Glutamine synthesized in the astroglial cells is a precursor of glutamate (an excitatory neurotransmitter) and GABA (an inhibitory neurotransmitter) in the neuronal cells (see Fig. 40.12). It is converted to glutamate by a neuronal glutaminase isozyme. In GABAergic neurons, glutamate is then decarboxylated to GABA, which is released during excitation of the neuron. GABA is one of the neurotransmitters that is recycled; a transaminase converts it to succinaldehyde, which is then oxidized to succinate. Succinate enters the TCA cycle.

 During hyperammonemia, ammonia (NH_3) can diffuse into the brain from the blood. The ammonia is able to inhibit the neural isozyme of glutaminase, thereby decreasing additional ammonia formation in the brain and inhibiting the formation of glutamate and its subsequent metabolism to GABA. This effect of ammonia might contribute to the lethargy associated with the hyperammonemia found in patients with hepatic disease.

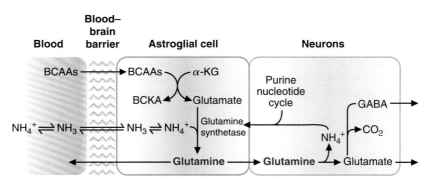

FIGURE 40.12 Role of glutamine in the brain. Glutamine serves as a nitrogen transporter in the brain for the synthesis of many different neurotransmitters. Different neurons convert glutamine to γ-aminobutyric acid (GABA) or to glutamate. Glutamine also transports excess NH_4^+ from the brain into the blood. *α-KG*, α-ketoglutarate; *BCAAs*, branched-chain amino acids; *BCKA*, branched-chain α-keto acids.

III. Changes in Amino Acid Metabolism with Dietary and Physiologic State

The rate and pattern of amino acid use by different tissues change with dietary and physiologic state. Two such states, the postprandial period following a high-protein meal and the hypercatabolic state produced by sepsis or surgical trauma, differ from the postabsorptive state with respect to the availability of amino acids and other fuels and the levels of different hormones in the blood. As a result, the pattern of amino acid use is somewhat different.

A. High-Protein Meal

After the ingestion of a high-protein meal, the gut and the liver use most of the absorbed amino acids (Fig. 40.13). Glutamate and aspartate are used as fuels by the gut, and very little enters the portal vein. The gut also may use some BCAAs. The liver takes up 60% to 70% of the amino acids present in the portal vein. These amino acids, for the most part, are converted to glucose in the gluconeogenic pathway.

After a pure protein meal, the increased levels of dietary amino acids reaching the pancreas stimulate the release of glucagon above fasting levels, thereby increasing amino acid uptake into the liver and stimulating gluconeogenesis. Insulin release is also stimulated but not nearly to the levels found after a high-carbohydrate meal. In general, the insulin released after a high-protein meal is sufficiently high that the uptake of BCAAs into skeletal muscle and net protein synthesis is stimulated, but gluconeogenesis in the liver is not inhibited. The higher the carbohydrate content of the meal, the higher is the insulin/glucagon ratio and the greater the shift of amino acids away from gluconeogenesis into biosynthetic pathways in the liver, such as the synthesis of plasma proteins.

Most of the amino acid nitrogen entering the peripheral circulation after a high-protein meal or a mixed meal is present as BCAAs. Because the liver has low levels of transaminases for these amino acids, it cannot oxidize them to a significant extent, and they enter the systemic circulation. The BCAAs are slowly taken up by

 The levels of transthyretin (also known as prealbumin and binds to vitamin A and thyroid hormones in the blood) and serum albumin in the blood may be used as indicators of the degree of protein malnutrition. In the absence of hepatic disease, decreased levels of these proteins in the blood indicate insufficient availability of amino acids to the liver for synthesis of serum proteins. The levels of transthyretin can be determined by immunologic means. The levels of albumin are rapidly determined using a hydrophobic dye-binding assay and determining the amount of colored dye bound to albumin. The dye that is used binds specifically to the hydrophobic pocket of albumin and not to other proteins in the serum.

 In what ways does liver metabolism after a high-protein meal resemble liver metabolism in the fasting state?

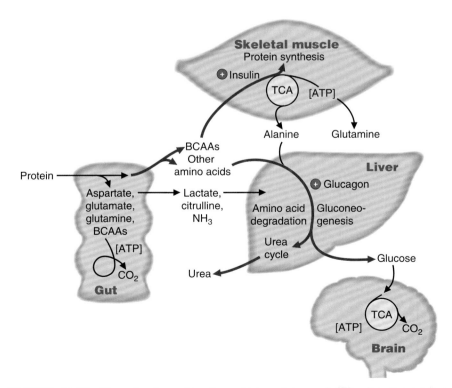

FIGURE 40.13 Flux of amino acids after a high-protein meal. *ATP*, adenosine triphosphate; *BCAAs*, branched-chain amino acids; *TCA*, tricarboxylic acid.

Both of these dietary states are characterized by an elevation of glucagon. Glucagon stimulates amino acid transport into the liver, stimulates gluconeogenesis through decreasing levels of fructose 2,6-bisphosphate, and induces the synthesis of enzymes in the urea cycle, the gluconeogenic pathway, and the pathways for degradation of some of the amino acids.

The degree of the body's hypercatabolic response depends on the severity and duration of the trauma or stress. After an uncomplicated surgical procedure in an otherwise healthy patient, the net negative nitrogen balance may be limited to about 1 week. The mild nitrogen losses are usually reversed by dietary protein supplementation as the patient recovers. With more severe traumatic injury or septic stress, the body may catabolize body protein and adipose tissue lipids for a prolonged period, and the negative nitrogen balance may not be corrected for weeks.

Katherine B.'s severe negative nitrogen balance was caused by both her malnourished state and her intraabdominal infection complicated by sepsis. The systemic and diverse responses the body makes to insults such as an acute febrile illness are termed the acute-phase response. An early event in this response is the stimulation of phagocytic activity (see Fig. 40.14). Stimulated macrophages release cytokines, which are regulatory proteins that stimulate the release of cortisol, insulin, and growth hormone. Cytokines also directly mediate the acute-phase response of the liver and skeletal muscle to sepsis.

skeletal muscle and other tissues. These peripheral nonhepatic tissues use the amino acids derived from the diet principally for net protein synthesis.

High-protein, low-carbohydrate diets are based on the premise that ingesting high-protein, low-carbohydrate meals will keep circulating insulin levels low, so that energy storage is not induced, and glucagon release will point the insulin/glucagon ratio to energy mobilization, particularly fatty acid release from the adipocyte and oxidation by the tissues. The lack of energy storage, coupled with the loss of fat, leads to weight loss.

B. Hypercatabolic States

Surgery, trauma, burns, and septic stress are examples of hypercatabolic states characterized by increased fuel use and a negative nitrogen balance. The mobilization of body protein, fat, and carbohydrate stores serves to maintain normal tissue function in the presence of a limited dietary intake as well as to support the energy and amino acid requirements for the immune response and wound healing. The negative nitrogen balance that occurs in these hypercatabolic states results from accelerated protein turnover and an increased rate of net protein degradation, primarily in skeletal muscle.

The catabolic state of sepsis (acute, generalized, febrile infection) is one of enhanced mobilization of fuels and amino acids to provide the energy and precursors required by cells of the immune system, host defense mechanisms, and wound healing. The amino acids must provide the substrates for new protein synthesis and cell division. Glucose synthesis and release are enhanced to provide fuel for these cells, and the patient may become mildly hyperglycemic.

In these hypercatabolic states, skeletal muscle protein synthesis decreases and protein degradation increases. Oxidation of BCAAs is increased and glutamine production enhanced. Amino acid uptake is diminished. Cortisol is the major hormonal mediator of these responses, although certain cytokines may also have direct effects on skeletal muscle metabolism. As occurs during fasting and metabolic acidosis, increased levels of cortisol stimulate ubiquitin-mediated proteolysis, induce the synthesis of glutamine synthetase, and enhance release of amino acids and glutamine from the muscle cells.

The amino acids released from skeletal muscle during periods of hypercatabolic stress are used in a prioritized manner, with the cellular components of the immune system receiving top priority. For example, the uptake of amino acids by the liver for the synthesis of acute-phase proteins, which are part of the immune system, is greatly increased. Conversely, during the early phase of the acute response, the synthesis of other plasma proteins (e.g., albumin) is decreased. The increased availability of amino acids and the increased cortisol levels also stimulate gluconeogenesis, thereby providing fuel for the glucose-dependent cells of the immune system (e.g., lymphocytes). An increase of urea synthesis accompanies the acceleration of amino acid degradation.

The increased efflux of glutamine from skeletal muscle during sepsis serves several functions (see Fig. 40.1). It provides the rapidly dividing cells of the immune system with an energy source. Glutamine is available as a nitrogen donor for purine synthesis, for NAD^+ synthesis (to convert nicotinic acid to nicotinamide), and for other biosynthetic functions that are essential to growth and division of the cells. Increased production of metabolic acids may accompany stress such as sepsis, so there is increased use of glutamine by the kidney.

Under the influence of elevated levels of glucocorticoids, epinephrine, and glucagon, fatty acids are mobilized from adipose tissue to provide alternate fuels for other tissues and spare glucose. Under these conditions, fatty acids are the major energy source for skeletal muscle, and glucose uptake is decreased. These changes may lead to a mild hyperglycemia.

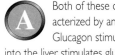
CLINICAL COMMENTS

Katherine B. The clinician can determine whether a patient such as **Katherine B.** is mounting an acute-phase response to some insult, however subtle, by determining whether several unique acute-phase proteins are being secreted by the liver. One such protein is C-reactive protein, so named because of its ability to interact with the C-polysaccharide of pneumococci. It is presently the most commonly used acute-phase protein used to show signs of an acute-phase response. Another, serum amyloid A protein, a precursor of the amyloid fibril found in secondary amyloidosis, is also elevated in patients undergoing the acute-phase response as compared with healthy individuals, although not used in practice. Other proteins normally found in the blood of healthy individuals are present in increased concentrations in patients undergoing an acute-phase response. These include haptoglobin, certain protease inhibitors, complement components, ceruloplasmin, and fibrinogen. The elevated concentration of these proteins in the blood increases the erythrocyte sedimentation rate (ESR), another laboratory measure used to show the presence of an acute-phase response.

To determine the ESR, the patient's blood is placed vertically in a small-bore glass tube. The speed with which the red blood cells sediment toward the bottom of the tube depends on what percentage of the red blood cells clump together and thereby become more dense. The degree of clumping is directly correlated with the presence of one or more of the acute-phase proteins listed previously. These proteins interfere with what is known as the *zeta-potential* of the red blood cells, which normally prevents the red blood cells from clumping. Because many different proteins can individually alter the zeta-potential, the ESR is a nonspecific test for the presence of acute inflammation.

The weight loss often noted in patients in sepsis is caused primarily by a loss of appetite resulting from the effect of certain cytokines on the medullary appetite center. Other causes include increased energy expenditure caused by fever, and enhanced muscle proteolysis.

BIOCHEMICAL COMMENTS

Amino Acid Metabolism in Trauma and Sepsis. After a catabolic insult such as injury, trauma, infection, or cancer, the interorgan flow of glutamine and fuels is altered dramatically. Teleologically, the changes in metabolism that occur give first priority to cells that are part of the immune system. Evidence suggests that the changes in glutamine and fuel metabolism are mediated by the insulin counterregulatory hormones, such as cortisol and epinephrine, and several different cytokines (see Chapter 11 for a review of cytokines). Cytokines appear to play a more important role than hormones during sepsis, although they exert their effects, in part, through hormones (Fig. 40.14). Although cytokines can be released from a variety of cells, macrophages are the principal source during trauma and sepsis.

Two cytokines that are important in sepsis are interleukin-1 (IL-1) and tumor necrosis factor (TNF). IL-1 and TNF affect amino acid metabolism both through regulation of the release of glucocorticoids and through direct effects on tissues. Although cytokines are generally considered to be paracrine, with their effects being exerted over cells in the immediate vicinity, TNF and IL-1 increase in the blood during sepsis. Other cytokines, such as interleukin-6 (IL-6), also may be involved.

During sepsis, TNF, IL-1, and possibly other cytokines, bacterial products, or mediators act on the brain to stimulate the release of glucocorticoids from the adrenal cortex (a process mediated by adrenocorticotropic hormone [ACTH]), epinephrine from the adrenal medulla, and both insulin and glucagon from the pancreas. Although insulin is elevated during sepsis, the tissues exhibit an insulin resistance that is similar to that of the patient with non–insulin-dependent diabetes mellitus, possibly resulting from the elevated levels of the insulin counterregulatory hormones (glucocorticoids, epinephrine, and glucagon). Changes in the rate of acute-phase protein synthesis are mediated, at least in part, by effects of TNF, IL-1, and IL-6 on the synthesis of groups of proteins in the liver.

The molecular mechanism whereby sepsis/trauma leads to reduced muscle protein synthesis involves, in part, mTOR (mammalian target of rapamycin; see

 Hypercatabolic states may be accompanied by varying degrees of insulin resistance caused, in part, by the release of counterregulatory hormones into the blood. Thus, patients with diabetes mellitus may require higher levels of exogenous insulin during sepsis.

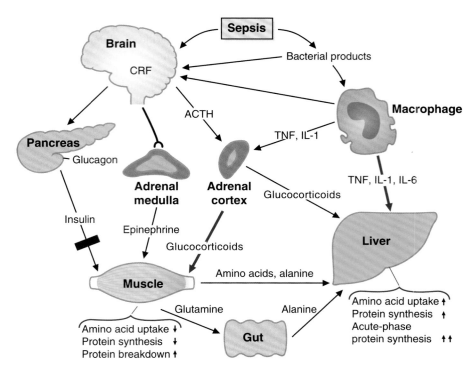

FIGURE 40.14 Cytokines and hormones mediate amino acid flux during sepsis. Bacterial products act on macrophages to stimulate the release of cytokines and on the brain to stimulate the sympathoadrenal response. The result is a stimulation of the release of the insulin counterregulatory hormones, epinephrine, glucagon, and glucocorticoids. The glucocorticoid cortisol may be the principal mediator of net muscle protein degradation during sepsis. Hepatic protein synthesis, particularly that of acute-phase proteins, is stimulated by both cortisol and cytokines. Amino acid metabolism in the gut is also probably affected by glucocorticoids and cytokines. Because of the release of the counterregulatory hormones, muscle and other tissues become resistant to insulin action, as indicated by the *bar* on the figure. *ACTH*, adrenocorticotropic hormone; *CRF*, corticotropin-releasing factor; *IL-1*, interleukin-1; *IL-6*, interleukin-6; *TNF*, tumor necrosis factor. (Adapted with permission from Fischer JE, Hasselgren PO. Cytokines and glucocorticoids in the regulation of the hepato-skeletal muscle axis in sepsis. *Am J Surg.* 1991;161:266–271.)

Chapter 34, Fig. 34.9). Sepsis reduces translational efficiency, primarily at the translation initiation step. Initiation is regulated by, and requires, specific eukaryotic initiation factors (eIFs; see Chapter 15). eIF4E is a multifactor complex required to assemble the charged initiator transfer RNA^{Met}–40S small ribosomal subunit complex onto the capped messenger RNA. The activity of eIF4E is regulated by the eIF4E-binding protein 4E-BP1. When eIF4E is bound to 4E-BP1, translation initiation is reduced. mTOR, when active, will phosphorylate 4E-BP1, causing the binding protein to dissociate from the eIF4E complex, thereby stimulating translation initiation. Sepsis and/or release of TNF-α leads to the inactivation of mTOR and reduced phosphorylation of 4E-BP1, resulting in a decrease in translation. The reduced translation, coupled with enhanced protein turnover, allows the muscle to export amino acids for use by other tissues.

KEY CONCEPTS

- The body maintains a large free amino acid pool in the blood, even during fasting, allowing tissues continuous access to these building blocks.
- Amino acids are used for gluconeogenesis by the liver, as a fuel source for the gut, and as neurotransmitter precursors in the nervous system. They are also required by all organs for protein synthesis.

- During an overnight fast, and during hypercatabolic states, degradation of labile protein (primarily from skeletal muscle) is the major source of free amino acids.
- The liver is the major site for urea synthesis. Nitrogen from other tissues travels to the liver in the form of glutamine and alanine.
- Branched-chain amino acids are oxidized primarily in the skeletal muscle.
- Glutamine in the blood serves several roles:
  - The kidney uses the ammonium ion carried by glutamine for excretion in the urine to act as a buffer against acidotic conditions.
  - The kidney and the gut use glutamine as a fuel source.
  - All tissues use glutamine for protein synthesis.
- The body can enter a catabolic state, characterized by negative nitrogen balance, under the following conditions:
  - Sepsis (the presence of various pathogenic organisms, or their toxins, in the blood or tissues)
  - Trauma
  - Injury
  - Burns
- The negative nitrogen balance results from increased net protein degradation in skeletal muscle, brought about by release of glucocorticoids. The released amino acids are used for protein synthesis and cell division in cells involved in the immune response and wound healing.
- Diseases discussed in this chapter are summarized in Table 40.3.

TABLE 40.3   Diseases Discussed in Chapter 40

DISEASE OR DISORDER	ENVIRONMENTAL OR GENETIC	COMMENTS
Catabolic state	Environmental	The body adapts to a catabolic state by degrading proteins to enhance survival. This change in metabolism is initiated through the stress response, as mediated by cortisol, epinephrine, and norepinephrine, among other signaling molecules.
Hyperammonemia	Both	Hyperammonemia can result from mutations in urea-cycle enzymes or from a failing liver as caused by a variety of conditions (one of which is alcohol abuse over many years).

REVIEW QUESTIONS—CHAPTER 40

1. Which one of the profiles indicated below would occur within 2 hours after eating a meal that was very high in protein and low in carbohydrates?

	Blood Glucagon Levels	Liver Gluconeogenesis	BCAA Oxidation in Muscle
A	↓	↓	↑
B	↑	↓	↑
C	↓	↑	↑
D	↑	↑	↑
E	↓	↓	↓
F	↑	↓	↓
G	↓	↑	↓
H	↑	↑	↓

2. The gut uses glutamine as an energy source, but it can also secrete citrulline, synthesized from the carbons of glutamine. Which one of the following compounds is an obligatory intermediate in this conversion (consider only the carbon atoms of glutamine while answering this question)?
   A. Aspartate
   B. Succinyl-CoA
   C. Glutamate
   D. Serine
   E. Fumarate

3. The signal that indicates to muscle that protein degradation needs to be initiated is which one of the following?
   A. Insulin
   B. Glucagon
   C. Epinephrine
   D. Cortisol
   E. Glucose

4. The skeletal muscles convert BCAA carbons to glutamine for export to the rest of the body. An obligatory intermediate, which carries carbons originally from the BCAAs, in the conversion of BCAAs to glutamine, is which one of the following?
   A. Urea
   B. Pyruvate
   C. Lactate
   D. Isocitrate
   E. PEP

5. An individual in sepsis will display which one of the following metabolic patterns?

	Nitrogen Balance	Gluconeogenesis	Fatty Acid Oxidation
A	Positive	↑	↓
B	Negative	↑	↑
C	Positive	↑	↓
D	Negative	↑	↓
E	Positive	↓	↑
F	Negative	↓	↓

6. Ammonia toxicity in the nervous system results, in part, from inhibition of which one of the following enzymes?
   A. Glutaminase
   B. Glutamate–α-ketoglutarate transaminase
   C. Glutamine synthetase
   D. Carbamoyl phosphate synthetase I
   E. Ornithine transcarbamoylase

7. The purine nucleotide cycle, which releases fumarate, is found primarily in which one of the following tissues?
   A. Liver
   B. Red blood cells
   C. Brain
   D. Gut
   E. Kidney

8. Which of the following occurs *primarily* in the liver? Choose the one best answer.

	Alanine Uptake	Urea Synthesis	Amino Acid Degradation	Gluconeogenesis From Amino Acid Precursors	BCAA Oxidation
A	No	Yes	No	No	No
B	Yes	Yes	Yes	Yes	Yes
C	No	No	Yes	No	No
D	Yes	Yes	No	Yes	Yes
E	No	No	No	Yes	Yes
F	Yes	Yes	Yes	Yes	No

9. The amino acid pool allows for constant substrates to be available for numerous bodily uses. Which statement below best describes this amino acid pool?
   A. Approximately 80% of the body's total protein is in the amino acid pool.
   B. Dietary proteins constitute most of the amino acid pool.
   C. The concentration of free amino acids is as rigidly controlled as blood glucose levels.
   D. The synthesis of new protein is the major use of amino acids in the amino acid pool.
   E. Changes in the rate of protein synthesis and degradation occur within seconds to minutes.

10. Which hormone(s) and action(s) are paired correctly regarding protein metabolism/catabolism? Choose the one best answer.
    A. Insulin stimulates uptake of amino acids into the liver.
    B. Glucocorticoid induces ubiquitin synthesis.
    C. Insulin induces ubiquitin-dependent proteolysis.
    D. Glucocorticoid and insulin induce gluconeogenesis.
    E. Glucagon suppresses alanine transport to the liver.

ANSWERS

1. **The answer is D.** High levels of amino acids in the blood stimulate the pancreas to release glucagon (thus, A, C, E, and G are incorrect). Insulin is also released, but the glucagon/insulin ratio is such that the liver still uses the carbons of amino acids to synthesize glucose (thus, A, E, and F are incorrect). However, the insulin levels are high enough to stimulate BCAA uptake into the muscle for oxidation (thus, E, F, G, and H are incorrect).

2. **The answer is C.** The pathway followed is glutamine to glutamate, to glutamate semialdehyde, to ornithine, and then, after condensation with carbamoyl phosphate, to citrulline. Aspartate, succinyl-CoA, serine, and fumarate are not part of this pathway.

3. **The answer is D.** Cortisol is released during fasting and times of stress, and signals muscle cells to initiate ubiquitin-mediated protein degradation. The other hormones listed do not have this effect on muscle protein metabolism. Insulin stimulates protein synthesis; glucagon has no effect on muscle because muscle has no glucagon receptors. Epinephrine initiates glycogen degradation but not protein degradation, and glucose is not a signaling molecule for muscle as it can be for the pancreas.

4. **The answer is D.** Glutamine is derived from glutamate, which is formed from α-ketoglutarate. Only isoleucine and valine can give rise to glutamine because leucine is strictly ketogenic. These amino acids give rise to succinyl-CoA, which goes around the TCA cycle to

form citrate (after condensing with acetyl-CoA), which then forms isocitrate (the correct answer), and the isocitrate is converted to α-ketoglutarate. Urea, pyruvate, PEP, and lactate are not required intermediates in the conversion of BCAA carbons to glutamine carbons.

5. **The answer is B.** An individual in sepsis will be catabolic; protein degradation exceeds protein intake (leading to negative nitrogen balance; thus, A, C, and E are incorrect). The liver is synthesizing glucose from amino acid precursors to raise blood glucose levels for the immune cells and the nervous system (thus, gluconeogenesis is active, and E and F must be incorrect). Fatty acid release and oxidation has also been stimulated to provide an energy source for the liver and skeletal muscle (indicating that C, D, and F are incorrect).

6. **The answer is A.** Elevated levels of ammonia in the nervous system inhibits the production of more ammonia by both glutaminase and glutamate dehydrogenase. This leads to high glutamine levels and low glutamate levels (because the glutamate has been converted to glutamine owing to the high ammonia levels). The high glutamine leads to an osmotic imbalance across the astrocyte membrane, leading to brain edema (swelling), and also leads to the opening of the mitochondrial permeability transition pore. The opening of this pore will lead to cell death. The low glutamate levels also interfere with glutamate acting as a neurotransmitter, as well as the synthesis of GABA, and brain signaling goes awry. Carbamoyl phosphate synthetase I and ornithine transcarbamoylase are not present in cells of the nervous system. High ammonia promotes the synthesis of glutamine and does not affect transaminase activity.

7. **The answer is C.** The purine nucleotide cycle is found in the brain and skeletal muscle but is absent in the liver and other tissues. It responds to the rapid use of ATP during exercise, which generates AMP. The AMP is deaminated to form IMP, which then reacts with aspartate (with the release of fumarate) to regenerate AMP. The fumarate can be used anaplerotically to allow the TCA cycle to operate more rapidly.

8. **The answer is F.** The liver is the major site of amino acid metabolism and degradation, urea synthesis (from the major nitrogen carriers alanine and glutamine released from muscle), and gluconeogenesis from amino acid substrates, but BCAAs are oxidized primarily in skeletal muscle and not in the liver.

9. **The answer is D.** The major use of the amino acid pool is to produce new proteins. Every day, 300 to 600 g of new proteins are produced, with only about 100 g originating from the diet. The rest are derived from the turnover of existing proteins, the majority of which are found in skeletal muscle (~80% of body's total protein is in skeletal muscle). The concentration of free amino acids is not as tightly controlled as blood glucose levels because changes in protein synthesis and degradation occur over a time span of hours, not minutes. Because the amino acid pool consists of free amino acids, the amino acids within proteins do not count as an amino acid pool.

10. **The answer is B.** Glucocorticoids induce ubiquitin synthesis and increase ubiquitin-dependent proteolysis in order to provide substrates for liver gluconeogenesis. Alanine transport into the liver is particularly enhanced by glucagon (again, to bring in carbons for gluconeogenesis). Glucagon and glucocorticoid stimulate amino acid uptake into the liver, gluconeogenesis, and ureagenesis. Insulin has the opposite effects of glucagon and glucocorticoids, which are considered insulin counterregulatory hormones. Insulin does not stimulate amino acid uptake into the liver (but it does in the muscle).

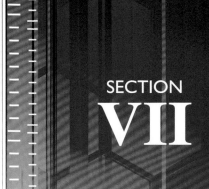

Tissue Metabolism

Although many of the pathways described previously are present in all tissues of the body, many tissues also carry out specialized functions and contain unique biochemical pathways. This section describes several such tissues and, in some cases, how the tissues interact with the rest of the body to coordinate their functions. Previous chapters have focused primarily on insulin and glucagon as the major mediators for regulating metabolic pathways; however, a large number of other hormones also regulate the storage and use of metabolic fuels (see Chapter 41). These hormones primarily counteract the effects of insulin and are called *counterregulatory hormones*. They include growth hormone; thyroid hormone; glucocorticoids, such as cortisol; small peptides, such as the somatostatins; and small molecules, such as the catecholamines. Growth hormone works, in part, by inducing the synthesis of the insulinlike growth factors. These hormones can exert their effects rapidly (through covalent modification of selected enzymes) or long-term (through alterations in the rate of synthesis of selected enzymes). The interplay of these hormones with insulin and glucagon is discussed, as are the synthesis, secretion, and conditions leading to secretion of each hormone.

The proteins and cells in the blood form their own tissue system (see Chapter 42). All blood cells are derived from a common precursor, the stem cell, in the bone marrow. Different cytokine signals trigger differentiation of a particular blood cell lineage. For example, when oxygen supply to the tissues is decreased, the kidney responds by releasing erythropoietin. This hormone specifically stimulates the production of red blood cells.

Red blood cells have limited metabolic functions, owing to their lack of internal organelles. Their main function is to deliver oxygen to the tissues through the binding of oxygen to hemoglobin. When the number of red blood cells is decreased, that, by definition, represents anemia. This can be attributable to many causes, including nutritional deficiencies or mutations (hereditary anemias). The morphology of the red blood cell can sometimes aid in distinguishing the various types of anemia.

Red blood cell metabolism is geared toward preserving the ability of these cells to transport oxygen, as well as to regulate oxygen binding to hemoglobin. Glycolysis provides energy and reduced nicotinamide adenine dinucleotide (NADH) to protect the oxidation state of the heme-bound iron. The hexose monophosphate shunt pathway generates NADPH to protect red blood cell membranes from oxidation. Heme synthesis, which uses succinyl coenzyme A (succinyl-CoA) and glycine for all of the carbon and nitrogen atoms in the structure, occurs in the precursors of red blood cells. Inherited defects in heme synthesis lead to a class of diseases known as the *porphyrias*. Because red blood cells normally pass through the very narrow capillaries, their membranes must be easily deformable. This deformability is, in part, attributable to the complex cytoskeletal structure that surrounds the erythrocyte. Mutations in these structural proteins can lead to less deformable cells, which are more easily lysed as they circulate in the bloodstream. This, in turn, can result in hemolytic anemia.

Among other functions, the hematologic system is responsible for hemostasis as well as for maintaining a constant blood volume (see Chapter 43). A tear in the wall of a vessel can lead to blood loss, which, when extensive, can be fatal. Repairing vessel damage, whether internal or external, is accomplished by a complicated series of zymogen activations of circulating blood proteins resulting in the formation of a fibrin clot (the coagulation cascade). Platelets play a critical role in hemostasis not only through their release of procoagulants but through their ability to form aggregates within the thrombus (clot) as well. Clots function as a plug, allowing defects or rents in vessel walls to repair and thereby preventing further blood loss. Conversely, inappropriate or accelerated clot formation in the lumen of vessels that supply blood to vital organs or tissues can cause an intraluminal obstruction to flow that may lead to an acute cerebral or myocardial infarction. Because clotting must be tightly controlled, intricate mechanisms exist that regulate this important hematologic function.

The liver is an altruistic organ that provides multiple services for other tissues (see Chapter 44). It supplies glucose and ketone bodies to the rest of the body when fuel stores are limited. It disposes of ammonia as urea when amino acid degradation occurs. It is the site of detoxification of xenobiotics, and it synthesizes many of the proteins found in the blood. The liver synthesizes triacylglycerols and cholesterol and distributes them to other tissues in the form of very-low-density lipoprotein (VLDL). The liver also synthesizes bile acids for fat digestion in the intestine. The liver recycles cholesterol and triglyceride through its uptake of intermediate-density lipoprotein (IDL), chylomicron and VLDL remnants, and low-density lipoprotein (LDL) particles. Because of its protective nature and its strategic location between the gut and the systemic circulation, the liver has "first crack" at all compounds that enter the blood through the enterohepatic circulation. Thus, xenobiotic compounds can be detoxified as they enter the liver, before they have a chance to reach other tissues.

Muscle cells contain unique pathways that allow them to store energy as creatine phosphate and to regulate closely their use of fatty acids as an energy source (see Chapter 45). The adenosine monophosphate (AMP)-activated protein kinase is an important regulator of muscle energy metabolism. Muscle is comprised of different types of contractile fibers that derive their energy from different sources. For example, the slow-twitch type I fibers use oxidative energy pathways, whereas the type II fast-twitch fibers use the glycolytic pathway for their energy requirements.

The nervous system consists of various cell types that are functionally interconnected to allow efficient signal transmission throughout the system (see Chapter 46). The cells of the central nervous system are protected from potentially toxic compounds by the blood–brain barrier, which restricts entry of potentially toxic compounds into the nervous system (ammonia, however, is a notable exception). The brain cells communicate with each other and with other organs through the synthesis of neurotransmitters and neuropeptides. Many of the neurotransmitters are derived from amino acids, most of which are synthesized within the nerve cells. Because the pathways of amino acid and neurotransmitter biosynthesis require cofactors (such as pyridoxal phosphate, thiamine pyrophosphate, and vitamin B_{12}), deficiencies of these cofactors can lead to neuropathies (dysfunction of specific neurons in the nervous system).

Because of the restrictions imposed by the blood–brain barrier, the brain also must synthesize its own lipids. An adequate supply of lipids is vital to the central nervous system because lipids are constituents of the myelin sheath that surrounds the neurons and allows them to conduct impulses normally. The neurodegenerative disorders, such as multiple sclerosis, are a consequence of varying degrees of demyelination of the neurons.

Connective tissue, which consists primarily of fibroblasts, produces extracellular matrix materials that surround cells and tissues, determining their appropriate position within the organ (see Chapter 47). These materials include structural proteins (collagen and elastin), adhesive proteins (fibronectin), and glycosaminoglycans (heparan sulfate, chondroitin sulfate). The unique structures of the proteins and carbohydrates in the extracellular matrix allow tissues and organs to carry out their many functions. Loss of these supportive and barrier functions of connective tissue sometimes leads to significant clinical consequences, such as those that result from the microvascular alterations that lead to blindness, renal failure, or peripheral neuropathies in patients with diabetes mellitus.

Actions of Hormones that Regulate Fuel Metabolism

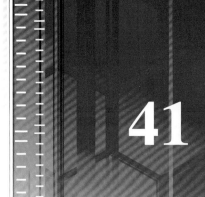

41

Many hormones affect fuel metabolism, including those that regulate appetite as well as those that influence absorption, transport, and oxidation of foodstuffs. The major hormones that influence nutrient metabolism and their actions on muscle, liver, and adipose tissue are listed in Table 41.1.

Insulin is the major **anabolic hormone**. It promotes the **storage** of **nutrients** as **glycogen** in liver and muscle and as **triacylglycerols** in adipose tissue. It also stimulates the **synthesis** of **proteins** in tissues such as muscle. At the same time, insulin acts to inhibit fuel mobilization.

Glucagon is the major **counterregulatory** hormone. The term *counterregulatory* means that its actions are generally opposed to those of insulin (**contrainsular**). The major action of glucagon is to **mobilize fuel reserves** by stimulating **glycogenolysis** and **gluconeogenesis**. These actions ensure that glucose will be available to glucose-dependent tissues between meals.

Epinephrine, **norepinephrine**, **cortisol**, **somatostatin**, and **growth hormone** also have contrainsular activity. **Thyroid hormone** also must be classified as an insulin-counterregulatory hormone because it **increases** the rate of **fuel consumption** and also increases the sensitivity of the target cells to other insulin-counterregulatory hormones.

Insulin and the counterregulatory hormones exert two types of metabolic regulation (see Chapter 19). The first type of control occurs within minutes to hours of the hormone–receptor interaction and usually results from changes in the catalytic activity or kinetics of key preexisting enzymes, caused by phosphorylation or dephosphorylation of these enzymes. The second type of control involves regulation of the **synthesis of key enzymes** by mechanisms that stimulate or inhibit transcription and translation of messenger RNA (mRNA). These processes are slow and require hours to days.

TABLE 41.1 Major Hormones that Regulate Fuel Metabolism

HORMONES	MUSCLE			GLUCOSE OUTPUT	LIVER					ADIPOSE TISSUE	
	GLUCOSE UPTAKE	GLUCOSE USE	PROTEIN SYNTHESIS		KETO-GENESIS	GLUCONEO-GENESIS	GLYCO-GENOLYSIS	GLYCO-GENESIS	PROTEIN SYNTHESIS	FAT SYNTHESIS	TISSUE LIPOLYSIS
Anabolic Hormones											
Insulin	⇈	⇈	⇈	⇊	⇊	⇊	⇊	↑	↑	⇈	⇊
Counterregulatory Hormones[a]											
Glucagon	–	–	–	⇈	↑	↑	⇈	↓	–	–	↑ (at large doses)
Epinephrine and norepinephrine	–	↓	–	⇈	–	↑	⇈ (initial)	↓	–	–	⇈
Glucocorticoid	↓	↓	↓	↑	↑	↑ (mainly permissive)	–	↑	↑	–	↑ (permissive)
Growth hormone	↓ (weakly)	↓ (weakly)	↑	↑	↑	↑	–	–	↑	–	↑ (mainly permissive)
Thyroid hormone	–	↑	↑	↑	↑	↑	↑	–	–	–	↑ (permissive)
Somatostatin[b]	–	–	–	–	–	–	–	–	–	–	–

⇈, pronounced increased effect; ↑, moderate increased effect; ↓, moderate decreased effect; –, no effect.

[a] Hormones with actions that are generally opposed to those of insulin.

[b] Somatostatin's effects on metabolism are indirect via suppression of secretion of insulin, glucagon, growth hormone, and thyroid hormone and by effects on gastric acid secretion, gastric emptying time, and pancreatic exocrine secretion (see text).

THE WAITING ROOM

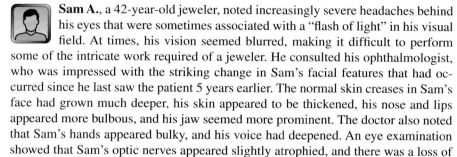

Otto S., now a third-year medical student, was assigned to do a history and physical examination on a newly admitted 47-year-old patient named **Chet S.** Mr. S. had consulted his physician for increasing weakness and fatigue and was found to have a severely elevated serum glucose level. While he was examining the patient, Otto noted marked redness of Mr. S.'s facial skin as well as reddish-purple stripes (striae) in the skin of his lower abdomen and thighs. The patient's body fat was unusually distributed in that it appeared to be excessively deposited centrally in his face, neck, upper back, chest, and abdomen, whereas the distal portions of his arms and legs appeared to be almost devoid of fat. Mr. S.'s skin appeared thinned and large bruises were present over many areas of his body, for which Mr. S. had no explanation. The neurologic examination showed severe muscle weakness, especially in the proximal arms and legs, where the muscles seemed to have atrophied.

Sam A., a 42-year-old jeweler, noted increasingly severe headaches behind his eyes that were sometimes associated with a "flash of light" in his visual field. At times, his vision seemed blurred, making it difficult to perform some of the intricate work required of a jeweler. He consulted his ophthalmologist, who was impressed with the striking change in Sam's facial features that had occurred since he last saw the patient 5 years earlier. The normal skin creases in Sam's face had grown much deeper, his skin appeared to be thickened, his nose and lips appeared more bulbous, and his jaw seemed more prominent. The doctor also noted that Sam's hands appeared bulky, and his voice had deepened. An eye examination showed that Sam's optic nerves appeared slightly atrophied, and there was a loss of the upper outer quadrants of his visual fields.

I. Physiologic Effects of Insulin and Amylin

The effects of insulin on fuel metabolism and substrate flux were considered in many of the earlier chapters of this book, particularly in Chapter 19. Insulin stimulates the storage of glycogen in liver and muscle and the synthesis of fatty acids and triacylglycerols and their storage in adipose tissue. In addition, insulin stimulates the synthesis in various tissues of >50 proteins, some of which contribute to the growth of the organism. In fact, it is difficult to separate the effects of insulin on cell growth from those of a family of proteins known as the somatomedins or the insulinlike growth factors 1 and 2 (IGF-1 and IGF-2) (see Section III.B.6).

Finally, insulin has paracrine actions within the pancreatic islet cells. When insulin is released from the β-cells, it suppresses glucagon release from the α-cells.

Amylin is a 37-amino-acid peptide that is synthesized in the β-cells of the pancreas and is cosecreted with insulin when blood glucose levels rise. Amylin has been demonstrated to suppress the postprandial glucagon secretion (thereby enhancing the effect of insulin by keeping the insulin:glucagon ratio high), to slow gastric emptying, which decreases the rate at which food reaches the intestine, and the bloodstream (thereby blunting a large increase in blood nutrient levels immediately after a meal), and to reduce food intake (and thereby body weight). All of amylin's actions are geared toward reducing blood glucose levels, just as insulin does when it is released from the pancreas. Individuals with type 1 diabetes, who experience destruction of the β-cells of the pancreas, lose the ability to secrete both insulin and amylin in response to an increase in blood nutrient levels, and this may partially explain why insulin therapy for individuals with type 1 diabetes often is inadequate in preventing the long-term complications of diabetes.

II. Physiologic Effects of Glucagon

Glucagon is one of several counterregulatory (contrainsular) hormones. It is synthesized as part of a large precursor protein called *proglucagon*. Proglucagon is produced in the α-cells of the islets of Langerhans in the pancreas and in the L-cells

The measurement of hormone levels in blood is best performed using immunologic reagents that specifically recognize the hormone being measured. Such techniques are further described in the "Biochemical Comments" in this chapter.

Pramlintide is an amylin analog that is used to treat individuals with either type 1 or type 2 diabetes. Pramlintide will bind to amylin receptors and elicit amylinlike responses. It can cause nausea in almost half of patients; less commonly, it causes vomiting. This can lead to discontinuing the drug.

of the intestine. It contains several peptides linked in tandem: glicentin-related peptide, glucagon, glucagon-related peptide 1 (GLP-1), and glucagon-related peptide 2 (GLP-2). Proteolytic cleavage of proglucagon releases various combinations of its constituent peptides. Glucagon is cleaved from proglucagon in the pancreas and constitutes 30% to 40% of the immunoreactive glucagon in the blood. The remaining immunoreactivity is caused by other cleavage products of proglucagon released from the pancreas and the intestine. Pancreatic glucagon has a plasma half-life of 3 to 6 minutes and is removed mainly by the liver and kidney.

Glucagon promotes glycogenolysis, gluconeogenesis, and ketogenesis by stimulating the generation of cyclic adenosine monophosphate (cAMP) in target cells. The liver is the major target organ for glucagon, in part because the concentrations of this hormone bathing the liver cells in the portal blood are higher than in the peripheral circulation. Levels of glucagon in the portal vein may reach concentrations as high as 500 pg/mL.

Finally, glucagon stimulates insulin release from the β-cells of the pancreas. Whether this is a paracrine effect or an endocrine effect has not been established. The pattern of blood flow in the pancreatic islet cells is believed to bathe the β-cells first and then the α-cells. Therefore, the β-cells may influence α-cell function by an endocrine mechanism, whereas the influence of α-cell hormone on β-cell function is more likely to be paracrine. The glucagon-stimulated insulin release is most likely necessary to maintain blood glucose levels in the physiologic range.

III. Physiologic Effects of Other Counterregulatory Hormones

A. Somatostatin

1. Biochemistry

Preprosomatostatin, a 116-amino-acid peptide, is encoded by a gene located on the long arm of chromosome 3. Somatostatin (SS-14), a cyclic peptide with a molecular weight of 1,600 Da, is produced from the 14 amino acids at the C terminus of this precursor molecule. SS-14 was first isolated from the hypothalamus and named for its ability to inhibit the release of growth hormone (GH, somatotropin) from the anterior pituitary. It also inhibits the release of insulin. In addition to the hypothalamus, somatostatin is also secreted from the D-cells (δ-cells) of the pancreatic islets, many areas of the central nervous system (CNS) outside of the hypothalamus, and gastric and duodenal mucosal cells. SS-14 predominates in the CNS and is the sole form secreted by the δ-cells of the pancreas. In the gut, however, prosomatostatin (SS-28), which has 14 additional amino acids extending from the C-terminal portion of the precursor, makes up 70% to 75% of the immunoreactivity (the amount of hormone that reacts with antibodies to SS-14). The prohormone SS-28 is 7 to 10 times more potent in inhibiting the release of GH and insulin than is SS-14.

2. Secretion of Somatostatin

The secretagogues for somatostatin are similar to those that cause secretion of insulin. The metabolites that increase somatostatin release include glucose, arginine, and leucine. The hormones that stimulate somatostatin secretion include glucagon, vasoactive intestinal polypeptide (VIP), and cholecystokinin (CCK). Insulin, however, does not influence somatostatin secretion directly.

3. Physiologic Effects of Somatostatin

Five somatostatin receptors have been identified and characterized, all of which are members of the G-protein–coupled receptor superfamily. Four of the five receptors do not distinguish between SS-14 and SS-28. Somatostatin binds to its plasma membrane receptors on target cells. These "activated" receptors interact with a variety of intracellular signaling pathways, depending on the cell type expressing the receptor

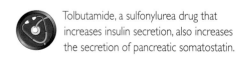 Tolbutamide, a sulfonylurea drug that increases insulin secretion, also increases the secretion of pancreatic somatostatin.

and which somatostatin receptor is being expressed. These pathways include inactivation of adenylate cyclase (via an inhibitory G-protein), regulation of phosphotyrosine phosphatases and mitogen-activated protein (MAP) kinases, and alterations of intracellular ion concentrations (calcium and potassium). The inactivation of adenylate cyclases reduces the production of cAMP, and protein kinase A is not activated. This inhibitory effect suppresses secretion of GH and thyroid-stimulating hormone (TSH) from the anterior pituitary gland as well as the secretion of insulin and glucagon from the pancreatic islets. If one were to summarize the action of somatostatin in one phrase, it would be "somatostatin inhibits the secretion of many other hormones." As such, it acts to regulate the effects of those other hormones. In addition to these effects on hormones that regulate fuel metabolism, somatostatin also reduces nutrient absorption from the gut by prolonging gastric emptying time (through a decrease in the secretion of gastrin, which reduces gastric acid secretion), by diminishing pancreatic exocrine secretions (i.e., digestive enzymes, bicarbonate, and water), and by decreasing visceral blood flow. Thus, somatostatin exerts a broad, albeit indirect, influence on nutrient absorption and, therefore, on the use of fuels.

Somatostatin and its synthetic analogs are used clinically to treat a variety of secretory neoplasms such as GH-secreting tumors of the pituitary. Such tumors can cause gigantism if GH is secreted in excess before the closure of the growth centers of the ends of long bones, or acromegaly if excess GH is chronically secreted after the closure of these centers (as in **Sam A.**).

B. Growth Hormone

1. Biochemistry

GH is a polypeptide that, as its name implies, stimulates growth. Many of its effects are mediated by IGFs, also known as *somatomedins*, that are produced by cells in response to the binding of GH to its cell membrane receptors (see Section III.B.6). However, GH also has direct effects on fuel metabolism.

Human GH is a water-soluble 22-kDa polypeptide with a plasma half-life of 20 to 50 minutes. It is composed of a single chain of 191 amino acids having two intramolecular disulfide bonds (Fig. 41.1). The gene for GH is located on chromosome 17. It is secreted by the somatotroph cells (the cells that synthesize and release GH) in the lateral areas of the anterior pituitary. GH is structurally related to human prolactin and to human chorionic somatomammotropin (hCS) from the placenta, a polypeptide that stimulates growth of the developing fetus. Yet, the hCS peptide has only 0.1% of the growth-inducing potency of GH. GH is the most abundant trophic hormone in the anterior pituitary, being present in concentrations of 5 to 15 mg per gram of tissue. The other anterior pituitary hormones are present in quantities of micrograms per gram of tissue.

 In addition to its effects on normal GH secretion, somatostatin also suppresses the pathologic increase in GH that occurs in acromegaly (caused by a GH-secreting pituitary tumor), diabetes mellitus, and carcinoid tumors (tumors that secrete serotonin). Somatostatin also suppresses the basal secretion of TSH, TRH, insulin, and glucagon. The hormone also has a suppressive effect on a wide variety of nonendocrine secretions.

The major limitation in the clinical use of native somatostatin is its short half-life of <3 minutes in the circulation. Analogs of native somatostatin, however, have been developed that are resistant to degradation and, therefore, have a longer half-life. One such analog is octreotide, an octapeptide variant of somatostatin with a half-life of approximately 110 minutes.

 A magnetic resonance imaging (MRI) scan of **Sam A.'s** brain showed a macroadenoma (a tumor >10 mm in diameter) in the pituitary gland, with superior extension that compressed the optic nerve as it crossed above the sella turcica, causing his visual problems. The skeletal and visceral changes noted by the ophthalmologist are characteristic of patients with acromegaly who have chronically elevated serum levels of GH and IGF-1.

Therapy for acromegaly caused by a GH-secreting tumor of the anterior pituitary gland includes surgery if the mass is amenable or, if not amendable to surgery, lifelong medical therapy. Medical therapy includes a somatostatin analog, such as octreotide, or a dopamine agonist that inhibits the secretion of GH, such as cabergoline. If a somatostatin analog is not tolerated or is not successful, a GH-receptor antagonist such as pegvisomant can be used. Another therapeutic option is stereotactic radiation therapy if other treatments are not successful. If the excessive secretion of GH is controlled successfully, some of the visceral or soft-tissue changes of acromegaly may slowly subside to varying degrees. The skeletal changes, however, cannot be reversed.

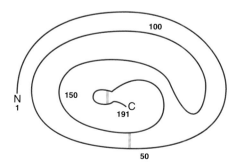

Human growth hormone

FIGURE 41.1   Structure of human growth hormone. (From Murray RK, Granner DK, Mayes PA, Rodwey VW. *Harper's Biochemistry*. 23rd ed. Stamford, CT: Appleton & Lange; 1993:502.)

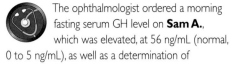

The ophthalmologist ordered a morning fasting serum GH level on **Sam A.**, which was elevated, at 56 ng/mL (normal, 0 to 5 ng/mL), as well as a determination of circulating IGF-1 levels.

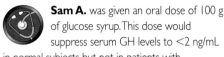

Sam A. was given an oral dose of 100 g of glucose syrup. This dose would suppress serum GH levels to <2 ng/mL in normal subjects but not in patients with acromegaly who have an autonomously secreting pituitary tumor making GH. Because Sam's serum GH level was 41 ng/mL after the oral glucose load, a diagnosis of acromegaly was made. The patient was referred to an endocrinologist for further evaluation.

GH stimulates *IGF-1* gene expression not only in the liver but in several extrahepatic tissues as well. In people with acromegaly, rising levels of IGF-1 cause a gradual generalized increase in skeletal, muscular, and visceral growth. As a consequence, a diffuse increase occurs in the bulk of all tissues (*megaly* means enlargement) especially in the *acral* (most peripheral) tissues of the body, such as the face, the hands, and the feet; hence, the term *acromegaly*.

Sam A.'s coarse facial features and bulky hands are typical of patients with acromegaly.

The actions of GH can be classified as those that occur as a consequence of the hormone's direct effect on target cells and those that occur indirectly through the ability of GH to generate other factors, particularly IGF-1.

The IGF-1–independent actions of GH are exerted primarily in hepatocytes. GH administration is followed by an early increase in the synthesis of 8 to 10 proteins, among which are IGF-1, α_2-macroglobulin, and the serine protease inhibitors Spi 2.1 and Spi 2.3. Expression of the gene for ornithine decarboxylase, an enzyme that is active in polyamine synthesis (and, therefore, in the regulation of cell proliferation), is also significantly increased by GH.

Muscle and adipocyte cell membranes contain GH receptors that mediate direct, rapid metabolic effects on glucose and amino acid transport as well as on lipolysis. These receptors use associated cytoplasmic tyrosine kinases for signal transduction (such as the janus kinases; see Chapter 11, Section III.C.). STAT (signal transducer and activator of transcription) transcription factors are activated, and, depending on the tissue, the MAP kinase pathway and/or the AKT pathway is also activated. For example, in adipose tissue, GH has acute insulinlike effects followed by increased lipolysis, inhibition of lipoprotein lipase, stimulation of hormone-sensitive lipase, decreased glucose transport, and decreased lipogenesis. In muscle, GH causes increased amino acid transport, increased nitrogen retention, increased fat-free (lean) tissue, and increased energy expenditure. GH also has growth-promoting effects. GH receptors are present on a variety of tissues in which GH increases *IGF-1* gene expression. The subsequent rise in IGF-1 levels contributes to cell multiplication and differentiation by autocrine or paracrine mechanisms. These, in turn, lead to skeletal, muscular, and visceral growth. These actions are accompanied by a direct anabolic influence of GH on protein metabolism with a diversion of amino acids from oxidation to protein synthesis and a shift to a positive nitrogen balance.

2. Control of Secretion of Growth Hormone

Although the regulation of GH secretion is complex, the major influence is hormonal (Fig. 41.2). The pulsatile pattern of GH secretion reflects the interplay of two hypothalamic regulatory peptides. Release is stimulated by GH-releasing hormone (GHRH, also called *somatocrinin*). The structure of GHRH was identified in 1982 (Fig. 41.3). It exists as both a 40- and a 44-amino-acid peptide encoded on chromosome 20 and produced exclusively in cells of the arcuate nucleus. Its *C*-terminal leucine residue is amidated. Full biologic activity of this releasing hormone resides in the first 29 amino acids of the *N*-terminal portion of the molecule. GHRH interacts with specific receptors on the plasma membranes of the somatotrophs. The intracellular signaling mechanisms that result in GH synthesis and release appear to be multiple because cAMP and calcium-calmodulin both stimulate GH release.

Conversely, GH secretion is suppressed by GH release–inhibiting hormone (GHRIH, the same as somatostatin, which has already been discussed). In addition, IGF-1, produced primarily in the liver in response to the action of GH on hepatocytes, feeds back negatively on the somatotrophs to limit GH secretion. Other physiologic factors (e.g., exercise and sleep) and many pathologic factors also control its release (Table S41.1 in the online supplement).

In addition, GH release is modulated by plasma levels of all of the metabolic fuels, including proteins, fats, and carbohydrates. A rising level of glucose in the blood normally suppresses GH release, whereas hypoglycemia increases GH secretion in normal subjects. Amino acids, such as arginine, stimulate release of GH when their concentrations rise in the blood. Rising levels of fatty acids may blunt the GH response to arginine or a rapidly dropping blood glucose level. However, prolonged fasting, in which fatty acids are mobilized in an effort to spare protein, is associated with a rise in GH secretion. Some of the physiologic, pharmacologic, and pathologic influences on GH secretion are given in Table S41.1. These modulators of GH secretion provide the basis for clinical suppression and stimulation tests in patients suspected of having excessive or deficient GH secretion.

3. Effects of Growth Hormone on Energy Metabolism

GH affects the uptake and oxidation of fuels in adipose tissue, muscle, and liver and indirectly influences energy metabolism through its actions on the islet cells of the pancreas. In summary, GH increases the availability of fatty acids, which are oxidized for energy. This and other effects of GH spare glucose and protein; that is, GH indirectly decreases the oxidation of glucose and amino acids (Fig. 41.4).

4. Effects of Growth Hormone on Adipose Tissue

GH increases the sensitivity of the adipocyte to the lipolytic action of the catecholamines and decreases its sensitivity to the lipogenic action of insulin. These actions lead to the release of free fatty acids and glycerol into the blood to be metabolized by the liver. GH also decreases esterification of fatty acids, thereby reducing triacylglycerol synthesis within the fat cell. Recent evidence suggests that GH may impair glucose uptake by both fat and muscle cells by a postreceptor inhibition of insulin action. As a result of the metabolic effects of GH, the clinical course of acromegaly (increased GH secretion) may be complicated by impaired glucose tolerance or even overt diabetes mellitus.

5. Effects of Growth Hormone on Muscle

The lipolytic effects of GH increase free fatty acid levels in the blood that bathes muscle. These fatty acids are used preferentially as fuel, indirectly suppressing glucose uptake by muscle cells. Through the effects on glucose uptake, the rate of glycolysis is proportionately reduced.

GH increases the transport of amino acids into muscle cells, providing substrate for protein synthesis. Through a separate mechanism, GH increases the synthesis of DNA and RNA. The positive effect on nitrogen balance is reinforced by the protein-sparing effect of GH-induced lipolysis that makes fatty acids available to muscle as an alternative fuel source.

6. Effects of Growth Hormone on the Liver

When plasma insulin levels are low, as in the fasting state, GH enhances fatty acid oxidation to acetyl-CoA. This effect, in concert with the increased flow of fatty

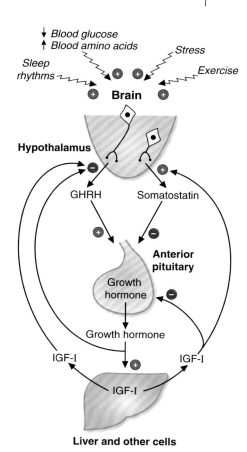

FIGURE 41.2 Control of growth hormone secretion. Various factors stimulate the release of growth hormone–releasing hormone (GHRH) from the hypothalamus. The hypothalamus also releases somatostatin in response to other stimuli. GHRH stimulates and somatostatin inhibits the release of growth hormone from the anterior pituitary. Growth hormone causes the release of insulinlike growth factor-1 (IGF-1) from liver and other tissues. IGF-1 inhibits GHRH release and stimulates somatostatin release.

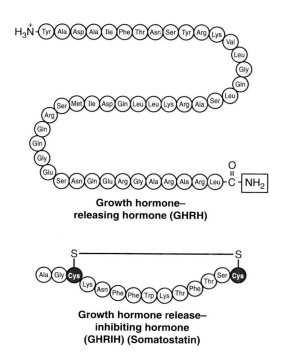

Growth hormone–releasing hormone (GHRH)

Growth hormone release–inhibiting hormone (GHRIH) (Somatostatin)

FIGURE 41.3 Structures of growth hormone–releasing hormone (GHRH) and growth hormone release–inhibiting hormone (GHRIH, the same as somatostatin). GHRH has an amide at the C terminus (in *box*).

 While **Sam A.** was trying to decide which of the major alternatives to choose for the treatment of his GH-secreting pituitary tumor, he noted progressive fatigue and the onset of increasing urinary frequency associated with a marked increase in thirst. In addition, he had lost 4 lb over the course of the last 6 weeks in spite of a good appetite. His physician suspected that Mr. A. had developed diabetes mellitus perhaps related to the chronic hypersecretion of GH. This suspicion was confirmed when Sam's serum glucose level, drawn before breakfast, was reported to be 236 mg/dL.

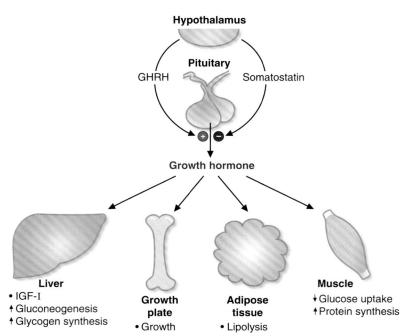

FIGURE 41.4 Anabolic effects of growth hormone on various tissues. *GHRH*, growth hormone–releasing hormone; *IGF-I*, insulinlike growth factor-1.

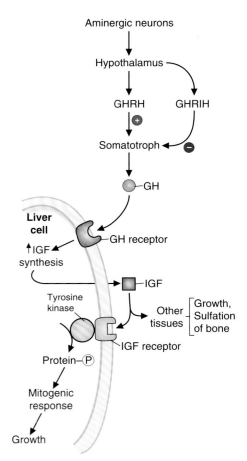

FIGURE 41.5 Production and action of insulinlike growth factors (IGFs). The hypothalamus produces growth hormone–releasing hormone (GHRH), which stimulates somatotrophs in the anterior pituitary to release growth hormone (GH). GH release–inhibiting hormone (GHRIH) inhibits GH release. GH binds to cell surface receptors and stimulates IGF production and release by liver and other tissues. IGF binds to cell-surface receptors and stimulates the phosphorylation of proteins that lead to cell division and growth.

acids from adipose tissue, enhances ketogenesis. The increased amount of glycerol reaching the liver as a consequence of enhanced lipolysis acts as a substrate for gluconeogenesis.

Hepatic glycogen synthesis is also stimulated by GH in part because of the increased gluconeogenesis in the liver. Finally, glucose metabolism is suppressed by GH at several steps in the glycolytic pathway.

A major effect of GH on liver is to stimulate production and release of IGFs. The IGFs are also known as *somatomedins*. The two somatomedins in humans share structural homologies with proinsulin, and both have substantial insulinlike growth activity—hence, the designations *insulinlike growth factor 1* (human IGF-1, or somatomedin-C) and *insulinlike growth factor 2* (human IGF-2, or somatomedin A). IGF-1 is a single-chain basic peptide that has 70 amino acids, and IGF-2 is slightly acidic, with 67 amino acids. These two peptides are identical to insulin in half of their residues. In addition, they contain a structural domain that is homologous to the C-peptide of proinsulin.

A broad spectrum of normal cells responds to high doses of insulin by increasing thymidine uptake and initiating cell propagation. In most instances, IGF-1 causes the same response as insulin in these cells but at significantly lower, more physiologic concentrations. Thus, the IGFs are more potent than insulin in their growth-promoting actions.

Evidence suggests that the IGFs exert their effects through either an endocrine or a paracrine/autocrine mechanism. IGF-1 appears to stimulate cell propagation and growth by binding to specific IGF-1 receptors on the plasma membrane of target cells rather than binding to GH receptors (Fig. 41.5).

Like insulin, the intracellular portion of the plasma membrane receptor for IGF-1 (but not IGF-2) has intrinsic tyrosine kinase activity. The fact that the receptors for insulin and several other growth factors have intrinsic tyrosine kinase activity indicates that tyrosine phosphorylation initiates the process of cellular replication and growth. Subsequently, a chain of kinases is activated, which include several protooncogene products (see Chapters 11 and 18).

Most cells of the body have messenger RNA (mRNA) for IGF, but the liver has the greatest concentration of these messages, followed by kidney and heart.

The synthesis of IGF-1 is regulated, for the most part, by GH, whereas hepatic production of IGF-2 is independent of GH levels in the blood.

C. Catecholamines (Epinephrine, Norepinephrine, Dopamine)

The catecholamines belong to a family of bioamines and are secretory products of the sympathoadrenal system. They are required for the body to adapt to a great variety of acute and chronic stresses. Epinephrine (80% to 85% of stored catecholamines) is synthesized primarily in the cells of the adrenal medulla, whereas norepinephrine (15% to 20% of stored catecholamines) is synthesized and stored not only in the adrenal medulla but also in various areas of the CNS and in the nerve endings of the adrenergic nervous system. Dopamine, another catecholamine, acts primarily as a neurotransmitter and has little effect on fuel metabolism.

The first total chemical synthesis of epinephrine was accomplished by Stolz et al. in 1904. In 1950, Sutherland was the first to demonstrate that epinephrine (and glucagon) induces glycogenolysis. This marked the beginning of our understanding of the molecular mechanisms through which hormones act.

1. Synthesis of the Catecholamines

Tyrosine is the precursor of the catecholamines. The pathway for the biosynthesis of these molecules is described in Chapter 46.

2. Secretion of the Catecholamines

Secretion of epinephrine and norepinephrine from the adrenal medulla is stimulated by a variety of stresses, including pain, hemorrhage, exercise, hypoglycemia, and hypoxia. Release is mediated by stress-induced transmission of nerve impulses emanating from adrenergic nuclei in the hypothalamus. These impulses stimulate the release of the neurotransmitter acetylcholine from preganglionic neurons that innervate the adrenomedullary cells. Acetylcholine depolarizes the plasma membranes of these cells, allowing the rapid entry of extracellular calcium (Ca^{2+}) into the cytosol. Ca^{2+} stimulates the synthesis and release of epinephrine and norepinephrine from the chromaffin granules into the extracellular space by exocytosis.

3. Physiologic Effects of Epinephrine and Norepinephrine

The catecholamines act through two major types of receptors on the plasma membrane of target cells, the α-adrenergic and the β-adrenergic receptors (see Chapter 19, Section IV.C).

The actions of epinephrine and norepinephrine in the liver, the adipocyte, the skeletal muscle cell, and the α- and β-cells of the pancreas directly influence fuel metabolism (Fig. 41.6). These catecholamines are counterregulatory hormones that have metabolic effects directed toward mobilization of fuels from their storage sites for oxidation by cells to meet the increased energy requirements of acute and chronic stress. They simultaneously suppress insulin secretion, which ensures that fuel fluxes will continue in the direction of fuel use rather than storage as long as the stressful stimulus persists.

In addition, norepinephrine works as a neurotransmitter and affects the sympathetic nervous system in the heart, lungs, blood vessels, bladder, gut, and other organs. These effects of catecholamines on the heart and blood vessels increase cardiac output and systemic blood pressure, hemodynamic changes that facilitate the delivery of bloodborne fuels to metabolically active tissues.

Epinephrine has a short half-life in the blood, and to be effective pharmacologically, it must be administered parenterally. It may be used clinically to support the beating of the heart, to dilate inflamed bronchial muscles, and even to decrease bleeding from organs during surgery.

High levels of circulating IGF-1 have been linked to the development of breast, prostate, colon, and lung cancer. In addition, experimental modulation of IGF-1 receptor activity can alter the growth of different types of tumor cells. Current research is aimed at targeting the interaction of IGF-1 and its receptor to reduce tumor cell proliferation. Clinical studies using monoclonal antibodies to the IFG-1 receptor, or specific IGF-1 receptor tyrosine kinase inhibitors, are under way, with promising results.

In patients suspected of having a neoplasm of the adrenal medulla that is secreting excessive quantities of epinephrine or norepinephrine (a pheochromocytoma), either the catecholamines themselves (epinephrine, norepinephrine, and dopamine) or their metabolites (the metanephrines and vanillylmandelic acid [VMA]), may be measured in a 24-hour urine collection, or the level of catecholamines in the blood may be measured. A patient who has consistently elevated levels in the blood or urine should be considered to have a pheochromocytoma, particularly if the patient has signs and symptoms of catecholamine excess, such as excessive sweating, palpitations, tremulousness, and hypertension.

A relatively rare form of secondary hypertension (high blood pressure) is caused by a catecholamine-secreting neoplasm of the adrenal medulla, known as a *pheochromocytoma*. Patients with this kind of tumor periodically secrete large amounts of epinephrine and norepinephrine into the bloodstream. Symptoms related to this secretion include a sudden and often severe increase in blood pressure, heart palpitations, a throbbing headache, and inappropriate and diffuse sweating. In addition, chronic hypersecretion of these catecholamines may lead to impaired glucose tolerance or even overt diabetes mellitus. Describe the actions of these hormones that lead to the significant rise in glucose levels.

The catecholamines are counterregulatory hormones that mobilize fuels from their storage sites for oxidation in target cells to meet the increased energy requirements that occur during acute or chronic stress or, in this case, the release of catecholamines by a tumor in the adrenal medulla. These actions provide the liver, for example, with increased levels of substrate needed for gluconeogenesis. Although in normal individuals, most of the glucose generated through this mechanism is oxidized, blood glucose levels rise in the process. In addition, the catecholamines suppress insulin secretion to ensure that fuels will continue to flow in the direction of use rather than into storage under these circumstances. Hence, blood glucose levels may rise in patients who have a pheochromocytoma.

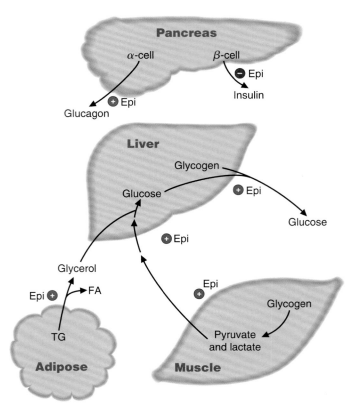

FIGURE 41.6 Effects of epinephrine on fuel metabolism and pancreatic endocrine function. Epinephrine (Epi) stimulates glycogen breakdown in muscle and liver, gluconeogenesis in liver, and lipolysis in adipose tissue. Epinephrine further reinforces these effects because it increases the secretion of glucagon, a hormone that shares many of the same effects as epinephrine. Epi also inhibits insulin release while stimulating glucagon release from the pancreas. *FA*, fatty acid; *TG*, triglyceride.

4. Metabolism and Inactivation of Catecholamines

Catecholamines have a relatively low affinity for both α- and β-receptors. After binding, the catecholamine disassociates from its receptor quickly, causing the duration of the biologic response to be brief. The free hormone is degraded in several ways, as outlined in Chapter 46.

D. Glucocorticoids

1. Biochemistry

Cortisol (hydrocortisone) is the major physiologic glucocorticoid (GC) in humans, although corticosterone also has some GC activity. GCs, such as cortisol, were named for their ability to raise blood glucose levels. These steroids are among the "counterregulatory" hormones that protect the body from insulin-induced hypoglycemia. The biosynthesis of steroid hormones and their basic mechanism of action has been described in Chapters 32 and 16.

2. Secretion of Glucocorticoids

The synthesis and secretion of cortisol are controlled by a cascade of neural and endocrine signals linked in tandem in the cerebrocortical–hypothalamic–pituitary–adrenocortical axis. Cerebrocortical signals to the midbrain are initiated in the cerebral cortex by "stressful" signals such as pain, hypoglycemia, hemorrhage, and exercise (Fig. 41.7). These nonspecific "stresses" elicit the production of monoamines in the cell bodies of neurons of the midbrain. Those that stimulate the

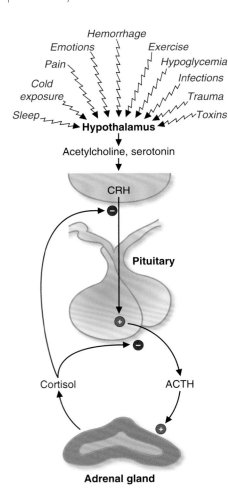

FIGURE 41.7 Regulation of cortisol secretion. Various factors act on the hypothalamus to stimulate the release of corticotropin-releasing hormone (CRH). CRH stimulates the release of adrenocorticotropic hormone (ACTH) from the anterior pituitary, which stimulates the release of cortisol from the adrenal cortex. Cortisol inhibits the release of CRH and ACTH via negative feedback loops.

synthesis and release of corticotropin-releasing hormone (CRH) are acetylcholine and serotonin. These neurotransmitters then induce the production of CRH by neurons originating in the paraventricular nucleus. These neurons discharge CRH into the hypothalamico-hypophyseal portal blood. CRH is delivered through these portal vessels to specific receptors on the cell membrane of the adrenocorticotropic hormone (ACTH)–secreting cells of the anterior pituitary gland (corticotrophs). This hormone–receptor interaction causes ACTH to be released into the general circulation, eventually to interact with specific receptors for ACTH on the plasma membranes of cells in the zona fasciculata and zona reticularis of the adrenal cortex. The major trophic influence of ACTH on cortisol synthesis is at the level of the conversion of cholesterol to pregnenolone, from which the adrenal steroid hormones are derived (see Chapter 32 for the biosynthesis of the steroid hormones).

Cortisol is secreted from the adrenal cortex in response to ACTH. The concentration of free (unbound) cortisol that bathes the CRH-producing cells of the hypothalamus and the ACTH-producing cells of the anterior pituitary acts as a negative feedback signal that has a regulatory influence on the release of CRH and ACTH (see Fig. 41.7). High cortisol levels in the blood suppress CRH and ACTH secretion, and low cortisol levels stimulate secretion. In severe stress, however, the negative feedback signal on ACTH secretion exerted by high cortisol levels in the blood is overridden by the stress-induced activity of the higher portions of the axis (see Fig. 41.7).

The effects of GCs on fuel metabolism in liver, skeletal muscle, and adipose tissue are outlined in Table 41.1 and in Figure 41.8. Their effects on other tissues are diverse and, in many instances, essential for life. Some of the nonmetabolic actions of GCs are listed in Table S41.2 of the online supplement.

3. Effects of Glucocorticoids

GCs have diverse actions that affect most tissues of the body. At first glance, some of these effects may appear to be contradictory (such as inhibition of glucose uptake by certain tissues), but taken together, they promote survival in times of stress.

When **Otto S.** was writing his list of differential diagnoses to explain the clinical presentation of **Chet S.**, he suddenly thought of a relatively rare endocrine disorder that could explain all of the presenting signs and symptoms. He made a provisional diagnosis of excessive secretion of cortisol secondary to an excess secretion of ACTH (Cushing disease) or by a primary increase of cortisol production by an adrenocortical tumor (Cushing syndrome).

Otto suggested that resting, fasting plasma cortisol and ACTH levels be measured at 8:00 the next morning. These studies showed that Mr. S.'s morning plasma ACTH and cortisol levels were both significantly above the reference range. Therefore, Otto concluded that Mr. S. probably had a tumor that was producing ACTH autonomously (i.e., not subject to normal feedback inhibition by cortisol). The high plasma levels of ACTH were stimulating the adrenal cortex to produce excessive amounts of cortisol. Additional laboratory and imaging studies indicated that the hypercortisolemia was caused by a benign ACTH-secreting adenoma of the anterior pituitary gland (Cushing disease).

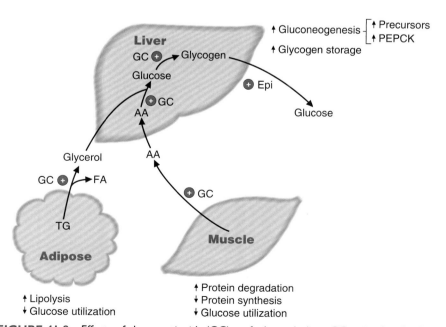

FIGURE 41.8 Effects of glucocorticoids (GC) on fuel metabolism. GCs stimulate lipolysis in adipose tissue and the release of amino acids from muscle protein. In liver, glucocorticoids stimulate gluconeogenesis and the synthesis of glycogen. The breakdown of liver glycogen is stimulated by epinephrine. *AA*, amino acid; *Epi*, epinephrine; *PEPCK*, phosphoenolpyruvate carboxykinase; *TG*, triglyceride.

Otto S. was now able to explain the mechanism for most of **Chet S.'s** signs and symptoms. For example, Otto knew the metabolic explanation for the patient's hyperglycemia. Some of Mr. S.'s muscle wasting and weakness were caused by the catabolic effect of hypercortisolism on protein stores, such as those in skeletal muscle, to provide amino acids as precursors for gluconeogenesis. This catabolic action also resulted in the degradation of elastin, a major supportive protein of the skin, as well as an increased fragility of the walls of the capillaries of the cutaneous tissues. These changes resulted in the easy bruisability and the torn subcutaneous tissues of the lower abdomen, which resulted in red striae (stripes). The plethora (redness) of Mr. S.'s facial skin was also caused in part by the thinning of the skin as well as by a cortisol-induced increase in the bone marrow production of red blood cells, which enhanced the redness of the subcutaneous tissues.

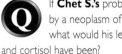

If **Chet S.'s** problem had been caused by a neoplasm of the adrenal cortex, what would his levels of blood ACTH and cortisol have been?

In many tissues, GCs inhibit DNA, RNA, and protein synthesis and stimulate the degradation of these macromolecules. In response to chronic stress, GCs act to make fuels available, so that when the acute alarm sounds and epinephrine is released, the organism can fight or flee. When GCs are elevated, glucose uptake by the cells of many tissues is inhibited, lipolysis occurs in peripheral adipose tissue, and proteolysis occurs in skin, lymphoid cells, and muscle. The fatty acids that are released are oxidized by the liver for energy, and the glycerol and amino acids serve in the liver as substrates for the production of glucose, which is converted to glycogen and stored. The alarm signal of epinephrine stimulates liver glycogen breakdown, making glucose available as fuel to combat the acute stress.

The mechanism by which GCs exert these effects involves binding of the steroid to intracellular receptors, interaction of the steroid–receptor complex with GC response elements on DNA, transcription of genes, and synthesis of specific proteins (see Chapter 16, Section III.C.2). In some cases, the specific proteins responsible for the GC effect are known (e.g., the induction of phosphoenolpyruvate carboxykinase that stimulates gluconeogenesis). In other cases, the proteins responsible for the GC effect have not yet been identified.

E. Thyroid Hormone

1. Biochemistry

The secretory products of the thyroid acinar cells are tetraiodothyronine (thyroxine, T_4) and triiodothyronine (T_3). Their structures are shown in Figure 41.9. The basic steps in the synthesis of T_3 and T_4 in these cells involve the transport or trapping of iodide from the blood into the thyroid acinar cell against an electrochemical gradient, the oxidation of iodide to form an iodinating species, the iodination of tyrosyl residues on the protein thyroglobulin to form iodotyrosines, and the coupling of residues of monoiodo- and diiodotyrosine (DIT) in thyroglobulin to form residues of T_3 and T_4 (Fig. 41.10). Proteolytic cleavage of thyroglobulin releases free T_3 and T_4. The steps in thyroid hormone synthesis are stimulated by TSH, a glycoprotein produced by the anterior pituitary. Approximately 35% of T_4 is deiodinated at the $5'$-position to form T_3, and 41% is deiodinated at the 5-position to form the inactive "reverse" T_3. Further deiodination or oxidative deamination leads to formation of compounds that have no biologic activity.

Iodide transport from the blood into the thyroid acinar cell is accomplished through an energy-requiring, iodide-trapping mechanism that requires symport with sodium. The sodium–iodide symporter (NIS, encoded by the *SLC5A5* gene) is driven by the electrochemical gradient across the membrane that is established by the Na^+,K^+-ATPase. For each iodide anion transported across the membrane, two sodium ions are cotransported to facilitate and drive the translocation of the ions. Loss of NIS activity leads to a congenital iodide transport defect.

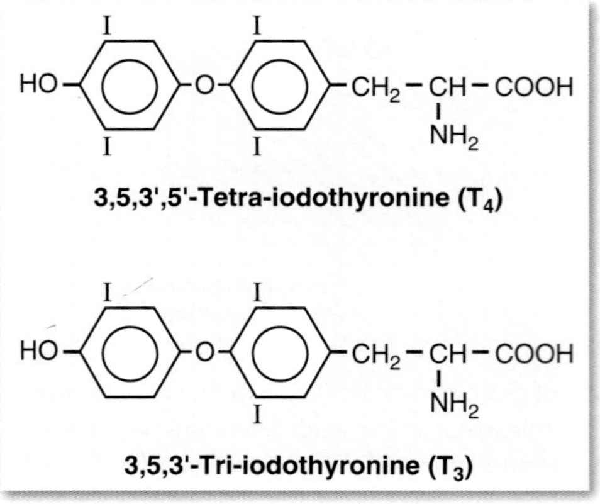

3,5,3',5'-Tetra-iodothyronine (T_4)

3,5,3'-Tri-iodothyronine (T_3)

FIGURE 41.9 Thyroid hormones, triiodothyronine (T_3) and tetraiodothyronine (T_4).

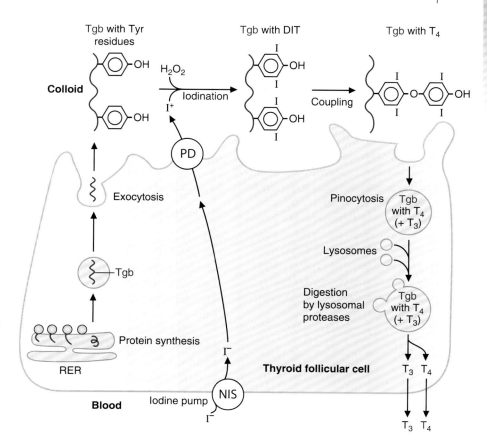

FIGURE 41.10 Synthesis of the thyroid hormones (triiodothyronine [T_3] and tetraiodothyronine [T_4]). The protein thyroglobulin (Tgb) is synthesized in thyroid follicular cells and secreted into the colloid. Iodination and coupling of tyrosine residues in Tgb produce T_3 and T_4 residues, which are released from Tgb by pinocytosis (endocytosis) and lysosomal action. The coupling of a monoiodotyrosine with a diiodotyrosine (DIT) to form T_3 is not depicted here. *NIS*, sodium–iodide symporter; *PD*, pendrin; *RER*, rough endoplasmic reticulum.

The rate of iodide transport is influenced by the absolute concentration of iodide within the thyroid cell. An internal autoregulatory mechanism decreases transport of iodide into the cell when the intracellular iodide concentration exceeds a certain threshold and increases transport when intracellular iodide falls below this threshold level. The iodide-concentrating or trapping process in the plasma membrane of thyroid acinar cells creates iodide levels within the thyroid cell that are several hundredfold greater than those in the blood, depending on the current size of the total body iodide pool and the present need for new hormone synthesis.

The oxidation of intracellular iodide is catalyzed by thyroid peroxidase (located at the apical border of the thyroid acinar cell) in what may be a two-electron oxidation step forming I^+ (iodinium ion). Iodinium ion may react with a tyrosine residue in the protein thyroglobulin to form a tyrosine quinoid and then a 3′-monoiodotyrosine (MIT) residue. It has been suggested that a second iodide is added to the ring by similar mechanisms to form a 3,5-DIT residue. Because iodide is added to these organic compounds, iodination is also referred to as the *organification of iodide*.

The biosynthesis of thyroid hormone proceeds with the coupling of an MIT and a DIT residue to form a T_3 residue or the coupling of two DIT residues to form a T_4 residue. T_3 and T_4 are stored in the thyroid follicle as amino acid residues in thyroglobulin. Under most circumstances, the T_4/T_3 ratio in thyroglobulin is approximately 13:1. Normally, the thyroid gland secretes 80 to 100 μg of T_4 and approximately 5 μg of T_3 per day. The additional 22 to 25 μg of T_3 "produced" daily is the result of the deiodination of the 5′-carbon of T_4 in peripheral tissues. T_3 is believed to be the predominant biologically active form of thyroid hormone in the body. The thyroid gland is unique in that it has the capacity to store large amounts of hormone as amino acid residues in thyroglobulin within its colloid space. This storage accounts for the low overall turnover rate of T_3 and T_4 in the body.

If **Chet S.'s** problem had resulted from primary hypersecretion of cortisol by a neoplasm of the adrenal cortex, his blood cortisol levels would have been elevated. The cortisol would have acted on the CRH-producing cells of the hypothalamus and the ACTH-secreting cells of the anterior pituitary by a negative feedback mechanism to decrease ACTH levels in the blood.

Because his cortisol and ACTH levels were both high, Mr. S.'s tumor was most likely in the pituitary gland or possibly in neoplastic extrapituitary tissue that was secreting ACTH "ectopically." (*Ectopic* means that the tumor or neoplasm is producing and secreting a substance that is not ordinarily made or secreted by the tissue from which the tumor developed.) Mr. S.'s tumor was in the anterior pituitary, not in an extrapituitary ACTH-producing site.

Once iodide anion enters the thyroid follicular cell, it must be transported across the apical membrane to react with thyroid peroxidase and thyroglobulin. The apical iodide transporter is pendrin (encoded by the *SLC26A4* gene), and mutations in pendrin lead to Pendred syndrome. Children with this syndrome display a total loss of hearing, goiter (swelling of the thyroid gland), and metabolic defects in iodide organification.

The "central" deposition of fat in patients such as **Chet S.** with Cushing disease or syndrome is not readily explained because GCs actually cause lipolysis in adipose tissue. The increased appetite caused by an excess of GC and the lipogenic effects of the hyperinsulinemia that accompanies the GC-induced chronic increase in blood glucose levels have been suggested as possible causes. Why the fat is deposited centrally under these circumstances, however, is not understood. This central deposition leads to the development of a large fat pad at the center of the upper back ("buffalo hump"), to accumulation of fat in the cheeks and jowls ("moon facies") and neck area, as well as a marked increase in abdominal fat. Simultaneously, there is a loss of adipose and muscle tissue below the elbows and knees, exaggerating the appearance of "central obesity" in Cushing disease or syndrome.

In areas of the world in which the soil is deficient in iodide, hypothyroidism is common. The thyroid gland enlarges (forms a goiter) in an attempt to produce more thyroid hormone. In the United States, table salt (NaCl) enriched with iodide (iodized salt) is used to prevent hypothyroidism caused by iodine deficiency.

The plasma half-life of T_4 is approximately 7 days, and that of T_3 is 1 to 1.5 days. These relatively long plasma half-lives result from binding of T_3 and T_4 to several transport proteins in the blood. Of these transport proteins, thyroid-binding globulin (TBG) has the highest affinity for these hormones and carries approximately 70% of bound T_3 and T_4. Only 0.03% of total T_4 and 0.3% of total T_3 in the blood are in the unbound state. This free fraction of hormone has biologic activity because it is the only form that is capable of diffusing across target cell membranes to interact with intracellular receptors. The transport proteins, therefore, serve as a large reservoir of hormone that can release additional free hormone as the metabolic need arises.

The thyroid hormones are degraded in liver, kidney, muscle, and other tissues by deiodination, which produces compounds with no biologic activity.

2. Secretion of Thyroid Hormone

The release of T_3 and T_4 from thyroglobulin is controlled by TSH from the anterior pituitary. TSH stimulates the endocytosis of thyroglobulin to form endocytic vesicles within the thyroid acinar cells (see Fig. 41.10). Lysosomes fuse with these vesicles, and lysosomal proteases hydrolyze thyroglobulin, releasing free T_4 and T_3 into the blood in a 10:1 ratio. In various tissues, T_4 is deiodinated, forming T_3, which is the active form of the hormone.

TSH is synthesized in the thyrotropic cells of the anterior pituitary. Its secretion is regulated primarily by a balance between the stimulatory action of hypothalamic thyrotropin-releasing hormone (TRH) and the inhibitory (negative feedback) influence of thyroid hormone (primarily T_3) at levels above a critical threshold in the blood bathing the pituitary thyrotrophs. TSH secretion occurs in a circadian pattern, a surge beginning late in the afternoon and peaking before the onset of sleep. In addition, TSH is secreted in a pulsatile fashion, with intervals of 2 to 6 hours between peaks.

TSH stimulates all phases of thyroid hormone synthesis by the thyroid gland, including iodide trapping from the plasma, organification of iodide, coupling of monoiodotyrosine and diiodotyrosine, endocytosis of thyroglobulin, and proteolysis of thyroglobulin to release T_3 and T_4 (see Fig. 41.10). In addition, the vascularity of the thyroid gland increases as TSH stimulates hypertrophy and hyperplasia of the thyroid acinar cells.

The predominant mechanism of action of TSH is mediated by binding of TSH to its G-protein–coupled receptor on the plasma membrane of the thyroid acinar cell, leading to an increase in the concentration of cytosolic cAMP (through $G_{\alpha s}$) and calcium (through $G_{\alpha q}$). The increase in calcium is brought about by activation of phospholipase C, eventually leading to the activation of the MAP kinase pathway.

The large protein thyroglobulin, which contains T_3 and T_4 in peptide linkage, is stored extracellularly in the colloid that fills the central space of each thyroid follicle. Each of the biochemical reactions that leads to the release and eventual secretion of T_3 and T_4, such as those that lead to their formation in thyroglobulins, is TSH-dependent. Rising levels of serum TSH stimulate the endocytosis of stored thyroglobulin into the thyroid acinar cell. Lysosomal enzymes then cleave T_3 and T_4 from thyroglobulin. T_3 and T_4 are secreted into the bloodstream in response to rising levels of TSH.

As the free T_3 level in the blood bathing the thyrotrophs of the anterior pituitary gland rises, the feedback loop is closed. Secretion of TSH is inhibited until the free T_3 levels in the systemic circulation fall just below a critical level, which once again signals the release of TSH. This feedback mechanism ensures an uninterrupted supply of biologically active free T_3 in the blood (Fig. 41.11). High levels of T_3 also inhibit the release of TRH from the hypothalamus.

3. Physiologic Effects of Thyroid Hormone

Only those physiologic actions of thyroid hormone that influence fuel metabolism are considered here. It is important to stress the term *physiologic* because the effects of supraphysiologic concentrations of thyroid hormone on fuel metabolism may not be simple extensions of their physiologic effects. For example, when T_3 is present in excess, it has severe catabolic effects that increase the flow of amino acids from muscle into the blood and eventually to the liver. In general, the following comments apply to the effects of thyroid hormone on energy metabolism in individuals who have normal thyroid hormone levels in their blood.

a. Effects of Thyroid Hormone on the Liver

Several actions of thyroid hormone affect carbohydrate and lipid metabolism in the liver. Thyroid hormone increases glycolysis and cholesterol synthesis and increases the conversion of cholesterol to bile salts. Through its action of increasing the sensitivity of the hepatocyte to the gluconeogenic and glycogenolytic actions of epinephrine, T_3 indirectly increases hepatic glucose production (permissive or facilitatory action). Because of its ability to sensitize the adipocyte to the lipolytic action of epinephrine, T_3 increases the flow of fatty acids to the liver and thereby indirectly increases hepatic triacylglycerol synthesis. The concurrent increase in the flow of glycerol to the liver (as a result of increased lipolysis) further enhances hepatic gluconeogenesis.

b. Effects of Thyroid Hormone on the Adipocyte

T_3 has an amplifying or facilitatory effect on the lipolytic action of epinephrine on fat cells. Yet, thyroid hormone has a bipolar effect on lipid storage because it increases the availability of glucose to the fat cells, which serves as a precursor for fatty acid and glycerol 3-phosphate synthesis. The major determinant of the rate of lipogenesis, however, is not T_3 but rather the amount of glucose and insulin available to the adipocyte for triacylglycerol synthesis.

c. Effects of Thyroid Hormone on Muscle

In physiologic concentrations, T_3 increases glucose uptake by muscle cells. It also stimulates protein synthesis, and, therefore, growth of muscle through its stimulatory actions on gene expression.

In physiologic concentrations, thyroid hormone sensitizes the muscle cell to the glycogenolytic actions of epinephrine. Glycolysis in muscle is increased by this action of T_3.

d. Effects of Thyroid Hormone on the Pancreas

Thyroid hormone increases the sensitivity of the β-cells of the pancreas to those stimuli that normally promote insulin release and is required for optimal insulin secretion.

4. Calorigenic Effects of Thyroid Hormone

The oxidation of fuels converts approximately 25% of the potential energy present in the foods ingested by humans to adenosine triphosphate (ATP). This relative inefficiency of the human "engine" leads to the production of heat as a consequence of fuel use. This inefficiency, in part, allows homeothermic animals to maintain a constant body temperature in spite of rapidly changing environmental conditions. The acute response to cold exposure is shivering, which is probably secondary to increased activity of the sympathetic nervous system in response to this "stressful" stimulus.

Thyroid hormone participates in this acute response by sensitizing the sympathetic nervous system to the stimulatory effect of cold exposure. The ability of T_3 to increase heat production is related to its effects on the pathways of fuel oxidation, which both generate ATP and release energy as heat. The effects of T_3 on the sympathetic nervous system increase the release of norepinephrine. Norepinephrine stimulates the uncoupling protein thermogenin in brown adipose tissue (BAT), resulting in increased heat production from the uncoupling of oxidative phosphorylation (see Chapter 24). Very little residual brown fat persists in normal adult human beings, however.

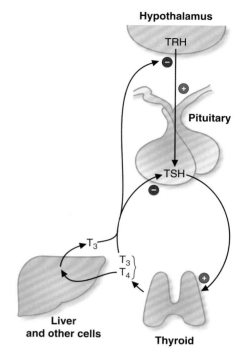

FIGURE 41.11 Feedback regulation of thyroid hormone levels. Thyrotropin-releasing hormone (TRH) from the hypothalamus stimulates the release of thyroid-stimulating hormone (TSH) from the anterior pituitary, which stimulates the release of triiodothyronine (T_3) and tetraiodothyronine (T_4) from the thyroid. T_4 is converted to T_3 in the liver and other cells. T_3 inhibit the release of TSH from the anterior pituitary and of TRH from the hypothalamus.

Q A patient presents with the following clinical and laboratory profile: the serum free and total T_3 and T_4 and the serum TSH levels are elevated, but the patient has symptoms of mild hypothyroidism, including a diffuse, palpable goiter. What single abnormality in the pituitary–thyroid–thyroid hormone target cell axis would explain all of these findings?

A generalized (i.e., involving all of the target cells for thyroid hormone in the body) but incomplete resistance of cells to the actions of thyroid hormone could explain the profile of the patient. In Refetoff disorder, a mutation in the portion of the gene that encodes the ligand-binding domain of the β-subunit of the thyroid hormone–receptor protein (expressed in all thyroid hormone–responsive cells) causes a relative resistance to the suppressive action of thyroid hormone on the secretion of TSH by the thyrotrophs of the anterior pituitary gland. Therefore, the gland releases more TSH than normal into the blood. The elevated level of TSH causes an enlargement of the thyroid gland (goiter) as well as an increase in the secretion of thyroid hormone into the blood. As a result, the serum levels of both T_3 and T_4 rise in the blood. The increase in the secretion of thyroid hormone may or may not be adequate to fully compensate for the relative resistance of the peripheral tissues to thyroid hormone. If the compensatory increase in the secretion of thyroid hormone is inadequate, the patient may develop the signs and symptoms of hypothyroidism.

In hypothyroid patients, insulin release may be suboptimal, although glucose intolerance on this basis alone is uncommon.

In hyperthyroidism, the degradation and the clearance of insulin are increased. These effects, plus the increased demand for insulin caused by the changes in glucose metabolism, may lead to varying degrees of glucose intolerance in these patients (a condition called *metathyroid diabetes mellitus*). A patient with uncomplicated hyperthyroidism, however, rarely develops significant diabetes mellitus.

Ghrelin, a hormone identified as a GH secretagogue, has recently been linked to appetite stimulation. The mechanism whereby this occurs is through the activation of the AMP-activated protein kinase in the hypothalamus. The activation of this kinase leads to the release of neuropeptide Y, which increases appetite. Research geared toward interrupting the ghrelin/ghrelin receptor signaling system is increasing in order to develop new anti-obesity agents.

Norepinephrine also increases the permeability of BAT and skeletal muscle to sodium. Because an increase of intracellular Na^+ is potentially toxic to cells, Na^+,K^+-ATPase is stimulated to transport Na^+ out of the cell in exchange for K^+. The increased hydrolysis of ATP by Na^+,K^+-ATPase stimulates the oxidation of fuels and the regeneration of more ATP and heat from oxidative phosphorylation. Over a longer time course, thyroid hormone also increases the level of Na^+,K^+-ATPase and many of the enzymes of fuel oxidation. Because even at normal room temperature, ATP use by Na^+,K^+-ATPase accounts for 20% or more of our basal metabolic rate (BMR), changes in its activity can cause relatively large increases in heat production.

Thyroid hormone also may increase heat production by stimulating ATP use in futile cycles (in which reversible ATP-consuming conversions of substrate to product and back to substrate use fuels and, therefore, produce heat).

F. Gastrointestinal-Derived Hormones that Affect Fuel Metabolism

In addition to insulin and the counterregulatory hormones discussed so far, a variety of peptides synthesized in the endocrine cells of the pancreatic islets, or the cells of the enteric nervous system, or the endocrine cells of the stomach, small bowel, and large bowel, as well as certain cells of the central and peripheral nervous system, influence fuel metabolism directly. Some of these peptides and their tissues of origin, their actions on fuel metabolism, and the factors that stimulate (or suppress) their secretion are listed in Table 41.2. In addition to these peptides, others, such as gastrin, motilin, pancreatic polypeptide (PP), peptide YY (PYY), and secretin may also influence fuel metabolism but by indirect effects on the synthesis or secretion of insulin or the counterregulatory hormones (Table S41.3, online supplement). For example, gastrin induces gastric acid secretion, which ultimately affects nutrient absorption and metabolism. Motilin, secreted by enteroendocrine M-cells of the proximal small bowel, stimulates gastric and pancreatic enzyme secretion, which, in turn, influences nutrient digestion. PP from the pancreatic islets reduces gastric emptying and slows upper intestinal motility. PYY from the α-cells in the mature pancreatic islets inhibits gastric acid secretion. Finally, secretin, produced by the enteroendocrine S-cells in the proximal small bowel, regulates pancreatic enzyme secretion and inhibits gastrin release and secretion of gastric acid. Although these "gut" hormones do not influence fuel metabolism directly, they have a significant impact on how ingested nutrients are digested and prepared for absorption. If digestion or absorption of fuels is altered through a disturbance in the delicate interplay among all of the peptides, fuel metabolism will be altered as well.

Several of these gastrointestinal peptides, such as glucagonlike peptide-1 (GLP-1) and gastric inhibitory polypeptide/glucose-dependent insulinotropic polypeptide (GIP), do not act as direct insulin secretagogues when blood glucose levels are normal but do so after a meal large enough to cause an increase in the blood glucose concentration. The release of these peptides may explain why the modest postprandial increase in serum glucose that is seen in normal subjects has a relatively robust stimulatory effect on insulin release, whereas a similar glucose concentration in vitro elicits a significantly smaller increase in insulin secretion. Likewise, this effect (certain factors potentiating insulin release), known as the *incretin effect*, could account for the greater β-cell response seen after an oral glucose load as opposed to that seen after the administration of glucose intravenously. This phenomenon is estimated to account for approximately 50% to 70% of the total insulin secreted after oral glucose administration. It is clear, then, that the gastrointestinal tract plays a critical role in peripheral energy homeostasis through its ability to influence the digestion, absorption, and assimilation of ingested nutrients. Importantly, the incretin hormones also regulate the amount of nutrients ingested, through their central action as satiety signals.

TABLE 41.2 Gastrointestinal-Derived Hormones Directly Affecting Fuel Metabolism

HORMONE	PRIMARY CELL/TISSUE OF ORIGIN	ACTIONS	SECRETORY STIMULI (AND INHIBITORS)
Amylin	Pancreatic β-cell, endocrine cells of stomach and small intestine	1. Inhibits arginine-stimulated and postprandial glucagon secretion 2. Inhibits insulin secretion	Cosecreted with insulin in response to oral nutrients
Calcitonin gene-related peptide (CGRP)	Enteric neurons and enteroendocrine cells of the rectum	Inhibits insulin secretion	Oral glucose intake and gastric acid secretion
Galanin	Nervous system, pituitary, neurons of gut, pancreas, thyroid, and adrenal gland	Inhibits secretion of insulin, somatostatin, enteroglucagon, pancreatic polypeptide, and others	Intestinal distension
Gastric inhibitory polypeptide/glucose-dependent insulinotropic polypeptide (GIP)	Neuroendocrine K-cells of duodenum and proximal jejunum	1. Increases insulin release via an "incretin" effect 2. Regulates glucose and lipid metabolism	Oral nutrient ingestion, especially long-chain fatty acids
Gastrin-releasing peptide (GRP)	Enteric nervous system and pancreas	Stimulates release of cholecystokinin; GIP, gastrin, glucagon, GLP-1, GLP-2, and somatostatin	
Ghrelin	Central nervous system, stomach, small intestine, and colon	Stimulates growth hormone release	Fasting
Glucagon	Pancreatic α-cell, central nervous system	Primary counterregulatory hormone that restores glucose levels in hypoglycemic state (increases glycogenolysis and gluconeogenesis as well as protein-lipid flux in liver and muscle)	Neural and humoral factors released in response to hypoglycemia
Glucagonlike peptide-1 (GLP-1)	Enteroendocrine L-cells in ileum, colon, and central nervous system	1. Enhances glucose disposal after meals by inhibiting glucagon secretion and stimulating insulin secretion 2. Acts through second messengers in β-cells to increase sensitivity of these cells to glucose (an incretin)	1. Oral nutrient ingestion 2. Vagus nerve 3. GRP and GIP 4. Somatostatin inhibits secretion
Glucagonlike peptide-2 (GLP-2)	Same as for GLP-1	Stimulates intestinal hexose transport	Same as GLP-1
Neuropeptide Y	Central and peripheral nervous system, pancreatic islet cells	Inhibits glucose-stimulated insulin secretion	Oral nutrient ingestion and activation of sympathetic nervous system
Neurotensin (NT)	Small intestine N-cells (especially ileum), enteric nervous system, adrenal gland, pancreas	In brain, modulates dopamine neurotransmission and anterior pituitary secretions	1. Luminal lipid nutrients 2. GRP 3. Somatostatin inhibits secretion
Pituitary adenylate cyclase activating peptide (PACAP)	Brain, lung, and enteric nervous system	Stimulates insulin and catecholamine release	Activation of central nervous system
Somatostatin	Central nervous system, pancreatic δ-cells, and enteroendocrine δ-cells	1. Inhibits secretion of insulin, glucagon and PP (islets), and gastrin, secretin, GLP-1, and GLP-2 (in gut) 2. Reduces carbohydrate absorption from gut lumen	1. Luminal nutrients 2. GLP-1 3. GIP 4. PACAP 5. VIP 6. β-Adrenergic stimulation
Vasoactive intestinal peptide (VIP)	Widely expressed in the central and peripheral nervous systems	May regulate release of insulin and pancreatic glucagon	1. Mechanical stimulation of gut 2. Activation of central and peripheral nervous systems

In Table 41.3 the actions of GLP-1 and GIP on key target organs that are important for the control of glucose homeostasis are given. Both GLP-1 and GIP enhance the synthesis and release of insulin as well as exerting a positive influence on the survival of pancreatic islet cells. In addition, GLP-1 contributes to the regulation of glucose homeostasis by inhibiting the secretion of glucagon from the α-cells of the pancreas as well as by slowing the rate of gastric emptying. GIP, but not GLP-1, interacts with GIP receptors on adipocytes, an interaction that is coupled to energy storage. Figure 41.12 summarizes the key effects of GLP-1 and GIP on energy metabolism.

TABLE 41.3 Actions of Glucagonlike Peptide-1 and Gastric Inhibitory Polypeptide/Glucose-Dependent Insulinotropic Polypeptide Relevant to Glucose Control

	GLP-1	GIP
Pancreas		
Stimulates glucose-dependent insulin release	+	+
Increase insulin biosynthesis	+	+
Inhibits glucagon secretion	+	−
Stimulates somatostatin secretion	+	−
Induces β-cell proliferation	+	+
Inhibits β-cell apoptosis	+	+
Gastrointestinal Tract		
Inhibits gastric emptying	+	−
Inhibits gastric acid secretion	+	+
Central nervous system		
Inhibits food and water intake	+	−
Promotes satiety and weight loss	+	−
Cardiovascular System		
Improves cardiovascular function after ischemia	+	−
Adipose tissue		
Insulinlike lipogenic actions	−	+
Lipid storage	−	+

GLP-1, glucagonlike peptide-1; GIP, gastric inhibitory polypeptide/glucose-dependent insulinotropic polypeptide.

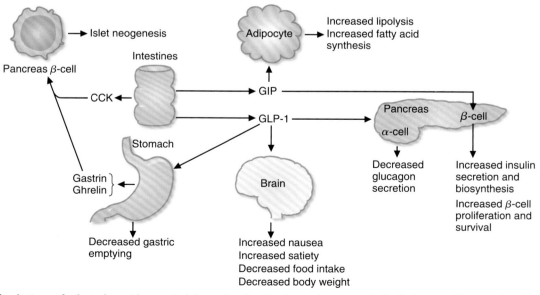

FIGURE 41.12 Actions of selected peptides on vital tissues involved in glucose homeostasis. Both glucagon-like peptide 1 (GLP-1) and gastric inhibitory polypeptide/glucose-dependent insulinotropic polypeptide (GIP) increase insulin secretion and β-cell survival. GLP-1 has additional actions related to glucose metabolism. In contrast, gastrin and cholecystokinin (CCK) do not acutely regulate plasma glucose levels but appear to increase β-cell proliferation.

As the biologic effects of the incretins were being discovered it was hypothesized that agents that would increase the levels of the incretins, or increase their half-life in circulation, may provide an effective means of treating type 2 diabetes by increasing insulin secretion from the pancreas. The half-lives of GIP and GLP-1 in the circulation are on the order of 2.5 minutes. The protease dipeptidyl peptidase 4 (DPP-4), found on the surface of kidneys, intestine, liver, and many other tissues, is responsible for inactivating GIP and GLP-1. In order to increase the efficacy of the incretins, synthetic incretin mimetics with longer half-lives, were developed, along with drugs which inhibit DPP-4, thereby increasing the serum half-lives of GIP and GLP-1. These types of medications are used for the treatment of type 2 diabetes mellitus. The first are potent GLP-1 receptor agonists. Exendin-4 or exenatide (Byetta) isolated from the venom of a lizard, *Heloderma suspectum*, was the first drug approved for such treatment. This agonist of the GLP-1 receptor must be administered subcutaneously, but because of its relative resistance to enzymatic cleavage by DPP-4 (unlike native GLP-1, which is rapidly cleaved by this enzyme), its biologic half-life in the plasma allows it to be administered only twice daily. DPP-4 cleaves GLP-1 after amino acid 2 (alanine) and breaks the alanine–glutamate peptide bond at that position. Exenatide has a glycine–glutamate sequence at amino acids 2 and 3, rendering this peptide more resistant to DPP-4 action than GLP-1. A second GLP-1 receptor agonist is liraglutide, which is a modified version of GLP-1. Liraglutide has a substitution, at position 34 of the peptide, of an arginine for a lysine (K34R), along with the addition of a palmitate at position K26 (covalently linked to the lysine side chain). Addition of the fatty acid to the peptide allows liraglutide to bind to albumin in the circulation, protecting it from DPP-4 and allowing just a single daily dosing.

The second class of agents (first marketed in October 2006 as sitagliptin [Januvia]) are orally administered inhibitors of DPP-4. Through this action, sitagliptin slows the rate of catalytic cleavage of GIP and of GLP-1 by DPP-4 and, therefore, prolongs their half-lives in the blood, allowing sitagliptin to be administered just twice daily. The contrasting actions of GLP-1 receptor agonists and the DPP-4 inhibitors are listed in Table 41.4. Since the introduction of sitagliptin, other DPP-4 inhibitors have been introduced, including alogliptin, linagliptin, saxagliptin, and vildagliptin. All have been approved by the FDA for use in the United States, and some are bundled in combinations with other drugs to treat type 2 diabetes.

Early estimates of their glucose-lowering efficacy in patients with type 2 diabetes mellitus suggest that the drugs that boost incretin action lower the blood hemoglobin A_{1c} level to approximately the same extent as do the other currently available oral antidiabetic agents (see the "Biochemical Comments" in Chapter 32) such as the sulfonylureas, metformin, and the thiazolidine diones (e.g., rosiglitazone [Avandia] and pioglitazone [Actos]).

 It has long been noted that when obese individuals with type 2 diabetes mellitus undergo gastric bypass procedure, their type 2 diabetes is resolved very shortly after surgery and before there is significant weight loss. This effect has been linked to a rapid and sustained increase in both amylin and GLP-1, which is greater than in individuals who have not had the procedure done. The incretin effect of GLP-1 leads to insulin and amylin release and to a reduction of high blood glucose levels in the patient.

TABLE 41.4 Similarities and Differences in Glucagonlike Peptide-1 Receptor Agonists and Dipeptidyl Peptidase 4 Inhibitors

CHARACTERISTIC	GLP-1 RECEPTOR AGONISTS	DPP-4 INHIBITORS
Administration	Injection	Oral
GLP-1 concentrations	Pharmacologic	Physiologic
Increased insulin secretion	Yes	Yes
Reduced glucagon secretion	Yes	Yes
Activation of portal glucose sensor	No	Yes
Gastric emptying inhibited	Yes	No
Weight loss	Yes	No
Loss of appetite, nausea	Yes	No
Proliferation of β-cells	Yes	Yes
Potential immunogenicity	Yes	No

GLP-1, glucagonlike peptide-1; DPP-4, dipeptidyl peptidase 4.

To establish the diagnosis of a secretory tumor of an endocrine gland, one must first demonstrate that basal serum levels of the hormone in question are regularly elevated. More important, one must show that the hypersecretion of the hormone (and hence, its elevated level in the peripheral blood) cannot be adequately inhibited by "maneuvers" that are known to suppress secretion from a normally functioning gland (i.e., one must show that the hypersecretion is "autonomous").

To ensure that both the basal and the postsuppression levels of the specific hormone to be tested will reflect the true secretory rate of the suspected endocrine tumor, all of the known factors that can stimulate the synthesis of the hormone must be eliminated. For GH, for example, the secretagogues (stimulants to secretion) include nutritional factors; the patient's level of activity, consciousness, and stress; and certain drugs. GH secretion is stimulated by a high-protein meal or by a low level of fatty acids or of glucose in the blood. Vigorous exercise, stage III–IV sleep, psychologic and physical stress, and levodopa, clonidine, and estrogens also increase GH release.

The suppression test used to demonstrate the autonomous hypersecretion of GH involves giving the patient an oral glucose load and measuring GH levels subsequently. A sudden rise in blood glucose suppresses serum GH to 2 ng/mL or less in normal subjects but not in patients with active acromegaly.

If one attempts to demonstrate autonomous hypersecretion of GH in a patient suspected of having acromegaly, therefore, before drawing the blood for both the basal (pre–glucose load) serum GH level and the post–glucose load serum GH level, one must be certain that the patient has not eaten for 6 to 8 hours, has not done vigorous exercise for at least 4 hours, remains fully awake during the entire testing period (in a nonstressed state to the extent possible), and has not taken any drugs known to increase GH secretion for at least 1 week.

Under these carefully controlled circumstances, if both the basal and postsuppression serum levels of the suspect hormone are elevated, one can conclude that autonomous hypersecretion is probably present. At this point, localization procedures (such as an MRI of the pituitary gland in a patient with suspected acromegaly) are performed to further confirm the diagnosis.

G. Neural Factors that Control Secretion of Insulin and Counterregulatory Hormones

Although a full treatment is beyond the scope of this text, the gastrointestinal neuroendocrine system is described briefly here with regard to its effects on fuel metabolism. The pancreatic islet cells are innervated by both the adrenergic and the cholinergic limbs of the autonomic nervous system. Although stimulation of both the sympathetic and the parasympathetic systems increases glucagon secretion, insulin secretion is increased by vagus nerve fibers and suppressed by sympathetic fibers via the α-adrenoreceptors. Evidence also suggests that the sympathetic nervous system regulates pancreatic β-cell function indirectly, through stimulation or suppression of the secretion of somatostatin, β_2-adrenergic receptor number, and the neuropeptides neuropeptide Y and galanin.

A tightly controlled interaction between the hormonal and neural factors that control nutrient metabolism is necessary to maintain normal fuel and hence energy homeostasis.

CLINICAL COMMENTS

Chet S. One of the functions of cortisol is to prepare the body to deal with periods of stress. In response to cortisol, the body re-sorts its fuel stores so that they can rapidly be made available for the "fight-or-flight" response to the alarm signal sounded by epinephrine. Cortisol causes gluconeogenic substrates to move from peripheral tissues to the liver, where they are converted to glucose and stored as glycogen. The release of epinephrine stimulates the breakdown of glycogen, increasing the supply of glucose to the blood. Thus, fuel becomes available for muscle to fight or flee.

Cushing syndrome is a prolonged and inappropriate increased level of cortisol. The most common cause is Cushing disease, the cause of **Chet S.'s** current problems. This results from prolonged hypersecretion of ACTH from a benign pituitary tumor. ACTH stimulates the adrenal cortex to produce cortisol, and blood levels of this steroid hormone rise.

Other nonpituitary causes of Cushing syndrome include a primary tumor of the adrenal cortex secreting excessive amounts of cortisol directly into the bloodstream. This disorder also can result from the release of ACTH from secretory nonendocrine, nonpituitary neoplasms ("ectopic" ACTH syndrome). Cushing syndrome often is caused by excessive doses of synthetic GCs used to treat a variety of disorders because of their potent antiinflammatory effects (iatrogenic Cushing syndrome).

Sam A. The diabetogenic potential of chronically elevated GH levels in the blood is manifest by the significant incidence of diabetes mellitus (25%) and impaired glucose tolerance (33%) in patients with acromegaly, such as **Sam A.** Under normal circumstances, however, physiologic concentrations of GH (as well as of cortisol and thyroid hormone) have a facilitatory or permissive effect on the quantity of insulin released in response to hyperglycemia and other insulin secretagogues. This "proinsular" effect is probably intended to act as a "brake" to dampen any potentially excessive "contrainsular" effects that increments in GH and the other counterregulatory hormones exert.

BIOCHEMICAL COMMENTS

Radioimmunoassays. Most hormones are present in body fluids in picomolar to nanomolar amounts, requiring highly sensitive assays to determine their concentration in the blood or urine. Radioimmunoassays (RIAs), developed in the 1960s, use an antibody, generated in animals, against a specific antigen (the hormone to be measured). Determining the concentration of the hormone in the sample involves incubating the plasma or urine sample with the antibody and then quantifying the level of antigen–antibody complex formed during the incubation by one of several techniques.

The classic RIA uses very high-affinity antibodies, which have been fixed (immobilized) on the inner surface of a test tube, a Teflon bead, or a magnetized particle. A standard curve is prepared using a set amount of the antibody and various known concentrations of the unlabeled hormone to be measured. In addition to a known concentration of the unlabeled hormone, each tube contains the same small, carefully measured amount of radiolabeled hormone. The labeled hormone and the unlabeled hormone compete for binding to the antibody. The higher the amount of unlabeled hormone in the sample, the less radiolabeled hormone is bound. A standard curve is plotted (Fig. 41.13). The sample from the patient's blood or urine, containing the unlabeled hormone to be measured, is incubated with the immobilized antibody in the presence of the same small, carefully measured amount of radiolabeled hormone. The amount of radiolabeled hormone bound to the antibody is determined, and the standard curve is used to quantitate the amount of unlabeled hormone in the patient sample.

The same principle is used in immunoradiometric assays (IRMAs), but with this technique, the antibody, rather than the antigen to be measured, is radiolabeled.

The sensitivity of RIAs can be enhanced using a "sandwich technique." This method uses two different monoclonal antibodies (antibodies generated by a single clone of plasma cells rather than multiple clones), each of which recognizes a different specific portion of the hormone's structure. The first antibody, attached to a solid support matrix such as a plastic culture dish, binds the hormone to be assayed. After exposure of the patient sample to this first antibody, the excess plasma is washed away, and the second antibody (which is radiolabeled) is then incubated with the first antibody–hormone complex. The amount of binding of the second (labeled) antibody to the first complex is proportional to the concentration of the hormone in the sample.

The sandwich technique can be improved even further if the second antibody is attached to an enzyme, such as alkaline phosphatase. The enzyme rapidly converts an added colorless substrate into a colored product, or a nonfluorescent substrate into a highly fluorescent product. These changes can be quantitated if the degree of change in color or fluorescence is proportional to the amount of hormone present in the patient sample. Less than a nanogram (10^{-9} g) of a protein can be measured by such an enzyme-linked immunosorbent assay (ELISA).

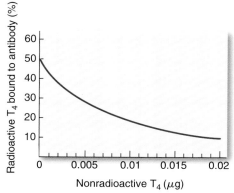

FIGURE 41.13 Standard curve for a radioimmunoassay. A constant amount of radioactive tetraiodothyronine (T_4) is added to a series of tubes, each of which contains a different amount of nonradioactive T_4. The amount of radioactive hormone that binds to an antibody that is specific for the hormone is measured and plotted against the nonradioactive hormone concentration. When more nonradioactive T_4 is present in the tube, less radioactive T_4 binds to the antibody.

KEY CONCEPTS

- Insulin is the major anabolic hormone of the body.
- Hormones that counteract the action of insulin are known as *counterregulatory* (*contrainsular*) *hormones.*
- Glucagon is the major counterregulatory hormone.
- Other contrainsular hormones are
  - Epinephrine
  - Norepinephrine
  - Cortisol
  - Somatostatin
  - Growth hormone
  - Thyroid hormone
- Somatostatin inhibits insulin secretion as well as the secretion of a large number of other hormones.
- Growth hormone (GH) exhibits a wide variety of effects.
  - GH increases lipolysis in adipose tissue, which increases the availability of fatty acids for oxidation, thereby reducing the oxidation of glucose and amino acids.
  - GH increases amino acid uptake into muscle cells, thereby increasing muscle protein synthesis.
  - GH stimulates gluconeogenesis (from amino acid substrates) and glycogen production in the liver.

- The catecholamines have metabolic effects directed toward mobilization of fuels from their storage sites for oxidation by cells while simultaneously suppressing insulin secretion.
- Cortisol (a glucocorticoid) promotes survival in times of stress, primarily via alteration of gene expression.
  - ATP-requiring processes, such as DNA, RNA, and protein synthesis, are inhibited.
- Fuels are made available.
- Fat-cell lipolysis is stimulated.
- Muscle proteolysis is stimulated.
- Glucose uptake by many tissues is inhibited to provide the nervous system with the glucose.
  - The liver uses the carbons of the amino acids for gluconeogenesis and glycogen storage.
- Thyroid hormone secretion is regulated by thyroid-stimulating hormone (TSH) and thyrotropin-releasing hormone (TRH).
- Thyroid hormone effects in the liver include
  - Increases in glycolysis and cholesterol synthesis
  - Increase in the synthesis of bile salts
  - Increase in triglyceride synthesis
- Thyroid hormone effects on fat cells include
  - Increased lipolysis
  - Increased glycerol release to the liver
- Thyroid hormone also stimulates heat production via a variety of mechanisms.
- The intestine and stomach (the gut) also secrete a variety of factors that affect fuel metabolism by working with (or against) the other hormones already described.
- The incretins glucagonlike peptide-1 (GLP-1) and glucose-dependent insulinotropic peptide (GIP) are synthesized in specialized cells of the gastrointestinal tract.
- GLP-1 and GIP influence nutrient homeostasis by increasing insulin release from the pancreatic β-cells in a glucose-dependent manner.
- Incretin action facilitates the uptake of glucose by muscle tissue and by the liver while simultaneously suppressing glucagon secretion by the α-cells of the pancreas.
- The incretins also increase the levels of cAMP in the islets, leading to expansion of β-cell mass and resistance to β-cell apoptosis.
- Diseases discussed in this chapter are summarized in Table 41.5.

TABLE 41.5 Diseases Discussed in Chapter 41		
DISEASE OR DISORDER	**ENVIRONMENTAL OR GENETIC**	**COMMENTS**
Hypercortisolemia	Both	Excessive cortisol secretion, leading to inappropriate catabolic responses
Acromegaly	Environmental	Excessive secretion of growth hormone, most often caused by ACTH- or GH-secreting neoplasms
Cushing disease	Environmental	A pituitary adenoma leading to excessive secretion of ACTH, which leads to excessive cortisol secretion
Cushing syndrome	Environmental or genetic (multiple endocrine neoplasia [MEN] I)	Exposure to high levels of cortisol for prolonged periods of time, with its subsequent effects
Hypothyroidism	Environmental or genetic	Reduced secretion of thyroid hormone, weight gain

ACTH, adrenocorticotropic hormone; GH, growth hormone.

REVIEW QUESTIONS—CHAPTER 41

1. As a third-year medical student, you examine your first patient. You find that he is 52 years old, has a round face, acne, and a large hump of fat on the back of his neck. He complains that he is too weak to mow his lawn. His fasting blood glucose level is 170 mg/dL (reference range, 80 to 100 mg/dL). His plasma cortisol levels are 62 μg/mL (reference range, 3 to 31 μg/mL). His plasma ACTH levels are 0 pg/mL (reference range, 0 to 100 pg/mL). Based on the information given, if the patient's problem is attributable to a single cause, the most likely diagnosis is which one of the following?
   A. Non–insulin-dependent diabetes mellitus
   B. Insulin-dependent diabetes mellitus
   C. A secretory tumor of the anterior pituitary
   D. A secretory tumor of the posterior pituitary
   E. A secretory tumor of the adrenal cortex

2. A woman was scheduled for a GH suppression test. If each of the following events occurred the morning of the test, which one of the events would be most likely to cause a decrease in GH levels?
   A. She ate four large doughnuts for breakfast.
   B. She was on estrogen replacement therapy and took her tablets after breakfast.
   C. While unlocking her car, she was chased by the neighbor's vicious dog.
   D. She fell asleep at the start of the test and slept soundly until it was completed 1.5 hours later.
   E. She forgot to eat breakfast before the test.

3. A dietary deficiency of iodine will lead to which one of the following?
   A. A direct effect on the synthesis of thyroglobulin on ribosomes
   B. An increased secretion of TSH
   C. Decreased production of TRH
   D. Increased heat production
   E. Weight loss

4. A woman whose thyroid gland was surgically removed was treated with 0.10 mg of thyroxine daily (tablet form). After 3 months of treatment, serial serum TSH levels ranged between 10 and 15 MIU/mL (reference range, 0.3 to 5.0 MIU/mL). She complained of fatigue, weight gain, and hoarseness. Her dose of thyroid hormone should be adjusted in which direction?
   A. Increased
   B. Decreased
   C. Remain the same

5. Which one of the insulin counterregulatory hormones stimulates both amino acid release from the muscle and glycogenesis?
   A. Glucagon
   B. Epinephrine
   C. Cortisol
   D. Growth hormone
   E. Thyroid hormone

6. Which of the following are hormones that would antagonize the actions of insulin (insulin counterregulatory hormones)? Choose the one best answer.

	Erythro-poietin	Epineph-rine	Norepi-nephrine	Soma-tostatin	Growth Hormone
A	Yes	No	No	No	Yes
B	Yes	Yes	Yes	Yes	No
C	Yes	No	No	No	Yes
D	No	Yes	Yes	Yes	Yes
E	No	No	Yes	No	No
F	No	Yes	Yes	Yes	No

7. A patient has been diagnosed with acromegaly caused by a GH-secreting tumor in the anterior pituitary. The patient is prescribed an analog of somatostatin to suppress GH secretion from the tumor in order to treat the condition. This treatment will also lead to the suppression of which one of the following hormones?
   A. Epinephrine
   B. Norepinephrine
   C. Glucocorticoid
   D. Thyroid hormone
   E. Erythropoietin

8. A patient had a recent history of headaches, sweating, and rapid heart palpitations. The physician ordered a 24-hour urine test that indicated greatly elevated levels of VMA. This finding strongly suggests that the patient has which type of tumor?
   A. Prolactinoma
   B. GH-secreting tumor
   C. Insulinoma
   D. Glucagonoma
   E. Pheochromocytoma

9. A new patient to your practice has been diagnosed with type 2 diabetes. Your treatment plan includes prescribing a drug that would be beneficial in lowering postprandial serum glucose levels. A class of such a drug is which one of the following?
   A. Drugs that decrease levels of GIP
   B. Drugs that decrease levels of GLP-1
   C. Drugs that increase levels of somatostatin
   D. Drugs that decrease levels of DPP-4
   E. Drugs that increase the levels of glucagon

10. When viewing the adrenal gland from external covering (capsule) through the cortex into the medulla, which one of the following is the correct order of hormone synthesis?
    A. Epinephrine, cortisol, dehydroepiandrosterone (DHEA), aldosterone
    B. Aldosterone, cortisol, DHEA, epinephrine
    C. Cortisol, DHEA, epinephrine, aldosterone
    D. Aldosterone, DHEA, cortisol, epinephrine
    E. DHEA, aldosterone, epinephrine, cortisol

ANSWERS

1. **The answer is E.** A tumor of the adrenal cortex is secreting excessive amounts of cortisol into the blood, which adversely affects glucose tolerance; suppresses pituitary secretion of ACTH; and, through chronic hypercortisolemia, causes the physical changes described in this patient. Uncomplicated non–insulin-dependent and insulin-dependent diabetes mellitus can be eliminated as possible diagnoses because they are not associated with elevated plasma cortisol levels and low plasma ACTH levels. In this patient, hyperglycemia resulted from the diabetogenic effects of chronic hypercortisolemia. An ACTH-secreting tumor of the anterior pituitary gland would cause hypercortisolemia, which, in turn, could adversely affect glucose tolerance; however, in this case, the plasma ACTH levels would have been high rather than 0 pg/mL. The posterior pituitary gland secretes oxytocin and vasopressin, neither of which influences blood glucose, cortisol, or ACTH levels.

2. **The answer is A.** High blood glucose levels cause a decrease in GH levels in the blood. This fact serves as the basis for the glucose suppression test for GH. Answers B, C, and D all would cause GH levels to increase, whereas answer E would have no effect on the test.

3. **The answer is B.** When iodine is deficient in the diet, the thyroid does not make normal amounts of T_3 and T_4. Consequently, there is less feedback inhibition of TSH production and release; hence, an increased secretion of TSH would be observed. There is no direct effect on thyroglobulin synthesis (thus, A is incorrect). TRH is released by the hypothalamus to release TSH from the pituitary; a lack of thyroid hormone would increase production of TRH, not decrease it (thus, C is incorrect). An overproduction of thyroid hormone leads to increased heat production and weight loss; lack of thyroid hormone does not lead to these symptoms (thus, D and E are incorrect).

4. **The answer is A.** The woman is experiencing hypothyroidism; TSH is elevated in an attempt to secrete more thyroid hormone because the existing dose is too low to suppress TSH release.

5. **The answer is C.** Glucagon, epinephrine, and norepinephrine decrease glycogenesis (the synthesis of glycogen). Growth and thyroid hormones have no effect on glycogenesis. The only counterregulatory hormone

to increase glycogenesis is cortisol, which is preparing the body for future needs by storing amino acid carbons (obtained from protein degradation in the muscle) as glycogen in the liver.

6. **The answer is D.** Counterregulatory hormones oppose the actions of insulin. Glucagon is the major counterregulatory hormone, but epinephrine, norepinephrine, cortisol, somatostatin, GH, and thyroid hormone are all classified as counterregulatory hormones because all affect fuel metabolism in a manner opposite that of insulin's action on fuel metabolism. Erythropoietin stimulates bone marrow production of red blood cells and does not oppose the actions of insulin.

7. **The answer is D.** Somatostatin leads to the inactivation of adenylate cyclase, thereby reducing cAMP levels. This reduces the secretion of GH, TSH, insulin, glucagon, serotonin, and TRH. The reduction of TRH and TSH would reduce thyroid hormone production. Somatostatin will not reduce the secretion of GCs, catecholamines (such as epinephrine and norepinephrine), and erythropoietin.

8. **The answer is E.** A pheochromocytoma is a catecholamine-producing tumor of the adrenal glands that overproduces and secretes epinephrine and other catecholamines. VMA and the metanephrines are the degradation products from these hormones. Because the levels of the degradation products are elevated, the tumor is secreting catecholamines, which also explains the symptoms. None of the other tumors listed will produce VMA as a degradation product.

9. **The answer is D.** GIP and GLP-1 accentuate insulin release after a meal large enough to cause an increase in blood glucose concentration (so they should be increased as a treatment for diabetes). Both GIP and GLP-1 have a very short half-life owing to inactivation by DPP-4. Reducing the levels of DPP-4 would allow more GLP-1 and GIP to stimulate insulin release and lower postprandial blood glucose levels. Somatostatin and glucagon are counterregulatory hormones and would antagonize the effects of insulin.

10. **The answer is B.** The outermost layer of the adrenal cortex produces mineralocorticoids (aldosterone). The intermediate layer produces GCs (cortisol). The inner most layer of the cortex produces adrenal androgens (DHEA). The adrenal medulla (inside the cortex) produces catecholamines such as epinephrine.

The Biochemistry of Erythrocytes and Other Blood Cells

42

The cells of the blood are classified as **erythrocytes**, **leukocytes**, or **thrombocytes**. The erythrocytes (**red cells**) carry oxygen to the tissues and are the most numerous cells in the blood. The leukocytes (**white cells**) are involved in defense against infection, and the thrombocytes (**platelets**) function in blood clotting. All of the cells in the blood can be generated from hematopoietic stem cells in the bone marrow on demand. For example, in response to infection, leukocytes secrete **cytokines** called **interleukins** that stimulate the production of additional leukocytes to fight the infection. Decreased supply of oxygen to the tissues signals the kidney to release **erythropoietin**, a hormone that stimulates the production of red cells.

The red cell has limited metabolic function, owing to its lack of internal organelles. **Glycolysis** is the main energy-generating pathway, with lactate production regenerating nicotinamide adenine dinucleotide (NAD^+) for glycolysis to continue. The NADH produced in glycolysis is also used to reduce the ferric form of hemoglobin, **methemoglobin**, to the normal ferrous state. Glycolysis also leads to a side pathway in which **2,3-bisphosphoglycerate (2,3-BPG)** is produced, which is a major allosteric effector for oxygen binding to hemoglobin (see Chapter 7). The **hexose monophosphate shunt** pathway generates **NADPH** to protect red cell membrane lipids and proteins from oxidation, through regeneration of reduced glutathione. **Heme synthesis** occurs in the precursors of red cells and is a complex pathway that originates from succinyl coenzyme A (succinyl-CoA) and glycine. Mutations in any of the steps of heme synthesis lead to a group of diseases known collectively as **porphyrias**.

The red cell membrane must be highly deformable to allow it to travel throughout the capillary system in the body. This is because of a complex **cytoskeletal** structure that consists of the major proteins spectrin, ankyrin, and **band 3 protein**. Mutations in these proteins lead to improper formation of the membrane cytoskeleton, ultimately resulting in malformed red cells, **spherocytes**, in the circulation. Spherocytes have a shortened life span, leading to loss of blood cells.

When the body does not have sufficient red cells, the patient is said to be **anemic**. Anemia can result from many causes. **Nutritional deficiencies** of iron, folate, or **vitamin B$_{12}$** prevent the formation of adequate numbers of red cells. **Mutations** in the genes that encode red cell metabolic **enzymes, membrane structural proteins**, and **globins** cause **hereditary anemias**. The appearance of red cells on a blood smear frequently provides clues to the cause of an anemia. Because the mutations that give rise to hereditary anemias also provide some protection against malaria, hereditary anemias are some of the most common genetic diseases known.

In human, globin gene expression is altered during development, a process known as **hemoglobin switching**. The switch between expression of one gene to another is regulated by transcription factor binding to the promoter regions of these genes. Current research is attempting to reactivate fetal hemoglobin genes to combat sickle cell disease and thalassemia.

THE WAITING ROOM

Lisa N., who has β^+-thalassemia, complains of pain in her lower spine (see Chapters 14 and 15). A quantitative computed tomogram (CT) of the vertebral bodies of the lumbar spine shows evidence of an area of early spinal cord compression in the upper lumbar region. She is suffering from severe anemia, resulting in stimulation of production of red blood cell (RBC) precursors (the erythroid mass) from the stem cells in her bone marrow. This expansion of marrow volume causes osteoporosis, leading to compression fractures in the lumbar spine area, which, in turn, cause pain. In addition to treatment of the osteoporosis, local irradiation to reduce the marrow volume in the lumbar spine is considered, as is a program of regular blood transfusions to maintain the oxygen-carrying capacity of circulating RBCs. The results of special studies related to the genetic defect underlying her thalassemia are pending, although preliminary studies have shown that she has elevated levels of fetal hemoglobin, which, in part, moderates the manifestations of her disease. **Lisa N.'s** parents have returned to the clinic to discuss the results of these tests.

Edward R. is a 21-year-old college student who complains of feeling tired all the time. Two years previously he had had gallstones removed, which consisted mostly of bilirubin. His spleen is palpable, and jaundice (icterus) is evidenced by yellowing of the whites of his eyes. His hemoglobin is low (8 g/dL; reference value, 13.5 to 17.5 g/dL). A blood smear showed dark, rounded, abnormally small red cells called *spherocytes* as well as an increase in the number of circulating immature RBCs known as *reticulocytes*.

I. Cells of the Blood

The blood, together with the bone marrow, composes the organ system that makes a significant contribution to achieving homeostasis, the maintenance of the normal composition of the body's internal environment. Blood can be considered a liquid tissue consisting of water, proteins, and specialized cells. The most abundant cells in the blood are the erythrocytes or RBCs, which transport oxygen to the tissues and contribute to buffering of the blood through the binding of protons by hemoglobin (see the material in Chapter 4, Section IV.B, and Chapter 7, Section VII). RBCs lose all internal organelles during the process of differentiation. The white blood cells (leukocytes) are nucleated cells present in blood that function in the defense against infection. The platelets (thrombocytes), which contain cytoplasmic organelles but no nucleus, are involved in the control of bleeding by contributing to normal thrombus (clot) formation within the lumen of the blood vessel. The average concentration of these cells in the blood of normal individuals is presented in Table 42.1.

A. Classification and Functions of Leukocytes and Thrombocytes

The leukocytes can be classified either as polymorphonuclear leukocytes (granulocytes) or mononuclear leukocytes, depending on the morphology of the nucleus in

TABLE 42.1	Normal Values of Blood Cell Concentrations in Adults
CELL TYPE	**MEAN (cells/mm³)**
Erythrocytes	5.2×10^6 (men) 4.6×10^6 women
Neutrophils	4,300
Lymphocytes	2,700
Monocytes	500
Eosinophils	230
Basophils	40

these cells. The mononuclear leukocyte has a rounded nucleus, whereas the polymorphonuclear leukocyte has a multilobed nucleus.

I. The Granulocytes

The granulocytes, so named because of the presence of secretory granules visible on staining, are the neutrophils, eosinophils, and basophils. When these cells are activated in response to chemical stimuli, the vesicle membranes fuse with the cell plasma membrane, resulting in the release of the granule contents (degranulation). The granules contain many cell-signaling molecules that mediate inflammatory processes. The granulocytes, in addition to displaying segmented nuclei (are polymorphonuclear), can be distinguished from each other by their staining properties (caused by different granular contents) in standard hematologic blood smears: Neutrophils stain pink, eosinophils stain red, and basophils stain blue.

Neutrophils are phagocytic cells that migrate rapidly to areas of infection or tissue damage. As part of the response to acute infection, neutrophils engulf foreign bodies and destroy them, in part, by initiating the respiratory burst (see Chapter 25). The respiratory burst creates oxygen radicals that rapidly destroy the foreign material found at the site of infection.

A primary function of eosinophils is to protect against parasites, such as worms, and to remove fibrin during inflammation. The eosinophilic granules are lysosomes containing hydrolytic enzymes and cationic proteins, which are toxic to parasitic worms. Increased eosinophils are also present in asthma and allergic responses, autoimmune diseases, and some cancers. Elucidating the function of eosinophils is currently an active area of research.

Basophils, the least abundant of the leukocytes, participate in hypersensitivity reactions, such as allergic responses. Histamine, produced by the decarboxylation of histidine, is stored in the secretory granules of basophils. Release of histamine during basophil activation stimulates smooth muscle cell contraction and increases vascular permeability. The granules also contain enzymes such as proteases, β-glucuronidase, and lysophospholipase. These enzymes degrade microbial structures and assist in the remodeling of damaged tissue.

2. Mononuclear Leukocytes

The mononuclear leukocytes consist of various classes of lymphocytes and the monocytes. Lymphocytes are small, round cells that were originally identified in lymph fluid. These cells have a high ratio of nuclear volume to cytoplasmic volume and are the primary antigen (foreign body)-recognizing cells. There are three major types of lymphocytes: T-cells, B-cells, and natural killer (NK)-cells. The precursors of T-cells (thymus-derived lymphocytes) are produced in the bone marrow and then migrate to the thymus, where they mature before being released to the circulation. Several subclasses of T-cells exist. These subclasses are identified by different surface membrane proteins, the presence of which correlate with the function of the subclass. Lymphocytes that mature in the bone marrow are the B-cells, which secrete antibodies in response to antigen binding. The third class of lymphocytes is the NK-cells, which target virally infected and malignant cells for destruction.

Circulatory monocytes are the precursors of tissue macrophages. Macrophages ("large eaters") are phagocytic cells that enter inflammatory sites and consume microorganisms and necrotic host cell debris left behind by granulocyte attack of the foreign material. Macrophages in the spleen play an important role in maintaining the oxygen-delivering capabilities of the blood by removing damaged RBCs that have a reduced oxygen-carrying capacity.

3. The Thrombocytes

Platelets are heavily granulated disclike cells that aid in intravascular clotting. Like the erythrocyte, platelets lack a nucleus. Their function is discussed in the following chapter. Platelets arise by budding of the cytoplasm of *megakaryocytes*, multinucleated cells that reside in the bone marrow.

A complete blood count (CBC) is ordered when a physician suspects a problem in the cellular composition of a patient's blood. The cells within the collected blood are counted and typed using an automated analyzer, based on flow cytometry (counting cells one at a time as they flow through a detector). As each cell flows through the machine, a laser shines light at the cell, which leads to predictable light-scattering and absorbance depending on the cell type. Based on the light-scattering and absorption pattern, the machine keeps track of the results of each cell that flows through the machine, leading to a very accurate count of each cell type present in the sample. The data from this analysis will include the total number of red cells per liter, the amount of hemoglobin in the red cells (in grams per liter), the hematocrit (the fraction of whole blood that consists of RBCs), the MCV, the total number of white blood cells, as well as a count of the different types of white blood cells (neutrophils, lymphocytes, monocytes, eosinophils, and basophils).

An inherited deficiency in erythrocyte pyruvate kinase leads to hemolytic anemia (an anemia caused by the destruction of RBCs; hemoglobin values typically drop to 4 to 10 g/dL in this condition, with normal values being 13.5 to 17.5 in males or 11.5 to 15.5 in females). Because the amount of ATP formed from glycolysis can be decreased by 50%, RBC ion transporters cannot function effectively. The RBCs tend to gain Ca^{2+} and lose K^+ and water. The water loss increases the intracellular hemoglobin concentration. With the increase in intracellular hemoglobin concentration, the internal viscosity of the cell is increased to the point that the cell becomes rigid and, therefore, more susceptible to damage by shear forces in the circulation. Once they are damaged, the RBCs are removed from circulation, leading to the anemia. However, the effects of the anemia are frequently moderated by the twofold to threefold elevation in 2,3-BPG concentration that results from the blockage of the conversion of phosphoenolpyruvate to pyruvate. Because 2,3-BPG binding to hemoglobin decreases the affinity of hemoglobin for oxygen, the RBCs that remain in circulation are highly efficient in releasing their bound oxygen to the tissues.

TABLE 42.2 Normal Hemoglobin Levels in Blood (g/dL)	
Adult	
Males	13.5–17.5
Females	11.5–15.5
Children	
Newborns	15.0–21.0
3–12 mo	9.5–12.5
1 y to puberty	11.0–13.5

B. Anemia

The major function of erythrocytes is to deliver oxygen to the tissues. To do this, a sufficient concentration of hemoglobin in the RBCs is necessary for efficient oxygen delivery to occur. When the hemoglobin concentration falls below normal values (Table 42.2), the patient is classified as anemic. Anemias can be categorized based on red cell size and hemoglobin concentration. Red cells can be of normal size (normocytic), small (microcytic), or large (macrocytic). Cells containing a normal hemoglobin concentration are termed *normochromic*; those with decreased concentration are *hypochromic*. This classification system provides important diagnostic tools (Table 42.3) that enable one to properly classify, diagnose, and treat the anemia.

Other measurements used to classify the type of anemia present include the mean corpuscular volume (MCV) and the mean corpuscular hemoglobin concentration (MCHC). The MCV is the average volume of the RBC, expressed in femtoliters (10^{-15} L). Normal MCV values range from 80 to 100 fL. The MCHC is the average concentration of hemoglobin in each individual erythrocyte, expressed in grams per liter. The normal range is 32 to 37 g/L; a value of <32 g/L indicates hypochromic cells. Thus, microcytic, hypochromic RBCs have an MCV of <80 fL and an MCHC of <32 g/L. Macrocytic, normochromic cells have an MCV of >100 fL, with an MCHC between 32 and 37 g/L.

II. Erythrocyte Metabolism

A. The Mature Erythrocyte

To understand how the erythrocyte can carry out its major function, a discussion of erythrocyte metabolism is required. Mature erythrocytes contain no intracellular organelles, so the metabolic enzymes of the RBC are limited to those found in the cytoplasm. In addition to hemoglobin, the cytosol of the RBC contains enzymes

TABLE 42.3 Classification of the Anemias on the Basis of Red Cell Morphology		
RED CELL MORPHOLOGY	**FUNCTIONAL DEFICIT**	**POSSIBLE CAUSES**
Microcytic, hypochromic	Impaired hemoglobin synthesis	Iron deficiency, mutation leading to thalassemia, lead poisoning
Macrocytic, normochromic	Impaired DNA synthesis	Vitamin B_{12} or folic acid deficiency, erythroleukemia
Normocytic, normochromic	Red cell loss	Acute bleeding, sickle cell disease, red cell metabolic defects, red cell membrane defects

necessary for the prevention and repair of damage done by reactive oxygen species (ROS; see Chapter 25) and the generation of energy (Fig. 42.1). Erythrocytes can only generate adenosine triphosphate (ATP) by glycolysis (see Chapter 22). The ATP is used for ion transport across the cell membrane (primarily Na^+, K^+, and Ca^{2+}), the phosphorylation of membrane proteins, and the priming reactions of glycolysis. Erythrocyte glycolysis also uses the Rapoport-Luebering shunt to generate 2,3-BPG. Red cells contain 4 to 5 mM 2,3-BPG, compared with trace amounts in other cells. The trace amounts of 2,3-BPG found in cells other than erythrocytes is required for the phosphoglycerate mutase reaction of glycolysis, in which 3-phosphoglycerate is isomerized to 2-phosphoglycerate. Because the 2,3-BPG is regenerated during each reaction cycle, it is required in only catalytic amounts. As has been discussed in more detail in Chapter 7, 2,3-BPG is a modulator of oxygen binding to hemoglobin that stabilizes the deoxy form of hemoglobin, thereby facilitating the release of oxygen to the tissues.

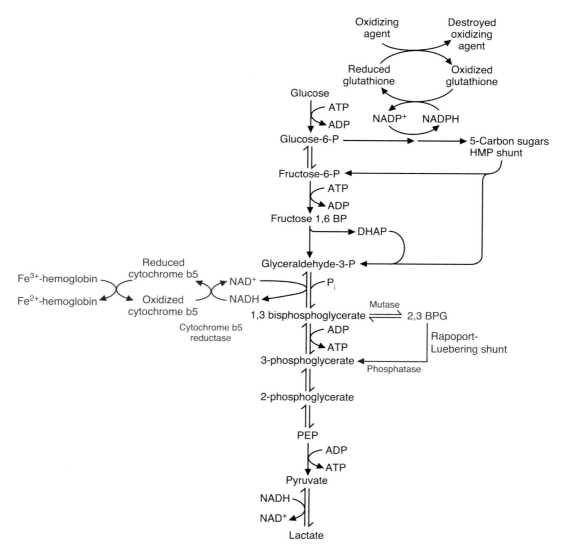

FIGURE 42.1 Overview of erythrocyte metabolism. Glycolysis is the major pathway, with branches for the hexose monophosphate (HMP) shunt (for protection against oxidizing agents) and the Rapoport-Luebering shunt (which generates 2,3-bisphosphoglycerate [2,3-BPG], which moderates oxygen binding to hemoglobin). The reduced nicotinamide adenine dinucleotide (NADH) generated from glycolysis can be used to reduce methemoglobin (Fe^{3+}) to normal hemoglobin (Fe^{2+}), or to convert pyruvate to lactate, so that NAD^+ can be regenerated and used for glycolysis. Pathways that are unique to the erythrocyte are indicated in *red*. *ADP*, adenosine diphosphate; *ATP*, adenosine triphosphate; *DHAP*, dihydroxyacetone phosphate; *Fructose 1,6-BP*, fructose 1,6-bisphosphate; *Fructose 6-P*, fructose 6-phosphate; *Glucose 6-P*, glucose 6-phosphate; *Glyceraldehyde 3-P*, glyceraldehyde 3-phosphate; P_i, inorganic phosphate; *PEP*, phosphoenolpyruvate.

Congenital methemoglobinemia, the presence of excess methemoglobin, is found in people with an enzymatic deficiency in cytochrome b_5 reductase or in people who have inherited hemoglobin M. In hemoglobin M, a single amino acid substitution in the heme-binding pocket stabilizes the ferric (Fe^{3+}) oxygen. Individuals with congenital methemoglobinemia appear cyanotic but have few clinical problems. Methemoglobinemia can be acquired by ingestion of certain oxidants such as nitrites, quinones, aniline, and sulfonamides. Acquired methemoglobinemia can be treated by the administration of reducing agents, such as ascorbic acid or methylene blue.

Glucose 6-PD deficiency is the most common enzyme deficiency in humans, probably, in part, because individuals with glucose 6-PD deficiency have resistance to malaria. The resistance to malaria counterbalances the deleterious effects of the deficiency. Glucose 6-PD–deficient red cells have a shorter life span and are more likely to lyse under conditions of oxidative stress. When soldiers during the Korean War were given the antimalarial drug primaquine prophylactically, approximately 10% of the soldiers of African ancestry developed spontaneous anemia. Because the gene for glucose 6-PD is found on the X chromosome, these men had only one copy of a variant *G6PD* gene.

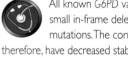

All known *G6PD* variant genes contain small in-frame deletions or missense mutations. The corresponding proteins, therefore, have decreased stability or lowered activity, leading to a reduced half-life or life span for the red cell. No mutations have been found that result in complete absence of glucose 6-PD. Based on studies with knockout mice, those mutations would be expected to result in embryonic lethality.

To bind oxygen, the iron of hemoglobin must be in the ferrous ($+2$) state. ROS can oxidize the iron to the ferric ($+3$) state, producing methemoglobin. Some of the reduced nicotinamide adenine dinucleotide (NADH) produced by glycolysis is used to regenerate hemoglobin from methemoglobin by the NADH–cytochrome b_5–methemoglobin reductase system. Cytochrome b_5 reduces the Fe^{3+} of methemoglobin. The oxidized cytochrome b_5 is then reduced by a flavin-containing enzyme, cytochrome b_5 reductase (also called *methemoglobin reductase*), using NADH as the reducing agent.

Approximately 5% to 10% of the glucose metabolized by RBCs is used to generate NADPH by way of the hexose monophosphate shunt. The NADPH is used to maintain glutathione in the reduced state. The glutathione cycle is the RBC's chief defense against damage to proteins and lipids by ROS (see Chapter 25).

The enzyme that catalyzes the first step of the hexose monophosphate shunt is glucose 6-phosphate (glucose 6-P) dehydrogenase (glucose 6-PD). The lifetime of the RBC correlates with glucose 6-P activity. Lacking ribosomes, the RBC cannot synthesize new glucose 6-PD protein. Consequently, as the glucose 6-PD activity decreases, oxidative damage accumulates, leading to lysis of the erythrocyte. When RBC lysis (hemolysis) substantially exceeds the normal rate of RBC production, the number of erythrocytes in the blood drops below normal values, leading to hemolytic anemia.

B. The Erythrocyte Precursor Cells and Heme Synthesis

1. Heme Structure

Heme consists of a porphyrin ring coordinated with an atom of iron (Fig. 42.2). Four pyrrole rings are joined by methylene bridges ($=CH-$) to form the porphyrin ring (see Fig. 7.12). Eight side chains serve as substituents on the porphyrin ring, two on each pyrrole. These side chains may be acetate (A), propionate (P), methyl (M), or vinyl (V) groups. In heme, the order of these groups is M V M V M P P M. This order, in which the position of the methyl group is reversed on the fourth ring, is characteristic of the porphyrins of the type III series, the most abundant in nature.

Heme is the most common porphyrin found in the body. It is complexed with proteins to form hemoglobin, myoglobin, and the cytochromes (see Chapters 7 and 24), including cytochrome P450 (see Chapter 25).

2. Synthesis of Heme

Heme is synthesized from glycine and succinyl-CoA (Fig. 42.3), which condense in the initial reaction to form δ-aminolevulinic acid (δ-ALA) (Fig. 42.4). The enzyme that catalyzes this reaction, δ-ALA synthase, requires the participation of pyridoxal

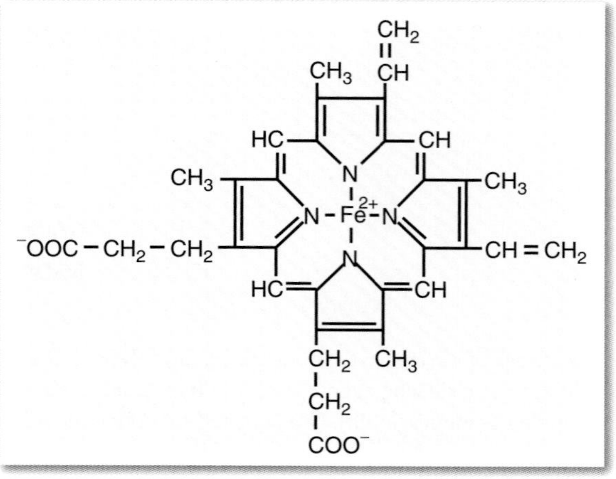

FIGURE 42.2 Structure of heme. The side chains can be abbreviated as MVMVMPPM: M, methyl ($-CH_3$); P, propionate ($-CH_2-CH_2-COO^-$); V, vinyl ($-CH=CH_2$).

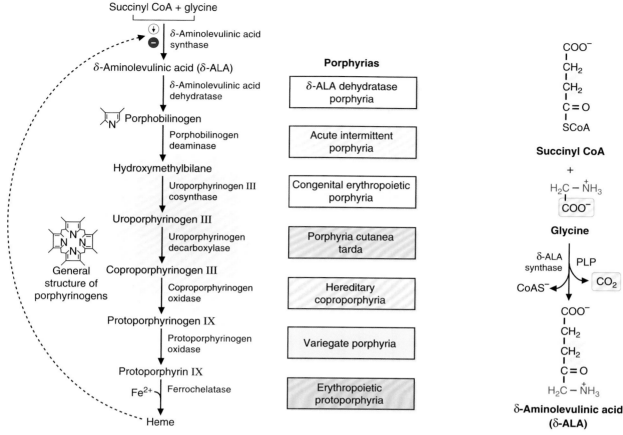

FIGURE 42.3 Synthesis of heme. To produce one molecule of heme, eight molecules each of glycine and succinyl coenzyme A (succinyl-CoA) are required. A series of porphyrinogens is generated in sequence. Finally, iron is added to produce heme. Heme regulates its own production by repressing the synthesis of δ-aminolevulinic acid (δ-ALA) synthase ⊕ and by directly inhibiting the activity of this enzyme ⊖. Deficiencies of enzymes in the pathway result in a series of diseases known as porphyrias (listed on the *right*, beside the deficient enzyme).

FIGURE 42.4 Synthesis of δ-aminolevulinic acid (δ-ALA). The atoms in *red* in δ-ALA are derived from glycine. *CoA*, coenzyme A; *PLP*, pyridoxal phosphate; *succinyl CoA*, succinyl coenzyme A.

phosphate because the reaction is an amino acid decarboxylation reaction (glycine is decarboxylated; see Chapter 37).

The next reaction of heme synthesis is catalyzed by δ-ALA dehydratase, in which two molecules of δ-ALA condense to form the pyrrole, porphobilinogen (Fig. 42.5). Four of these pyrrole rings condense to form a linear chain and then a series of porphyrinogens. The side chains of these porphyrinogens initially contain acetate (A) and propionate (P) groups. The acetyl groups are decarboxylated to form methyl groups. Then, the first two propionyl side chains are decarboxylated and oxidized to vinyl groups, forming a protoporphyrinogen. The methylene bridges are subsequently oxidized to form protoporphyrin IX (see Fig. 42.3). Heme is red, and it is responsible for the color of RBCs and of muscles that contain a large number of mitochondria.

In the final step of the pathway, iron (as Fe^{2+}) is incorporated into protoporphyrin IX in a reaction catalyzed by ferrochelatase (also known as *heme synthase*).

3. Source of Iron

Iron, which is obtained from the diet, has a US Recommended Dietary Allowance (RDA) of 10 mg for men and postmenopausal women and 15 mg for premenopausal women. The average daily US diet contains 10 to 50 mg of iron. However, only 10% to 15% is normally absorbed, and iron deficiencies are fairly common. The iron in meats is in the form of heme, which is readily absorbed. The nonheme iron

Pyridoxine (vitamin B_6) deficiencies are often associated with a microcytic, hypochromic anemia. Why would a vitamin B_6 deficiency result in small (microcytic), pale (hypochromic) RBCs?

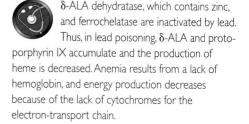

δ-ALA dehydratase, which contains zinc, and ferrochelatase are inactivated by lead. Thus, in lead poisoning, δ-ALA and protoporphyrin IX accumulate and the production of heme is decreased. Anemia results from a lack of hemoglobin, and energy production decreases because of the lack of cytochromes for the electron-transport chain.

In a vitamin B₆ deficiency, the rate of heme production is slow because the first reaction in heme synthesis requires pyridoxal phosphate (see Fig. 42.4). Thus, less heme is synthesized, causing RBCs to be small and pale. Iron stores are usually elevated.

 Porphyrias are a group of rare inherited disorders resulting from deficiencies of enzymes in the pathway for heme biosynthesis (see Fig. 42.3). Intermediates of the pathway accumulate and may have toxic effects on the nervous system that cause neuropsychiatric symptoms. When porphyrinogens accumulate, they may be converted by light to porphyrins, which react with molecular oxygen to form oxygen radicals. These radicals may cause severe damage to the skin. Thus, individuals with excessive production of porphyrins are photosensitive. The scarring and increased growth of facial hair seen in some porphyrias may have contributed to the rise of the werewolf legends.

An inherited mutation in *SLC11A2* (the gene encoding DMT-1) leads to an iron deficiency anemia, as indicated by a refractory hypochromic microcytic anemia. The iron is trapped in endosomal vesicles and cannot be released to bind to ferritin or used in other necessary biosynthetic reactions. This leads to reduced heme synthesis, reduced globin synthesis, and anemia.

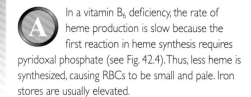

FIGURE 42.5 Two molecules of δ-aminolevulinic acid (δ-ALA) condense to form porphobilinogen.

in plants is not as readily absorbed, in part because plants often contain oxalates, phytates, tannins, and other phenolic compounds that chelate or form insoluble precipitates with iron, preventing its absorption. Conversely, vitamin C (ascorbic acid) increases the uptake of nonheme iron from the digestive tract. The uptake of iron is also increased in times of need by mechanisms that are not yet understood. Iron is absorbed in the ferrous (Fe^{2+}) state (Fig. 42.6) but is oxidized to the ferric state by a ferroxidase known as *ceruloplasmin* (a copper-containing enzyme) for transport through the body.

Because free iron is toxic, it is usually found in the body bound to proteins (see Fig. 42.6). Iron is carried in the blood (as Fe^{3+}) by the protein apotransferrin, with which it forms a complex known as *transferrin*. Transferrin is usually only one-third saturated with iron. The total iron-binding capacity of blood, owing mainly to its content of transferrin, is approximately 300 μg/dL. Transferrin, with bound iron, binds to the transferrin receptor on the cell surface, and the complex is internalized into the cell. The internalized membrane develops into an endosome, with a slightly acidic pH. The iron is reduced by a membrane-bound oxidoreductase, and the ferrous iron is transported out of the endosome into the cytoplasm via the divalent metal ion transporter 1 (DMT-1). Once in the cytoplasm, the iron is shunted to necessary enzymes, or it can be oxidized and bind to ferritin for long-term storage.

Storage of iron occurs in most cells but especially those of the liver, spleen, and bone marrow. In these cells, the storage protein apoferritin forms a complex with iron (Fe^{3+}), known as *ferritin*. Normally, ferritin is present in the blood in small amounts. The level increases, however, as iron stores increase. Therefore, the amount of ferritin in the blood is the most sensitive indicator of the amount of iron in the body's stores.

Iron can be drawn from ferritin stores, transported in the blood as transferrin, and taken up via receptor-mediated endocytosis by cells that require iron (e.g., by

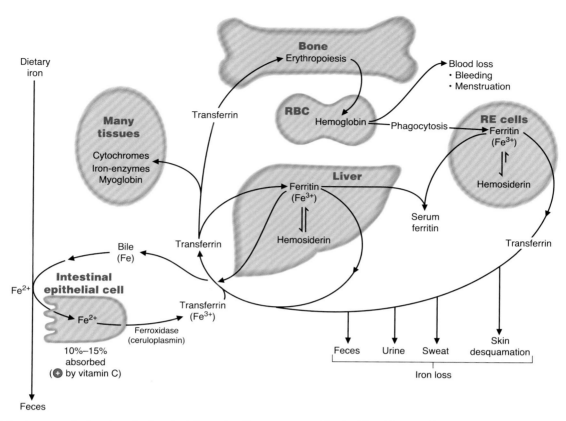

FIGURE 42.6 Iron metabolism. Iron is absorbed from the diet, transported in the blood by transferrin, stored in ferritin, and used for the synthesis of cytochromes, iron-containing enzymes, hemoglobin, and myoglobin. It is lost from the body with bleeding and sloughed-off cells, sweat, urine, and feces. Hemosiderin is the protein in which excess iron is stored. Small amounts of ferritin enter the blood and can be used to measure the adequacy of iron stores. *RBC*, red blood cells; *RE*, reticuloendothelial.

reticulocytes that are synthesizing hemoglobin). When excess iron is absorbed from the diet, it is stored as hemosiderin, a form of ferritin complexed with additional iron that cannot be readily mobilized.

4. Regulation of Heme Synthesis

Heme regulates its own synthesis by mechanisms that affect the first enzyme in the pathway, δ-ALA synthase (see Fig. 42.3). Heme represses the synthesis of this enzyme and also directly inhibits the activity of the enzyme (an allosteric modifier). Thus, heme is synthesized when heme levels fall. As heme levels rise, the rate of heme synthesis decreases.

Heme also regulates the synthesis of hemoglobin by stimulating synthesis of the protein globin. Heme maintains the ribosomal initiation complex for globin synthesis in an active state (see Chapter 15).

5. Degradation of Heme

Heme is degraded to form bilirubin, which is conjugated with glucuronic acid and excreted in the bile (Fig. 42.7). Although heme from cytochromes and myoglobin also undergoes conversion to bilirubin, the major source of this bile pigment is hemoglobin. After RBCs reach the end of their life span (~120 days), they are phagocytosed by cells of the reticuloendothelial system. Globin is cleaved to its constituent amino acids, and iron is returned to the body's iron stores. Heme is oxidized and cleaved to produce carbon monoxide and biliverdin (Fig. 42.8). Biliverdin is reduced to bilirubin, which is transported to the liver complexed with serum albumin.

 The iron lost by adult men (~1 mg/day) by desquamation of the skin and in bile, feces, urine, and sweat is replaced by iron absorbed from the diet. Men are not as likely to suffer from iron deficiencies as premenopausal adult women, who also lose iron during menstruation and who must supply iron to meet the needs of a growing fetus during pregnancy. If a man eating a Western diet has iron deficiency anemia, his physician should suspect bleeding from the gastrointestinal tract as a result of ulcers or colon cancer.

 Drugs, such as phenobarbital, induce enzymes of the drug-metabolizing systems of the endoplasmic reticulum that contain cytochrome P450. Because heme is used for synthesis of cytochrome P450, free heme levels fall and δ-ALA synthase is induced to increase the rate of heme synthesis.

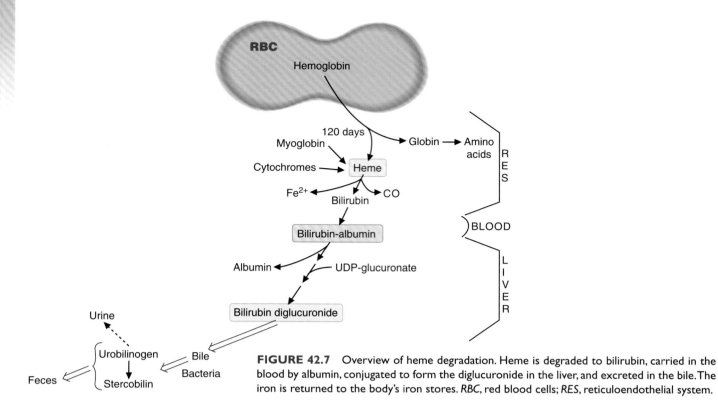

FIGURE 42.7 Overview of heme degradation. Heme is degraded to bilirubin, carried in the blood by albumin, conjugated to form the diglucuronide in the liver, and excreted in the bile. The iron is returned to the body's iron stores. *RBC*, red blood cells; *RES*, reticuloendothelial system.

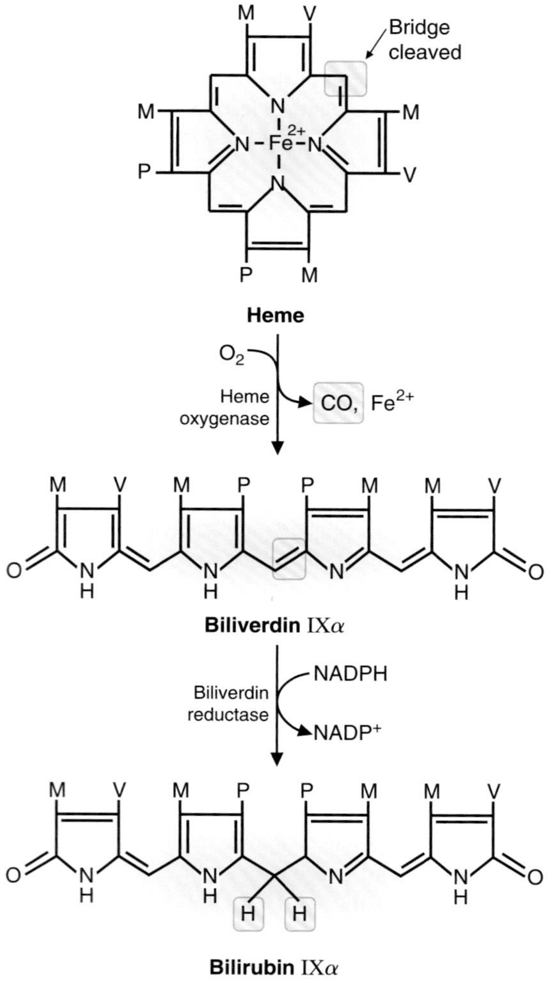

FIGURE 42.8 Conversion of heme to bilirubin. A methylene bridge in heme is cleaved, releasing carbon monoxide (CO) and iron. Then, the center methylene bridge is reduced. *NADP*, nicotinamide adenine dinucleotide phosphate.

In the liver, bilirubin is converted to a more water-soluble compound by reacting with uridine diphosphate (UDP)-glucuronate to form bilirubin monoglucuronide, which is converted to the diglucuronide (see Fig. 27.12). This conjugated form of bilirubin is excreted into the bile.

In the intestine, bacteria deconjugate bilirubin diglucuronide and convert the bilirubin to urobilinogens (see Fig. 42.7). Some urobilinogen is absorbed into the blood and excreted in the urine. However, most of the urobilinogen is oxidized to urobilins, such as stercobilin, and excreted in the feces. These pigments give feces their brown color.

III. The Red Blood Cell Membrane

Under the microscope, the RBC appears to be a red disc with a pale central area (biconcave disc) (Fig. 42.9). The biconcave disc shape (as opposed to a spherical shape) serves to facilitate gas exchange across the cell membrane. The membrane proteins that maintain the shape of the RBC also allow the RBC to traverse the capillaries with very small luminal diameters to deliver oxygen to the tissues. The interior diameters of many capillaries are smaller than the approximately 7.5-μm diameter of the red cell. Furthermore, in passing through the kidney, RBCs traverse hypertonic areas that are up to 6 times the normal isotonicity and back again, causing the red cell to shrink and expand during its travels. The spleen is the organ responsible for determining the viability of the RBCs. Erythrocytes pass through the spleen 120 times per day. The elliptical passageways through the spleen are approximately 3 μm in diameter, and normal red cells traverse them in approximately 30 seconds. Thus, to survive in the circulation, the red cell must be highly deformable. Damaged red cells that are no longer deformable become trapped in the passages in the spleen, where they are destroyed by macrophages. The reason for the erythrocyte's deformability lies in its shape and in the organization of the proteins that make up the RBC membrane.

The surface area of the red cell is approximately 140 μm^2, which is greater than the surface of a sphere needed to enclose the contents of the red cell (98 μm^2). The presence of this extra membrane and the cytoskeleton that supports it allows the red cell to be stretched and deformed by mechanical stresses as the cell passes through narrow vascular beds. On the cytoplasmic side of the membrane, proteins form a two-dimensional lattice that gives the red cell its flexibility (Fig. 42.10). The major proteins are spectrin, actin, band 4.1, band 4.2, and ankyrin. Spectrin, the major protein, is a heterodimer composed of α- and β-subunits wound around each other. The dimers self-associate at the heads. At the opposite end of the spectrin dimers, actin and band 4.1 bind near to each other. Multiple spectrins can bind to each actin filament, resulting in a branched membrane cytoskeleton.

The spectrin cytoskeleton is connected to the membrane lipid bilayer by ankyrin, which interacts with β-spectrin and the integral membrane protein band 3. Band 4.2 helps to stabilize this connection. Band 4.1 anchors the spectrin skeleton with the membrane by binding the integral membrane protein glycophorin C and the actin complex, which has bound multiple spectrin dimers.

When the RBC is subjected to mechanical stress, the spectrin network rearranges. Some spectrin molecules become uncoiled and extended; others become compressed, thereby changing the shape of the cell but not its surface area.

The mature erythrocyte cannot synthesize new membrane proteins or lipids. However, membrane lipids can be freely exchanged with circulating lipoprotein lipids. The glutathione system protects the proteins and lipids from oxidative damage.

The unusual names for some erythrocyte membrane proteins, such as band 4.1, arose through analysis of RBC membranes by polyacrylamide gel electrophoresis. The stained bands observed in the gel were numbered according to molecular weight

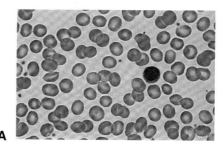

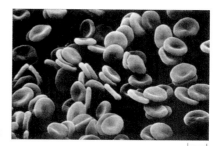

A

B

5 μm

FIGURE 42.9 The shape of the RBC. **A.** Wright-stained cells, displaying the pale staining in the *center*. **B.** Scanning electron micrograph, showing the biconcave disc structure of the cells. The stacks of erythrocytes in this preparation (collected from a blood tube) are not unusual. (These photographs were obtained, with permission, from Cohen BJ, Wood DL. *Memmler's the Human Body in Health and Disease.* 9th ed. Philadelphia, PA: Lippincott Williams & Wilkins, 2000:230 [Panel A]; and Alberts B, Johnson A, Lewis J, et al. *Molecular Biology of the Cell.* 4th ed. New York, NY: Garland Science, 2002:600 [Panel B].)

In an iron deficiency, what characteristics will be evident in the blood?

Defects in erythrocyte cytoskeletal proteins lead to hemolytic anemia. Shear stresses in the circulation result in the loss of pieces of the red cell membrane. As the membrane is lost, the RBC becomes more spherical and loses its deformability. As these cells become more spherical, they are more likely to lyse in response to mechanical stresses in the circulation or to be trapped and destroyed in the spleen.

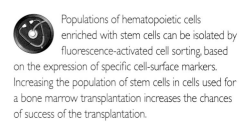

Iron deficiency will result in a microcytic, hypochromic anemia. RBCs will be small and pale. In contrast to a vitamin B_6 deficiency, which also results in a microcytic, hypochromic anemia, iron stores are low in an iron deficiency anemia.

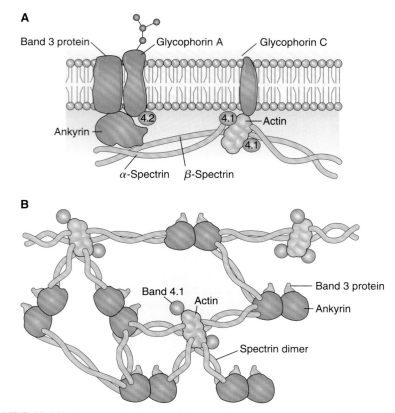

FIGURE 42.10 A generalized view of the erythrocyte cytoskeleton. **A.** The major protein, spectrin, is linked to the plasma membrane either through interactions with ankyrin and band 3, or with actin, band 4.1, and glycophorin. Other proteins in this complex, not shown, are tropomyosin and adducin. **B.** A view from inside the cell, looking up at the cytoskeleton. This view displays the cross-linking of the spectrin dimers to actin and band 3 anchor sites.

(e.g., band 1, band 2), and as functions were assigned to the proteins, more common names were assigned to the proteins (e.g., spectrin is actually band 1).

IV. Hematopoiesis

The various types of cells (lineages) that make up the blood are constantly being produced in the bone marrow. All cell lineages are descended from hematopoietic stem cells—cells that are renewable throughout the life of the host. The population of hematopoietic stem cells is quite small. Estimates vary between 1 and 10 per 10^5 bone marrow cells. In the presence of the appropriate signals, hematopoietic stem cells proliferate, differentiate, and mature into any of the types of cells that make up the blood (Fig. 42.11).

Hematopoietic differentiation is hierarchical. The number of fates a developing blood cell may adopt becomes progressively restricted. Hematopoietic progenitors are designated *colony-forming unit–lineage*, or *colony-forming unit–erythroid* (CFU-E). Progenitors that form very large colonies are termed *burst-forming units*.

Populations of hematopoietic cells enriched with stem cells can be isolated by fluorescence-activated cell sorting, based on the expression of specific cell-surface markers. Increasing the population of stem cells in cells used for a bone marrow transplantation increases the chances of success of the transplantation.

A. Cytokines and Hematopoiesis

Developing progenitor cells in the marrow grow in proximity with marrow stromal cells. These include fibroblasts, endothelial cells, adipocytes, and macrophages. The

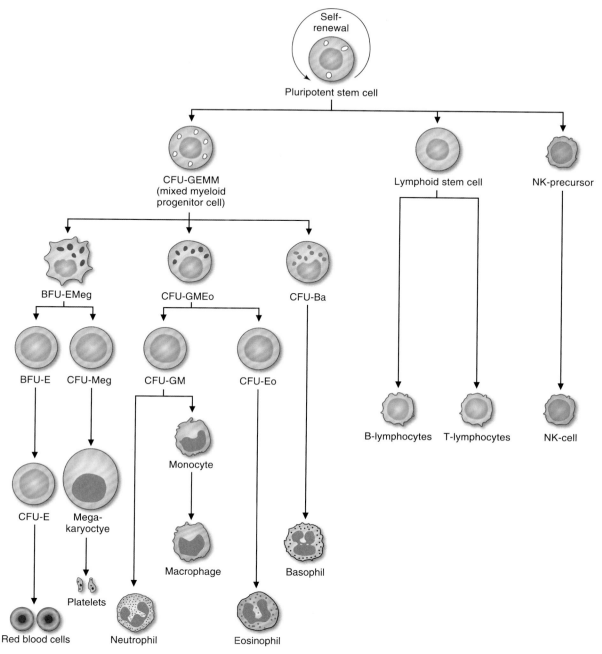

FIGURE 42.11 The hematopoietic tree. All blood cells arise from the self-renewing pluripotent stem cell. Different cytokines are required at each step for these events to occur. *BFU*, burst-forming unit; *CFU*, colony-forming unit.

stromal cells form an extracellular matrix and secrete growth factors that regulate hematopoietic development.

The hematopoietic growth factors have multiple effects. An individual growth factor may stimulate proliferation, differentiation, and maturation of the progenitor cells and also may prevent apoptosis. These factors also may activate various functions within the mature cell. Some hematopoietic growth factors act on multiple lineages, whereas others have more limited targets.

Most hematopoietic growth factors are recognized by receptors belonging to the cytokine receptor superfamily. Binding of ligand to receptor results in

 Leukemias, malignancies of the blood, arise when a differentiating hematopoietic cell does not complete its developmental program but remains in an immature, proliferative state. Leukemias have been found in every hematopoietic lineage.

In X-linked severe combined immunodeficiency disease (SCID), the most common form of SCID, circulating mature T-lymphocytes are not formed, and therefore, B-lymphocytes are not active. The affected gene encodes the γ-chain of the interleukin 2 receptor. Mutant receptors are unable to activate JAK3, and the cells are unresponsive to the cytokines that stimulate growth and differentiation. Recall also that adenosine deaminase deficiency (see Chapter 39), which is not X-linked, also leads to a form of SCID but for different reasons.

Families have been identified whose members have a mutant erythropoietin (Epo) receptor that is unable to bind SHP-1. Erythropoietin is the hematopoietic cytokine that stimulates production of RBCs. Individuals with the mutant Epo receptor have a higher-than-normal percentage of RBCs in the circulation because the mutant Epo receptor cannot be deactivated by SHP-1. Erythropoietin causes sustained activation of JAK2 and STAT 5 in these cases.

receptor aggregation, which induces phosphorylation of janus kinases (JAKs). The JAKs are a family of cytoplasmic tyrosine kinases that are active when phosphorylated (see Chapter 11, Section III.C and Fig. 11.15). The activated JAKs then phosphorylate the cytokine receptor. Phosphorylation of the receptor creates docking regions where additional signal transduction molecules bind, including members of the signal transducer and activator of transcription (STAT) family of transcription factors. The JAKs phosphorylate the STATs, which dimerize and translocate to the nucleus, where they activate target genes. Additional signal transduction proteins bind to the phosphorylated cytokine receptor, leading to activation of the Ras/Raf/mitogen-activated protein (MAP) kinase pathways. Other pathways are also activated, some of which lead to an inhibition of apoptosis (see Chapter 18).

The response to cytokine binding is usually transient because the cell contains multiple negative regulators of cytokine signaling. The family of *silencer of cytokine signaling* (SOCS) proteins is induced by cytokine binding. One member of the family binds to the phosphorylated receptor and prevents the docking of signal transduction proteins. Other SOCS proteins bind to JAKs and inhibit them. Whether SOCS inhibition of JAKs is a consequence of steric inhibition or whether SOCS proteins recruit phosphatases that then dephosphorylate the JAKs (Fig. 42.12) is uncertain.

SHP-1 is a tyrosine phosphatase found primarily in hematopoietic cells that is necessary for proper development of myeloid and lymphoid lineages. Its function is to dephosphorylate JAK2, thereby inactivating it.

STATs are also inactivated. The *protein inhibitors of activated STAT* (PIAS) family of proteins bind to phosphorylated STATs and prevent their dimerization or promote the dissociation of STAT dimers. STATs also may be inactivated by dephosphorylation, although the specific phosphatases have not yet been identified, or by targeting activated STATs for proteolytic degradation.

B. Erythropoiesis

The production of red cells is regulated by the demands of oxygen delivery to the tissues. In response to reduced tissue oxygenation, the kidney releases the hormone erythropoietin, which stimulates the multiplication and maturation of erythroid

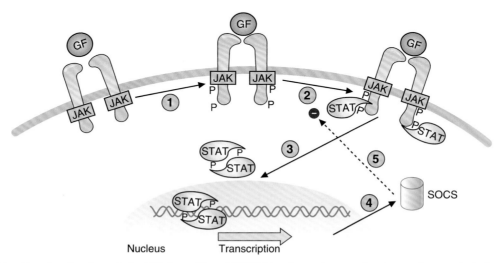

FIGURE 42.12 Cytokine signaling through the JAK (janus kinase)/STAT (signal transducer and activator of transcription) pathway. (*1*) Cytokine binding to receptors initiates dimerization and activation of the JAK kinase, which phosphorylates the receptor on tyrosine residues. (*2*) STAT proteins bind to the activated receptors and are themselves phosphorylated. (*3*) Phosphorylated STAT proteins dimerize, travel to the nucleus, and initiate gene transcription. (*4*) One family of proteins whose synthesis is stimulated by STATs is the SOCS (suppressor of cytokine signaling) family, which inhibits further activation of STAT proteins (*5*) by a variety of mechanisms. *GF*, growth factor.

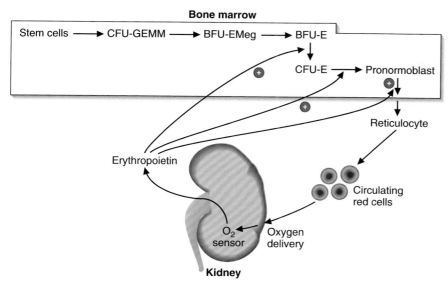

FIGURE 42.13 Erythropoietin stimulation of erythrocyte maturation. The abbreviations are described further in the text. *BFU*, burst-forming unit; *CFU*, colony-forming unit; *CFU-GEMM*, colony-forming unit—granulocyte, erythroid, monocyte, megakaryocyte.

progenitors. The progression along the erythroid pathway begins with the stem cell and passes through the mixed myeloid progenitor cell (colony-forming unit–granulocyte, erythroid, monocyte, megakaryocyte [CFU-GEMM]), burst-forming unit–erythroid (BFU-E), CFU-E, and to the first recognizable red cell precursor, the normoblast. Each normoblast undergoes four more cycles of cell division. During these four cycles, the nucleus becomes smaller and more condensed. After the last division, the nucleus is extruded. The red cell at this state is called a *reticulocyte*. Reticulocytes still retain ribosomes and messenger RNA (mRNA) and are capable of synthesizing hemoglobin. They are released from the bone marrow and circulate for 1 to 2 days. Reticulocytes mature in the spleen, where the ribosomes and mRNA are lost (Fig. 42.13).

 Perturbed JAK/STAT signaling is associated with development of lymphoid and myeloid leukemias, severe congenital neutropenia (a condition in which levels of circulating neutrophils are severely reduced), and Fanconi anemia, which is characterized by bone marrow failure and increased susceptibility to malignancy.

C. Nutritional Anemias

Each person produces approximately 10^{12} RBCs per day. Because so many cells must be produced, nutritional deficiencies in iron, vitamin B_{12}, and folate prevent adequate RBC formation. The physical appearance of the cells in the case of a nutritional anemia frequently provides a clue as to the nature of the deficiency.

In the case of iron deficiency, the cells are smaller and paler than normal. The lack of iron results in decreased heme synthesis, which in turn affects globin synthesis. Maturing red cells following their normal developmental program divide until their hemoglobin has reached the appropriate concentration. Iron- (and hemoglobin)-deficient developing RBCs continue dividing past their normal stopping point, resulting in small (microcytic) red cells. The cells are also pale because of the lack of hemoglobin, compared with normal cells (thus, a pale microcytic anemia results).

Deficiencies of folate or vitamin B_{12} can cause megaloblastic anemia, in which the cells are larger than normal. Folate and vitamin B_{12} are required for DNA synthesis (see Chapters 38 and 39). When these vitamins are deficient, DNA replication and nuclear division do not keep pace with the maturation of the cytoplasm. Consequently, the nucleus is extruded before the requisite number of cell divisions has taken place, and the cell volume is greater than it should be, and fewer blood cells are produced.

 A complication of sickle cell disease is an increased formation of gallstones. A sickle cell crisis accompanied by the intravascular destruction of RBCs (hemolysis) experienced by patients with sickle cell disease, such as **Will S.**, increases the amount of unconjugated bilirubin that is transported to the liver. If the concentration of this unconjugated bilirubin exceeds the capacity of the hepatocytes to conjugate it to the more soluble diglucuronide through interaction with hepatic UDP-glucuronate, both the total and the unconjugated bilirubin levels in the blood increase. More unconjugated bilirubin is then secreted by the liver into the bile. The increase in unconjugated bilirubin (which is not very water-soluble) results in its precipitation within the gallbladder lumen, leading to the formation of pigmented (calcium bilirubinate) gallstones.

HbC is found in high frequency in West Africa, in regions with a high frequency of HbS. Consequently, compound heterozygotes for HbS and HbC are not uncommon both in some African regions and among African Americans. HbS/HbC individuals have significantly more hematopathology than individuals with sickle cell trait (HbA/HbS). Polymerization of deoxygenated HbS is dependent on the HbS concentration within the cell. The presence of HbC in the compound heterozygote increases the HbS concentration by stimulating K$^+$ and water efflux from the cell. Because the HbC globin tends to precipitate, the proportion of HbS tends to be higher in HbS/HbC cells than in the cells of individuals with sickle cell trait (HbS/HbA). The way in which multiple mutations ameliorate or exacerbate hematologic diseases has provided insights into the molecular mechanisms of hemoglobin function and developmental regulation.

There are two ways in which an individual might have two α-globin genes deleted. In one case, one copy of chromosome 16 might have both α-globin genes deleted, whereas the other copy had two functional α-globin genes. In the second case, both chromosomes might have lost one of their two copies of the α-globin gene. The former possibility is more common among Asians, the latter among Africans.

V. Hemoglobinopathies, Hereditary Persistence of Fetal Hemoglobin, and Hemoglobin Switching

A. Hemoglobinopathies: Disorders in the Structure or Amount of the Globin Chains

More than 700 different mutant hemoglobins have been discovered. Most arise from a single base substitution, resulting in a single amino acid replacement. Many have been discovered during population screenings and are not clinically significant. However, in patients with hemoglobin S (HbS; sickle cell anemia), the most common hemoglobin mutation, the amino acid substitution has a devastating effect in the homozygote (see **Will S.** in Chapter 6). Another common hemoglobin variant, HbC, results from a Glu-to-Lys replacement in the same position as the HbS mutation. This mutation has two effects. It promotes water loss from the cell by activating the K$^+$ transporter by an unknown mechanism, resulting in a higher-than-normal concentration of hemoglobin within the cell. The amino acid replacement also substantially lowers the hemoglobin solubility in the homozygote, resulting in a tendency of the mutant hemoglobin to precipitate within the red cell, although, unlike sickle cells, the cell does not become deformed. Homozygotes for the HbC mutation have a mild hemolytic anemia. Heterozygous individuals are clinically unaffected.

B. Thalassemias

For optimal function, the hemoglobin α- and β-globin chains must have the proper structure and be synthesized in a 1:1 ratio. A large excess of one subunit over the other results in the class of diseases called *thalassemias*. These anemias are clinically very heterogeneous because they can arise by multiple mechanisms. Like sickle cell anemia, the thalassemia mutations provide resistance to malaria in the heterozygous state.

Hemoglobin single amino acid replacement mutations that give rise to a globin subunit of decreased stability is one mechanism by which thalassemia arises. More common, however, are mutations that result in decreased synthesis of one subunit. The α-thalassemias usually arise from complete gene deletions. Two copies of the α-globin gene are found on each chromosome 16, for a total of four α-globin genes per precursor cell. If one copy of the gene is deleted, the size and hemoglobin concentration of the individual RBCs is minimally reduced. If two copies are deleted, the RBCs are of decreased size (microcytic) and reduced hemoglobin concentration (hypochromic). However, the individual usually does not have an anemia. The loss of three α-globin genes causes a moderately severe microcytic hypochromic anemia (hemoglobin, 7 to 10 g/dL) with splenomegaly (enlarged spleen). The absence of four α-globin genes (hydrops fetalis) is usually fatal in utero.

As discussed in Chapter 14, β-thalassemia is a very heterogeneous genetic disease. Insufficient β-globin synthesis can result from deletions, promoter mutations, and splice-junction mutations. Heterozygotes for β$^+$ (some globin chain synthesis) or β-null (β^0, no globin chain synthesis) are generally asymptomatic, although they typically have microcytic, hypochromic RBCs and may have mild anemia. β$^+$/β$^+$ homozygotes have anemia of variable severity, β$^+$/β^0 compound heterozygotes tend to be more severely affected, and β^0/β^0 homozygotes have severe disease. In general, diseases of β-chain deficiency are more severe than diseases of α-chain deficiency. Excess β-chains form a homotetramer, hemoglobin H (HbH), which is ineffective for delivering oxygen to the tissues because of its high oxygen affinity. As RBCs age, HbH precipitates in the cells, forming inclusion bodies. RBCs with inclusion bodies have shortened life spans because they are more likely to be trapped and destroyed in the spleen. Excess α-chains are unable to form a stable tetramer. However, excess α-chains precipitate in erythrocytes at every developmental stage. The α-chain precipitation in erythroid precursors results in their widespread destruction, a process called *ineffective erythropoiesis*. The precipitated α-chains also damage RBC membranes through the heme-facilitated lipid oxidation by ROS. Both lipids and proteins, particularly band 4.1, are damaged.

C. Hereditary Persistence of Fetal Hemoglobin

Fetal hemoglobin (HbF), the predominant hemoglobin of the fetal period, consists of two α-chains and two γ-chains, whereas adult Hb consists of two α-chains and two β-chains. The process that regulates the conversion of HbF to HbA is called *hemoglobin switching*. Hemoglobin switching is not 100%; most individuals continue to produce a small amount of HbF throughout life. However, some people, who are clinically normal, produce abnormally high levels (up to 100%) of HbF in place of HbA. Patients with hemoglobinopathies such as β-thalassemia or sickle cell anemia frequently have less severe illnesses if their levels of HbF are elevated. One goal of much research on hemoglobin switching is to discover a way to reactivate transcription of the γ-globin genes to compensate for defective β-globin synthesis. Individuals who express HbF past birth have hereditary persistence of HbF (HPFH).

 The difference in amino acid composition between the β-chains of HbA and the γ-chains of HbF results in structural changes that cause HbF to have a lower affinity for 2,3-BPG than HbA and thus a greater affinity for oxygen. Therefore, the oxygen released from the mother's hemoglobin (HbA) is readily bound by HbF in the fetus. Thus, the transfer of oxygen from the mother to the fetus is facilitated by the structural difference between the hemoglobin molecule of the mother and that of the fetus.

1. Nondeletion Forms of HPFH

The nondeletion forms of HPFH are those that derive from point mutations in the Aγ and Gγ promoters. When these mutations are found with sickle cell or β-thalassemia mutations, they have an ameliorating effect on the disease because of the increased production of γ-chains.

2. Deletion Forms of HPFH

In deletion HPFH, both the entire δ- and β-genes have been deleted from one copy of chromosome 11, and only HbF can be produced. In some individuals, the fetal globins remain activated after birth, and enough HbF is produced that the individual is clinically normal. Other individuals with similar deletions that remove the entire δ- and β-genes do not produce enough HbF to compensate for the deletion and are considered to have δ^{0}β^0-thalassemia. The difference between these two outcomes is believed to be the site at which the deletions end within the β-globin gene cluster. In deletion HPFH, powerful enhancer sequences 3′ of the β-globin gene are resituated because of the deletion so that they activate the γ-promoters. In individuals with δ^{0}β^0-thalassemia, the enhancer sequences have not been relocated so that they can interact with the γ-promoters.

D. Hemoglobin Switching: A Developmental Process Controlled by Transcription Factors

In humans, embryonic megaloblasts (the embryonic RBC is large and is termed a *blast* because it retains its nucleus) are first produced in the yolk sac approximately 15 days after fertilization. After 6 weeks, the site of erythropoiesis shifts to the liver. The liver, and to a lesser extent the spleen, are the major sites of fetal erythropoiesis. In the last few weeks before birth, the bone marrow begins producing RBCs. By 8 to 10 weeks after birth, the bone marrow is the sole site of erythrocyte production. The composition of the hemoglobin also changes with development because both the α-globin locus and the β-globin locus have multiple genes that are differentially expressed during development (Fig. 42.14).

E. Structure and Transcriptional Regulation of the α- and β-Globin Gene Loci

The α-globin locus on chromosome 16 contains the embryonic ζ (zeta) gene and two copies of the α-gene, α$_2$ and α$_1$. The β-globin locus on chromosome 11 contains the embryonic ε-gene; two copies of the fetal β-globin gene, Gγ and Aγ (which differ by one amino acid); and two adult genes, δ and β. The order of the genes along

A Chromosome 16

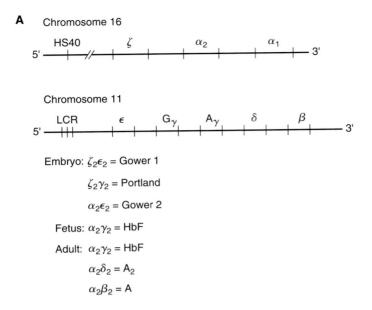

Embryo: $\zeta_2\epsilon_2$ = Gower 1

$\zeta_2\gamma_2$ = Portland

$\alpha_2\epsilon_2$ = Gower 2

Fetus: $\alpha_2\gamma_2$ = HbF

Adult: $\alpha_2\gamma_2$ = HbF

$\alpha_2\delta_2$ = A$_2$

$\alpha_2\beta_2$ = A

B

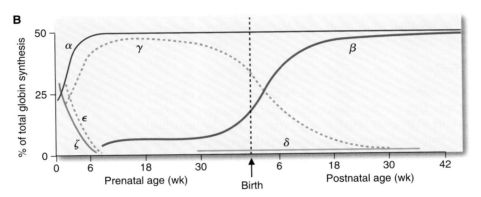

FIGURE 42.14 Globin gene clusters and expression during development. **A.** The globin gene clusters with the α-genes on chromosome 16 and the β-genes on chromosome 11. *HbF*, fetal hemoglobin; *LCR*, locus control region. **B.** The switching of globin chain synthesis during development.

the chromosome parallels the order of expression of the genes during development (see Fig. 42.14). The embryonic hemoglobins are $\zeta_2\varepsilon_2$ (Gower 1), $\zeta_2\gamma_2$ (Portland), and $\alpha_2\gamma_2$ (Gower 2). HbF is predominantly α_2Gγ_2. The major adult species is $\alpha_2\beta_2$ (hemoglobin A); the minor adult species is $\alpha_2\delta_2$ (hemoglobin A$_2$). The HbF found in adult cells is α_2Aγ_2. The timing of hemoglobin switching is controlled by a developmental clock that is not significantly altered by environmental conditions and is related to changes in expression of specific transcription factors. Premature newborns convert from HbF to HbA on schedule with their gestational ages.

CLINICAL COMMENTS

Edward R. Edward R.'s RBCs are deficient in spectrin. This deficiency impairs the ability of his erythrocytes to maintain the redundant surface area necessary to maintain deformability. Mechanical stresses in the circulation cause progressive loss of pieces of membrane. As membrane components are lost, Edward R.'s RBCs become spherical and unable to deform. His spleen is enlarged because of the large number of RBCs that have become trapped within it. His erythrocytes are lysed by mechanical stresses in the circulation and by macrophages in the spleen. Consequently, this hemolytic process results in anemia. His gallstones were the result of the large amounts of bilirubin that were produced and stored in the gallbladder as a result of the hemolysis. The abnormally rounded red cells seen on a blood smear are characteristic of hereditary spherocytosis.

Mutations in the genes for ankyrin, β-spectrin, or band 3 account for three-quarters of the cases of hereditary spherocytosis, whereas mutations in the genes for α-spectrin or band 4.2 account for the remainder. The defective synthesis of any of the membrane cytoskeletal proteins results in improper formation of the membrane cytoskeleton. Excess membrane proteins are catabolized, resulting in a net deficiency of spectrin. **Edward R.** underwent a splenectomy. Because the spleen was the major site of destruction of his RBCs, his anemia improved significantly after surgery. He was discharged with the recommendation to take a folate supplement daily. It was explained to Mr. R. that because the spleen plays a major role in protection against certain bacterial agents, he would require immunizations against pneumococcus, meningococcus, and *Haemophilus influenzae* type b.

 Lisa N. Lisa N. was found to be a compound heterozygote for mutations in the β-globin gene. On one gene, a mutation in position 6 of intron 1 converted a T to a C. The presence of this mutation, for unknown reasons, raises HbF production. The other β-globin gene had a mutation in position 110 of exon 1 (a C-to-T mutation). Both β-globin chains have reduced activity, but combined with the increased expression of HbF, the result is a β⁺-thalassemia.

BIOCHEMICAL COMMENTS

 Control of Hemoglobin Switching. How is hemoglobin switching controlled? Although there are still many unanswered questions, some of the molecular mechanisms have been identified. The α-globin locus covers approximately 100 kb (kilobases). The major regulatory element, HS40, is a nuclease-sensitive region of DNA that lies 5′ of the ζ-gene (see Fig. 42.14). HS40 acts as an erythroid-specific enhancer that interacts with the upstream regulatory regions of the ζ- and α-genes and stimulates their transcription. The region immediately 5′ of the ζ-gene contains the regulatory sequences responsible for silencing ζ-gene transcription. However, the exact sequences and transcription factors responsible for this silencing have not yet been identified. Even after silencing, low levels of ζ-gene transcripts are still produced after the embryonic period; however, they are not translated. This is because both the ζ-globin and α-globin transcripts have regions that bind to a messenger ribonucleoprotein (mRNP) stability-determining complex. Binding to this complex prevents the mRNA from being degraded. The α-globin mRNA has a much higher affinity for the mRNP than the ζ-globin message, which leads to the ζ-globin message being rapidly degraded.

The β-globin locus covers approximately 100 kb. From 5 to 25 kb upstream of the ε-gene is the locus control region (LCR), containing five DNase hypersensitive sites. The LCR is necessary for the function of the β-globin locus. It maintains the chromatin of the entire locus in an active configuration and acts as an enhancer and entry point for the factors that transcribe the genes of the β-globin locus. One model of the control of hemoglobin switching postulates that proteins bound at the promoters of the ε-, γ-, and β-globin genes compete to interact with the enhancers of the LCR.

Each gene in the β-globin locus has individual regulatory elements—a promoter, silencers, or enhancers that control its developmental regulation. The promoters

A.

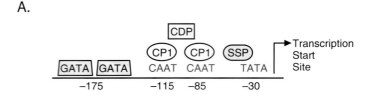

B.

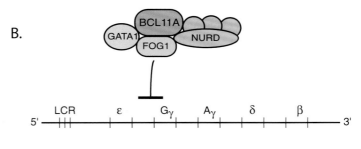

Chromosome 11

FIGURE 42.15 A. The γ-globin gene promoter, indicating some of the transcription factor–binding sites associated with hereditary persistence of fetal hemoglobin. **B.** The β-globin gene locus. When BCL11A is expressed, the interaction between the locus control region (LCR) and the γ-gene promoter is blocked, turning off γ-gene expression. NURD is a chromatin-remodeling complex containing histone deacetylase activity. *CDP*, CAAT displacement protein; *SSP*, stage-selector protein-binding.

that control the γ- and β-globin genes have been intensively studied because of their clinical relevance.

The ε-globin gene, like the ζ-globin gene, has silencers in the 5′-regulatory region. Binding of proteins to these regions turns off the ε-gene.

The proximal region of the γ-globin gene promoter has multiple transcription factor–binding sites (Fig. 42.15). Many HPFH mutations map to these transcription factor–binding sites, either by destroying a site or by creating a new one, but the exact mechanisms are still not understood. Two sites (out of many) that appear to be significant in the control of hemoglobin switching are the stage-selector protein–binding (SSP) site and the CAAT box region. When the SSP complex (consisting of the transcription factors CP2 and NFE4) is bound to the promoter, the γ-globin gene has a competitive advantage over the β-globin promoter for interaction with the LCR. A second transcription factor, Sp1, also binds at the SSP-binding site, where it may act as a repressor, and competition between these two protein complexes for the SSP-binding site helps to determine the activity of the γ-globin gene. A similar mechanism appears to be operating at the CAAT box. CP1, thought to be a transcription activator, binds at the CAAT box. CAAT displacement protein (CDP) is a repressor that binds at the CAAT site and displaces CP1. Part of the mechanism of hemoglobin switching appears to be the binding of repressors at the ε-globin and γ-globin upstream regulatory regions.

The β-globin gene also has binding sites for multiple transcription factors in its regulatory regions. Mutations that affect binding of transcription factors can produce thalassemia by reducing the activity of the β-globin promoter. There is also an enhancer 3′ of the poly(A) signal that seems to be required for stage-specific activation of the β-globin promoter.

Further insights into the control of hemoglobin switching indicate that the transcription factor BCL11A is a strong repressor of γ-globin gene expression. BCL11A interacts with a variety of other transcription factors (GATA-1, FOG1, and the NURD [nucleosome remodeling and histone deacetylase] repressor complex) to repress γ-globin expression. This appears to be caused by BCL11A interfering with LCR interactions with the γ-globin gene promoter. Experiments that reduce, or eliminate, BCL11A expression lead to an increase in γ-globin synthesis. BCL11A expression is regulated by the transcription factor KLF1, which is essential for β-globin expression. KLF1 increases BCL11A expression, which blocks γ-globin gene expression, whereas KLF1 stimulates β-globin gene expression. These recent results suggest that drugs which interfere with KLF1 action would enhance and activate fetal globin gene expression in individuals with either β-thalassemia or sickle cell disease (see Fig. 42.15B).

KEY CONCEPTS

- The blood contains a wide variety of distinct cell types, each of whose function is necessary for maintaining the body's internal environment.
- Erythrocytes transport oxygen throughout the body and return carbon dioxide back to the lung.
  - Erythrocytes lack nuclei and carry out limited metabolic reactions.
    - Glycolysis provides energy and NADH.
    - The NADH maintains the iron in hemoglobin in the ferrous state.
    - The hexose monophosphate shunt provides NADPH to regenerate reduced glutathione to protect the membrane from oxidative damage.
    - 1,3-Bisphosphoglycerate (1,3-BPG) is converted to 2,3-BPG as a by-product of glycolysis in order to regulate oxygen binding to hemoglobin.
  - Heme synthesis occurs in the erythrocyte precursor, using succinyl-CoA and glycine. Inherited defects in heme synthesis lead to porphyrias.
  - Iron, a critical part of heme, is carried throughout the body on protein carriers, because free iron is toxic.
  - The erythrocyte membrane is flexible as a result of its unique cytoskeletal structure, which allows erythrocytes to deform in order to travel through narrow capillaries.
- Hematopoiesis is the generation of the unique blood cell types from a single precursor stem cell in the bone marrow.
- Polymorphonuclear leukocytes consist of a variety of cells types that release chemical signals when activated (granulocytes), phagocytose foreign bodies (neutrophils), destroy parasites (eosinophils), and are involved in the allergic response (basophils).
- Mononuclear leukocytes include the lymphocytes (necessary for the immune response) and monocytes (which develop into macrophages, which engulf debris left behind after granulocytes attack foreign material).
- A wide variety of mutations can lead to alterations in hemoglobin function (hemoglobinopathies):
  - Sickle cell anemia
  - Thalassemias
  - Hereditary persistence of HbF (hemoglobin switching and its regulation)
- Diseases discussed in this chapter are summarized in Table 42.4.

TABLE 42.4	Diseases Discussed in Chapter 42	
DISEASE OR DISORDER	**ENVIRONMENTAL OR GENETIC**	**COMMENTS**
Thalassemias	Genetic	Unbalanced synthesis of α- and β-chains of hemoglobin, leading to anemia
Pyruvate kinase deficiency	Genetic	Red cell hemolysis, leading to fewer red cells. An increase in 2,3-bisphosphoglycerate levels often masks the effects of the anemia.
Congenital methemoglobinemia	Genetic	Oxidation of the iron in heme to the ferric state, which will not bind oxygen, although many individuals with this disorder are asymptomatic
Glucose 6-phosphate dehydrogenase deficiency	Genetic	Affects red blood cell (RBC) membrane stability through an inability to protect membrane proteins and lipids against oxidation
Porphyrias	Genetic	Inherited defects in almost any step of heme synthesis, leading to a series of diseases with different symptoms and outcomes
Iron deficiency	Both	Reduced iron leads to reduced heme synthesis and reduced oxygen delivery to the tissues
X-linked severe combined immunodeficiency syndrome	Genetic	Loss of a cytokine receptor subunit, leading to a complete loss of B- and T-cell maturation and proliferation and no functional immune system
Defective erythropoietin receptor	Genetic	RBC formation is reduced under conditions in which RBC production should be increased (such as reduced oxygen delivery to the tissues).
Hemoglobin C	Genetic	A point mutation in hemoglobin, leading to a lysine for a glutamic acid at position 6 of the β-chain (E6K), leading to hemolytic anemia in the homozygous state
Hereditary persistence of fetal hemoglobin	Genetic	Mutations in promoter and enhancer regions, leading to misexpression of the globin γ-gene and constant expression of the gene
Spherocytosis	Genetic	Mutations in any of several RBC membrane proteins (such as spectrin), leading to instability of the red cells, destruction of the RBCs, and an anemia

REVIEW QUESTIONS—CHAPTER 42

1. A compensatory mechanism to allow adequate oxygen delivery to the tissues at high altitudes, where oxygen concentrations are low, is which one of the following?
   A. An increase in 2,3-BPG synthesis by the red cell
   B. A decrease in 2,3-BPG synthesis by the red cell
   C. An increase in hemoglobin synthesis by the red cell
   D. A decrease in hemoglobin synthesis by the red cell
   E. Decreasing the blood pH

2. A 2-year-old boy of normal weight and height is brought to a clinic because of excessive fatigue. Blood work indicates anemia, with microcytic hypochromic red cells. The boy lives in a 100-year-old apartment building and has been seen ingesting paint chips. His parents indicate that the child eats a healthy diet and takes a Flintstones vitamin supplement every day. His anemia is most likely attributable to a deficiency in which one of the following?
   A. Iron
   B. Vitamin B_{12}
   C. Folate
   D. Heme
   E. Vitamin B_6

3. Drugs are being developed that will induce the transcription of certain globin genes, which are normally silent in patients affected with sickle cell disease. A good target gene for such therapy in this disease would be which one of the following?
   A. The α_1-gene
   B. The α_2-gene
   C. The γ-gene
   D. The β-gene
   E. The ζ-gene

4. A mature blood cell that lacks a nucleus is which one of the following?
   A. Lymphocyte
   B. Basophil
   C. Eosinophil
   D. Platelet
   E. Neutrophil

5. A family has two children, one with a mild case of thalassemia, and a second with a severe case of thalassemia that requires frequent blood transfusions as part of the treatment plan. One parent is of Mediterranean descent; the other is of Asian descent. Neither parent exhibits clinical signs of thalassemia. Both children express 20% of the expected level of β-globin; the more severely affected child expresses normal levels of α-globin, whereas the less severely affected child expresses only 50% of the normal levels of α-globin. Why is the child who has a deficiency in α-globin expression less severely affected?
   A. Thalassemia is caused by a mutation in the α-gene, and the more severely affected child expresses more of it.
   B. The less severely affected child must be synthesizing the ζ-gene to make up for the deficiency in α-chain synthesis.
   C. The more severely affected child also has HPFH.
   D. The more severely affected child produces more inactive globin tetramers than the less severely affected child.
   E. Thalassemia is caused by an iron deficiency, and when the child is synthesizing normal levels of α-globin, there is insufficient iron to populate all of the heme molecules synthesized.

6. An individual displays an anemic condition and upon molecular analysis is shown to be a compound heterozygote for HbS/HbC. The symptoms exhibited by the patient are more severe than those exhibited by patients with sickle cell trait (HbA/HbS) owing primarily to which one of the following?
   A. Increased concentration of HbC molecules in the patient's RBCs
   B. Increased volume of the patient's RBCs
   C. Increased concentration of HbS in the patient's RBCs
   D. Alterations in the patient's RBC morphology
   E. Precipitation of HbS molecules within the patient's RBCs

7. A young boy has been observed to have bluish fingertips and toes. Blood work indicates a mild anemia, and molecular analysis indicates the child has an inherited erythrocyte pyruvate kinase deficiency. This enzyme mutation leads to an increase in the 2,3-BPG levels in the erythrocyte, which helps to ameliorate the effects of the mutation. The increase in 2,3-BPG levels occurs because of which one of the following?
   A. The lack of pyruvate kinase leads to an increase in 1,3-BPG levels, which is used to form 2,3-BPG by the Rapoport-Luebering shunt pathway.
   B. The increase in phosphoenolpyruvate levels leads to the phosphorylation of 3-phosphoglycerate, forming 2,3-BPG.
   C. The increase in phosphoenolpyruvate levels leads to the phosphorylation of 2-phosphoglycerate, forming 2,3-BPG.
   D. The increase in phosphoenolpyruvate levels leads to an increase in 3-phosphoglycerate, which is phosphorylated by ATP to produce 2,3-BPG.
   E. The lack of pyruvate kinase activity leads to an increase of glyceraldehyde 3-phosphate, which is oxidized by an isozyme of glyceraldehyde 3-phosphate dehydrogenase to form 2,3-BPG.

8. A young boy was recently diagnosed with anemia, and further analysis demonstrated that he had hereditary spherocytosis. This disease leads to anemia through which one of the following mechanisms?
   A. Lack of NADPH to protect cell membrane lipids and proteins from oxidation
   B. Nutritional deficiency of iron, folate, or vitamin B_{12}
   C. Inability to reduce ferric hemoglobin to the normal ferrous state
   D. Improper formation of the RBC membrane cytoskeleton
   E. A mutation in heme synthesis

9. A patient is a strict vegetarian and, as such, is concerned about getting sufficient iron in his diet. Which suggestion below could increase his dietary iron absorption?
   A. Never peel potatoes when preparing a potato dish.
   B. Squeeze fresh lemon juice on spinach salad.
   C. Reassure him that iron in plants is readily absorbed.
   D. Meat is the only dietary source of iron.
   E. Taking a vitamin with vitamin B_{12} would help iron absorption.

10. The pluripotent stem cell of the bone marrow produces all blood cells through different lineages via induction of different differentiation pathways. Which one of the following is produced from the same cell line as RBCs?
    A. NK-cells
    B. B-lymphocytes
    C. T-lymphocytes
    D. Basophils
    E. Platelets

ANSWERS

1. **The answer is A.** Increased 2,3-BPG in the red cell will favor the deoxy conformation of hemoglobin and thus allow more oxygen to be released in the tissues. This is useful because the hemoglobin is not as saturated at high altitudes as at low elevations because of the lower concentration of oxygen at high altitudes. Answers C and D are incorrect because the red cells do not synthesize proteins. Answer E is incorrect because reducing the blood pH will not aid in oxygen delivery; the Bohr effect works best when tissue pH is lower than blood pH in order to stabilize the deoxy form of hemoglobin. If the pH of both the blood and the tissue are the same, the Bohr effect will not be able to occur.

2. **The answer is D.** The boy is suffering from lead poisoning, which interrupts heme synthesis at the ALA dehydratase and ferrochelatase steps. Without heme, the oxygen-carrying capability of blood is reduced, and the flow of electrons through the electron-transfer chain is reduced because of the lack of functional cytochromes. Together, these lead to an inability to generate energy, and fatigue results. Answer A is incorrect because although an iron deficiency would lead to the same symptoms, this would not be expected in the patient because of his daily vitamin uptake. Lead ingestion will not lead to an iron loss. Answers B and C are incorrect because vitamin B_{12} and folate deficiencies will lead to macrocytic anemia, owing to disruption of DNA synthesis. Answer E is incorrect because the ingestion of paint chips is unlikely to lead to a vitamin B_6 deficiency in a child, particularly one who is taking daily vitamins.

3. **The answer is C.** Turning on a gene that would provide a functional alternative to the β-gene would enable the defective β-protein to be bypassed. Only the γ-chain can do this, but it is normally only found in HbF. The δ-chain is also a β-replacement globin, but it was not listed as a potential answer. Answer D is incorrect because it is the β-chain that is mutated, and it is already being expressed. Unlike the α-gene, of which there are two copies per chromosome, there is only one copy of the β-gene per chromosome. The other genes listed (answers A, B, and E) are α-chain replacements, and expression of these genes will not alleviate the problem inherent in the β-gene.

4. **The answer is D.** The only two types of blood cells that lack nuclei are the mature RBC and the platelet. Platelets arise from membrane budding from megakaryocytes and are essentially membrane sacs containing the cytoplasmic contents of their precursor cell. All of the other cell types listed contain a nucleus.

5. **The answer is D.** Thalassemias result from an imbalance in the synthesis of α- and β-chains. Excessive synthesis of α-chains results in their precipitation in developing red cells, which often kills the developing cell. The more severely affected child has an α/β ratio of 1:5, whereas the less severely affected child has a ratio of 1:2.5. When β-chains are in excess, they form stable tetramers that bind but do not release oxygen, thus reducing the red cell's ability to deliver oxygen. Thus, this difference in chain ratio makes an important difference in the functioning of the red cell.

6. **The answer is C.** HbC forms an insoluble tetramer that precipitates in RBCs. Because of this, the concentration of HbS is increased in the RBCs, leading to enhanced sickling as compared to someone who has a mixture of HbS and HbA molecules. The enhanced sickling is not directly the result of the precipitation of the HbC molecules, nor is it a result of an increased volume of RBCs (an increased volume would reduce the concentration of HbS, which would reduce sickling). The HbS molecules will form rods under low-oxygen conditions, but they do not precipitate in the cell as do the HbC molecules. Alterations in RBC morphology are a result of the sickling, not a cause of the sickling.

7. **The answer is A.** When pyruvate kinase activity is reduced, phosphoenolpyruvate (PEP) will accumulate. PEP is in equilibrium with 2-phosphoglycerate, which is in equilibrium with 3-phosphoglycerate (3-PG). As 3-PG accumulates, the phosphoglycerate kinase reaction will be inhibited, increasing the levels of 1,3-BPG. As 1,3-BPG levels accumulate, some of it will be shunted to produce 2,3-BPG via 1,3-BPG mutase. The increase in 2,3-BPG levels will then affect the release of oxygen to the tissues from hemoglobin. PEP is not used as a phosphate donor in phosphorylation reactions in the generation of higher levels of 2,3-BPG. ATP is used in the conversion of 3-PG to 1,3-BPG but not to form 2,3-BPG. The oxidation of glyceraldehyde 3-phosphate (glyceraldehyde 3-P) does not generate 2,3-BPG; there is no isozyme of glyceraldehyde 3-P dehydrogenase which will produce 2,3-BPG from glyceraldehyde 3-P.

8. **The answer is D.** Mutations in spectrin, ankyrin, and band 3 proteins lead to improper formation of the RBC membrane cytoskeleton, resulting in malformed RBCs (spherocytes) which have a shortened life span, thus leading to anemia. Mutations in heme synthesis lead to porphyrias. Lack of NAPDH (such as in glucose 6-P dehydrogenase deficiency) leads to anemia via cell membrane oxidation and lysis. Oxidation of the heme iron to the ferric state results in reduced oxygen binding to hemoglobin. Nutritional deficiencies of iron, folate, or vitamin B_{12} would lead to a megaloblastic anemia (folate and vitamin B_{12} deficiencies) or a microcytic anemia (iron deficiency).

9. **The answer is B.** Meats, green leafy vegetables, and fortified cereals and grains are all sources of dietary iron, whereas potatoes are not. Plant nonheme iron is not readily absorbed from the diet, but the presence of vitamin C (citrus fruits) increases the uptake of nonheme iron from the digestive tract. Vitamin B_{12} is not involved in iron absorption.

10. **The answer is E.** Both platelets and RBCs are derived from the BFU-EMeg lineage. Basophils are derived from the CFU-Ba lineage, B- and T-lymphocytes from the lymphoid stem cell lineage, and NK-cells from NK-precursor.

Blood Plasma Proteins, Coagulation, and Fibrinolysis

The blood is the body's main transport system. Although the transport and delivery of oxygen to the cells of the tissues is carried out by specialized cells, other vital components such as nutrients, metabolites, electrolytes, and hormones are all carried in the noncellular fraction of the blood, the **plasma**. Some components, such as glucose, are dissolved in the plasma; others—for example, lipids and steroid hormones—are bound to carrier proteins for transport. The **osmotic pressure** exerted by the plasma proteins regulates the distribution of water between the blood and the tissues. Plasma proteins in conjunction with platelets maintain the integrity of the circulatory system through the process of clotting.

Blood normally circulates through endothelium-lined blood vessels. When a blood vessel is severed, a **blood clot** (called a **thrombus**, which is formed by the process of **thrombosis**) forms as part of **hemostasis**, the physiologic response that stops bleeding. Blood clots also form to repair damage to the endothelial lining, in which components of the **subendothelial layer** become accessible to plasma proteins.

In hemostasis and thrombosis, a primary hemostatic plug, consisting of **aggregated platelets** and a **fibrin clot**, forms at the site of injury. Platelets are attached to the subendothelial layer of the vessel principally through the protein **von Willebrand factor** (vWF) and are activated to bind fibrinogen. **Fibrinogen** binds the platelets to each other to form a platelet aggregate. The platelet aggregate is rapidly covered with layers of **fibrin**, which are formed from fibrinogen by the proteolytic enzyme **thrombin**.

Injury to the endothelium and exposure of **tissue factor** on the **subendothelial layer** to plasma proteins also activate the blood coagulation cascade, which ultimately activates thrombin and **factor XIII**. Factor XIII **cross-links** strands of polymerized fibrin monomers to form a stable clot (the **secondary hemostatic plug**). The blood coagulation cascade consists of a series of enzymes (such as **factor X**), which are inactive until they are proteolytically cleaved by the preceding enzyme in the cascade. Other proteins (**factor V** and **factor VIII**) serve as binding proteins, which assemble factor complexes at the site of injury. Ca^{2+} and **γ-carboxyglutamate** residues in the proteins (formed by a vitamin K–dependent process in the liver) attach the factor complexes to **phospholipids** exposed on platelet membranes. Consequently, thrombus formation is rapidly accelerated and localized to the site of injury.

Regulatory mechanisms within the blood coagulation cascade and **antifibrinolytic mechanisms** prevent random coagulation within blood vessels that might obstruct blood flow. Impairments in these mechanisms lead to thrombosis.

There are two basic assays for measuring the activity of factor VIII in a blood sample. The first is a functional (clotting) assay; the second is a coupled (to factor X activation) enzyme system leading to the cleavage of a chromogenic substrate, generating a colored product.

For the functional assay, a sample of the patient's plasma is added to a factor VIII–deficient sample of plasma (which can be obtained commercially), and the time to generate clot formation is determined. Although clot formation is the end-product of this assay, one is measuring the eventual activation of factor II to IIa, which allows clot formation to initiate.

In the automated chromogenic assay, a sample of the unknown is mixed with purified factor IXa, Ca^{2+}, phospholipid vesicles, the chromogenic substrate, and purified factor X. If the unknown sample contains factor VIII, factors VIII and IXa will synergize and activate factor X to Xa. Factor Xa will cleave the chromogenic substrate, forming a colored product whose concentration can be determined spectrophotometrically. Comparison to a standard curve of factor VIII addition enables an accurate estimate of the level of active factor VIII in the sample.

In cases of severe protein malnutrition (kwashiorkor), the concentration of the plasma proteins decreases, as a result of which the osmotic pressure of the blood decreases. As a result, fluid is not drawn back to the blood and instead accumulates in the interstitial space (edema). The distended bellies of famine victims are the result of fluid accumulation in the extravascular tissues because of the severely decreased concentration of plasma proteins, particularly albumin. Albumin synthesis decreases fairly early under conditions of protein malnutrition.

In spite of the importance of albumin in the maintenance of osmotic pressure in the blood, individuals who lack albumin (analbuminemia) have only moderate edema. Apparently, the concentration of other plasma proteins is increased to compensate for the lack of albumin. The frequency of analbuminemia is < I per million individuals.

THE WAITING ROOM

Peter K., a 6-month-old male infant, was brought to his pediatrician's office with a painful, expanding mass in his right upper thigh that was first noted just hours after he fell down three uncarpeted steps in his home. The child appeared to be in severe distress.

A radiograph showed no fractures, but a soft tissue swelling, consistent with a hematoma (bleeding into the tissues), was noted. Peter's mother related that soon after he began to crawl, his knees occasionally became swollen and seemed painful.

The pediatrician suspected a disorder of coagulation. A screening coagulation profile suggested a possible deficiency of factor VIII, a protein involved in the formation of blood clots. Peter's plasma factor VIII level was found to be only 3% of the average level found in normal subjects. A diagnosis of hemophilia A was made.

I. Plasma Proteins Maintain Proper Distribution of Water between Blood and Tissues

When cells are removed from the blood, the remaining plasma is composed of water, nutrients, metabolites, hormones, electrolytes, and proteins. Plasma has essentially the same electrolyte composition as other extracellular fluids and constitutes approximately 25% of the body's total extracellular fluid. The plasma proteins serve several functions, including maintaining the proper distribution of water between the blood and the tissues; transporting nutrients, metabolites, and hormones throughout the body; defending against infection; and maintaining the integrity of the circulation through clotting. Many diseases alter the amounts of plasma proteins produced and hence their concentration in the blood. These changes can be determined by electrophoresis of plasma proteins over the course of a disease.

A. Body Fluid Maintenance between Tissues and Blood

As the arterial blood enters the capillaries, fluid moves from the intravascular space into the interstitial space (that surrounding the capillaries) owing to Starling's forces. The hydrostatic pressure in the arteriolar end of the capillaries (~37 mm Hg) exceeds the sum of the tissue pressure (~1 mm Hg) and the osmotic pressure of the plasma proteins (~25 mm Hg). Thus, water tends to leave the capillaries and enter extravascular spaces. At the venous end of the capillaries, the hydrostatic pressure falls to approximately 17 mm Hg, whereas the osmotic pressure and the tissue pressure remain constant, resulting in movement of fluid back from the extravascular (interstitial) spaces and into the blood. Thus, most of the force bringing water back from the tissues into the plasma is the osmotic pressure mediated by the presence of proteins in the plasma.

B. The Major Serum Protein, Albumin

As indicated in Table 43.1, the liver produces several transport or binding proteins and secretes them into the blood. The major protein synthesized is albumin, which constitutes approximately 60% of the total plasma protein, but because of its relatively small size (69 kDa), it is thought to contribute 70% to 80% of the total osmotic pressure of the plasma. Albumin, like most plasma proteins, is a glycoprotein (GP) and is a carrier of free fatty acids, calcium, zinc, steroid hormones, copper, and bilirubin. Many drugs also bind to albumin, which may have important pharmacologic implications. For example, when a drug binds to albumin, such binding will likely lower the effective concentration of that drug and may lengthen its lifetime in the circulation. Drug dosimetry may need to be recalculated if a patient's plasma protein concentration is abnormal.

TABLE 43.1	Specific Plasma-Binding Proteins Synthesized in the Liver
Albumin	Binds free fatty acids, calcium, zinc, steroid hormones, copper, bilirubin
Ceruloplasmin	Binds copper; appears to be more important as a copper storage pool than as a transport protein; integrates iron and copper homeostasis
Corticosteroid-binding globulin	Binds cortisol
Haptoglobin	Binds extracorpuscular heme
Lipoproteins	Transport cholesterol and fatty acids
Retinol-binding protein	Binds vitamin A
Sex hormone–binding globulin	Binds estradiol and testosterone
Transferrin	Transports iron
Transthyretin	Binds tetraiodothyronine (thyroxine; T_4); also forms a complex with retinol-binding protein

II. The Plasma Contains Proteins that Aid in Immune Defense

Two different sets of proteins aid in the immune response, the immunoglobulins and the complement proteins. The immunoglobulins are secreted by a subset of differentiated B-lymphocytes termed *plasma cells* and bind antigens at binding sites formed by the hypervariable regions of the proteins (see Chapter 7). Once the antibody–antigen complex is formed, it must be cleared from the circulation. The complement system participates in this function. The complement system, consisting of approximately 20 proteins, becomes activated in either of two ways. The first is interaction with antigen–antibody complexes, and the second, specific for bacterial infections, is through interaction of bacterial cell polysaccharides with complement protein C3b. Activation of the complement system by either trigger results in a proteolytic activation cascade of the proteins of the complement system, resulting in the release of biologically active peptides or polypeptide fragments. These peptides mediate the inflammatory response, attract phagocytic cells to the area, initiate degranulation of granulocytes, and promote clearance of antigen–antibody complexes.

Protease inhibitors in plasma serve to carefully control the inflammatory response. Activated neutrophils release lysosomal proteases from their granules that can attack elastin, the various types of collagen, and other extracellular matrix proteins. The plasma proteins α_1-antiproteinase (α_1-antitrypsin) and α_2-macroglobulin limit proteolytic damage by forming noncovalent complexes with the proteases, thereby inactivating them. However, the product of neutrophil myeloperoxidase, HOCl, inactivates the protease inhibitors, thereby ensuring that the proteases are active at the site of infection.

III. Plasma Proteins Maintain the Integrity of the Circulatory System

Blood is lost from the circulation when the endothelial lining of the blood vessels is damaged and the vessel wall is partly or wholly severed. When this occurs, the subendothelial cell layer is exposed, consisting of the basement membrane of the endothelial cells and smooth muscle cells. In response to the damage, a barrier (the hemostatic plug, a fibrin clot), initiated by platelet binding to the damaged area, is formed at the site of injury. Regulatory mechanisms limit clot formation to the site of injury and control its size and stability. As the vessel heals, the clot is degraded (fibrinolysis). Plasma proteins are required for these processes to occur.

 α_1-Antiproteinase (AAP), also known as α_1-*antitrypsin*, is the main serine protease inhibitor of human plasma. Individuals with a point mutation in exon 5 of the AAP gene, which results in a single amino acid substitution in the protein, have diminished secretion of AAP from the liver. These individuals are at increased risk for developing emphysema. When neutrophils degranulate in the lungs as part of the body's defense against microorganisms, insufficient levels of AAP are present to neutralize the elastase and other proteases released. The excess proteolytic activity damages lung tissue, leading to loss of alveolar elasticity and the development of emphysema.

Methionine 358 of AAP is necessary for AAP binding to the proteases. Oxidation of this methionine destroys the protease-binding capacity of AAP. Chemicals within cigarette smoke lead to the oxidation of Met-358, thereby increasing the risk of emphysema through the inactivation of AAP.

Idiopathic thrombocytopenic purpura (ITP) is an autoimmune disease in which antibodies to platelet GPs are produced. Antibody binding to platelets results in their clearance by the spleen. An early symptom of the disorder is the appearance of small red spots on the skin (petechial hemorrhages) caused by blood leakage from capillaries. Minor damage to vascular endothelial cells is constantly being caused by mechanical forces related to blood flow. In patients with ITP, few platelets are available to repair the damage.

vWF is a large multimeric GP with a subunit molecular weight of 220,000 Da. Its size in the circulation ranges between 500 and 20,000 kDa, and its role in circulation is to stabilize factor VIII and protect it from degradation. The high-molecular-weight forms are concentrated in the endothelium of blood vessels and are released in response to stress hormones and endothelial damage. High-molecular-weight vWF released by the endothelium is cleaved by a specific metalloprotease in the serum, reducing the size of the circulating vWF. Large vWF multimers are more effective at forming complexes with platelets than are small vWF multimers.

vWF deficiency is the most common cause of inherited bleeding disorders. Both platelet adherence and the clotting cascade are affected because levels of factor VIII are low. In the absence of vWF, factor VIII is rapidly cleared from the system. The vWF gene is large, covering approximately 180 kb, and contains 52 exons. Multiple mutations are known, with varying clinical presentations.

A. Formation of the Hemostatic Plug

1. The Platelet

Platelets are nonnucleated cells in the blood whose major role is to form mechanical plugs at the site of vessel injury and to secrete regulators of the clotting process and vascular repair. In the absence of platelets, leakage of blood from rents in small vessels is common. Platelets are derived from megakaryocytes in the bone marrow. Megakaryocytes differentiate from the hematopoietic stem cell. As the megakaryocyte matures, it undergoes synchronous nuclear replication without cellular division, to form a cell with a multilobed nucleus and enlarged cytoplasm. At approximately the eight-nucleus stage, the cytoplasm becomes granular, and the platelets are budded off the cytoplasm. A single megakaryocyte gives rise to approximately 4,000 platelets.

In the nonactivated platelet (a platelet that is not involved in forming a clot), the plasma membrane invaginates extensively into the interior of the cell, forming an open membrane (canalicular) system. Because the plasma membrane contains receptors and phospholipids that accelerate the clotting process, the canalicular structure substantially increases the membrane surface area that is potentially available for clotting reactions. The platelet interior contains microfilaments and an extensive actin/myosin system. Platelet activation in response to endothelial injury causes Ca^{2+}-dependent changes in the contractile elements, which, in turn, substantially change the architecture of the plasma membrane. Long pseudopodia are generated, increasing the surface area of the membrane as clot formation is initiated.

Platelets contain three types of granules. The first are electron-dense granules, which contain calcium, adenosine diphosphate (ADP), adenosine triphosphate (ATP), and serotonin. The second type of granule is the α-granule, which contains a heparin antagonist (heparin interferes with blood clotting; see "Biochemical Comments"), platelet-derived growth factor, β-thromboglobulin, fibrinogen, vWF, and other clotting factors. The third type of granule is the lysosomal granule, which contains hydrolytic enzymes. During activation, the contents of these granules, which modulate platelet aggregation and clotting, are secreted.

2. Platelet Activation

Three fundamental mechanisms are involved in platelet function during blood coagulation: adhesion, aggregation, and secretion. Adhesion sets off a series of reactions termed platelet activation, which leads to platelet aggregation and secretion of platelet granule contents.

The *adhesion step* refers primarily to the platelet–subendothelial interaction that occurs when platelets initially adhere to the sites of blood vessel injury (Fig. 43.1). Blood vessel injury exposes collagen, subendothelial matrix-bound vWF, and other

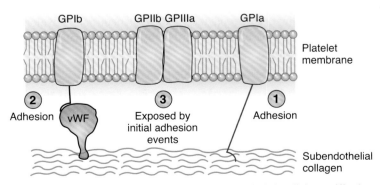

FIGURE 43.1 Adhesion of platelets to the subendothelial cell layer. (*1*) glycoprotein la (GPIa) initially binds to the exposed collagen, which results in changes in the three-dimensional configuration of the complex, allowing GPIb to bind to von Willebrand factor (vWF) (*2*). (*3*) This second binding event exposes the GPIIb–GPIIIa complex, which also can bind to vWF and fibrinogen.

matrix components. vWF is a protein synthesized in endothelial cells and megakaryocytes and is located in the subendothelial matrix, in specific platelet granules, and in the circulation bound to factor VIII. The platelet cell membrane contains GPs that bind to collagen and to vWF, causing the platelet to adhere to the subendothelium. Binding to collagen by GPIa ($\alpha_2\beta_1$ integrin) causes the platelet to change its shape from a flat disc to a spherical cell. The latter extrudes long pseudopods, which promote platelet–platelet interactions. Binding of subendothelial vWF by GPIb causes changes in the platelet membrane that expose GPIIb-IIIa ($\alpha_{IIb}\beta_3$ integrin)–binding sites to fibrinogen and vWF.

The initial adherence of platelets sets off a series of reactions (platelet activation) that results in more platelets being recruited and aggregated at the site of injury. After initial adherence, some of the platelets release the contents of their dense granules and their α-granules, with ADP release being of particular importance because ADP is a potent platelet activator. ADP released from the platelets and from damaged red blood cells binds to a receptor on the platelet membrane, which leads to the further unmasking of GPIIb-IIIa–binding sites. Aggregation of platelets cannot take place without ADP stimulation because ADP induces swelling of the activated platelets, promoting platelet–platelet contact and adherence.

Fibrinogen is a protein that circulates in the blood and is also found in platelet granules. It consists of two triple helices held together with disulfide bonds (Fig. 43.2). Binding of fibrinogen to activated platelets is necessary for aggregation, providing, in part, the mechanism by which platelets adhere to one another. Cleavage of fibrinogen by thrombin (a protease that is activated by the coagulation cascade) produces fibrin monomers that polymerize and, together with platelets, form a "soft" clot. Thrombin itself is a potent activator of platelets, through binding to a specific receptor on the platelet surface.

B. The Blood Coagulation Cascade

Thrombus (clot) formation is enhanced by thrombin activation, which is mediated by the complex interaction that constitutes the blood coagulation cascade. This cascade (Fig. 43.3) consists primarily of proteins that serve as enzymes or cofactors, which function to accelerate thrombin formation and localize it at the site of injury. These proteins are listed in Table 43.2. All of these proteins are present in the plasma as proproteins (zymogens). These precursor proteins are activated by cleavage of the polypeptide chain at one or more sites. The key to successful and appropriate thrombus formation is the regulation of the proteases that activate these zymogens.

The proenzymes (factors VII, XI, IX, X, and prothrombin) are serine proteases that, when activated by cleavage, cleave the next proenzyme in the cascade. Because of the sequential activation, great acceleration and amplification of the response is achieved. That cleavage and activation have occurred is indicated by the addition of an "a" to the name of the proenzyme (e.g., factor IX is cleaved to form the active factor IXa).

The cofactor proteins (tissue factor, factors V and VIII) serve as binding sites for other factors. Tissue factor is not related structurally to the other blood coagulation cofactors and is an integral membrane protein that does not require cleavage for active function. Factors V and VIII serve as procofactors, which, when activated by cleavage, function as binding sites for other factors.

Two additional proteins that are considered part of the blood coagulation cascade, protein S and protein C, are regulatory proteins. Only protein C is regulated by proteolytic cleavage, and when it is activated, it is itself a serine protease.

In addition, in response to collagen and thrombin, platelets release vasoconstrictors. Serotonin is released from the dense granules of the platelets, and the synthesis of thromboxane A_2 is stimulated. This reduces blood flow to the damaged area. Platelet-derived growth factor, which stimulates proliferation of vascular cells, is also released into the environment surrounding the damage.

Mutations in GPIb cause a bleeding disorder known as *Bernard-Soulier syndrome*. Platelet aggregation is affected because of the inability of GPIb to adhere to subendothelial vWF.

Thrombotic thrombocytopenic purpura (TTP) is a disease characterized by the formation in the circulation of microclots (microthrombi) consisting of aggregated platelets. The microthrombi collect in the microvasculature and damage red blood cells, resulting in hemolytic anemia. They also damage vascular endothelium, exposing collagen and releasing high-molecular-weight vWF, promoting more platelet aggregation. The subsequent depletion of platelets renders the patient susceptible to internal hemorrhage. Mortality in untreated TTP can approach 90%.

Familial TTP, which is a less common cause of TTP, is associated with mutations in the vWF-specific metalloprotease, although not all individuals with defective protease develop TTP. Sporadic cases of TTP are associated with the development of an antibody to the metalloprotease.

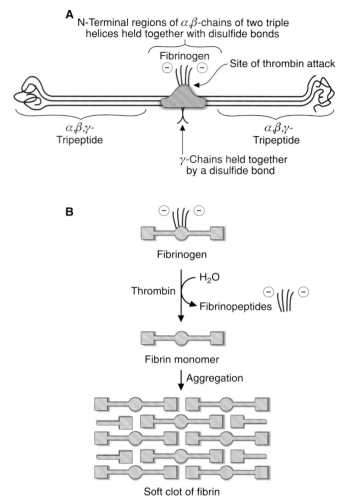

FIGURE 43.2 Cleavage of fibrinogen results in clot formation. **A.** Fibrinogen, the precursor protein of fibrin, is formed from two triple helices joined together at their N-terminal ends. The α,β-peptides are held together by disulfide bonds, and the γ-peptides are joined to each other by disulfide bonds. The terminal α,β-peptide regions, shown in *red*, contain negatively charged glutamate and aspartate residues that repel each other and prevent aggregation. **B.** Thrombin, a serine protease, cleaves the terminal portions of fibrinogen that contain negative charges. The fibrin monomers can then aggregate and form a "soft" clot. The soft clot is subsequently cross-linked by another enzyme.

C. The Process of Blood Coagulation

Activation of the blood coagulation cascade is triggered by the reaction of plasma proteins with the subendothelium at the same time that platelets are adhering to the subendothelial layer. Historically, two different pathways were discovered, one dependent on external stimuli (such as blunt trauma, which initiates the extrinsic pathway) and one using internal stimuli (the intrinsic pathway). As our understanding of blood clotting has expanded, it has become obvious that these distinctions are no longer correct because there is overlap between the pathways, but the terms have persisted in the description of the pathways.

In the case of external trauma, damaged tissues present tissue factor to the blood at the injured site, thereby triggering the extrinsic phase of blood coagulation. Circulating factor VII binds to tissue factor, which autocatalyzes its own activation to factor VIIa. Factor VIIa then activates factor X (to Xa) in the extrinsic pathway and factor IX (to IXa) in the intrinsic pathway. Factor IXa, as part of the intrinsic pathway, also activates factor X. Therefore, activation of both the extrinsic and

The use of an active-site serine to cleave a peptide bond is common to a variety of enzymes referred to as *serine proteases*. Serine proteases are essential for activating the formation of a blood clot from fibrin. Fibrin and many of the other proteins involved in blood coagulation are present in the blood as inactive precursors or zymogens, which must be activated by proteolytic cleavage. Thrombin, the serine protease that converts fibrinogen to fibrin, has the same aspartate–histidine–serine catalytic triad found in chymotrypsin and trypsin.

Thrombin is activated by proteolytic cleavage of its precursor protein, prothrombin. The sequence of proteolytic cleavages leading to thrombin activation requires factor VIII, the blood-clotting protein that is deficient in **Peter K.**

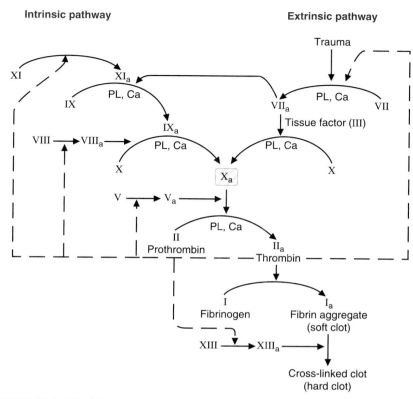

FIGURE 43.3   The blood coagulation cascade. Activation of clot formation occurs through interlocking pathways, termed the *intrinsic* and *extrinsic* pathways. The intrinsic pathway is activated when factor XI is converted to factor XIa by thrombin. The extrinsic pathway (external damage, such as a cut) is activated by tissue factor. The reactions designated by *PL, Ca* are occurring through cofactors bound to phospholipids (PL) on the platelet and blood vessel endothelial cell surface in a Ca^{2+}–coordination complex. Factors XIa, IXa, VIIa, Xa, and thrombin are serine proteases. Note the positive feedback regulation of thrombin on the activation of proteases earlier in the cascade sequence (indicated by the *dashed lines*).

TABLE 43.2 **Proteins of Blood Coagulation**		
FACTOR	**DESCRIPTIVE NAME**	**FUNCTION/ACTIVE FORM**
Coagulation Factors		
I	Fibrinogen	Fibrin
II	Prothrombin	Serine protease
III	Tissue factor	Receptor and cofactor
IV	Ca^{2+}	Cofactor
V	Proaccelerin, labile factor	Cofactor
VII	Proconvertin	Serine protease
VIII	Antihemophilia factor A	Cofactor
IX	Antihemophilia factor B, Christmas factor	Serine protease
X	Stuart-Prower factor	Serine protease
XI	Plasma thromboplastin antecedent	Serine protease
XIII	Fibrin-stabilizing factor	Ca^{2+}-dependent transglutaminase
Regulatory Proteins		
Thrombomodulin	Endothelial cell receptor, binds thrombin	
Proteins C and S	Activated by thrombomodulin-bound thrombin; is a serine protease cofactor; binds activated protein C	

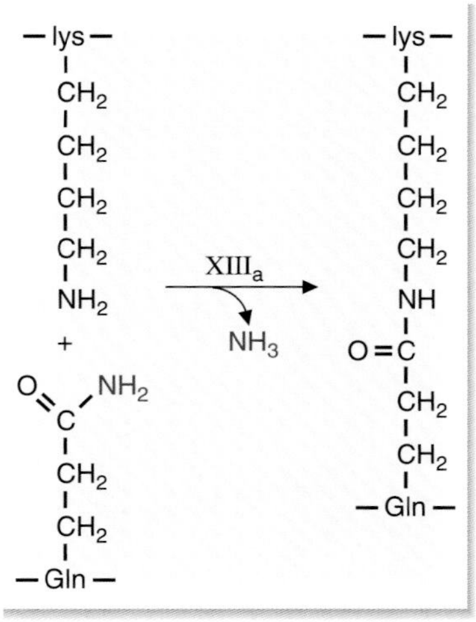

FIGURE 43.4 The transamidation reaction catalyzed by factor XIIIa, transglutaminase. This reaction cross-links fibrin monomers, allowing "hard" clots to form.

Warfarin (Coumadin) is a slow- and long-acting blood anticoagulant with a structure resembling that of vitamin K. The structural similarity allows the compound to compete with vitamin K and prevent γ-carboxylation of glutamate residues in factors II, VII, IX, and X and proteins C and S. The noncarboxylated blood clotting protein precursors increase in both the blood and plasma, but they are unable to promote blood coagulation because they cannot bind calcium and thus cannot bind to their phospholipid membrane sites of activation.

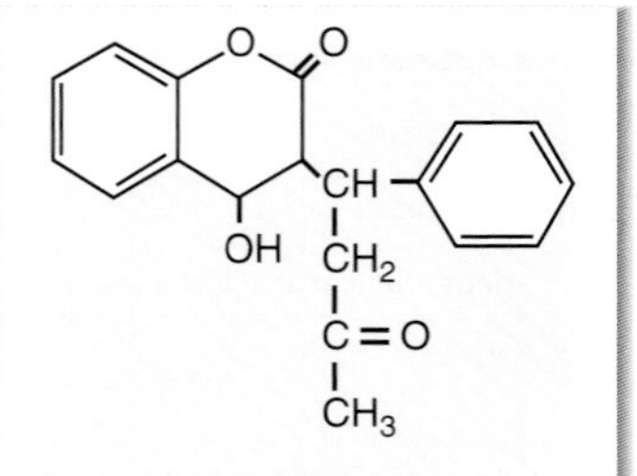

Warfarin

intrinsic pathways results in the conversion of factor X to factor Xa. All of these conversions require access to membranes and calcium; the platelet membrane, which had adhered to the damaged site, is used as a scaffold for the activation reactions to occur. The γ-carboxylated clotting proteins are chelated to membrane surfaces via electrostatic interactions with calcium and negatively charged phospholipids of the platelet membrane. The protein cofactors VIIIa and Va serve as sites for assembling enzyme–cofactor complexes on the platelet surface, thereby accelerating and localizing the reaction. The result is thrombin formation, which augments its own formation by converting factors V, VIII, and XI into activated cofactors and stimulating platelet degranulation. The initial activation of prothrombin is slow because the activator cofactors, VIIIa and Va, are present only in small amounts. However, once a small amount of thrombin is activated, it accelerates its own production by cleaving factors V and VIII to their active forms. Note that these factors are in the intrinsic pathway. The intrinsic pathway is thought to sustain the coagulation response initiated by the extrinsic pathway. The major substrate of thrombin is fibrinogen, which is hydrolyzed to form fibrin monomers that undergo spontaneous polymerization to form the fibrin clot. This is considered a "soft" clot because the fibrin monomers are not cross-linked. Cross-linking requires factor XIIIa, which is activated by thrombin cleavage of factor XIII.

1. Cross-Linking of Fibrin

Factor XIIIa catalyzes a transamidation reaction between glutamine and lysine side chains on adjacent fibrin monomers. The covalent cross-linking takes place in three dimensions, creating a strong network of fibers that is resistant to mechanical and proteolytic damage. This network of fibrin fibers traps the aggregated platelets and other cells, forming the clot that plugs the vent in the vascular wall (Fig. 43.4). Factor XIIIa is the only enzyme in the blood coagulation cascade that is not a serine protease.

2. Factor Complexes

In several of the essential steps in the blood coagulation cascade, the activated protease is bound in a complex attached to the surfaces of the platelets that have aggregated at the site of injury. Factors VII, IX, X, and prothrombin contain a domain in which one or more glutamate residues are carboxylated to γ-carboxyglutamate in a reaction that requires vitamin K (Fig. 43.5). Prothrombin and factor X both contain 10 or more γ-carboxyglutamate residues that bind Ca^{2+}. The Ca^{2+} forms a coordination complex with the negatively charged platelet membrane phospholipids and the γ-carboxyglutamates, thereby localizing the complex assembly and thrombin formation to the platelet surface.

Cofactor Va contains a binding site for both factor Xa and prothrombin, the zymogen substrate of factor Xa. Upon binding to the factor Va–platelet complex, prothrombin undergoes a conformational change, rendering it more susceptible to enzymatic cleavage. Binding of factor Xa to the factor Va–prothrombin–platelet complex allows the prothrombin-to-thrombin conversion. Complex assembly accelerates the rate of this conversion 10,000- to 15,000-fold as compared with non–complex formation.

Factor VIIIa forms a similar type of complex on the surface of activated platelets but binds factor IXa and its zymogen substrate, factor X. Tissue factor works slightly differently because it is an integral membrane protein. However, once it is exposed by injury, it also binds factor VIIa and initiates complex formation.

Complex assembly has two physiologically important consequences. First, it enhances the rate of thrombin formation by as much as several hundred thousand-fold, enabling the clot to form rapidly enough to preserve hemostasis. Second, such explosive thrombin formation is localized to the site of vascular injury at which the negatively charged phospholipids are exposed. From our knowledge of the location of such phospholipids in cellular and subcellular organelle membranes, these surface binding sites are only exposed at an injury site in which cell rupture exposes

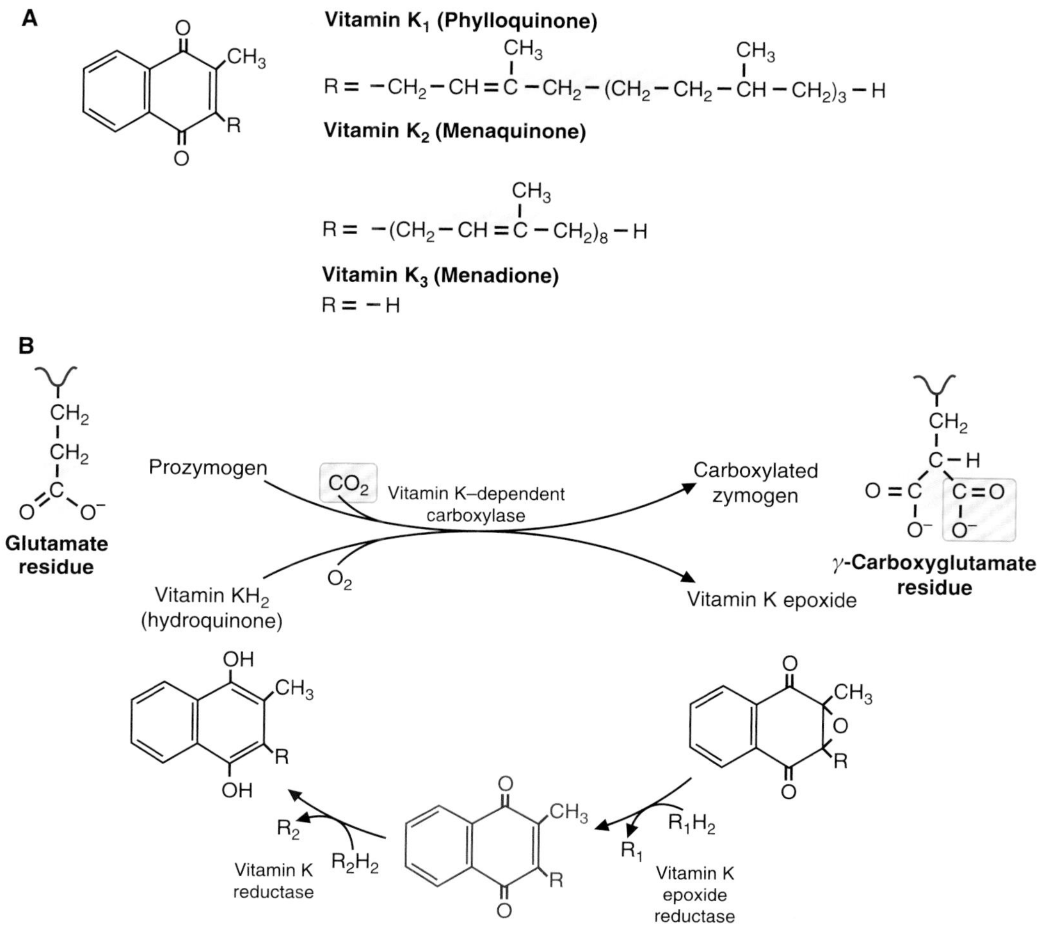

A

Vitamin K₁ (Phylloquinone)

$$R = -CH_2 - CH = C - CH_2 - (CH_2 - CH_2 - CH - CH_2)_3 - H$$

with CH_3 groups

Vitamin K₂ (Menaquinone)

$$R = -(CH_2 - CH = C - CH_2)_8 - H$$

with CH_3 group

Vitamin K₃ (Menadione)

$$R = -H$$

B

Glutamate residue → (Prozymogen, CO_2, Vitamin K–dependent carboxylase, Vitamin KH₂ (hydroquinone), O_2) → Carboxylated zymogen, Vitamin K epoxide → γ-Carboxyglutamate residue

Vitamin K reductase (R_2, R_2H_2) — Vitamin K — Vitamin K epoxide reductase (R_1, R_1H_2)

FIGURE 43.5   A. Structures of vitamin K derivatives. Phylloquinone is found in green leaves, and intestinal bacteria synthesize menaquinone. Humans convert menadione to a vitamin K active form. **B.** Vitamin K–dependent formation of γ-carboxyglutamate residues. Thrombin and factors VII, IX, and X are bound to their phospholipid activation sites on cell membranes by Ca^{2+}. The vitamin K–dependent carboxylase, which adds the extra carboxyl group, uses a reduced form of vitamin K (KH_2) as the electron donor and converts vitamin K to an epoxide. Vitamin K epoxide is reduced, in two steps, back to its active form by the enzymes vitamin K epoxide reductase and vitamin K reductase.

the internal membrane surface (recall that certain phospholipids face only the cytoplasm; if these lipids are now exposed to the environment, substantial cell damage must have occurred).

3. Vitamin K Requirement for Blood Coagulation

The formation of the γ-carboxyglutamate residues on blood coagulation factors takes place in the hepatocyte before release of the protein. Within the hepatocyte, vitamin K (which is present in the quinone form) is reduced to form vitamin KH_2 by a microsomal quinone reductase (see Fig. 43.5). Vitamin KH_2 is a cofactor for carboxylases that add a carboxyl group to the appropriate glutamate residues in the proenzyme to form the carboxylated proenzyme (e.g., prothrombin). In the same reaction, vitamin K is converted to vitamin K epoxide. To recover active vitamin KH_2, vitamin K is first reduced to the quinone form by vitamin K epoxide reductase, and then to the active hydroquinone form.

D. Regulation through Feedback Amplification and Inhibition

Once the formation of the clot (thrombus) begins, clot formation is accelerated in an almost explosive manner by several processes that are collectively termed feedback amplification.

Warfarin is a commonly used rat poison and thus is occasionally encountered in emergency departments in cases of accidental poisoning. It is effective as a rat poison because it takes many hours to develop pathologic symptoms, which allows one poisoned trap to kill more than one rat.

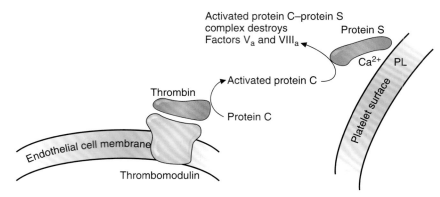

FIGURE 43.6   Antithrombotic effects of thrombin. Thrombin, bound to thrombomodulin on the endothelial cell surface, activates protein C. Activated protein C, in complex with protein S, binds to the platelet membrane, and the activated complex destroys factors Va and VIIIa, thereby inhibiting the coagulation cascade. *PL*, phospholipids.

1. The Role of Thrombin in Regulation

Thrombin has both a prothrombotic regulatory role (feedback amplification) and an antithrombotic regulatory role (feedback inhibition). The prothrombotic action is initiated when thrombin stimulates its own formation by activating factors V, VIII, and XI, thereby accelerating the rate of clot formation (see Fig. 43.3). Thrombin also promotes clot formation by activating platelet aggregation, stimulating the release of factor VIII from vWF, and cleaving factor XIII to factor XIIIa.

Antithrombotic effects of thrombin result from its binding to an endothelial cell receptor called *thrombomodulin* (Fig. 43.6). Thrombomodulin abolishes the clotting function of thrombin and allows thrombin to activate protein C, which has anticoagulant effects.

2. Proteins S and C

Protein C and its cofactor protein S serve to suppress the activity of the coagulation cascade. After activation, protein C forms a complex with protein S. Protein S anchors the activated protein C complex (APC) to the clot through Ca^{2+}/γ-carboxyglutamate binding to platelet phospholipids. The APC destroys the active blood coagulation cofactors factor VIIIa and Va by proteolytic cleavage, decreasing the production of thrombin. The APC also stimulates endothelial cells to increase secretion of the prostaglandin I_2 (PGI_2), which reduces platelet aggregation.

3. Serpins

Many proteases of the blood coagulation enzyme system are serine proteases. Because uncontrolled proteolytic activity would be destructive, modulating mechanisms control and limit intravascular proteolysis. The serpins (*ser*ine *p*rotease *in*hibitors) are a group of naturally occurring inhibitory proteins that are present in the plasma at high concentration ($\sim$10% of the plasma proteins are serpins). At least eight major inhibitors have been found that share a common mechanism of action and inhibit proteases involved in coagulation and clot dissolution (fibrinolysis). Each inhibitor possesses a reactive site that appears to be an ideal substrate for a specific serine protease and thus acts as a trap for that protease. The bound serine protease attacks a peptide bond located at a critical amino acid residue within the serpin and forms a tight enzyme–inhibitor complex.

The activity of thrombin is controlled by the serpin antithrombin III (ATIII). Regulation of blood coagulation at the level of thrombin is critical because this enzyme affects the pathways of both coagulation and fibrinolysis (see Section III.F). One molecule of ATIII irreversibly inactivates one molecule of thrombin through reaction of an arginine residue in ATIII with the active-site serine residue of thrombin.

Deficiency in the amount or functionality of protein C or protein S increases the risk of venous thromboembolism. Individuals who are homozygous for these mutations do not survive the neonatal period unless they are given replacement therapy.

In European populations, a point mutation in the factor V gene (factor V Leiden) causes the replacement of an Arg with a Gln in the preferred site for cleavage by activated protein C, rendering factor Va Leiden resistant to APC. Heterozygous individuals have a sixfold to eightfold increased risk of deep vein thromboses, and homozygous individuals have a 30- to 140-fold increased risk. The factor V Leiden mutation does not appear to be associated with increased risk of arterial thrombosis, such as myocardial infarction, except in young women who smoke.

Genetic studies suggest that the factor V Leiden mutation arose after the separation of the European, Asian, and African populations. The frequency of this variant indicates that it conferred some selective advantage at one time. In the developed world, inherited APC. resistance is the most prevalent risk factor for familial thrombotic disease.

ATIII–thrombin complex formation is markedly enhanced in the presence of heparin. Heparin is a glycosaminoglycan (see Chapter 47) found in the secretory granules of mast cells and in the loose connective tissue around small vascular beds. Heparin binds to lysyl residues on ATIII and dramatically accelerates its rate of binding to thrombin. This is because of an allosteric alteration in ATIII such that the position of the critical arginine residue of ATIII is more readily available for interaction with thrombin. The formation of the ATIII–thrombin complex releases the heparin molecule so that it can be reused, and, therefore, the function of heparin is catalytic. Thrombin that is attached to a surface—for example, to thrombomodulin on the endothelial cell membrane—is no longer participating in clot formation and is not readily attacked by ATIII or the ATIII–heparin complex. The ATIII–heparin complex can also inactivate the serine protease factors XIIIa, XIa, IXa, and Xa but has no effect on factor VIIa or activated protein C.

E. Thromboresistance of Vascular Endothelium

Endothelial cells of blood vessels provide a selectively permeable barrier between the circulating blood and the tissues. The normal endothelial cell lining neither activates coagulation nor supports platelet adhesion; thus, it is called a *nonthrombogenic surface*. The thromboresistance of normal vascular endothelium is contributed to by several properties. Endothelial cells are highly negatively charged, a feature that may repel the negatively charged platelets. Endothelial cells synthesize PGI_2 and nitric oxide, vasodilators and powerful inhibitors of platelet aggregation. PGI_2 synthesis is stimulated by thrombin, epinephrine, and local vascular injury. Endothelial cells also synthesize two cofactors that each inhibit the action of thrombin: thrombomodulin and heparan sulfate. Heparan sulfate is a glycosaminoglycan similar to heparin that potentiates ATIII, but not as efficiently. The inactivation of thrombin is accelerated by heparan sulfate present on the endothelial cell surface. Thus, the intact endothelium has the capability of modifying thrombin action and inhibiting platelet aggregation.

F. Fibrinolysis

After successful formation of a hemostatic plug, further propagation of the clot must be prevented. This is accomplished in part by switching off blood coagulation and in part by turning on fibrinolysis. Fibrinolysis involves the degradation of fibrin in a clot by plasmin, a serine protease that is formed from its zymogen, plasminogen. Plasminogen is a circulating serum protein that has a high affinity for fibrin, promoting the incorporation of plasminogen in the developing clot. The activity of plasminogen is mediated by proteins known as *plasminogen activators*. The conversion of plasminogen to plasmin by plasminogen activators can occur both in the liquid phase of the blood and at the clot surface; however, the latter process is by far more efficient. Activated protein C (APC), in addition to turning off the blood coagulation cascade, also stimulates the release of plasminogen activator from tissues (tissue plasminogen activator [tPA]) and simultaneously inactivates an inhibitor of plasminogen activator, PAI-1.

Plasminogen activator release can lead to plasmin formation in the circulation. However, the circulating plasmin is rapidly inactivated by binding with α_2-antiplasmin, a circulating protease inhibitor. Clot-bound plasmin is not readily inactivated by α_2-antiplasmin. Thus, plasminogen binding to fibrin facilitates its activation to plasmin, protects it from blood serpins, and localizes it on the fibrin substrate for subsequent efficient proteolytic attack. This mechanism allows for dissolution of fibrin in pathologic thrombi or oversized hemostatic plugs, and at the same time it prevents degradation of fibrinogen in the circulating blood.

Two endogenous plasminogen activators are most important; both are synthesized in a variety of cells. tPA is produced chiefly by the vascular endothelial cells, has a high binding affinity for fibrin, and plays a major role in fibrinolysis.

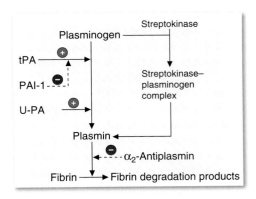

FIGURE 43.7 Regulation of plasmin activation. Plasminogen can be activated by either tissue plasminogen activator (tPA) or urokinase (uPA) (⊕). Plasminogen activator inhibitor I (PAI-1) blocks tPA action (⊖). Streptokinase binding to plasminogen allows autocatalysis to form plasmin. Circulating α_2-antiplasmin blocks (⊖) the activity of any soluble plasmin that may be in the blood.

 Both streptokinase and tPA have been approved for the treatment of myocardial infarction but have been used less frequently over the last several years. If there is cardiac catheterization available, this procedure will be used to treat a myocardial infarction. tPA can also be used to dissolve clots in an acute cerebral vascular accident (CVA; or stroke) or a massive pulmonary embolus (lung clot). Owing to the availability of newer drugs, streptokinase is rarely used at this time.

Single-chain urokinase (uPA) is synthesized in most cells and tissues and has a moderate affinity for fibrin. Streptokinase, the bacterial exogenous plasminogen activator from β-hemolytic streptococci, is not an enzyme but an allosteric modifier of human plasminogen that allows an autocatalytic reaction such that plasmin is formed. In vivo, physical stress, hypoxia, and large numbers of low-molecular-weight organic compounds promote increased synthesis and release of tPA and uPA from tissues into the blood. The balance between release of plasminogen activators, the availability of fibrin, and inhibitors of the activators and plasmin determines regulation of the fibrinolytic response, as indicated in Figure 43.7.

G. Regulation of Fibrinolysis

Antiactivators regulate interaction of plasminogen in blood with plasminogen activators in a dynamic equilibrium. Even if minute amounts of plasmin are generated (e.g., after stress-induced release of vascular plasminogen activator), the enzyme is probably inactivated by antiplasmin. Upon activation of the blood coagulation system, a fibrin clot is formed, which not only strongly binds tPA and plasminogen from blood but also accelerates the rate of plasmin activation. The clot-bound plasmin is protected from inhibitors while attached to fibrin. The enzyme is inactivated by α_2-antiplasmin and α_2-macroglobulin after proteolytic dissolution of fibrin and its liberation into the liquid phase of blood. Thus, the fibrin network catalyzes both initiation and regulation of fibrinolysis.

CLINICAL COMMENTS

 Peter K. Peter K. has hemophilia A, the most frequently encountered serious disorder of blood coagulation in humans, occurring in 1 in every 10,000 males. The disease is transmitted with an X-linked pattern of inheritance.

The most common manifestations of hemophilia A are those caused by bleeding into soft tissues (hematomas) such as muscle or into body spaces like the peritoneal cavity, joint spaces, or the lumen of the gastrointestinal tract. When bleeding occurs repeatedly into joints (hemarthrosis), the joint may eventually become deformed and immobile.

In the past, bleeding episodes have been managed primarily by administration of factor VIII, sometimes referred to as *antihemophilia cofactor*. Unfortunately, the concentration of factor VIII in plasma is quite low (0.3 nM, compared with 8,800 nM for fibrinogen), requiring that it be prepared from multiple human donors.

Before donor screening and virus-inactivation procedures during preparation essentially eliminated transmission with blood transfusions, >50% of patients with hemophilia who were treated with factor VIII during the 1980s in Western Europe or North America became infected with HIV and hepatitis C. Recombinant factor VIII is now available for clinical use and mitigates the threat of HIV/hepatitis C transmission in these patients.

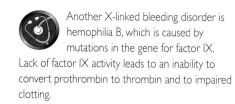

Another X-linked bleeding disorder is hemophilia B, which is caused by mutations in the gene for factor IX. Lack of factor IX activity leads to an inability to convert prothrombin to thrombin and to impaired clotting.

BIOCHEMICAL COMMENTS

Drugs that Inhibit Blood Coagulation. Several drugs have been developed that inhibit the blood coagulation cascade. Such drugs are useful in cases in which patients develop spontaneous thrombi, which, if left untreated, would result in a fatal pulmonary embolism. There are several major classes of such drugs: the heparins, vitamin K antagonists, specific inhibitors of thrombin, and P2Y12 inhibitors.

Heparin binds to and activates ATIII, which leads to thrombin inactivation. ATIII also blocks the activity of factors VIIIa, IXa, Xa, and XIa. Heparin can be administered in either of two forms: unfractionated, or high-molecular-weight (HMW) heparin; and fractionated, or low-molecular-weight (LMW) heparin. HMW heparin is a heterogenous mixture of glycosaminoglycans that have an average chain length of 43 monosaccharides with an average molecular weight of 15 kDa (range, 3 to 30 kDa). LMW heparins are fragments of HMW heparin, containing fewer than 18 monosaccharides with an average molecular weight of 4 to 5 kDa.

HMW heparin binds to plasma proteins and cell surfaces in addition to its prime target, ATIII. Because different individuals synthesize different levels of plasma proteins, the use of this form of heparin as an anticoagulant requires constant monitoring of the patient to ensure that the correct dosage has been given so that spontaneous thrombi do not develop but not so much that spontaneous bleeding occurs. LMW heparin has fewer nonspecific interactions than HMW heparin, and its effects are easier to predict on patients, so constant monitoring is not required.

A major complication of heparin therapy is heparin-induced thrombocytopenia (HIT; excessive blood clotting with a reduction in the number of circulating platelets). This unexpected result of heparin treatment is caused by heparin binding to a platelet protein, platelet factor 4 (PF4), which induces a conformational change in PF4 such that the immune system believes the complex is foreign. Thus, antibodies are developed against the heparin–PF4 complex. When the antibodies bind to the platelets, the platelets become activated, and thrombi develop. Treatment consists of removing the heparin and using a different form of antithrombotic agent.

The classic vitamin K antagonist is warfarin. Warfarin acts by blocking the vitamin K reductase enzymes required to regenerate active vitamin K (see Fig. 43.5). This results in reduced γ-carboxylation of factors II, VII, IX, and X. In the absence of γ-carboxylation, the factors cannot bind calcium or form the complexes necessary for the coagulation cascade to be initiated. However, warfarin also blocks the activity of proteins S and C, so both blood clotting and the regulation of clotting are impaired by warfarin administration.

Both heparin and warfarin therapy suffer from their lack of specificity, so drugs specific for single steps in the blood coagulation pathway have been sought and identified. Analysis of heparin potentiation of factor Xa binding to ATIII showed that a unique pentasaccharide sequence was required. An appropriate pentasaccharide, named *fondaparinux*, was developed that would specifically enhance ATIII interactions with factor Xa. Fondaparinux stimulates the binding of ATIII to factor Xa by 300-fold and is specific for factor Xa inhibition. Fondaparinux does not affect thrombin or platelet activity, and it is not an activating agent of platelets. Because fondaparinux does not bind to PF4, HIT is not a complication with this therapy.

Direct thrombin inhibitors are based on the hirudin molecules, which were initially discovered in leeches and other blood-sucking organisms. These organisms would not be able to feed if the blood clotted at the site of the puncture wound, so the organisms secrete thrombin inhibitors to prevent clotting from occurring. Hirudin treatment itself is dangerous in that formation of the hirudin–thrombin complex is irreversible, and use of the drug requires constant monitoring of the patient. Thus, to overcome this problem, rational drug design based on the hirudin structure was used, and a synthetic 20-amino-acid peptide known as *bivalirudin* was synthesized. This agent has a high binding affinity and specificity for thrombin, although its effects on thrombin are transient (not irreversible), making this a safer agent for long-term use. More recently, there have been multiple other direct-acting anticoagulants developed that inhibit either thrombin or factor Xa.

The P2Y12 receptor inhibitors (examples of which are clopidogrel [Plavix] and ticagrelor [Brilinta]) inhibit platelet aggregation by binding tightly to the ADP receptor on the platelet surface. These drugs are used in patients to prevent strokes and heart attacks in patients who have had a previous stroke or heart attack as well as in patients with cardiovascular disease who have had stents placed to correct narrowed coronary arteries. The use of the drugs prevents platelet aggregation on the newly placed stent. The P2Y12 receptor is coupled to an inhibitory G-protein. ADP is found in the platelet-dense granule, and when the platelet encounters an appropriate agent (such as thrombin), the granular contents are released and ADP binds to its receptor, which amplifies the platelet response and contributes to platelet aggregation. Blocking ADP binding to its receptor will prevent efficient platelet aggregation.

KEY CONCEPTS

- The plasma contains water, nutrients, metabolites, hormones, electrolytes, and proteins.
- Plasma proteins provide osmotic pressure to maintain fluid balance between the tissues and the blood.
- The plasma proteins provide transport for many molecules and also aid in immune defense.
- The plasma proteins, in association with platelets, maintain the integrity of the circulatory system.
  - Platelets form mechanical plugs at the site of vessel injury and secrete regulators of the blood-clotting process.
  - Platelets become activated when bound to a site of injury, which leads to more platelet binding and aggregation at the injured site.
  - Circulating fibrinogen also binds to the activated platelets at sites of injury.
- Clot formation is carefully regulated such that overclotting (thrombosis) or underclotting (bleeding) does not occur.
  - The clotting cascade consists of a series of protease activation steps leading to the activation of thrombin, which converts fibrinogen to fibrin.
  - Thrombin also activates transglutaminase, which cross-links the fibrin and leads to "hard" clot formation.
  - Proteins S and C regulate the clotting cascade and are activated by thrombin.
  - In order to form a clot, protein complexes must adhere to the activated platelets, which occurs via γ-carboxyglutamate binding to calcium and platelet membranes.
  - Serpins are serine protease inhibitors; the serpin antithrombin III (ATIII) aids in regulating blood coagulation by modulating thrombin activity.
  - Heparin enhances the interaction of thrombin with ATIII.
  - Plasmin, the active product of plasminogen, is the only protease that can dissolve fibrin clots.
  - Hemophilia A is caused by a lack of factor VIII, an essential factor required for thrombin activation.
- Diseases discussed in this chapter are summarized in Table 43.3.

TABLE 43.3   Diseases Discussed in Chapter 43

DISEASE OR DISORDER	ENVIRONMENTAL OR GENETIC	COMMENTS
Factor V Leiden	Genetic	Factor V is altered such that it cannot be inactivated by activated protein C, leading to hypercoagulation and deep vein thrombosis (excessive clotting).
Hemophilia B	Genetic	Lack of factor IX in the blood clotting cascade, such that clots cannot be formed
Hemophilia A	Genetic	Lack of factor VIII in the blood clotting cascade, leading to a bleeding disorder (reduced clot formation)
α_1-Antiproteinase deficiency	Genetic	Lack of α_1-antitrypsin leads to elastase destruction of lung tissue, progressing to emphysema and chronic obstructive pulmonary disease (COPD).
Kwashiorkor	Environmental	Protein deficiency in a calorie-sufficient diet leads to a reduction in circulating blood proteins, resulting in edema.
Thrombocytopenic purpura	Both	Formation of microscopic thrombi which lead to hemolysis and organ failure, if untreated. The idiopathic type may be caused by autoimmune destruction of platelets.
von Willebrand factor deficiency	Both	A defect in von Willebrand factor (vWF), a necessary factor for initiation of the blood clotting cascade. In its absence, clotting will not occur and bleeding disorders will result.
Bernard-Soulier syndrome	Genetic	Lack of glycoprotein 1b, the receptor for vWF. Leads to lack of function of vWF and a bleeding disorder because the coagulation cascade cannot be fully initiated.

REVIEW QUESTIONS—CHAPTER 43

1. The edema observed in patients with non–calorie-protein malnutrition is caused by which of the following?
   A. Loss of muscle mass
   B. Ingestion of excess carbohydrates
   C. Increased fluid uptake
   D. Reduced protein synthesis in the liver
   E. Increased production of ketone bodies

2. A recent surgery patient receiving warfarin therapy was found to be bleeding internally. The clotting process is impaired in this patient primarily because of which one of the following?
   A. Inability of the liver to synthesize clotting factors
   B. Specific inhibition of factor XIII activation
   C. Inability to form clotting factor complexes on membranes
   D. Reduction of plasma calcium levels
   E. Enhancement of protein C activity

3. An inactivating mutation in which one of the following proenzymes would be expected to lead to thrombosis (uncontrolled blood clotting)?
   A. Factor XIII
   B. Prothrombin
   C. Protein C
   D. Factor VIII
   E. Tissue factor

4. Classic hemophilia A results in an inability to directly activate which one of the following factors?
   A. Factor II
   B. Factor IX
   C. Factor X
   D. Protein S
   E. Protein C

5. Hemophilia B results in an inability to directly activate which one of the following factors?
   A. Factor II
   B. Factor IX
   C. Factor X
   D. Protein S
   E. Protein C

6. An infant is born with a severe bleeding disorder. It is quickly determined via analysis of blood components that the patient has greatly decreased levels of circulating vWF. The bleeding disorder most likely results from which one of the following as a primary cause?
   A. Inability to activate factor II
   B. Inability of platelets to bind to blood vessel walls
   C. Inability to activate factor IX
   D. Inability to activate protein C
   E. Inability of platelets to bind fibrinogen

7. An individual has a family history of factor V Leiden. Factor V Leiden leads to an increased risk of deep vein thrombosis owing to which one of the following?
   A. The activated form of factor V Leiden is resistant to protein C cleavage.
   B. Factor V Leiden does not need to be cleaved to be activated.
   C. Factor V Leiden enhances factor XIIIa formation.
   D. Factor V Leiden has a reduced need for phospholipids and calcium to activate other factors.
   E. Factor V Leiden directly converts fibrinogen to fibrin.

8. An individual accidently ingested rat poison that interfered with vitamin K action. The activity of which one of the following clotting factors is vitamin K-dependent?
   A. Factor II
   B. Factor III
   C. Factor V
   D. Factor VIII
   E. Factor XIII

9. A patient had a stroke (a cerebrovascular accident [CVA]) caused by a clot in the carotid circulation and received "clot busters" intravenously as emergency treatment. Which clot buster below is not normally found in the human body?
   A. APC
   B. PAI-1
   C. tPA
   D. Streptokinase
   E. uPA

10. A patient had a deep vein thrombosis complicated by a pulmonary embolus and was placed on an anticoagulant as prevention of future clots. He decided to adopt a healthier lifestyle and changed his diet from primarily meat and potatoes to strict vegetarian. This change in diet could affect the efficiency of which one of his following medications?
    A. Unfractionated heparin
    B. LMW heparin
    C. Warfarin
    D. Fondaparinux
    E. Direct thrombin inhibitor

ANSWERS

1. **The answer is D.** Under conditions of reduced protein ingestion, essential amino acids are scarce and the liver reduces protein synthesis, including circulating plasma proteins. The reduction of protein in the plasma results in a lower osmotic pressure, so excess fluid in the extravascular spaces cannot return to the blood and remains outside of the circulation, collecting in tissues.

2. **The answer is C.** Warfarin inhibits the reduction of vitamin K epoxide, so active vitamin K levels decrease. The reduction in active vitamin K levels reduces the γ-carboxylation of clotting factors. In the absence of γ-carboxylation, the clotting factors cannot bind to calcium to form membrane-associated complexes with other clotting factors. Warfarin has no effect on the liver's ability to synthesize the clotting factor (the synthesized factor is not modified), nor does warfarin specifically inhibit the activation of factor XIII. The inhibition is more global than just attacking one step in the coagulation cascade. Plasma calcium levels are not altered by warfarin, and protein C activity is actually decreased in the presence of warfarin because protein C is one of the proteins that is γ-carboxylated in a vitamin K–dependent reaction.

3. **The answer is C.** APC turns off the clotting cascade; in the absence of protein C, regulation of clotting is impaired and clots can develop when not required. Mutations in any of the other answers listed would lead to excessive bleeding, because an essential component of the clotting cascade would be inactivated.

4. **The answer is C.** Classic hemophilia is absence of factor VIII, which is a necessary cofactor for the activation of factor X by factor IXa. Factor II is directly activated by factor Xa, and factor IX is directly activated by factor XIa. Proteins and S are directly activated by thrombin, factor IIa.

5. **The answer is B.** Hemophilia B is an inactivating mutation in factor IX, such that factor IXa cannot be formed. Factor XIa is formed but its substrate, factor IX, is defective, and a nonactive protein results.

6. **The answer is B.** GPIb on the platelet membrane binds to vWF exposed on the subendothelial cell layer. In this patient, vWF levels are reduced and the initial platelet adhesion event is disturbed. Inability of platelets to adhere to the sites of injury leads to blockage of platelet aggregation, fibrinogen deposition, and clot formation. Owing to this problem, most clotting factors will not be activated, but the inability to activate these factors is not the primary cause of the disorder.

7. **The answer is A.** Factor V Leiden still needs to be converted to factor Va to be active, but once active, it is not inactivated by APC. Continued Va activity leads to dysregulation of the clotting cascade and the potential for thrombi formation when none is required. Factor Va aids in factor II activation, not factor XIII activation, and factor V Leiden does not have an altered phospholipid or calcium requirement for complex formation. Factor V Leiden also cannot convert fibrinogen to fibrin, which is the function of thrombin (factor IIa).

8. **The answer is A.** Factors VII, IX, X, and prothrombin (factor II) contain a domain in which glutamate residues are carboxylated to γ-carboxyglutamate in a reaction that requires vitamin K (vitamin K–dependent). The carboxylation is required to allow the factors to bind to positive charges on the forming clot surface, many times aided by the presence of calcium. Factors III, V, VIII, and XIII are not carboxylated in a vitamin K–dependent reaction.

9. **The answer is D.** Streptokinase is produced by β-hemolytic streptococci but has the ability to activate plasminogen to plasmin. All the other proteins listed are produced in the human body. PAI-1 is an inhibitor of plasminogen activator promoting clot retention instead of "clot busting." uPA activates plasminogen to plasmin, as does tPA. Protein C is a normal component of the body and when activated works with protein S to inhibit the clotting cascade.

10. **The answer is C.** Warfarin acts as a vitamin K antagonist. Green leafy vegetables are high in vitamin K and are a staple in vegetarian diets. The increased vitamin K in the patient's diet, and subsequently in his circulation, would greatly reduce warfarin's action and could put the patient at risk for further clots. Both types of heparin bind to and activate ATIII, which, when activated, directly inhibits thrombin. Direct thrombin inhibitors bind to thrombin directly to inhibit clotting. Fondaparinux enhances ATIII interaction with factor Xa, inhibiting Xa and blocking the clotting cascade. The mechanism of action of the heparins, fondaparinux, and direct thrombin inhibitors would not be influenced by a vegetarian diet and an increase in vitamin K levels.

Liver Metabolism

The liver is strategically interposed between the general circulation and the digestive tract. It receives 20% to 25% of the volume of blood leaving the heart each minute (the cardiac output) through the portal vein (which delivers absorbed nutrients and other substances from the gastrointestinal tract to the liver) and through the hepatic artery (which delivers blood from the general circulation back to the liver). Potentially toxic agents absorbed from the gut or delivered to the liver by the hepatic artery must pass through this **metabolically active organ** before they can reach the other organs of the body. The liver's relatively large size (~3% of total body weight) allows extended residence time in the liver for nutrients to be properly metabolized as well as for potentially harmful substances to be detoxified and prepared for excretion into the urine or feces. Among other functions, therefore, the liver, along with the kidney and gut, is an **excretory organ**, equipped with a broad spectrum of detoxifying mechanisms. It can, for example, carry out **metabolic conversion pathways** and use **secretory systems** that allow the excretion of potentially toxic compounds. Concurrently, the liver contains highly specific and selective **transport mechanisms** for essential nutrients that are required not only to sustain its own energy but also to provide physiologically important substrates for the systemic needs of the organism. In addition to the myriad transport processes within the sinusoidal and canalicular plasma membrane sheets (see below), intracellular hepatocytic transport systems exist in organelles such as **endosomes, mitochondria,** and **lysosomes** as well as the **nucleus**. The sequential transport steps carried out by these organelles include (1) **uptake**, (2) **intracellular binding and sequestration**, (3) **metabolism**, (4) **sinusoidal secretion**, and (5) **biliary excretion**. The rate of hepatobiliary transport is determined, in part, by the rate of activity of each of these steps. The overall transport rate is also determined by such factors as hepatic blood flow, plasma protein binding, and the rate of canalicular reabsorption. The various aspects of the major metabolic processes performed by the liver have been discussed in greater detail elsewhere in this text. These previous sources will be referred to as the broad spectrum of the liver's contributions to overall health and diseases are described.

THE WAITING ROOM

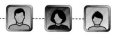

Jean T.'s family difficulties continued, and, in spite of a period of sobriety that lasted 6 months, she eventually started drinking increasing amounts of gin again in an effort to deal with her many anxieties. Her appetite for food declined slowly as well. She gradually withdrew from much of the social support system that her doctors and friends had attempted to build during her efforts for rehabilitation. Upper midabdominal pain became almost constant, and she noted increasing girth and distention of her abdomen. Early one morning, she was awakened with pain in her upper abdomen. She vomited dark-brown "coffee ground" material followed by copious amounts of bright red blood. She called a friend, who rushed her to the hospital emergency department.

Amy B., a 23-year-old missionary, was brought to the hospital emergency department complaining of the abrupt onset of fever, chills, and severe pain in the right upper quadrant of her abdomen. The pain was constant and radiated to her right shoulder top. She vomited undigested food twice in the hour before arriving at the emergency department. This did not relieve her pain.

Her medical history indicated that, while serving as a missionary in western Belize, Central America, 2 months earlier, she had a 3-day illness that included fever, chills, and mild but persistent diarrhea. A friend of Amy's there, a medical missionary, had given her an unidentified medication for 7 days. Amy's diarrhea slowly resolved, and she felt well again until her current abdominal symptoms began.

On physical examination, she appeared toxic and had a temperature of 101°F. She was sweating profusely. Her inferior anterior liver margin was palpable three fingerbreadths below the right rib cage, suggestive of an enlarged liver. The liver edge was rounded and tender. Gentle fist percussion of the lower posterior right rib cage caused severe pain. Routine laboratory studies were ordered, and a computed tomogram (CT) of the upper abdomen was scheduled to be done immediately.

I. Liver Anatomy

The human liver consists of two lobes, each containing multiple lobules and sinusoids. The liver receives 75% of its blood supply from the portal vein, which carries blood returning to the heart from the small intestine, stomach, pancreas, and spleen. The remaining 25% of the liver's blood supply is arterial, carried to the liver by the hepatic artery.

Blood from both the portal vein and hepatic artery empty into a common conduit, mixing their contents as they enter the liver sinusoids (Fig. 44.1). The sinusoids are expandable vascular channels that run through the hepatic lobules. They are lined with endothelial cells that have been described as "leaky" because, as blood flows through the sinusoids, the contents of the plasma have relatively free access to the hepatocytes, which are located on the other side of the endothelial cells.

The liver is also an exocrine organ, secreting bile into the biliary drainage system. The hepatocytes secrete bile into the bile canaliculus, whose contents flow parallel to that in the sinusoids, but in the opposite direction. The canaliculi empty into the bile ducts. The lumina of the bile ducts then fuse, forming the common bile duct. The common duct then releases bile into the duodenum. Some of the liver's effluent is stored in the gallbladder and discharged into the duodenum postprandially to aid in digestion.

The entire liver surface is covered by a capsule of connective tissue that branches and extends throughout the liver. This capsule provides support for the blood vessels, lymphatic vessels, and bile ducts that permeate the liver. In addition, this connective tissue sheet subdivides the liver lobes into the smaller lobules.

Liver lobule

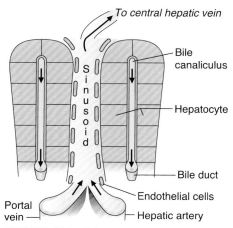

FIGURE 44.1 Schematic view of liver anatomy.

II. Liver Cell Types

The primary cell type of the liver is the hepatocyte. Hepatocytes, also known as *hepatic parenchymal cells*, form the liver lobules. Eighty percent of the liver volume is composed of hepatocytes, but only 60% of the total number of cells in the liver are hepatocytes. The other 40% of the cells are nonparenchymal cells and constitute the lining cells of the walls of the sinusoids. The lining cells comprise the endothelial cells, Kupffer cells, and hepatic stellate cells. In addition, intrahepatic lymphocytes, which include pit cells (liver-specific natural killer cells), are also present in the sinusoidal lining.

A. Hepatocytes

The reports of **Amy B.'s** initial laboratory studies showed an elevation in her serum hepatic transaminases, her serum alkaline phosphatases, as well as her serum total bilirubin level.

The hepatocyte is the cell that carries out the many functions of the liver. Almost all pathways of metabolism are represented in the hepatocyte, and these pathways are controlled through the actions of hormones that bind to receptors located on the plasma membrane of their cells. Although hepatocytes are normally quiescent cells with low turnover and a long life span, they can be stimulated to grow if damage occurs to other cells in the liver. The liver mass has a relatively constant relationship to the total body mass of adult individuals. Deviation from the normal or optimal ratio (e.g., caused by a partial hepatectomy or significant hepatic cell death or injury) is rapidly corrected by hepatic growth caused by a proportional increase in hepatocyte replication.

B. Endothelial Cells

The sinusoidal endothelial cells constitute the lining cells of the sinusoid. Unlike endothelial cells in other body tissues, these cells contain fenestrations with a mean diameter of 100 nm. They do not, therefore, form a tight basement membrane barrier between themselves and the hepatocytes. In this way, they allow for free diffusion of small molecules to the hepatocytes but not of particles the size of chylomicrons (chylomicron remnants, however, which are smaller than chylomicrons, do have free passage to the hepatocyte). The endothelial cells are capable of endocytosing many ligands and also may secrete cytokines when appropriately stimulated. Because of their positioning, lack of tight junctions, and absence of a tight basement membrane, the liver endothelial cells do not present a significant barrier to the movement of the contents of the sinusoids into hepatocytes. Their fenestrations or pores further promote the free passage of blood components through this membrane into the liver parenchymal cells.

C. Kupffer Cells

Kupffer cells are located within the sinusoidal lining. They contain almost one-quarter of all the lysosomes of the liver. The Kupffer cells are tissue macrophages with both endocytotic and phagocytic capacity. They phagocytose many substances such as denatured albumin, bacteria, and immune complexes. They protect the liver from gut-derived particulate materials and bacterial products. On stimulation by immunomodulators, these cells secrete potent mediators of the inflammatory response and play a role in liver immune defense through the release of cytokines that lead to the inactivation of substances considered foreign to the organism. The Kupffer cells also remove damaged erythrocytes from the circulation.

D. Hepatic Stellate Cells

The stellate cells are also called *perisinusoidal* or *Ito cells*. There are approximately 5 to 20 of these cells per 100 hepatocytes. The stellate cells are lipid-filled cells and also serve as the primary storage site for vitamin A. They also control the turnover of hepatic connective tissue and extracellular matrix and regulate the contractility of the sinusoids. When cirrhosis of the liver is present, the stellate cells are stimulated by various signals to increase their synthesis of extracellular matrix material. This, in turn, diffusely infiltrates the liver, eventually interfering with the function of the hepatocytes.

E. Pit Cells

The hepatic pit cells, also known as *liver-associated lymphocytes*, are natural killer cells, which are a defense mechanism against the invasion of the liver by potentially toxic agents, such as tumor cells or viruses.

III. Major Functions of the Liver

A. The Liver Is a Central Receiving and Recycling Center for the Body

The liver can carry out a multitude of biochemical reactions. This is necessary because of its role in constantly monitoring, recycling, modifying, and distributing all of the various compounds absorbed from the digestive tract and delivered to the liver. If any portion of an ingested compound is potentially useful to that organism, the liver retrieves this portion and converts it to a substrate that can be used by hepatic and nonhepatic cells. At the same time, the liver removes many of the toxic compounds that are ingested or produced in the body and targets them for excretion in the urine or in the bile.

As mentioned previously, the liver receives nutrient-rich blood from the enteric circulation through the portal vein; thus, all of the compounds that enter the blood from the digestive tract pass through the liver on their way to other tissues. The enterohepatic circulation allows the liver first access to nutrients to fulfill specific functions (such as the synthesis of blood coagulation proteins, heme, purines, and pyrimidines) and first access to ingested toxic compounds (such as ethanol) and to such potentially harmful metabolic products (such as NH_4^+ produced from bacterial metabolism in the gut).

In addition to the blood supply from the portal vein, the liver receives oxygen-rich blood through the hepatic artery; this arterial blood mixes with the blood from the portal vein in the sinusoids. This unusual mixing process gives the liver access to various metabolites ingested and produced in the periphery and secreted into the peripheral circulation, such as glucose, individual amino acids, certain proteins, iron–transferrin complexes, and waste metabolites as well as potential toxins produced during substrate metabolism. As mentioned, fenestrations in the endothelial cells, combined with gaps between the cells, the lack of a basement membrane between the endothelial cells and the hepatocytes, and low portal blood pressure (which results in slow blood flow), contribute to the efficient exchange of compounds between sinusoidal blood and the hepatocyte and clearance of unwanted compounds from the blood. Thus, large molecules targeted for processing, such as serum proteins and chylomicron remnants, can be removed by hepatocytes, degraded, and their components recycled. Similarly, newly synthesized molecules, such as very-low-density lipoprotein (VLDL) and serum proteins, can be easily secreted into the blood. In addition, the liver can convert all of the amino acids found in proteins into glucose, fatty acids, or ketone bodies. The secretion of VLDL by the liver not only delivers excess calories to adipose tissue for storage of fatty acids in triacylglycerol but also delivers phospholipids and cholesterol to tissues that are in need of these compounds for synthesis of cell walls as well as other functions. The secretion of glycoproteins by the liver is accomplished through the liver's gluconeogenic capacity and its access to a variety of dietary sugars to form the oligosaccharide chains as well as its access to dietary amino acids with which it synthesizes proteins. Thus, the liver has the capacity to carry out a large number of biosynthetic reactions. It has the biochemical wherewithal to synthesize a myriad of compounds from a broad

 The CT scan of **Amy B.'s** upper abdomen showed an elevated right hemidiaphragm as well as several cystic masses in her liver, the largest of which was located in the superior portion of the right lobe. Her clinical history as well as her history of possible exposure to various parasites while working in a part of Belize, Central America, that is known to practice substandard sanitation, prompted her physicians to order a titer of serum antibodies against the parasite *Entamoeba histolytica*, in addition to measuring serum antibodies against other invasive parasites.

A knowledge of functional characteristics of liver cells has been used to design diagnostic agents to determine the normalcy of specific biochemical pathways of the hepatocytes. These "tailor-made" pharmaceuticals can be designed to be taken up by one or more of the transport mechanisms available to the liver. For example, receptor-related endocytic processes can be used as targets to probe specific receptor-mediated transport functions of the liver cells. The asialoglycoprotein receptor, also known as the *hepatic binding protein*, has been used in this diagnostic approach. The substrate $^{99}Tc^m$-galactosyl-neoglycoalbumin (NGA) was developed as a specific ligand for selective uptake via this hepatic receptor. The timing and extent of the assimilation of this probe into the hepatocytes, as determined by imaging the liver at precise intervals after the administration of this isotope, yields an estimate of hepatic blood flow as well as the transport capacity of this particular hepatic transporter protein.

Antibody titers against *Entamoeba histolytica* by use of an enzyme immunoassay were strongly reactive in **Amy B.'s** blood. A diagnosis of *amoebiasis* was made. Her physicians started a nitroimidazole amoebicide (metronidazole) orally in a dose of 750 mg every 8 hours for 10 days. By the third day of treatment, Amy began to feel noticeably better. Her physicians told her that they expected a full clinical response in 95% of patients with amoebic liver abscesses treated in this way, although her multiple hepatic abscesses adversely affected her prognosis to a degree. After her response to oral therapy for the liver abscess, she was also treated with a "luminal agent" (a drug which acts primarily in the lumen of the intestine) to clear the organism from her intestine.

spectrum of precursors. At the same time, the liver metabolizes compounds into biochemically useful products. Alternatively, it has the ability to degrade and excrete those compounds presented to it that cannot be further used by the body.

Each of the liver cells described contains specialized transport and uptake mechanisms for enzymes, infectious agents, drugs, and other xenobiotics that specifically target these substances to certain liver cell types. These are accomplished by linking these agents covalently by way of biodegradable bonds to their specific carrier. The latter then determines the particular fate of the drug by using specific cell recognition, uptake, transport, and biodegradation pathways.

B. Inactivation and Detoxification of Xenobiotic Compounds and Metabolites

Xenobiotics are compounds that have no nutrient value (cannot be used by the body for energy requirements) and are potentially toxic. They are present as natural components of foods or they may be introduced into foods as additives or through processing. Pharmacologic and recreational drugs are also xenobiotic compounds. The liver is the principal site in the body for the degradation of these compounds. Because many of these substances are lipophilic, they are oxidized, hydroxylated, or hydrolyzed by enzymes in phase I reactions. Phase I reactions introduce or expose hydroxyl groups or other reactive sites that can be used for conjugation reactions (the phase II reactions). The conjugation reactions add a negatively charged group such as glycine, sulfate, or glucuronic acid to the molecule. Many xenobiotic compounds are transformed through several different pathways. A general scheme of inactivation is shown in Figure 44.2.

The conjugation and inactivation pathways are similar to those used by the liver to inactivate many of its own metabolic waste products. These pathways are intimately related to the biosynthetic cascades that exist in the liver. The liver can synthesize the precursors that are required for conjugation and inactivation reactions from other compounds. For example, sulfation is used by the liver to clear steroid hormones from the circulation. The sulfate used for this purpose can be obtained from the degradation of cysteine or methionine.

The liver, kidney, and intestine are the major sites in the body for biotransformation of xenobiotic compounds. Many xenobiotic compounds contain aromatic rings (such as benzopyrene in tobacco smoke) or heterocyclic ring structures (such as the nitrogen-containing rings of nicotine or pyridoxine) that we are unable to degrade or recycle into useful components. These structures are hydrophobic, causing the molecules to be retained in adipose tissue unless they are sequestered by the liver, kidney, or intestine for biotransformation reactions. Sometimes, however, the phase I and II reactions backfire, and harmless hydrophobic molecules are converted to toxins or potent chemical carcinogens.

I. Cytochrome P450 and Xenobiotic Metabolism

The toxification/detoxification of xenobiotics is accomplished through the activity of a group of enzymes with a broad spectrum of biologic activity. Some examples of enzymes involved in xenobiotic transformation are described in Table 44.1. Of the

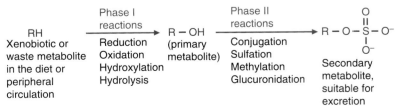

FIGURE 44.2 General scheme of xenobiotic detoxification. The toxic compound RH has been converted to a sulfated derivative suitable for excretion. *RH*, a general xenobiotic.

TABLE 44.1 Examples of Enzymes Used in Biotransformation of Xenobiotic Compounds

Acetyl transferase
Amidase-esterase
Dehydrogenase
Flavin-containing monooxygenase
Glutathione S-transferase
Methyl transferase
Mixed-function oxidase
Reductase
Sulfotransferase
UDP-glucosyltransferase
UDP-glucuronosyltransferase

UDP, uridine diphosphate.

wide variety of enzymes that are involved in xenobiotic metabolism, only the cytochrome P450–dependent monooxygenase system is discussed here (see Chapter 33). The cytochrome P450–dependent monooxygenase enzymes are determinants in oxidative, peroxidative, and reductive degradation of exogenous (e.g., chemicals, carcinogens, pollutants) and endogenous (e.g., steroids, prostaglandins, retinoids) substances. The key enzymatic constituents of this system are the flavoprotein reduced nicotinamide adenine dinucleotide phosphate (NADPH)–cytochrome P450 oxidoreductase and cytochrome P450 (see Fig. 33.5). The latter is the terminal electron acceptor and substrate-binding site of the microsomal mixed-function oxidase complex, a very versatile catalytic system. The system got its name in 1962, when Omura and Sato found a pigment with unique spectral characteristics that was derived from liver microsomes of rabbits. When reduced and complexed with carbon monoxide, it exhibited a spectral absorbance maximum at 450 nm.

The major role of the cytochrome P450 enzymes (see Chapter 33) is to oxidize substrates and introduce oxygen to the structure. Similar reactions can be carried out by other flavin monooxygenases that do not contain cytochrome P450.

The human cytochrome P450 enzyme family contains 57 functional genes, which produce proteins with at least 40% sequence homology. These isozymes have different but overlapping specificities. The human enzymes are generally divided into nine major subfamilies, and each of these is further subdivided. For example, in the naming of the principal enzyme involved in the oxidation of ethanol to acetaldehyde, CYP2E1, the *CYP* denotes the cytochrome P450 family, the *2* denotes the subfamily, the *E* denotes ethanol, and the *1* denotes the specific isozyme.

The CYP3A4 isoform accounts for 30% to 40% of CYP450 enzymes in the liver and 70% of cytochrome enzymes in gut-wall enterocytes. It metabolizes the greatest number of drugs in humans. Specific drugs are substrates for CYP3A4. The concomitant ingestion of two CYP3A4 substrates could potentially induce competition for the binding site, which, in turn, could alter the blood levels of these two agents. The drug with the highest affinity for the enzyme will be preferentially metabolized, whereas the metabolism (and degradation) of the other drug will be reduced. The latter drug's concentration in the blood will then rise.

Moreover, many substances or drugs impair or inhibit the activity of the CYP3A4 enzyme, thereby impairing the body's ability to metabolize a drug. Some of the lipid-lowering agents known as the *statins* (hydroxymethylglutaryl coenzyme A [HMG-CoA] reductase inhibitors) require CYP3A4 for degradation. Appropriate drug treatment and dosing takes into account the normal degradative pathway of the drug. However, a component of grapefruit juice is a potent inhibitor of CYP3A4-mediated drug metabolism. Evidence suggests that if certain statins are regularly taken with grapefruit juice, its level in the blood may increase as much as 15-fold. This marked increase in plasma concentration could increase the muscle and liver toxicity of the statin in question because side effects of the statins appear to be dose-related.

The cytochrome P450 isozymes all have certain features in common:

1. They all contain cytochrome P450, oxidize the substrate, and reduce oxygen.
2. They all have a flavin-containing reductase subunit that uses NADPH, and not NADH, as a substrate.
3. They are all found in the smooth endoplasmic reticulum and are referred to as *microsomal enzymes* (e.g., CYP2E1 is also referred to as the *microsomal ethanol-oxidizing system* [MEOS]).
4. They are all bound to the lipid portion of the membrane, probably to phosphatidylcholine.
5. They are all inducible by the presence of their own best substrate and somewhat less inducible by the substrates for other P450 isozymes.
6. They all generate a reactive free radical compound as an intermediate in the reaction.

2. Examples of Cytochrome P450 Detoxification Reactions

a. Vinyl Chloride

The detoxification of vinyl chloride provides an example of effective detoxification by a P450 isozyme (ethanol detoxification is discussed in Chapter 33). Vinyl chloride is used in the synthesis of plastics and can cause angiosarcoma in the liver of exposed workers. It is activated in a phase I reaction to a reactive epoxide by a hepatic P450 isozyme (CYP2E1), which can react with guanine in DNA or other cellular molecules. However, it also can be converted to chloroacetaldehyde, conjugated with reduced glutathione, and excreted in a series of phase II reactions (Fig. 44.3).

b. Aflatoxin B$_1$

Aflatoxin B$_1$ is an example of a compound that is made more toxic by a cytochrome P450 reaction (CYP2A1). Current research suggests that ingested aflatoxin B$_1$ in contaminated food (it is produced by a fungus [*Aspergillus flavus*] that grows on peanuts that may have been stored in damp conditions) is directly involved in hepatocarcinogenesis in humans by introducing a G $\rightarrow$ T mutation into the *p53* gene. Aflatoxin is metabolically activated to its 8,9-epoxide by two different isozymes of cytochrome P450. The epoxide modifies DNA by forming covalent adducts with guanine residues. In addition, the epoxide can combine with lysine residues in proteins and thus is also a hepatotoxin.

c. Acetaminophen

Acetaminophen (Tylenol) is an example of a xenobiotic that is metabolized by the liver for safe excretion; however, it can be toxic if ingested in high doses. The pathways for acetaminophen metabolism are shown in Figure 44.4. As shown in the figure, acetaminophen can be glucuronylated or sulfated for safe excretion by the kidney. However, a cytochrome P450 enzyme produces the toxic intermediate *N*-acetyl-*p*-benzoquinoneimine (NAPQI), which can be excreted safely in the urine after conjugation with glutathione.

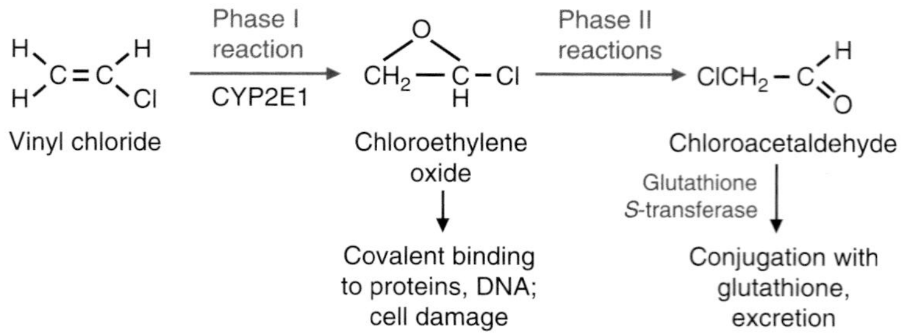

FIGURE 44.3 Detoxification of vinyl chloride.

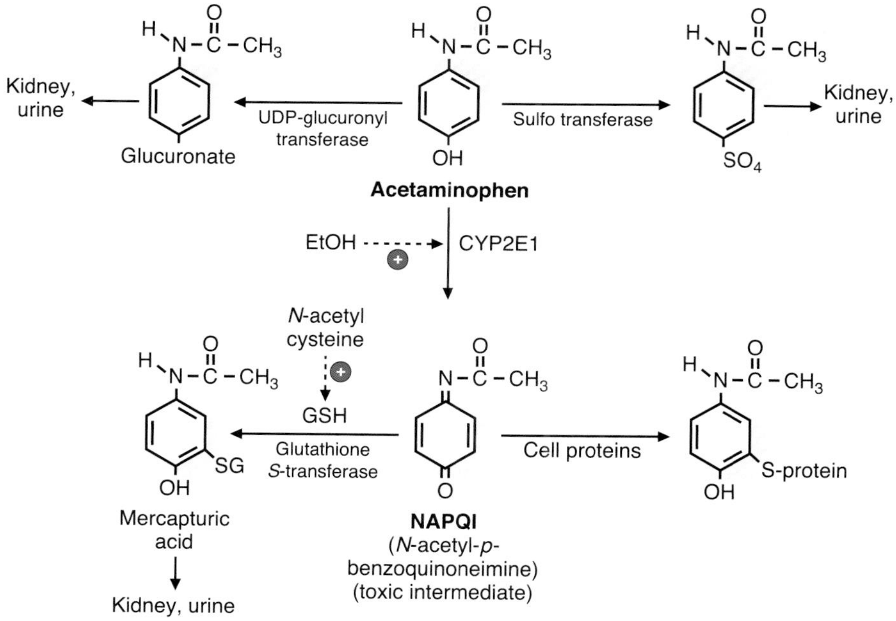

FIGURE 44.4 Pathways of acetaminophen detoxification. *N*-Acetylcysteine stimulates the production of glutathione, thereby reducing the levels of NAPQI, which can damage cellular proteins. Ethanol upregulates CYP2E1 activity (the microsomal ethanol-oxidizing system [MEOS]). *GSH*, reduced glutathione; *UDP*, uridine diphosphate.

NAPQI is a dangerous and unstable metabolite that can damage cellular proteins and lead to death of the hepatocyte. Under normal conditions, when acetaminophen is taken in the correct therapeutic amounts, <10% of the drug forms NAPQI, an amount that can be readily handled by the glutathione detoxifying system (phase II reactions). However, when taken in doses that are potentially toxic, the sulfotransferase and glucuronyl transferase systems are overwhelmed, and more acetaminophen is metabolized through the NAPQI route. When this occurs, the levels of glutathione in the hepatocyte are insufficient to detoxify NAPQI, and hepatocyte death can result.

The enzyme that produces NAPQI, CYP2E1, is induced by alcohol (see Chapter 33; MEOS). Thus, individuals who chronically abuse alcohol have increased sensitivity to acetaminophen toxicity, because a higher percentage of acetaminophen metabolism is directed toward NAPQI, compared with an individual with low levels of CYP2E1. Therefore, even recommended therapeutic doses of acetaminophen can be toxic to these individuals.

An effective treatment for acetaminophen poisoning involves the use of *N*-acetylcysteine. This compound supplies cysteine as a precursor for increased glutathione production, which, in turn, enhances the phase II reactions, which reduces the levels of the toxic intermediate.

C. Regulation of Blood Glucose Levels

One of the primary functions of the liver is to maintain blood glucose concentrations within the normal range. The manner in which the liver accomplishes this has been the subject of previous chapters (Chapters 19, 28, and 34). In brief, the pancreas monitors blood glucose levels and secretes insulin when blood glucose levels rise and glucagon when such levels decrease. These hormones initiate regulatory cascades that affect liver glycogenolysis, glycogen synthesis, glycolysis, and gluconeogenesis. In addition, sustained physiologic increases in growth hormone, cortisol, and catecholamine secretion help to sustain normal blood glucose levels during fasting (see Chapter 41).

When blood glucose levels drop, glycolysis and glycogen synthesis are inhibited, and gluconeogenesis and glycogenolysis are activated. Concurrently, fatty acid oxidation is activated to provide energy for glucose synthesis. During an overnight fast, blood glucose levels are maintained primarily by glycogenolysis and, if gluconeogenesis is required, the energy (six ATP molecules are required to produce one molecule of glucose from two molecules of pyruvate) is obtained by fatty acid oxidation. On insulin release, the opposing pathways are activated such that excess fuels can be stored either as glycogen or fatty acids. The pathways are regulated by the activation or inhibition of two key kinases, the cyclic adenosine monophosphate (cAMP)–dependent protein kinase, and the AMP-activated protein kinase (see Fig. 34.8 for a review of these pathways). Recall that the liver can export glucose because it is one of only two tissues that express glucose 6-phosphatase.

D. Synthesis and Export of Cholesterol and Triacylglycerol

When food supplies are plentiful, hormonal activation leads to fatty acid, triacylglycerol, and cholesterol synthesis. High dietary intake and intestinal absorption of cholesterol compensatorily reduces the rate of hepatic cholesterol synthesis, in which case the liver acts as a recycling depot for sending excess dietary cholesterol to the peripheral tissue when needed as well as accepting cholesterol from these tissues when required. The pathways of cholesterol metabolism were discussed in Chapter 32.

E. Ammonia and the Urea Cycle

The liver is the primary organ for synthesizing urea and thus is the central depot for the disposition of ammonia in the body. Ammonia groups travel to the liver on glutamine and alanine, and the liver converts these ammonia nitrogens to urea for excretion in the urine. The reactions of the urea cycle were discussed in Chapter 36.

Table 44.2 lists some of the important nitrogen-containing compounds that are primarily synthesized or metabolized by the liver.

F. Formation of Ketone Bodies

The liver is the only organ that can produce ketone bodies, yet it is one of the few that cannot use these molecules for energy production. Ketone bodies are produced when the rate of glucose synthesis is limited (i.e., substrates for gluconeogenesis are limited) and fatty acid oxidation is occurring rapidly. Ketone bodies can cross the blood–brain barrier and become a major fuel for the nervous system under conditions of starvation. Synthesis and metabolism of ketone bodies have been described in Chapter 30.

G. Nucleotide Biosynthesis

The liver can synthesize and salvage all ribonucleotides and deoxyribonucleotides for other cells to use. Certain cells have lost the capacity to produce nucleotides de novo but can use the salvage pathways to convert free bases to nucleotides. The liver can secrete free bases into the circulation for these cells to use for this purpose. Nucleotide synthesis and degradation are discussed in Chapter 39.

H. Synthesis of Blood Proteins

The liver is the primary site of the synthesis of circulating proteins such as albumin and the clotting factors. When liver protein synthesis is compromised, the protein levels in the blood are reduced. Hypoproteinemia may lead to edema because of a decrease in the protein-mediated osmotic pressure in the blood. This, in turn, causes plasma water to leave the circulation and enter (and expand) the interstitial space, causing edema.

Cirrhosis of the liver results in portal hypertension, which, because of increasing back pressure into the esophageal veins, promotes the development of dilated thin-walled esophageal veins (varices). At the same time, synthesis of blood coagulation proteins by the liver and required vitamin K–dependent reactions are greatly diminished (resulting in a prolonged prothrombin time; which, in turn, increases clotting time). When the esophageal varices rupture, massive bleeding into the thoracic or abdominal cavity as well as the stomach may occur. Much of the protein content of the blood entering the gastrointestinal tract is metabolized by intestinal bacteria, releasing ammonium ion, which enters the portal vein. Because hepatocellular function has been compromised, the urea-cycle capacity is inadequate, and the ammonium ion enters the peripheral circulation, thereby contributing to hepatic encephalopathy (brain toxicity owing to elevated ammonia levels).

TABLE 44.2   Nitrogen-Containing Products Produced by the Liver

PRODUCT	PRECURSORS	TISSUES	FUNCTION
Creatine	Arginine, glycine, and S-adenosylmethionine (SAM)	Liver	Forms creatine phosphate in muscle for energy storage. Excreted as creatinine.
Glutathione	Glutamate, cysteine, glycine	All tissues, but highest use in the liver	Protection against free-radical injury by reduction of hydrogen peroxide and lipid peroxides. In liver and kidney, forms mercapturic acids.
Purines	Glycine, glutamine, aspartate, carbon dioxide, tetrahydrofolate, phosphoribosyl pyrophosphate (PRPP)	Liver, small amounts in brain and cells of the immune system	Adenine and guanine nucleosides and nucleotides. DNA, RNA, and coenzymes, and energy-transferring nucleotides.
Pyrimidines	Aspartate, glutamine, carbon dioxide	Liver, small amounts in brain and cells of the immune system	Uracil, thymine, and cytosine
Sialic acid (N-acetylneuraminic acid [NANA]), other amino sugars	Glutamine	Most cells	In the liver, synthesis of oligosaccharide chains on secreted proteins. Most cells, glycoproteins, proteoglycans, and glycolipids.
Sulfated compounds	Cysteine	Liver and kidney produce sulfate	Many cells use sulfate in blood for formation of phosphoadenosine phosphosulfate (PAPS), which transfers sulfate to proteoglycans, drugs, and xenobiotics.
Taurine	Cysteine	Liver	Conjugated bile salts
Glycocholic acid, and glycochenodeoxycholic acid	Glycine, bile salts	Liver	Conjugated bile salts are excreted into the bile and assist in the absorption of lipids and fat-soluble vitamins through the formation of micelles.
Sphingosine	Serine and palmitoyl-CoA	Liver, brain, and other tissues	Precursor of sphingolipids found in myelin and other membranes.
Heme	Glycine and succinyl-CoA	Liver, bone marrow cytochromes. Heme from bone marrow	Heme from liver is incorporated into hemoglobin.
Glycine conjugates of xenobiotic compounds	Glycine, medium-size hydrophobic carboxylic acids	Liver, kidney	Inactivation and targeting toward urinary excretion.
Niacin	Tryptophan, glutamine	Liver	NAD, NADP coenzymes for oxidation reactions.
One-carbon methyl donors for tetrahydrofolate and SAM	Glycine, serine, histidine, methionine	Most cells, but highest in liver	Choline, phosphatidylcholine, purine and pyrimidine synthesis, inactivation of waste metabolites and xenobiotics through methylation.

NAD, nicotinamide adenine dinucleotide; palmitoyl-CoA, palmitoyl coenzyme A; succinyl-CoA, succinyl coenzyme A.

Most circulating plasma proteins are synthesized by the liver. Therefore, the hepatocyte has a well-developed endoplasmic reticulum, Golgi system, and cellular cytoskeleton, all of which function in the synthesis, processing, and secretion of proteins. The most abundant plasma protein produced by the liver is albumin, which represents 55% to 60% of the total plasma protein pool. Albumin serves as a carrier for a large number of hydrophobic compounds, such as fatty acids, steroids, hydrophobic amino acids, vitamins, and pharmacologic agents. It is also an important osmotic regulator in the maintenance of normal plasma osmotic pressure. The other proteins synthesized by the liver are, for the most part, glycoproteins. They function in hemostasis, transport, protease inhibition, and ligand binding, and as secretogogues for hormone release. The acute-phase proteins that are part of the immune response and the body's response to many forms of "injury" are also synthesized in the liver.

I. The Synthesis of Glycoproteins and Proteoglycans

The liver, because it is the site of synthesis of most of the blood proteins (including the glycoproteins), has a high requirement for the sugars that go into the oligosaccharide portion of glycoproteins. (The synthesis of glycoproteins was discussed in Chapter 27.) These include mannose, fructose, galactose, and amino sugars.

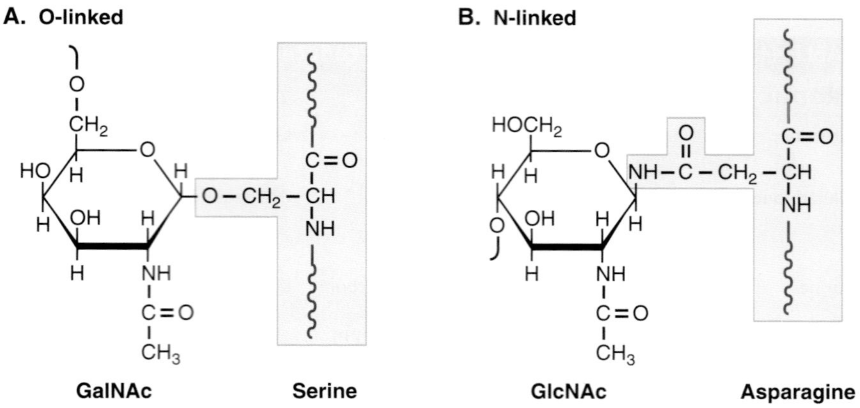

A. O-linked　　　　　　　　　　　　　　**B. N-linked**

FIGURE 44.5 The general configuration of O-linked and N-linked glycoproteins. GalNAc, N-acetylgalactosamine.

One of the intriguing aspects of the hepatic biosynthetic pathways that use carbohydrate in the synthesis of these compounds is that the liver is not dependent on either dietary glucose or hepatic glucose to generate the precursor intermediates for these pathways. This is because the liver can generate carbohydrates from dietary amino acids (which enter gluconeogenesis generally as pyruvate or an intermediate of the tricarboxylic acid [TCA] cycle), lactate (generated from anaerobic glycolysis in other tissues), and glycerol (generated by the release of free fatty acids from the adipocyte). Of course, if dietary carbohydrate is available, the liver can use that source as well.

Most of the sugars secreted by the liver are O-linked; that is, the carbohydrate is attached to the protein at its anomeric carbon through a glycosidic link to the –OH of a serine or a threonine residue. This is in contrast to the N-linked arrangement in which there is an N-glycosyl link to the amide nitrogen of an asparagine residue (Fig. 44.5). A particularly important O-linked sugar is N-acetylneuraminic acid (NANA or sialic acid), a nine-carbon sugar that is synthesized from fructose 6-phosphate and phosphoenolpyruvate (see Fig. 27.15). As circulating proteins age, NANA (sialic acid) residues are lost from the serum proteins. This change signals their removal from the circulation and their eventual degradation. An asialoglycoprotein receptor on the liver cell surface binds such proteins, and the receptor–ligand complex is endocytosed and transported to the lysosomes. The amino acids from the degraded protein are then recycled within the liver.

J. The Pentose Phosphate Pathway

The major functions of the pentose phosphate pathway (see Chapter 27) are the generation of NADPH and five-carbon sugars. All cell types, including red blood cells, can carry out this pathway because they need to generate NADPH so that the activity of glutathione reductase, the enzyme that catalyzes the conversion of oxidized glutathione (GSSG) back to reduced glutathione (GSH) can be maintained. Without the activity of this enzyme, the protection against free-radical injury is lost. All cells also need this pathway for the generation of ribose, especially those cells that are dividing rapidly or that have high rates of DNA synthesis.

The liver has a much greater demand for NADPH than do most other organs. It uses NADPH for the biosynthesis of fatty acids (which are needed to produce phospholipids) and cholesterol, and for the synthesis of VLDL and bile salts. It also uses NADPH for other biosynthetic reactions, such as proline synthesis. NADPH is also used by mixed-function oxidases such as cytochrome P450 that are involved in the metabolism of xenobiotics and of a variety of pharmaceuticals. Because the liver participates in so many reactions that are capable of generating free radicals, the liver uses more glutathione and NADPH to maintain glutathione reductase and catalase activity than any other tissue. Consequently, the concentration of glucose 6-phosphate dehydrogenase (the rate-limiting and regulated enzyme in the pentose phosphate pathway) is high in the liver, and the rate of flux through this pathway may be as high as 30% of the rate of flux through glycolysis.

IV. Fuels for the Liver

The reactions used to modify and inactivate dietary toxins and waste metabolites are energy-requiring, as are the reactions used by anabolic (biosynthetic) pathways, such as gluconeogenesis and fatty acid synthesis. Thus, the liver has a high energy requirement and consumes approximately 20% of the total oxygen used by the body. The principal forms in which energy is supplied to these reactions are the high-energy phosphate bonds of adenosine triphosphate (ATP), uridine triphosphate (UTP), and guanosine triphosphate (GTP), reduced NADPH, and acyl coenzyme A (acyl-CoA) thioesters. The energy for the formation of these compounds is obtained directly from oxidative metabolism, the TCA cycle, or the electron-transport chain and oxidative phosphorylation. After a mixed meal containing carbohydrate, the major fuels used by the liver are glucose, galactose, and fructose. If ethanol is consumed, the liver is the major site of ethanol oxidation, yielding principally acetate and then acetyl coenzyme A (acetyl-CoA). During an overnight fast, fatty acids become the major fuel for the liver. They are oxidized to carbon dioxide or ketone bodies. The liver also can use all of the amino acids as fuels (although its use of branched-chain amino acids [BCAAs] is small compared to the muscles), converting many of them to glucose. The urea cycle disposes of the ammonia that is generated from amino acid oxidation.

A. Carbohydrate Metabolism in the Liver

After a carbohydrate-containing meal, glucose, galactose, and fructose enter the portal circulation and flow to the liver. This organ serves as the major site in the body for the use of dietary galactose and fructose. It metabolizes these compounds by converting them to glucose and intermediates of glycolysis. Their fate is essentially the same as that of glucose (Table 44.3).

B. Glucose as a Fuel

The entry of glucose into the liver is dependent on a high concentration of glucose in the portal vein after a high-carbohydrate meal. Because the K_m for both the glucose transporter (GLUT2) and glucokinase is so high ($\sim$10 mM), glucose enters the liver principally after its concentration rises to 10 to 40 mM in the portal blood and

---

TABLE 44.3 Major Fates of Carbohydrates in the Liver

Storage as glycogen
Glycolysis to pyruvate
Followed by oxidation to carbon dioxide in the TCA cycle
Precursors for the synthesis of glycerol 3-phosphate (the backbone of triacylglycerols and other glycolipids), sialic acid, and serine
Entry into the TCA cycle and exit as citrate, followed by conversion to acetyl-CoA, malonyl-CoA, and entry into fatty acid synthesis and secretion as VLDL
Synthesis of phospholipids and other lipids from triacylglycerols
Conversion to mannose, sialic acid, and other sugars necessary for the synthesis of oligosaccharides for glycoproteins, including those secreted into blood
Synthesis of acid sugars for proteoglycan synthesis and formation of glucuronides
Oxidation in the pentose phosphate pathway for the formation of NADPH (necessary for biosynthetic reactions such as fatty acid synthesis, glutathione reduction, and other NADPH-using detoxification reactions)

acetyl-CoA, acetyl coenzyme A; malonyl-CoA, malonyl coenzyme A; NADPH, reduced nicotinamide adenine dinucleotide phosphate; TCA, tricarboxylic acid; VLDL, very-low-density lipoprotein.

not at the lower 5 mM concentration in the hepatic artery. The increase in insulin secretion that follows a high-carbohydrate meal promotes the conversion of glucose to glycogen. In addition, the rate of glycolysis is increased (phosphofructokinase-2 [PFK-2] kinase activity is active; thus, phosphofructokinase-1 [PFK-1] is activated by fructose 2,6-bisphosphate) so that acetyl-CoA can be produced for fatty acid synthesis (acetyl-CoA carboxylase is activated by citrate; see Chapter 31). Thus, after a high-carbohydrate meal, the liver uses glucose as its major fuel while activating the pathways for glycogen and fatty acid synthesis.

The rate of glucose use by the liver is determined, in part, by the level of activity of glucokinase. Glucokinase activity is regulated by a glucokinase regulatory protein (RP), which is located in the nucleus. In the absence of glucose, glucokinase is partially sequestered within the nucleus, bound to RP, in an inactive form. High concentrations of fructose 6-phosphate promote the interaction of glucokinase with RP, whereas high levels of either glucose or fructose 1-phosphate (fructose 1-P) block glucokinase from binding to RP and promote the dissociation of the complex. Thus, as glucose levels rise in the cytoplasm and nucleus (e.g., because of increased blood glucose levels after a meal), there is a significant enhancement of glucose phosphorylation as glucokinase is released from the nucleus, travels to the cytoplasm, and phosphorylates glucose.

The major regulatory step for liver glycolysis is the PFK-1 step. Even under fasting conditions, the ATP concentration in the liver ($\sim$2.5 mM) is sufficiently high to inhibit PFK-1 activity. Thus, liver glycolysis is basically controlled by modulating the levels of fructose 2,6-bisphosphate, the product of the PFK-2 reaction. As fructose 2,6-bisphosphate levels increase (which will occur in the presence of insulin), the rate of glycolysis increases; when glucagon levels increase and protein kinase A is activated so that PFK-2 is phosphorylated and its kinase activity is inactive, glycolysis slows down and gluconeogenesis is enhanced (see Chapters 22 and 28).

Why would you expect fructose 1-P levels to promote the dissociation of glucokinase from RP?

C. Lipid Metabolism

Long-chain fatty acids are a major fuel for the liver during periods of fasting, when they are released from adipose tissue triacylglycerols and travel to the liver as fatty acids bound to albumin. In the liver, they bind to fatty acid–binding proteins and are then activated on the outer mitochondrial membrane, the peroxisomal membrane, and the smooth endoplasmic reticulum by fatty acyl-CoA synthetases. The fatty acyl group is transferred from coenzyme A (CoA) to carnitine for transport through the inner mitochondrial membrane, where it is reconverted back into fatty acyl-CoA and oxidized to acetyl-CoA in the β-oxidation spiral (see Chapter 30).

The enzymes in the pathways of fatty acid activation and β-oxidation (the synthetases, the carnitine acyl transferases, and the dehydrogenases of β-oxidation) are somewhat specific for the length of the fatty acid carbon chain. The chain-length specificity is divided into enzymes for very-long-chain fatty acids (C20 to $\sim$C12), medium-chain ($\sim$C12 to C4), and short-chain (C4 to C2). The major lipids oxidized in the liver as fuels are the long-chain fatty acids (palmitic, stearic, and oleic acids), because these are the lipids that are synthesized in the liver, are the major lipids ingested from meat or dairy sources, and are the major form of fatty acids present in adipose tissue triacylglycerols. The liver, as well as many other tissues, uses fatty acids as fuels when the concentration of the fatty acid–albumin complex is increased in the blood.

1. Medium-Chain-Length Fatty Acid Oxidation

The liver and certain cells in the kidney are the major sites for the oxidation of medium-chain-length fatty acids. These fatty acids usually enter the diet of infants in maternal milk as medium-chain-length triacylglycerols (MCTs). In the intestine, the MCTs are hydrolyzed by gastric lipase, bile salt–dependent lipases, and pancreatic lipase more readily than long-chain triacylglycerols. In the enterocytes, they are neither reconverted to triacylglycerols nor incorporated into chylomicrons.

Instead, they are released directly into the portal circulation (fatty acids of approximately eight-carbon chain lengths or less are water-soluble). In the liver, they diffuse through the inner mitochondrial membrane and are activated to acyl-CoA derivatives by medium-chain-length fatty acid–activating enzyme (MMFAE), a family of similar isozymes present only in liver and kidney. The medium-chain fatty acyl-CoA is then oxidized by the normal route, beginning with medium-chain-length acyl-CoA dehydrogenase (MCAD; see Chapter 30).

2. Peroxisomal Oxidation of Very-Long-Chain Fatty Acids

Peroxisomes are present in greater numbers in the liver than in other tissues. Liver peroxisomes contain the enzymes for the oxidation of very-long-chain fatty acids such as C24:0 and phytanic acid, for the cleavage of the cholesterol side chain necessary for the synthesis of bile salts, for a step in the biosynthesis of ether lipids, and for several steps in arachidonic acid metabolism. Peroxisomes also contain catalase and are capable of detoxifying hydrogen peroxide.

Very-long-chain fatty acids of C20 to C26 or greater are activated to CoA derivatives by very-long-chain acyl-CoA synthetase present in the peroxisomal membrane. The very-long-chain acyl-CoA derivatives are then oxidized in liver peroxisomes to the eight-carbon octanoyl coenzyme A (octanoyl-CoA) level. In contrast to mitochondrial β-oxidation, the first enzyme in peroxisomal β-oxidation introduces a double bond and generates hydrogen peroxide instead of reduced flavin adenine dinucleotide (FAD[2H]). The remainder of the cycle, however, remains the same, releasing NADH and acetyl-CoA. Peroxisomal catalase inactivates the hydrogen peroxide, and the acetyl-CoA can be used in biosynthetic pathways such as those of cholesterol and dolichol synthesis.

The octanoyl-CoA that is the end-product of peroxisomal oxidation leaves the peroxisomes and the octanoyl group is transferred through the inner mitochondrial membrane by medium-chain-length acylcarnitine transferase. In the mitochondria, it enters the regular β-oxidation pathway, beginning with MCAD.

3. Peroxisome Proliferator–Activated Receptors

The peroxisome proliferator–activated receptors (PPARs) play an important role in liver metabolism. These receptors obtained their name from the finding that certain agonists were able to induce the proliferation of peroxisomes in liver. These agonists included hypolipidemic agents, nonsteroidal antiinflammatory agents, and environmental toxins. The receptors that bind these agents, the PPARs, are members of a nuclear receptor family and, when activated, stimulate new gene transcription. In the liver, the major form of PPAR regulates directly the activity of genes that are involved in fatty acid uptake and β- and ω-oxidation of fatty acids.

Although the roles of the PPARs have been discussed previously (see Section V of this text), it is worth reviewing them here. There are three major PPAR isoforms: α, δ/β, and γ. The major form found in the liver is the α-form. Fatty acids are an endogenous ligand for PPARα, such that when the level of fatty acids in the circulation is increased (with a concurrent increase in the fatty acid content of hepatocytes), there is increased gene transcription for those proteins involved in regulating fatty acid metabolism (Table 44.4). Genetically altered mice have been generated that lack PPARα. These knockout mice exhibit no abnormal phenotype when they are fed a normal diet. When they are fasted, however, or when they are fed a high-fat diet, these mice develop severe fatty infiltration of the liver. The inability to increase the rate of fatty acid oxidation in this organ leads to excessive fatty acid buildup in the hepatocytes. It also leads to an insufficient energy supply with which to make glucose (leading to hypoglycemia) as well as an inability to produce ketone bodies. In normal fasted mice or mice fed a high-fat diet, fatty acids will eventually stimulate their own oxidation via peroxisome proliferation and by induction of other enzymes needed for their oxidation. The knockout mice cannot make these compensations.

Fructose 1-P is produced from fructose metabolism. The major dietary source of fructose, the ingestion of which would lead to increased fructose 1-P levels, is sucrose. Sucrose is a disaccharide of glucose and fructose. Thus, an elevation of fructose 1-P usually indicates an elevation of glucose levels as well.

MCTs are important components of nutritional supplements used in patients with digestive disorders. They, therefore, can be used as an easily absorbed source of calories in patients who have a gastrointestinal disorder that may result in malabsorption of nutrients. These diseases include pancreatic insufficiency, intraluminal bile salt deficiency owing to cholestatic liver disease, biliary obstruction, ileal disease or resection, and disease that causes obstruction of intestinal lymphatics. Remember, however, that MCTs do not contain polyunsaturated fatty acids that can be used for synthesis of eicosanoids (see Chapter 31).

Zellweger (cerebrohepatorenal) syndrome occurs in individuals with a rare inherited absence of peroxisomes in all tissues. Patients accumulate C26 to C38 polyenoic acids in brain tissue because of defective peroxisomal oxidation of the very-long-chain fatty acids synthesized in the brain for myelin formation. In liver, bile acid and ether lipid synthesis are affected, as is the oxidation of very-long-chain fatty acids.

The fibrates (e.g., clofibrate) are a class of drugs that bind to PPARs to elicit changes in lipid metabolism. They are typically prescribed for individuals with elevated triglyceride levels because they increase the rate of triglyceride oxidation. This, in turn, leads to a reduction in serum triacylglycerol levels. Fibrates, through PPARα stimulation, also suppress apolipoprotein CIII (apoCIII) synthesis and stimulate LPL activity. ApoCIII normally inhibits LPL activity, so by reducing CIII synthesis overall, LPL activity is increased. ApoCIII also blocks apolipoprotein E on intermediate-density lipoprotein (IDL) particles, causing the IDL particles to accumulate because they cannot be taken up by the apoE receptor in the liver. The suppression of apoCIII levels allows more IDL to be endocytosed, thereby also reducing circulating triacylglycerol levels.

TABLE 44.4	Genes Regulated by Activation of PPARα
Fatty acid transport proteins (upregulated)	
The mitochondrial and peroxisomal enzymes of fatty acid oxidation (upregulated)	
Carnitine palmitoyl transferase I (upregulated)	
Lipoprotein lipase (upregulated)	
Apoproteins AI and A2 (upregulated, leading to increased high-density lipoprotein production)	
Apoprotein CIII (downregulated)	
Acyl coenzyme A synthetase (upregulated)	

PPARα, α isoform of peroxisome proliferator–activated receptor.

Reye syndrome is characterized clinically by vomiting with signs of progressive central nervous system damage. In addition, there are signs of hepatic injury and hypoglycemia. There is mitochondrial dysfunction, with decreased activity of hepatic mitochondrial enzymes. Hepatic coma may occur as serum ammonia levels rise. It is associated epidemiologically with the consumption of aspirin by children during a viral illness, but it may occur in the absence of exposure to salicylates. The incidence in the United States has decreased dramatically since the 1980s, when parents were made aware of the dangers of giving aspirin to children to reduce fever. Reye syndrome is not necessarily confined to children. In patients who die of this disease, the liver at autopsy shows swollen and disrupted mitochondria and extensive accumulation of lipid droplets with fatty vacuolization of cells in both the liver and the renal tubules.

4. Xenobiotics Metabolized as Fatty Acids

The liver uses the pathways of fatty acid metabolism to detoxify very hydrophobic and lipid-soluble xenobiotics that, like fatty acids, either have carboxylic acid groups or can be metabolized to compounds that contain carboxylic acids. Benzoate and salicylate are examples of xenobiotics that are metabolized in this way. Benzoate is naturally present in plant foods and is added to foods such as sodas as a preservative. Its structure is similar to that of salicylic acid (which is derived from the degradation of aspirin). Salicylic acid and benzoate are similar in size to medium-chain-length fatty acids and are activated to an acyl-CoA derivative by MMFAE (Fig. 44.6). The acyl group is then conjugated with glycine, which targets the compound for urinary excretion. The glycine derivatives of salicylate and benzoate are called *salicylurate* and *hippurate*, respectively. Salicylurate is the major urinary metabolite of aspirin in humans. Benzoate has been administered to treat hyperammonemia associated with congenital defects because urinary hippurate excretion tends to lower the free ammonia pool. Aspirin cannot be used for this purpose because it is toxic in the large doses required.

5. The Metabolism of Lipids in Liver Disease

Chronic parenchymal liver disease is associated with relatively predictable changes in plasma lipids and lipoproteins. Some of these changes are related to a reduction in the activity of lecithin–cholesterol acyltransferase (LCAT). This plasma enzyme is synthesized and glycosylated in the liver; then, it enters the blood, where it catalyzes

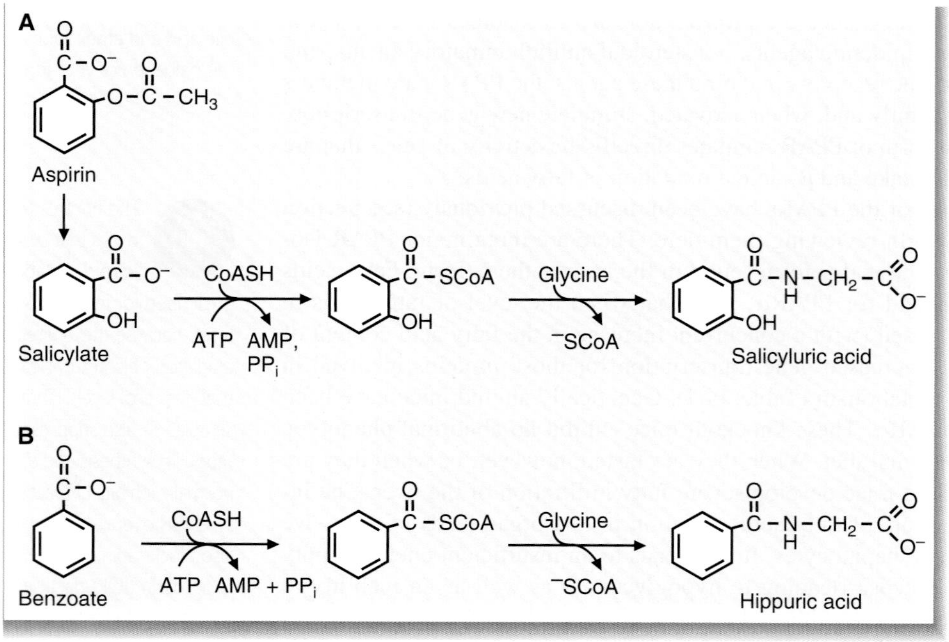

FIGURE 44.6 Benzoate and salicylate metabolism. *AMP*, adenosine monophosphate; *ATP*, adenosine triphosphate; *CoA*, coenzyme A; *PPi*, pyrophosphate.

the transfer of a fatty acid from the 2-position of lecithin to the 3β-OH group of free cholesterol to produce cholesterol ester and lysolecithin. As expected, in severe parenchymal liver disease, in which LCAT activity is decreased, plasma levels of cholesterol ester are reduced and free cholesterol levels are normal or increased.

Plasma triacylglycerols are normally cleared by peripheral lipases (lipoprotein lipase [LPL] and hepatic triglyceride lipase [HTGL]). Because the activities of both LPL and HTGL are reduced in patients with hepatocellular disease, a relatively high level of plasma triacylglycerols may be found in both acute and chronic hepatitis, in patients with cirrhosis of the liver, and in patients with other diffuse hepatocellular disorders.

With low LCAT activity and the elevated triacylglycerol level described, low-density lipoprotein (LDL) particles have an abnormal composition. They are relatively triacylglycerol-rich and cholesterol ester–poor.

High-density lipoprotein (HDL) metabolism may be abnormal in chronic liver disease as well. For example, because the conversion of HDL_3 (less antiatherosclerotic) to HDL_2 (more antiatherosclerotic) is catalyzed by LCAT, the reduced activity of LCAT in patients with cirrhosis leads to a decrease in the HDL_2/HDL_3 ratio. Conversely, the conversion of HDL_2 to HDL_3 requires hepatic lipases. If the activity of this lipase is reduced, one would expect an elevation in the HDL_2/HDL_3 ratio. Because the HDL_2/HDL_3 ratio is usually elevated in cirrhosis, the lipase deficiency appears to be the more dominant of the two mechanisms. These changes may result in an overall increase in serum total HDL levels. How this affects the efficiency of the reverse cholesterol transport mechanism and the predisposition to atherosclerosis is not fully understood.

With regard to triacylglycerol levels in patients with severe parenchymal liver disease, the hepatic production of the triacylglycerol-rich, VLDL particle is impaired. Yet, the total level of plasma triacylglycerols remains relatively normal because the LDL particle in such patients is triacylglycerol-rich, for reasons that have not been fully elucidated.

Nonesterified fatty acid (NEFA) levels are elevated in patients with cirrhosis. This change might be expected because basal hepatic glucose output is low in these patients. As a result, more NEFA are presumably required (via increased lipolysis) to meet the fasting energy requirements of peripheral tissues.

The level of NEFA levels in blood samples can be determined using enzyme-coupled reactions. The unknown sample is incubated with CoA and acyl-CoA synthetase, which adds the coenzyme to the NEFAs, creating acyl-CoA. The acyl-CoA produced is oxidized by acyl-CoA oxidase, which generates hydrogen peroxide. The hydrogen peroxide is used as a source of electrons by peroxidase to reduce a chromogenic substrate, which produces a colored reaction product. The concentration of the reaction product is determined spectrophotometrically and is directly proportional to the level of NEFA in the sample.

D. Amino Acid Metabolism in the Liver

The liver is the principal site of amino acid metabolism in humans. It essentially balances the free amino acid pool in the blood through the metabolism of amino acids supplied by the diet after a protein-containing meal and through metabolism of amino acids supplied principally by skeletal muscles during an overnight fast. In an adult who is no longer growing linearly, the total protein content of the body on a daily basis is approximately constant, so the net degradation of amino acids (either to other compounds or used for energy) is approximately equal to the amount consumed. The key points concerning hepatic amino acid metabolism are the following:

1. The liver contains all the pathways for catabolism of all of the amino acids (although its metabolism of the BCAAs is low) and can oxidize most of the carbon skeletons to carbon dioxide. A small proportion of the carbon skeletons is converted to ketone bodies. The liver also contains the pathways for converting amino acid carbon skeletons to glucose (gluconeogenesis) that can be released into the blood.

2. Because the liver is the principal site of amino acid catabolism, it also contains the urea cycle, the pathway that converts toxic ammonium ion to nontoxic urea. The urea is then excreted in the urine.

3. After a mixed or high-protein meal, the gut uses dietary aspartate, glutamate, and glutamine as fuel (during fasting, the gut uses glutamine from the blood as a major fuel). Thus, the ingested acidic amino acids do not enter the general circulation. The nitrogen from gut metabolism of these amino acids is passed to the liver as citrulline or ammonium ion via the portal vein.

Unlike **Amy B.**, whose hepatic amoebic disorder was more localized (abscesses), **Jean T.** had a diffuse hepatic disease, known as *alcohol-induced cirrhosis* (referred to historically as *Laennec cirrhosis*). The latter is characterized by diffuse fine scarring, a fairly uniform loss of hepatic cells, and the formation of small regenerative nodules (sometimes referred to as *micronodular cirrhosis*). With continued alcohol intake, fibroblasts and activated stellate cells deposit collagen at the site of persistent injury. This leads to the formation of weblike septa of connective tissue in periportal and pericentral zones. These eventually connect portal triads and central veins. With further exposure to alcohol, the liver shrinks and then becomes nodular and firm as end-stage cirrhosis develops. Unless they are successfully weaned from alcohol, these patients eventually die of liver failure. **Amy B.**, however, can probably look forward to enjoying normal liver function after successful amebicidal therapy without evidence of residual hepatic scarring.

4. The BCAAs (valine, leucine, and isoleucine) can be used as a fuel by most cell types, including cells of the gut and skeletal muscle. After a high-protein meal, most of the BCAAs are not oxidized by the liver (because of very low activity of the BCAA transaminase) and instead enter the peripheral circulation to be used as a fuel by other tissues or for protein synthesis (these amino acids are essential amino acids). The liver does, however, take up whatever amino acids it needs to carry out its own protein synthesis.

5. Most tissues transfer the amino acid nitrogen to the liver to dispose of as urea. They, therefore, produce either alanine (from the pyruvate–glucose–alanine cycle in skeletal muscle, kidney, and intestinal mucosa) or glutamine (skeletal muscle, lungs, neural tissues) or serine (kidney), which are released into the blood and taken up by the liver.

6. The liver uses amino acids for the synthesis of proteins that it requires as well as for the synthesis of proteins to be used elsewhere. For example, the liver uses the carbon skeletons and nitrogens of amino acids for the synthesis of nitrogen-containing compounds such as heme, purines, and pyrimidines. The amino acid precursors for these compounds are all nonessential because they can be synthesized in the liver.

E. Amino Acid Metabolism in Liver Disease

The concentration of amino acids in the blood of patients with liver disease is often elevated. This change is, in part, attributable to a significantly increased rate of protein turnover (a general catabolic effect seen in severely ill patients) as well as to impaired amino acid uptake by the diseased liver. It is unlikely that the increased levels are the result of degradation of liver protein and the subsequent release of amino acids from the failing hepatocyte into the blood. This is true because the total protein content of the liver is only approximately 300 g. To account for the elevated amino acid levels in the blood, the entire protein content of the liver would have to be degraded within 6 to 8 hours to account for the increased protein turnover rates found. Because 18 to 20 times more protein is present in skeletal muscle (greater mass), the muscle is probably the major source of the elevated plasma levels of amino acids seen in catabolic states such as cirrhosis of the liver.

In cirrhotic patients, such as **Jean T.**, the fasting blood α-amino nitrogen level is elevated as a result of reduced clearance. Urea synthesis is reduced as well.

The plasma profile of amino acids in cirrhosis characteristically shows an elevation in aromatic amino acids, phenylalanine and tyrosine, and in free tryptophan and methionine. The latter changes may be caused by impaired hepatic use of these amino acids as well as by portosystemic shunting. Although the mechanism is not known, a reduction in fasting plasma levels of the BCAAs is also seen in cirrhotic patients. These findings, however, must be interpreted with caution because most of the free amino acid pool in humans is found in the intracellular space. Therefore, changes seen in their plasma concentrations do not necessarily reflect their general metabolic fate. Yet the elevation in aromatic amino acids and the suppression of the level of BCAAs in the blood of patients with cirrhosis have been implicated in the pathogenesis of hepatic encephalopathy.

V. Diseases of the Liver

Diseases of the liver can be clinically and biochemically devastating because no other organ can compensate for the loss of the multitude of functions that the liver normally performs. Alcohol-induced liver disease has been discussed in Chapter 33. Several diseases can lead to hepatic fibrosis (see "Biochemical Comments") and cirrhosis. When this occurs to a great enough extent, liver function becomes inadequate for life. Signs and symptoms of liver disease include elevated levels of the enzymes alanine aminotransferase (ALT) and aspartate aminotransferase (AST) in the plasma (owing to hepatocyte injury or death with a consequent release of these enzymes into the blood), jaundice (an accumulation of bilirubin in the blood caused by inefficient bilirubin glucuronidation by the liver; see Chapter 43), increased clotting times (the liver has difficulty producing clotting factors for secretion), edema (reduced albumin synthesis by the liver leads to a reduction in osmotic pressure in the blood), and hepatic encephalopathy (reduced urea cycle activity leading to excessive levels of ammonia and other toxic compounds in the central nervous system).

CLINICAL COMMENTS

Jean T. Patients with cirrhosis of the liver who have no known genetic propensity to glucose intolerance, such as **Jean T.**, tend to have higher blood glucose levels than do normal subjects in both fasting and fed states. The mechanisms that may increase glucose levels in the fasting state include a reduction in the metabolic clearance rate of glucose by 25% to 40% compared with normal subjects. This reduction in glucose clearance results, in part, from increased oxidation of fatty acids and ketone bodies and the consequent decrease in glucose oxidation by peripheral tissues in cirrhosis patients. This is suggested by the discovery that plasma NEFA levels are high in many patients with hepatocellular dysfunction, in part because of decreased hepatic clearance of NEFA and in part because of increased adipose tissue lipolysis. Another possible explanation for the reduction in whole-body glucose use in patients with cirrhosis relates to the finding that ketone body production is increased in some patients with cirrhosis. This could lead to enhanced use of ketone bodies for fuel by the central nervous system in such patients, thereby reducing the need for glucose oxidation by the highly metabolically active brain.

After glucose ingestion (fed state), many patients with liver disease have abnormally elevated blood glucose levels ("hepatogenous diabetes"). Using World Health Organization (WHO) criteria, 60% to 80% of cirrhotic patients have varying degrees of glucose intolerance, and overt diabetes mellitus occurs 2 to 4 times as often in cirrhotics than it does in subjects without liver disease. The proposed mechanisms include a degree of insulin resistance in peripheral tissues; however, as the cirrhotic process progresses, these patients develop a marked impairment of insulin secretion as well. Although the mechanisms are not well understood, this decrease in insulin secretion leads to increased hepatic glucose output (leading to fasting hyperglycemia) and reduced suppression of hepatic glucose output after meals, leading to postprandial hyperglycemia as well. If the patient has an underlying genetic predisposition to diabetes mellitus, the superimposition of the mechanisms outlined previously will lead to an earlier and more significant breakdown in glucose tolerance in these specific patients.

BIOCHEMICAL COMMENTS

Hepatic Fibrosis. Extensive and progressive fibrosis of the hepatic parenchyma leads to cirrhosis of the liver, a process that has many causes. The development of fibrosis requires the activities of hepatic stellate cells, cytokines, proteases, and protease inhibitors.

A major change that occurs when fibrosis is initiated is that the normally "sparse" or "leaky" basement membrane between the endothelial cell and the hepatocyte is replaced with a high-density membrane containing fibrillar collagen. This occurs because of both increased synthesis of a different type of collagen than is normally produced and a reduction in the turnover rate of existing extracellular matrix components.

The supportive tissues of the normal liver contain an extracellular matrix that, among other proteins, includes type IV collagen (which does not form fibers), glycoproteins, and proteoglycans. After a sustained insult to the liver, a threefold to eightfold increase occurs in extracellular matrix components, some of which contain fibril-producing collagen (types I and III), glycoproteins, and proteoglycans. The accumulation of these fibril-producing compounds leads to a loss of endothelial cell fenestrations and, therefore, a loss of the normal sievelike function of the basement membranes. These changes interfere with normal transmembrane metabolic exchanges between the blood and hepatocytes.

The hepatic stellate cell is the source of the increased and abnormal collagen production. These cells are activated by growth factors whose secretion is induced by injury to the hepatocytes or endothelial cells. Growth factors involved in cellular activation include transforming growth factor β_1 (which is derived from the endothelial cells, Kupffer cells, and platelets) and platelet-derived growth factor (PDGF) and epidermal growth factor (EGF) from platelets. The release of PDGF stimulates stellate cell proliferation and, in the process, increases their synthesis and release of extracellular matrix materials and remodeling enzymes. These enzymes include matrix metalloproteinases (MMPs) and tissue inhibitors of MMPs as well as converting (activating) enzymes. This cascade leads to the degradation of the normal extracellular matrix and replacement with a much denser and more rigid type of matrix material. These changes are in part the result of an increase in the activity of tissue inhibitors of MMPs for the new collagen relative to the original collagen in the extracellular matrix.

One consequence of the increasing stiffness of the hepatic vascular channels through which hepatic blood must flow is a greater resistance to the free flow of blood through the liver as a whole. Resistance to intrahepatic blood flow is also increased by a loss of vascular endothelial cell fenestrations, loss of free space between the endothelial cells and the hepatocytes (space of Disse), and even loss of vascular channels per se. This increased vascular resistance leads to an elevation of intrasinusoidal fluid pressure. When this intrahepatic (portal) hypertension reaches a critical threshold, the shunting of portal blood away from the liver (portosystemic shunting) contributes further to hepatic dysfunction. If the portal hypertension cannot be reduced, portal blood will continue to bypass the liver and return to the heart through the normally low-pressure esophageal veins. When this increasing intraesophageal venous pressure becomes severe enough, the walls of these veins thin dramatically and expand to form varices, which may burst suddenly, causing life-threatening esophageal variceal hemorrhage. This is a potentially fatal complication of cirrhosis of the liver.

KEY CONCEPTS

- The liver consists of a variety of cell types, each with a different function.
  - Hepatocytes carry out the bulk of the metabolic pathways of the liver.
  - Endothelial cells line the sinusoids and release growth factors.
  - Kupffer cells are tissue macrophages that protect the liver from gut-derived particulate materials and bacterial products.
  - Stellate cells store vitamin A and regulate the contractility of the sinusoids.
  - Pit cells are liver-associated lymphocytes, which act as a defense mechanism against potentially toxic agents.
- The liver is the body's central receiving and recycling center:
  - Inactivation and detoxification of xenobiotic compounds and metabolites via cytochrome P450 systems
  - Regulation of blood glucose levels
  - Synthesis and export of cholesterol and triglyceride via VLDL
  - Synthesis and excretion of urea
  - Formation of ketone bodies from fatty acid oxidation
  - Nucleotide biosynthesis
  - Synthesis of blood proteins
- The liver highly coordinates its use of fuels versus that of the body. This is, in part, controlled by modulation of the activity of PPARα.
- Liver disease affects amino acid, carbohydrate, and lipid metabolism, leading to abnormalities in virtually all aspects of metabolism.
- Diseases discussed in this chapter are summarized in Table 44.5.

TABLE 44.5 Diseases Discussed in Chapter 44		
DISEASE OR DISORDER	**GENETIC OR ENVIRONMENTAL**	**COMMENTS**
Liver failure	Both, though primarily environmental	Destruction of hepatocyte function, leading to hyperammonemia, edema, and jaundice
Amoebiasis	Environmental	Infection by amoeba *Entamoeba histolytica*
Cirrhosis	Environmental	Destruction of hepatocytes via inappropriate collagen and other fibrous protein deposition within the liver, usually in response to environmental insult
Zellweger syndrome	Genetic	Lack of functional peroxisomes in all cells of the liver, kidney, and brain
Reye syndrome	Environmental	Both the brain and liver primarily affected, with progressive loss of nervous system function

REVIEW QUESTIONS—CHAPTER 44

1. Drinking grapefruit juice while taking statins can lead to potentially devastating side effects. This is owing to a component of grapefruit juice doing which one of the following?
   A. Interfering with hepatic uptake of statins
   B. Accelerating the conversion of the statin to a more toxic form
   C. Inhibiting the inactivation of statins
   D. Upregulating the HMG-CoA reductase
   E. Downregulating the HMG-CoA reductase

2. Which one of the following characteristics of cytochrome P450 enzymes is correct?
   A. They are all found in the Golgi apparatus and are referred to as *microsomal enzymes.*
   B. They all contain a flavin-containing reductase unit that uses NADH and not NADPH as a source of electrons.
   C. They are all inducible by oxygen, which binds to the iron of the cytochrome.
   D. They all oxidize the substrate on which they act.
   E. They all generate a free-radical compound as a final product of the reaction.

3. Fairly predictable changes occur in the various metabolic pathways of lipid metabolism in patients with moderately advanced hepatocellular disease. Which one of the following changes would you expect to see under these conditions?
   A. The activity of plasma LCAT is increased.
   B. Serum cholesterol esters are increased.
   C. HTGL activity is increased.
   D. Serum triacylglycerol levels are increased.
   E. Serum NEFA levels are decreased.

4. After a 2-week alcoholic binge, Ms. T. ingested some acetaminophen (Tylenol) to help her with a severe headache. She took three times the suggested dose because of the severity of the pain. Within 24 hours, Ms. T. became very lethargic, vomited frequently, and developed severe abdominal pain. The symptoms Ms. T. is experiencing are attributable to a reaction to the acetaminophen caused by which one of the following?
   A. The hypoglycemia experienced by the patient
   B. Ethanol-induced inhibition of acetaminophen metabolism
   C. The hyperglycemia experienced by the patient
   D. Ethanol-induced acceleration of acetaminophen metabolism
   E. Acetaminophen inhibition of VLDL secretion by the liver

5. An individual displays impaired glucose tolerance; blood glucose levels remain elevated after a meal for a longer time than is normal, although they do eventually go down to fasting levels. The patient has a normal release of insulin from the pancreas in response to elevated blood glucose levels. Hepatocytes obtained from the patient display normal levels of insulin binding to its receptor, and normal activation of the intrinsic tyrosine kinase activity associated with the insulin receptor. Analysis of glucose 6-phosphate formation within the hepatocytes, however, indicates a much slower rate of formation than in hepatocytes obtained from a normal control. A possible mutation that could lead to these results is which one of the following?
   A. A decrease in the K_m of glucokinase
   B. An increase in the V_{max} of glucokinase
   C. A nonfunctional glucokinase-regulatory protein
   D. An increase in hexokinase activity
   E. A decrease in hexokinase activity

6. Individuals with cirrhosis frequently display elevated levels of amino acids in the blood. The source of these amino acids is predominantly which one of the following?
   A. Red blood cell turnover
   B. Liver protein turnover
   C. Enterocyte degradation and turnover
   D. Muscle protein turnover
   E. Plasma protein turnover

7. Phase I reactions for xenobiotic detoxification require a reduced cofactor to donate electrons to oxygen as one atom of oxygen is incorporated into the substrate and the other atom of oxygen is incorporated into water. The reduced cofactor for the phase I reactions is derived primarily from which one of the following pathways?
   A. Hexose monophosphate shunt
   B. Glycolysis
   C. Fatty acid biosynthesis
   D. TCA cycle
   E. Fatty acid oxidation

8. A patient with chronic alcoholism presents to his physician with complaints of lethargy. Physical exam displays a malnourished individual with yellow sclera. Bloodwork indicates elevation of prealbumin, AST, and ALT. The yellow sclera is most likely caused by which one of the following?
   A. Reduction in amino acid metabolism
   B. Reduction in glycosylation reactions
   C. Reduction in fatty acid oxidation
   D. Reduction in VLDL production
   E. Reduction in urea synthesis

9. Liver disease exhibits which of the following? Choose the one best answer.

	Elevated Blood Levels of ALT and AST	Elevated Blood Levels of Bilirubin	Elevated Levels of Blood Clotting Factors	Edema	Elevated Levels of Blood Ammonia
A	No	No	Yes	No	No
B	No	Yes	Yes	Yes	Yes
C	No	No	Yes	No	No
D	Yes	Yes	No	Yes	No
E	Yes	No	No	No	Yes
F	Yes	Yes	No	Yes	Yes

10. A person with chronic alcoholism has developed cirrhosis of the liver. The liver is filled with a type of collagen that interferes with appropriate liver function. Under these conditions, which liver cell type has been stimulated to produce fibril-producing collagen?
    A. Kupffer cells
    B. Stellate cells
    C. Endothelial cells
    D. Hepatocytes
    E. Pit cells

ANSWERS

1. **The answer is C.** Grapefruit juice contains a component that blocks CYP3A4 activity, which is the cytochrome P450 isozyme that converts statins to an inactive form. If the degradative enzyme is inhibited, statin levels rise above normal, accelerating their damage of muscle cells. Grapefruit juice does not affect hepatic uptake of the drug (thus, A is incorrect), nor does it accelerate statin metabolism (thus, B is also incorrect). Although HMG-CoA reductase is the target of the statins, grapefruit juice neither up- or downregulates the amount of enzyme present in the cell (thus, D and E are incorrect).

2. **The answer is D.** Cytochrome P450 enzymes oxidize their substrates, transferring the electrons to molecular oxygen to form water and a hydroxylated product. The enzymes require NADPH (thus, B is incorrect) and are located in the endoplasmic reticulum membrane (thus, A is incorrect). Oxygen does not induce all cytochrome P450 members (although it is a substrate for all of these isozymes; thus, C is incorrect), and although these enzymes proceed through a free-radical mechanism, the final products are not radicals (thus, E is incorrect).

3. **The answer is D.** Hepatocellular disease reduces protein synthesis in the liver, which leads to reduced levels of both LCAT and HTGL being produced (thus, A and C are incorrect). Because LCAT activity is reduced, cholesterol ester formation in circulating particles is reduced (thus, B is incorrect). Because a diseased liver has trouble synthesizing glucose, fatty acid release from adipocytes is increased to provide energy (thus, E is incorrect). Serum triacylglycerol levels are increased as a result of the reduced HTGL activity; LPL activity is also reduced in liver disease.

4. **The answer is D.** Ethanol induces the CYP2E1 system, which converts acetaminophen to NAPQI, a toxic intermediate. Under normal conditions (noninduced levels of CYP2E1), the conversion of acetaminophen to NAPQI results in low levels of NAPQI being produced, which can easily be detoxified. However, when CYP2E1 is induced, the excessive levels of NAPQI being produced when acetaminophen is taken in greater than recommended amounts cannot be readily detoxified, and NAPQI binds to proteins and inactivates them, leading to hepatocyte death. The toxicity is not related to blood glucose levels (thus, A and C are incorrect) or to secretion of VLDL (thus, E is incorrect). Ethanol does not inhibit the detoxification of acetaminophen per se but rather accelerates one of its potential metabolic fates (thus, B is also incorrect).

5. **The answer is C.** The glucokinase regulatory protein regulates glucokinase expression at a posttranscriptional level. A lack of appropriate regulation of the regulatory protein activity results in less glucokinase being present in the cell and a reduced overall rate of glucose phosphorylation by the liver. This results in less circulating glucose being removed by the liver and a longer clearance time for glucose levels to return to fasting levels.

A decrease in the glucokinase K_m, or an increase in the V_{max} for glucokinase, would lead to the opposite effect, enhanced glucose phosphorylation by the liver and an accelerated clearance from the circulation (thus, A and B are incorrect). The liver does not express hexokinase, so D and E are also incorrect.

6. **The answer is D.** The large increase in circulating amino acid levels in an individual with cirrhosis is the result of two things: reduced uptake of amino acids by the liver and enhanced muscle protein turnover owing to the catabolic state of the patient. Liver contains much less protein than muscle, and the entire liver would have to have its protein content degraded in order to provide the high levels of amino acids seen in the circulation under these conditions. In addition, red blood cells, enterocytes, and circulating proteins in the blood do not provide for sufficient protein turnover for the large increase in free amino acids seen when the liver is not functioning.

7. **The answer is A.** The cofactor required for the phase I reactions is NADPH, which is derived from either malic enzyme (a minor pathway) or the oxidative reactions of the HMP shunt pathway (glucose 6-phosphate dehydrogenase and 6-phosphogluconate dehydrogenase). For each glucose 6-phosphate entering these oxidative reactions, two molecules of NADPH are produced, along with carbon dioxide and ribulose 5-phosphate. Neither glycolysis nor the TCA cycle produce NADPH (both will produce NADH). Fatty acid biosynthesis requires NADPH for the two reduction reactions along the pathway, whereas fatty acid oxidation generates NADH and FAD(2H) but not NADPH.

8. **The answer is B.** The patient is exhibiting signs of liver failure (release of prealbumin, AST, and ALT) as the result of many years of drinking. The yellow sclera are signs of jaundice, owing to bilirubin precipitation. Normally, bilirubin would be glucuronylated (using UDP-glucuronic acid) to increase its solubility, via a reaction carried out in the liver. With the failing liver, however, this reaction efficiency is reduced, and more unconjugated bilirubin (which is less soluble than the conjugated form) is found in circulation. The increased levels of free bilirubin are not caused by alterations in either fatty acid or amino acid metabolism within the liver. It is also not related to VLDL production or urea biosynthesis.

9. **The answer is F.** ALT and AST, along with transaminases, are released by damaged hepatocytes. Elevated bilirubin causes jaundice, and a damaged liver cannot process bilirubin appropriately. The damaged liver has trouble synthesizing proteins, including serum albumin. Decreased blood albumin levels lead to low intravascular osmotic pressure and leakage of fluid into interstitial spaces, causing edema. The liver is the site of urea synthesis, and reduced urea synthesis leads to elevated blood ammonia levels. The liver also produces the blood clotting factors, so a damaged liver produces a reduced amount of clotting factors, leading to increased clotting time and bleeding.

10. **The answer is B.** In cirrhosis, stellate cells increase their synthesis of extracellular matrix components including fibril-producing collagen types I and III instead of type IV collagen, which does not form fibrils. The synthesis of the fibril-forming collagen leads to a loss of endothelial cell fenestrations and continuing fibrosis, eventually leading to cirrhosis. The other cells listed do not produce hepatic connective tissue and extracellular matrix material.

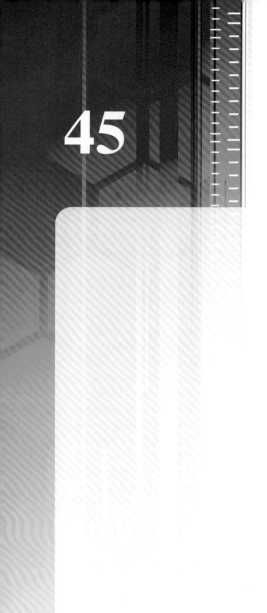

45

Metabolism of Muscle at Rest and during Exercise

There are three types of muscle cells: **smooth**, **skeletal**, and **cardiac**. In all types of muscle, contraction occurs via an actin/myosin sliding filament system, which is regulated by oscillations in **intracellular calcium levels**.

Muscle cells use stored glycogen and circulating glucose, fatty acids, and amino acids as energy sources. Muscle glycolysis is regulated differently from the liver, with the key difference being the regulation of **phosphofructokinase-2** (**PFK-2**). Muscle PFK-2 is not inhibited by phosphorylation; cardiac PFK-2 is actually activated by phosphorylation by several protein kinases. Thus, under conditions in which liver PFK-2 is inactive, and glycolysis is running slowly, muscle glycolysis is either unaffected, or even stimulated, depending on the isoform of PFK-2 being expressed.

Although muscle cells do not synthesize fatty acids, they do contain an isozyme of **acetyl coenzyme A carboxylase** (**ACC-2**) to regulate the **rate of fatty acid oxidation**. ACC-2 produces malonyl coenzyme A (malonyl-CoA), which inhibits carnitine palmitoyltransferase I (CPTI), thereby blocking fatty acid entry into the mitochondria. Muscle also contains **malonyl-CoA decarboxylase**, which catalyzes the conversion of malonyl-CoA to acetyl coenzyme A (acetyl-CoA) and carbon dioxide. Thus, both the synthesis and degradation of malonyl-CoA is carefully regulated in muscle cells to balance glucose and fatty acid oxidation. Both allosteric and covalent means of regulation are used. Citrate activates ACC-2, and phosphorylation of ACC-2 by the adenosine monophosphate (AMP)–activated protein kinase inhibits ACC-2 activity. Phosphorylation of malonyl-CoA decarboxylase by the AMP-activated protein kinase (AMPK) activates the enzyme, further enhancing fatty acid oxidation when energy levels are low.

Muscles use **creatine phosphate** to store high-energy bonds. Creatine is derived from arginine and glycine in the kidney, and the guanidinoacetate formed is methylated (using S-adenosylmethionine) in the liver to form creatine. The enzyme **creatine phosphokinase** (**CPK**) then catalyzes the reversible transfer of a high-energy phosphate from adenosine triphosphate (ATP) to creatine, forming creatine phosphate and adenosine diphosphate (ADP). Creatine phosphate is unstable and spontaneously cyclizes to form **creatinine**, which is excreted in the urine. The spontaneous production of creatinine occurs at a constant rate and is proportional to body muscle mass. Thus, the amount of creatinine excreted each day (the creatinine clearance rate) is constant and can be used as an indicator of the normalcy of the excretory function of the kidneys.

Skeletal muscle cells can be subdivided into **type I** and **type II fibers**. Type I fibers are **slow-twitch** fibers that use primarily **oxidative metabolism** for energy, whereas the type II fibers (**fast-twitch**) use **glycolysis** as their primary energy-generating pathway.

Glucose transport into muscle cells can be stimulated during exercise because of the activity of the **AMPK**. Fatty acid uptake into exercising muscle is dependent on the levels of circulating fatty acids, which are increased by **epinephrine** release.

THE WAITING ROOM

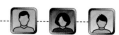

Renee F., a 9-year-old girl, complained of a severe pain in her throat and difficulty in swallowing. She had chills, sweats, headache, and a fever of 102.4°F. When her symptoms persisted for several days, her mother took her to her pediatrician, who found diffuse erythema (redness) in her posterior pharynx (throat), with yellow exudates (patches) on her tonsils. Large, tender lymph nodes were present under her jaw on both sides of her neck. A throat culture was taken, and therapy with penicillin was begun.

Although the sore throat and fever improved, 10 days after the onset of the original infection, Renee's eyes and legs became swollen and her urine suddenly turned the color of cola. Her blood pressure was elevated. Protein and red blood cells were found in her urine. Her serum creatinine level (see Chapter 3 for how creatinine is measured) was elevated at 1.8 mg/dL (reference range, 0.3 to 0.7 for a child). Because the throat culture grew group A β-hemolytic streptococci, the doctor ordered an antistreptolysin O titer, which was positive. As a result, a diagnosis of acute poststreptococcal glomerulonephritis (PSGN) was made. Supportive therapy, including bed rest and treatment for hypertension, was initiated.

Damaged muscle cells release myoglobin, which can be observed clinically as a reddish tint to the urine. The primary measurement for myoglobin is via a sandwich technique immunoassay. The primary antibody is linked to an insoluble support, whereas the second antibody is linked to alkaline phosphatase. Using a fluorescent substrate for the phosphatase allows low levels of myoglobin to be detected. If high in the urine, muscle damage and potential renal failure could be the culprits.

I. Muscle Cell Types

Muscle consists of three different types: skeletal, smooth, and cardiac (Fig. 45.1). The metabolism of each is similar, but the functions of the muscles are quite different.

A. Skeletal Muscle

Skeletal muscles are those muscles that are attached to bone and facilitate the movement of the skeleton. Skeletal muscles are found in pairs, which are responsible for opposing, coordinated directions of motion on the skeleton. The muscles appear striated under the microscope and are controlled voluntarily (you think about moving a specific muscle group, and then it happens).

Skeletal muscle cells are long, cylindrical fibers that run the length of the muscle. The fibers are multinucleated because of cell fusion during embryogenesis. The cell membrane surrounding the fibers is called the *sarcolemma*, and the sarcoplasm is the intracellular milieu, which contains the proteins, organelles, and contractile apparatus of the cell. The sarcoplasmic reticulum is analogous to the endoplasmic reticulum in other cell types and is an internal membrane system that runs throughout the length of the muscle fiber. Another membrane structure, the transverse tubules (T-tubules), are thousands of invaginations of the sarcolemma that tunnel from the surface toward the center of the muscle fiber to make contact with the terminal cisterns of the sarcoplasmic reticulum. Because the T-tubules are open to the outside of the muscle fiber and are filled with extracellular fluid, the muscle action potential that propagates along the surface of the muscle fiber's sarcolemma travels into the T-tubules and to the sarcoplasmic reticulum.

The striations in skeletal muscle are attributable to the presence and organization of myofibrils in the cells. Myofibrils are threadlike structures consisting of thin and thick filaments. The contractile proteins actin and myosin are contained within the filaments—myosin in the thick filaments and actin in the thin filaments. The sliding of these filaments relative to each other, using myosin-catalyzed ATP hydrolysis as an energy source, allows for the contraction and relaxation of the muscle (see Fig. 20.4).

Muscle fibers can be classified as either fast-twitch or slow-twitch. The slow-twitch fibers, or type I fibers (also called *slow-oxidative fibers*), contain large amounts of mitochondria and myoglobin (giving them a red color), use respiration and oxidative phosphorylation for energy, and are relatively resistant

Duchenne muscular dystrophy is caused by the absence of the protein dystrophin, which is a structural protein located in the sarcolemma. Dystrophin is required to maintain the integrity of the sarcolemma, and when it is absent, there is a loss of muscle function, which is caused by breakdown of the sarcolemma. The gene is X-linked, and mutations that lead to Duchenne muscular dystrophy generally result from large deletions of the gene, such that dystrophin is absent from the membrane. Becker muscular dystrophy, a milder form of disease, is caused by point mutations in the dystrophin gene. In Becker muscular dystrophy, dystrophin is present in the sarcolemma but in a mutated form.

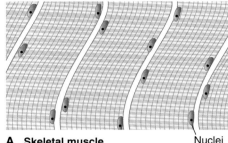

A. Skeletal muscle   Nuclei

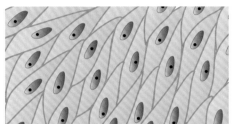

B. Smooth muscle
                                                Nuclei

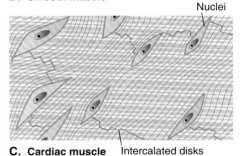

C. Cardiac muscle   Intercalated disks

FIGURE 45.1   Structures of the three different muscle types. (Adapted from Junqueira LC, Carneiro S. *Basic Histology, Text and Atlas.* 10th ed. New York, NY: Lange, McGraw-Hill; 2002.)

TABLE 45.1 **Properties of Muscle Fiber Types**		
	TYPE II FIBERS	
TYPE I FIBERS	**TYPE IIA**	**TYPE IIB**
Slow-twitch (slow speed of contraction)	Intermediate-twitch (fast speed of contraction)	Fast-twitch (fast speed of contraction)
Slow-oxidative (low glycogen content)	Fast-oxidative glycolytic fibers (intermediate glycogen levels)	Fast-glycolytic (high glycogen content)
High myoglobin content (appear red)	High myoglobin content (appear red)	Low myoglobin content (appear white)
Small fiber diameter	Intermediate fiber diameter	Large fiber diameter
Increased concentration of capillaries surrounding muscle (greater oxygen delivery)	Increased oxidative capacity on training	Limited aerobic metabolism Low mitochondrial content
High capacity for aerobic metabolism	Intermediate resistance to fatigue	More sensitive to fatigue compared with other fiber types
High resistance to fatigue		Least efficient use of energy, primarily glycolytic pathway
Used for prolonged aerobic exercise		Used for sprinting and resistance tasks

to fatigue. Compared with fast-twitch fibers, their glycogen content is low. The slow-twitch fibers develop force slowly but maintain contractions longer than fast-twitch muscles.

The fast-twitch fibers, or type II, can be subdivided as type IIa or type IIb. Type IIb fibers (also called *fast-glycolytic fibers*) have few mitochondria and low levels of myoglobin (hence, they appear white). They are rich in glycogen and use glycogenolysis and glycolysis as their primary energy source. These muscles are prone to fatigue because continued reliance on glycolysis to produce ATP leads to an increase in lactic acid levels, resulting in a drop in the intracellular pH. As the pH drops, the ability of the muscle to produce ATP also diminishes. However, fast-twitch muscle can develop greater force than slow-twitch muscle, so contractions occur more rapidly. Type IIa fibers (also called *fast-oxidative glycolytic fibers*) have properties of both type I and IIb fibers and thus display functional characteristics of both fiber types. The properties of types I, IIa, and IIb fibers are summarized in Table 45.1.

Muscles are a mixture of the different fiber types, but depending on the function, a muscle may have a preponderance of one fiber type over another. Type I fibers are found in postural muscles such as the psoas in the back musculature or the soleus in the leg. The ratio of type I to type II varies with the muscle. The triceps, which functions phasically, has 32.6% type I, whereas the soleus, which functions tonically, has 87.7% type I. Type II fibers are more prevalent in the large muscles of the limbs that are responsible for sudden, powerful movements. Extraocular muscles would also have more of these fibers than type I.

B. Smooth Muscle Cells

Smooth muscle cells are found in the digestive system, blood vessels, bladder, airways, and uterus. The cells have a spindle shape with a central nucleus (see Fig. 45.1B). The designation *smooth* refers to the fact that these cells, which contain a single nucleus, display no striations under the microscope. The contraction of smooth muscle is controlled involuntarily (the cells contract and relax without any conscious attempt to have them do so; examples of smooth muscle activity include moving food along the digestive tract, altering the diameter of the blood vessels, and expelling urine from the bladder). In contrast to skeletal muscle, these cells have the ability to maintain tension for extended periods, and do so efficiently, with a low use of energy.

C. Cardiac Muscle Cells

The cardiac cells are similar to skeletal muscle in that they are striated (contain fibers), but like smooth muscle cells, they are regulated involuntarily (we do not have to think about making our heart beat). The cells are quadrangular in shape (see Fig. 45.1C) and form a network with multiple other cells through tight membrane junctions and gap junctions. The multicellular contacts allow the cells to act as a common unit and to contract and relax synchronously. Cardiac muscle cells are designed for endurance and consistency. They depend on aerobic metabolism for their energy needs because they contain many mitochondria and very little glycogen. These cells thus generate only a small amount of their energy from glycolysis using glucose derived from glycogen. A reduced flow of oxygen-rich blood to the heart muscle may lead to a myocardial infarction (heart attack). The amount of ATP that can be generated by glycolysis alone is not sufficient to meet the energy requirements of the contracting heart.

II. Neuronal Signals to Muscle

For an extensive review of how muscle contracts or a detailed view of the signaling to allow muscle contraction, consult a medical physiology book. Only a brief overview is presented here.

The nerve–muscle cell junction is called the *neuromuscular junction* (Fig. 45.2). When appropriately stimulated, the nerve cell releases acetylcholine at the junction, which binds to acetylcholine receptors on the muscle membrane. This binding stimulates the opening of sodium channels on the sarcolemma. The massive influx of sodium ions results in the generation of an action potential in the sarcolemma at the edges of the motor end plate of the neuromuscular junction. The action potential sweeps across the surface of the muscle fiber and down the transverse tubules to the sarcoplasmic reticulum, where it initiates the release

 The ryanodine receptors are calcium release channels found in the endoplasmic reticulum and sarcoplasmic reticulum of muscle cells. One type of receptor can be activated by a depolarization signal (depolarization-induced calcium release). Another receptor type is activated by calcium ions (calcium-induced calcium release). The proteins received their name because they bind ryanodine, a toxin obtained from the stem and roots of the plant *Ryania speciosa*. Ryanodine inhibits sarcoplasmic reticulum calcium release and acts as a paralytic agent. It was first used commercially in insecticides.

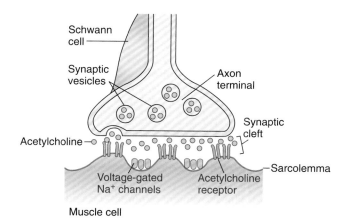

FIGURE 45.2   The neuromuscular junction. When they are stimulated appropriately, the synaptic vesicles, containing acetylcholine, fuse with the axonal membrane and release acetylcholine into the synaptic cleft. The acetylcholine binds to its receptors on the muscle cells, which initiate signaling for muscle contraction.

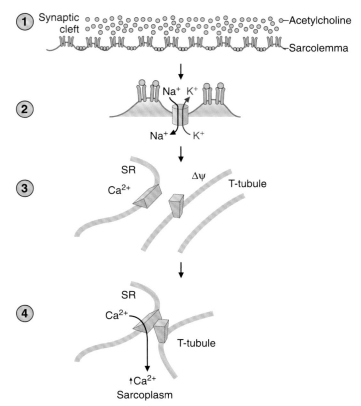

FIGURE 45.3 Events leading to sarcoplasmic reticulum (SR) calcium release in skeletal muscle. (*1*) Acetylcholine, released at the synaptic cleft, binds to acetylcholine receptors on the sarcolemma, leading to a change of conformation of the receptors so that they now act as an ion pore. This allows sodium to enter the cell and potassium to leave. (*2*) The membrane depolarization that results from these ion movements is transmitted throughout the muscle fiber by the T-tubule system. (*3*) A receptor in the T-tubules (the dihydropyridine receptor [DHPR]) is activated by membrane depolarization (a voltage-gated activation) so that activated DHPR binds physically to and activates the ryanodine receptor in the SR (depolarization-induced calcium release). (*4*) The activation of the ryanodine receptor, which is a calcium channel, leads to calcium release from the SR into the sarcoplasm. In cardiac muscle, activation of DHPR leads to calcium release from the T-tubules, and this small calcium release is responsible for the activation of the cardiac ryanodine receptor (calcium-induced calcium release) to release large amounts of calcium into the sarcoplasm.

Acetylcholine levels in the neuromuscular junction are rapidly reduced by the enzyme acetylcholinesterase. Several nerve-gas poisons act to inhibit acetylcholinesterase (such as sarin and VX), so that muscles are continuously stimulated to contract. This leads to blurred vision, bronchoconstriction, seizures, respiratory arrest, and death. The poisons are covalent modifiers of acetylcholinesterase; therefore, recovery from exposure to such poisons requires the synthesis of new enzyme. Acetylcholinesterase inhibitors, which act reversibly (i.e., they do not form covalent bonds with the enzyme), are used to treat dementia.

of calcium from its lumen, via the ryanodine receptor (Fig. 45.3). The calcium ion binds to troponin, resulting in a conformational change in the troponin–tropomyosin complexes so that they move away from the myosin-binding sites on the actin. When the binding site becomes available, the myosin head attaches to the myosin-binding site on the actin. The binding is followed by a conformational change (pivoting) in the myosin head, which shortens the sarcomere. After the pivoting, ATP binds the myosin head, which detaches from the actin and is available to bind another myosin-binding site on the actin. As long as calcium ion and ATP remain available, the myosin heads will repeat this cycle of attachment, pivoting, and detachment (Fig. 45.4). This movement requires ATP, and when ATP levels are low (such as occurs during ischemia), the ability of the muscle to relax or contract is compromised. As the calcium release channel closes, the calcium is pumped back into the sarcoplasmic reticulum against its concentration gradient using the energy-requiring protein sarcoplasmic reticulum Ca^{2+} ATPase (SERCA), and contraction stops. This basic process occurs in all muscle cell types, with some slight variations between cell types.

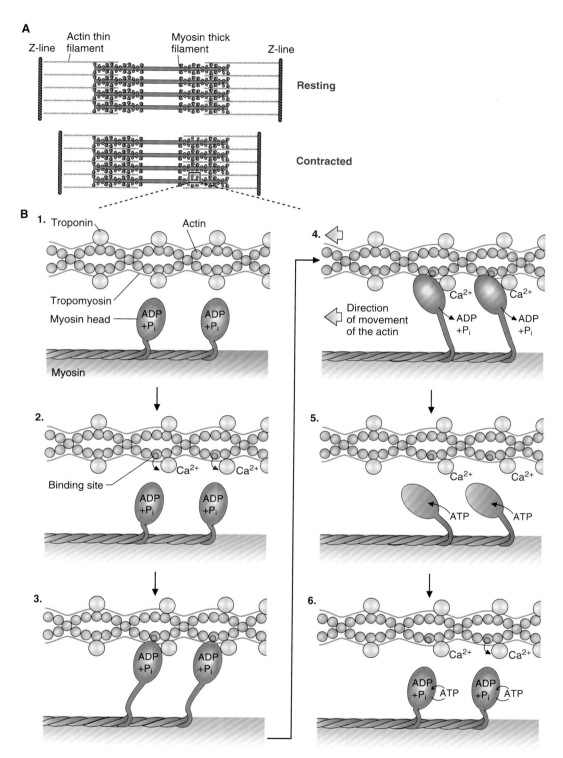

FIGURE 45.4   An overview of muscle contraction. **A.** Muscle contraction. During muscle contraction, the myosin head binds to the actin thin fila-ment. Pivoting of the myosin head toward the center of the sarcomere pulls the Z-lines closer together, with subsequent shortening of the sarcomere. **B.** A closer look at myosin–actin interactions. (*1*) A resting sarcomere. The troponin–tropomyosin complex is blocking the myosin-binding sites on the actin. The myosin head is already energized to power a contraction. (*2*) Exposure of the active site. After calcium binding to troponin, a conforma-tional change in the troponin molecule pulls the troponin away from the binding site. (*3*) Cross-bridge attachment. Once the binding sites on the actin are exposed, the myosin head binds to it. (*4*) Myosin head pivoting. After cross-bridge attachment, the energy stored in the myosin head is released, and the myosin head pivots toward the center of the sarcomere (power stroke). Now the adenosine diphosphate (ADP) and phosphate bound to the myosin head are released. (*5*) Detachment of the cross-bridge. Now a molecule of adenosine triphosphate (ATP) binds to the myosin head with simultaneous detachment of the myosin head from the binding site on the actin molecule. (*6*) Reactivation of the myosin head. The ATPase activity of the myosin head hydrolyzes the ATP into ADP and phosphate. The energy released from the hydrolysis of this high-energy bond is used to reenergize the myosin head, and the entire cycle can be repeated as long as calcium is present and there are sufficient ATP reserves. P_i, inorganic phosphate.

III. Glycolysis and Fatty Acid Metabolism in Muscle Cells

The pathways of glycolysis and fatty acid oxidation in muscle are the same, as has been described previously (see Chapters 22 and 30). The difference between muscles and other tissues is how these pathways are regulated.

PFK-2 is negatively regulated by phosphorylation in the liver (the enzyme that catalyzes the phosphorylation is the cyclic adenosine monophosphate [cAMP]–dependent protein kinase). However, in skeletal muscle, PFK-2 is not regulated by phosphorylation. This is because the skeletal muscle isozyme of PFK-2 lacks the regulatory serine residue, which is phosphorylated in the liver. However, the cardiac isozyme of PFK-2 is phosphorylated and activated by a kinase cascade initiated by insulin. This allows the heart to activate glycolysis and to use blood glucose when blood glucose levels are elevated. The AMPK also activates cardiac PFK-2 (kinase activity) as a signal that energy is low.

Fatty acid uptake by muscle requires the participation of fatty acid–binding proteins and the usual enzymes of fatty acid oxidation. Fatty acyl coenzyme A (fatty acyl-CoA) uptake into the mitochondria is controlled by malonyl-CoA, which is produced by an isozyme of ACC-2 (the ACC-1 isozyme is found in liver and adipose tissue cytosol and is used for fatty acid biosynthesis). ACC-2 (a mitochondrial protein, linked to CPTI in the outer mitochondrial membrane) is inhibited by phosphorylation by the AMPK so that when energy levels are low, the levels of malonyl-CoA drop, allowing fatty acid oxidation by the mitochondria. In addition, muscle cells also contain the enzyme malonyl-CoA decarboxylase, which is activated by phosphorylation by the AMPK. Malonyl-CoA decarboxylase converts malonyl-CoA to acetyl-CoA, thereby relieving the inhibition of CPTI and stimulating fatty acid oxidation (Fig. 45.5). Muscle cells do not synthesize fatty acids; the presence of acetyl-CoA carboxylase in muscle is exclusively for regulatory purposes. Mice that have been bred to lack ACC-2 have a 50% reduction of fat stores compared with control mice. This was shown to be attributable to a 30% increase in skeletal muscle fatty acid oxidation resulting from dysregulation of CPTI, brought about by the lack of malonyl-CoA inhibition of CPTI.

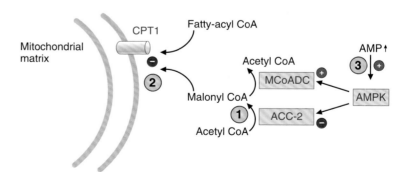

FIGURE 45.5 Regulation of fatty acyl coenzyme A (fatty acyl-CoA) entry into muscle mitochondria. (*1*) Acetyl coenzyme A carboxylase-2 (ACC-2) converts acetyl coenzyme A (acetyl-CoA) to malonyl coenzyme A (malonyl-CoA), which inhibits carnitine palmitoyltransferase I (CPTI), thereby blocking fatty acyl-CoA entry into the mitochondria. (2) However, as energy levels drop, adenosine monophosphate (AMP) levels rise because of the activity of the adenylate kinase reaction. (3) The increase in AMP levels activates the AMP-activated protein kinase (AMPK), which phosphorylates and inactivates ACC-2 and also phosphorylates and activates malonyl-CoA decarboxylase (MCoADC). The decarboxylase converts malonyl-CoA to acetyl-CoA, thereby relieving the inhibition of CPTI and allowing fatty acyl-CoA entry into the mitochondria. This allows the muscle to generate adenosine triphosphate (ATP) via the oxidation of fatty acids.

IV. Fuel Use in Cardiac Muscle

A. Normal Conditions

The heart uses primarily fatty acids (60% to 80%), lactate, and glucose (20% to 40%) as its energy sources. Ninety-eight percent of cardiac ATP is generated by oxidative means; 2% is derived from glycolysis. The lactate used by the heart is taken up by a monocarboxylate transporter in the cell membrane that is also used for the transport of ketone bodies. However, ketone bodies are not a preferred fuel for the heart; the heart prefers to use fatty acids.

Lactate is generated by red blood cells and working skeletal muscle. When the lactate is used by the heart, it is oxidized to carbon dioxide and water, following the pathway lactate to pyruvate, pyruvate to acetyl-CoA, acetyl-CoA oxidation in the tricarboxylic acid (TCA) cycle, and ATP synthesis through oxidative phosphorylation. An alternative fate for lactate is its use in the reactions of the Cori cycle in the liver.

Glucose transport into the cardiocyte occurs via both GLUT 1 and GLUT 4 transporters, although approximately 90% of the transporters are GLUT 4. Insulin stimulates an increase in the number of GLUT 4 transporters in the cardiac cell membrane, as does myocardial ischemia. This ischemia-induced increase in GLUT 4 transporter number is additive to the effect of insulin on the translocation of GLUT 4 transporters to the plasma membrane.

Fatty acid uptake into cardiac muscle is similar to that for other muscle cell types and requires fatty acid–binding proteins and CPTI for transfer into the mitochondria. Fatty acid oxidation in cardiac muscle cells is regulated by altering the activities of ACC-2 and malonyl-CoA decarboxylase. Under conditions in which ketone bodies are produced, fatty acid levels in the plasma are also elevated. Because the heart preferentially burns fatty acids as a fuel rather than the ketone bodies produced by the liver, the ketone bodies are spared for use by the nervous system.

B. Ischemic Conditions

When blood flow to the heart is interrupted, the heart switches to anaerobic metabolism. The rate of glycolysis increases, but the accumulation of protons (via lactate formation) is detrimental to the heart. Ischemia also increases the levels of free fatty acids in the blood and, surprisingly, when oxygen is reintroduced to the heart, the high rate of fatty acid oxidation in the heart is detrimental to the recovery of the damaged heart cells. Fatty acid oxidation occurs so rapidly that nicotinamide adenine dinucleotide (NADH) accumulates in the mitochondria, leading to a reduced rate of NADH shuttle activity, an increased cytoplasmic NADH level, and lactate formation, which generates more protons. In addition, fatty acid oxidation increases the levels of mitochondrial acetyl-CoA, which inhibits pyruvate dehydrogenase, leading to cytoplasmic pyruvate accumulation and lactate production. As lactate production increases and the intracellular pH of the heart drops, it is more difficult to maintain ion gradients across the sarcolemma. ATP hydrolysis is required to repair these gradients, which are essential for heart function. However, the use of ATP for gradient repair reduces the amount of ATP available for the heart to use in contraction, which, in turn, compromises the ability of the heart to recover from the ischemic event.

 A class of drugs known as *partial fatty acid oxidation (pFOX) inhibitors* has been developed to reduce the extensive fatty acid oxidation in heart after an ischemic episode. The reduction in fatty acid oxidation induced by the drug will allow glucose oxidation to occur and reduce lactate buildup in the damaged heart muscle. An example of a pFOX is trimetazidine (TMZ), which partially inhibits mitochondrial long-chain β-ketoacyl coenzyme A thiolase (the enzyme that catalyzes the release of acetyl-CoA from the oxidized fatty acid chain). It can be used to decrease symptoms of angina with chronic coronary artery disease. Other possible targets of such drugs, which have yet to be developed, include ACC-2, malonyl-CoA decarboxylase, and CPTI.

V. Fuel Use in Skeletal Muscle

Skeletal muscles use many fuels to generate ATP. The most abundant immediate source of ATP is creatine phosphate. ATP also can be generated from glycogen stores, either anaerobically (generating lactate) or aerobically, in which case pyruvate is converted to acetyl-CoA for oxidation via the TCA cycle. All human skeletal muscles have some mitochondria and thus are capable of fatty acid and ketone body oxidation. Skeletal muscles are also capable of completely oxidizing the carbon skeletons of alanine, aspartate, glutamate, valine, leucine, and isoleucine, but not other amino acids. Each of these fuel oxidation pathways plays a particular role in skeletal muscle metabolism.

A. ATP and Creatine Phosphate

ATP is not a good choice as a molecule to store in quantity for energy reserves. Many reactions are allosterically activated or inhibited by ATP levels, especially those that generate energy. Muscle cells solve this problem by storing high-energy phosphate bonds in the form of creatine phosphate. When energy is required, creatine phosphate donates a phosphate to ADP, to regenerate ATP for muscle contraction (Fig. 45.6).

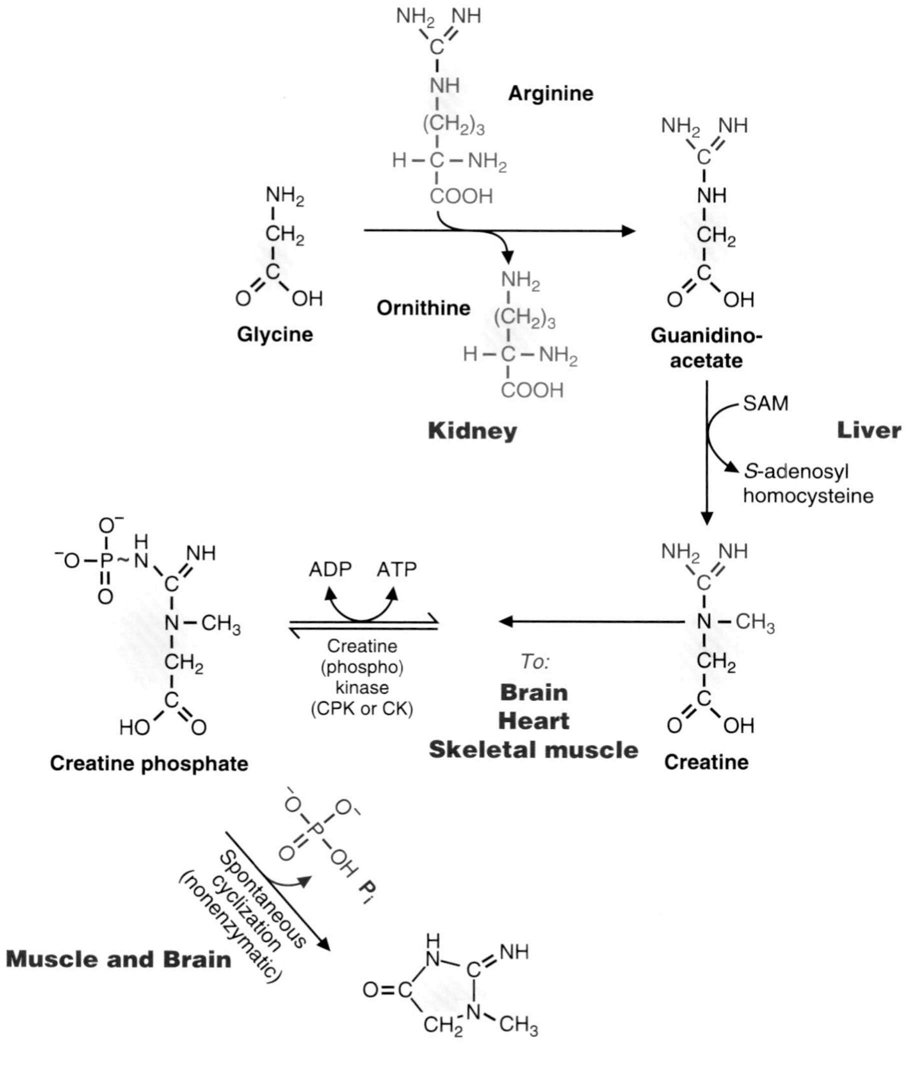

FIGURE 45.6 The synthesis of creatine and the generation of creatinine. The creatine phosphokinase reaction transfers a high-energy bond from ATP to creatine, conserving the high-energy bond. The high-energy bond is the unusual nitrogen–phosphate bond, as indicated by the *red squiggle*. Creatine is synthesized from arginine, glycine, and S-adenosylmethionine (SAM). The synthesis originates in the kidney and is completed in the liver. Creatine phosphate (and creatine) spontaneously cyclize, forming creatinine, which is excreted in the urine. *ADP*, adenosine diphosphate; *ATP*, adenosine triphosphate; P_i, inorganic phosphate.

Creatine synthesis begins in the kidney and is completed in the liver. In the kidney, glycine combines with arginine to form guanidinoacetate. In this reaction, the guanidinium group of arginine (the group that also forms urea) is transferred to glycine, and the remainder of the arginine molecule is released as ornithine. Guanidinoacetate then travels to the liver, where it is methylated by *S*-adenosylmethionine to form creatine (see Fig. 45.6).

The creatine formed is released from the liver and travels through the bloodstream to other tissues, particularly brain, heart, and skeletal muscle, where it reacts with ATP to form the high-energy compound creatine phosphate (see Fig. 45.6). This reaction, catalyzed by creatine phosphokinase (CK, also abbreviated as CPK), is reversible. Therefore, cells can use creatine phosphate to regenerate ATP.

Creatine phosphate serves as a small reservoir of high-energy phosphate that can readily regenerate ATP from ADP. As a result, it plays a particularly important role in muscle during exercise. It also carries high-energy phosphate from mitochondria, where ATP is synthesized, to myosin filaments, where ATP is used for muscle contraction.

Creatine phosphate is an unstable compound. It spontaneously cyclizes, forming creatinine (see Fig. 45.6). Creatinine cannot be further metabolized and is excreted in the urine. The amount of creatinine excreted each day is constant and depends on body muscle mass. Therefore, it can be used as a gauge for determining the amounts of other compounds excreted in the urine and as an indicator of renal excretory function. The daily volume of urine is determined by such factors as the volume of blood reaching the renal glomeruli and the amount of renal tubular fluid reabsorbed from the tubular urine back into the interstitial space of the kidneys over time. At any given moment, the concentration of a compound in a single urine specimen does not give a good indication of the total amount that is being excreted on a daily basis. However, if the concentration of the compound is divided by the concentration of creatinine, the result provides a better indication of the true excretion rate.

B. Fuel Use at Rest

Muscle fuel use at rest is dependent on the serum levels of glucose, amino acids, and fatty acids. If blood glucose and amino acids are elevated, glucose will be converted to glycogen, and branched-chain amino acid (BCAA) metabolism will be high. Fatty acids will be used for acetyl-CoA production and will satisfy the energy needs of the muscle under these conditions.

There is a balance between glucose oxidation and fatty acid oxidation, which is regulated by citrate. When the muscle cell has adequate energy, citrate leaves the mitochondria and activates ACC-2, which produces malonyl-CoA. The malonyl-CoA inhibits CPTI, thereby reducing fatty acid oxidation by the muscle. Malonyl-CoA decarboxylase is also inactive because the AMPK is not active in the resting state. Thus, the muscle regulates its oxidation of glucose and fatty acids in part through monitoring of cytoplasmic citrate levels.

C. Fuel Use during Starvation

As blood glucose levels drop, insulin levels drop. This reduces the levels of GLUT 4 transporters in the muscle membrane, and glucose use by muscle drops significantly. This conserves glucose for use by the nervous system and red blood cells. In cardiac muscle, PFK-2 is phosphorylated and activated by insulin. The lack of insulin results in a reduced use of glucose by these cells as well. Pyruvate dehydrogenase is inhibited by the high levels of acetyl-CoA and NADH being produced by fatty acid oxidation.

Fatty acids become the muscle's preferred fuel under starvation conditions. The AMPK is active because of lower-than-normal ATP levels, ACC-2 is inhibited, and malonyl-CoA decarboxylase is activated, thereby retaining full activity of CPTI. The lack of glucose reduces the glycolytic rate, and glycogen synthesis does not occur because of the inactivation of glycogen synthase by epinephrine-stimulated phosphorylation.

Each kidney normally contains approximately 1 million glomerular units. Each unit is supplied by arterial blood via the renal arteries and acts as a "filter." Metabolites such as creatinine leave the blood by passing through pores or channels in the glomerular capillaries and enter the fluid within the proximal kidney tubule for eventual excretion in the urine. When they are functionally intact, these glomerular tissues are impermeable to all but the smallest of proteins. When they are acutely inflamed; however, this barrier function is lost to varying degrees, and albumin and other proteins may appear in the urine.

The marked inflammatory changes in the glomerular capillaries that accompany PSGN significantly reduce the flow of blood to the filtering surfaces of these vessels. As a result, creatinine, urea, and other circulating metabolites that are filtered into the urine at a normal rate (the glomerular filtration rate [GFR]) in the absence of kidney disease now fail to reach the filters, and, therefore, they accumulate in the plasma. These changes explain **Renee F.'s** laboratory profile during her acute inflammatory glomerular disease (glomerulonephritis). In most patients, prognosis is excellent, although in some patients, recovery may not occur. Such patients may progress to chronic renal insufficiency and even renal failure.

Recall that in prolonged starvation, muscle proteolysis is induced (in part by cortisol release) for gluconeogenesis by the liver. This does not, however, alter the use of fatty acids by the muscle for its own energy needs under these conditions.

D. Fuel Use during Exercise

The rate of ATP use in skeletal muscle during exercise can be as much as 100 times greater than that in resting skeletal muscles; thus, the pathways of fuel oxidation must be rapidly activated during exercise to respond to the much greater demand for ATP. ATP and creatine phosphate would be rapidly used up if they were not continuously regenerated. The synthesis of ATP occurs from glycolysis (either aerobic or anaerobic) and oxidative phosphorylation (which requires a constant supply of oxygen).

Anaerobic glycolysis is especially important as a source of ATP in three conditions. The first is during the initial period of exercise, before exercise-stimulated increase in blood flow and substrate and oxygen delivery begin, allowing aerobic processes to occur. The second condition in which anaerobic glycolysis is important is exercise by muscle containing predominately fast-twitch glycolytic muscle fibers because these fibers have low oxidative capacity and generate most of their ATP through glycolysis. The third condition is during strenuous activity, when the ATP demand exceeds the oxidative capacity of the tissue, and the increased ATP demand is met by anaerobic glycolysis.

1. Anaerobic Glycolysis at the Onset of Exercise

During rest, most of the ATP required in all types of muscle fibers is obtained from aerobic metabolism. However, as soon as exercise begins, the demand for ATP increases. The amount of ATP present in skeletal muscle could sustain exercise for only 1.2 seconds if it were not regenerated, and the amount of phosphocreatine could sustain exercise for only 9 seconds if it were not regenerated. It takes longer than 1 minute for the blood supply to exercising muscle to increase significantly as a result of vasodilation and, therefore, oxidative metabolism of bloodborne glucose and fatty acids cannot increase rapidly at the onset of exercise. Thus, for the first few minutes of exercise, the conversion of glycogen to lactate provides a considerable portion of the ATP requirement.

2. Anaerobic Glycolysis in Type IIb Fast-Twitch Glycolytic Fibers

Although humans have no muscles that consist entirely of fast-twitch fibers, many other animals do. Examples are white abdominal muscles of fish and the pectoral muscles of game birds (turkey white meat). These muscles contract rapidly and vigorously (*fast twitch* refers to the time to peak tension), but only for short periods. Thus, they are used for activities such as flight by birds and for sprinting and weightlifting by humans.

In such muscles, the glycolytic capacity is high because the enzymes of glycolysis are present in large amounts (thus, the overall V_{max} [maximum velocity] is large). The levels of hexokinase, however, are low, so very little circulating glucose is used. The low levels of hexokinase in fast-twitch glycolytic fibers prevent the muscle from drawing on blood glucose to meet this high demand for ATP, thus avoiding hypoglycemia. Glucose 6-phosphate, formed from glycogenolysis, further inhibits hexokinase. The tissues rely on endogenous fuel stores (glycogen and creatine phosphate) to generate ATP, following the pathway of glycogen breakdown to glucose 1-phosphate, the conversion of glucose 1-phosphate to glucose 6-phosphate, and the metabolism of glucose 6-phosphate to lactate. Thus, anaerobic glycolysis is the main source of ATP during exercise of these muscle fibers.

3. Anaerobic Glycolysis from Glycogen

Glycogenolysis and glycolysis during exercise are activated together because both PFK-1 (the rate-limiting enzyme of glycolysis) and glycogen phosphorylase b (the inhibited form of glycogen phosphorylase) are allosterically activated by AMP.

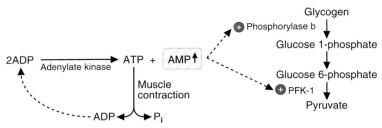

FIGURE 45.7 Activation of muscle glycogenolysis and glycolysis by adenosine monophosphate (AMP). As muscle contracts, adenosine triphosphate (ATP) is converted to adenosine diphosphate (ADP) and inorganic phosphate (P_i). In the adenylate kinase reaction, two ADP molecules react to form ATP and AMP. The ATP is used for contraction. As AMP accumulates, it activates glycogenolysis and glycolysis. *PFK-1*, phosphofructokinase.

AMP is an ideal activator because its concentration is normally kept low by the adenylate kinase (also called *myokinase* in muscle) equilibrium (2ADP $\leftrightarrow$ AMP + ATP). Thus, whenever ATP levels decrease slightly, the AMP concentration increases manyfold (Fig. 45.7).

Starting from a molecule of glucose 1-phosphate derived from glycogenolysis, three ATP molecules are produced in anaerobic glycolysis, as compared with 31 to 33 molecules of ATP in aerobic glycolysis. To compensate for the low ATP yield of anaerobic glycolysis, fast-twitch glycolytic fibers have a much higher content of glycolytic enzymes, and the rate of glucose 6-phosphate use is more than 12 times as fast as in slow-twitch fibers.

Muscle fatigue during exercise generally results from a lowering of the pH of the tissue to approximately 6.4. Both aerobic and anaerobic metabolism lowers the pH. Both the lowering of pH and lactate production can cause pain.

Metabolic fatigue also can occur once muscle glycogen is depleted. Muscle glycogen stores are used up in <2 minutes of anaerobic exercise. If you do pushups, you can prove this to yourself. The muscle used in pushups, a high-strength exercise, is principally fast-twitch glycolytic fibers. Time yourself from the start of your pushups. No matter how well you have trained, you probably cannot do pushups for as long as 2 minutes. Furthermore, you will feel the pain as the muscle pH drops as lactate production continues.

The regulation of muscle glycogen metabolism is complex. Recall that glycogen degradation in muscle is not sensitive to glucagon (muscles lack glucagon receptors), so there is little change in muscle glycogen stores during overnight fasting or long-term fasting, if the individual remains at rest. Glycogen synthase is inhibited during exercise but can be activated in resting muscle by the release of insulin after a high-carbohydrate meal. Unlike the liver form of glycogen phosphorylase, the muscle isozyme contains an allosteric site for AMP binding. When AMP binds to muscle glycogen phosphorylase b, the enzyme is activated even though it is not phosphorylated. Thus, as muscle begins to work and the myosin-ATPase hydrolyzes existing ATP stores to ADP, AMP begins to accumulate (because of the adenylate kinase reaction), and glycogen degradation is enhanced. The activation of muscle glycogen phosphorylase b is further enhanced by the release of Ca^{2+} from the sarcoplasmic reticulum, which occurs when muscles are stimulated to contract. The increase in sarcoplasmic Ca^{2+} also leads to the allosteric activation of glycogen phosphorylase kinase (through binding to the calmodulin subunit of the enzyme), which phosphorylates muscle glycogen phosphorylase b, fully activating it. And, finally, during intense exercise, epinephrine release stimulates the activation of adenylate cyclase in muscle cells, thereby activating the cAMP-dependent protein kinase (see Fig. 26.9). Protein kinase A phosphorylates and fully activates glycogen phosphorylase kinase so that continued activation of muscle glycogen phosphorylase can occur. The hormonal signal is slower than the initial activation events triggered by AMP and calcium (Fig. 45.8).

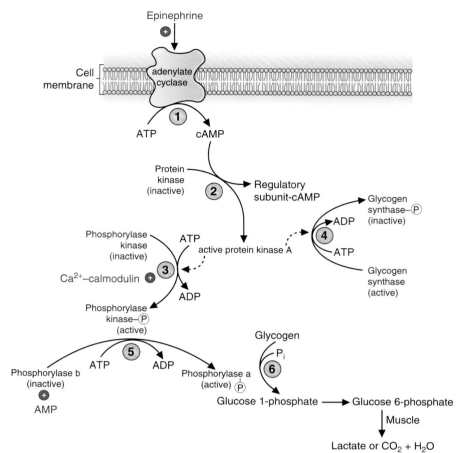

FIGURE 45.8 Stimulation of glycogenolysis in muscle by epinephrine. (*1*) Epinephrine binding to its receptor leads to the activation of adenylate cyclase, which increases cyclic adenosine monophosphate (cAMP) levels. (*2*) cAMP binds to the regulatory subunits of protein kinase A (PKA), thereby activating the catalytic subunits. (*3*) Active PKA phosphorylates and activates phosphorylase kinase. Phosphorylase kinase also can be activated partially by the Ca^{2+}–calmodulin complex as Ca^{2+} levels increase as muscles contract. (*4*) PKA phosphorylates and inactivates glycogen synthase. (*5*) Active phosphorylase kinase converts glycogen phosphorylase b to glycogen phosphorylase a. (*6*) Glycogen degradation forms glucose 1-phosphate, which is converted to glucose 6-phosphate, which enters the glycolytic pathway for energy production. *ADP*, adenosine diphosphate; *ATP*, adenosine triphosphate.

4. Anaerobic Glycolysis during High-Intensity Exercise

Once exercise begins, the electron-transport chain, the TCA cycle, and fatty acid oxidation are activated by the increase of ADP and the decrease of ATP. Pyruvate dehydrogenase remains in the active, nonphosphorylated state as long as NADH can be reoxidized in the electron-transport chain and acetyl-CoA can enter the TCA cycle. However, even though mitochondrial metabolism is working at its maximum capacity, additional ATP may be needed for very strenuous, high-intensity exercise. When this occurs, ATP is not being produced rapidly enough to meet the muscle's needs, and AMP begins to accumulate. Increased AMP levels activate PFK-1 and glycogenolysis, thereby providing additional ATP from anaerobic glycolysis (the additional pyruvate produced does not enter the mitochondria but rather is converted to lactate so that glycolysis can continue). Thus, under these conditions, most of the pyruvate formed by glycolysis enters the TCA cycle, whereas the remainder is reduced to lactate to regenerate NAD^+ for continued use in glycolysis.

Q If **Otto S.** runs at a pace at which his muscles require approximately 500 calories per hour, how long could he run on the amount of glucose that is present in circulating blood? Assume that the blood volume is 5 L.

5. Fate of Lactate Released during Exercise

The lactate that is released from skeletal muscles during exercise can be used by resting skeletal muscles or by the heart, a muscle with a large amount of mitochondria and very high oxidative capacity. In such muscles, the NADH/NAD$^+$ ratio is lower than in exercising skeletal muscle, and the lactate dehydrogenase reaction proceeds in the direction of pyruvate formation. The pyruvate that is generated is then converted to acetyl-CoA and oxidized in the TCA cycle, producing energy by oxidative phosphorylation.

The second potential fate of lactate is that it will return to the liver through the Cori cycle, where it is converted to glucose (see Fig. 22.12).

VI. Mild- and Moderate-Intensity Long-Term Exercise

A. Lactate Release Decreases with Duration of Exercise

Mild- to moderate-intensity exercise can be performed for longer periods than can high-intensity exercise. This is because of the aerobic oxidation of glucose and fatty acids, which generates more energy per fuel molecule than anaerobic metabolism, and which also produces lactic acid at a slower rate than anaerobic metabolism. Thus, during mild- and moderate-intensity exercise, the release of lactate diminishes as the aerobic metabolism of glucose and fatty acids becomes predominant.

B. Blood Glucose as a Fuel

At any given time during fasting, the blood contains only approximately 5 g of glucose, enough to support a person running at a moderate pace for a few minutes. Therefore, the blood glucose supply must be constantly replenished. The liver performs this function by processes similar to those used during fasting. The liver produces glucose by breaking down its own glycogen stores and by gluconeogenesis. The major source of carbon for gluconeogenesis during exercise is, of course, lactate, produced by the exercising muscle, but amino acids and glycerol are also used (Fig. 45.9). Epinephrine released during exercise stimulates liver glycogenolysis and gluconeogenesis by causing cAMP levels to increase.

During long periods of exercise, blood glucose levels are maintained by the liver through hepatic glycogenolysis and gluconeogenesis. The amount of glucose that the liver must export is greatest at higher workloads, in which case the muscle is using a greater proportion of the glucose for anaerobic metabolism. With increasing duration of exercise, an increasing proportion of blood glucose is supplied by gluconeogenesis. For up to 40 minutes of mild exercise, glycogenolysis is mainly responsible for the glucose output of the liver. However, after 40 to 240 minutes of exercise, the total glucose output of the liver decreases. This is caused by the increased use of fatty acids, which are being released from adipose tissue triacylglycerols (stimulated by epinephrine release). Glucose uptake by the muscle is stimulated by the increase in AMP levels and the activation of the AMPK, which stimulates the translocation of GLUT 4 transporters to the muscle membrane.

The hormonal changes that direct the increased hepatic glycogenolysis, hepatic gluconeogenesis, and adipose tissue lipolysis include a decrease in insulin and an increase in glucagon, epinephrine, and norepinephrine. Plasma levels of growth hormone, cortisol, and thyroid-stimulating hormone (TSH) also increase and may contribute to fuel mobilization as well (see Chapter 41). The activation of hepatic glycogenolysis occurs through glucagon and epinephrine release. Hepatic gluconeogenesis is activated by the increased supply of precursors (lactate, glycerol, amino acids, and pyruvate), the induction of gluconeogenic enzymes by glucagon and cortisol (this occurs only during prolonged exercise), and the increased supply of fatty acids to provide the ATP and NADH needed for gluconeogenesis and the regulation of gluconeogenic enzymes.

 Remember from Chapter 1 that a food calorie (cal) is equivalent to 1 kilocalorie (kcal) of energy. One gram of glucose can give rise to 4 kcal of energy, so at a rate of consumption of 500 cal/hour, we have

$$(500 \text{ cal/h}) \times (1 \text{ g of glucose/4 cal of energy}) \times (1 \text{ h/60 min}) = 2 \text{ g of glucose/min}$$

Thus, Otto must use 2 g of glucose per minute to run at his current pace. In the fasting state, blood glucose levels are approximately 90 mg/dL, or 900 mg/L. Because blood volume is estimated at 5 L, Otto has 4.5 g of glucose available. If it is not replenished, that amount of glucose will support only 2.25 minutes of running at 2 g of glucose per minute.

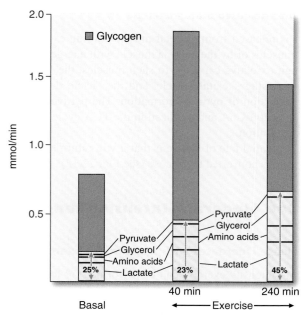

FIGURE 45.9 Production of blood glucose by the liver from various precursors during rest and during prolonged exercise. The *green area* represents the contribution of liver glycogen to blood glucose, and the *lighter area* represents the contribution of gluconeogenesis. (From Wahren J, et al. In: Howald H, Poortmans JR, eds. *Metabolic Adaptation to Prolonged Physical Exercise.* Cambridge, MA: Birkhauser; 1973:148.)

C. Free Fatty Acids as a Source of ATP

The longer the duration of the exercise, the greater the reliance of the muscle on free fatty acids for the generation of ATP (Fig. 45.10). Because ATP generation from free fatty acids depends on mitochondria and oxidative phosphorylation, long-distance running uses muscles that are principally slow-twitch oxidative fibers, such as the gastrocnemius. It is also important to realize that resting skeletal muscle uses free fatty acids as a principal fuel. At almost any time except the postprandial state (right after eating), free fatty acids are the preferred fuel for skeletal muscle.

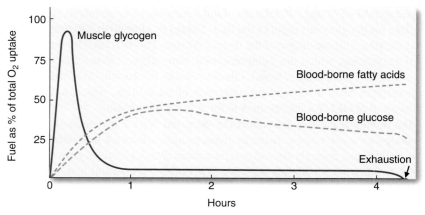

FIGURE 45.10 Fuels used during exercise. The pattern of fuel use changes with the duration of the exercise. (From Felig P, Baxter JD, Broadus AE, Frohman LA. *Endocrinology & Metabolism.* New York, NY: McGraw-Hill; 1981:796.)

The preferential use of fatty acids over glucose as a fuel in skeletal muscle depends on the following factors:

1. The availability of free fatty acids in the blood, which depends on their release from adipose tissue triacylglycerols by lipases. During prolonged exercise, the small decrease of insulin, and increases of glucagon, epinephrine and norepinephrine, cortisol, and possibly growth hormone all activate adipocyte tissue lipolysis.

2. Inhibition of glycolysis by products of fatty acid oxidation. Pyruvate dehydrogenase activity is inhibited by acetyl-CoA, NADH, and ATP, all of which are elevated as fatty acid oxidation proceeds. As AMP levels drop, and ATP levels rise, PFK-1 activity is decreased (see Chapter 22).

3. Glucose transport may be reduced during long-term exercise. Glucose transport into skeletal muscles via the GLUT 4 transporter is greatly activated by either insulin or exercise. During long-term exercise, the effect of falling insulin levels or increased fatty acid levels may counteract the stimulation of glucose transport by the exercise itself.

4. Oxidation of ketone bodies also increases during exercise. Their use as a fuel is dependent on their rate of production by the liver. Ketone bodies are never, however, a major fuel for skeletal muscle (muscles prefer free fatty acids).

5. Acetyl-CoA carboxylase (isozyme ACC-2) must be inactivated for the muscle to use fatty acids. This occurs as the AMPK is activated and phosphorylates ACC-2, rendering it inactive, and activates malonyl-CoA decarboxylase, to reduce malonyl-CoA levels and allow full activity of CPTI.

D. Branched-Chain Amino Acids

BCAA oxidation has been estimated to supply a maximum of 20% of the ATP supply of resting muscle. Oxidation of BCAAs in muscle serves two functions. The first is the generation of ATP, and the second is the synthesis of glutamine, which effluxes from the muscle. The highest rates of BCAA oxidation occur under conditions of acidosis, in which there is a higher demand for glutamine to transfer ammonia to the kidney and to buffer the urine as ammonium ion during proton excretion. Recall that glutamine synthesis occurs from the carbon skeletons of BCAA oxidation (valine and isoleucine) after the initial five steps of the oxidative pathway.

E. The Purine Nucleotide Cycle

Exercise increases the activity of the purine nucleotide cycle, which converts aspartate to fumarate plus ammonia (see Fig. 39.12). The ammonia is used to buffer the proton production and lactate production from glycolysis, and the fumarate is recycled and can form glutamine.

F. Acetate

Acetate is an excellent fuel for skeletal muscle. It is treated by the muscle as a very-short-chain fatty acid. It is activated to acetyl-CoA in the cytosol and then transferred into the mitochondria via acetylcarnitine transferase, an isozyme of carnitine palmitoyltransferase. Sources of acetate include the diet (vinegar is acetic acid) and acetate produced in the liver from alcohol metabolism. Certain commercial power bars for athletes contain acetate.

VII. Metabolic Effects of Training on Muscle Metabolism

The effect of training depends, to some extent, on the type of training. In general, training increases the muscle glycogen stores and increases the number and size of mitochondria. The fibers thus increase their capacity for generation of ATP from oxidative metabolism and their ability to use fatty acids as a fuel. The winners in marathon races seem to use muscle glycogen more efficiently than others.

Training to improve strength, power, and endurance of muscle performance is called *resistance training*. Its goal is to increase the size of the muscle fibers (hypertrophy of the muscle). Muscle fibers can develop a maximal force of 3 to 4 kg/cm^2 of muscle area. Thus, if we could increase our muscle size from 80 to 120 cm^2, the maximum resistance that could be lifted would increase from 240 to 360 kg. Hypertrophy occurs by increased protein synthesis in the muscle and a reduction in existing protein turnover.

CLINICAL COMMENTS

 Renee F. Poststreptococcal glomerulonephritis (PSGN) may follow pharyngeal or cutaneous infection with one of a limited number of "nephritogenic" strains of group A β-hemolytic streptococci. The pathogenesis of PSGN involves a host immune (antibody) response to one or more of the enzymes secreted by the bacterial cells. The antigen–antibody complexes are deposited on the tissues of glomerular units, causing a local acute inflammatory response. Hypertension may occur as a consequence of sodium and water retention caused by an inability of the inflamed glomerular units to filter sodium and water into the urine. Proteinuria is usually mild if the immune response is self-limited.

Overall, one of the most useful clinical indicators of GFR in both health and disease is the serum creatinine concentration. The endogenous production of creatinine, which averages approximately 15 mg/kg of body weight per day, is correlated with muscle mass and, therefore, tends to be constant for a given individual if renal function is normal. Any rise in serum creatinine in a patient such as **Renee F.**, therefore, can be assumed to result from decreased excretion of this metabolite into the urine. The extent of the rise in the blood is related directly to the severity of the pathologic process involving the glomerular units in the kidneys.

BIOCHEMICAL COMMENTS

The SERCA Pump. The SERCA pump is a transmembrane protein of 110 kDa that is present in several different isoforms throughout the body. Three genes encode SERCA proteins, designated SERCA1, SERCA2, and SERCA3. The *SERCA1* gene produces two alternatively spliced transcripts, *SERCA1a* and *SERCA1b*. SERCA1b is expressed in the fetal and neonatal fast-twitch skeletal muscles and is replaced by SERCA1a in adult fast-twitch muscles. The *SERCA2* gene also undergoes alternative splicing, producing the SERCA2a and SERCA2b isoforms. The SERCA2b isoform is expressed in all cell types and is associated with inositol trisphosphate (IP$_3$)–regulated calcium stores. SERCA2a is the primary isoform expressed in cardiac tissue. *SERCA3* produces at least five different alternatively spliced isoforms, which are specifically expressed in different tissues.

SERCA2a plays an important role in cardiac contraction and relaxation. Contraction is initiated by the release of calcium from intracellular stores, whereas relaxation occurs as the calcium is resequestered in the sarcoplasmic reticulum, in part mediated by the SERCA2a protein. The SERCA2a pump is regulated, in part, by its association with the protein phospholamban (PLN). PLN is a pentameric molecule consisting of five identical subunits of molecular weight 22,000 Da. PLN associates with SERCA2a in the sarcoplasmic reticulum and reduces its pumping activity. Because new contractions cannot occur until cytosolic calcium has been resequestered into the sarcoplasmic reticulum, a reduction in SERCA2a activity increases the relaxation time. However, when called on, the heart can increase its rate of contractions by inhibiting the activity of PLN. This is accomplished by phosphorylation of PLN by protein kinase A (PKA). Epinephrine release stimulates the heart to beat faster. This occurs through epinephrine binding to its receptor, activating a G-protein, which leads to adenylate cyclase activation, elevation of cAMP levels, and activation of PKA. PKA phosphorylates PLN, thereby reducing its association with SERCA2a and relieving the inhibition of pumping activity. This results in reduced relaxation times and more frequent contractions.

Mutations in PLN lead to cardiomyopathies, primarily an autosomal-dominant form of dilated cardiomyopathy. This particular mutation substitutes an arginine in place of cysteine at position 9 in PLN, which forms an inactive complex with PKA and blocks PKA phosphorylation of PLN. Individuals with this form of PLN develop cardiomyopathy in their teens. In this condition, the cardiac muscle does not pump well (because of the constant inhibition of SERCA2a) and becomes enlarged (dilated). Because of the poor pumping action of the heart, fluid can build up in the lungs (left heart failure). The pulmonary congestion results in a sense of breathlessness (dyspnea). Eventually, progressive left heart failure leads to right heart failure and fluid accumulation in other tissues and organs of the body, such as the legs and ankles (edema).

KEY CONCEPTS

- Muscle comprises three different types: skeletal, smooth, and cardiac.
  - Skeletal muscle facilitates movement of the skeleton.
- Slow-twitch fibers contain large amounts of mitochondria and myoglobin, and generate energy primarily via oxidative means.
- Fast-twitch fibers have few mitochondria, low levels of myoglobin, and are rich in glycogen. These fibers generate energy primarily via glycolysis.
  - Smooth muscle cells display no striations and aid in maintaining the shape and movement of the blood vessels, airways, uterus, and digestive systems.
  - Cardiac muscle cells contain striations but are regulated involuntarily. They use aerobic metabolism, oxidizing fatty acids, glucose, and lactate, and they contain many mitochondria, with very little glycogen.
- Acetylcholine release at the neuromuscular junction leads to muscle contraction.
- Fatty acid oxidation in muscle is controlled by the levels of malonyl-CoA produced by a muscle-specific isozyme of acetyl-CoA carboxylase (ACC-2).
- Skeletal muscle uses many fuels to generate ATP, storing excess high-energy phosphate bonds as creatine phosphate.
- Muscle fuel use is regulated carefully.
  - At rest, the muscle uses what is available in the blood (glucose, amino acids, fatty acids).
  - During starvation, fatty acids are the preferred energy source (even over ketone bodies).
  - During exercise, stored glycogen, blood glucose, and blood fatty acids are the primary sources of energy for the skeletal muscles.
- Diseases discussed in this chapter are summarized in Table 45.2.

TABLE 45.2 Diseases Discussed in Chapter 45		
DISEASE OR DISORDER	**GENETIC OR ENVIRONMENTAL**	**COMMENTS**
Renal failure	Both	The lack of kidney function can lead to encephalopathy, owing to the buildup of toxic metabolites in the blood.
Duchenne muscular dystrophy	Genetic	The lack of dystrophin, owing to deletions in the *DMD* gene on the X-chromosome, leads to muscle dysfunction at an early age.

REVIEW QUESTIONS—CHAPTER 45

1. The process of stretching before exercise has which one of the following biochemical benefits?
   A. Stimulates the release of epinephrine
   B. Activates glycolysis in the liver
   C. Increases blood flow to the muscles
   D. Activates glycolysis in the muscles
   E. Stimulates glycogenolysis in the liver

2. The major metabolic fuel for participating in a prolonged aerobic exercise event is which of the following?
   A. Liver glycogen
   B. Muscle glycogen
   C. Brain glycogen
   D. Adipose triacylglycerol
   E. Red blood cell–produced lactate

3. A 24-hour urine collection showed that an individual's excretion of creatinine was much lower than normal. Decreased excretion of creatinine could be caused by which one of the following?
   A. A decreased dietary intake of creatine
   B. A higher-than-normal muscle mass resulting from weight lifting
   C. A genetic defect in the enzyme that converts creatine phosphate to creatinine
   D. Kidney failure
   E. A vegetarian diet

4. In the biosynthetic pathways for the synthesis of heme, creatine, and guanine, which one of the following amino acids directly provides carbon atoms that appear in the final product?
   A. Serine
   B. Aspartate
   C. Cysteine
   D. Glutamate
   E. Glycine

5. In skeletal muscle, increased hydrolysis of ATP during muscular contraction leads to which one of the following?
   A. A decrease in the rate of palmitate oxidation to acetyl-CoA
   B. A decrease in the rate of NADH oxidation by the electron-transport chain
   C. Activation of PFK-1
   D. An increase in the proton gradient across the inner mitochondrial membrane
   E. Activation of glycogen synthase

6. A new drug is being developed which can specifically inhibit the ACC-2 isozyme in muscle. This drug could potentially be used for which one of the following purposes?
   A. To accelerate weight loss
   B. To reduce the severity of a myocardial infarction
   C. To enhance high-intensity exercise performance
   D. To increase ketone body synthesis in a patient with hypoglycemia
   E. To increase fatty acid synthesis in muscle

7. Insulin release stimulates the heart's glycolytic rate because increased levels of glucose are present in the circulation. The increase in glycolytic rate occurs owing to which one of the following?
   A. An increase in ATP levels
   B. A decrease in ATP levels
   C. A decrease in fructose 2,6-bisphosphate levels
   D. An increase in lactate levels
   E. An increase in fructose 2,6-bisphosphate levels
   F. A decrease in lactate levels

8. An athlete is actively training for her 1,500-meter race. She runs a series of sprints, followed by longer distances at a slower pace. Which statement correctly describes her muscle energy production and usage during a training session?
   A. Muscle cells synthesize fatty acids for energy.
   B. Skeletal muscle uses lactate and glucose for energy needs.
   C. The heart uses glycolysis to meet 10% to 20% of its energy needs.
   D. Fatty acids are the preferred fuel for the heart.
   E. Ketone bodies are a preferred fuel for skeletal muscle.

9. A person had an ischemic cardiac event caused by a clot lodged in a coronary artery. He then received tissue plasminogen activator (tPA; a clot buster) and worsened when the ischemia was relieved (ischemia reperfusion injury). This occurred because of which one of the following after the ischemia was relieved?
   A. Increased glycolysis
   B. Increased fatty acid oxidation
   C. Increased levels of NADPH in mitochondria
   D. Decreased levels of NADH in mitochondria
   E. Decreased lactate production

10. Muscle cells use creatine phosphate to store high-energy phosphate bonds instead of ATP. Creatine can be best described by which one of the following?
    A. Creatine is synthesized in the kidney.
    B. Creatine reacts with ATP to produce CPK.
    C. Creatine cannot be further metabolized and is excreted in the urine.
    D. Creatine excretion in the urine is constant each day.
    E. Creatine is used by the brain, heart, and skeletal muscle.

ANSWERS

1. **The answer is C.** Stretching aids in stimulating blood flow to the muscles, which enhances oxidative muscle metabolism (by allowing for better oxygen delivery). Stretching, per se, does not stimulate epinephrine release (thus, A is incorrect), nor does it activate glycolysis in either the liver or muscle.

2. **The answer is D.** Triacylglycerol is the largest energy store in the body and is the predominant fuel in long-term aerobic exercise. During exercise, muscle glycogen is used for bursts of speed but not for long-term energy requirements. Liver glycogen is used to maintain blood glucose levels for use by the nervous system and as a supplement for use by muscle when rapid speed is required; however, it is not designed to be a long-term energy source. The brain does not contain significant levels of glycogen, and lactic acid produced by the red blood cells is used as a gluconeogenic precursor by liver but not as a fuel for muscle.

3. **The answer is D.** Creatine is synthesized from glycine, arginine, and *S*-adenosylmethionine (thus, intake of dietary creatine is not relevant). In muscle, creatine is converted to creatine phosphate, which is nonenzymatically cyclized to form creatinine (thus, C is incorrect). The amount of creatinine excreted by the kidneys each day depends on body muscle mass but is constant for each individual (therefore, if there is an increase in body muscle mass, there would be an increase in creatinine excretion). In kidney failure, the excretion of creatinine into the urine is low, and an elevation of serum creatinine would be observed.

4. **The answer is E.** Glycine is required for the synthesis of heme (combining with succinyl-CoA in the initial step), for the synthesis of purine rings (the entire glycine molecule is incorporated into adenine and guanine) and for creatine, where glycine reacts with arginine in the first step.

5. **The answer is C.** A decrease in the concentration of ATP (which occurs as muscle contracts) stimulates processes that generate ATP. The proton gradient across the inner mitochondrial membrane decreases as protons enter the matrix via the ATPase in order to synthesize ATP; NADH oxidation by the electron-transport chain increases to reestablish the proton gradient; fuel use also increases in order to generate more ATP. Glycogen synthesis is inhibited because of phosphorylation of glycogen synthase as induced by epinephrine. Palmitate is oxidized and glycolysis increases because of the activation of PFK-1 by AMP. As ATP decreases, AMP rises as a result of the myokinase reaction (2ADP → ATP + AMP).

6. **The answer is A.** ACC-2 produces malonyl-CoA in the muscle for the purpose of regulating fatty acid oxidation via inhibition of CPTI. When malonyl-CoA cannot be synthesized through inhibition of ACC-2, fatty acid oxidation in the muscle is rapid and not regulated. Skeletal muscle then oxidizes fatty acids instead of glucose, leading to a drop in stored fatty acids in the adipocyte. After a myocardial infarction, fatty acid oxidation must be regulated such that glucose oxidation can also occur; otherwise, lactic acid is produced (via anaerobic glycolysis), which further damages the heart. High-intensity exercise requires very rapid ATP synthesis, which can only occur by anaerobic glycolysis; as a result, increasing the rate of fatty acid oxidation by drug use will not aid in high-intensity exercise. Muscle cells do not produce either ketone bodies or fatty acids; thus, inhibition of ACC-2 would not lead to those effects.

7. **The answer is E.** Insulin release leads to the activation of protein kinase B (Akt), which, in the heart, will phosphorylate PFK-2. The phosphorylation of the heart isozyme of PFK-2 leads to activation of its kinase activity, thereby producing increased amounts of fructose 2,6-bisphosphate, a potent activator of PFK-1 activity. Simultaneously, the phosphatase activity of cardiac PFK-2 is inhibited, thereby allowing the increased levels of fructose 2,6-bisphosphate to stay elevated. The activation of PFK-1 leads to an increased glycolytic rate within the heart, taking advantage of the high glucose levels in the blood. High levels of ATP will inhibit glycolysis as an allosteric inhibitor, and high levels of lactate reduce glycolysis, owing to a reduction in intracellular pH. Low levels of ATP do not stimulate glycolysis (AMP will activate PFK-1), nor will low levels of lactate.

8. **The answer is D.** The heart uses primarily fatty acids (60% to 80% of energy needs) for its energy needs but can use lactate and glucose. Only 2% of its energy requirement is derived from glycolysis. Muscles do not synthesize fatty acids. Exercising skeletal muscles use glucose and fatty acids preferentially for their energy needs (glucose during sprints, and a mixture of fatty acids and glucose during longer distances). Ketone bodies are not produced when adults exercise. The lactate generated by the muscle during exercise can also be used by the heart as an energy source. The muscle, when generating lactate, does not use the lactate as a fuel.

9. **The answer is B.** During ischemia, glycolysis increases, creating lactate. However, after ischemia is relieved, the high rate of fatty acid oxidation is damaging to already-damaged heart cells by rapidly increasing NADH levels in the mitochondria. This leads to even more lactate production in the cytoplasm as the high intramitochondrial NADH levels inhibit the shuttle systems that transfer

electrons from cytoplasmic NADH to mitochondrial NAD^+. The increased cytoplasmic NADH levels lead to increased lactate production, reducing the pH of the cardiac cells. The high acetyl-CoA levels in the mitochondria (owing to fatty acid oxidation) inhibit pyruvate dehydrogenase, which leads to increased pyruvate in the cytoplasm and increased lactate production. NADPH is not involved in the increase in cardiac damage after ischemia.

10. **The answer is E.** Creatine synthesis begins in the kidney and is completed in the liver. It is then released into the blood and travels particularly to brain, heart, and skeletal muscle, where it is used to react with ATP to form creatine phosphate (catalyzed by CPK). Creatine phosphate is unstable and spontaneously cyclizes to creatinine, which is excreted in the urine. The amount of creatinine excreted each day is constant and proportional to muscle mass.

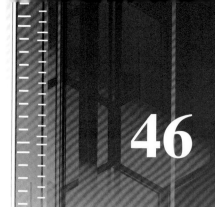

Metabolism of the Nervous System

46

The nervous system consists of various cell types. The most abundant cell in the nervous system is the **glial cell**, which consists of **astrocytes** and **oligodendrocytes** in the **central nervous system** (**CNS**), and **Schwann cells** in the **peripheral nervous system** (**PNS**). These cells provide support for the neurons and synthesize the protective **myelin sheath** that surrounds the axons emanating from the neurons. **Microglial cells** in the nervous system act as immune cells, destroying and ingesting foreign organisms that enter the nervous system. The interface between the brain parenchyma and the **cerebrospinal fluid** (**CSF**) compartment is formed by the **ependymal cells**, which line the cavities of the brain and spinal cord. These cells use their cilia to allow for the circulation of the CSF, which bathes the cells of the CNS.

The cells of the brain are separated from free contact with the rest of the body by the **blood–brain barrier**. The capillaries of the brain exhibit features, such as tight endothelial cell junctions, that restrict their permeability to metabolites in the blood. This protects the brain from compounds that might be toxic or otherwise interfere with nerve impulse transmission. It also affects the entry of precursors for brain metabolic pathways such as fuel metabolism and neurotransmitter synthesis.

Neurotransmitters can be divided structurally into two categories: **small nitrogen-containing neurotransmitters** and **neuropeptides**. The small nitrogen-containing neurotransmitters are generally synthesized in the **presynaptic terminal** from amino acids and intermediates of glycolysis and the tricarboxylic acid (TCA) cycle. They are retained in storage vesicles until the neuron is depolarized. The **catecholamine** neurotransmitters (**dopamine**, **norepinephrine**, and **epinephrine**) are derived from tyrosine. **Serotonin** is synthesized from **tryptophan**. **Acetylcholine** is synthesized from **choline**, which can be supplied from the diet or is synthesized and stored as part of **phosphatidylcholine**. **Glutamate** and its neurotransmitter derivative, **γ-aminobutyric acid** (**GABA**), are derived from **α-ketoglutarate** in the TCA cycle. **Glycine** is synthesized in the brain from **serine**. The synthesis of the neurotransmitters is regulated to correspond to the rate of depolarization of the individual neurons. A large number of cofactors are required for the synthesis of neurotransmitters, and deficiencies of **pyridoxal phosphate**, **thiamin pyrophosphate**, and **vitamin B$_{12}$** result in a variety of neurologic dysfunctions.

Brain metabolism has a high **requirement for glucose and oxygen. Deficiencies of either** (**hypoglycemia** or **hypoxia**) affect brain function because they influence adenosine triphosphate (ATP) production and the supply of precursors for neurotransmitter synthesis. **Ischemia** elicits a condition in which increased **calcium levels**, **swelling**, **glutamate excitotoxicity**, and **nitric oxide** generation affect brain function and can lead to a stroke. The generation of **free radicals** and abnormalities in nitric oxide production are important players in the pathogenesis of a variety of **neurodegenerative** diseases.

Because of the restrictions posed by the blood–brain barrier to the entry of a variety of substances into the CNS, the brain generally synthesizes and degrades its own lipids. Essential fatty acids can enter the brain, but the more common fatty acids do not. The turnover of lipids at the synaptic membrane is very rapid, and the neuron must replace those lipids lost during exocytosis. The glial cells produce the **myelin**

sheath, which is composed primarily of lipids. These lipids are of a different composition than those of the neuronal cells. Because there is considerable lipid synthesis and turnover in the brain, this organ is sensitive to **disorders of peroxisomal function** (Refsum disease; interference in very-long-chain fatty acid oxidation and α-oxidation) and **lysosomal diseases** (mucopolysaccharidoses; inability to degrade complex lipids and glycolipids).

THE WAITING ROOM

 Katie C., a 34-year-old dress designer, developed alarming palpitations of her heart while bending forward to pick up her cat. She also developed a pounding headache and sweated profusely. After 5 to 10 minutes, these symptoms subsided. One week later, her aerobic exercise instructor, a registered nurse, noted that Katie grew very pale and was tremulous during exercise. The instructor took Katie's blood pressure, which was 220 mm Hg systolic (normal, up to 120 at rest) and 132 mm Hg diastolic (normal, up to 80 at rest). Within 15 minutes, Katie recovered, and her blood pressure returned to normal. The instructor told Katie to see her physician the next day.

The doctor told Katie that her symptom complex coupled with severe hypertension strongly suggested the presence of a tumor in the medulla of one of her adrenal glands (a pheochromocytoma) that was episodically secreting large amounts of catecholamines, such as norepinephrine (noradrenaline) and epinephrine (adrenaline). Her blood pressure was normal until moderate pressure to the left of her umbilicus caused Katie to suddenly develop a typical attack, and her blood pressure rose rapidly. In addition to ordering several biochemical tests, Katie also was scheduled for a magnetic resonance imaging (MRI) study of her abdomen and pelvis. The MRI showed a 3.5 × 2.8 × 2.6 cm mass in the left adrenal gland, with imaging characteristics typical of a pheochromocytoma.

 Ivan A.'s brother, **Evan A.**, was 6 ft tall and weighed 425 lb (body mass index [BMI] = 57.6 kg/m²). He had only been successful in losing weight once in his life, in 1977, when he had lost 30 pounds through a combination of diet and exercise with the support of a registered dietitian. However, he quickly regained this weight over the next year. Evan's weight was not usually a concern for him, but in 1997, he became worried when it became difficult because of joint pain in his knees, for him to take walks or go fishing. He was also suffering from symptoms suggestive of a peripheral neuropathy, manifesting primarily as tingling in his legs. In 1997, Evan approached his physician, desperate for help to lose weight. The physician placed Evan on a new drug, Redux, which had just been approved for use as a weight-loss agent, and a low-fat, low-calorie diet along with physical therapy to help increase his activity level. In 4 months, Evan's weight dropped from 425 to 375 lb, his total cholesterol dropped from 250 to 185, and his serum triglycerides dropped from 375 to 130. However, Redux was withdrawn from the market by its manufacturer late in 1997 because of its toxicity. Evan was then placed on Prozac, a drug used primarily as an antidepressant but which may cause mild weight loss.

I. Cell Types of the Nervous System

The nervous system consists of neurons, the cells that transmit signals, and supporting cells, the neuroglia. The neuroglia consist of oligodendrocytes and astrocytes (known collectively as *glial cells*), microglial cells, ependymal cells, and Schwann cells. The neuroglia are designed to support and sustain the neurons and do so by surrounding neurons and holding them in place, supplying nutrients and oxygen to the neurons, insulating neurons so their electrical signals are more rapidly propagated, and cleaning up any debris that enters the nervous system. The CNS consists of the brain and spinal cord. This system integrates all signals emanating from the PNS. The PNS is composed of all neurons that lie outside the CNS.

A. Neurons

Neurons consist of a cell body (soma) from which long (axons) and short (dendrites) extensions protrude. Dendrites receive information from the axons of other neurons, whereas the axons transmit information to other neurons. The axon–dendrite connection is known as a *synapse* (Fig. 46.1). Most neurons contain multiple dendrites, each of which can receive signals from multiple axons. This configuration allows a single neuron to integrate information from multiple sources. Although neurons also contain just one axon, most axons branch extensively and distribute information to multiple targets (divergence). The neurons transmit signals by changes in the electrical potential across their membrane. Signaling across a synapse requires the release of neurotransmitters that, when bound to their specific receptors, initiate an electrical signal in the receiving or target cell. Neurons are terminally differentiated cells and, as such, have little capability for division. As a result, injured neurons have a limited capacity to repair themselves and frequently undergo apoptosis (programmed cell death) when damaged.

B. Neuroglial Cells

1. Astrocytes

The astrocytes are found in the CNS and are star-shaped cells that provide physical and nutritional support for neurons. During development of the CNS, the astrocytes guide neuronal migration to their final adult position and form a matrix that keeps neurons in place. These cells serve several functions, including phagocytosing debris left behind by cells, providing lactate (from glucose metabolism) as a carbon source for the neurons, and controlling the brain extracellular ionic environment. Astrocytes help to regulate the content of the extracellular fluid (ECF) by taking up, processing, and metabolizing nutrients and waste products.

2. Oligodendrocytes

Oligodendrocytes provide the myelin sheath that surrounds the axon, acting as "insulation" for many of the neurons in the CNS. The myelin sheath is the lipid–protein covering of the axons (see Section V.B for a description of the composition and

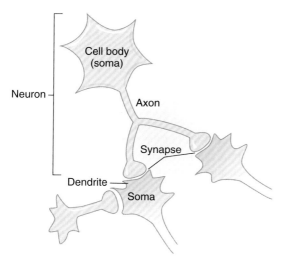

FIGURE 46.1   A neuron consists of a cell body (soma) with short extensions (dendrites) and a long extension (axon). The axon–dendrite interface is the synapse. A soma may receive input from multiple axons.

synthesis of the myelin sheath). Oligodendrocytes can form myelin sheaths around multiple neurons in the CNS by sending out processes that bind to the axons on target neurons. The speed with which a neuron conducts its electric signal (action potential) is directly proportional to the degree of myelination. Oligodendrocytes, along with the astrocytes, form a supporting matrix for the neurons. Oligodendrocytes have a limited capacity for mitosis and, if damaged, do not replicate. If this occurs, demyelination of the axons may occur, resulting in abnormalities in signal conduction along that axon (see "Biochemical Comments").

3. Schwann Cells

Schwann cells are the supporting cells of the PNS. Like oligodendrocytes, Schwann cells form myelin sheaths around the axons, but unlike the oligodendrocytes, Schwann cells myelinate only one axon; they also clean up cellular debris in the PNS. In addition, Schwann cells provide a means for peripheral axons to regenerate if damaged. There is a synergistic interaction among the Schwann cells, secreted growth factors, and the axon that allows damaged axons to reconnect to the appropriate target axon.

4. Microglial Cells

The microglial cells are the smallest glial cells in the nervous system. They serve as immunologically responsive cells that function similarly to the action of macrophages in the circulation. Microglial cells destroy invading microorganisms and phagocytose cellular debris.

5. Ependymal Cells

The ependymal cells are ciliated cells that line the cavities (ventricles) of the CNS and the spinal cord. In some areas of the brain, the ependymal cells are functionally specialized to elaborate and secrete CSF into the ventricular system. The beating of the ependymal cilia allows for efficient circulation of the CSF throughout the CNS. The CSF acts as both a shock absorber protecting the CNS from mechanical trauma and as a system for the removal of metabolic wastes. The CSF can be aspirated from the spinal canal and analyzed to determine whether disorders of CNS function, with their characteristic CSF changes, are present.

For many years, it had been believed that damaged neurons in the CNS could not regenerate because it was thought that there are no pluripotent stem cells (cells that can differentiate into various cell types found in the CNS) in the CNS. However, recent data suggest that cells found within the ependymal layer can act as neural stem cells, which under appropriate stimulation can regenerate cells within the nervous system. Such a finding opens up a large number of potential treatments for diseases that alter neuronal cell function.

II. The Blood–Brain Barrier

A. Capillary Structure

In the capillary beds of most organs, rapid passage of molecules occurs from the blood through the endothelial wall of the capillaries into the interstitial fluid. Thus, the composition of interstitial fluid resembles that of blood, and specific receptors or transporters in the plasma membrane of the cells being bathed by the interstitial fluid may interact directly with amino acids, hormones, or other compounds from the blood. In the brain, transcapillary movement of substrates in the peripheral circulation into the brain is highly restricted by the blood–brain barrier. This barrier limits the accessibility of bloodborne toxins and other potentially harmful compounds to the neurons of the CNS.

The blood–brain barrier begins with the endothelial cells that form the inner lining of the vessels supplying blood to the CNS (Fig. 46.2). Unlike the endothelial cells of other organs, these cells are joined by tight junctions that do not permit the

Inside of capillary

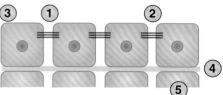

1. Tight junctions between endothelial cells

2. Narrow intercellular spaces

3. Lack of pinocytosis

4. Continuous basement membrane

5. Astrocyte extension

FIGURE 46.2 The blood–brain barrier. Compounds in the blood cannot pass freely into the brain; they must traverse the endothelial cells, basement membrane, and astrocytes, using specific carriers to gain access to the brain. Very lipophilic molecules may pass through all of these membranes in the absence of a carrier.

movement of polar molecules from the blood into the interstitial fluid bathing the neurons. They also lack mechanisms for transendothelial transport that are present in other capillaries of the body. These mechanisms include fenestrations ("windows" or pores that span the endothelial lining and permit the rapid movement of molecules across membranes) or transpinocytosis (vesicular transport from one side of the endothelial cell to another).

The endothelial cells serve actively, as well as passively, to protect the brain. Because they contain a variety of drug-metabolizing enzyme systems similar to the drug-metabolizing enzymes found in the liver, the endothelial cells can metabolize neurotransmitters and toxic chemicals and, therefore, form an enzymatic barrier to entry of these potentially harmful substances into the brain. They actively pump hydrophobic molecules that diffuse into endothelial cells back into the blood (especially xenobiotics) with P-glycoproteins, which act as transmembranous, ATP-dependent efflux pumps. Although lipophilic substances, water, oxygen, and carbon dioxide can readily cross the blood–brain barrier by passive diffusion, other molecules depend on specific transport systems. Differential transporters on the luminal and abluminal endothelial membranes can transport compounds into, as well as out of, the brain.

Further protection against the free entry of bloodborne compounds into the CNS is provided by a continuous collagen-containing basement membrane that completely surrounds the capillaries. The basement membrane appears to be surrounded by the foot processes of astrocytes. Thus, compounds must pass through endothelial cell membranes, the enzymatic barrier in the endothelial cells, the basement membrane, and possibly additional cellular barriers formed by the astrocytes to reach the neurons in the brain.

B. Transport through the Blood–Brain Barrier

Many nonpolar substances, such as drugs and inert gases, probably diffuse through the endothelial cell membranes. A large number of other compounds are transported through the endothelial capillaries by facilitative transport, whereas others, such as nonessential fatty acids, cannot cross the blood–brain barrier. Essential fatty acids, however, are transported across the barrier.

I. Fuels

Glucose, which is the principal fuel of the brain, is transported through both endothelial membranes by facilitated diffusion via the GLUT 1 transporter (see Fig. 21.9). GLUT 3 transporters present on the neurons then allow the neurons to transport the glucose from the ECF. Glial cells express GLUT 1 transporters. Although the rate of glucose transport into the ECF normally exceeds the rate required for energy metabolism by the brain, glucose transport may become rate-limiting as blood glucose levels fall below the normal range. Thus, individuals begin to experience hypoglycemic symptoms at glucose levels of approximately 60 mg/dL, as the glucose levels are reduced to the K_m, or below the K_m values of the GLUT 1 transporters in the endothelial cells of the barrier.

Monocarboxylic acids, including L-lactate, acetate, pyruvate, and the ketone bodies acetoacetate and β-hydroxybutyrate, are transported by a separate stereospecific system that is slower than the transport system for glucose. During starvation, when the level of ketone bodies in the blood is elevated, this transporter is upregulated. Ketone bodies are important fuels for the brain of both adults and neonates during prolonged starvation (>46 hours).

2. Amino Acids and Vitamins

Large neutral amino acids (LNAAs) (such as phenylalanine, leucine, tyrosine, isoleucine, valine, tryptophan, methionine, and histidine) enter the CSF rapidly via a single amino acid transporter (L [leucine preferring] system amino acid transporter). Many of these compounds are essential in the diet and must be imported for protein

 Several disorders of glucose transport across the blood–brain barrier are known. The most common of these is facilitated glucose transporter protein type 1 (GLUT 1) deficiency syndrome. In this disorder, GLUT 1 transporters are impaired, which results in a low glucose concentration in the CSF (a condition known as *hypoglycorrhachia*). A diagnostic indication of this disorder is that in the presence of normal blood glucose levels the ratio of CSF glucose to blood glucose levels is <0.4. Clinical features are variable but include seizures, developmental delay, and a complex motor disorder. These symptoms are the result of inadequate glucose levels in the brain. The disorder can be treated by prescribing a ketogenic diet (high-fat, low-carbohydrate). This will force the patient to produce ketone bodies, which are easily transported into the CNS and can partially spare the brain's requirement for glucose as an energy source.

The finding that the LNAAs have a common carrier system across the blood–brain barrier suggests that if one amino acid is in excess, it can, by competitive inhibition, result in lower transport of the other amino acids. This suggests that the mental retardation that results from untreated phenylketonuria (PKU) and maple syrup urine disease (see Chapter 37) may be attributable to the high levels of either phenylalanine or branched-chain amino acids in the blood. These high levels overwhelm the LNAA carrier so that excessive levels of the damaging amino acid enter the CNS. In support of this theory is the finding that treatment of patients with PKU with large doses of LNAAs that lack phenylalanine resulted in a decrease of phenylalanine levels in the CSF and brain, with an improvement in the patients' cognitive functions as well.

synthesis or as precursors of neurotransmitters. Because a single transporter is involved, these amino acids compete with each other for transport into the brain.

The entry of small neutral amino acids, such as alanine, glycine, proline, and GABA, is markedly restricted because their influx could dramatically change the content of neurotransmitters (see Section III). They are synthesized in the brain, and some are transported out of the CNS and into the blood via the A (alanine-preferring) system carrier. Vitamins have specific transporters through the blood–brain barrier, just as they do in most tissues.

3. Receptor-Mediated Transcytosis

Certain proteins, such as insulin, transferrin, and insulin-like growth factors, cross the blood–brain barrier by receptor-mediated transcytosis. Once the protein binds to its membrane receptor, the membrane containing the receptor–protein complex is endocytosed into the endothelial cell to form a vesicle. It is released on the other side of the endothelial cell. Absorption-mediated transcytosis also can occur. This differs from receptor-mediated transcytosis in that the protein binds nonspecifically to the membrane and not to a distinct receptor.

III. Synthesis of Small Nitrogen-Containing Neurotransmitters

Molecules that serve as neurotransmitters fall into two basic structural categories: (1) small nitrogen-containing molecules and (2) neuropeptides. The major small nitrogen-containing molecule neurotransmitters include glutamate, GABA, glycine, acetylcholine, dopamine, norepinephrine, serotonin, and histamine. Additional neurotransmitters that fall into this category include epinephrine, aspartate, and nitric oxide. In general, each neuron synthesizes only those neurotransmitters that it uses for transmission through a synapse or to another cell. The neuronal tracts are often identified by their neurotransmitter; for example, a dopaminergic tract synthesizes and releases the neurotransmitter dopamine.

Neuropeptides are usually small peptides that are synthesized and processed in the CNS. Some of these peptides have targets within the CNS (such as endorphins, which bind to opioid receptors and block pain signals), whereas others are released into the circulation to bind to receptors on other organs (such as growth hormone and thyroid-stimulating hormone). Many neuropeptides are synthesized as a larger precursor, which is then cleaved to produce the active peptides. Until recently, the assumption was that a neuron synthesized and released only a single neurotransmitter. More recent evidence suggests that a neuron may contain (1) more than one small-molecule neurotransmitter, (2) more than one neuropeptide neurotransmitter, or (3) both types of neurotransmitters. The differential release of the various neurotransmitters is the result of the neuron altering its frequency and pattern of firing.

A. General Features of Neurotransmitter Synthesis

Several features are common to the synthesis, secretion, and metabolism of most small nitrogen-containing neurotransmitters (Table 46.1). Most of these neurotransmitters are synthesized from amino acids, intermediates of glycolysis and the TCA cycle, and O_2 in the cytoplasm of the presynaptic terminal. The rate of synthesis is generally regulated to correspond to the rate of firing of the neuron. Once they are synthesized, the neurotransmitters are transported into storage vesicles by an ATP-requiring pump linked with the proton gradient. Release from the storage vesicle is triggered by the nerve impulse that depolarizes the postsynaptic membrane and causes an influx of Ca^{2+} ions through voltage-gated calcium channels. The influx of Ca^{2+} promotes fusion of the vesicle with the synaptic membrane and release of the neurotransmitter into the synaptic cleft. The transmission across the synapse is completed by binding of the neurotransmitter to a receptor on the postsynaptic membrane (Fig. 46.3).

TABLE 46.1	**Features Common to Neurotransmitters**[a]

- Synthesis from amino acid and common metabolic precursors usually occurs in the cytoplasm of the presynaptic nerve terminal. The synthetic enzymes are transported by fast axonal transport from the cell body, where they are synthesized, to the presynaptic terminal.
- The synthesis of the neurotransmitter is regulated to correspond to the rate of firing of the neuron, both acutely and through long-term enhancement of synaptic transmission.
- The neurotransmitter is actively taken up into storage vesicles in the presynaptic terminal.
- The neurotransmitter acts at a receptor on the postsynaptic membrane.
- The action of the neurotransmitter is terminated through reuptake into the presynaptic terminal, diffusion away from the synapse, or enzymatic inactivation. The enzymatic inactivation may occur in the postsynaptic terminal, the presynaptic terminal, or an adjacent astrocyte or microglial cell.
- The blood–brain barrier affects the supply of precursors for neurotransmitter synthesis.

[a]Not all neurotransmitters exhibit all of these features. Nitric oxide is an exception to most of these generalities. Some neurotransmitters (epinephrine, serotonin, and histamine) are also secreted by cells other than neurons. Their synthesis and secretion by nonneuronal cells follows other principles.

The action of the neurotransmitter is terminated through reuptake into the presynaptic terminal, uptake into glial cells, diffusion away from the synapse, or enzymatic inactivation. The enzymatic inactivation may occur in the postsynaptic terminal, the presynaptic terminal or an adjacent astrocyte microglia cell, or in endothelial cells in the brain capillaries.

Not all neurotransmitters exhibit all of these features. Nitric oxide, because it is a gas, is an exception to most of these generalities. Some neurotransmitters are synthesized and secreted by both neurons and other cells (e.g., epinephrine, serotonin, histamine).

B. Dopamine, Norepinephrine, and Epinephrine

1. Synthesis of the Catecholamine Neurotransmitters

The three neurotransmitters dopamine, norepinephrine, and epinephrine are synthesized in a common pathway from the amino acid L-tyrosine. Tyrosine is supplied in the diet or is synthesized in the liver from the essential amino acid phenylalanine by phenylalanine hydroxylase (see Chapter 37). The pathway of catecholamine biosynthesis is shown in Figure 46.4.

 Drugs have been developed that block neurotransmitter uptake into storage vesicles. Reserpine, which blocks catecholamine uptake into vesicles, had been used as an antihypertensive and antiepileptic drug for many years, but it was noted that a small percentage of patients on the drug became depressed and even suicidal. Animals treated with reserpine showed signs of lethargy and poor appetite, similar to depression in humans. Thus, a link was forged between monoamine release and depression in humans.

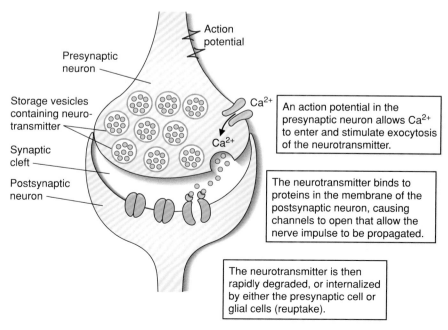

FIGURE 46.3 Action of neurotransmitters.

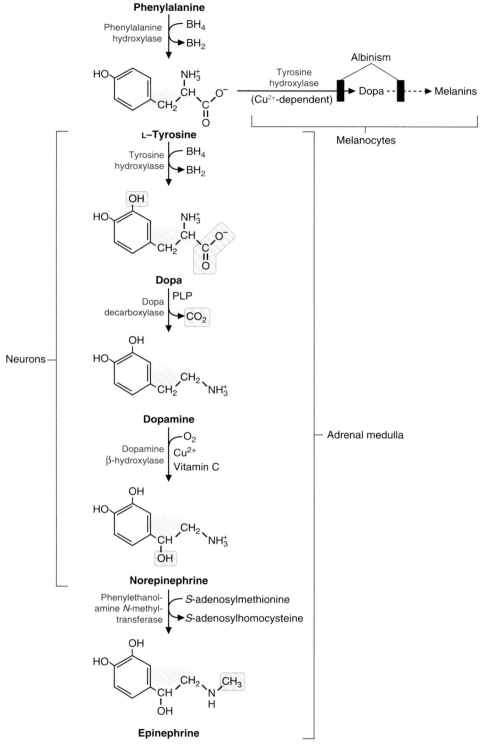

FIGURE 46.4 The pathways of catecholamine and melanin biosynthesis. The *dark boxes* indicate the enzymes, which, when defective, lead to albinism. BH_2, dihydrobiopterin; BH_4, tetrahydrobiopterin; *Dopa*, dihydroxyphenylalanine; *PLP*, pyridoxal phosphate.

The first and rate-limiting step in the synthesis of these neurotransmitters from tyrosine is the hydroxylation of the tyrosine ring by tyrosine hydroxylase, a tetrahydrobiopterin (BH_4)-requiring enzyme. The product formed is dihydroxyphenylalanine (L-DOPA). The phenyl ring with two adjacent –OH groups is a catechol; hence, dopamine, norepinephrine, and epinephrine are called *catecholamines*.

The second step in catecholamine synthesis is the decarboxylation of L-DOPA to form dopamine. This reaction, like many decarboxylation reactions of amino acids, requires pyridoxal phosphate. Dopaminergic neurons (neurons that use dopamine as a neurotransmitter) stop the synthesis at this point because these neurons do not synthesize the enzymes required for the subsequent steps.

Neurons that secrete norepinephrine synthesize it from dopamine in a hydroxylation reaction catalyzed by dopamine β-hydroxylase (DBH). This enzyme is present only within the storage vesicles of these cells. Like tyrosine hydroxylase, it is a mixed-function oxidase that requires an electron donor. Ascorbic acid (vitamin C) serves as the electron donor and is oxidized in the reaction. Copper (Cu^{2+}) is a bound cofactor that is required for the electron transfer.

Although the adrenal medulla is the major site of epinephrine synthesis, epinephrine is also synthesized in a few neurons that use it as a neurotransmitter. These neurons contain the above pathway for norepinephrine synthesis and in addition contain the enzyme that transfers a methyl group from *S*-adenosylmethionine (SAM) to norepinephrine to form epinephrine. Thus, epinephrine synthesis is dependent on the presence of adequate levels of vitamin B_{12} and folate in order to produce the SAM (see Chapter 38).

2. *Storage and Release of Catecholamines*

Ordinarily, only low concentrations of catecholamines are free in the cytosol, whereas high concentrations are found within the storage vesicles. Conversion of tyrosine to L-DOPA and that of L-DOPA to dopamine occurs in the cytosol. Dopamine is then taken up into the storage vesicles. In norepinephrine-containing neurons, the final β-hydroxylation reaction occurs in the vesicles.

The catecholamines are transported into vesicles by the protein VMAT2 (*vesicle monoamine transporter 2*) (Fig. 46.5). The vesicle transporters contain 12 transmembrane domains and are homologous to a family of bacterial drug-resistance transporters, including P-glycoprotein. The mechanism that concentrates the catecholamines in the storage vesicles is an ATP-dependent process linked to a proton pump (secondary active transport). Protons are pumped into the vesicles by a vesicular ATPase (V-ATPase). The protons then exchange for the positively charged catecholamine via the transporter VMAT2. The influx of the catecholamine is thus driven by the H^+ gradient across the vesicular membrane. The intravesicular concentration of catecholamines is approximately 0.5 M, roughly 100 times the cytosolic concentration. In the vesicles, the catecholamines exist in a complex with ATP and acidic proteins known as *chromogranins*.

The vesicles play a dual role: They maintain a ready supply of catecholamines at the nerve terminal that is available for immediate release, and they mediate the process of release. When an action potential reaches the nerve terminal, Ca^{2+} channels open, allowing an influx of Ca^{2+}, which promotes the fusion of vesicles with the neuronal membrane. The vesicles then discharge their soluble contents, including the neurotransmitters, ATP, chromogranins, and DBH, into the extraneuronal space by the process of exocytosis. In some cases, the catecholamines affect other neurons. In other cases, they circulate in the blood and initiate responses in peripheral tissues.

3. *Inactivation and Degradation of Catecholamine Neurotransmitters*

The action of catecholamines is terminated through reuptake into the presynaptic terminal and diffusion away from the synapse. Degradative enzymes are present in the presynaptic terminal and in adjacent cells, including glial cells and endothelial cells.

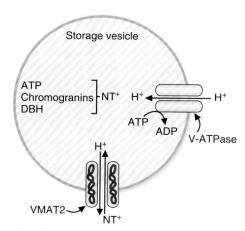

FIGURE 46.5 Transport of catecholamines into storage vesicles. This is a secondary active transport based on the generation of a proton gradient across the vesicular membrane. *ADP, adenosine diphosphate; ATP, adenosine triphosphate; DBH, dopamine β-hydroxylase; NT^+, positively charged neurotransmitter (catecholamine); V-ATPase, vesicular ATPase; VMAT2, vesicle monoamine transporter 2.*

 Chromogranins are required for the biogenesis of the secretory vesicles. When chromogranins are released from the vesicles, they can be proteolytically clipped to form bioactive peptides. Elevated levels of chromogranins in the circulation may be found in patients who have neuroendocrine tumors, such as pheochromocytomas.

In albinism, either the copper-dependent tyrosine hydroxylase of melanocytes (which is distinct from the tyrosine hydroxylase found in the adrenal medulla) or other enzymes that convert tyrosine to melanins may be defective. Individuals with albinism suffer from a lack of pigment in the skin, hair, and eyes; have vision problems; and are sensitive to sunlight.

Tyramine is a degradation product of tyrosine that can lead to headaches, palpitations, nausea and vomiting, and elevated blood pressure if it is present in large quantities. Tyramine stimulates norepinephrine release, which binds to norepinephrine receptors, stimulating them. Tyramine is inactivated by MAO-A, but if a person is taking an MAO inhibitor, foods containing tyramine should be avoided.

Two of the major reactions in the process of inactivation and degradation of catecholamines are catalyzed by monamine oxidase (MAO) and catechol O-methyltransferase (COMT). MAO is present on the outer mitochondrial membrane of many cells and oxidizes the carbon containing the amino group to an aldehyde, thereby releasing ammonium ion (Fig. 46.6). In the presynaptic terminal, MAO inactivates catecholamines that are not protected in storage vesicles. (Thus, drugs that deplete storage vesicles indirectly increase catecholamine degradation.) There are two isoforms of MAO with different specificities of action: MAO-A preferentially deaminates norepinephrine and serotonin, whereas MAO-B acts on a wide spectrum of phenylethylamines (*phenylethyl* refers to a –CH_2– group linked to a phenyl ring). MAO in the liver and other sites protects against the ingestion of dietary biogenic amines such as the tyramine found in many cheeses.

COMT is also found in many cells, including erythrocytes. It works on a broad spectrum of extraneuronal catechols and those that have diffused away from the synapse. COMT transfers a methyl group from SAM to a hydroxyl group on the catecholamine or its degradation product (see Fig. 46.6). Because the inactivation reaction requires SAM, it is indirectly dependent on vitamin B_{12} and folate. The action of MAO and COMT can occur in almost any order, resulting in a large number of degradation products and intermediates, many of which appear in the urine. Cerebrospinal homovanillylmandelic acid (HVA) is an indicator of dopamine degradation. Its concentration is decreased in the brains of patients with Parkinson disease.

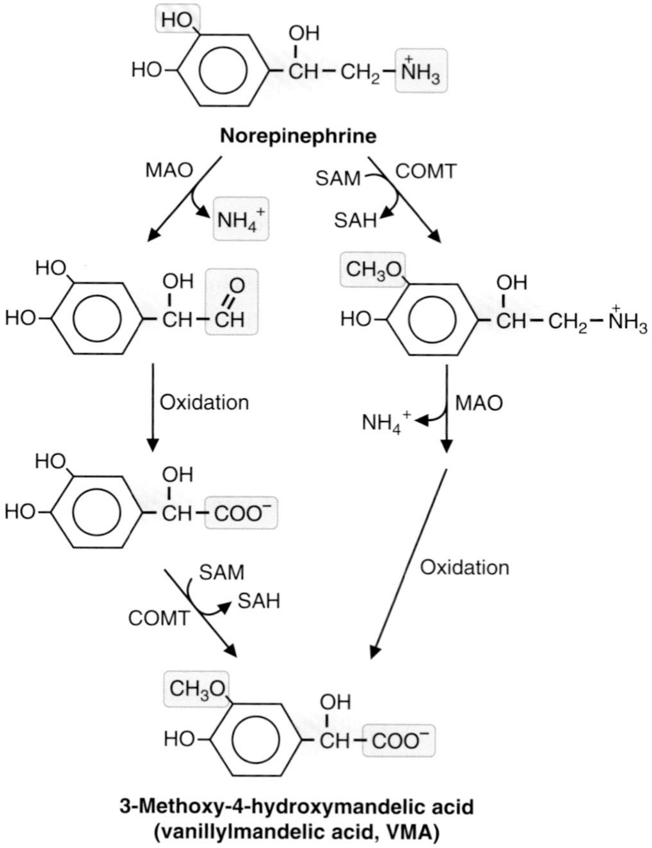

FIGURE 46.6 Inactivation of catecholamines. Methylation and oxidation may occur in any order. Methylated and oxidized derivatives of norepinephrine and epinephrine are produced, and 3-methoxy-4-hydroxymandelic acid is the final product. These compounds are excreted in the urine. *COMT*, catechol O-methyltransferase; *MAO*, monoamine oxidase; *SAH*, S-adenosylhomocysteine; *SAM*, S-adenosylmethionine.

4. Regulation of Tyrosine Hydroxylase

Efficient regulatory mechanisms coordinate the synthesis of catecholamine neurotransmitters with the rate of firing. Tyrosine hydroxylase, the first committed step and rate-limiting enzyme in the pathway, is regulated by feedback inhibition that is coordinated with depolarization of the nerve terminal. Tyrosine hydroxylase is inhibited by free cytosolic catecholamines that compete at the binding site on the enzyme for the pterin cofactor (BH_4; see Chapter 37).

Depolarization of the nerve terminal activates tyrosine hydroxylase. Depolarization also activates several protein kinases (including protein kinase C, protein kinase A [the cAMP-dependent protein kinase], and Ca^{2+}–calmodulin–dependent [CAM] kinases) that phosphorylate tyrosine hydroxylase. These activation steps result in an enzyme that binds BH_4 more tightly, making it less sensitive to end-product inhibition.

In addition to these short-term regulatory processes, a long-term process involves alterations in the amounts of tyrosine hydroxylase and DBH present in nerve terminals. When sympathetic neuronal activity is increased for a prolonged period, the amounts of messenger RNA that code for tyrosine hydroxylase and DBH are increased in the neuronal perikarya (the cell body of the neuron). The increased gene transcription may be the result of phosphorylation of *c*AMP *r*esponse *e*lement–*b*inding protein [CREB]; see Chapter 19) by protein kinase A or by other protein kinases. CREB then binds to the *c*AMP *r*esponse *e*lement [CRE]) in the promoter region of the gene (similar to the mechanism for the induction of gluconeogenic enzymes in the liver). The newly synthesized enzyme molecules are then transported down the axon to the nerve terminals. The concentration of dopamine decarboxylase in the terminal does not appear to change in response to neuronal activity.

C. Metabolism of Serotonin

The pathway for the synthesis of serotonin from tryptophan is very similar to the pathway for the synthesis of norepinephrine from tyrosine (Fig. 46.7). The first enzyme of the pathway, tryptophan hydroxylase, uses an enzymatic mechanism similar to that of tyrosine and phenylalanine hydroxylase and requires BH_4 to hydroxylate the ring structure of tryptophan. The second step of the pathway is a decarboxylation reaction catalyzed by the same enzyme that decarboxylates DOPA. Serotonin, like the catecholamine neurotransmitters, can be inactivated by MAO.

The neurotransmitter melatonin is also synthesized from tryptophan (see Fig. 46.7). Melatonin is produced in the pineal gland in response to the light–dark cycle, its level in the blood rising in a dark environment. It is probably through melatonin that the pineal gland conveys information about light–dark cycles to the body, organizing seasonal and circadian rhythms. Melatonin also may be involved in regulating reproductive functions.

Katie C.'s doctor ordered plasma fractionated metanephrine (methylated epinephrine) levels and also had Katie collect a 24-hour urine specimen for the determination of catecholamines and their degradation products (in particular, metanephrine). All of these tests showed unequivocal elevations of these compounds in Katie's blood and urine. Katie was placed on phenoxybenzamine, an α_1- and α_2-adrenergic receptor antagonist that blocks the pharmacologic effect of the elevated catecholamines on these receptors. Once stable on the α-blockers, Katie was started on an agent that blocked β-adrenergic receptors (propranolol). After ruling out evidence to suggest metastatic disease to the liver or other organs (in case Katie's tumor was malignant), the doctor referred Katie to a surgeon with extensive experience in adrenal surgery. Katie's doctor also ordered diagnostic studies to rule out multiple endocrine neoplasm syndrome (MEN). The tests for the presence of MEN were negative.

In addition to the catecholamines, serotonin is also inactivated by MAO. The activity of several antipsychotic drugs is based on inhibiting MAO. The first generation of drugs (exemplified by iproniazid, which was originally developed as an antituberculosis drug and was found to induce mood swings in patients) were irreversible inhibitors of both the A and B forms of MAO. Although they did reduce the severity of depression (by maintaining higher levels of serotonin), these drugs suffered from the "cheese" effect. Cheese and other foods that are processed over long periods (such as red wine) contain tyramine, a degradation product of tyrosine. Usually, tyramine is inactivated by MAO-A, but if an individual is taking an MAO inhibitor, tyramine levels increase. Tyramine induces the release of norepinephrine from storage vesicles, which leads to potentially life-threatening hypertensive episodes. When it was realized that MAO existed in two forms, selective irreversible inhibitors were developed; examples include clorgyline for MAO-A, and deprenyl for MAO-B. Deprenyl has been used to treat Parkinson disease (which is caused by a lack of dopamine, which is also inactivated by MAO). Deprenyl, however, is not an antidepressant. Clorgyline is an antidepressant but suffers from the "cheese" effect. This led to the development of the third generation of MAO inhibitors, which are reversible inhibitors of the enzyme, as typified by moclobemide. Moclobemide is a specific, reversible inhibitor of MAO-A and is effective as an antidepressant. More important, because of the reversible nature of the drug, the "cheese" effect is not observed, because as tyramine levels increase, they displace the drug from MAO and the tyramine is safely inactivated. However, it has not been approved for use in the United States.

Tyramine

A potential complication of using heparin as an anticoagulant is the generation of antiheparin antibodies in the patients. The production of such antibodies leads to the patient developing heparin-induced thrombocytopenia (HIT). The antiheparin antibodies bind to the heparin platelet factor 4 complex and also to the platelet surface. The antibody-induced binding leads to platelet activation, serotonin release, and thrombin activation. The platelet number drops (the thrombocytopenia), but thrombus formation (owing to thrombin activation) increases. To determine whether a patient has developed HIT, the serotonin-release assay has emerged as the gold standard. Platelets store serotonin in granules and release the serotonin upon activation. Antiheparin antibody–sensitive platelets are obtained from donors and incubated with radioactively labeled serotonin, in order for the platelets to incorporate the serotonin. The treated platelets are then incubated with two samples of the patient's sera: one with a high level of exogenous heparin and the second with a low level of heparin. Serotonin release is then measured by determining the percentage of total radioactivity released by the platelets into the assay buffer. A positive result is obtained if, when using a low concentration of heparin, >20% of the radioactivity incorporated into the platelets is released and, when using the high concentration of heparin, <20% of the incorporated radioactivity is released. The rationale behind the use of high heparin levels is to titrate out the antibody in the sera such that it cannot bind to the platelet cell surface and to demonstrate that the release is caused by antibody binding to platelets.

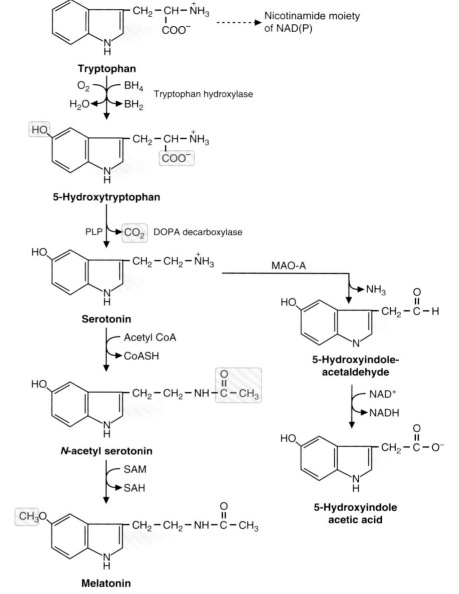

FIGURE 46.7 Synthesis and inactivation of serotonin. *Acetyl CoA*, acetyl coenzyme A; *CoA*, coenzyme A; DOPA, dihydroxyphenylalanine; *MAO*, monoamine oxidase; *NAD*, nicotinamide adenine dinucleotide; *PLP*, pyridoxal phosphate; *SAH*, S-adenosylhomocysteine; *SAM*, S-adenosylmethionine.

The catecholamines exert their physiologic and pharmacologic effects by circulating in the bloodstream to target cells whose plasma membranes contain catecholamine receptors. This interaction initiates a biochemical cascade leading to responses that are specific for different types of cells. Patients such as **Katie C.** experience palpitations, excessive sweating, hypertensive headaches, and a host of other symptoms when a catecholamine-producing tumor of the adrenal medulla suddenly secretes supraphysiologic amounts of epinephrine and/or norepinephrine into the venous blood draining from the neoplasm.

D. Metabolism of Histamine

Within the brain, histamine is produced both by mast cells and by certain neuronal fibers. Mast cells are a family of bone marrow–derived secretory cells that store and release high concentrations of histamine. They are prevalent in the thalamus, hypothalamus, dura mater, leptomeninges, and choroid plexus. Histaminergic neuronal cell bodies in the human are found in the tuberomammillary nucleus of the posterior basal hypothalamus. The fibers project into nearly all areas of the CNS, including the cerebral cortex, the brainstem, and the spinal cord.

Histamine is synthesized from histidine in a single enzymatic step. The enzyme histidine decarboxylase requires pyridoxal phosphate, and its mechanism is very similar to that of DOPA decarboxylase (Fig. 46.8).

Like other neurotransmitters, newly synthesized neuronal histamine is stored in the nerve terminal vesicles. Depolarization of nerve terminals activates the

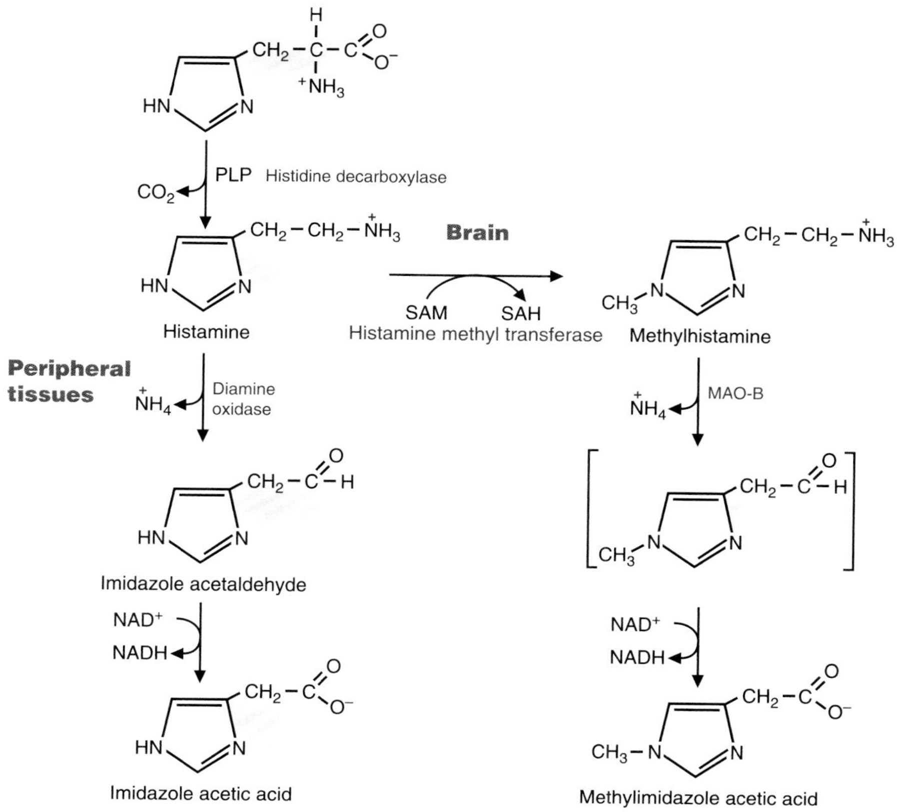

Evan A. was placed on Redux (dexfenfluramine hydrochloride), which increased the secretion of serotonin. Serotonin has been implicated in many processes, including mood control and appetite regulation. Serotonin agonists are thought to exert their hypophagic actions via stimulation of receptors located on proopiomelanocortin (POMC)-containing neurons within the arcuate (ARC) nucleus of the hypothalamus. When serotonin levels are high, satiety results; when serotonin levels are low, increased appetite, or depression, or both, can occur. Thus, drugs that can increase serotonin levels may be able to control appetite and depression. Redux was a second-generation drug developed from fenfluramine, a known appetite suppressant. When it was first used, fenfluramine could not be resolved between two distinct optical isomers (D versus L). The L-isomer induced sleepiness, so to counteract this effect, fenfluramine was often given with phentermine, which elevated norepinephrine levels to counteract the drowsiness (the combination of drugs was known as *fen/phen*). Once the two isomers of fenfluramine could be resolved, Redux—dexfenfluramine—was developed. Because levels of serotonin have been linked to mood, many antidepressant drugs were developed that affect serotonin levels. The first of these is the MAO inhibitors, a second class is the tricyclics, and the third class is known as selective serotonin reuptake inhibitors (SSRIs). The SSRIs block reuptake of serotonin from the synapse, leading to an elevated response to serotonin. Redux not only acted as an SSRI but also increased the secretion of serotonin, leading to elevated levels of this compound in the synapse. None of the other drugs that affect serotonin levels has this effect.

Histamine elicits several effects on different tissues. Histamine is the major mediator of the allergic response, and when it is released from mast cells (a type of white blood cell found in tissues), it leads to vasodilation and an increase in the permeability of blood vessel walls. This leads to the allergic symptoms of a runny nose and watering eyes. When histamine is released in the lungs, the airways constrict in an attempt to reduce the intake of the allergic material. The ultimate result of this, however, is bronchospasm, which can lead to difficulty in breathing. In the brain, histamine is an excitatory neurotransmitter. Antihistamines block histamine from binding to its receptor. In the tissues, this counteracts histamine's effect on vasodilation and blood vessel wall permeability, but in the brain, the effect is to cause drowsiness. The new generation of "nondrowsy" antihistamines have been modified so that they cannot pass through the blood–brain barrier. Thus, the effects on the peripheral tissues are retained, with no effect on CNS histamine response.

FIGURE 46.8 Synthesis and inactivation of histamine; note the different pathways for brain and peripheral tissues. *MAO*, monoamine oxidase; *NAD*, nicotinamide adenine dinucleotide; *PLP*, pyridoxal phosphate; *SAH*, S-adenosylhomocysteine; *SAM*, S-adenosylmethionine.

exocytotic release of histamine by a voltage-dependent as well as a calcium-dependent mechanism.

Once it is released from neurons, histamine is thought to activate both postsynaptic and presynaptic receptors. Unlike other neurotransmitters, histamine does not appear to be recycled into the presynaptic terminal to any great extent. However, astrocytes have a specific high-affinity uptake system for histamine and may be the major sites of the inactivation and degradation of this monoamine.

The first step in the inactivation of histamine in the brain is methylation (see Fig. 46.8). The enzyme histamine methyltransferase transfers a methyl group from SAM to a ring nitrogen of histamine to form methylhistamine. The second step is oxidation by MAO-B, followed by an additional oxidation step. In peripheral tissues, histamine undergoes deamination by diamine oxidase, followed by oxidation to a carboxylic acid (see Fig. 46.8).

E. Acetylcholine

I. Synthesis

The synthesis of acetylcholine from acetyl coenzyme A (acetyl-CoA) and choline is catalyzed by the enzyme choline acetyltransferase (ChAT) (Fig. 46.9). This synthetic step occurs in the presynaptic terminal. The compound is stored in vesicles and later released through calcium-mediated exocytosis. Choline is taken up by the presynaptic terminal from the blood via a low-affinity transport system (high K_m) and from the synaptic cleft via a high-affinity transport mechanism (low K_m). It is also derived from the hydrolysis of phosphatidylcholine (and possibly sphingomyelin) in membrane lipids. Thus, membrane lipids may form a storage site for choline, and their hydrolysis, with the subsequent release of choline, is highly regulated.

It is believed that the vitamin B_{12} requirement for choline synthesis contributes to the neurologic symptoms of vitamin B_{12} deficiency. The methyl groups for choline synthesis are donated by SAM, which is converted to S-adenosylhomocysteine in the reaction. Recall that formation of SAM through recycling of homocysteine requires both FH_4 and vitamin B_{12} (unless extraordinary amounts of methionine are available to bypass the vitamin B_{12}–dependent methionine synthase step).

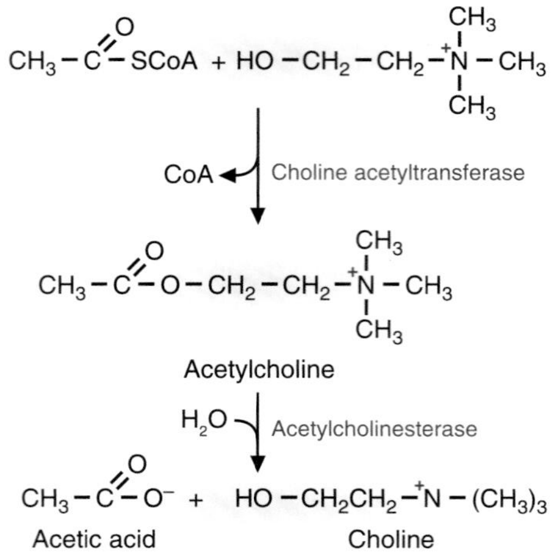

The supply of choline in the brain can become rate-limiting for acetylcholine synthesis, and supplementation of the diet with lecithin (phosphatidylcholine) has been used (although without clear effects) to increase brain acetylcholine in patients suffering from *tardive dyskinesia* (often persistent involuntary movements of the facial muscles and tongue). The neonate has a very high demand for choline, for both brain lipid synthesis (phosphatidylcholine and sphingomyelin) and acetylcholine biosynthesis. High levels of phosphatidylcholine in maternal milk and a high activity of a high-affinity transport system through the blood–brain barrier for choline in the neonate help to maintain brain choline concentrations. The fetus also has a high demand for choline, and there is a high-affinity transport system for choline across the placenta. The choline is derived from maternal stores, maternal diet, and synthesis primarily in the maternal liver. Because choline synthesis is dependent on folate and vitamin B_{12}, the high fetal demand may contribute to the increased maternal requirement for both vitamins during pregnancy.

An inherited pyruvate dehydrogenase deficiency, a thiamin deficiency, or hypoxia deprives the brain of a source of acetyl-CoA for acetylcholine synthesis, as well as a source of acetyl-CoA for ATP generation from the TCA cycle.

$$CH_3-\overset{O}{\overset{\|}{C}}-SCoA \;+\; HO-CH_2-CH_2-\overset{CH_3}{\overset{|}{\overset{+}{N}}}-CH_3$$
$$\underset{CH_3}{}$$

CoA — Choline acetyltransferase

$$CH_3-\overset{O}{\overset{\|}{C}}-O-CH_2-CH_2-\overset{CH_3}{\overset{|}{\overset{+}{N}}}-CH_3$$

Acetylcholine

H_2O — Acetylcholinesterase

$$CH_3-\overset{O}{\overset{\|}{C}}-O^- \;+\; HO-CH_2CH_2-\overset{+}{N}-(CH_3)_3$$
Acetic acid   Choline

FIGURE 46.9 Acetylcholine synthesis and degradation. *CoA*, coenzyme A.

Choline is a common component of the diet but also can be synthesized in humans as part of the pathway for the synthesis of phospholipids (see Chapter 31). The only route for choline synthesis is via the sequential addition of three methyl groups from SAM to the ethanolamine portion of phosphatidylethanolamine to form phosphatidylcholine. Phosphatidylcholine is subsequently hydrolyzed to release choline or phosphocholine. Conversion of phosphatidylethanolamine to phosphatidylcholine occurs in many tissues, including liver and brain. This conversion is folate- and vitamin B_{12}–dependent.

The acetyl group used for acetylcholine synthesis is derived principally from glucose oxidation to pyruvate and decarboxylation of pyruvate to form acetyl-CoA via the pyruvate dehydrogenase reaction. This is because neuronal tissues have only a limited capacity to oxidize fatty acids to acetyl-CoA, so glucose oxidation is the major source of acetyl groups. Pyruvate dehydrogenase is found only in mitochondria. The acetyl group is probably transported to the cytoplasm as part of citrate, which is then cleaved in the cytosol to form acetyl-CoA and oxaloacetate.

2. Inactivation of Acetylcholine

Acetylcholine is inactivated by acetylcholinesterase, which is a serine esterase that forms a covalent bond with the acetyl group. The enzyme is inhibited by a wide range of compounds (pharmacologic agents and neurotoxins) that form a covalent bond with this reactive serine group. Neurotoxins such as sarin (the gas used in Japanese subways by a terrorist group) and the nerve gas in the movie *The Rock* work through this mechanism. Acetylcholine is the major neurotransmitter at the neuromuscular junctions; inability to inactivate this molecule leads to constant activation of the nerve–muscle synapses, a condition that leads to varying degrees of paralysis.

F. Glutamate and γ-Aminobutyric Acid

1. Synthesis of Glutamate

Glutamate functions as an excitatory neurotransmitter within the CNS, leading to the depolarization of neurons. Within nerve terminals, glutamate is generally synthesized de novo from glucose rather than taken up from the blood because its plasma concentration is low and it does not readily cross the blood–brain barrier.

Glutamate is synthesized primarily from the TCA cycle intermediate α-ketoglutarate (Fig. 46.10). This process can occur via either of two routes. The first is via the enzyme glutamate dehydrogenase, which reduces α-ketoglutarate to glutamate, thereby incorporating free ammonia into the carbon backbone. The ammonia pool is provided by amino acid/neurotransmitter degradation or by diffusion of ammonia across the blood–brain barrier. The second route is through transamination reactions in which an amino group is transferred from other amino acids to α-ketoglutarate to form

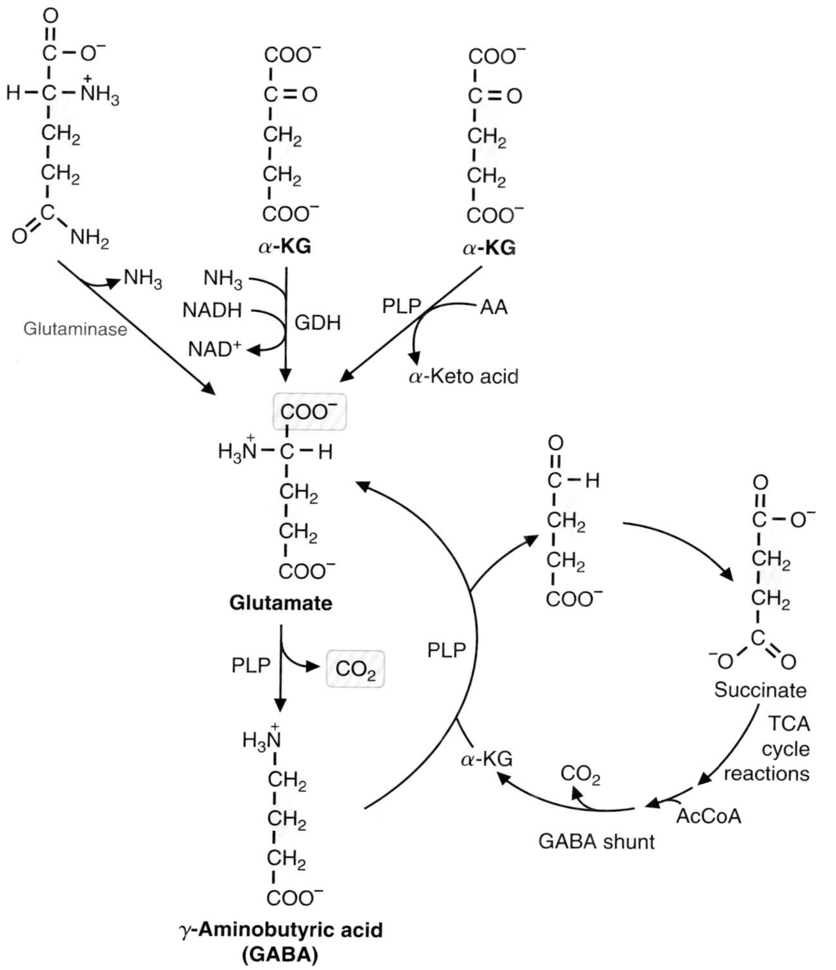

FIGURE 46.10 Synthesis of glutamate and γ-aminobutyric acid (GABA), and the GABA shunt. *AA*, amino acid; *AcCoA*, acetyl coenzyme A; *α-KG*, α-ketoglutarate; *GDH*, glutamate dehydrogenase; *NAD*, nicotinamide adenine dinucleotide; *PLP*, pyridoxal phosphate; *TCA*, tricarboxylic acid.

glutamate. Glutamate also can be synthesized from glutamine, using glutaminase. The glutamine is derived from glial cells, as described in Section III.F.2.

Like other neurotransmitters, glutamate is stored in vesicles, and its release is Ca^{2+}-dependent. It is removed from the synaptic cleft by high-affinity uptake systems in nerve terminals and glial cells.

2. γ-Aminobutyric Acid

GABA is the major inhibitory neurotransmitter in the CNS. Its functional significance is far-reaching, and altered GABAergic function plays a role in many neurologic and psychiatric disorders.

GABA is synthesized by the decarboxylation of glutamate (see Fig. 46.10) in a single step catalyzed by the enzyme glutamic acid decarboxylase (GAD). GABA is recycled in the CNS by a series of reactions called the *GABA shunt*, which conserves glutamate and GABA (see Fig. 46.10).

Much of the uptake of GABA occurs in glial cells. The GABA shunt in glial cells produces glutamate, which is converted to glutamine and transported out of the glial cells to neurons, where it is converted back to glutamate. Glutamine thus serves as a transporter of glutamate between cells in the CNS (see Chapter 40). Glial cells lack GAD and cannot synthesize GABA.

 Tiagabine is a drug that inhibits the reuptake of GABA from the synapse, and it has been used to treat epilepsy as well as other convulsant disorders. Because GABA is an inhibitory neurotransmitter in the brain, its prolonged presence can block neurotransmission by other agents, thereby reducing the frequency of convulsions.

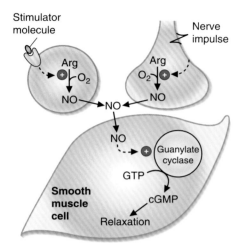

FIGURE 46.11 Action of nitric oxide (NO) in vasodilation. The synthesis of NO occurs in response to a stimulator binding to a receptor on some cells or to a nerve impulse in neurons. NO enters smooth muscle cells, stimulating guanylate cyclase to produce cGMP, which causes smooth muscle cell relaxation. When the smooth muscle cells relax, blood vessels dilate. *GTP*, guanosine triphosphate.

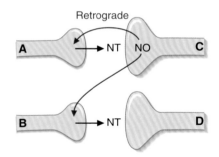

FIGURE 46.12 Nitric oxide (NO) as a retrograde messenger. Cell *A* releases a neurotransmitter, which stimulates cell *C* to produce NO. NO, being a gas, can diffuse back and regulate cell *A*'s production and release of neurotransmitters. NO can also diffuse to cell *B*, and stimulate cell *B* to produce a different neurotransmitter to elicit a response from cell *D*. *NT*, neurotransmitter.

G. Other Amino Acid Neurotransmitters

I. Aspartate

Aspartate, like glutamate, is an excitatory neurotransmitter, but it functions in far fewer pathways. It is synthesized from the TCA cycle intermediate oxaloacetate via transamination reactions. Like glutamate synthesis, aspartate synthesis uses oxaloacetate that must be replaced through anaplerotic reactions. Aspartate cannot pass through the blood–brain barrier.

2. Glycine

Glycine is the major inhibitory neurotransmitter in the spinal cord. Most of the glycine in neurons is synthesized de novo within the nerve terminal from serine by the enzyme serine hydroxymethyltransferase, which requires folic acid. Serine, in turn, is synthesized from the intermediate 3-phosphoglycerate in the glycolytic pathway. The action of glycine is probably terminated via uptake by a high-affinity transporter.

3. Conversion of Arginine to Nitric Oxide

Nitric oxide (NO) is a biologic messenger in a variety of physiologic responses, including vasodilation, neurotransmission, and the ability of the immune system to kill tumor cells and parasites. NO is synthesized from arginine in a reaction catalyzed by NO synthase (see Fig. 25.10).

NO synthase exists as tissue-specific forms of two families of enzymes. The form present in macrophages is responsible for overproduction of NO, leading to its cytotoxic actions on parasites and tumor cells. The enzyme present in nervous tissue, vascular endothelium, platelets, and other tissues is responsible for the physiologic responses to NO such as vasodilation and neural transmission. In target cells, NO activates a soluble guanylate cyclase, which results in increased cellular levels of $3',5'$-cyclic guanosine monophosphate (cGMP) (Fig. 46.11). In smooth muscle cells, cGMP, like cyclic adenosine monophosphate (cAMP), activates one or more protein kinases, which are responsible for the relaxation of smooth muscle and the subsequent dilation of vessels. NO stimulates penile erection by acting as a neurotransmitter, stimulating smooth muscle relaxation that permits the corpus cavernosum to fill with blood. Nitric oxide can readily cross cell membranes because it is a gas. As a result, its effect may not necessarily be limited to the neuron that synthesizes it (Fig. 46.12). There is ample evidence that NO may function as a retrograde messenger that can influence neurotransmitter release from the presynaptic terminal after diffusing from the postsynaptic neuron (where it is synthesized). There is also evidence supporting retrograde messenger roles for both arachidonic acid and carbon monoxide in the CNS.

IV. Metabolic Encephalopathies and Neuropathies

The brain has an absolute dependence on the blood for its supply of glucose and oxygen. It uses approximately 20% of the oxygen supply of the body. During the developmental period and during prolonged fasting, ketone bodies can be used as a fuel, but they cannot totally substitute for glucose. Glucose is converted to pyruvate in glycolysis, and the pyruvate is oxidized in the TCA cycle. Anaerobic glycolysis, with a yield of two molecules of ATP per molecule of glucose, cannot sustain the ATP requirement of the brain, which can be provided only by the complete oxidation of glucose to CO_2, which yields approximately 32 ATP/glucose. However, during periods of mild hypoglycemia or mild hypoxia, decreased neurotransmitter synthesis contributes as much, if not more, to the development of symptoms, as does an absolute deficiency of ATP for energy needs.

A. Hypoglycemic Encephalopathy

Hypoglycemia is sometimes encountered in medical conditions such as malignancies that produce insulin or insulinlike growth factors, or chronic alcoholism. Early clinical signs in hypoglycemia reflect the appearance of physiologic protective mechanisms initiated by hypothalamic sensory nuclei, such as sweating, palpitations, anxiety, and hunger. If these symptoms are ignored, they proceed to a more serious CNS disorder, progressing through confusion and lethargy to seizures and, eventually, coma. Prolonged hypoglycemia can lead to irreversible brain damage.

During the progression of hypoglycemic encephalopathy, as blood glucose falls to <2.5 mM (45 mg/dL), the brain attempts to use internal substrates such as glutamate and TCA cycle intermediates as fuels. Because the pool size of these substrates is quite small, they are quickly depleted. If blood glucose levels continue to fall to <1 mM (18 mg/dL), ATP levels become depleted.

As the blood glucose level drops from 2.5 to 2.0 mM (45 to 36 mg/dL, before electroencephalographic [EEG] changes are observed), the symptoms appear to arise from decreased synthesis of neurotransmitters in particular regions of the brain rather than a global energy deficit. The oxidation of glucose in glycolysis provides 3-phosphoglycerate, a precursor for the neurotransmitter glycine. Pyruvate entry into the mitochondria and conversion to acetyl-CoA can generate α-ketoglutarate (for glutamate and GABA synthesis) and oxaloacetate, for the synthesis of the neurotransmitter aspartate. A lack of glucose could disrupt the synthesis of these neurotransmitters.

As hypoglycemia progresses below 1 mM (18 mg/dL) and high-energy phosphate levels are depleted, the EEG becomes isoelectric, and neuronal cell death ensues. As is the case in some other metabolic encephalopathies, cell death is not global in distribution; rather, certain brain structures—in particular, hippocampal and cortical structures—are selectively vulnerable to hypoglycemic insult. Pathophysiologic mechanisms responsible for neuronal cell death in hypoglycemia include the involvement of glutamate excitotoxicity. Glutamate excitotoxicity occurs when the cellular energy reserves are depleted. The failure of the energy-dependent reuptake pumps results in a buildup of glutamate in the synaptic cleft and overstimulation of the postsynaptic glutamate receptors. The prolonged glutamate receptor activation leads to prolonged opening of the receptor ion channel and the influx of lethal amounts of Ca^{2+} ion, which can activate cytotoxic intracellular pathways in the postsynaptic neuron.

B. Hypoxic Encephalopathy

Experimental studies with human volunteers show that cerebral energy metabolism remains normal when mild to moderate hypoxia (partial pressure of oxygen [PaO_2] = 25 to 40 mm Hg) results in severe cognitive dysfunction. The diminished cognitive function is believed to result from impaired neurotransmitter synthesis. In mild hypoxia, cerebral blood flow increases to maintain oxygen delivery to the brain. In addition, anaerobic glycolysis is accelerated, resulting in maintenance of ATP levels. This occurs, however, at the expense of an increase of lactate production and a fall of pH. Acute hypoxia ($PaO_2 \leq 20$ mm Hg) generally results in a coma.

Hypoxia can result from insufficient oxygen reaching the blood (e.g., at high altitudes), severe anemia (e.g., iron deficiency), or a direct insult to the oxygen-using capacity of the brain (e.g., cyanide poisoning). All forms of hypoxia result in diminished neurotransmitter synthesis. Inhibition of pyruvate dehydrogenase diminishes acetylcholine synthesis, which is acutely sensitive to hypoxia. Glutamate and GABA synthesis, which depend on a functioning TCA cycle, are decreased as a result of elevated reduced nicotinamide adenine dinucleotide (NADH) levels, which inhibit TCA-cycle enzymes. NADH levels are increased when oxygen is unavailable to accept electrons from the electron-transport chain and NADH cannot be readily converted back into NAD^+. Even the synthesis of catecholamine neurotransmitters may be decreased because the hydroxylase reactions require O_2.

C. Relationship between Glutamate Synthesis and the Anaplerotic Pathways of Pyruvate Carboxylase and Methylmalonyl Coenzyme A Mutase

Synthesis of glutamate removes α-ketoglutarate from the TCA cycle, thereby decreasing the regeneration of oxaloacetate in the TCA cycle. Because oxaloacetate is necessary for the oxidation of acetyl-CoA, oxaloacetate must be replaced by anaplerotic reactions. There are two major types of anaplerotic reactions: (1) pyruvate carboxylase and (2) the degradative pathway of the branched-chain amino acids valine and isoleucine, which contribute succinyl coenzyme A (succinyl-CoA) to the TCA cycle. This pathway uses vitamin B_{12} (but not folate) in the reaction catalyzed by methylmalonyl coenzyme A (methylmalonyl-CoA) mutase.

V. Lipid Synthesis in the Brain and Peripheral Nervous System

Several features of lipid synthesis and degradation in the nervous system distinguish it from most other tissues. The first is that the portion of the neuronal cell membrane involved in synaptic transmission has a unique role and a unique composition. At the presynaptic terminal, the lipid composition changes rapidly as storage vesicles containing the neurotransmitter fuse with the cell membrane and release their contents. Portions of the membrane are also lost as endocytotic vesicles. On the postsynaptic terminal, the membrane contains the receptors for the neurotransmitter as well as a high concentration of membrane signaling components, such as phosphatidylinositol. A second important feature of brain lipid metabolism is that the blood–brain barrier restricts the entry of nonessential fatty acids, such as palmitate, that are released from adipose tissue or present in the diet. Conversely, essential fatty acids are taken up by the brain. Because of these considerations, the brain is constantly synthesizing those lipids (cholesterol, fatty acids, glycosphingolipids, and phospholipids), which it needs for various neurologic functions. Neuronal signaling also requires that nonneuronal glial cells synthesize myelin, a multilayered membrane that surrounds the axons of many neurons. Myelin is lipid-rich and has a different lipid composition than the neuronal membranes. The white matter in the brain contains significantly more myelin than the gray matter; it is the presence of myelin sheaths that is responsible for the characteristic color differences that exist between the two types of brain tissue.

A. Brain Lipid Synthesis and Oxidation

Because the blood–brain barrier significantly inhibits the entry of certain fatty acids and lipids into the CNS, virtually all lipids found there must be synthesized within the CNS. The exceptions are the essential fatty acids (linoleic and linolenic acid), which do enter the brain, where they are elongated or further desaturated. The uptake of fatty acids into the CNS is insufficient to meet the energy demands of the CNS—hence, the requirement for aerobic glucose metabolism. Thus, cholesterol, glycerol, sphingolipids, glycosphingolipids, and cerebrosides are all synthesized using pathways discussed previously in this text. Of particular note is that very-long-chain fatty acids are synthesized in the brain, where they play a major role in myelin formation.

Oxidation and turnover of brain lipids occurs as described previously (see Chapter 30). Peroxisomal fatty acid oxidation is important in the brain because the brain contains very-long-chain fatty acids and phytanic acid (from the diet), both of which are oxidized in the peroxisomes by α-oxidation. Thus, disorders that affect peroxisome biogenesis (such as Refsum disease) severely affect brain cells because of the inability to metabolize both branched-chain and very-long-chain fatty acids. If there is a disorder in which the degradation of glycosphingolipids or mucopolysaccharides is impaired, lysosomes in brain cells become engorged with partially digested glycolipids, leading to varying degrees of neurologic dysfunction.

B. Myelin Synthesis

A rapid rate of nerve conduction in the peripheral and central motor nerves depends on the formation of myelin, a multilayered lipid and protein structure that is formed from the plasma membrane of glial cells. In the PNS, the Schwann cell is responsible for myelinating one portion of an axon of one nerve cell. The Schwann cell does this by wrapping itself around the axon multiple times so that a multilayered sheath of membrane surrounds the axon. In the CNS, the oligodendrocyte is responsible for myelination. Unlike the Schwann cell, oligodendrocytes can myelinate portions of numerous axons (up to 40), and do so by extending a thin process that wraps around the axon multiple times. Thus, CNS axons are surrounded only by the membranes of oligodendrocytes, whereas axons in the PNS are surrounded by the entire Schwann cell. A generalized view of myelination is depicted in Figure 46.13. To maintain the myelin structure, the oligodendrocyte synthesizes four times its own weight in lipids per day.

1. Myelin Lipids

As the plasma membrane of the glial cell is converted into myelin, the lipid composition of the brain changes (Table 46.2). The lipid-to-protein ratio is greatly increased, as is the content of sphingolipids. The myelin is a tightly packed structure, and there are significant hydrophobic interactions between the lipids and proteins to allow this to occur. Cerebrosides constitute approximately 16% of total myelin lipid and are almost completely absent from other cell-type membrane lipids. The predominant cerebroside, galactosylcerebroside, has a single sugar attached to the hydroxyl group of the sphingosine. In contrast, sphingomyelin, which one might guess is the predominant lipid of myelin, is present in roughly the same low concentration

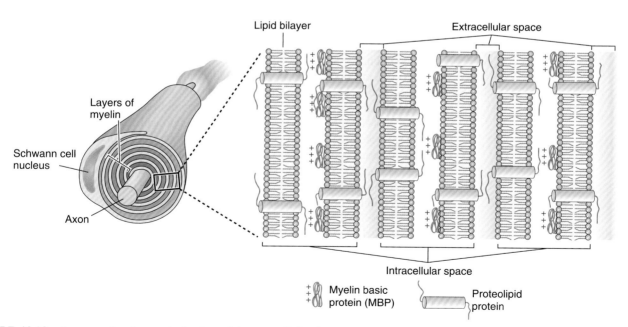

FIGURE 46.13 A composite diagram indicating a Schwann cell that has wrapped around a portion of an axon, forming the myelin sheath. The expansion represents a portion of the myelin sheath. Central nervous system myelin is shown, although it is similar to peripheral nervous system myelin except that P0 replaces proteolipid protein. Recall that there are multiple layers of membrane surrounding the axon; proteolipid protein protrudes into the extracellular space and aids in compaction of the membranes through hydrophobic interactions. Myelin basic proteins help to stabilize the structure from within the membrane.

TABLE 46.2   Protein and Lipid Composition of Central Nervous System Myelin and Human Brain

SUBSTANCE[a]	MYELIN	WHITE MATTER	GRAY MATTER
Protein	30.0	39.0	55.3
Lipid	70.0	54.9	32.7
Cholesterol	27.7	27.5	22.0
Cerebroside	22.7	19.8	5.4
Sulfatide	3.8	5.4	1.7
Total galactolipid	27.5	26.4	7.3
Ethanolamine phosphatides	15.6	14.9	22.7
Phosphatidylcholine	11.2	12.8	26.7
Sphingomyelin	7.9	7.7	6.9
Phosphatidylserine	4.8	7.9	8.7
Phosphatidylinositol	0.6	0.9	2.7
Plasmalogens	12.3	11.2	8.8
Total phospholipids	43.1	45.9	69.5

[a]Protein and lipid figures in percent dry weight; all others in percent total lipid weight.
Data from Norton W. In: Siegel GJ, Albers RW, Agranoff BW, Katzman R, eds. *Basic Neurochemistry*. 3rd ed. Boston, MA: Little, Brown; 1981:77.

in all membranes. Galactocerebrosides pack more tightly together than phosphatidylcholine; the sugar, although polar, carries no positively charged amino group or negatively charged phosphate. The brain synthesizes very-long-chain fatty acids (>20 carbons long); these long uncharged side chains develop strong hydrophobic associations, allowing close packing of the myelin sheath. The high cholesterol content of the membrane also contributes to the tight packing, although the myelin proteins are also required to complete the tightness of the packing process.

2. Myelin Structural Proteins

The layers of myelin are held together by protein–lipid and protein–protein interactions, and any disruption can lead to demyelination of the membrane (see "Biochemical Comments"). Although numerous proteins are found in both the CNS and PNS, only the major proteins are discussed here. The major proteins in the CNS and PNS are different. In the CNS, two proteins constitute between 60% and 80% of the total proteins—proteolipid protein and myelin basic proteins (MBPs). The proteolipid protein is a very hydrophobic protein that forms large aggregates in aqueous solution and is relatively resistant to proteolysis. Its molecular weight, based on sequence analysis, is 30,000 Da. Proteolipid protein is highly conserved in sequence among species. Its role is thought to be one of promoting the formation and stabilization of the multilayered myelin structure.

The MBPs are a family of proteins. Unlike proteolipid protein, MBPs are easily extracted from the membrane and are soluble in aqueous solution. The major MBP has no tertiary structure and has a molecular weight of 15,000 Da. MBP is located on the cytoplasmic face of myelin membranes. Antibodies directed against MBPs elicit experimental allergic encephalomyelitis (EAE), which has become a model system for understanding multiple sclerosis, a demyelinating disease. A model of how proteolipid protein and MBPs aid in stabilizing myelin is shown in Figure 46.13.

In the PNS, the major myelin protein is P0, a glycoprotein that accounts for >50% of the PNS myelin protein content. The molecular weight of P0 is 30,000 Da, the same as proteolipid protein. P0 is thought to play a similar structural role in maintaining myelin structure as proteolipid protein does in the CNS. MBPs are also found in the PNS, with some similarities and differences to the MBPs found in the CNS. The major PNS-specific MBP has been designated P2.

CLINICAL COMMENTS

Katie C. Catecholamines affect nearly every tissue and organ in the body. Their integrated release from nerve endings of the sympathetic (adrenergic) nervous system plays a critical role in the reflex responses we make to sudden changes in our internal and external environment. For example, under stress, catecholamines appropriately increase heart rate, blood pressure, myocardial (heart muscle) contractility, and conduction velocity of the heart.

Episodic, inappropriate secretion of catecholamines in supraphysiologic amounts, such as occurs in patients with pheochromocytomas, like **Katie C.**, causes an often acute and alarming array of symptoms and signs of a hyperadrenergic state.

Most of the signs and symptoms related to catecholamine excess can be masked by phenoxybenzamine, a long-acting α_1- and α_2-adrenergic receptor antagonist, combined with a β_1- and β_2-adrenergic receptor blocker such as propranolol. Pharmacologic therapy alone is reserved for patients with inoperable pheochromocytomas (e.g., patients with malignant tumors with metastases and patients with severe heart disease). Because of the sudden, unpredictable, and sometimes life-threatening discharges of large amounts of catecholamines from these tumors, definitive therapy involves surgical resection of the neoplasms after appropriate preoperative preparation of the patient with the agents mentioned above. Katie's tumor was resected without intraoperative or postoperative complications. After surgery, she remained free of symptoms and her blood pressure decreased to normal levels.

Evan A. Evan A., after stopping Redux, was placed on Prozac, an antidepressant that acts as an SSRI but does not lead to increased synthesis or secretion of serotonin, as did the dexfenfluramine in Redux. Thus, the mechanism of action of these two drugs is different, even if the end result (elevated levels of serotonin) is the same. Unfortunately, Prozac did not work as well for Mr. A. as did Redux, and he regained his 50 lb within 1 year after switching medications. Redux was withdrawn from the market by its manufacturer because of reports of heart valve abnormalities in a small percentage of patients who had taken either fenfluramine and phentermine (phen/fen) or Redux. Since then, the US Food and Drug Administration (FDA) has banned the use of Redux for weight loss because of the undesirable side effects. Mr. A. now has several other options. Other medical treatments include orlistat, a partial inhibitor of dietary fatty acid absorption from the gastrointestinal tract; phentermine alone (described previously); and several medications used to treat other conditions, including diabetes, seizures, and depression, that also lead to weight loss. These latter agents are not FDA-approved for weight loss, and thus, Evan's physician did not want to try any more medications with him. Instead, the physician referred Evan for bariatric surgery.

BIOCHEMICAL COMMENTS

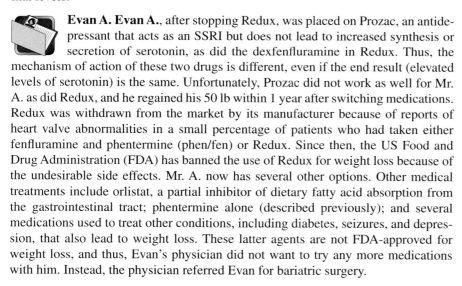

Demyelinating Diseases of the Central Nervous System. The importance of myelin in nerve transmission is underscored by the wide variety of demyelinating diseases, all of which lead to neurologic symptoms. The best-known disease in this class is multiple sclerosis (MS). MS can be a progressive disease of the CNS in which demyelination of CNS neurons is the key anatomic and pathologic finding. The cause of MS has yet to be determined, although it is believed that an event occurs that triggers the formation of autoimmune antibodies directed against components of the nervous system. This event could be a bacterial or viral infection that stimulates the immune system to fight off the invaders. Unfortunately, this stimulus may also trigger the autoimmune response that leads to the antibody-mediated demyelinating process. The unusual geographic distribution of MS is of interest. Patients are concentrated in northern and southern latitudes, yet its incidence is almost nil at the Equator. Clinical presentation of MS varies widely. It can be a mild disease that has few or no obvious clinical manifestations. At the other end of the spectrum, is a rapidly progressive and fatal disease. The most well-known presentation is the relapsing–remitting type. In this type, early in the course of the disease, the natural history is one of exacerbations followed by remission. Eventually, the CNS cannot repair the damage that has accumulated through the years, and remissions occur less and less frequently. Available treatments for MS target the relapsing–remitting type of disease.

The primary injury to the CNS in MS is the loss of myelin in the white matter, which interferes with nerve conduction along the demyelinated area (the insulator is lost). The CNS compensates by stimulating the oligodendrocyte to remyelinate the damaged axon, and when this occurs, remission is achieved. Often remyelination leads to a slowing in conduction velocity because of a reduced myelin thickness (speed is proportional to myelin thickness) or a shortening of the internodal distances (the action potential has to be propagated more times). Eventually, when it becomes too difficult to remyelinate large areas of the CNS, the neuron adapts by upregulating and redistributing along its membrane ion pumps to allow nerve conductance along demyelinated axons. Eventually, this adaptation also fails and the disease progresses.

Treatment of MS is now based on blocking the action of the immune system. Because antibodies directed against cellular components appear to be responsible for the progression of the disease (regardless of how the autoantibodies were first generated), agents that interfere with immune responses have had various levels of success in keeping patients in remission for extended periods.

Other demyelinating diseases also exist, and their cause is much more straightforward. These are relatively rare disorders. In all of these diseases, there is no fully effective treatment for the patient. Inherited mutations in P0 (the major PNS myelin protein) leads to a version of Charcot-Marie-Tooth polyneuropathy syndrome. The inheritance pattern for this disease is autosomal-dominant, indicating that the expression of one mutated allele leads to expression of the disease. Mutations in proteolipid protein (the major myelin protein in the CNS) lead to Pelizaeus-Merzbacher disease and X-linked spastic paraplegia type 2 disease. These diseases display a wide range of phenotypes, from a lack of motor development and early death (most severe) to mild gait disturbances. The phenotype displayed depends on the precise location of the mutation within the protein. An altered function of either P0 or proteolipid protein leads to demyelination and its subsequent clinical manifestations.

KEY CONCEPTS

- The nervous system consists of a variety of cell types with different functions.
  - Neurons transmit and receive signals from other neurons at synaptic junctions.
  - Astrocytes, found in the CNS, provide physical and nutritional support for the neurons.
  - Oligodendrocytes provide the myelin sheath that coats the axon, providing insulation for the electric signal that is propagated along the axon.
    - Myelin has a lipid composition that is distinct from that of cellular membranes.
    - A lack of myelin leads to demyelinating diseases as a result of impaired signal transmission across the axon.
  - Schwann cells are the supporting cells (and myelin-producing cells) of the PNS.
  - Microglial cells destroy invading microorganisms and phagocytose cellular debris.
  - Ependymal cells line the cavities of the CNS and spinal cord.

- The brain is protected against bloodborne toxic agents by the blood–brain barrier.
  - Glucose, amino acids, vitamins, ketone bodies, and essential fatty acids (but not other fatty acids) can all be transported across the blood–brain barrier.
  - Proteins, such as insulin, can cross the blood–brain barrier by receptor-mediated transcytosis.
- Neurotransmitters are synthesized primarily from amino acids in the nervous system; others are derived from intermediates of glycolysis and the TCA cycle.
  - Neurotransmitters are synthesized in the cytoplasm of the presynaptic terminal and then transported into storage vesicles for release upon receiving the appropriate signal.
  - Neurotransmitter action is terminated by reuptake into the presynaptic terminal, by diffusion away from the synapse, or by enzymatic inactivation.
  - MAO is a key enzyme for the inactivation of the catecholamines and serotonin.
- An encephalopathy will develop if the nervous system cannot generate sufficient ATP:
  - Hypoglycemic encephalopathy (lack of glucose to the brain)
  - Hypoxic encephalopathy (lack of oxygen to the brain)
- Diseases discussed in this chapter are summarized in Table 46.3.

TABLE 46.3	Diseases Discussed in Chapter 46	
DISEASE OR DISORDER	**GENETIC OR ENVIRONMENTAL**	**COMMENTS**
Albinism	Genetic	A lack of melanocyte tyrosinase leads to the inability to produce dihydroxyphenylalanine (DOPA), a required precursor to melanin production, such that pigment formation is inhibited.
Hypercholesterolemia	Both	Elevated cholesterol levels in the blood may be regulated by appropriate pharmacologic agents.
Multiple sclerosis	Environmental/may have genetic predisposition	An autoimmune-induced loss of myelin sheath formation around neurons
Pheochromocytoma	Both	Tumor of the adrenal gland, leading to episodic and excessive epinephrine and norepinephrine release
Facilitated glucose transporter protein type I deficiency syndrome	Genetic	Infantile seizures related to low glucose levels in the nervous system (low glucose in the cerebrospinal fluid)
Tyramine poisoning	Environmental	Tyramine, a compound found in aged cheeses (for example), is degraded by monoamine oxidase (MOA). In the presence of MOA inhibitors, tyramine levels can accumulate, triggering the release of high levels of norepinephrine, leading to a hypertensive crisis.
Depression	Both	Drugs used to elevate serotonin levels may alleviate depression and may also lead to appetite suppression.
Appetite suppression	Both	A variety of drugs have been used to treat obesity, although many have side effects that need to be monitored carefully.

1. A patient with a tumor of the adrenal medulla experienced palpitations, excessive sweating, and hypertensive headaches. His urine contained increased amounts of vanillylmandelic acid. His symptoms are probably caused by an overproduction of which of the following?
   A. Acetylcholine
   B. Norepinephrine and epinephrine
   C. DOPA and serotonin
   D. Histamine
   E. Melatonin

2. The two lipids found in highest concentration in myelin are which of the following?
   A. Cholesterol and cerebrosides such as galactosylceramide
   B. Cholesterol and phosphatidylcholine
   C. Galactosylceramide sulfatide and sphingomyelin
   D. Plasmalogens and sphingomyelin
   E. Triacylglycerols and lecithin

3. MBP can be best described by which one of the following?
   A. It is synthesized in Schwann cells but not in oligodendrocytes.
   B. It is a transmembrane protein found only in peripheral myelin.
   C. It attaches the two extracellular leaflets together in central myelin.
   D. It contains basic amino acid residues that bind the negatively charged extracellular sides of the myelin membrane together.
   E. It contains lysine and arginine residues that bind the negatively charged intracellular sides of the myelin membrane together.

4. A patient presented with dysmorphia and cerebellar degeneration. Analysis of his blood indicated elevated levels of phytanic acid and very-long-chain fatty acids but no elevation of palmitate. His symptoms are consistent with a defect in an enzyme involved in which of the following?
   A. α-Oxidation
   B. Mitochondrial β-oxidation
   C. Transport of enzymes into lysosomes
   D. Degradation of mucopolysaccharides
   E. Elongation of fatty acids

5. One of the presenting symptoms of vitamin B_6 deficiency is dementia. This may result from an inability to synthesize serotonin, norepinephrine, histamine, and GABA from their respective amino acid precursors. This is because vitamin B_6 is required for which type of reaction?
   A. Hydroxylation
   B. Transamination
   C. Deamination
   D. Decarboxylation
   E. Oxidation

6. In a patient with a damaged blood–brain barrier, such that the barrier is now leaky, which one of the following substances would be able to cross this damaged barrier which normally could not cross an intact blood–brain barrier?
   A. Ammonia
   B. Pyruvate
   C. LNAAs
   D. Nonessential fatty acids
   E. Ketone bodies

7. A patient is deficient in vitamin B_{12} and folate. The production of which one of the following would therefore be expected to be impaired in this patient, as compared to a patient with no vitamin deficiencies?
   A. GABA
   B. Serotonin
   C. Dopamine
   D. Norepinephrine
   E. Epinephrine

8. Lack of vitamin B_{12} leads to neuropathy. Which one of the following neurotransmitters will exhibit reduced synthesis when this vitamin is deficient?
   A. Serotonin
   B. Glycine
   C. GABA
   D. Nitric oxide
   E. Norepinephrine

9. A patient presents with headaches, palpitations, nausea and vomiting, and elevated blood pressure. These symptoms appear after the person has eaten a large meal containing aged cheeses and wine. The patient's history indicates that they are on a medication for a different condition. Assuming that the medication is in some way involved in these symptoms, which enzyme might be the target of this drug?
   A. COMT
   B. Tyrosine hydroxylase
   C. Glutamate decarboxylase
   D. MAO
   E. DOPA decarboxylase

10. A 2-year-old patient presents with a history of frequent seizures, developmental delay, and difficulty in moving her arms and legs. Analysis of the CSF demonstrated a ratio of CSF glucose to blood glucose of 0.25. A potential treatment for this disorder would be which one of the following?
    A. A high-fat, low-carbohydrate diet to produce ketone bodies as a fuel for the brain
    B. A high-carbohydrate diet to increase glucose transport into the brain
    C. A high-protein diet to enhance gluconeogenesis and increase blood glucose levels
    D. Insulin therapy to increase the number of glucose transporters in the endothelial cells lining the blood–brain barrier
    E. A high-fat, high-carbohydrate diet to increase free fatty acid levels in the blood for use by the nervous system

ANSWERS

1. **The answer is B.** The symptoms exhibited by the patient are caused by excessive release of epinephrine or norepinephrine. Vanillylmandelic acid is also the degradation product of norepinephrine; thus, these hormones are being overproduced. Acetylcholine degradation leads to the formation of acetic acid and choline, which are not observed (thus, A is incorrect). Although DOPA degradation could lead to vanillylmandelic acid production, serotonin degradation does not (it leads to 5-hydroxyindole acetic acid), and the symptoms exhibited by the patient are not consistent with DOPA or serotonin overproduction (thus, C is incorrect). Histamine and melatonin also do not produce the symptoms exhibited by the patient (thus, D and E are incorrect).

2. **The answer is A.** Myelin contains very high levels of cholesterol and cerebrosides, particularly galactosylcerebrosides.

3. **The answer is E.** MBP is a basic protein, indicating that it must contain a significant number of lysine and arginine residues. MBP is found on the intracellular side of the myelin membrane, and its role is to compact the membrane by binding to negative charges on both sides of it, thereby reducing the "width" of the membrane. Both Schwann cells and oligodendrocytes synthesize myelin (thus, A is incorrect). MBP is not a transmembrane protein (proteolipid protein in the CNS and P0 in the PNS are, so B is incorrect), and because MBP is found intracellularly, answers C and D cannot be correct.

4. **The answer is A.** The accumulation of both phytanic acid and very-long-chain fatty acids indicates a problem in peroxisomal fatty acid oxidation, which is where α-oxidation occurs. Lysosomal transport is, therefore, not required to metabolize these fatty acids (thus, C is incorrect). The finding that palmitate levels are low indicates that β-oxidation is occurring; therefore, answer B is incorrect. The compounds that accumulate are not mucopolysaccharides, nor is fatty acid elongation required in the metabolism of these compounds (thus, D and E are incorrect).

5. **The answer is D.** Vitamin B_6 participates in transamination and decarboxylation reactions (and indirectly in deamination reactions). The one common feature in the synthesis of serotonin, GABA, norepinephrine, and histamine is decarboxylation of an amino acid, which requires vitamin B_6. The other reactions are not required in the biosynthesis of these neurotransmitters.

6. **The answer is D.** Normally, only essential fatty acids can be transported across the blood–brain barrier, whereas nonessential fatty acids do not cross the barrier to any appreciable extent. Ammonia, in its uncharged form, can freely diffuse across the blood–brain barrier. Pyruvate can cross the barrier through the monocarboxylic acid transport protein. LNAAs are transported through the L system of amino acid transport. Ketone bodies can also cross the blood–brain barrier when their concentration is increased in the blood, as under fasting conditions.

7. **The answer is E.** In order to form epinephrine, a methyl group from SAM is transferred to norepinephrine. SAM production is dependent on adequate levels of both vitamin B_{12} and folate. Without B_{12} and folate (and therefore SAM), epinephrine synthesis is blocked. Inactivation of catecholamines (and serotonin) is also dependent on SAM, so a lack of vitamin B_{12} and folate (and therefore, SAM) would result in a higher level of serotonin, dopamine, and norepinephrine. GABA synthesis is not affected by a B_{12} or folate deficiency.

8. **The answer is B.** A vitamin B_{12} deficiency leads to tetrahydrofolate (FH_4) being trapped as N^5-methyl-FH_4, thereby producing a functional folate deficiency. Folate is required for the synthesis of glycine from serine. Glycine in the circulation cannot pass through the blood–brain barrier, so it must be synthesized from serine within the brain. In the absence of vitamin B_{12}, this reaction will not occur. In addition, owing to the lack of vitamin B_{12} and the functional folate deficiency, levels of SAM will drop. Thus, although norepinephrine synthesis is normal, epinephrine synthesis would be reduced. There is no effect on serotonin synthesis (from tryptophan), nor for GABA and NO synthesis, because none of their biosynthetic steps requires either vitamin B_{12} or a folate derivative.

9. **The answer is D.** Aged cheese contains a degradation product of tyrosine, tyramine, which stimulates catecholamine release if not degraded. MAO-B inactivates the tyramine, but if the patient is taking an MAO inhibitor for another reason, the tyramine would not be degraded and symptoms of catecholamine excess will be exhibited. None of the other enzymes listed as answers inactivates or metabolizes tyramine.

10. **The answer is A.** The patient exhibits hypoglycorrhachia, a deficiency of the GLUT 1 transporters in the endothelial cells lining the blood–brain barrier. This results in insufficient glucose in the CSF and a lack of energy for the brain to function properly. Ingesting a high-fat, low-carbohydrate diet will force ketone body production (a ketogenic diet), a fuel source that the brain can use in place of glucose. Such a diet will aid in alleviating the symptoms brought about by the lack of the glucose transporter. Any diet that increases glucose levels (high carbohydrate, or high protein) will not increase the amount of glucose entering the CSF because the transporter is defective. Insulin will increase the number of GLUT 4 transporters, but those transporters are not expressed in the nervous system. The brain also cannot transport most fatty acids across the blood–brain barrier, so increasing fat content in the diet to increase fatty acid levels will not increase the levels of fatty acids in the brain.

47

The Extracellular Matrix and Connective Tissue

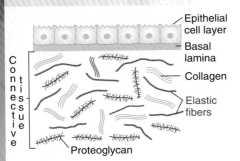

Epithelial cell layer

Basal lamina

Collagen

Elastic fibers

Proteoglycan

Connective tissue

FIGURE 47.1 An overview of connective tissue extracellular matrix. Supporting the epithelial cell layer is a basal lamina, beneath which are collagen, elastic fibers, and proteoglycans. The cell types present in connective tissue, such as fibroblasts and macrophages, have been removed from the diagram for clarity.

Many of the cells in tissues are embedded in an **extracellular matrix** (**ECM**) that fills the spaces between cells and binds cells and tissue together. In so doing, the ECM aids in determining the shape of tissues as well as the nature of the partitioning between tissue types. In the skin, loose connective tissue beneath epithelial cell layers consists of an ECM in which fibroblasts, blood vessels, and other components are distributed (Fig. 47.1). Other types of connective tissue, such as tendon and cartilage, consist largely of ECM, which is principally responsible for their structure and function. This matrix also forms the sheetlike **basal laminae**, or basement membranes, on which layers of epithelial cells rest and which act as supportive tissue for muscle cells, adipose cells, and peripheral nerves.

Basic components of the ECM include fibrous structural proteins, such as **collagens**, **proteoglycans** containing long glycosaminoglycan chains attached to a protein backbone, and **adhesion proteins** linking components of the matrix to each other and to cells.

These **fibrous structural proteins** are composed of repeating elements that form a linear structure. **Collagens**, **elastin**, and **laminin** are the principal structural proteins of connective tissue.

Proteoglycans consist of a core protein covalently attached to many long, linear chains of **glycosaminoglycans**, which contain repeating disaccharide units. The repeating disaccharides usually contain a **hexosamine** and a **uronic acid**, and these sugars are frequently **sulfated**. Synthesis of the proteoglycans starts with the attachment of a sugar to a serine, threonine, or asparagine residue of the protein. Additional sugars, donated by **UDP-sugar precursors**, add sequentially to the nonreducing end of the molecule.

Proteoglycans, such as glycoproteins and glycolipids, are **synthesized in the endoplasmic reticulum** (**ER**) and the **Golgi complex**. The glycosaminoglycan chains of proteoglycans are **degraded by lysosomal enzymes** that cleave one sugar at a time from the nonreducing end of the chain. An inability to degrade proteoglycans leads to a set of diseases known as the **mucopolysaccharidoses**.

Adhesion proteins, such as **fibronectin** and **laminin**, are extracellular glycoproteins that contain separate distinct binding domains for proteoglycans, collagen, and fibrin. These domains allow these adhesion proteins to bind the various components of the ECM. They also contain specific binding domains for cell surface receptors known as **integrins**. These integrins bind to **fibronectin** on the external surface, span the plasma membrane of cells, and adhere to proteins, which, in turn, bind to the intracellular **actin** filaments of the **cytoskeleton**. Integrins also provide a mechanism for signaling between cells via both internal signals and through signals generated via the ECM.

Cell movement within the ECM requires remodeling of the various components of the matrix. This is accomplished by a variety of **matrix metalloproteinases** (**MMPs**) and regulators of the MMPs, **tissue inhibitors of matrix metalloproteinases** (**TIMPs**). Dysregulation of this delicate balance of the regulators of cell movement allows cancer cells to travel to other parts of the body (**metastasize**) as well as to spread locally to contiguous tissues.

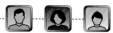

 Sarah L. (first introduced in Chapter 14) noted a moderate reduction in pain and swelling in the joints of her fingers while she was taking her immunosuppressant medication. At her next checkup, her rheumatologist described to Sarah the underlying inflammatory tissue changes that her systemic lupus erythematosus (SLE) was causing in the joint tissues.

 Deborah S. complained of a declining appetite for food as well as severe weakness and fatigue. The reduction in her kidneys' ability to maintain normal daily total urinary net acid excretion contributed to her worsening metabolic acidosis. This, plus her declining ability to excrete nitrogenous waste products, such as creatinine and urea, into her urine ("azotemia"), was responsible for many of her symptoms. Her serum creatinine level was rising steadily. As it approached a level of 5 mg/dL, she developed a litany of complaints caused by the multisystem dysfunction associated with her worsening metabolic acidosis and retention of nitrogenous waste products ("uremia"). Her physicians discussed with Deborah the need to consider peritoneal dialysis or hemodialysis.

I. Composition of the Extracellular Matrix

A. Fibrous Proteins

1. Collagen

Collagen, a family of fibrous proteins, is produced by a variety of cell types but principally by fibroblasts (cells found in interstitial connective tissue), muscle cells, and epithelial cells. Type I collagen, collagen(I), the most abundant protein in mammals, is a fibrous protein that is the major component of connective tissue. It is found in the ECM of loose connective tissue, bone, tendons, skin, blood vessels, and the cornea of the eye. Collagen(I) contains approximately 33% glycine and 21% proline and hydroxyproline. Hydroxyproline is an amino acid produced by posttranslational modification of peptidyl proline residues.

Procollagen(I), the precursor of collagen(I), is a triple helix composed of three polypeptide (pro-α) chains that are twisted around each other, forming a ropelike structure. Polymerization of collagen(I) molecules forms collagen fibrils, which provide great tensile strength to connective tissues (see Fig. 7.22). The individual polypeptide chains each contain approximately 1,000 amino acid residues. The three polypeptide chains of the triple helix are linked by interchain hydrogen bonds. Each turn of the triple helix contains three amino acid residues, such that every third amino acid is in close contact with the other two strands in the center of the structure. Only glycine, which lacks a side chain, can fit in this position, and indeed, every third amino acid residue of collagen is glycine. Thus, collagen is a polymer of (Gly-X-Y) repeats, where Y is frequently proline or hydroxyproline and X is any other amino acid found in collagen.

Procollagen(I) is an example of a protein that undergoes extensive posttranslational modifications. Hydroxylation reactions produce hydroxyproline residues from proline residues and hydroxylysine from lysine residues. These reactions occur after the protein has been synthesized (Fig. 47.2) and require vitamin C (ascorbic acid) as a cofactor of the enzymes prolyl hydroxylase and lysyl hydroxylase. Hydroxyproline residues are involved in hydrogen bond formation that helps to stabilize the triple helix, whereas hydroxylysine residues are the sites of attachment of disaccharide moieties (galactose–glucose). The role of carbohydrates in collagen structure is still controversial. In the absence of vitamin C (scurvy), the melting temperature of collagen drops from 42°C to 24°C because of the loss of interstrand hydrogen bond formation, which is in turn caused by the lack of hydroxyproline residues.

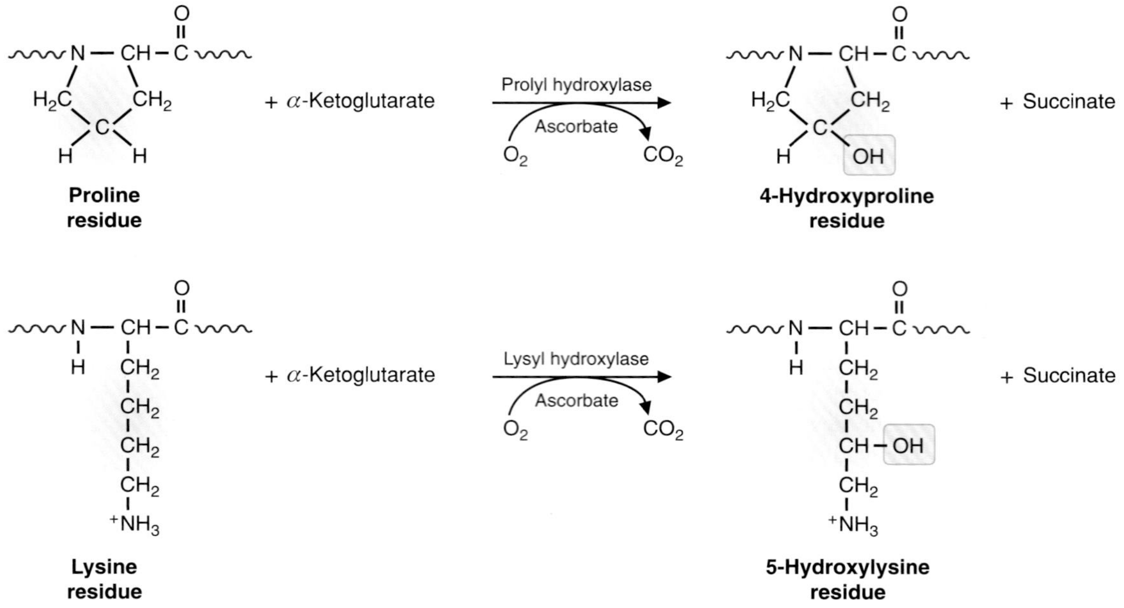

FIGURE 47.2 Hydroxylation of proline and lysine residues in collagen. Proline and lysine residues within the collagen chains are hydroxylated by reactions that require vitamin C.

The side chains of lysine residues also may be oxidized to form the aldehyde allysine. These aldehyde residues produce covalent cross-links between collagen molecules (Fig. 47.3). An allysine residue on one collagen molecule reacts with the amino group of a lysine residue on another molecule, forming a covalent Schiff base that is converted to more stable covalent cross-links. Aldol condensation also may occur between two allysine residues, which forms the structure lysinonorleucine.

a. Types of Collagen

At least 28 different types of collagen have been characterized (Table 47.1). Although each type of collagen is found only in particular locations in the body, more than one type may be present in the ECM at a given location. The various types of collagen can be classified as fibril-forming (types I, II, III, V, XI, XXIV, and XXVII), network-forming (types IV, VIII, and X), those that associate with fibril surfaces (types IX, XII, XIV, XXI, and XXII), those that are transmembrane proteins (types XIII, XVII, XXIII. and XXV), endostatin-forming (types XV and XVIII), and those that form periodic beaded filaments (type VI).

All collagens contain three polypeptide chains with at least one stretch of triple helix. The non–triple-helical domains can be short (as in the fibril-forming collagens), or they can be rather large, such that the triple helix is actually a minor component of the overall structure (examples are collagen types XII and XIV). The fibril-associated collagens with interrupted triple helices (FACITs; collagen types IX, XII, and XIV) collagen types associate with fibrillar collagens, without themselves forming fibers. The endostatin-forming collagens are cleaved at their C terminus to form endostatin, an inhibitor of angiogenesis. The network-forming collagens (type IV) form a meshlike structure because of large ($\sim$230 amino acids) noncollagenous domains at the carboxyl terminus (Fig. 47.4). And finally, several collagen types are actually transmembrane proteins (XIII, XVII, XXIII, and XXV) found on epithelial or epidermal cell surfaces, which play a role in several cellular processes, including adhesion of components of the ECM to cells embedded within it. Type XXV collagen has been associated with the neuronal plaques that develop during Alzheimer disease.

Endostatins block angiogenesis (new blood vessel formation) by inhibiting endothelial cell migration. Because endothelial cell migration and proliferation are required to form new blood vessels, inhibiting this action blocks angiogenesis. Tumor growth is dependent on a blood supply; inhibiting angiogenesis can reduce tumor-cell proliferation.

TABLE 47.1	**Types of Collagen**		
COLLAGEN TYPE	**GENE**	**STRUCTURAL DETAILS**	**LOCALIZATION**
I	Col1A1–Col1A2	Fibrils	Skin, tendon, bone, cornea
II	Col2A1	Fibrils	Cartilage, vitreous humor
III	Col3A1	Fibrils	Skin, muscle, associates with type I collagen
IV	Col4A1–Col4A6	Nonfibrillar, mesh collagen	All basal laminae (basement membranes)
V	Col5A1–Col5A3	Small fibers, N-terminal globular domains	Associates with type I collagen in most interstitial tissues
VI	Col6A1–Col6A3	Microfibrils, with both N- and C-terminal globular domains	Associates with type I collagen in most interstitial tissues
VII	Col7A1	An anchoring collagen	Epithelial cells; dermal–epidermal junction
VIII	Col8A1–Col8A2	Nonfibrillar, mesh collagen	Cornea, some endothelial cells
IX	Col9A1–Col9A3	Fibril-associated collagens with interrupted triple helices (FACIT); N-terminal globular domain	Associates with type II collagen in cartilage and vitreous humor
X	Col10A1	Nonfibrillar, mesh collagen, with C-terminal globular domain	Growth plate, hypertrophic and mineralizing cartilage
XI	Col11A1–Col11A3	Small fibers	Cartilage, vitreous humor
XII	Col12A1	FACIT	Interacts with types I and II collagen in soft tissues
XIII	Col13A1	Transmembrane collagen	Cell surfaces, epithelial cells
XIV	Col14A1	FACIT	Soft tissue
XV	Col15A1	Endostatin-forming collagen	Endothelial cells
XVI	Col16A1	Other	Ubiquitous
XVII	Col17A1	Transmembrane collagen	Epidermal cell surface
XVIII	Col18A1	Endostatin-forming	Endothelial cells
XIX	Col19A1	Other	Ubiquitous
XXI	Col21A1	FACIT	Heart, skeletal muscle, stomach, kidney, placenta
XXII	Col22A1	FACIT	Tissue junctions
XXIII	Col23A1	Transmembrane collagen	Lung, skin, cornea, brain, kidney, tendon
XXIV	Col24A1	Fibrils	Bone
XXV	Col25A1	Transmembrane collagen	Brain
XXVI	EMID2	Other	Mesenchymal cells
XXVII	Col27A1	Fibrils	Stomach, lung, gonads, skin, tooth
XXVIII	Col28A1	Other	Nervous system

See the text for descriptions of the differences in types of collagen. Type XX collagen is not present in humans.

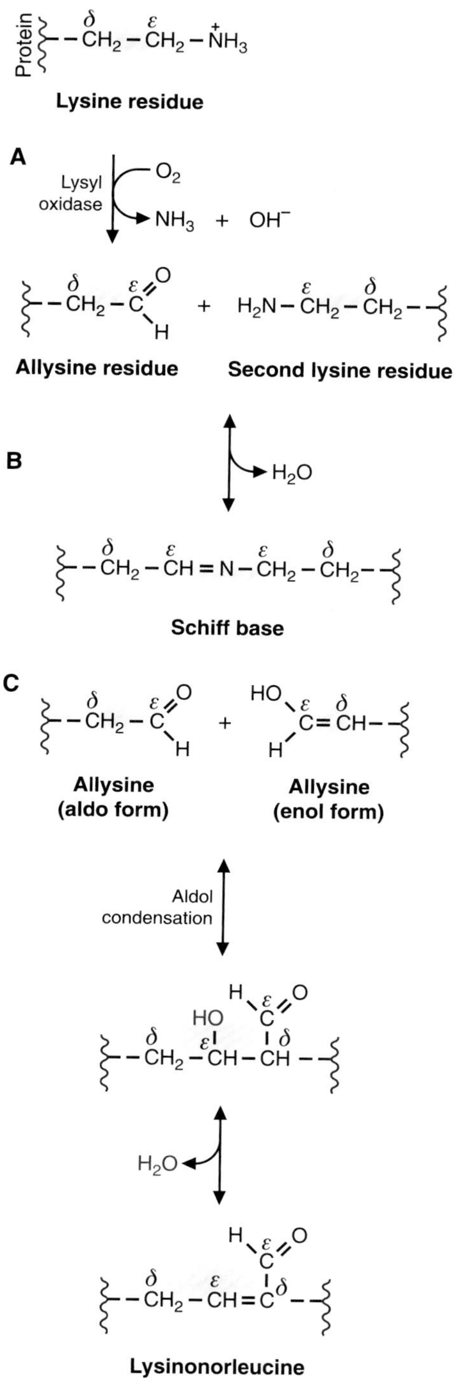

FIGURE 47.3 Formation of cross-links in collagen. **A.** Lysine residues are oxidized to allysine (an aldehyde). Allysine may react with an unmodified lysine residue to form a Schiff base (**B**), or two allysine residues may undergo an aldol condensation (**C**).

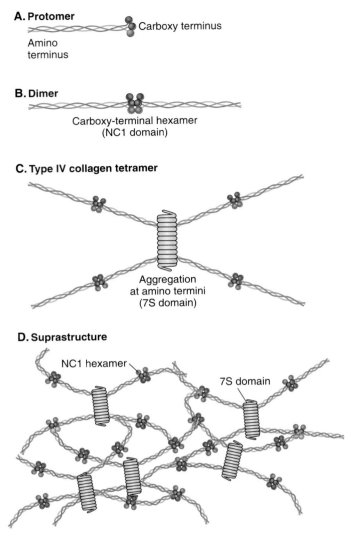

A. Protomer

Amino terminus

Carboxy terminus

B. Dimer

Carboxy-terminal hexamer
(NC1 domain)

C. Type IV collagen tetramer

Aggregation
at amino termini
(7S domain)

D. Suprastructure

NC1 hexamer

7S domain

FIGURE 47.4 Type IV collagen contains a globular carboxyl-terminal domain **(A)**, which forms tropocollagen dimers (hexamers of collagen, **B**). Four dimers associate at the amino-terminal domains to form a 7S domain **(C)**, and the tetramers form a lattice **(D)**, which provides structural support to the basal lamina.

One form of osteogenesis imperfecta (OI) is caused by a mutation in a gene that codes for collagen. The phenotype of affected individuals varies greatly, depending on the location and type of mutation. See the "Biochemical Comments" for more information concerning this type of OI.

Types I, II, and III collagens form fibrils that assemble into large insoluble fibers. The fibrils (see below) are strengthened through covalent cross-links between lysine residues on adjacent fibrils. The arrangement of the fibrils gives individual tissues their distinct characteristics. Tendons, which attach muscles to bones, contain collagen fibrils aligned parallel to the long axis of the tendon, thus giving the tendon tremendous tensile strength.

The types of collagen that do not form fibrils perform a series of distinct roles. Fibril-associated collagens bind to the surface of collagen fibrils and link them to other matrix-forming components. The transmembrane collagens form anchoring fibrils that link components of the ECM to underlying connective tissue. The network-forming collagens (type IV) form a flexible collagen that is part of the basement membrane and basal lamina that surround many cells.

b. Synthesis and Secretion of Collagen

Collagen is synthesized within the ER as a precursor known as preprocollagen. The presequence acts as the signal sequence for the protein and is cleaved, forming procollagen within the ER. From there, it is transported to the Golgi apparatus (Table 47.2). Three procollagen molecules associate through formation of inter- and

TABLE 47.2 Steps in Collagen Biosynthesis

LOCATION	PROCESS
Rough endoplasmic reticulum	Synthesis of preprocollagen; insertion of the procollagen molecule into the lumen of the ER
Lumen of ER	Hydroxylation of proline and lysine residues; glycosylation of selected hydroxylysine residues
Lumen of ER and Golgi apparatus	Self-assembly of the tropocollagen molecule, initiated by disulfide bond formation in the carboxyl-terminal extensions; triple-helix formation
Secretory vesicle	Procollagen prepared for secretion from cell
Extracellular	Cleavage of the propeptides, removing the amino- and carboxyl-terminal extensions, and self-assembly of the collagen molecules into fibrils, and then fibers

ER, endoplasmic reticulum.

intrastrand disulfide bonds at the carboxyl terminus; once these disulfides are formed, the three molecules can align properly to initiate formation of the triple helix. The triple helix forms from the carboxyl end toward the amino end, forming tropocollagen. The tropocollagen contains a triple-helical segment between two globular ends, the amino- and carboxyl-terminal extensions. The tropocollagen is secreted from the cell, the extensions are removed using extracellular proteases, and the mature collagen takes its place within the ECM. The individual fibrils of collagen line up in a highly ordered fashion to form the collagen fiber.

2. Elastin

Elastin is the major protein found in elastic fibers, which are located in the ECM of connective tissue of smooth muscle cells, endothelial and microvascular cells, chondrocytes, and fibroblasts. Elastic fibers allow tissues to expand and contract; this is of particular importance to blood vessels, which must deform and reform repeatedly in response to the changes in intravascular pressure that occur with the contraction of the left ventricle of the heart. It is also important for the lungs, which stretch each time a breath is inhaled and return to their original shape with each exhalation. In addition to elastin, the elastic fibers contain microfibrils, which are composed of several acidic glycoproteins, the major ones being fibrillin-1 and fibrillin-2.

a. Tropoelastin

Elastin has a highly cross-linked, insoluble, amorphous structure. Its precursor, tropoelastin, is a molecule of high solubility, which is synthesized on the rough endoplasmic reticulum (RER) for eventual secretion. Tropoelastin contains two types of alternating domains. The first domain consists of a hydrophilic sequence that is rich in lysine and alanine residues. The second domain consists of a hydrophobic sequence that is rich in valine, proline, and glycine, which frequently occur in repeats of VPGVG or VGGVG. The protein contains approximately 16 regions of each domain, alternating throughout the protein (Fig. 47.5).

Upon secretion from the cell, the tropoelastin is aligned with the microfibrils, and lysyl oxidase initiates the reactions that cross-link elastin molecules, using lysine residues within the hydrophilic alternating domains in the proteins. This cross-linking reaction is the same as that which occurs in collagen. In this reaction, two, three, or four lysine residues are cross-linked to form a stable structure. The net result of the cross-linking is the generation of a fibrous mesh that encircles the cells.

b. Elastic Properties of Elastin

Elastic fibers have the ability to stretch and then to reform without requiring an obvious energy source with which to do so. The mechanism by which this stretching and relaxing actively occurs is still controversial but does relate to the basic principles of protein folding described in Chapter 7. When the elastic fibers are stretched (such as when a breath is taken in and the lung fills up with air), the amorphous elastin structure

 Supravalvular aortic stenosis (SVAS) results from an insufficiency of elastin in the vessel wall, leading to a narrowing of the large elastic arteries. Current theory suggests that the levels of elastin in the vessel walls may regulate the number of smooth muscle cell rings that encircle the vessel. If the levels of elastin are low, smooth muscle hypertrophy results, leading to a narrowing and stenosis of the artery.

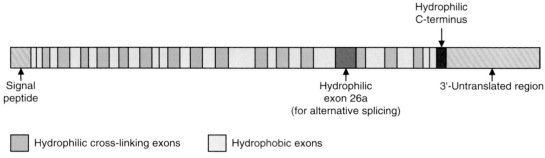

Hydrophilic
C-terminus

Signal peptide

Hydrophilic exon 26a
(for alternative splicing)

3'-Untranslated region

Hydrophilic cross-linking exons   Hydrophobic exons

FIGURE 47.5   The complementary DNA structure of elastin, indicating the repeating cross-linking and hydrophobic domains.

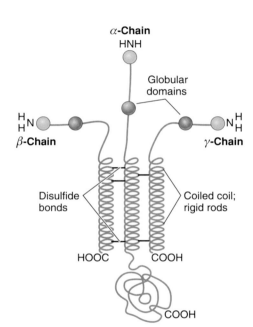

FIGURE 47.6   The structure of laminin.

Defects in the structures of laminin 5 or laminin 6 (proteins that contribute to the cohesion of the dermis and epidermis) lead to the disorder referred to as *junctional epidermolysis bullosa* (JEB). In this disorder, there can be severe spontaneous blistering of the skin and mucous membranes. A severe form of the disease, JEB gravis, is often fatal early in life. Death occurs as a result of epithelial blistering of the respiratory, digestive, and genitourinary systems.

Congenital muscular dystrophy (CMD) results from a defect in laminin 2, which is a component of the bridge that links the muscle cell cytoskeleton to the ECM. Lack of this bridge triggers muscle cell apoptosis, which results in weakened muscles.

is stretched. This stretching exposes the repeating hydrophobic regions of the molecule to the aqueous environment. This, in turn, leads to a decrease in the entropy of water, because the water molecules need to rearrange to form cages about each hydrophobic domain. When this stretching force within the lung is removed (e.g., when the subject exhales), the elastin takes on its original structure because of the increase in entropy that occurs because the water no longer needs to form cages about hydrophobic domains. Thus, the hydrophobic effect is the primary force that allows this stretched structure to reform. Elastin is inherently stable, with a half-life of up to 70 years.

3. Laminin

After type IV collagen, laminin is the most abundant protein in basal laminae. Laminin provides additional structural support for the tissues through its ability to bind to type IV collagen, to other molecules present in the ECM, and also to cell surface–associated proteins (the integrins; see Section II).

a. Laminin Structure

Laminin is a heterotrimeric protein that is shaped, for the most part, like a cross (Fig. 47.6). The trimer is composed of α-, β-, and γ-subunits. There are five possible α-proteins (designated α_1 through α_5), three different versions of the β-subunit (β_1 through β_3), and three different γ-forms (γ_1 through γ_3). Thus, there is a potential for the formation of as many as 45 different combinations of these three subunits. However, only 18 have been discovered. Laminin 111, composed of $\alpha_1\beta_1\gamma_1$, is typical of this class of proteins. The major feature of the laminin structure is a coiled α-helix, which joins the three subunits together and forms a rigid rod. All three chains have extensions at the amino-terminal end. Only the α-chain has a significant carboxyl-terminal extension past the rodlike structure. It is the laminin extensions that allow laminin to bind to other components within the ECM and to provide stability for the structure. Components of the ECM that are bound by laminin include collagen, sulfated lipids, and proteoglycans.

b. Laminin Biosynthesis

Like other secreted proteins, laminin is synthesized with a leader sequence that targets the three chains to the ER. Chain association occurs within the Golgi apparatus before secretion from the cell. After laminin is secreted by the cell, the amino-terminal extensions promote self-association as well as the binding to other ECM components. Disulfide linkages are formed to stabilize the trimer, but there is much less posttranslational processing of laminin than there is of collagen and elastin.

B. Proteoglycans

The fibrous structural proteins of the ECM are embedded in gels formed from proteoglycans. Proteoglycans consist of polysaccharides called *glycosaminoglycans* (GAGs) linked to a core protein. The GAGs are composed of repeating units of disaccharides (Fig. 47.7). One sugar of the disaccharide is either *N*-acetylglucosamine

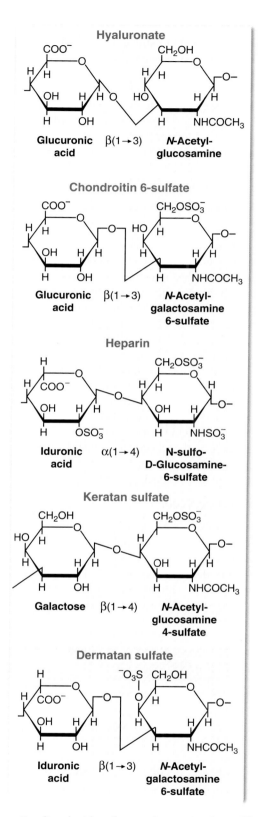

FIGURE 47.7   Repeating disaccharides of some glycosaminoglycans. These repeating disaccharides usually contain an N-acetylated sugar and a uronic acid, which usually is glucuronic acid or iduronic acid. Sulfate groups are often present and are included in the sugar names in this figure. Iduronic acid and glucuronic acid are epimers at position 5 of the sugar.

The ECM is not simply a glue that holds cells together; it also serves to keep cells from moving to other locations and to prevent large molecules and other particles, such as microorganisms, from reaching contiguous and distant cells. This confining property of the matrix is medically important. For example, infections spread, in part, because the infectious agent alters the "containing" capacity of the ECM. Cancer cells that metastasize (migrate to other tissues) can do so only by altering the integrity of the matrix. Diseases such as rheumatoid arthritis (an autoimmune destruction of articular and periarticular tissues) and osteoarthritis (degenerative joint disease often associated with aging) involve damage to the functional capacity of the matrix. Alterations in the structural characteristics of the matrix of the renal glomerulus may allow proteins to be excreted into the urine, an indication of inexorable decline in renal function. Genetic defects may cause components of the matrix to be structurally and functionally abnormal, resulting in connective tissue disorders such as Ehlers-Danlos syndrome (caused by several mutations that affect specific collagen genes) and Marfan syndrome (a defect in the protein, fibrillin, in which >330 different mutations, many of which give rise to different phenotypes, have been identified). Deficiencies of lysosomal enzymes involved in normal degradation of molecules of the matrix result in diseases such as the mucopolysaccharidoses.

or *N*-acetylgalactosamine, and the second is usually acidic (either glucuronic acid or iduronic acid). These sugars are modified by the addition of sulfate groups to the parent sugar. A proteoglycan may contain greater than 100 GAG chains and consist of up to 95% carbohydrate by weight.

The negatively charged carboxylate and sulfate groups on the proteoglycan bind positively charged ions and form hydrogen bonds with trapped water molecules, thereby creating a hydrated gel. The gel provides a flexible mechanical support for the ECM. The gel also acts as a filter that allows the diffusion of ions (e.g., Ca^{2+}), H_2O, and other small molecules, but slows diffusion of proteins and movement of cells. The gel also acts as a lubricant. Hyaluronan is the only GAG that occurs as a single long polysaccharide chain and is the only GAG that is not sulfated.

1. Structure and Function of the Proteoglycans

Proteoglycans are found in interstitial connective tissues—for example, the synovial fluid of joints, the vitreous humor of the eye, arterial walls, bone, cartilage, and cornea. They are major components of the ECM in these tissues. The proteoglycans interact with a variety of proteins in the matrix, such as collagen and elastin, fibronectin (which is involved in cell adhesion and migration), and laminin.

Proteoglycans are proteins that contain many chains of GAGs (formerly called *mucopolysaccharides*). After synthesis, proteoglycans are secreted from cells; thus, they function extracellularly. Because the long, negatively charged GAG chains repel each other, the proteoglycans occupy a very large space and act as "molecular sieves," determining which substances enter or leave cells (Table 47.3). Their properties also give resilience and a degree of flexibility to substances such as cartilage, permitting compression and reexpansion of the molecule to occur.

At least seven types of GAGs exist, which differ in the monosaccharides present in their repeating disaccharide units: chondroitin sulfate, dermatan sulfate, heparin, heparan sulfate, hyaluronic acid, and keratan sulfates I and II. Except for hyaluronic acid, the GAGs are linked to proteins, usually attached covalently to serine or threonine residues. Keratan sulfate I is attached to asparagine.

2. Synthesis of the Proteoglycans

The protein component of the proteoglycans is synthesized on the ER. It enters the lumen of this organelle, where the initial glycosylations occur. Uridine diphosphate (UDP)-sugars serve as the precursors that add sugar units, one at a time, first to the protein and then to the nonreducing end of the growing carbohydrate chain (Fig. 47.8). Glycosylation occurs initially in the lumen of the ER and subsequently in the Golgi complex. Glycosyltransferases, the enzymes that add sugars to the chain,

GLYCOSAMINOGLYCAN	FUNCTION
Hyaluronic acid	Cell migration in: Embryogenesis Morphogenesis Wound healing
Chondroitin sulfate proteoglycans	Formation of bone, cartilage, cornea
Keratan sulfate proteoglycans	Transparency of cornea
Dermatan sulfate proteoglycans	Transparency of cornea Binds low-density lipoprotein to plasma walls
Heparin	Anticoagulant (binds antithrombin III) Causes release of lipoprotein lipase from capillary walls
Heparan sulfate (syndecan)	Component of skin fibroblasts and aortic wall; commonly found on cell surfaces

TABLE 47.3 Some Specific Functions of the Glycosaminoglycans and Proteoglycans

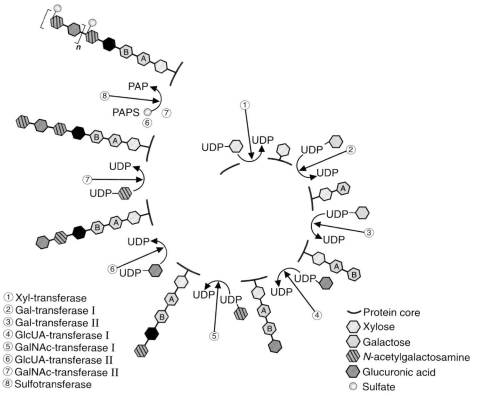

① Xyl-transferase
② Gal-transferase I
③ Gal-transferase II
④ GlcUA-transferase I
⑤ GalNAc-transferase I
⑥ GlcUA-transferase II
⑦ GalNAc-transferase II
⑧ Sulfotransferase

⌒ Protein core
⬡ Xylose
⬡ Galactose
⬡ N-acetylgalactosamine
⬡ Glucuronic acid
○ Sulfate

FIGURE 47.8 Synthesis of chondroitin sulfate. Sugars are added to the protein one at a time, with uridine diphosphate (UDP)-sugars serving as the precursors. Initially a xylose residue is added to a serine in the protein. Then, two galactose residues are added, followed by a glucuronic acid (GlcUA) and an *N*-acetylglucosamine (GalNAc). Subsequent additions occur by the alternating action of two enzymes that produce the repeating disaccharide units. One enzyme ⑥ adds GlcUA residues, and the other ⑦ adds GalNAc. As the chain grows, sulfate groups are added by phosphoadenosine phosphosulfate (PAPS). (Modified from Roden L. In: Fishman WH, ed. *Metabolic Conjugation and Metabolic Hydrolysis.* Vol. II. Orlando, FL: Academic Press; 1970:401.)

are specific for the sugar being added, the type of linkage that is formed, and the sugars already present in the chain. Once the initial sugars are attached to the protein, the alternating action of two glycosyltransferases adds the sugars of the repeating disaccharide to the growing GAG chain. Sulfation occurs after addition of the sugar. 3′-Phosphoadenosine 5′-phosphosulfate (PAPS), also called *active sulfate*, provides the sulfate groups (see Fig. 31.34). An epimerase converts glucuronic acid residues to iduronic acid residues.

After synthesis, the proteoglycan is secreted from the cell. Its structure resembles a bottle brush, with many GAG chains extending from the core protein (Fig. 47.9). The proteoglycans may form large aggregates, noncovalently attached by a "link" protein to hyaluronic acid (Fig. 47.10). The proteoglycans interact with the adhesion protein, fibronectin, which is attached to the cell membrane protein integrin. Cross-linked fibers of collagen also associate with this complex, forming the ECM (Fig. 47.11).

The long polysaccharide side chains of the proteoglycans in cartilage contain many anionic groups. This high concentration of negative charges attracts cations that create a high osmotic pressure within cartilage, drawing water into this specialized connective tissue and placing the collagen network under tension. At equilibrium, the resulting tension balances the swelling pressure caused by the proteoglycans. The complementary roles of this macromolecular organization give cartilage its resilience. Cartilage can thus withstand the compressive load of weight bearing and then reexpand to its previous dimensions when that load is relieved.

 The functional properties of a normal joint depend, in part, on the presence of a soft, well-lubricated, deformable, and compressible layer of cartilaginous tissue covering the ends of the long bones that constitute the joint.

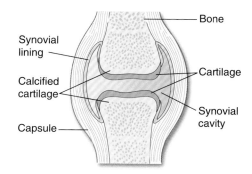

In **Sarah L.'s** case, the pathologic process that characterizes SLE disrupted the structural and functional integrity of her articular (joint) cartilage.

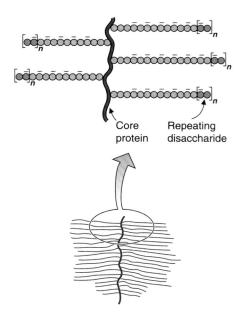

FIGURE 47.9 "Bottle brush" structure of a proteoglycan, with a magnified segment.

3. Degradation of Proteoglycans

Lysosomal enzymes degrade proteoglycans, glycoproteins, and glycolipids, which are brought into the cell by the process of endocytosis. Lysosomes fuse with the endocytic vesicles, and lysosomal proteases digest the protein component. The carbohydrate component is degraded by lysosomal glycosidases.

Lysosomes contain both endoglycosidases and exoglycosidases. The endoglycosidases cleave the chains into shorter oligosaccharides. Then, exoglycosidases, specific for each type of linkage, remove the sugar residues, one at a time, from the nonreducing ends.

Deficiencies of lysosomal glycosidases cause partially degraded carbohydrates from proteoglycans, glycoproteins, and glycolipids to accumulate within membrane-enclosed vesicles inside cells. These "residual bodies" can cause marked enlargement of the organ, with impairment of its function.

In the clinical disorders known as the *mucopolysaccharidoses* (caused by accumulation of partially degraded GAGs), deformities of the skeleton may occur (Table 47.4). Developmental delay and impaired cognitive abilities often accompany these skeletal changes.

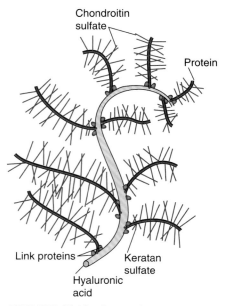

FIGURE 47.10 Proteoglycan aggregate.

Chondroitin sulfate

Protein

Link proteins

Keratan sulfate

Hyaluronic acid

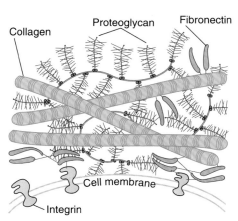

Collagen

Proteoglycan

Fibronectin

Cell membrane

Integrin

FIGURE 47.11 Interactions between the cell membrane and the components of the extracellular matrix.

TABLE 47.4	Defective Enzymes in the Mucopolysaccharidoses	
DISEASE	**ENZYME DEFICIENCY**	**ACCUMULATED PRODUCTS**
Hunter	Iduronate sulfatase	Heparan sulfate, dermatan sulfate
Hurler + Scheie	α-L-Iduronidase	Heparan sulfate, dermatan sulfate
Maroteaux-Lamy	N-Acetylgalactosamine sulfatase	Dermatan sulfate
Mucolipidosis VII	β-Glucuronidase	Heparan sulfate, dermatan sulfate
Sanfilippo A	Heparan sulfamidase	Heparan sulfate
Sanfilippo B	N-Acetylglucosaminidase	Heparan sulfate
Sanfilippo D	N-Acetylglucosamine 6-sulfatase	Heparin sulfate

These disorders share many clinical features, although there are significant variations between disorders, and even within a single disorder, based on the amount of residual activity remaining. In most cases, multiple organ systems are affected (with bone and cartilage being a primary target). For some disorders, there is significant neuronal involvement, leading to impaired cognitive abilities.

II. Integrins

Integrins are the major cellular receptors for ECM proteins and provide a link between the internal cytoskeleton of cells (primarily the actin microfilament system) and extracellular proteins, such as fibronectin, collagen, and laminin. Integrins consist of an α- and a β-subunit. There are 18 distinct α- and 10 distinct β-gene products. Twenty-four unique α/β-dimers have been discovered. Mice have been genetically engineered to be unable to express many of the integrin genes (one gene at a time), and the phenotypes of these knockout mice vary from embryonic lethality (the α_5 gene is an example) to virtually no observable defects (as exemplified by the α_1 gene). In addition to anchoring the cell's cytoskeleton to the ECM, thereby providing a stable environment in which the cell can reside, the integrins are also involved in a wide variety of cell signaling options.

Certain integrins, such as those associated with white blood cells, are normally inactive because the white cell must circulate freely in the bloodstream. However, if an infection occurs, cells located in the area of the infection release cytokines, which activate the integrins on the white blood cells, allowing them to bind to vascular endothelial cells (leukocyte adhesion) at the site of infection. Leukocyte adhesion deficiency (LAD) is a genetic disorder that results from mutations in the β_2-integrin such that leukocytes cannot be recruited to the sites of infection. Conversely, drugs are now being developed to block either the β_2- or α_4-integrins (on lymphocytes) to treat inflammatory and autoimmune disorders by interfering with the normal white blood cell response to cytokines.

Integrins can be activated by "inside-out" mechanisms, whereby intracellular signaling events activate the molecule, or by "outside-in" mechanisms, in which a binding event with the extracellular portion of the molecule initiates intracellular signaling events. For those integrins that bind cells to ECM components, activation of specific integrins can result in migration of the affected cell through the ECM. This mechanism is operative during growth, during cellular differentiation, and in the process of metastasis of malignant cells to neighboring tissues.

III. Adhesion Proteins

Adhesion proteins are found in the ECM and link integrins to ECM components. Adhesion proteins, of which fibronectin is a prime example, are large multidomain proteins that allow binding to many different components simultaneously. In addition to integrin-binding sites, fibronectin contains binding sites for collagen and GAGs.

The movement of tumor cells from its tissue of origin (metastasis) through the blood or lymph system, and colonization of a target tissue, requires degradation of the ECM to allow for cell movement. This is accomplished by a family of proteins known as *matrix metalloproteinases* (MMPs). The MMPs degrade specific ECM components (such as collagen or elastin), thereby allowing cells access through this compartment. One assay for determining whether MMPs are present in a biologic sample is the gelatin zymography assay; a newer, more sensitive assay is based on fluorescence resonance energy transfer (FRET). In the zymography assay, polyacrylamide gels containing the protein gelatin are prepared, and the enzyme samples are run through the gel in the presence of SDS. After the gel has run, enzyme activity is reconstituted by substituting Triton X-100 for the SDS. An assay buffer is then placed over the gel, which is left overnight. During this part of the procedure, if a lane on the gel contained MMP activity, the MMP would be digesting the gelatin in the area of the gel where the MMP resided. After the activity phase is complete, the gel is developed with Coomassie stain, which binds to the proteins in the gel, including the gelatin. A positive result would appear as white bands on a blue background. The white bands are caused by the absence of gelatin in that region of the gel, as the MMPs present at that region have digested the gelatin such that Coomassie stain has nothing to bind to in that area of the gel. The FRET assay uses a peptide substrate that contains both a fluorophore and a quencher in close proximity. When excited, the quencher blocks fluorescence emittance from the fluorophore owing to the close proximity of the two molecules on the peptide. After MMP treatment, however, the peptide is cleaved between the fluorophore and quencher, such that the quencher is no longer in close proximity to the fluorophore. This results in a strong fluorescence emittance. Thus, fluorescence intensity will increase as the peptide is cleaved in the presence of the MMP. This is a very sensitive assay, detecting subnanogram levels of a wide variety of members of the MMP family.

As the integrin molecule is bound to intracellular cytoskeletal proteins, the adhesion proteins provide a bridge between the actin cytoskeleton of the cell and the cells' position within the ECM. Loss of adhesion protein capability can lead to either physiologic or abnormal cell movement. Alternative splicing of fibronectin allows many different forms of this adhesion protein to be expressed, including a soluble form (vs. cell-associated forms), which is found in the plasma. The metabolic significance of these products remains to be determined.

Fibronectin was first discovered as a large external transformation-sensitive (LETS) protein, which was lost when fibroblasts were transformed into tumor cells. Many tumor cells secrete less-than-normal amounts of adhesion protein material, which allows for more movement within the extracellular milieu. This, in turn, increases the potential for the tumor cells to leave their original location and take root at another location within the body (metastasis).

IV. Matrix Metalloproteinases

The ECM contains a series of proteases known as the *matrix metalloproteinases*, or *MMPs*. These are zinc-containing proteases that use the zinc to appropriately position water to participate in the proteolytic reaction. More than 20 different types of human MMPs exist, and they cleave all proteins found in the ECM, including collagen and laminin.

Because MMPs degrade ECM components, their expression is important to allow cell migration and tissue remodeling during growth and differentiation. In addition, many growth factors bind to ECM components and, as bound components, do not exhibit their normal growth-promoting activity. Destruction of the ECM by the MMPs releases these growth factors, allowing them to bind to cell surface receptors to initiate growth of tissues. Thus, coordinated expression of the MMPs is required for appropriate cell movement and growth. Cancer cells that metastasize require extensive ECM remodeling and usually use MMP activity to spread throughout the body.

A propeptide is present in newly synthesized MMPs that contains a critical cysteine residue. The cysteine residue in the propeptide binds to the zinc atom at the active site of the protease and prevents the propeptide from exhibiting proteolytic activity. Removal of the propeptide is required to activate the MMPs. Once they are activated, certain MMPs can activate other forms of MMP.

Regulation of MMP activity is quite complex. These regulatory processes include transcriptional regulation, proteolytic activation, inhibition by the circulating protein α_2-macroglobulin, and regulation by a class of inhibitors known as *tissue inhibitors of metalloproteinases*, or *TIMPs*. It is important that the synthesis of TIMPs and MMPs be coordinately regulated because dissociation of their expression can facilitate various clinical disorders, such as certain forms of cancer and atherosclerosis.

CLINICAL COMMENTS

Sarah L. Articular cartilage is a living tissue with a turnover time determined by a balance between the rate of its synthesis and that of its degradation (Fig. 47.12). The chondrocytes that are embedded in the matrix of intraarticular cartilage participate in both its synthesis and its enzymatic degradation. The latter occurs as a result of cleavage of proteoglycan aggregates by enzymes produced and secreted by the chondrocytes.

SLE, the condition that affects **Sarah L.**, involves an autoimmune-induced inflammation. The inflammation can damage the kidneys, skin, and several other parts of the body. Joint pain is very common and results from inflammation around the joint. The inflammatory process excites the local release of cytokines such as

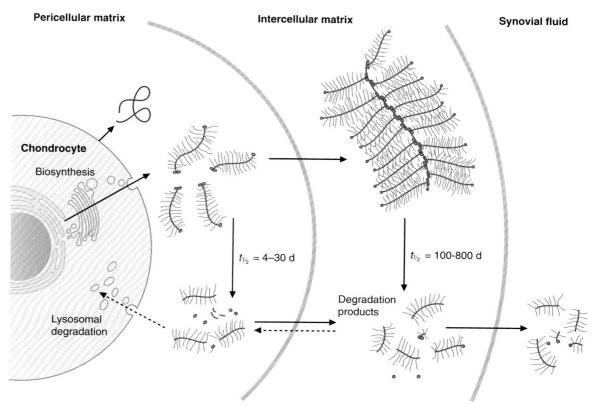

Pericellular matrix   **Intercellular matrix**   **Synovial fluid**

FIGURE 47.12 Synthesis and degradation of proteoglycans by chondrocytes. (From Cohen RD, et al. *The Metabolic Basis of Acquired Disease.* Vol. 2. London: Bailliere Tindall; 1990:1859.)

interleukin-1 (IL-1), which can increase the proteolytic activity of the chondrocytes, causing loss of articular proteins such as the proteoglycans. This can result in joint damage and pain.

 Deborah S. The microvascular complications of both type 1 and type 2 diabetes mellitus involve the small vessels of the retina (diabetic retinopathy), the renal glomerular capillaries (diabetic nephropathy), and the vessels that supply blood to the peripheral nerves (autonomic neuropathy). The lack of adequate control of **Deborah S.'s** diabetic state over many years caused a progressive loss of the filtering function of the approximately 1.5 million glomerular capillary–mesangial units that are present in her kidneys.

Chronic hyperglycemia is postulated to be a major metabolic initiator or inducer of diabetic microvascular disease, including those renal glomerular changes that often lead to end-stage renal disease ("glucose toxicity").

For a comprehensive review of the four postulated molecular mechanisms by which chronic hyperglycemia causes these vascular derangements, the reader is referred to several excellent reviews suggested in the online references.

Regardless of which of the postulated mechanisms (increased flux through the aldose reductase or polyol pathway [see Chapter 27], the generation of advanced glycosylation end-products [AGEs], the generation of reactive oxygen intermediates [see Chapter 25], or excessive activation of protein kinase C [see Chapter 18]) will eventually be shown to be the predominant causative mechanism, each can lead to the production of critical intracellular and extracellular signaling molecules (e.g., cytokines). These, in turn, can cause pathologic changes within the glomerular filtration apparatus that reduce renal function. These changes include increased

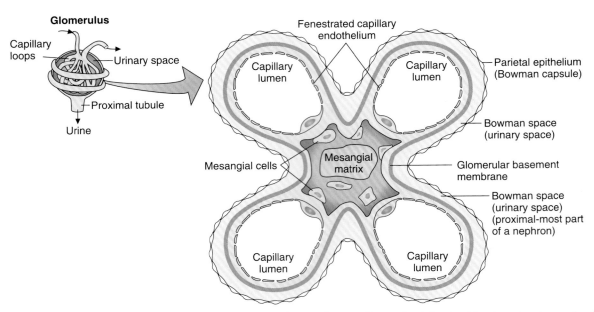

FIGURE 47.13 A cross-section of a normal renal glomerulus showing four capillary tufts delivering blood to the glomerulus for filtration across the fenestrated capillary endothelium, then through the glomerular basement membrane into the Bowman space to form urine. The urine then enters the proximal tubule of the nephron. This filtration removes potentially toxic metabolic end-products from the blood. The mesangium, by contracting and expanding, controls the efficiency of these filtering and excretory functions by regulating the hydraulic filtration pressures in the glomerulus. An intact basement membrane must be present to maintain the integrity of the filtering process.

synthesis of type IV collagen, fibronectin, and some of the proteoglycans, causing the glomerular basement membrane (GBM; Fig. 47.13) to become diffusely thickened throughout the glomerular capillary network. This membrane thickening alters certain specific filtration properties of the GBM, preventing some of the metabolites that normally enter the urine from the glomerular capillary blood (via the fenestrated capillary endothelium) from doing so (a decline in glomerular filtration rate [GFR]). As a result, these potentially toxic substances accumulate in the blood and contribute to the overall clinical presentation of advancing uremia. In spite of the thickening of the GBM, this membrane becomes "leaky" for some macromolecules (e.g., albumin) that normally do not enter the urine from the glomerular capillaries (microalbuminuria). Suggested mechanisms for this increased permeability or leakiness include reduced synthesis of the specific proteoglycan heparan sulfate, as well as increased basement membrane production of vascular endothelium growth factor (VEGF), a known angiogenic and permeability factor; and expansion of the ECM in the mesangium. The mesangium consists of specialized tissue containing collagen, proteoglycans, and other macromolecules that surround the glomerular capillaries and that, through its gel-like and sieving properties, determine, in part, the glomerular capillary hydraulic filtration pressure as well as the functional status of the capillary endothelium–mesangial GBM filtration apparatus (see Fig. 47.13). As the mesangial tissue expands, the efficiency of glomerular filtration diminishes proportionately. The cause of these mesangial changes is, in part, the consequence of increased expression of certain growth factors, especially transforming growth factor β (TGF-β) and connective tissue growth factor (CTGF). Future therapeutic approaches in patients with early diabetic nephropathy may include the use of antibodies that neutralize TGF-β.

BIOCHEMICAL COMMENTS

Osteogenesis Imperfecta. OI is a heterogenous group of genetic diseases that have in common a defect in collagen production. This defect can be either of two types: The first type is associated with a reduction in the synthesis of normal collagen (resulting from a gene deletion or splice-site mutation). The second type is associated with the synthesis of a mutated form of collagen. Most of the mutations have a dominant-negative effect, leading to an autosomal-dominant mode of transmission.

In the second type of OI, many of the known mutations involve substitutions of another amino acid for glycine. This results in an unstable collagen molecule because glycine is the only amino acid that can fit between the other two chains within the triple helix of collagen. If the mutation is near the carboxyl-terminal end of the molecule, the phenotype of the disease is usually more severe than if the mutation is near the amino-terminal end (recall that triple helix formation proceeds from the carboxyl- to the amino-terminal end of the molecule). Of interest are mutations that replace glycine with either serine or cysteine. Such mutations are more stable than expected because of the hydrogen-bonding capabilities of serine and the ability of cysteine to form disulfide bonds. Both would aid in preventing the strands of the triple helix from unwinding.

Children with OI can be treated with a class of compounds known as *bisphosphonates*, which consist of two phosphates linked by a carbon or nitrogen bridge (thus, they are analogs of pyrophosphate, in which the two phosphates are linked by oxygen). Normal bone remodeling is the result of a coordinated "coupling" between osteoclast activity (cells that resorb bone) and osteoblast activity (cells that form bone). In OI, bone resorption outpaces bone formation because osteoclast activity is enhanced (perhaps because of the reduced levels of normal collagen present to act as nucleating sites for bone formation). This leads to a net loss of bone mass and fragility of the skeleton. Bisphosphonates inhibit osteoclast action with the potential to increase bone mass and its tensile strength.

 OI can occur owing to mutations in genes other than collagen. Mutations in cartilage-associated protein (CRTAP) or prolyl 3-hydroxylase 1 or PH3-1 (LEPRE1) lead to defective collagen fibers being produced. CRTAP forms a complex with PH3-1 and cyclophilin to hydroxylate a specific proline residue in types I and II collagen. Failure to hydroxylate this proline residue leads to unstable collagen and moderate to severe forms of OI. The pattern of inheritance for both *CRTAP* and *LEPRE1* mutations is autosomal-recessive.

KEY CONCEPTS

- The extracellular matrix (ECM) consists of fibrous structural proteins, proteoglycans, and adhesion proteins.
- The ECM provides support to the tissues and restricts movement of cells.
- Collagen is the most abundant fibrous protein, and it consists of a triple helix stabilized by hydrogen bonds and intramolecular cross-links. There are >25 different types of collagen.
- Elastin is the major protein found in elastic fibers, and it is responsible for the contractility exhibited by these fibers.
- Laminin provides structural support to tissues via binding to various components of the ECM.
- Proteoglycans consist of polysaccharides (glycosaminoglycans) bound to a core protein.
  - The polysaccharides are usually a repeating disaccharide unit, containing negative charges.
  - Because of charge repulsion, the proteoglycans form a hydrated gel that provides flexible mechanical support to the ECM.
- Integrins are cellular membrane receptors for ECM proteins, and they link the cellular cytoskeleton to extracellular proteins.
- Integrins are also signaling proteins when they are bound to appropriate components.
- Adhesion proteins link the integrins to ECM components.
- Matrix metalloproteinases (MMPs) are the only proteases that can degrade ECM components, and they are carefully regulated by the tissue inhibitors of matrix metalloproteinases (TIMPs).
- Diseases discussed in this chapter are summarized in Table 47.5.

TABLE 47.5	Diseases Discussed in Chapter 47	
DISEASE OR DISORDER	**GENETIC OR ENVIRONMENTAL**	**COMMENTS**
Lupus	Both (genetic predisposition)	Alterations in cell matrix components owing to an autoimmune-induced trigger
Type 2 diabetes	Both	Cell matrix interactions can be altered because of elevated glucose levels and nonenzymatic glycosylation.
Osteogenesis imperfecta	Genetic	Inherited mutations in collagen genes that disrupt the function of the altered collagen
Supravalvular aortic stenosis (William-Beuren syndrome)	Genetic	An inherited mutation in the elastin gene, leading to abnormal heart function
Junctional epidermolysis bullosa	Genetic	A blistering skin condition caused by a mutation in either one form of collagen or laminin
Mucopolysaccharidoses	Genetic	Defects in the breakdown of mucopolysaccharides found primarily in the extracellular matrix. See Table 47.4 for more details on these diseases.

REVIEW QUESTIONS—CHAPTER 47

1. Individuals who develop scurvy suffer from sore and bleeding gums and loss of teeth. This is a result, in part, of the synthesis of a defective collagen molecule. The step that is affected in collagen biosynthesis attributable to scurvy is which one of the following?
   A. The formation of disulfide bonds, which initiates tropocollagen formation
   B. The formation of lysyl cross-links between collagen molecules
   C. Transcription of the collagen genes
   D. The formation of collagen fibrils
   E. The hydroxylation of proline residues, which stabilizes the collagen structure

2. The underlying mechanism that allows elastin to exhibit elastic properties (expand and contract) is which one of the following?
   A. Proteolysis during expansion, and resynthesis during contraction
   B. Breaking of disulfide bonds during expansion, and reformation of these bonds during contraction
   C. A decrease in entropy during expansion, and an increase in entropy during contraction
   D. The breaking of salt bridges during expansion, and reformation of the salt bridges during contraction
   E. Hydroxylation of elastin during expansion, and decarboxylation of elastin during contraction

3. The underlying mechanism by which GAGs allow for the formation of a gel-like substance in the ECM is which one of the following?
   A. Charge attraction between GAG chains
   B. Charge repulsion between GAG chains
   C. Hydrogen bonding between GAG chains
   D. Covalent cross-linking between GAG chains
   E. Hydroxylation of adjacent GAG chains

4. The movement of tumor cells from their site of origin to other locations within the body requires the activity of which one of the following proteins?
   A. Collagen
   B. Laminin
   C. Proteoglycans
   D. Elastin
   E. MMPs

5. Fibronectin is frequently absent in malignant fibroblast cells. One of the major functions of fibronectin is which one of the following?
   A. To inhibit the action of MMPs
   B. To coordinate collagen deposition within the ECM
   C. To fix the position of cells within the ECM
   D. To regulate GAG production
   E. To extend GAG chains using nucleotide sugars

6. Which one of the following alterations would reduce the ability of cartilage to cushion weight-bearing activities at joints?
   A. Loss of negative charges on the proteoglycans
   B. Loss of positive charges on the proteoglycans
   C. Gain of negative charges on the proteoglycans
   D. Increased concentration of glucuronic acid residues
   E. Increased concentration of sulfated sugars on the proteoglycans

7. A newborn displays the symptoms of a moderate case of OI. Analysis of the child's collagen by sodium dodecyl sulfate–polyacrylamide gel electrophoresis (SDS-PAGE) indicates a molecular species with a greater-than-normal molecular weight. Treatment of the child's collagen with β-mercaptoethanol prior to SDS-PAGE results in a normal-sized collagen. The mutation in this child is most likely which one of the following?
   A. Proline to hydroxyproline
   B. Glycine to cysteine
   C. Proline to glycine
   D. Glycine to proline
   E. Serine to proline

8. Bisphosphonate treatment of children with OI is based on which one of the following?
   A. Stimulation of osteoclast activity
   B. Inhibition of osteoclast activity
   C. Stimulation of osteoblast activity
   D. Inhibition of osteoblast activity
   E. Stimulation of laminin synthesis
   F. Inhibition of laminin synthesis

9. Collagen provides great tensile strength to connective tissue by its structure as a triple helix. Which amino acid is critical in allowing triple-helix formation?
   A. Proline
   B. Hydroxyproline
   C. Lysine
   D. Glycine
   E. Elastin

10. A common feature of the mucopolysaccharidoses is the accumulation of heparin sulfate. Which of the following disorders leads to an accumulation of that particular GAG? Choose the one best answer.

	Maroteaux-Lamy	Hunter	Sanfilippo A	Mucolipidosis VII	Sanfilippo D
A	Yes	Yes	Yes	Yes	Yes
B	No	No	Yes	Yes	Yes
C	Yes	No	No	Yes	Yes
D	No	Yes	Yes	Yes	No
E	Yes	Yes	No	Yes	No
F	No	Yes	Yes	Yes	Yes

ANSWERS

1. **The answer is E.** Scurvy is caused by a deficiency of vitamin C. Vitamin C is a required cofactor for the hydroxylation of both proline and lysine residues in collagen. The hydroxyproline residues that are formed stabilize the collagen fiber through the formation of hydrogen bonds with other collagen triple helices within the fiber. The loss of this stabilizing force greatly reduces the strength of the collagen fibers. The hydroxylation of lysine allows carbohydrates to be attached to collagen, which appear to be necessary for efficient transport of tropocollagen from the cell to the ECM. Vitamin C is not required for disulfide bond formation, the formation of lysyl cross-links (that enzyme is lysyl oxidase), transcription of the collagen genes, or the formation of collagen fibrils. Thus, all the other choices are incorrect.

2. **The answer is C.** When elastin expands as a result of outside forces (such as the respiratory muscles causing the lungs to expand with air), hydrophobic regions of elastin are exposed to the aqueous environment, resulting in a decrease in the entropy of water. When the outside force is removed (by relaxation of the respiratory muscles), the driving force for contraction of elastin is an increase in the entropy of water, so that the hydrophobic residues of elastin are again shielded from the environment. The expansion and contraction of elastin does not involve covalent modifications (thus, A, B, and E are incorrect), nor does it involve extensive changes in salt bridge formation (thus, D is also incorrect).

3. **The answer is B.** GAG chains contain negative charges, resulting from the presence of acidic sugars and the sulfated sugars in the molecule. Thus, in their characteristic bottleneck structure, the chains repel each other (thus, A is incorrect), yet they also attract positively charged cations and water into the spaces between the chains. The water forms hydrogen bonds with the sugars and a gel-like space is created. This gel acts as a diffusion sieve for materials that leave, or enter, this space. Hydroxylation and cross-linking of chains does not occur (thus, D and E are incorrect), nor does hydrogen bonding between chains (they are too far apart because of the charge repulsion, but they do form hydrogen bonds with water).

4. **The answer is E.** In order for cells to migrate, they must free themselves from the ECM material, which requires remodeling of the matrix components. Because of the unique structural aspects of these components, only a small subset of proteases, the metalloproteinases, is capable of doing this. The other answers listed are all components of the matrix, which must be remodeled in order for cell migration to occur.

5. **The answer is C.** Fibronectin binds to integrins on the cell surface as well as to various ECM components (collagen and GAGs). This binding fixes the position of the cell within the matrix. Loss of these binding components can lead to undesirable cell movement. Fibronectin plays no role in any of the other functions listed as possible answers.

6. **The answer is A.** The proteoglycans, containing the GAGs, are highly negatively charged. The sugars often contain a carboxylic acid group (glucuronic and iduronic acids) and are often sulfated. This high level of negative charges attracts cations to the proteoglycans, bringing with the cations water through an osmotic effect. When weight is placed on the joint the water in the space cushions the force generated, and when the weight is removed, water can return to the space. Losing negative charges would reduce the amount of water in the joint and the ability of the joint to prevent bone–bone interactions. The proteoglycans are not positively charged and do not attract anions. Increasing the negative charges exhibited by the proteoglycans would enhance the cushioning effect, as would increasing the concentration of glucuronic acid residues and sulfated sugars (because both of those changes increase the concentration of negative charges in the joint).

7. **The answer is B.** Glycine is present at every third residue within a collagen monomer because it is the only amino acid side chain that can fit in the triple helix when the three chains wind about each other. Substitution of glycine with any other amino acid can lead to a weakened collagen structure. However, when cysteine is present instead of a glycine, the cysteine has the capability of forming disulfide bonds, which can stabilize the unstable collagen triple helix. A glycine-to-cysteine substitution requires the change of only one nucleotide in the DNA sequence. When the child's collagen is run on an SDS-PAGE gel, the molecular weight is greater than native collagen because of the cross-links in the collagen. Mercaptoethanol will break those links, so after treating with mercaptoethanol the molecular weight of collagen would appear normal in the gel. Conversion of proline to hydroxyproline is a normal event in collagen biosynthesis and allows for hydrogen bonding to occur, which will stabilize the collagen triple helix. Proline to glycine will not lead to cross-links in collagen, nor will glycine or serine to proline. The latter mutations may disrupt triple-helix formation and lead to a form of osteogenesis imperfecta, but they would not lead to the biochemical findings of cross-linking.

8. **The answer is B.** Osteoclasts resorb bone, whereas osteoblasts produce bone. Normally, there is a balance between osteoclast and osteoblast activity within bones, allowing the appropriate amount of bone tissue to be generated and then turned over and resynthesized. However, certain conditions can lead to enhanced osteoclast activity, such as reduced levels of collagen being produced or altered collagen molecules being produced. Under these conditions, the osteoclasts resorb more bone than the osteoblasts can synthesize, leading to weak and fragile bones. Bisphosphonates inhibit osteoclast activity, thereby allowing more bone to be produced, even if the collagen being produced is not normal. Laminin is not involved in bone formation. Inhibition of osteoblast activity would lead to reduced bone formation, which is the opposite of what one wants to occur under these conditions.

9. **The answer is D.** The three polypeptide chains of the triple helix are linked by interchain hydrogen bonds. Each turn of the helix contains three amino acid residues with every third amino acid in close contact with the other two strands in the center of the structure. Only glycine, which lacks a side chain, can fit in this position. The other amino acids listed are important amino acids in collagen but cannot fit into the central position critical for the triple helix. Elastin is a protein, not an amino acid. The proline is required for each chain to form a polyprolyl helix, but the glycine is essential for allowing triple-helix formation.

10. **The answer is F.** Maroteaux-Lamy is deficient in *N*-acetylgalactosamine sulfatase and accumulates dermatan sulfate. All the others listed accumulate heparin sulfate ($+/-$ dermatan sulfate).

Patient Index

NOTE: Page numbers followed by *f* denote figures; page numbers followed by *t* denote tables.

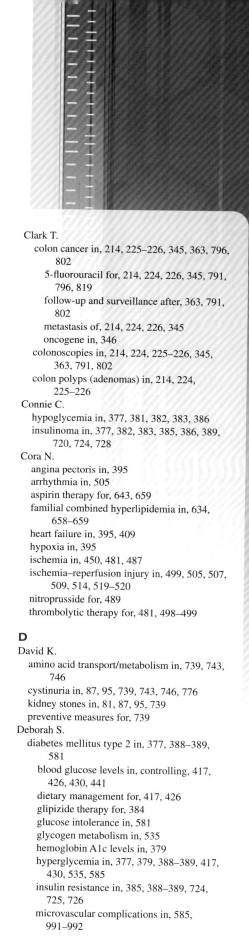

Subject Index

NOTE: Page numbers followed by *f* denote figures; page numbers followed by *t* denote tables.